Linguistic Disorders and Pathologies

HSK 8

Handbücher zur Sprach- und Kommunikationswissenschaft

Handbooks of Linguistics and Communication Science

Manuels de linguistique et des sciences de communication

Mitbegründet von
Gerold Ungeheuer

Herausgegeben von / Edited by / Edités par
Hugo Steger
Herbert Ernst Wiegand

Band 8

Walter de Gruyter · Berlin · New York
1993

Linguistic Disorders and Pathologies

An International Handbook

Edited by
Gerhard Blanken · Jürgen Dittmann
Hannelore Grimm · John C. Marshall
Claus-W. Wallesch

Walter de Gruyter · Berlin · New York
1993

⊗ Gedruckt auf säurefreiem Papier, das die
US-ANSI-Norm über Haltbarkeit erfüllt.

Library of Congress Cataloging-in-Publication Data

Linguistic disorders and pathologies : an international handbook /
edited by Gerhard Blanken ... [et al.].
p. cm. — (Handbücher zur Sprach- und Kommunikations
-wissenschaft ; Bd. 8)
Includes bibliographical references and index.
ISBN 3-11-011324-4 (Germany : acid-free paper)
1. Language disorders. 2. Neurolinguistics. 3. Psychotherapy
patients—Language. I. Blanken, Gerhard. II. Series.
RC423.L56 1993
616.85'5—dc20 93-34475
CIP

Die Deutsche Bibliothek — Cataloging-in-Publication Data

Handbücher zur Sprach- und Kommunikationswissenschaft /
mitbegr. von Gerold Ungeheuer. Hrsg. von Hugo Steger ;
Herbert Ernst Wiegand. — Berlin ; New York : de Gruyter.
Teilw. mit Parallelt.: Handbooks of linguistics and communication
science. — Teilw. mit Nebent.: HSK. — Früher hrsg. von Gerold
Ungeheuer und Herbert Ernst Wiegand
NE: Ungeheuer, Gerold [Begr.]; Steger, Hugo [Hrsg.]; PT; NT

Bd. 8. Linguistic disorders and pathologies. — 1993

Linguistic disorders and pathologies : an international
handbook / ed. by Gerhard Blanken ... — — BerBerlin ; New York :
de Gruyter, 1993
(Handbücher zur Sprach- und Kommunikationswissenschaft ; Bd. 8)
ISBN 3-11-011324-4
NE: Blanken, Gerhard [Hrsg.]

Printed in Germany
Satz und Druck: Arthur Collignon GmbH, Berlin
Buchbinderische Verarbeitung: Lüderitz & Bauer, Berlin

Preface

Language Processing, its Development and the Brain – Focussing on Errors and Disturbances

1. Motivations and Aims

The present handbook on 'Linguistic Disorders and Pathologies' is geared towards the following aims:

- a state of the art review of research on disordered language production and perception in adults and children;
- the description and discussion of current attempts at modelling human language processing by using linguistic disorders and pathologies as a data base;
- the presentation of diagnostic and therapeutic concepts;
- pointing out gaps and inconsistencies in current knowledge and theories.

Collaborating for more than seven years in order to produce this handbook, the editors were guided by many and diverse motivations. One of the strongest, shared by all of us, was the attempt to bring together knowledge from different sources and disciplines under one common roof and to achieve a comprehensive overview of the state of the art in the field of language pathology. Parts of the field are dominated by special disciplines such as psychology, speech-language pathology and therapy, neurology and psychiatry, others by psycho- and neurolinguistics or neurophonetics, to name but a few. Consequently, theories and methodologies and, of course, their empirical bases differ among the contributions of the subfields involved. Nevertheless, an important goal of this handbook is to clarify the common and interdisciplinary concern about linguistic disorders and pathologies and, furthermore, to demonstrate the extent of interdisciplinary interaction that is still required. According to this motivation and these aims of the editors, the title of the handbook was chosen to encompass as broadly as possible the disturbances, abnormalities and alterations of language production, perception and comprehension in adults and children.

2. Organization of the Handbook

2.1. Overview

In keeping with our goals, the handbook is organized in the following manner: The first chapter describes processes and sporadic disturbances of language in normal adult speakers. It is followed by two chapters on acquired organic pathologies of language in adults. Chapter IV describes pathologies of language in adults' psychiatric disorders. The final chapter discusses pathologies of language development.

2.2. Language Use in Normal Speakers and its Disorders

The reader may wonder why a handbook on pathology begins with an analysis of normal language use and likely speech errors. First of all, it is our conviction that prior to any theories of pathological function normal linguistic behavior should be defined as precisely as possible. Indeed, speech errors and slips of the tongue are omnipresent in normal language use, and the abstract norms of school grammars fail to serve as a valid scientific tool for distinguishing between normality and pathology. Fortunately, the last decades have witnessed dramatic progress in psycholinguistics including a number of theoretical models developed on empirical grounds. These serve to focus our view on what 'normal language processing' and, consequently, 'language pathology' are supposed to mean. A second reason for our drawing on psycholinguistic data and theories is the progress of the cognitive enterprise of neuro- and patholinguistics which has become one of the major scientific directions in the study of language pathologies, such as aphasia and developmental disorders. Models of normal language processing form a cornerstone of this approach, and it is the friction of hypotheses derived from these models and the patients' constellation of symptoms that make this approach successful. Thus, the editors believe that data and theories referring to normal language behavior are essential if an information source such as this handbook is to have lasting validity.

2.3. Acquired Organic Pathologies of Language Behavior: Neurolinguistic Disorders

In this volume, the field of acquired organic pathologies of language behavior in adults is divided into neurolinguistic disorders (e. g. aphasias; chpt. II) and neurophonetic disorders (e. g. dysarthrias; chpt. III). Although not regarded as completely distinct, these disorders are treated separately, since their investigation is based on different methodologies and theories.

Aphasic language disturbances and related disorders are the object of contemporary research in neurolinguistics, neuropsychology, speech-language pathology/therapy, and behavioral neurology. Besides clear-cut aphasic symptoms typically due to focal left-hemisphere damage, other and more subtle disorders of communication have received growing attention. In particular, observations of language behavior in dementing disease have recently had increasing implications for neurolinguistic theory, and related research is rapidly accumulating.

The whole field of research on neurolinguistic disorders has evolved into roughly five mutually related subfields:

(i) Issues of the cerebral representation and the neurobiological organization of human language functions dominated the beginning of scientific aphasiology in the last century, and they have since continued to be a central topic of research.

(ii) Similarly, the clinical-diagnostic classification of patients with neurolinguistic disorders into symptom-complexes or syndromes on the basis of test results continues to be an important aid in the assessment of aphasic disturbances.

(iii) Studies of aphasic disturbances can reveal a number of associations with and dissociations from other higher mental functions. These relations between different cognitive functions form an exciting window onto the role of language within the more general architecture of human cognition.

(iv) There is an increasing demand for improved treatment and rehabilitation approaches for patients suffering from aphasia and its consequences. Both psychosocial effects and therapeutic strategies are fields of research with direct clinical implications and applications.

(v) The neurolinguistic description of aphasic symptoms and their confrontation with psycholinguistic models of normal language processing have become one of the main streams of today's aphasia research. Much room has been allocated in this handbook to the cognitive approach to aphasia. In all contributions related to this approach, the authors refer to psycholinguistic theories and models and take into account this knowledge in their analyses of aphasic, alexic or agraphic symptoms on different levels of language processing. In many cases, the results obtained will have an important impact on the further development of the cognitive sciences of language.

2.4. Acquired Organic Pathologies of Language Behavior: Neurophonetic Disorders

Neurophonetics is an emerging field, and chapter III of this handbook gives an account of its potential. The editors acknowledge that a strict distinction between the subjects and methods of neurolinguistics, as outlined in chapter II, and neurophonetics is artificial both for theoretical and practical reasons. The proximity of the realms is exemplified by the topics of speech apraxia, speech tics and verbal agnosia, including both linguistic and phonetic aspects.

The chapter begins with an account of the dynamic properties of the articulatory apparatus, outlining future directions of investigation and explanation. Current approaches to the dysarthrias are rooted in neurology and neurophysiology, a fact which is reflected in the chapters of this section.

The articles on dysarthria demonstrate the rich data base, refined methodology and potential of clinical neurophonetics. Throughout, the contributions demonstrate that explanatory accounts are developing from anatomical to neurophysiological and further to dynamic models.

A survey of neurophonetics would be incomplete if it was restricted to the classical disorders of dysarthria and speech apraxia. Therefore, the editors have invited brief contributions on disorders of phonation, on the effects of anatomical alterations and on central auditory disorders affecting the analysis of speech signals (verbal agnosia).

2.5. Pathologies of Language Use in Psychiatric Disorders

Language pathology in psychiatric disorders is a field still requiring intensive cooperation between psychiatrists, psychologists, and linguists. Articles on language pathology in alexithymia, schizophrenia and affective psychoses have been included in this handbook, and we hope that they will contribute to renewed interdisciplinary effort and joint research enterprises.

That linguistic components bear relevance for psychiatric disorders is illustrated by the following examples: There is considerable agreement that schizophrenic patients have problems with metaphorical expressions, the organization of texts ('incoherence') and with communicative interactions. For many years it remained unclear, however, whether the utterances of these patients show pathological morpho-syntactic abnormalities. Recent research indicates that this is indeed the case. Further studies are required to clarify the consequences of these findings in terms of neurolinguistic modelling as well as for nosology and diagnosis. Linguistic abnormalities in affective psychoses, such as mania and depression, can vary considerably. Whereas in depression the syntax of utterances seems reduced in complexity and vocabulary is restricted, in mania the converse appears to be the case. The most impressive abnormalities are seen in the domains of fluency, prosody and articulation. Future research should be guided by psycholinguistic modelling of speech production and comprehension, which could lead to explanatory hypotheses about the deficits of these patients.

2.6. Pathologies and Disorders of Language Development

The most extensive chapter, with 31 articles, is chapter V. It covers the most important developmental language disorders and indicates new directions for future research. The chapter starts with a comprehensive overview on important landmarks in the language development of normal children. This overview is intended to furnish a framework in which the following articles on speech and language disorders may be organized for a better understanding. Of these disorders specific language impairment has been the subject of especially intensive investigation during the last few years. The reason is that this developmental disorder is found in the absence of any apparent cognitive, emotional and motor problems, hearing disability or evident profound neurological insult. Thus, such factors that could directly account for disordered language development in mentally retarded or hearing-impaired children as well as in children showing elective mutism or acquired aphasia do not play a primary causal role in specific language impairment.

Along with speech and language disorders, problems with written language are described, where the recurring question is which disordered language and cognitive processes might be responsible for reading problems. Fluency disorders, e. g. stuttering, fall at the intersection of impaired language development, neurolinguistics, neurophonetics, and psychopathology. As a result, the research on these disorders can draw upon the theories and methodologies of each discipline involved.

The chapter ends with an article on language changes in old age. Espousing a broad concept of development which encompasses the whole life span, this is certainly an important topic. The regression hypothesis, for example, claims that the breakdown of language is the inverse of its acquisition.

3. Target audience

This handbook will be of interest to all who are involved with disordered language and/or language and speech disturbances. This will include linguists and psychologists working in related research or teaching related subjects, scientists analyzing and modelling linguistic and cognitive processes (e. g. in Cognitive Psychology, Psycholinguistics, Neurolinguistics, Neuropsychology, Behavioral Neurology, Artificial Intelligence Research, and Cognitive Science), clinicians dealing with acquired or developmental language disorders, and speech pathologists and therapists. Besides presenting the state of the art, the handbook provides bibliographical information for researchers, clinicians, and advanced students.

4. Acknowledgements

For valuable suggestions during the preparation of this handbook, we would like to thank Evelyn R. Abberton, A. Castro-Caldas, Ernst G. de Langen, Rose A. Fehrenbach, Victoria A. Fromkin, Klaus Frühauf, Trevor A. Harley, Peter Hill, Ralph E. Hoffman, Thomas Jechle, Yves Joanette, B. L. J. Kaczmarek, Eric Keller, Susan Kemper, Raymond D. Kent, Uwe Koch-Gromus, André R. Lecours, Yvan Lebrun, Willem J. M. Levelt, Brendan A. Maher, Godehard Oepen, Wolfgang Raible, Susanne Schmidt-Knaebel, Michael von Rad, Diana Van Lancker and Harry A. Whitaker.

At the planning stage, Katrin Aderhold helped us with all kinds of practical matters, and Peter Tosic and Ashrav Noor gave us language assistance, for which we are grateful. The task of translating contributions into English and of editing those submissions written by non-English speakers was carried out meticulously by Debbie Johnson in Freiburg and by Elisabeth Wolter in Bielefeld. With their competence and their extraordinary efforts, both have played a decisive role in ensuring that the language quality of the translated chapters is of a good standard. Our gratitude also extends to Elisabeth Wolter, Bielefeld, and Peter Baier, Freiburg, for their invaluable help in the painstaking job of editing the entire volume and compiling the subjects' and authors' indexes.

We are expecially indebted to our publisher, Heinz Wenzel from de Gruyter: Although the conception and target audience of this volume diverge from the previously published volumes of the series 'Handbooks of Linguistics and Communication Science' he remained sensitive to our concerns and ideas which did not always correspond to his. Brigitte Schöning, successor of Heinz Wenzel, and Susanne Rade from de Gruyter were patient, helpful and encouraging consultants. We gratefully acknowledge their advice on all matters of organization and planning.

Last but not least, we wish to thank the series editors, Hugo Steger and Herbert Ernst Wiegand, who offered us the opportunity to edit a volume on language and speech pathology in their series. We are grateful to them for giving us the opportunity to compile this handbook and for their harmonious collaboration every step of the sometimes arduous way.

Gerhard Blanken, Freiburg /Br. (Germany)
Jürgen Dittmann, Freiburg/Br. (Germany)
Hannelore Grimm, Bielefeld (Germany)
John C. Marshall, Oxford (United Kingdom)
Claus-W. Wallesch, Freiburg/Br. (Germany)

Contents

V. Pathologies and Disorders of Language Development

I. Language Use in Normal Speakers and its Disorders

1. The Architecture of Normal Spoken Language Use

1. Introduction

The normal language user's production and understanding of speech involves the highly skilled coordination of myriad processes. When a speaker conceives of some communicative intention, he will select and order information whose expression may realize that intention. He will also formulate that information, i. e., give it linguistic shape. This includes retrieving the appropriate words from memory and assigning them their proper grammatical roles and syntactic positions. The speaker will further compute a phonetic specification for the developing utterance, and use it to guide the articulatory execution that produces overt speech. The addressee will normally try to reconstruct the speaker's communicative intentions. She will perform an acoustic-phonetic analysis on the continuous speech signal in order to segment it into recognizable words and phrases. She will retrieve the syntactic properties and meanings of successive words and parse the string into meaningful phrases and sentences. And she will interpret this information in terms of the context of interaction, the purpose of the exchange, the presuppositions about the speaker's intentions, etc.

This complex system operates largely unawares. A speaker concentrates his attention on what is to be said, not on how it is to be done. The rate of fluent speech, some 2 to 3 words per second, is too high for a speaker to ponder over each and every word or syntactic construction. And there is no way for a speaker to consciously prepare some fifteen speech sounds per second. Similarly, the listener normally attends to the content of what is said, not to the phonetic shape of words or the syntactic complexities of the utterance. Like in all other skills, the lower level processes are automatic. They don't use central resources; they come for free.

In the following I will outline the architecture of this skill. This involves the dissection of the speech processing system into component subsystems. It also involves a characterization of the representations computed by the processing components as well as the manner in which these representations are computed. And it requires a specification of how the processing components cooperate in producing their joint product. These matters will be discussed in reference to Figure 1.1. It is a 'blueprint' of the language user, depicting the main processing components and their connections. We will proceed anticlockwise through the system, beginning at the highest conceptual level at which the speaker generates information to be expressed. We will follow the flow of information down to articulation, the generation of overt speech. We will then turn to the perception and parsing of speech, back to the conceptual interpretative level. After this grand tour some remarks will be made about the modes of cooperation between the various components, in particular about incrementality and autonomy of processing.

2. Speaking

2.1. Conceptual Preparation

The conceptual preparation of speech (see Figure 1.1, 'conceptualizer') begins with the conception of an illocutionary intention, i. e., a communicative intention the speaker decides to express by means of language. A communicative intention is one the speaker wants to be recognized as such by the addressee (Grice 1968). The speaker may want to refer to something, to express some belief or expectation, to commit the addressee or himself to some course of action, etc. In order

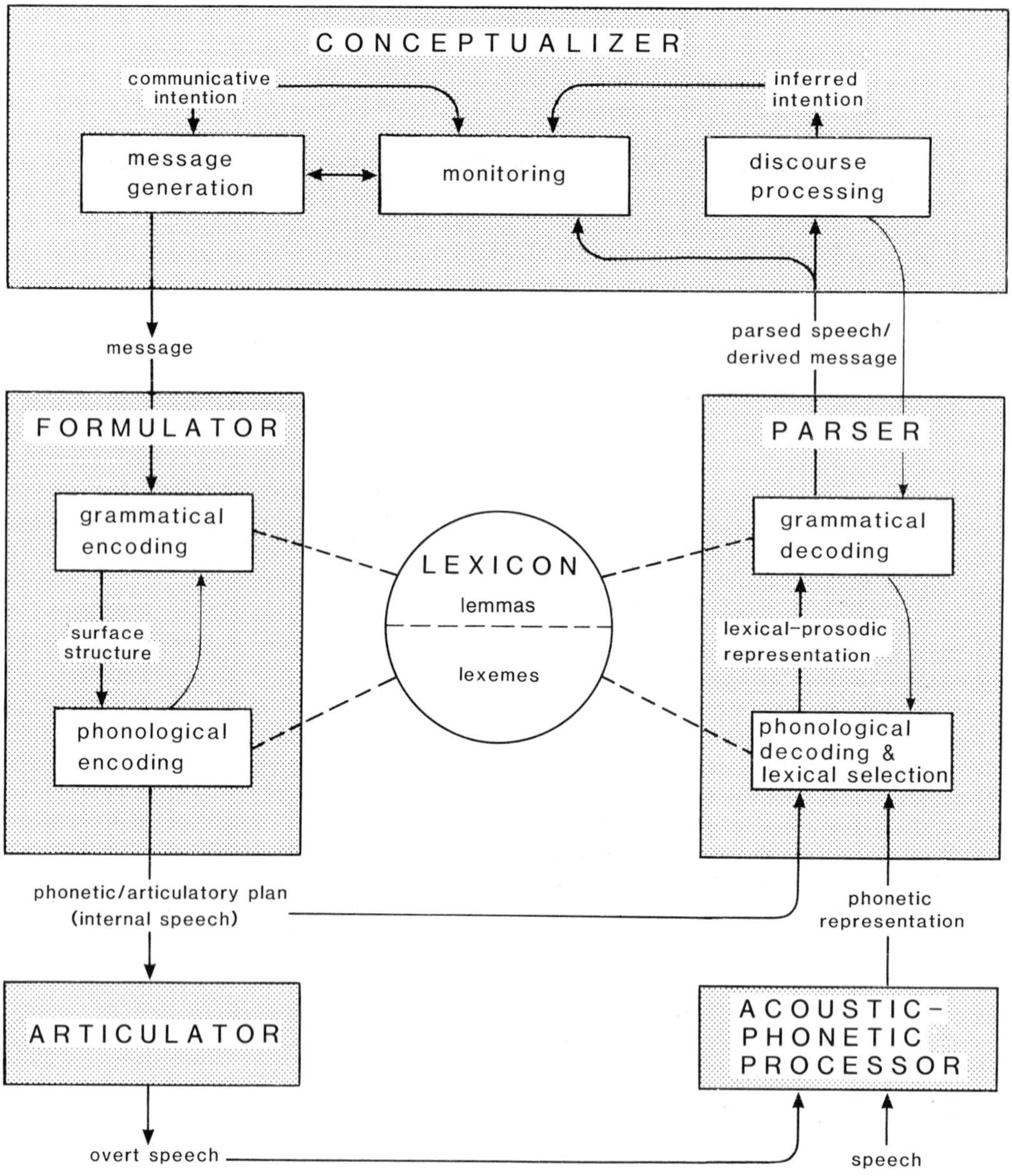

Fig. 1.1: Schematic representation of the processing components involved in spoken language use.

to make such intentions recognizable by the addressee, the speaker will decide on a speech act and select information whose expression can realize that purpose. So, for instance, if the illocutionary intention is that the addressee will believe X, then one way is to state that X is the case. Or if the intention is that the addressee performs action Y, then the speaker may request that Y be performed. Often the information expressed indicates the illocutionary intention indirectly. *It is cold in here* may express the request to close the window (Clark 1979). Such indirect speech acts convey an intention that is not literally expressed (as in *close the window*). It is the rule rather than the exception that the information selected for expression entertains an indirect relation to the intention to be conveyed. This is a powerful means to regulate personal relations in verbal interaction, to be polite, ironical, or whatever the situation might call for (Clark/Gerrig 1984). The information expressed invites the addressee to infer the intention, and this may be based on conventions (as in the request interpretation of *please*) and on the mutual knowledge of the interlocutors in a discourse situation (Grice 1975; Clark/Chunk 1980). Meanings are not so much expressed as negotiated between interlocutors. A simple intention to refer to a particular object may take several turns between interlocutors to become realized (*The newspaper — Which newspaper? — The one on the table — On the small table? — Yes*, cf. Clark/Wilkes-Gibbs 1986).

Conveying an intention may involve the planning of a sequence of speech acts. If a speaker decides to comply with a request to describe his apartment in some detail, he will have to retrieve from memory a complex spatial arrangement of spaces and objects. It will involve several statements of fact to express this information. In such cases speakers have to solve the 'linearization problem', i. e., what to say first, what to express next, etc. When the complex information to be expressed is spatial, speakers solve the problem by making an imaginary tour — a body tour or a gaze tour — through the scene. When the information is temporal, as in the description of events, speakers tend to adhere to the chronological order (For an analysis of speakers' linearization principles see Levelt 1989, 138 ff). The speaker's planning of a speech act, his selection of information to be expressed, and his linearization of that information are called 'macroplanning' (Butterworth 1980; Levelt 1989, 123 ff).

In addition there is 'microplanning' to be done. First, the information to be expressed should be given 'propositional shape' and 'perspective'. An image of an apartment is not enough for an apartment description: something should be said *about* that image, for instance that the table is in front of the window. The speaker decides what predications have to be made about what referents, and this usually involves taking perspective. Is the spatial relation to be expressed as a property of the table (being in front of the window) or as a property of the window (being behind the table)? Taking perspective is governed by various principles, among them Gestalt principles. Objects tend to be related to backgrounds, not inversely (i. e., the table being in front of the window, rather than the window being behind the table). Small objects are related to big objects, not inversely (a pen on the table, not a table under the pen), etc.

Likewise, the expression of an event requires a predication to be made, and that predication should have a certain perspective. One and the same event can be propositionalized as the mother giving an ice cream to the child, or as the child receiving an ice cream from the mother. The proposition involves the same three arguments: mother, child, and ice cream, but in the first case the mother is the topic of the event, in the second case the child is topic. These perspective relations have to be specified in the speaker's conceptual preparation of speech, because they are important determinants of word choice (*give, receive*), and of the assignment of grammatical roles (*the mother* as subject of the sentence or *the child*).

Microplanning also involves the assignment of an 'accessibility status' to the referents in a proposition. If the mother in the above proposition had already been mentioned in the previous sentence, she is likely to be in the focus of the addressee's attention. Knowing this, the speaker gives her a high accessibility status, which means that reduced or anaphoric reference can be made (*She gave the ice cream to the child*). There are various possible degrees of accessibility, each leading to a different choice of referring expression (cf. Levelt 1989, 144 ff). Related to accessibility is the assignment of 'prominence' to a referent. Something that may have particular 'news value' for the addressee can be marked in the message, so it will eventually be prosodically stressed in the utterance. Finally, microplanning involves certain language-specific decisions. When a language (such as English) has a tense system, it is obligatory to specify the relevant temporal relations, even if they don't contribute to conveying the speaker's intention. A speaker of a tenseless language (such as Chinese) will only plan for the expression of temporal relations where they are relevant for conveying his intentions. Languages may require conceptual prespecifications of various sorts, such as the number (singular, plural) of referents, the degree of distance of objects to the speaker (proximal, medial, distal), the form or material of referents (fork-shaped, clay), etc. Any of these quite arbitrary properties may be 'grammaticized' in a language, i. e., have an effect on morphology or syntax.

The eventual output of a speaker's conceptual preparation is technically called a 'message' (see Figure 1.1); in cases of linearized information it is a series of messages. It is the information to be expressed, in propositional format, and supplied with perspectives, accessibility statuses and language-specific conceptual information. Such messages form the characteristic input to the Formulator (see Figure 1.1).

The Formulator maps messages onto linguistic form. It performs two relatively independent operations: grammatical encoding and phonological encoding.

2.2. Grammatical Encoding

Grammatical encoding takes a message as input and delivers a surface structure as output. A surface structure is a hierarchical organization of syntactic phrases. Its lowest-level elements are 'lemmas'. These are lexical elements as yet unspecified for phonological form (That specification takes place during phonological encoding). The surface structure is a syntactic, not a conceptual representation. It represents syntactic relations or functions such as 'head of phrase', 'subject of', 'direct object of', etc. In so far, it is what Garrett (1975) called the 'functional level representation'.

The generation of surface structure is lexically driven. Each lemma requires a particular syntactic environment. Grammatical encoding is like solving a set of simultaneous equations: the surface structure must be such that for all lemmas the required syntactic environments are realized.

Lemmas can become available prior to syntactic construction. How are they retrieved? Lemmas are entries in the 'mental lexicon' (see Figure 1.1). That is the repository of knowledge about the words in one's language. Most lemmas have a semantic specification. This is the set of conceptual conditions under which the lemma can be appropriately used. So, for instance, the semantic specification for the lemma *give* is something like 'an event in which agent X causes object Y to be transferred from agent X to recipient Z' (This can, of course, be given formal expression in some logical language). So, if the speaker's message is that the mother gives the child an ice cream, the conceptual condition for the appropriate use of the lemma *give* is fulfilled: There is an agent X (the mother), who causes the transfer of an object or theme Y (the ice cream) to some recipient Z (the child). This being the case, the lemma *give* is retrieved from the lexicon. How does this take place? This is controversial, or rather unknown. Theories of lexical selection do exist (i.e., Morton's 1969 Logogen theory and Miller and Johnson-Laird's 1976 decision table theory), but they are seriously inadequate and underspecified (cf. Levelt 1989, 198 ff). Research on speech errors (cf. Garrett, this volume) and experimental studies (Levelt/Schriefers/Vorberg et al. 1991) indicate that a single concept can (temporarily) trigger the activation of two or more semantically related lemmas (the lemma lexicon is clearly organized according to semantic principles). In most cases, however, a single lemma is selected and determines the further progress of grammatical encoding. (For a further discussion of these issues, see the special issue of 'Cognition' on lexical access in speech production, Levelt 1992.)

Each retrieved lemma contains two kinds of syntactic information: First, information specifying the lemma's syntactic category (major category, such as Noun, Verb, Adjective, Preposition, or minor category, such as Auxiliary, Determiner). Second, information determining the lemma's mapping of conceptual arguments (also called 'thematic roles') onto grammatical functions. The lemma *give*, for instance, specifies that the conceptual agent (X) should be assigned the grammatical role of subject in the surface structure, that the theme (Y) should be realized as a direct object, and the recipient (Z) as an oblique object. These mapping conditions are met in a sentence such as *The mother gave an ice cream to the child.* The lemma *give* also allows for another argument-to-function mapping, the so-called dative, which figures in a sentence like *The mother gave the child an ice cream.* Many transitive verbs also have a passive mapping, as in *The child was given an ice cream by the mother*. Which of these mappings is chosen during grammatical encoding depends on what the speaker has chosen for the topic of discourse (mother or child in the example); the topic is preferably realized as the subject. It also depends on the order in which the various lemmas become available from the mental lexicon. The dative will be preferred if the recipient lemma (*child* in the example) is available before the theme lemma (*ice cream*). Hence, temporal ordering in grammatical encoding is multiply determined. Three forces compete in this ordering process: the syntactic ordering restrictions set by the grammar; the schedule of lemma retrieval which, in turn, depends on the timing and saliency of the concepts in the message (cf.

Bock/Warren 1985); and the topicalization the speaker has decided to achieve.

Various mechanisms of grammatical encoding have been proposed, in particular Kempen and Hoenkamp's Incremental Procedural Grammar (1987), Kempen and Vosse's incremental syntactic tree formation (1989), and MacWhinney and Bates' competition model (1989). See Levelt (1989, 235 ff) for a review.

The output of grammatical encoding is a surface structure, that is, a hierarchical phrase or tree structure with lemmas as terminal nodes. Each phrase corresponds to some predicate, argument or modifier in the message. And each lemma's syntactic environment is an appropriate realization of the lemmas syntax (its syntactic category and its argument-to-function mapping). Finally, lemmas may be marked for prosodic focus, dependent on the prominence of concepts in the message. The (developing) surface structure forms the input to the process of phonological encoding.

2.3. Phonological Encoding

Phonological encoding is the construction of a phonetic or articulatory plan, given the surface structure. The first step here is to retrieve each lemma's phonological specification, its 'lexeme', from the mental lexicon. These lexemes are not fully specified phonetic templates or motor programs, ready to be executed. In connected speech the shape of words is heavily dependent on their environment. For instance, the words *want* and *to* may become encoded as *wanna* in an utterance such as *Where d'you wanna go*? The context-dependent shape of words has to be created time and again from abstract phonological specifications. The units *d'you* and *wanna* in the example are called 'phonological words'. They consist of a head word and one or more clitics that are phonological traces of full words.

When the retrieval of a lemma's lexeme is momentarily blocked, the speaker is in a 'tip-of-the-tongue' (TOT) state (cf. Kohn/Wingfield/Menn et al. 1987). The speaker may then know the word's initial segment(s) or its accent structure. Normally, however, access to lexeme information is quite fast. But there is evidence that even then segmental information is retrieved 'from left to right' (Meyer 1990; 1991).

This segmental information is to be inserted into metrical frames. The basic metrical frame corresponds to a phonological word. In producing the utterance *Dick gave it*, two phonological word frames are set up, one for *Dick* and one for *gave it*. The first one is a one-syllable frame, the second one is a two-syllable frame. As the segments /d/, /I/ and /k/ become successively available, they fill the one-syllable frame. The segments of the *gave* and *it* lexemes, namely /g/, /eI/, /v/, /I/, and /t/, are successively inserted in the second phonological word frame. The first two segments, /g/ and /eI/, complete the first syllable; /v/, /I/ and /t/ compose the second syllable. The resulting syllabification (/geI – vIt/) thus 'straddles' the lexeme boundary. The output of this 'slot-filling' phase of phonological encoding is a string of syllable specifications. Crompton (1982) suggested that each syllable thus composed is in turn the address of a stored phonetic or articulatory plan for that syllable. As soon as a syllable address is composed, the corresponding phonetic plan can be retrieved. This model has been adopted and further developed by Levelt (1989), but there are highly respectable alternative views on the transition from phonological to phonetic representations (cf. Browman/Goldstein 1990).

Thus, three processes cooperate in phonological encoding. First metrical frames are generated, whose basic units are phonological words. Very little is known about the mechanisms generating such frames (cf. Levelt 1989, 318 ff for a review). In the second process, segmental information is spelled out and is inserted into the frames. This has been the subject of extensive empirical and theoretical research. Most of this research is based on the analysis of naturally observed and experimentally elicited speech errors. Shattuck-Hufnagel (1979) proposed the slot/filler model from which all subsequent work is derived. Dell (1986) added an activation spreading model of segmental spell-out, which provides a unified account of a large range of speech error phenomena. The third process is the mapping of syllabified and metrically specified phonological strings onto phonetic or articularly programs.

The articulatory plan's metrical specification is part of a larger p r o s o d i c specification. Phonological words are grouped together into 'phonological phrases'. They have their boundaries right after lexical heads-of-phrase (in particular after nouns in noun phrases, after main verbs in verb phrases and after adjectives in adjective phrases), as in

The detective/ suddenly remembered/ that the station/ could be entered/ from the other side/ (slashes mark ends of phonological phrases). In their turn, phonological phrases concatenate into 'intonational phrases', i. e., phrases over which a particular intonation contour is realized. Speakers have great freedom in partitioning an utterance in intonational phrases. The above example can be spoken either as a single intonational phrase; or a break could be made between *remembered* and *that*, so that two phrases result. Intonational phrases are characterized by their *tone*, and each language has a repertoire of meaningful tones. So, for instance, the 'high-fall' as in *Peter has come* has a serious declarative intention, the 'low-rise' as in *Peter has come* has something reassuring to it, whereas the 'high-rise' as in *Peter has come* mildly invites confirmation. But a speaker's intonational repertoire is not limited to these conventional tones. Nothing in speech is so directly expressive of emotion as intonation and prosody in general (cf. Scherer 1986). It is as yet unknown by what mechanisms the formal-representational planning of speech is merged with its directly expressive use.

2.4. Articulation

There is no reason to suppose that the pace at which the phonetic plan is generated is always completely synchronous with the pace of articulation. In fact, there is good evidence for the existence of an 'articulatory buffer' which temporarily stores successive bits of phonetic plan (at least the size of phonological words) until they are to be executed (Morton 1969). The time needed to retrieve a unit from the buffer depends on the total number of units it contains, each additional unit adding some 10 milliseconds to the retrieval time (Sternberg/Monsell/Knoll/Wright 1978). It is, therefore, most efficient for the buffer to be relatively empty. A retrieved motor program first has to be 'unpacked', making the whole hierarchy of motor commands available. The more complex a unit, the more time it takes to unpack it (Sternberg/Wright/Knoll/Monsell 1980). Buffered speech is subjectively experienced as 'internal speech'. Internal speech can to some extent be monitored by the speaker (see section 2.5.).

The articulatory program is executed by a motor system consisting of three major parts. The respiratory system provides the acoustic energy for speech by controlling the steady outflow of air. The respiratory cycle during speech is quite different from the normal breathing cycle; inhalation takes no more than 15 percent of the total cycle, and the air pressure gradient is almost constant during the outflow of air. The laryngeal system, with the vocal folds as their central part, controls voicing and loudness in speech. During voicing the laryngeal system provides a periodic string of puffs with a wide range of high-frequency components. The supralaryngeal system or vocal tract contains three cavities in which this frequency spectrum is modulated, the nasal, the oral and the pharyngeal cavities. They control the timbre of vowels and consonants. The vocal tract can be constricted in different places (dental, palatal, alveolar, velar, uvular, glottal), and there are different manners in which these constrictions can be released (plosive, fricative, affricative, lateral, etc.). The combinations of places and manners provide the wide variety of speech sounds that the world's languages display.

One of the most striking features of speech motor control is its context-dependency. The same speech sound can be produced in different ways, and speakers almost instantly adapt to changing physical contingencies in the vocal tract. Speech produced by a speaker with a pipe in his mouth hardly differs from unhampered speech. It is, therefore, unlikely that phonetic programs are detailed description of articularly gestures. Rather, they are 'tasks' for the articulators to perform; they prescribe the speech sounds to be generated. Recent theories of articulation suppose the existence of 'model-referenced' control (Arbib 1981). There is an internal model which relates an equivalence class of articulatory gestures to a particular target sound. Through proprioceptive feedback the model is also informed about the contingencies in force. It then automatically chooses the least energy consuming way to produce the sound structure dictated by the 'task'. The set of muscles that cooperate as a unit in the context-dependent execution of a particular phonetic task is called a 'synergism' (Lenneberg 1967) or a 'coordinative structure' (Saltzman/Kelso 1987).

2.5. Self-monitoring and Repair

Speakers are their own hearers. They can monitor anything in their own speech that they can monitor in the speech of others. They can attend to both the meaning and the form of their utterances. And when they detect trouble, they may interrupt themselves and make a repair, such as in *Left to pink – er straight to pink* (speaker tries to describe a pattern of colored dots) where a lexical error is repaired or in *What are this kid – is this kid going to say incorrectly?* where syntactic agreement is reestablished.

How is this self-monitoring performed? There are three loci of self-control in Figure 1.1. First, the speaker can attend to his own message planning. He may revise a planned message before it gets formulated. This probably happened in *Tell me, er what – d'you need a hot sauce?* Whatever the speaker intended to say here was revised before it was fully delivered. Hesitations in speech are often due to such preformulating revisions. Second, the speaker can attend to his internal speech. Speech in the articulatory buffer is accessible to attention in just the same way as overt speech. It can be parsed by the speaker's own language comprehension system. The speaker may then become aware of trouble (i. e., at the conceptual level) and decide to interrupt himself. This is the 'internal monitoring loop'. As long as the buffered internal speech has not been articulated, such an interruption can prevent the production of an error. This probably happened in *A v- ... a horizontal line*, where the speaker was on the verge of uttering *vertical* instead of *horizontal*. Third, the speaker can attend to his own overt speech, using his normal speech understanding system. This is the 'external monitoring loop'. The internal loop is faster than the external loop (cf. Lackner/Tuller 1979; Levelt 1989, 467 ff), but research on close shadowing (Marslen-Wilson 1985) shows that the external loop can, in exceptional cases, work in as few as 250 milliseconds, i. e., a syllable's duration.

There is good evidence that speakers interrupt their speech as soon as serious trouble is detected (Levelt 1983). But detection can be late because the speaker attends mainly to the planning of speech, not to his output. This means that one or more words can follow the trouble item before the speaker detects it. This happened in the utterance *And from green left to pink – er from blue left to pink*. Here *green* was wrong, but the speaker delivered three more words before interrupting his speech. The place of interruption is unprincipled; it can violate any clause, phrase, word, or syllable boundary. There is a tendency, however, to complete a word that is not itself the trouble item (Levelt 1983).

After interruption, the speaker often utters some 'editing expression'. When the occasion for repair is a real error, the dominant editing term is *er*, especially when the interruption is immediate. But it can also indicate a more explicit rejection of what was said, such as *no* or *sorry*. The use of editing terms is different when the repair is for appropriateness, not for error. In *To the right – further to the right is yellow* the repair involves a further specification, not a rejection of what was said. In such cases editing terms are used infrequently and they are of a different type, not indicating rejection, such as *I mean*.

Though there is no linguistic systematicity in where a speaker interrupts his speech, resuming speech is, in fact, systematic. It is governed by a linguistic well-formedness rule (Levelt 1983; 1989, 486) which says that repairing follows the rules of coordination. A repair like *Is the doctor seeing – er – the doctor interviewing patients?* is linguistically ill-formed, and so is the corresponding coordination *Is the doctor seeing patients or the doctor interviewing patients?* The repair *is the nurse – er – the doctor interviewing patients?*, however, is well-formed and so is the corresponding coordination *Is the nurse or the doctor interviewing patients?* Linguistically ill-formed repairs are probably as infrequent in spontaneous speech as are other linguistic deviances, but they can be experimentally elicited (van Wijk/Kempen 1987). The linguistic systematicity of repairing shows that the speaker keeps the interrupted formulation in abeyance during the planning of repair. The repair proper is then grafted on this still available grammatical structure.

Repairs are also often elicited by the interlocutor. She can make the speaker aware of some error or unclarity by saying *what?*, by raising her eyebrows, or by other signals to the speaker. In normal conversation, speakers capitalize on this cooperative feedback. They do not have to be too precise in planning their speech, since the interlocutor will react when necessary.

3. Speech Understanding

In normal conversation the listener's objective is to discover the speaker's communicative intentions. Several speech understanding mechanisms cooperate to accomplish this. There are, first, the mechanisms that perform an acoustic-phonetic analysis of the speech signal; they produce a phonetic representation of the signal. It is the code for accessing the lexicon and for deriving the metrical structure of the utterance. The recognized words and the prosodic information are then used to perform syntactic and semantic parsing of the utterance. And finally, the listener will interpret this linguistic structure in terms of the ongoing discourse in order to derive the speaker's communicative intentions.

We will consider these processes by following the right side of Figure 1.1 from bottom to top.

3.1. Acoustic-Phonetic Analysis

Most theories of speech perception assume the existence of a 'front end' processor that receives the acoustic signal as input and that delivers some kind of featural representation as output. Opinions differ about the character of these features. Liberman/Mattingly (1986) suggest that they are representations of the speaker's intended articulatory gestures. This would bring the output of acoustic-phonetic analysis quite close to what we called above the speaker's articulatory plan. Others stay closer to the spectral properties of the speech signal, and suggest the existence of detectors for onsets and spectral peaks, and for frequencies and motions of formants. These, in turn, are used to derive the presence, absence, or degree of phonetic features such as voicing, nasality, coronality, vowel height, stridency, sonorance, etc., as well as their temporal distribution (see especially Stevens 1986). These patterns of features are the access codes to words in the lexicon (Lahiri/Jongman 1990). They are called 'phonetic representations' in Figure 1.1.

There is still much controversy about the character of the phonetic representations and the way they are derived from the speech signal; see the two excellent reviews of acoustic-phonetic processing by Pisoni/Luce (1987) and Klatt (1989). A major problem to be dealt with is the huge variability in the speech signal. A word's acoustic shape depends on its linguistic context (e. g., the phonological word and phrase in which it partakes, its stress and its intonation), the rate of speech, the dialect and sex of the speaker, the reverberation and noise in the room, and so on. Still, there is an increasing conviction that there are relational patterns in the speech signal that are robust and from which the presence of phonetic features can be reliably derived (cf. Stevens/Blumstein 1981; Stevens 1986; Zue 1986).

Whatever the precise nature of the phonetic representation, it must be such that the listener's linguistic parsing can be based on it. The parser contains two major processing components. One deals with phonological decoding and lexical access, the other one with grammatical (both syntactic and semantic) decoding.

3.2. Phonological Decoding and Lexical Selection

The phonetic representation of an utterance forms the access code to the lexicon. When the listener is exposed to connected speech, a first major problem is how to segment it. To recognize a word, one must know where it begins. But connected speech does not have the nice spaces between words that we encounter in written language. And there is no reason to suppose that phonetic representations, i. e., temporal distributions of phonetic features, make this task any easier. There are two ways in which the listener can approach the segmentation problem. The first one is to use cues in the signal itself. Cutler/Ladd (1983) reviewed studies showing that English listeners prefer to perceive word boundaries before strong syllables (i. e., syllables that carry word accent). There is, for instance, Taft's (1984) finding that listeners dominantly perceive such speech strings as [lettuce] as a single word, *lettuce*, not as two words *let us*, whereas words such as [invests] are preferably heard as two words, *in vests*, not *invests*. Cutler (1989) computed that this segmentation strategy will be about 85% correct for English open class or content words. Other cues could be of a phonotactic nature. Frazier (1987 a) argued that certain strings can only be word-final, such as [-arpt] in English. That would tell the listener that what is about to follow must be a new word. A second approach is to recognize a word before it ends. The listener can then predict the end of the word, and hence the beginning of the next one. This would be a powerful strategy given the cohort theory, to which we will presently turn. Still, the perennial problems in automatic speech segmentation show that a satisfactory theory of segmentation is still long in coming.

But assuming that the listener knows where in the phonetic representation a new word is about to begin, how is that word identified? Dominant here is Marslen-Wilson's 'cohort theory' (for recent publications, see Marslen-

Wilson 1987; 1989). For each lexical item the recognition lexicon contains an abstract phonological code (probably not unlike the phonological code in the production lexicon. Notice that Figure 1.1 does not distinguish between a perception and a production lexicon; opinions differ as to whether such a distinction has to be made). This phonological code specifies a word's non-redundant distinctive features. For English, a phonetic feature like [+aspiration], as after [p] in *pot*, will not appear in the lexicon because it is not distinctive (there are no two different words *p'ot* and *pot*). Similarly, for a nasal consonant the feature [+voice] will not be specified, because it is redundant: all nasals are voiced (but not inversely). Finally, a feature is only specified in the word's representation if it is marked. Thus, nasality is marked and needs specification. But non-nasality is the default case; it needs no specification in the lexicon. See Lahiri/Marslen-Wilson (1991) for further details of this representational theory.

After a small stretch of sensory input (corresponding to about two segments of the input word) has been received, its phonetic feature pattern activates all lexical items whose word-initial phonological specification matches the input. So, if the input word is *trespass*, and the phonetic features of [tr] have become available, not only the lexical item *trespass* will be activated, but also items such as *tree, tremble, trestle, trombone*, etc. This set of initially activated items is called the 'word-initial cohort'.

As the incoming speech signal proceeds, the word-initial cohort is successively reduced. As soon as a feature appears that contradicts the specification of /o/ in *trombone* or /i/ in *tree*, *trombone* and *tree* disappear from the cohort. Next, the fricative feature of /s/ will exclude a candidate like *tremble*. The reduction of the cohort proceeds until a single candidate is left. In the example case this happens when the initial stretch *tresp-* has been received. The item *trespass* is the only one in the recognition lexicon whose phonological specification matches the phonetic pattern of that initial stretch.

The time course of word recognition is jointly determined by the developing information in the speech signal, and by the ensemble of competitors to the target word. The ensemble of competitor items determines a word's 'uniqueness point', the point at which it becomes different from all competitors in the lexicon. For *trespass* the uniqueness point is at /p/. The empirical issue is whether listeners in fact recognize a word when its uniqueness point is reached, i. e., does the recognition point coincide with the uniqueness point? The experimental evidence is surprisingly assuring here (cf. Marslen-Wilson 1987), though certain factors such as semantic/syntactic context (Zwitserlood 1989) or word frequency can additionally affect the position of the recognition point. Contrary to predictions of alternative theories, such as the connectionist model TRACE by Elman/McClelland (1984), there is no evidence that activated competitors actively inhibit one another (Frauenfelder/Segui/Dijkstra 1990).

Though accessing the lexicon is the main target of phonological decoding, another major task is prosodic decoding. In particular, the listener will have to recognize the metrical groupings of the words recognized. This will facilitate subsequent syntactic processing. For instance, the last element in a phonological phrase is usually the head of a syntactic phrase. Also, the listener will have to recognize the tone of an intonational phrase because this carries important communicative information. Little is known about these aspects of prosodic recognition, but see the volume edited by Cutler/Ladd (1983).

The final output of phonological decoding/lexical selection is what has been called a 'lexical/prosodic representation' in Figure 1.1. It forms the input to the higher-order interpretative processes.

3.3. Grammatical Decoding

As lexical items and metrical structure become successively available, the listener will immediately try to interpret these materials. The incrementality of this process (see section 4) implies that syntactic and semantic processing proceed 'on-line' with the incoming information. There is solid experimental evidence that this in fact the case in speech understanding (Marslen-Wilson/Tyler 1980; Tyler/Warren 1987).

Though syntactic analysis and semantic interpretation develop hand in hand, each follows its own principles. And there is a certain degree of autonomy in syntactic processing; it proceeds even in the face of semantic implausibility or anomaly. Let us first consider some aspects of syntactic processing.

The time pressure under which a listener must perform her syntactic analysis of the incoming materials, makes her follow a principle of syntactic analysis that Frazier

(1987b) called 'minimal attachment'. It means that new materials are syntactically attached in such a way that a minimum number of nodes is to be added to the existing syntactic structure. For example, when the listener has heard *The spy saw the cop* and now takes in *with binoculars*, then she will preferably attach the latter prepositional phrase to the already existing verb phrase node. This would lead to the interpretation that seeing the cop (by the spy) was done with binoculars. The non-preferred alternative, however, is that the noun phrase *the cop* is deleted from the verb phrase node, a new additional noun phrase node is created for *the cop with binoculars*, which then in turn gets attached to the verb phrase node. This would imply the interpretation that the cop was equipped with binoculars. The minimal attachment principle predicts that listeners will tend to 'garden path' on sentences where minimal attachment leads to the wrong solution. According to this assumption, a sentence like *The horse raced passed the barn fell in a puddle* must be harder to understand than *The horse raced past the barn and fell in a puddle*, and in fact it is (Ferreira/Clifton 1986). Regrettably, the minimal attachment principle has almost exclusively been studied in reading tasks. Whether it is equally valid for spoken language comprehension, where prosody provides important cues, is an open issue.

That speech is syntactically processed even if it is semantically anomalous was demonstrated by Marslen-Wilson/Tyler (1980). In a more recent experiment, Tyler/Warren (1987) confirmed and extended this finding. They used a word monitoring task, in which the listener had to push a button as soon as she heard a given target word. For example, the listener is given KITCHEN as target word, and is presented with the following normally spoken sentence: *The maid / was carefully peeling / the potatoes / in the garden / because during the summer / a hot KITCHEN / is unbearable to work in* (here the slashes mark phonological phrase boundaries). For such sentences listeners push the button about 300 milliseconds after onset of the target word. When a semantically anomalous text was presented (such as *An orange dream / was loudly watching / the house / during smelly nights / because within these signs / a slow KITCHEN / snored / with crashing leaves*) reaction times were, not surprisingly, slower (by some 60 milliseconds). If, however, the local syntax around *KITCHEN* was also disrupted (by replacing *a slow KITCHEN* by *slow very KITCHEN*), latencies increased (by another 45 milliseconds). Thus, local syntactic parsing apparently proceeds where it can, even when the speech is semantically anomalous.

However, this is not the case for global syntactic parsing. When the phonological phrases in the anomalous sentence are scrambled (as in *Because within these signs / during smelly lights / was loudly watching / the house / an orange dream / a slow KITCHEN / snored / with crashing leaves*) so that global (but not local) syntax is disrupted, the reaction times are the same as for the original semantically anomalous text. Tyler and Warren could show that global syntax is only effective when the text is meaningful. And this should not be surprising. The eventual output of global syntactic parsing is a conceptual structure whose thematic roles (see section 2.2. above) correspond to the function-argument mappings of the retrieved lexical items. If these mappings are violated, as in semantically anomalous text, global parsing will be blocked.

The following picture emerges: First, as words are successively recognized, their syntactic and semantic information becomes available to the parser. The syntactic information is concerned with a word's category (Noun, Verb, etc.) and its argument-to-function mapping (see section 2.2. above). Of these, the category information is probably enough to initiate a second process, local syntactic analysis (Frazier 1989). We have no difficulty in parsing nonsense such as *The beer slept the guitar*. Here we construct a verb phrase, *slept the guitar*, with *the guitar* as direct object of *slept*, in spite of the fact that this contradicts the argument-to-function mapping of *sleep* (an intransitive verb which does not take a direct object). The initial syntactic parsing can also ignore semantics (the meaning of *sleep* dictates that the verb requires an animate subject, but *beer* is inanimate). However, initial local parsing is very dependent on the intactness of phonological phrases. Tyler/Warren (1987) found a dramatic increase of reaction times when the phonological phrase was broken up (e. g., *the slow KITCHEN* being distributed over two phrases, with a break after *the slow*). In short, initial local syntactic analysis uses the metrical output of the acoustic-phonetic component plus the syntactic category information of the recognized words. But a third process, global syntactic parsing is, at least in part, based on semantic analysis. Grammatical functions such as 'subject', 'direct object', or 'indirect object' are translated into the thematic roles they are attached to in the lexical representations. For instance, the indirect object of the verb *give* in a sentence will be interpreted as the recipient of the action of transfer denoted by *give*. This is syntactically based semantic interpretation. The final output of global parsing, then, is a conceptual structure, akin to the speaker's 'message' (see section 2.1.). It is therefore referred to as a 'derived message' in Figure 1.1.

Only one aspect of global parsing has been studied in some detail for spoken language: the resolution of anaphora. Syntax can restrict the interpretation of an anaphor. In the sentence (i) *The boxer told the skier that the doctor of the team would blame himself for the recent injury*, the reflexive pronoun *himself* can only refer back to *the doctor*, not to *the boxer* or *the skier*. Will the listener reactivate *the doctor* at encountering the anaphor, in correspondence with syntax, or will the other referents also be reactivated, ignoring syntax? Nicol (1988) studied this question in a so-called cross-modal priming experiment. The subject listened to a sentence of this kind. Right after the pronoun, either a word (like *nurse*) or a non-word (like *murve*) was presented visually. The subject's task was to decide whether the visual probe was a word or a non-word, and to indicate this by pushing either a yes- or a no-button, accordingly. The latency of this lexical decision was measured. If the pronoun reactivates the syntactically indicated antecedent (e. g., *the doctor*), this may lead to a more rapid response to an associate probe (e. g., *nurse*) as compared to a neutral probe (e. g., *house*), and in fact it did. In contrast, no facilitation was obtained for associates of the other potential antecedents (e. g., *the boxer* or *the skier*).

What happens when there is no syntactic restriction on the interpretation of a pronoun? Consider sentence (ii), *The boxer told the skier that the doctor for the team would blame him for the recent injury*. Here the pronoun *him* can refer back to *the boxer* or *the skier* (but not to *the doctor*). And Nicol now found reactivation of both *the boxer* and *the skier* (but not of *the doctor*), in complete agreement with the syntax.

Even null-anaphors produce essentially the same effect. In *The policeman saw the boy that the crowd at the party accused t of the crime*, *t* stands for a null-anaphor (or *trace*) that refers back to *the boy*. And indeed, by probing at this position Swinney/Ford/Frauenfelder/Bresnan (unpublished) showed that *the boy* was reactivated there, but not *the crowd*. For an excellent review of this and related work, see Nicol/Swinney (1989). Notice also that in examples like these the listener is making essential use of the verb's function-argument structure. The verb *accuse* requires a direct object, so the listener knows that there must be a direct object trace after *accuse*. Global syntactic processing takes the verb-argument structure into account (i. e., different from local syntactic processing).

Though apparently automatically restricted by syntax, the listener's binding of anaphors is a semantic activity. Cloitre/Bever (1988), for instance, found that when the syntactic antecedent is a concrete noun it is easier reactivated by a pronoun than when it is an abstract noun.

Though the derived message is a conceptual interpretation of the utterance, it is one at a rather shallow level. As a rule, it will not be the ultimate interpretation. In example (ii) above, for instance, the derived message does not specify whether the anaphor refers back to *the boxer*, *the skier*, or somebody else mentioned earlier in the discourse. Solving such problems of interpretation, as well as many others, are part of 'discourse processing', to be discussed after a final remark on the output of the parser.

Though derived messages form the parser's main output, they are not the only information it makes available to the conceptualizer. The parser can also transmit certain intermediary results. The listener can, for instance, attend to phonetic or syntactic properties of the utterance. She can, for instance, notice the speaker's dialect, or grammatical errors. The term 'parsed speech' in Figure 1.1 includes these aspects, as well as the main output of parsing, the derived message.

3.4. Discourse Processing

The last step towards deriving the speaker's communicative intention is called discourse processing. It is the subject of extensive research; here we can touch on a few aspects only. The first one is 'identifying referents' and refers to the listener's attempt to determine what entities the speaker is talking about. Clark/Schreuder/Buttrick (1983) showed subjects a photograph depicting president Reagan and David Stockman (a high, but not well-known official). When they asked *You know who this man is, don't you?*, most subjects answered that it was Reagan. But when asked *Do you have any idea at all who this man is?*, nobody said Reagan; they all made guesses about the other person on the photograph. The referent chosen for *this man* depends on the listener's presupposition about the speaker's knowledge, namely that Reagan is better known than the other depicted person.

An important mechanism in the interpretation of discourse, and in particular in the assignment of reference, is the construction of a 'discourse model'. It is a mental model (Johnson-Laird 1983) about the state of affairs discussed. Typically, when the listener encounters an indefinite description (as in *There is a baby here*), she will set up a new address in the model (in this case an address for the baby entity). However, when she encounters a definite description (as in *The baby is crying*, or *It is crying*), she will infer that the address is already present, and the predication is interpreted as being about the entity at that address (cf. Seuren 1993 for a theory of reference assignment in discourse models).

Earlier we saw that anaphoric reference can still be undecided in the derived message (as was the case for *him* in example (ii) above). The listener can then choose the most salient entity in the discourse model as a referent for the pronoun (Clark/Schreuder/Buttrick 1983; Morrow 1986). Alternatively, the listener may select the entity mentioned last (*the skier* in example (ii)). This is also dependent on the 'genre' of the discourse, as Morrow established.

Inferring referents is devilishly complicated. How does a listener (waitress in a restaurant) compute the person referent for her colleague's remark *The hamburger wants the bill* (Nunberg 1979)? It must be the person who was served a hamburger. Nunberg argued that there is some 'referring function' that maps the demonstratum (*the hamburger*) onto the intended referent (see also Fauconnier 1985). But how does the listener compute such arbitrary referring functions?

Such cases of indirect reference are by no means the only instances of non-literal interpretation in speech understanding. Other paramount cases are the interpretation of indirect requests (see section 2.1.), the interpretation of metaphor (Sperber/Wilson 1986), irony (Clark/Gerrig 1984), hyperbole (Grice 1975) and other figures of speech. In these latter cases prosody, and especially the tones of intonational phrases, may cue the listener to infer the speaker's intention.

Finally, the 'denotation of words' surpasses the shallow semantic interpretation of the derived message. Hörmann (1983) showed that quantifiers such as *some* or *many* are interpreted in relationship to what they quantify. For example, there are less people in *some people* than grains of sand in *some grains of sand*. Morrow and Clark (1988) extended this study by showing that the distance denoted by the verb *approach* depends on what is approaching and what is being approached. A tractor approaching a farmhouse, for instance, is at a greater distance than a mouse approaching a farmhouse. The distance is even smaller, when a mouse approaches a piece of cheese. In all these cases the listener's discourse model, or image of the situation is decisive for the inference.

Discourse processing requires the listener's full attention. The derived message, which comes rather automatically with the incoming speech, is only a cue to the interlocutor's intentions. There is no limit to the variety of discourse situations, and every utterance is to be interpreted in the light of the current situation, the knowledge the interlocutors share, the social relation they are engaged in, the lay-out of their physical environment, and so on. Recovering the speaker's intentions, not speech perception or parsing, is the listener's ultimate goal.

4. Incrementality, Autonomy and Interaction

It is not the intention of Figure 1.1 to suggest that processing components work one after another. On the contrary, parallel processing does take place both in speaking and in listening. However, it occurs in a specific way that Kempen and Hoenkamp (1982) called 'incremental'. Though all components work in parallel, they work on different bits and pieces. Concretely, as soon as the speaker has conceived of an initial concept to be expressed, it is delivered to the Formulator. Instead of waiting until the whole message has been planned, the first concept is grammatically encoded — a word is retrieved from the lexicon and receives case. That bit of surface structure is then subjected to phonological encoding, and so on. Meanwhile other fragments follow the same route. As a consequence, a speaker can begin articulating a sentence long before he has completed the planning of his message. It is a 'roofing tile' organization of processing. Similarly in speech perception, as soon as the initial fragment of the speech signal has been received, acoustic-phonetic processing of that bit of signal begins. And as soon as its first two or three segments have been phonetically analyzed a word-initial cohort is activated. Syntactic local parsing can start as soon as the first word is recognized, and so can semantic processing and discourse interpretation. Each processor works incrementally on successive fragments it receives from the previous one. Thus, there is both staging and parallelness of computation.

Parallel computation is only possible because most components are fully automatic. If the language user were to pay attention to all component processes, parallel processing would be infeasible. Language users can normally limit their attention to conceptual processing: planning messages, selfmonitoring, and discourse interpretation. The fluency of speech production and the 'on-line' character of speech comprehension are essentially based on a combination of automaticity and incremental production.

The staging inherent in the notion of incremental processing is ultimately an empirical issue. And indeed, it has been, and still is a topic of much debate (cf. Garfield 1987). In the ideal case of staging, a later processing component down the line cannot affect the mode of processing of an earlier component. There is only feedforward of information, no interaction between components.

Research in speech production has produced evidence of feedback from phonological to grammatical encoding (Dell 1986; Bock 1987), but this feedback is highly limited (Levelt 1989, 275 ff.; Levelt/Schriefers/Vorberg et al. 1991). There is at present no hard evidence for any other direct feedback interaction between speech production components.

The picture for speech understanding is less straightforward. Though there is good evidence that a word's acoustic-phonetic processing is not affected by lexical or higher level processes (Frauenfelder/Segui/Dijkstra 1990), the effects of context on word recognition have been heavily debated. It is rather safe now to say that when a speaker hears an ambiguous word (like *bank*), both of its meanings are temporarily retrieved from the lexicon, even if one is ruled out by the context (as in *I withdrew my money from the bank*) (Seidenberg/Tanenhaus/Leiman/Bienkowski 1982). The inappropriate reading is then quickly lost (at least within 200 milliseconds, cf. Jones 1989). In other words, there is no feedback from semantic parsing to lexical access here. The story is more complicated for context effects on the recognition of non-ambiguous words. Using the cross-modal priming technique, Zwitserlood (1989) showed that (i) the structure of the word-initial cohort is independent of biasing semantic or syntactic context, but also that (ii) context begins to have an effect on lexical selection just before the stimulus information has reached the word's uniqueness point (cf., section 3.2. above). This finding contradicts Marslen-Wilson's (1989) claim that not only lexical activation but also lexical selection is exclusively stimulus driven.

As far as grammatical decoding is concerned, it probably involves a relatively autonomous syntactic subcomponent. Whereas the initial, local syntactic analysis proceeds independent of semantic context, global syntactic parsing seems to interact with both semantic and discourse interpretation.

5. References

Arbib, M. A. (1981). Perceptual structures and distributed motor control. In V. Brooks (Ed.), *Handbook of physiology. The nervous system: Vol. 2. Motor control.* 1449–1480. Bethesda, MD: American Physiological Society.

Bock, J. K. (1987). An effect of the accessibility of word forms on sentence structures. *Journal of Memory and Language, 26*, 119–137.

Bock, J. K. & Warren, R. K. (1985). Conceptual accessibility and syntactic structure in sentence formulation. *Cognition, 21*, 47–67.

Browman, C. P. & Goldstein, L. (1990). Articulatory gestures as phonological units. *Haskins Laboratories Status Report on Speech Research, SR-99/100*, 69–101.

Butterworth, B. (1980). Evidence from pauses in speech. In B. Butterworth (Ed.), *Language production: Vol. 1. Speech and talk. 155–176.* London: Academic Press.

Clark, H. H. (1979). Responding to indirect speech acts. *Cognitive Psychology, 4*, 430–477.

Clark, H. H. & Gerrig, R. J. (1984). On the pretense theory of irony. *Journal of Experimental Psychology: General, 133*, 121–126.

Clark, H. H., Schreuder, R. & Buttrick, S. (1983). Common ground and the understanding of demonstratives. *Journal of Verbal Learning and Verbal Behavior, 22*, 245–258.

Clark, H. H. & Schunk, D. H. (1980). Polite responses to polite requests. *Cognition, 8*, 111–143.

Clark, H. H. & Wilkes-Gibbs. D. L. (1986). Referring as a collaborative process. *Cognition, 22*, 1–39.

Cloitre, M. & Bever, T. G. (1988). Linguistic anaphors, levels of representation, and discourse. *Language and Cognitive Processes, 3*, 293–322.

Crompton, A. (1982). Syllables and segments in speech production. In A. Cutler (Ed.), *Slips of the tongue and language production. 109–162.* Berlin: Mouton.

Cutler, A. (1989). Auditory lexical access: Where do we start? In W. D. Marslen-Wilson (Ed.), *Lexical representation and process. 342–356.* Cambridge, Mass.: MIT Press.

Cutler, A. & Ladd, D. R. (Eds.) (1983). *Prosody: Models and measurements.* Heidelberg: Springer.

Dell, G. S. (1986). A spreading activation theory of retrieval in sentence production. *Psychological Review, 93*, 283–321.

Elman, J. L. & McClelland, J. L. (1984). Speech perception as a cognitive process: The interactive activation model. In N. Lass (Ed.), *Speech and language, vol. 10. 337–374.* New York: Academic Press.

Fauconnier, G. (1985). *Mental spaces: Aspects of meaning construction in natural language.* Cambridge, Mass.: MIT Press.

Ferreira, F. & Clifton, C. (1986). The independence of syntactic processing. *Journal of Memory and Language, 25*, 75–87.

Frauenfelder, U. H., Segui, J., & Dijkstra, T. (1990). Lexical effects in phoneme processing: Facilitatory or inhibitory? *Journal of Experimental Psychology: Human Perception and Performance, 16*, 77–91.

Frazier, L. (1987 a). Structure in auditory word recognition. *Cognition, 25*, 157–187.

Frazier, L. (1987 b). Sentence processing: A tutorial review. In M. Coltheart (Ed.), *Attention and performance XII. 559–586.* Hillsdale, N. J.: Lawrence Erlbaum.

Frazier, L. (1989). Against lexical generation. In W. D. Marslen-Wilson (Ed.), *Lexical representation and process. 505–528.* Cambridge, Mass.: MIT Press.

Garfield, J. L. (Ed.) (1987). *Modularity in knowledge representation and natural-language understanding.* Cambridge, Mass.: MIT Press.

Garrett, M. F. (1975). The analysis of sentence production. In G. Bower (Ed.), *Psychology of learning and motivation Vol. IX. 133–177.* New York: Academic Press.

Grice, H. P. (1968). Utterer's meaning, sentence meaning and word meaning. *Foundations of Language, 4*, 25–242.

Grice, H. P. (1975). Logic and conversation. In P. Cole & J. L. Morgan (Eds.), *Syntax and semantics: 3. Speech acts. 41–58.* New York: Academic Press.

Hörmann, H. (1983). The calculating listener or how many are *einige, mehrere*, and *ein paar* (*some, several* and *a few*)? In R. Bäuerle, C. Schwarze, & A. von Stechow (Eds.), *Meaning, use, and interpretation of language. 221–234.* Berlin: De Gruyter.

Johnson-Laird, P. N. (1983). *Mental models.* Cambridge: Cambridge University Press.

Jones, J. L. (1989). Multiple access of homonym meanings: An artifact of backward priming? *Journal of Psycholinguistic Research, 18*, 417–432.

Kempen, G. & Hoenkamp, E. (1982). Incremental sentence generation: Implications for the structure of a syntactic processor. In J. Horecky (Ed.), *Proceedings of the Ninth International Conference on Computational Linguistics. 151–156.* Amsterdam: North-Holland.

Kempen, G. & Hoenkamp, E. (1987). An incremental procedural grammar for sentence formulation. *Cognitive Science, 11*, 201–258.

Kempen, G. & Vosse, T. (1989). Incremental syntactic tree formation in human sentence processing: An interactive architecture based on activation decay and simulated annealing. *Cahiers de la Fondation Archives Jean Piaget.* Geneva.

Klatt, D. H. (1989). Review of selected models of speech perception. In W. D. Marslen-Wilson (Ed.), *Lexical representation and process. 169–226.* Cambridge, Mass.: MIT Press.

Kohn, S. E., Wingfield, A., Menn, L., Goodglass, H., Berko Gleason, J., & Hyde, M. (1987). Lexical retrieval: The tip of the tongue phenomenon. *Applied Psycholinguistics, 8*, 245–266.

Lackner, J. R. & Tuller, B. H. (1979). Role of efference monitoring in the detection of self-produced speech errors. In W. E. Cooper, E. C. T. Walker (Eds.), *Sentence processing: Psycholinguistic studies presented to Merrill Garrett. 281–294.* Hillsdale, N. J.: Lawrence Erlbaum.

Lahiri, A. & Jongman, A. (1990). Intermediate levels of analysis: features or segments? *Journal of Phonetics, 18*, 435–443.

Lahiri, A. & Marslen-Wilson, W. D. (1991). The mental representation of lexical form: A phonological approach to the recognition lexicon. *Cognition, 38*, 245–294.

Lenneberg, E. H. (1967). *Biological foundations of language.* New York: Wiley.

Levelt, W. J. M. (1983). Monitoring and self-repair in speech. *Cognition, 14*, 41–104.

Levelt, W. J. M. (1989). *Speaking: From intention to articulation.* Cambridge, Mass.: MIT Press.

Levelt, W. J. M. (Ed.) (1992). Lexical access in speech production. Special issue of *Cognition, 42.*

Levelt, W. J. M., Schriefers, H., Vorberg, D., Meyer, A. S., Pechmann, T., & Havinga, J. (1991). The time course of lexical access in speech production. A study of picture naming. *Psychological Review, 98*, 122–142.

Liberman, A. M. & Mattingly, I. G. (1968). The motor theory of speech perception revised. *Cognition, 21*, 1–36.

MacWhinney, B. & Bates, E. (1989). *The crosslinguistic study of sentence processing*. Cambridge: Cambridge University Press.

Marslen-Wilson, W. D. (1985). Speech shadowing and speech comprehension. *Speech Communication, 4*, 55–73.

Marslen-Wilson, W. D. (1987). Functional parallelism in spoken word-recognition. *Cognition, 25*, 71–102.

Marslen-Wilson, W. D. (1989). Access and integration: Projecting sound onto meaning. In W. D. Marslen-Wilson (Ed.), *Lexical representation and process. 3–24*. Cambridge, Mass.: MIT Press.

Marslen-Wilson, W. D. & Tyler, L. (1980). The temporal structure of spoken language understanding. *Cognition, 8*, 1–71.

Meyer, A. S. (1990). The time course of phonological encoding in language production: The encoding of successive syllables of a word. *Journal of Memory and Language, 29*, 524–545.

Meyer, A. S. (1991). The time course of phonological encoding in language production: Phonological encoding inside a syllable. *Journal of Memory and Language, 30*, 69–89.

Miller, G. A. & Johnson-Laird, P. N. (1976). *Language and perception*. Cambridge, Mass.: Harvard University Press.

Morrow, D. G. (1986). Places as referents in discourse. *Journal of Memory and Language, 25*, 676–690.

Morrow, D. G. & Clark, H. H. (1988). Interpreting words in spatial descriptions. *Language and Cognitive Processes, 3*, 275–291.

Morton, J. (1969). The interaction of information in word recognition. *Psychological Review, 76*, 165–178.

Nicol, J. (1988). *Coreference processing during sentence comprehension*. Ph. D. Dissertation. Cambridge, Mass.: M.I.T.

Nicol, J. & Swinney, D. (1989). The role of structure in coreference assignment during sentence comprehension. *Journal of Psycholinguistic Research, 18*, 5–19.

Nunberg, G. (1979). The non-uniqueness of semantic solutions: Polysemy. *Linguistics and Philosophy, 3*, 143–184.

Pisoni, D. B. & Luce, P. A. (1987). Acoustic-phonetic representations in word recognition. *Cognition, 25*, 21–52.

Saltzman, E. & Kelso, J. A. S. (1987). Skilled actions: A task-dynamic approach. *Psychological Review, 94*, 84–106.

Scherer, K. (1986). Vocal affect expression: A review and a model for future research. *Psychological Bulletin, 99*, 143–165.

Seidenberg, M. S., Tanenhaus, M. K., Leiman, J. M., & Bienkowski, M. (1982). Automatic access of the meanings of ambiguous words in context: Some limitations of knowledge-based processing. *Cognitive Psychology, 14*, 489–537.

Seuren, P. M. (1993). Principles of discourse semantics. *Behavioral and Brain Sciences, 16* (in press).

Shattuck-Hufnagel, S. (1979). Speech errors as evidence for a serial order mechanism in sentence production. In W. E. Cooper & E. C. T. Walker (Eds.), *Sentence processing: Psycholinguistic studies presented to Merrill Garrett. 295–342*. Hillsdale, NJ: Lawrence Erlbaum.

Sperber, D. & Wilson, D. (1986). *Relevance: Communication and cognition*. Oxford: Blackwell.

Sternberg, S., Monsell, S., Knoll, R. L., & Wright, C. E. (1978). The latency and duration of rapid movement sequences: Comparisons of speech and typewriting. In G. E. Stelmach (Ed.), *Information processing in motor control and learning. 118–152*. New York: Academic Press.

Sternberg, S., Wright, C. E., Knoll, R. L., & Monsell, S. (1980). Motor programs in rapid speech: Additional evidence. In R. A. Cole (Ed.), *Perception and production of fluent speech. 507–534*. Hillsdale, N. J.: Lawrence Erlbaum.

Stevens, K. N. (1986). Models of phonetic recognition II: A feature-based model of speech recognition. In P. Mermelstein (Ed.), *Proceedings of the Montreal Satellite Symposium on Speech Recognition*, Twelfth International Congress of Acoustics.

Stevens, K. N. & Blumstein, S. E. (1981). The search for invariant acoustic correlates of phonetic features. In P. D. Eimas & J. L. Miller (Eds.), *Perspectives on the study of speech. 1–38*. Hillsdale: Lawrence Erlbaum.

Taft, L. (1984). *Prosodic constraints and lexical parsing strategies*. Ph. D. thesis. University of Massachusetts.

Tyler, L. & Warren, P. (1987). Local and global structure in spoken Language comprehension. *Journal of Memory and Language, 26*, 638–657.

Van Wijk, C. & Kempen, G. (1987). A dual system for producing self-repairs in spontaneous speech: Evidence from experimentally elicited corrections. *Cognitive Psychology, 19*, 403–440.

Zue, V. W. (1986). Models of speech recognition III: The role of analysis by synthesis in phonetic recognition. In P. Mermelstein (Ed.), *Proceedings of the Montreal Satellite Symposium on Speech Recognition*. Twelfth International Congress on Acoustics.

Zwitserlood, P. (1989). The effects of sentential-semantic context in spoken-word processing. *Cognition, 32*, 25–64.

Willem J. M. Levelt, Nijmegen (The Netherlands)

2. Morphosyntactic Characteristics of Spoken Language

1. Introduction

Within a psycholinguistic model of normal language use, the present chapter fills the slot 'generation of surface structure' (see Levelt 1989, ch. 7), that is, the conversion of a message ready for expression into an utterance representation ready for phonological encoding. In short, the topic of this chapter is 'syntax in production'. It is undeniable that the major break throughs in modern theoretical linguistics and in our thinking about language have been achieved on the basis of thorough, deep, and abstract investigations of syntax. And it was mainly in the context of syntax research that the ghost of F. Gall and his doctrine of 'organology' was conjured up and that the idea was put forward that the human species is bestowed with a special language organ stigmatizing us as unique and qualitatively distinct from animals. This organ might be conceived of as an indivisible whole (Chomsky 1980) or as divisible into further organs or 'modules' (Fodor 1983). However, (leaving speech aside) it has almost always and primarily been syntax on which arguments of our uniqueness are based: it is maintained that syntax is not present in animal communication systems and that it is due to syntax that human language cannot be learnt by apes (even if the problem of speech is circumvented). One might very well assume a less discriminatory attitude towards our biological ancestors and brethren (as does Lieberman 1991, despite the title of his book); one might also reject the idea of a 'discontinuity' between the cognitive abilities of apes and humans (Greenfield/Savage-Rumbaugh 1990); furthermore, one might emphatically reject that the language 'organ' evolved out of nothing, but is rather an extension of an earlier system in our evolution with which language is still functionally related (Kimura 1979, with respect to the system of fine movements control). Nevertheless, despite all these possible reservations, it is undeniable that syntax (and speech) in man arrived at such a level of complexity that qualitatively new types of behaviour became possible (see again Lieberman 1991). Given this absolutely central position of syntax in modern linguistics, it is a bit surprising that within psycholinguistics 'syntax in production' is somewhat underdeveloped territory – or to be more polite and more realistic: territory under development. Thus, in this chapter, little more can be done than to present a sort of reference model of production and to indicate some problems and trends which in all likelihood will determine and dominate research in the next future.

The keywords in the title of this chapter, however, invite us to touch on at least two other topics. 'Spoken' suggests a brief discussion of the 'oral-written'-dimension, and, in my view, 'spoken' also refers to the fact that language use takes place in interpersonal social interaction. I shall include these topics, but only under the perspective of their consequences for the morphosyntactic form of utterances.

A last introductory remark concerns the fact that this chapter is part of a handbook on language pathology. It is my conviction that pathologies can be dealt with in a meaningful way only by relating them to models of normal language use. I shall not refrain from occasional excursions into particular fields of pathology in order to make this point precise.

2. Language as an Interpersonal Activity

2.1. The 'Grammarians' Approach'

2.1.1. Speech Acts, Pragmatics

It is taken for granted by almost everybody that the primeval situation of language use is oral face-to-face interaction between at least two participants. Throughout this chapter I shall refer to them by the terms 'interlocutor A' (InA) and 'interlocutor B' (InB), InA denoting the one who makes the first move. From an interactional perspective, the speaking human being is not a sentence-producing system. Rather he produces verbal actions such as demands, requests, complaints, statements (including lies), etc. Since Austin (1962) and Searle (1969), these actions have been called speech acts. The meaning of a speech act is its propositional content plus its illocutionary force – the latter indicating the type of action intended by the locutionary act, that is, the utterance itself (for the perlocutionary force see below). Since the introduction of speech act theory, there has been a keen interest in the possible direct relationship between syntactic form and illocutionary force. It has been a commonly held view that all languages have a limited number of sentence-type forms with a very direct and straightforward relation to illocutionary forces. Most often cited are: declaratives – statements, interrogatives – questions, imperatives – orders. Wunderlich (1976) argues for the existence of only two such transparent pairs (imperatives – orders, interrogatives – questions), the transparency being necessitated by the fact that these are typical interaction-opening moves so that there is no context which could otherwise help InB to infer the force. Sadock/Zwicky (1985) give a comprehensive overview of the possible form–force relations in the languages of the world, including the consideration of the distribution and the morphological properties of so-called performative verbs, i.e. verbs denoting exactly a specific act (*to order, to promise, to sentence, to christen*, etc.).

Sentence forms with a direct relation to their force can be said to have a 'literal meaning'. Altmann (1987) speaks of basic propositional attitudes expressed by these forms. The basic attitude can be modified and differentiated by the complex interplay of a variety of means. In spoken German, particles are used excessively in this respect. Their occurrence obeys specifiable restrictions: for example the particle *ja* – '*yes*' can occur only in declaratives and orders, but not in questions:

(1) Du rauchst ja – 'you smoke yes' (adding a nuance of reproach to the statement)
(2) Rauch' hier ja nicht – 'smoke here yes not' (adding a nuance of warning to the order)
(3) *Warum rauchst du ja? – 'why smoke you yes?'

The enterprise of establishing direct form–force relations meets its unsurmountable barriers when confronted with the so-called indirect speech acts (see Searle 1975) in which the syntactically suggested force is not identical with the actual force. The use of question forms for requests is notorious. I shall give a few more spectacular cases which I shall use again for illustrations in later paragraphs:

(4) Why paint your house purple (not just a question, but a suggestion to apply a different colour) from Gordon/Lakoff 1975)
(5) Mein Gott, es ist schon Mitternacht – 'My God, it is already midnight' (not just a statement, but – potentially – an announcement of InA to leave InB)
(6) Geh' mal ins Bett – 'go PARTICLE to bed' (not just an order, but – potentially – simply an initiation of closing the conversation, cf. Schegloff/Sacks 1973).

Even the highly flexible system of German particles cannot contribute to handling the problem of indirect speech acts. The particle *ja* remains ungrammatical in interrogatives even if they express an order:

(7) *Wie kannst du es ja wagen, hier zu rauchen?! – 'how can you it yes dare here to smoke?!'

An approach, particularly popular in the seventies, tried to come to grips with the form–force problem in indirect speech acts by abandoning the traditional delineation of syntax, semantics, and pragmatics, by creating a component 'pragmantax' (Ross 1975). Here rules of syntax and pragmatic regularities are intermingled. A syntactic rule can take a pragmatic specification as a contextual restriction for its application. In this sense, Gordon and Lakoff consider (4) as derived from the structure *Why do you paint your house purple* by a deletion rule 'WHY YOU TENSE x > WHY x' which can apply only relative to a conversational context specifiable as '*unless you have some good reason fo doing x, you should not do x*'. The pragmantax approach has lost favour and pragmatics has taken a different course. The mainstream of pragmatics is constructed – in some way or other – on the Gricean framework with its basic notions of maxims, background knowledge, and inferential rules (Grice 1957; 1968; 1975; for an elaboration of the Gricean framework representative of the development of 'mainstream pragmatics' see Sperber/Wilson 1986). The essential feature of this approach is the fact that pragmatics is placed outside linguistics *stricto sensu*. Nevertheless, there remains the emphasis on the single sentence (or its utterance) as the primary analytic category (which – for me – reflects the maintenance of a general spirit also evident in pragmantax). Even more surprising is the emergence of a school (discourse analysis – DA) which shifts the emphasis from the single utterance to the conversation, while still operating with notions inherited from linguistics in the narrow sense of the term, specifically with 'rules' and the notions of ill- and wellformedness. In discussing DA, I shall disregard 'text grammar', which sometimes allows itself to be assigned under this rubric as well.

2.1.2. Discourse Analysis (DA)

A major stream of DA has been developed within one tradition of British linguistics ('systemic linguistics', see Halliday 1976). Within limits, one may say that DA considers a conversation as a concatenation of acts which can be ill- or wellformed, respectively, dependent on whether it obeys or violates the rules of concatenation. The analogy to the linguistic treatment of a sentence is obvious. The presentation of a specific example might be more enlightening here than an abstract characterization. Berry (1981) investigates structural properties of a special type of discourse, an 'exchange', which is defined as 'the unit concerned with negotiating the transmission of information' (Coulthart/Brazil 1981, 101). In particular, she deals with the phenomena of increasing ellipticity over the course of an exchange and with the restrictions on the occurrence of the various formal types of queries within an exchange. She distinguishes queries seeking primary information and queries concerning the status of knowledge of the addressee (certainty, uncertainty). After a detailed discussion of the slots for such queries, she presents examples of illformed exchanges one of which will be quoted here:

(8) Son: is Salisbury the English cathedral with the tallest spire?
Father: yes
Son: well, is it
Father: yes
Son: that's right

As I understand Berry, the second query of the son constitutes the illformedness provided that the father's first *yes* was given in such a resolute fashion that it indicated the father's status of knowledge as very definite. Thus, the son's query (with a certain intonation) asks inappropriately (or could one even say: ungrammatically?) for information which is already given. I suppose that most readers will have problems with this example, and I shall indeed readdress it in the following section.

The conception of a set of acts which can be concatenated in an ill- or wellformed manner in a conversation is also inherent in the work of Labov (maybe not his most central, but most illustrative work is Labov/Fanshel 1977). In all fairness, it must be mentioned that there are many more directions and trends in DA than presented by the 'British School' and Labov, not all explicitly subscribing to the notions of concatenation and ill- and wellformedness. For an overview of other developments in discourse analysis, see van Dijk (1985).

2.2. Conversational Analysis (CA)

CA originated in a series of lectures by H. Sacks around 1970. From its inception on CA levelled serious criticisms against speech act theory. The fundamental criticism concerns the analytic primacy of the single act and the neglect of the fact that speech acts occur in first instance as parts of a sequentially ordered activity, namely conversation. The meaning of an utterance (its force) is determined by its position within the sequence, by its interactional consequences. The vexing problem of the form–force relation disappears in this approach. Schegloff (1984) argues that in actual conversation there normally is no ambiguity of an utterance with respect to its force (irrespective of the multiple possibilities of interpreting the syntactic form). To be sure, in a conversation there do occur occasionally ambiguities and subsequent misunderstanding, but then they do not have their source in the syntactic form of the utterances, but in their specific sequential positions.

CA also stands in opposition to DA (see Levinson 1983, ch. 6). To me, the most convincing argument of Levinson is that interlocutors can respond not only to the illocutionary force of a preceding act, but also to its perlocutionary force. Within speech act theory, perlocutionary force is defined as the effect brought about on the audience given the concrete circumstances. In the examples for indirect speech acts (4) – (6), I have already smuggled in two indications of perlocutionary forces (5 and 6). As the perlocutionary force of an act can by definition vary infinitely (see '*given the concrete circumstances*'), there can be no finite set of acts over which rules of concatenation can operate. As a consequence, the notion of ill- or wellformedness of a conversation becomes vacuous.

Seemingly, CA drives us far away from the consideration of formal properties of sentences as used in conversation – more so than any other approach. Interestingly, however, it is exactly CA which provides us with a host of observations most relevant to the impact of the interactional aspects of an utterance on its morphosyntactic form. The basic notions of CA will be briefly considered from this perspective.

A conversation is organized in terms of turns. Ideally, a turn is simply the uninterrupted speech of an interlocutor. During a turn, an interlocutor is said to 'keep the floor'. Such a purely observational definition of a turn is not without its horrors for a linguist: a turn can be anything from a *hm* to a fully fledged story. However, meticulous observation and strictly empirical analysis of conversations reveal that there exist preferred points for InB to take over the floor (so-called turn-transition relevant places – TRP's) so that turn-taking is organized in an orderly fashion (Sacks/Schegloff/Jefferson 1974). An optimal TRP is at the potential end of the syntacticians' pet, namely the sentence. A sentence can signal its own end by syntatic and prosodic means – some of them being better than others, and some languages more efficient in this respect than others. Let us consider the use of the perfect and preterite tense in modern spoken German. For most speakers, the semantic difference between preterite and perfect has – by and large – disappeared, but they prefer to use the perfect. According to German word order rules, the verb in a perfect construction has to appear at the end of the sentence, the verb in a preterite construction in second position:

(9) Perfect: Gestern habe ich unseren gemeinsamen Freund Peter in der Oper gesehen – 'yesterday have I our mutual friend Peter in the opera seen'

(10) Preterite: Gestern sah ich unseren gemeinsamen Freund Peter in der Oper – 'yesterday saw I our mutual friend Peter in the opera'

Let us for the sake of illustration disregard prosody. Then (10) is potentially finished already after *Peter*, while (9) is only potentially finished at the 'real' end. The perfect tense makes it more difficult for InB to take over before InA has delivered everything he had wanted to say. The use of the perfect tense has obvious interactional advantages. This is not to say that German speakers exploit the perfect intentionally, but there might very well be a conversational pressure for the deployment of the perfect in spoken German (in stark contrast to written German, see below).

Excursion 1

In adaptation theory as originated by Kolk/van Grunsven (1985) and Kolk/van Grunsven/Keyser (1985) and elaborated by Kolk/Heeschen (1992) it is argued that Broca's aphasics adapt to their syntactic deficit by systematically simplifying their utterances. A key feature of adaption is the substitution of inflected verbs by the infinitive which – in accordance with the German and Dutch word order rules – appears at the end of the Broca's utterance. It must be stressed that Broca's are not unable to use inflected verb forms. Thus, they could also simplify their utterances by resorting to very short subject – inflected verb – X constructions (and indeed they do so sometimes). But the prevailing method of simplification is the use of the infinitive. Again without imputing any intentions, there remains the fact that the way in which Broca's actually adapt has interactional advantages over other conceivable methods of adaptation – in particular, if one takes into account how difficult it is for the Broca's, anyway, to keep the floor given their dysfluency and the intonational problems (at least) most of them have.

Conversations do not always follow an orderly turn-taking system. Often interlocutors try to 'steal' the floor which as a rule leads to a certain period of simultaneous speech until finally one of the interlocutors wins. As of late, this phenomenon of interruptions has been under investigation from the perspective of dominance (including dominance relations between men and women). Leaving this aside, even such 'disorderly' acts as interruptions respect (at least minimally) the structure of the utterance the interrupting partner wants to invade. Mühlemann/Foppa (1989) have shown that the majority of interruptions occur after a predicate rather than before, and that interruptions after are more often successful than interruptions before.

Errors and repairs are natural ingredients of conversations, and as already noted by Schegloff in 1979, repairs are made in ways that respect the formal structure of turns. This idea was extended by Levelt (1983) who was able to show that the form and place of a repair – irrespective of what is repaired – obeys strict syntactic constraints, basically the constraints which also hold for coordinations. But from the standpoint of CA, there is more to say about repairs. A repair does not 'wipe out' the repaired stretch of speech. It can be readdressed in the following turn of InB, lexically as well as syntactically as illustrated by the following example (in agreement with the methodological postulate of strict empiricism within CA, I present a conversation which actually occurred; it is not constructed on the basis of intuition).

(11) *InA and InB, both being gay, converse about a premiere at the opera. Background is the notorious addiction of gays to opera. The word 'Schwester — sister' is frequently used by gays to refer to their brethren.*
InA: Eine Masse von den Schwestern — äh also man traf eigentlich tout Berlin (*the last words facetiously pronounced in French*) — 'A mass of the sisters — uh PARTICLE one met virtually tout Berlin'
InB: Natürlich, jeder von uns Schwestern will natürlich gesehen werden — 'of course, each MASC. of us sisters wants of course seen be'

This example does not only illustrate the lexical and syntactical 'survival' of the aborted stretch of speech, but also that InB takes, it up in order to shift the topic. Thus, the repaired error became an interactional resource, which makes the terms 'error' and 'repairs' a bit misleading (cf. Schegloff 1979; and Jefferson 1975, for the potential interactional power of repairs).

Excursion 2

Schegloff (1979) mentions a syntactically very interesting form of repair: the repair is a grammatical continuation of the last element(s) of the aborted stretch of speech. He gives a German example pointed out to him by J. Bergmann: 'Ja, nun gibt's ja offenbar / *apparently pending intonation*, 1.0/ ist Ihr Mann nicht ganz der gleichen Meinung — Yes, now gives it yes obviously/1.0/ is your husband not entirely of the same opinion' (simplified transcription and remark in italics by C.H.). The repair beginning with *ist* can be considered as a continuation of *offenbar* by virtue of the fact that otherwise the verb would be in the incorrect position. The element *offenbar* serves as a sort of 'pivot' between the aborted piece and the repair. In a sense, the pivot constructions 'mask' the break-off point and make it difficult for the other interlocutor to take over the floor. These pivot constructions are extremely frequent in the speech of German Wernicke's, and very often the transition point is not even prosodically marked. Whether we consider these constructions as break-off's plus new starts or as direct expressions of an insufficient suppression of a competing utterance plan (Huber/Schlenck 1988), the constructions 'guarantee' the Wernicke's the floor. The 'normality' of these constructions suggests that they should be reconsidered from the perspective of their interactional advantages. Admittedly, this necessitates the close inspection of where in the conversation they are used and what the interactional consequences really are. Up to now, they have only been investigated in isolation, and not with respect to their sequential position — a serious failure I feel.

There is a preference for organizing turns in terms of adjacency pairs (Schegloff/Sacks 1973). The prototype of such a pair is question-answering. Others are *invitation — acceptance/rejection* or *accusations — admission/denial.* A 'first' projects into the 'next' in terms of preferred types of acts. If the relevant 'next' consists of alternatives, it can be observed that there is preference for one of them. Thus, the preferred 'next' for an invitation is *acceptance* rather than *rejection.* This is the point where it must be emphasized that 'preference' in CA is a purely technical term within structural sociology. It does not have anything to do with psychological 'predilection' nor with frequency of occurence (Bilmes 1988). 'Preference' is established on the basis of the observed consequences of the absence of a response type. Thus, if an invitation is responded to by neither an acceptance nor a rejection, but by a conditionally irrelevant 'next', then the response is interpreted by InA as rejection (e. g. InA: Would you like to come to dinner with me? — InB: Did you hear the latest news about Gorbatchev? — a fairly impolite rejection, indeed). In such a case, the acceptance is said to be relevantly absent, and relevant absence then serves as the basis for defining preferences. As pointed out by Levinson (1983, 336), there are not only preferred acts for a 'next', but also preferred formats. This point is not further elaborated by Levinson. However, it is highly persuasive to assume that there are indeed 'hard core' syntactic correspondences between members of an adjacency pair. Levelt/Kelter (1982) have shown that people in answering a question like to take over some surface material of the question. Similarly, Tannen (1987) deals with the phenomenon of repetitions in conversations, and Schenkein (1980) presents some spectacular examples of echoing syntactic structures across turns. One should also mention the programmatic title 'polite responses to polite requests' (Clark/Schunk 1980). And, finally, in a totally different context ('laboratory' investigations of sentence production), Bock has shown that the syntactic structure of a sentence spoken by the experimenter can determine the structure of a subsequent picture description by a subject despite the fact that the priming sentence is semantically totally unrelated to the picture to be described (the priming procedure was first applied by Bock 1986). This issue, however, becomes a bit more complicated by the interference with another psycholinguistic problem: do listeners dispose of a verbatim recall? Since Jarvella (1971) it is a widespread view that structural aspects of an utterance are not very long-lived in the working memory: they 'die' as soon as the listener has arrived at the meaning. Potter/Lombardi (1990) deny radically the possibility of a verbatim recall, and Clark/Gerrig (1990) demonstrate that even for quotations (in conversations) a perfect verbatim repetition is not really essential and – as a rule – does not occur (though they do not explicitly deny its possibility). Seemingly verbatim recalls are explained by Potter and Lombardi as regenerations on the basis of meaning, and the priming effect found by Bock can be reinterpreted as 'procedural' priming. Neither of these stances however forces us to discard the expectation of formal syntactic correspondences between adjaceny pairs: they can very well arise on the basis of meaning or as a result of procedural priming. Thus, the question of syntactic pair relations remains an interesting *desideratum*. Formal syntactic correspondences have been observed between presequences and the next move of the same interlocutor. By means of a presequence an InA prefigures his next move (see Levinson 1983, 345). Levinson does not really elaborate this point, but Gibbs/Mueller (1988) present fairly rich and convincing data showing how a prerequest determines the form of the actually following request.

To conclude, let us reconsider the 'illformed' conversation (ex. 8). This conversation never occurred in reality. Thus, it is not particularly interesting for CA. However, let us assume that the conversation actually happened until and including the son's second (allegedly inappropriate) query. In all likelihood, it would give rise to further negotiations between son and father (e. g. Father: *What do you mean by this? Are you teasing me?*). In any case, the conversation would go on in a non-absurd manner so that the notion of illformedness is rendered meaningless.

2.3. Collaboration Between Interlocutors

Interlocutors normally share some knowledge (the 'common ground'). By uttering a sentence, InA adds something to the common ground ('accumulation'); he makes a contribution. How InB can understand what InA meant by his sentence, is the object of investigations within pragmatics or philosophy of language (the disciplines I alluded to in section 2.1.1.). However, this cannot be the whole story: it is not only that the speaker wants to be understood and that the listener wants to understand – the speaker also wants to know whether he was understood correctly, and the listener wants to know whether his understanding is accepted by the speaker. Clark/Schaefer (1989) formulate this in their 'grounding criterion': "The contributor and the partners mutually believe that the partners have understood what the contributor meant to a criterion sufficient for current purposes" (Clark/Schaefer, 262). The central term here is 'mutual belief', implying that a successful contribution is a collective act: the original contribution of InA (his first utterance or turn) can be considered as successfully finished only after InB has signalized his understanding and InA has accepted InB's understanding. (It will be noted that the term 'contribution' is ambiguous: it can refer to InA's first act as well as to the whole collective enterprise.) The way to a justified 'mutual belief' is full of pitfalls: InB might simply not understand what InA said or meant; InB understood correctly, but believes that he did not do so; InB might signalize that he believes that he understood, but InA believes that InB's belief is unjustified, etc. All these pitfalls necessitate either reiteration of the original contribution of InA or creation of new contributions which in turn require signalizing actions on the part of InB (which, by definition, are also contributions). From this it follows that contributions in conversations are hierarchically organized: contributions can be multiply embedded within each other. Particularly perilous are extended turns consisting of many contributions such as a formal talk where the speaker forestalls signalizing actions of the listener(s) before having finished the whole turn. In a sense, these contributions are noncollective. How a conversation can proceed in successful contributions is discussed and analyzed in luxuriant detail by Clark/Schaefer (1989), where also ample references to other relevant papers are made.

The introduction of the collaborative aspect into the analysis of discourse does not stand in opposition to the stances taken by CA; Clark and Schaefer make substantial use of the conceptual apparatus of CA. Thus, their approach does not reject, but enriches the CA-approach. In this context, I should like to readdress the open problem of formal correspondences between adjacency pairs: by adjusting his response to the form of the preceding act, InB can provide InA with relevant clues as to his understanding of InA's act. Thus, formal correspondences can be a powerful means to achieve the grounding criterion.

If there is one aspect in conversation that requires particularly high cooperativity, then this is reference (Clark/Wilkes-Gibbs 1986). With respect to the form of referential expressions (best demonstrated for NP's), interlocutors painstakingly try to take into consideration the partner's present state of knowledge, and the partner painstakingly tries to indicate his state of knowledge. Consequently, the forms of the referential expressions vary over the course of a conversation. As a rule of thumb, they become increasingly shorter (from fully fledged descriptions down to names and/or pronouns). Obviously, interlocutors find it completely natural that in establishing definite reference they have to share responsibility and that the burden is not entirely on the shoulders of the speaker. However, the 'percentage' of responsibility can vary depending (1) on differences with respect to the initial state of knowledge of the interlocutors, and (2) on external circumstances or settings for the conversation. As to (1), it has been shown by Isaacs/Clark (1987) that experts on a given topic adjust the form of the referential expressions according to the state of knowledge of their nonexpert partners. They are obviously perfectly willing and prepared to take over more responsibility for establishing reference than their partners – at least in the initial phases of conversation. As to (2), circumstances might be of such a kind that the partner has difficulties to provide the speaker with information about his state of knowledge, and, accordingly, the speaker again accepts more responsibility and adjusts the forms of his referential expressions. This source of variation has been investigated in various studies by Krauss/Weinheimer (1966; 1967) who manipulated experimentally the interactional setting, specifically the amount and type of feedback the speaker got from the recipient. A most drastic manipulation was carried out by the authors in 1964 (referred to in Krauss/Weinheimer 1967) where the speakers had to produce messages which were taperecorded for later decoding by some other person. Under this condition, the expressions became excessively long. The dependent variable in Krauss and Weinheimer's experiments was always the length of the referential expressions. Length almost invariably implies explicitness, and in terms of Clark's approach it can safely be assumed that greater explicitness is an indicator of the acceptance of greater responsibility.

There are additional factors influencing the form of referential expressions, most notably the social relations between the interlocutors (for familiarity see Redeker 1986). The whole field has exploded a bit recently, specifically through the introduction of the role of sex differences. This, however, takes me definitely beyond the scope of my chapter.

Excursion 3

Broca's aphasics do not always speak in telegraphic style. As demonstrated by Kolk/Heeschen (1992), they sometimes attempt complete sentences (successfully or not) so that Kolk and Heeschen claim telegraphic style to be an option. This has been an object of sustained criticism because Kolk and Heeschen give only vague indications of the factors on which this option depends. Within the framework of CA and the cooperation approach by Clark, however, the problem can be solved. The key features of telegraphic style are the omissions of the determiner (Det) and the finiteness of the verb (Infl). Both Det and Infl are reference establishing devices *par excellence*. If the patient can rely on anything, then on the interlocutor's preparedness to cooperate in arriving at definite reference. Thus, Det and Infl are just the most appropriate candidates for omissions. The more responsibility the interlocutor assumes, the more the patient can afford to omit them. The situation where the patient has a minimum and the interlocutor a maximum of responsibility is face-to-face conversation proceeding in short turns (each consisting of only one or very few contributions) and if the interlocutor is an 'expert'. This is exactly the situation of an aphasic conversing with an aphasiologist who is usually considered by the patient as an expert not only for language problems, but for almost every topic (be it justified or not). If the situation changes, for example if the patient has to speak on tape for later decoding by others, or if in the conversation a misunderstanding occurs, then more responsibility must be assumed by the patient. As a consequence, he must become more explicit which as a rule necessitates abandoning telegraphic style. In terms of CA, in the minimal responsibility situation telegraphic style is preferred, in a more marked situation it is dispreferred. Thus, the notion of 'option' can be reinterpreted as a purely technical term closely related to 'preference' which has the advantage that one does not have to attribute to the patients conscious intentions.

3. The 'Oral-Written' Dimension

The emergence of literacy has undeniably drastic consequences for the social organization of a society and for man's way of thinking, not only about language, but in general, see Goody (1978), Ong (1982). The ability to write might also be a prerequisite for our ability to conceive of our speech as consisting of discrete elements and to identify them. This appears to be well attested with respect to sounds (Morais/Bertelson/Cary/Alegria 1986), although with respect to larger units such as morphemes the experiences of V. Heeschen in a completely illiterate society tell a different story (Heeschen 1992, ch. 5). Writing is the manipulation of symbols *par excellence* so that Scheerer (in press) goes so far as to maintain that the symbolic-representational approach to language and cognition as put forward most resolutely by Fodor (1987) and Pylyshyn (1984) could arise only under the seductive influence of the properties of written language while an unprejudiced approach to oral language would call for connectionist models of language processing.

In the sixties and seventies some large projects were launched to explore the formal differences between written and spoken language (WL, SL), (see Betten 1977; 1978) for an overview of German projects and Akinnaso (1982) for a review of research carried out in English-speaking countries). With respect to morphosyntax, the collected observations converge on some fundamental points:

- preferential use of coordinate (paratactic) rather than subordinate structures in SL
- preferential use of deictic terms rather than nominal expressions with a definite article in SL
- preferential use of active rather than passive constructions in SL
- in general, preferential use of a less elaborate syntax in SL (though in such generality this has been contested by several authors)
- Preferential use of indirect speech acts in SL

Much effort has been spent on finding out the reasons for these phenomena. Chafe (1982) proposes that writers and speakers have different relations to their audience: writing has a distancing effect. The writer is more 'detached' than a speaker (who is more 'involved'). So the overuse of passives in WL reflects detachment (*it is said*) while the overuse of actives in SL reflects involvement (*I say*). Ochs (1979) elaborates the point that WL is more 'planned' than SL. And Olson/Hildyard (1983) claim that understanding direct speech acts (the 'literal' meaning of an utterance) would require recall of the 'very words' which in SL only have an elusive life (see discussion in section 2.2.).

However, in the first half of the eighties a major paradigm shift took place in the approach to the WL-SL dimension. More and larger corpora and a greater variety of discourse were investigated. These investigations brought to the fore the idea that certain types of written discourse could be abundant in means previously considered prototypically oral (e. g. ritual communication, see Akinnaso 1985), and vice versa. The categorial distinction WL-SL was replaced by the notion of an written-oral-continuum. Furthermore, one became more and more aware of the fact that the WL-SL-dimension is hopelessly confounded with co-varying factors (conversational style, topic, formality, interactional setting). As a consequence, more and more attention was paid to the similarities than to the differences between WL and SL. Major promoters of this trend were Tannen (1982 a; 1982 b; 1984) and Biber (1988).

Following this trend, I should like to come back to the use of the preterite and perfect tense in German. As mentioned above, in spoken German the preterite is almost completey thrust aside by the perfect despite the fact that semantic differences do indeed exist between the two tenses (Ehrich 1992), although they are fairly subtle. In writing, the floor of the writer is not threatened. Thus, there is no longer an interactional advantage for the perfect tense. As a consequence, even naive writers reintroduce the distinction between preterite and perfect even in fairly informal texts (post cards to friends). In terms of the model of Clark/Schaefer (1989), a text is an extended turn consisting of many noncollective contributions addressed to absent and sometimes even unknown partners. However, a formal talk is of the same nature, and one can safely assume that the differences between written texts and formal talks are minimal, if there are any at all.

Admittedly, in some languages constructions are accepted in SL which would be fairly unacceptable in WL. An oft-cited example is word order in French (see Klein 1985), and clitisation in German falls into the same category (*haste* [= contraction of *hast du* – *have you*] is certainly never found in written German). However, these differences show only that the power of the notoriously authoritarian prescriptive French and German grammarians is strong enough to regulate WL, but does not extend to what people say. If all differences between WL and SL could be reduced to covariables (including the institutionalization of prescriptive grammar), then we would have little reason to question the tenets of the grand old men of linguistics Saussure and Bloomfield (and indeed Aristotle): letters are only symbols for sounds, WL is only a secondary derivation of SL so that nothing beyond the grapheme-phoneme distinction needs to be said.

In all fairness, I have trivialized the problem, and I have done exactly what is unpermitted according to Ludwig (1983): I have reduced 'language in writing' to 'written speech'. Hopefully, my illegal doings have helped the reader to discover what the real issues are.

4. Generation of Surface Structure

A message must contain innumerable specifications: the event structure (commonly characterized in terms of thematic roles), topic, perspective, informational weight, etc. A frequently neglected factor ist the content itself and to whom this content is conveyed: Collier/Kuiken/Enzle (1982) have shown that the type of emotions one is speaking about and the relation of speaker and addressee have a strong interactive effect on the grammatical complexity of the resulting sentence. All these aspects have to be built into the message to trigger the appropriate process of the formulator. However, as things are, only a few of these aspects have thus far been dealt with in experimental psycholinguistic research. Most attention has been paid to: (1) lexical access and grammatical role assignment and (2) retrieval of the morphologically appropriate word forms (which is already on the borderline between syntax and phonology).

4.1. The Constructional Part

I intend to present a sort of 'reference model' based on the works of Garrett (1975; 1988), Levelt (1989), and various works by Bock and colleagues (summarized in Bock 1990). There are differences between these authors, but I shall emphasize more the communalities. The reference model is a typical serial stage model in the tradition of the 'symbolic representational' approach: Distinct sets of rules are operating over specified types of symbolic representations, or in more psychological terms: distinct sets of processes are triggered by specific types of information; they convert a given informational format into another serving as the input of the next set of processes. Processes are 'blind' with respect to the consequences of their output: there is little, if any, feedback from lower levels of representations (see Levelt in this volume).

Given the conceptual structure of a message, one might ask whether this can be converted *directly* into a surface structure. This stance is taken by among others McNeill (1987) and Stemberger (1982). In Stemberger's model sentence frames have a meaning *per se* which reminds one of the notion of 'Satzbauplan – sentence building plan' in traditional German linguistics (see Duden-Grammatik; Drosdowsky 1984) and of the notion of 'sentence schema' in traditional German psychology (Seltz 1922). The idea of sentence frames logically existing prior to the words used to fill them is not without problems. Bock/Loebell (1990) have shown that, in a picture description task, a passive construction (with a *by*-phrase for the agent) could be primed by a preceding sentence containing a *by*-phrase denoting location. It could be ruled out that the effect was brought about by the closed-class word similarity or by rhythmic similarities. These results demonstrate clearly a sort of autonomy of surface constituent structure and provide straightforward evidence against the direct mapping approach. Some sort of grammatical categorization is necessary as an intermediate step.

The next question then is whether thematic roles are directly mapped onto grammatical functions along the lines 'agent > subject, theme > direct object, etc.'. The answer is again negative. There is little evidence that an agent requires subjecthood (see Bock/Loebell/Morey 1992, also for a review of earlier experiments). A direct role-function mapping is also highly unlikely *vis a vis* such oft-cited examples as the German verb *helfen* – *to help*, which requires as its theme an indirect object, and such an innocuous verb as the Russian *vladet'* – *to govern*, which requires its theme to be in the instrumental case. This is a case – to make the picture completley bewildering – usually reserved for the agent in a passive sentence. The relevance of thematic roles for grammatical functions might be a bit different in language acquisition and language comprehension, and also for production one shoud keep in mind that thematic roles are construed in different, and sometimes fairly sophisticated ways. However, at least if we take the thematic roles as conceptual primitives in a straightforward sense, they appear not to be crucial for grammatical functions.

An alternative is suggested by Bock/Loebell/Morey (1992); Levelt (1989); cf. art. 1: it is the semantic content of a noun that determines its assignment to a given function. Most notably, an animate noun claims subjecthood. To be a bit more precise: first the message has to be inspected for appropriate lemmas, in particular the verb has to be selected together with its argument structure constraints. It is then the syntactic properties of the verb plus the semantic content of the nouns which determine the latter's status as arguments along these lines: there is a hierarchy of grammatical functions (or cases) (see Keenan 1975) and there is a hierarchy in terms of animateness (modified and differentiated by factors such as powerfulness, concreteness, etc.). It is then that the highest lemma in the animacy hierarchy claims the highest function in terms of Keenan's system. Thus, a human noun is a first-class candidate for subjecthood. Unfortunately, this brings about another problem: subject in a deep structure or in a surface structure? Bock/Loebell/Morey have convincingly shown that it is subjecthood in the surface structure which is claimed by the animates. With respect to argument-function assignment one can do without a level of deep structure. This claim hinges critically on the lexicalist-functional linguistic theory as initiated by Bresnan (1978; 1982). In this theory, verbs are already represented in the lexicon as either [+ active] or [+ passive] and, accordingly, are already specified as to their argument-structure requirements as well. The generalizations holding for the systematic relations between active and passive are then captured by lexical rules.

In addition to 'functional integration', the syntactic processor has to fulfill the job of ordering the words and/or phrases, serially as well as in terms of constituency, of handling phenomena such as agreement and government, and finally of finding the actual word forms for the lemmas. There is good reason to distinguish between the processes of functional integration and the processes regulating the formal aspects of the utterance. Analysis of speech errors are of considerable importance here; experimental evidence comes from Bock/Miller (1991) where it could be shown that the processes responsible for subject-verb agreement are oblivious to the semantic content of the subject noun: in a sentence completion task, the number of provoked agreement errors was the same for animate and inanimate subjects. Thus, the generation of surface structure falls into two stages: the first is semantic based, the second purely form based – a conception closely related to Garrett's distinction between functional and positional level representation, the latter being created by a component 'selection of positional level planning frames' (and indeed retrieval of word forms, see below). The distinction between two stages in the generation of surface structure does not necessarily imply that all processes of one component have to be finished before the other component can get started (see the notion of incremental production by Kempen/Hoenkamp 1987). However, logically, in terms of the type of information being processed, the components have to be kept apart.

The product of the syntactic processor is not simply a chain of (still abstractly represented) words forms, but a genuinely hierarchical phrasal structure. This is indirectly evidenced by certain phonetic properties of the sentence, in particular word and pause durations, which depend on the prosodic structure of the sentence (i. e. its division into intonational and phonological phrases) which, in turn, can hardly be derived from anything else than a phrasally organized syntactic structure (cf. (Ferreira 1991; Cooper/Paccia-Cooper 1980).

Excursion 4

I feel that I should also emphasize already here that within the framework of the reference model there is little space, if any, for two notions frequently used in explaining aphasiological data: Sentence forms/plans: In discussing agrammatism, it is often said that agrammatics prefer 'canonical sentence forms', thus the active sentence in SVO order. By this, one could indeed conveniently account for 'paradoxical' actives. Take the following example (stemming from material of the author):

(12) *A patient had to describe a picture of a dog biting a postman. The patient was prompted into a passive by the preceding question* 'What happens to the postman?' *The patient produced*:
Der Postbote beißt den Hund — 'the postman bites the dog'

Very similar misconstructions can be found in Stemberger (1982) for normals. It is convenient to say that the patient was pressed to assign subjecthood to *the postman* by the question, but then his preference for the 'canonical' active sentence comes through. Indeed this is the way Stemberger accounts for some of his examples. However, the reference model requires a different explanation: the *postman* claims subjecthood due to its high rank in the order of animacy and certainly through the support given by the question. The patient then retrieves the incorrect verb lemma — *beiß* [active] instead of *beiß* [passive]. There might be a preference for the active verb lemma; however, in any case, the misconstruction is due to a lexical access problem rather than to the incorrect selection of a 'sentence plan'. Sentence frames/plans arise from processes operating over lexically specified representations, they are not pre-existing in the sense of the 'Satzbauplan' or the 'Satzschema'. It may be that this interpretation is neither cogent nor correct. The objective of this little exercise is to demonstrate that an aphasiologist — implicitly or explicitly — subscribes to given psycholinguistic models in explaining his phenomena. Nobody is forced to accept the reference model, but in any case, aphasiologists should be aware of their committment to making their models explicit and to abiding by them consistently.

Trade-off between components: Martin/Frederick Wetzel/Blossom-Stach/Feher (1989) explain the fact that agrammatics' syntax was better in picture descriptions than in story telling by assuming that "... the presence of pictures reduced the capacity needed for the retrieval of content words, leaving more capacity for the development of syntactic structure or the retrieval of function words and inflections" (Martin/Frederick Wetzel/Blossom-Stach/Feher, 171). This implies the assumption of a working memory being shared by the lexical and the syntactic component. Thus, the unburdening of one component makes the job easier for the other component. The reference model is soaked with the spirit of modularity: processing components operate fairly independently of each other. The incorporation of a 'trade-off' and of shared buffers is — to say the least — fairly problematic. Again, nobody is obliged to subscribe to the reference model, but aphasiological explanations should be explicit and consistent in this respect.

The last question of this subsection concerns the basic planning units of the sentence processor. To make a long story short, one can safely assume that the clause is the main candidate. This does not at all exclude the possibility that two or more clauses are planned and processed simultaneously; otherwise it would be hard to account for sentences with multiple subordinations. A different issue, however, is whether sometimes two or more competing alternatives for a specific clause or even two or more rivalling messages and/or intentions can be processed in parallel all the way down until one finally wins. Butterworth (1982) postulates the possibility of such parallel processing in order to account for the occurrence of sentence blends. But this is exactly the problem: does the processor as a rule indulge in the luxury of parallel processing, being 'confident' that this only occasionally leads to blends, or does such a parallel processing as a rule lead to blends so that it must be considered as fairly exceptional?

With respect to 'syntax in production', the reference model is the most elaborated and most explicit one for the time being. However, it can be expected that rivalling models will enter the stage soon. I am thinking of the 'competition' model designed by Bates and MacWhinney and applied so far mainly to language acquisition and comprehension, but first steps have been taken to extend it to production (see MacWhinney/Bates 1990). Furthermore, we can be sure that connectionist models of syntax in production will be put forward. The way has already been paved (see McClelland/John/Taraban 1989).

4.2. Morphology

At the end of the generation of surface structure the lemmas must be fully specified for relevant morphological aspects so that the actual word forms can be inserted. On a first approach, one can conceive of these specifications as being expressed in terms of diacritical markers. Some of them are inherited from the message (e. g. plural), others are inherent to the lemmas themselves (e. g. syntactic gender), and others are accrued by the lemmas from processes of sentence construction (e. g. agreement features on the verb, case on nouns). Morphology here is split over various processing components, which resembles the situation in early generative grammar. In linguistics, however, Aronoff (1976) marked a turning point: he assigned the task of word derivation to the lexicon, following the general trend of these years to enrich the tasks of the lexicon and to abandon the view of the lexicon as a mere depository for idiosyncratic aspects of the language. Selkirk (1982) also assigned inflectional morphology to the lexicon within the framework set out by Bresnan (1978; 1982). Over the last few years, two trends have been promoted in generative grammar: (a) a more or less strong lexicalist position, and (b) a syntactic position. The distinction is confounded with the problem how far morphology constitutes an autonomous component of linguistic organization. For the lexicalist I refer to Di Sciullo/Williams (1987), and for the syntacticians to Baker's incorporation theory for word derivation (1988). An excellent overview of the linguistic approaches to morphology is given by Spencer (1991).

For a psycholinguistic model of production the key issue can be brought down to a straightforward question: anticipating that the lemmas are in some way appropriately specified, are then the concrete word forms created by rule-governed processes or are they directly retrieved from the lexical store? For regularly inflected forms Stemberger/MacWhinney (1986) argue that high frequency forms are stored as separate ready-made entries while low frequency forms are created. A similar stance is taken by Anshen/Aronoff (1988) for word derivations. However, they enrich the model by assuming that for certain forms three simultaneous processes might be "racing for the honor of being the first to present the speaker with a needed word" (Anshen/Aronoff, 648): word forming by rules, word forming by analogy, or a direct lexical lookup. Even if one assumes that all word forms are stored as units in the lexicon, this would not preclude the possibility that systematic relations holding between word forms are reflected in the organization of the mental lexicon. Lukatela/Gligorijevic/Kostic/Turvey (1980) have shown that the forms of inflected nouns are housed as families in the lexicon, with one form (the nom. sing.) being the head of the family. This comes very close to the traditional notions of paradigms and citation forms. The relation between word forms are accounted for by Bybee (1988) in a radically different way: relations are established exclusively by links and their relative strengths. In such a connectionistic model Bybee can do without any symbolic notions as stem, affix, inflection, case, etc., and furthermore the links can be based on formal as well as on semantic similarities.

Recently, the whole problem has become the object of a sustained controversy between connectionists and 'symbolists'. The debate focusses on the formation of the English past tense verb forms. It was originated by Rumelhart/McClelland (1986) proposing a model in which the distinction between regular and irregular forms becomes a matter of gradedness rather than a matter of two distinct symbolic categories. This ignited into a heated debate summarized by Pinker (1991), who proposes the alternative that regular past tense forms are created by rules (irrespective of their frequency) while irregular forms are stored and thus subject to the laws of associative memory. The controversy is still ongoing and is built mainly on observations from language acquisition so that I must leave things here as they are.

I should only add that the issue of 'whole' versus 'decomposed' forms is dealt with in much more detail for language comprehension than for production. It goes without saying that results obtained for comprehension are always also relevant for production (in principle at least), but discussing them here is beyond my brief.

5. 'Anomalies' in Spoken Language

5.1. Errors

As mentioned in section 2.2., errors and repairs are natural ingredients in conversation and spoken language in general. The significance of errors for the construction of models of language use is discussed in article 7 of this volume. Thus, I confine myself to commenting on an alleged *desideratum*.

For language pathologists, it is certainly an important question how many errors can be considered as 'normal'. Furthermore, this frequency question should be differentiated with respect to the type of errors so that a sort of probability profile for the various types of errors can be established. In approaching this question in a meaningful way, one first has to eliminate two types of phenomena:

- many of the repairs considered by conversational analysts are actually revisions (see the example of Schegloff in excursion 2, and the ex. 11). What is aborted is not a *reparandum*, but a *revidendum*, and this holds also for such deceptively clear errors as discussed by Jefferson (1975): a defendant in court says ... *the co- uh the officer* .... Jefferson interprets this as an act of self-determination. Of course, as a good CA'ist she avoids the term 'intention'. But is it really too farfetched to assume that the defendant intentionally used first *cop* in order to assert *I usually speak of cops, but I am aware that this would be inappropriate in court*?

– many 'errors' have to be accepted as normal at least relative to certain speaker varieties. Senft (1982) investigated the doubling of the finite part of the verb plus subject in a West German working class community. Example:

(13) Das sind schon drei Jahre sind das – 'that are already three years are that'

Senft has shown that these constructions occur so massively that we simply have to accept them as 'grammatical' in this community (and probably in many others in Germany).

Real errors appear to occur very rarely (cf. art. 5). The data of Garnham/Shillock/Brown/Mill/Cutler (1982) show that word as well as sound errors occur far below 1% relative to the number of words. With respect to syntactic errors Deese (1984) found 77 cases of sentences which could not be parsed sensibly in a corpus of approximately 15,000 sentences. This sounds incredible. A rough check carried out by myself, however, confirms this number: overhearing three live comments on sports events broadcast by German TV yielded 759 clauses (I excluded elliptic expressions even if they were of considerable length). Note that these comments are particularly error-prone because they are spoken fairly fast and the reporter must permanently adjust his commentary to what is going on the screen. Furthermore, the comments were dialogue-like; the reporters had famous sportsmen as co-commentators with whom they literally conversed. There was one change of a demonstrative (sing. > plur.) which could have been a revision, one doubling construction which is on the borderline of being ungrammatical (see above), one case error and two clear constructional errors. Even if we do not want to argue *pro domu* and include the alleged revision and the alleged (un)grammaticality, there remain five morphosyntactic errors for 749 fully fledged clauses (!) (minimally = 5200 words). So, even relative to clauses, the error rate remains below 1%.

Contrary to common wisdom, errors are a *quantité négligeable* in spoken language. This does not necessarily affect Schegloff's position because in actual conversations there might be many abortions and revisions.

Counts of classified errors are currently available only for such broad classes as sound versus word errors. Counts of syntactic errors specified for subtle types of them are not available yet, and I feel that this is for good reasons.We have no use for superficial classifications of errors in the manner of school teachers. What we want is to identify the psycholinguistic source of an error, its location at a specific stage of processing. An attempt to count such 'located' errors would be enmeshed in a host of methodological problems:

– an error surfacing as a sound error can have its source at a higher level (see the celebrated example of *clear* for the target *near*, commonly interpreted as a blend of *near* and *close*, that is as an error having its source in semantic aspects of the lexicon)
– the location of an error is theory or model dependent, see the above example of the paradoxical active. The situation becomes hopeless (for the attempt of an 'objective' count), if one allows for interactive effects of various levels of processing conspiring to cause an error (Dell 1986).
– even within a given model, many errors remain ambiguous. Consider the following naturalistic example:

(14) Boris Becker traf das letzte mal auf Michael Chang im Semifinale der Australian Opens, das er mit 6:4, 6:4, 6:4 bezwang – 'B. B. met the last time at M. C. in-the semi-final of the Australian OpenPLUR that (can only refer to 'das Semifinale') he with 6:4, 6:4, 6:4 defeated'
The verb *bezwang* requires Michael Chang as direct object (so that the relative pronoun should have been *den*). The 'semi-final' could be the direct object of the phonologically and semantically related verb form *gewann* – 'won'.

Within the reference model, there are 3 possible 'locations' of the error:
(a) the form *das* is simply a misselection

from the lexicon
(b) the intended verb was *gewann*, but due to phonological and semantic similarity the form *bezwang* intruded
(c) the verb *bezwang* was intended, but the assignment of the nouns to the grammatical functions went wrong.
Thus, even strictly abiding by one model, the 'location' of an error can become a conundrum. The only way out of the dilemma is to specify alternative explanations within a given model and then to check them by controlled experiments. I think that also for language pathology there is no other meaningful way.

Another aspect of errors is how often are they corrected and how far is correction dependent on the type of error. For word and sound errors (including prosodic errors) Nooteboom (1980), Cutler (1983), and Levelt (1983) converge on roughly 50% corrections. For syntactic errors, data obtained by Lackner (1980) in a shadowing task show 15% for complex syntactic errors (word transpositions) as opposed to 60% for phonological errors. The data come from a restrictive experimental arrangement so that their generalizability to spontaneous speech is problematic. Nevertheless, I feel that the general trend revealed by them (by far less corrections for syntactic than for word and/or sound errors) fits in very well with our everyday life experience..

Excursion 5

Even aphasaiologists sometimes cannot help but have the impression that Wernicke's speech sounds so normal (with respect to morphosyntax). One is seduced into assuming that this is based on the fact that the errors Wernicke's make are sort of normal (in particular the doublings and blends). Given the (admittedly) rough estimation of what and how much is normal, such an assumption would be patently wrong. However, CA forces us to look at errors not as mere technical accidents, but at the way in which the speaker and hearer deal with errors, and to ask what are the interactional consequences of errors. It might be that not the speech of Wernicke's is normal, but our conversations with them. A minimalistic first statement in this respect could be something like this: there is good evidence that morphosyntactic errors are very seldom repaired by normals — in contrast to sound and lexical errors. Thus, what is normal about Wernicke's, is not their syntactic errors, but the fact that they do not attempt to repair them.

5.2. Ellipsis

Notwithstanding my reservations with respect to the 'oral-written' distinction, it has to be admitted that the use of incomplete utterances is 'prototypically' bound to spoken language (disregarding highly restricted written text types such as headlines, encyclopedic entries, or postal telegramms). I have in mind the so-called 'contextual' ellipses in the sense of Clark/Clark (1977), not sentential ellipses. Within theoretical linguistics, predominantly sentential ellipsis has been dicussed. However, the principle problems extend to contextual ellipsis as well: are the incomplete structures derived from complete structures by means of deletion rules (Ross 1967) or can they be directly generated (Chao 1987)? Klein (in press) advocates a third alternative: in elliptic parts, everything is present, it is only that it is phonologically not realized. The problem for contextual ellipsis is totally analogous as evidenced by languages with case markings: In German, a physician can say to his receptionist *den nächsten — the next* ACC, but if the receptionist goes to the waiting room in order to call the 'next' patient, she has to say *der nächste, bitte — the next* NOM *please*. Where do the case markings come from? They cannot come from concrete and complete sentence structures. Assuming this, we would run into a problem with the following example from Shopen (1972) quoted in Kolk (1987):

(15) Three persons A, B, C, are in a room. C leaves, and A says to B 'der Idiot — the idiot NOM' referring to C.

There is n o complete sentence plausibly imaginable where the definite article could be used. Where does it come from?

Nevertheless, given examples such as the German physician and his receptionist, we must assume that case in elliptic utterances is somehow or other governed by some abstract element. Further convincing examples are constituted by slogans such as 'die Kunst dem Volke — the art to-the DAT people DAT'. Present-day psycholinguistics does not suggest any convincing solution to the problem.

Excursion 6

Kolk/Heeschen (1992) argue (see above) that agrammatics adapt to their syntactic problems by resorting to contextual elliptic utterances. Though formally perfect and interactionally meaningful (see exc. 1 and 3), the agrammatics' speech sounds hopelessly incoherent and incohesive. This impression cannot originate in the sheer mass of the elliptic expressions. Even normals can produce fairly long chains of elliptic utterances, but on the condition that they belong to the same 'script' (e. g. a report on the weather). Once the 'script' is abandoned, or the interlocutor introduces another topic, it would be highly abnormal to go on with elliptic utterances. But this is what agrammatics do. (I should like to thank B. Hofstede who brought this point to my attention.) The price for coping with their deficit by adaptation is discourse incoherence. Wernicke's do not adapt. Is that the reason why conversing with them is so much drastically more pleasant than conversing with Broca's?

5.3. Adjustments: Conversation Analysis Once Again

As discussed by Goodwin (1981, ch. 2), a speaker is able to adjust his utterance on the fly if during his utterance circumstances change. If InA, for example, is speaking to InB, and becomes aware of the fact that InB is not paying attention to him, but then an InC directs his gaze to InA during his speech, he can change his message, but encode it in such a way that the piece he has already produced while speaking to InB is directly syntactically continued.

Lerner (1991) points out that an InB often completes an utterance of InA in a syntactically perfect way. This and the observations by Goodwin constitute a challenge for the production model of Levelt (1989) and maybe to the whole reference model. What InB has to do is incredibly complicated: in Lerner's case, he has to understand the intention of InA as expressed so far, he then has to anticipate the intention of InA not expressed yet, make it into his own intention and then encode it so that it fits in syntactically with the piece already spoken by InA. This is not a logical problem for Levelt's model; it is an empirical problem of how all this can be achieved in real time. Thus, what we need and hopefully shall be provided with in the near future is a 'psycholinguistics-for-conversation' just as Schegloff (1979) postulated a 'syntax-for-conversation'.

6. Concluding Remarks

Throughout this chapter I have argued that research on disorders has to commit itself strictly and consistently to models of normal language use. Accounting for the deficit and errors (to the extent that they reflect the deficit) requires application of psycholinguistic models. For the other part – how are the deficit and the errors dealt with – I have proposed CA as a stringent conceptual framework. Given the fact that the relations between psycholinguistics and CA on the one hand and theoretical linguistics on the other hand are anything but clear, my position also means *a fortiori* that I consider it as precarious (if not even totally mistaken) to relate pathological data directly to linguistic theory without mediation of psycholinguistic theory.

Author's note: I thank my colleagues at the MPI für Psycholinguistik and the Forschungsgruppe Kognitive Anthropologie (members and guests) for many helpful discussions. I hope that nobody is offended if I mention only a few: K. Bock, V. Ehrich, A. S. Meyer, W. Levelt. I feel particularly indebted to H. Kolk. The longstanding cooperation with him was crucial for my approach to aphasia.

7. References

Akinnaso, F. N. (1982). On the differences between spoken and written language. *Language and Speech*, *25*, 97–125.

Akinnaso, F. N. (1985). On the similarities between spoken and written language. *Language and Speech*, *28*, 323–359.

Altmann, H. (1987). Zur Problematik der Konstitution von Satzmodi als Formtypen. In J. Meibauer (Ed.), *Satzmodus zwischen Grammatik und Pragmatik. 22–56*. Tübingen: Niemeyer.

Anshen, F. & Aronoff, M. (1988). Producing morphologically complex words. *Linguistics*, *26*, 641–655.

Aronoff, M. (1976). *Word Formation in Generative Grammar*. Cambridge, MA: MIT Press.

Austin, J. L. (1962). *How to Do Things with Words*. Oxford: Clarendon Press.

Baker, M. (1988). *Incorporation: a Theory of Grammatical Function Changing*. Chicago: University of Chicago Press.

Berry, M. (1981). Systemic linguistics and discourse analysis: a multi-layered approach to exchange structure. In M. Coulthard & M. Montgomery (Eds.), *Studies in Discourse Analysis. 120–145*. London: Routledge and Kegan Paul.

Betten, A. (1977). Erforschung gesprochener deutscher Sprache. *Deutsche Sprache*, *5*, 335–361.

Betten, A. (1978). Erforschung gesprochener deutscher Sprache. *Deutsche Sprache*, *6*, 21–44.

Biber, D. (1988). *Variations across Speech and Writing*. Cambridge: Cambridge University Press.

Bilmes, J. (1988). The concept of preference in conversation analysis. *Language in Society*, *17*, 161–181.

Bock, K. (1986). Syntactic persistence in language production. *Cognitive Psychology*, *18*, 355–387.

Bock, K. (1990) Structure in language: creating form in talk. *American Psychologist*, *45*, 1221–1236.

Bock, K. & Loebell, H. (1990). Framing sentences. *Cognition*, *35*, 1–39.

Bock, K., Loebell, H., & Morey, R. (1992). From conceptual roles to structural relations: bridging the syntactic cleft. *Psychological Review, 99,* 150–170.

Bock, K. & Miller, C. A. (1991). Broken agreement. *Cognitive Psychology, 23,* 45–93.

Bresnan, J. (1978). A realistic transformational grammar. In M. Halle, J. Bresnan, & G. A. Miller (Eds.), *Linguistic Theory and Psychological Reality. 1–59.* Cambridge, MA: MIT Press.

Bresnan, J. (1982). *The Mental Representation of Grammatical Relations.* Cambridge, MA: MIT Press.

Butterworth, B. (1982). Speech errors: old data in search of new theories. In A. Cutler (Ed.), *Slips of the Tongue and Language Production. 73–108.* Berlin: Mouton Publishers.

Bybee, J. L. (1988). Morphology as a lexical organization. In M. Hammond & M. Noonan (Eds.), *Theoretical Morphology: Approaches in Modern Linguistics. 119–141.* San Diego etc.: Academic Press.

Chafe, W. L. (1982). Integration and involvement in speaking, writing and oral literature. In D. Tannen (Ed.), *Spoken and Written Language: Exploring Orality and Literacy. 35–53.* Norwood, NJ: Ablex Publishing Corporation.

Chao, W. (1987). *On Ellipsis.* Doctoral dissertation, Amherst.

Chomsky, N. (1980). *Rules and Representations.* N. Y.: Columbia University Press.

Clark, H. H. & Clark, E. V. (1977). *Psychology and Language.* N. Y.: Harcourt Brace Jovanovich.

Clark, H. H. & Gerrig, R. J. (1990). Quotations as demonstrations. *Language, 66,* 764–805.

Clark, H. H. & Schaefer, E. F. (1989). Contributing to discourse. *Cognitive Science, 13,* 259–294.

Clark, H. H. & Schunk, D. H. (1980). Polite responses to polite requests. *Cognition, 8,* 111–143.

Clark, H. H. & Wilkes-Gibbs, D. (1986). Referring as a collaborative process. *Cognition, 22,* 1–39.

Cole, P. & Morgan, J. L. (Eds.) (1975). *Syntax and Semantics 3: Speech Acts.* N.Y. etc.: Academic Press.

Collier, G., Kuiken, D., & Enzle, M. E. (1982). The role of grammatical qualification in the expression and perception of emotion. *Journal of Psycholinguistic Research, 11,* 631–650.

Cooper, W. E. & Paccia-Cooper, J. (1980). *Syntax and Speech.* Cambridge, MA: Harvard University Press.

Coulthard, M. & Brazil, D. (1981). Exchange structure. In M. Coulthard & M. Montgomery (Eds.), *Studies in Discourse Analysis. 82–106.* London etc.: Routledge and Kegan Paul.

Coulthard, M. & Montgomery, M. (Eds.) (1981). *Studies in Discourse Analysis.* London etc.: Routledge and Kegan Paul.

Coulmas, F. & Ehlich, K. (Eds.) (1983). *Writing in Focus.* Berlin etc.: Mouton Publishers.

Cutler, A. (Ed.) (1982). *Slips of the Tongue and Language Production.* Berlin etc.: Mouton Publishers.

Cutler, A. (1983). Speakers' conceptions of the function of prosody. In A. Cuttler & D. R. Ladd (Eds.), *Prosody: Models and Measurements. 79–91.* Berlin etc.: SpPringer-Verlag.

Deese, J. (1984). *Thought into Speech: The Psychology of a Language.* Englewood Cliffs, NJ: Prentice-Hall.

Dell, G. S. (1986). A spreading activation theory of retrieval in sentence production. *Psychological Review, 93,* 283–321.

Di Sciullo, A.-M. & Williams, E. (1987). *On the Definition of Word.* Cambridge, MA: MIT Press.

van Dijk, T. A. (Ed.) (1985). *Handbook of Discourse Analysis, Vol. 1–4.* London etc.: Academic Press.

Drosdowski, G. (Ed.) (1984). *Duden: Grammatik der deutschen Gegenwartssprache.* Mannheim: Bibliographisches Institut.

Ehrich, V. (1992). Hier *und* Jetzt. *Studien zur positionalen und temporalen Deixis im Deutschen.* Tübingen: Niemeyer.

Ferreira, F. (1991). Effects of length and syntactic complexity on initiation times for prepared utterances. *Journal of Memory and Language, 30,* 210–233.

Fodor, J. A. (1983). *The Modularity of Mind.* Cambridge, MA: MIT Press.

Fodor, J. A. (1987). *Psychosemantics: The Problem of Meaning in the Philosophy of Mind.* Cambridge, MA: MIT Press.

Garnham, A., Shillock, R. C., Brown, G. D. A., Mill, A. I. D., & Cutler, A. (1982). Slips of the tongue in the London-Lund corpus of spontaneous conversation. In A. Cutler (Ed.), *Slips of the Tongue and Language Production. 251–264.* Berlin etc.: Mouton Publishers.

Garrett, M. F. (1975). The analysis of sentence production. In G. Bower (Ed.), *The Psychology of Learning and Motivation: Advances in Research and Theory, Vol. 9. 133–177.* N.Y.: Academic Press.

Garrett, M. F. (1988). Processes in language production. In F. J. Newmeyer (Ed.), *Language: Psychological and Biological Aspects. 69–96.* Cambridge etc.: Cambridge University Press.

Gibbs, R. W. Jr. & Mueller, R. A. G. (1988). Conversational sequences and preference for indirect speech acts. *Discourse Processes, 11,* 101–116.

Givon, T. (Ed.) (1979). *Syntax and Semantics 12: Discourse and Syntax.* N.Y. etc.: Academic Press.

Goodwin, Ch. (1981). *Conversational Organisation. Interaction between Speakers and Hearers.* N.Y. etc: Academic Press.

Goody, J. (1978). *The Domestication of the Savage Mind.* Cambridge: Cambridge University Press.

Gordon, D. & Lakoff, G. (1975). Conversational postulates. In P. Cole & J. L. Morgan (Eds.), *Syntax and Semantics 3: Speech Acts. 83–106.* N.Y. etc.: Academic Press.

Greenfield, P. M. & Savage-Rumbaugh, E. S. (1990). Grammatical combination in *Pan paniscus*: processes of learning and invention in the evolution and development of language. In S. T. Parker & K. R. Gibson (Eds.), *Language and Intelligence in Monkeys and Apes. Comparative Developmental Perspectives. 540–578.* Cambridge etc.: Cambridge University Press.

Grice, H. P. (1957). Meaning. *Philosophical Review, 66,* 377–388.

Grice, H. P. (1975). Logic and conversation. In P. Cole & J. L. Morgan (Eds.), *Syntax and Semantics 3: Speech Acts. 41–58.* N.Y. etc.: Academic Press.

Grice, H. P. (1968). Utterer's meaning, sentence meaning and word meaning. *Foundations of Language, 4,* 225–242.

Halliday, M. A. K. (1976). *System and Function in Language.* Selected Papers ed. by G. R. Kress. London: Oxford University Press.

Heeschen, V. (1992). *Prolegomena zu einer Grammatik des Eipo.* Habilitationsschrift, TU Berlin.

Huber, W. & Schlenck, K.-J. (1988). Satzverschränkungen bei Wernicke-Aphasie. In G. Blanken, J. Dittmann, & C.-W. Wallesch (Eds.), *Sprachproduktionsmodelle. Neuro- und psycholinguistische Modelle der menschlichen Spracherzeugung. 111–149.* Freiburg i. Br.: HochschulVerlag.

Isaacs, E. A. & Clark, H. H. (1987). References in conversation between experts and novices. *Journal of Experimental Psychology: General, 116,* 26–37.

Jarvella, R. J. (1971). Syntactic processing of connected speech. *Journal of Verbal Learning and Verbal Behavior, 10,* 409–416.

Jefferson, G. (1975). Error correction as an interactional resource. *Language in Society, 3,* 181–199.

Keenan, E. L. (1975). Variation in universal grammar. In R. Fasold & R. Shuy (Eds.), *Analyzing Variation in Language. 136–148.* Washington: Georgetown University Press.

Kempen, G. & Hoenkamp, E. (1987). An incremental procedural grammar for sentence formulation. *Cognitive Science, 11,* 201–258.

Kimura, D. (1979). Neuromotor mechanisms in the evolution of human communication. In H. D. Steklis & M. J. Raleigh (Eds.), *Neurobiology of Social Communication in Primates. 197–219.* N.Y.: Academic Press.

Klein, W. (1985). Gesprochene Sprache – geschriebene Sprache. *Zeitschrift für Literaturwissenschaft und Linguistik, 59,* 9–35.

Klein, W. (in press). Ellipse. In J. Jacobs, A. von Stechow, W. Sternefeld, & Th. Vennemann (Eds.), *Syntax. An international Handbook.* Berlin etc.: de Gruyter.

Kolk, H. (1987). A theory of grammatical impairment in aphasia. In G. Kempen (Ed.), *Natural Language Generation. 377–391.* Dordrecht etc.: Martinus Nijhoff Publishers.

Kolk, H. & van Grunsven, M. J. F. (1985). Agrammatism as a variable phenomenon. *Cognitive Neuropsychology, 2,* 347–384.

Kolk, H., van Grunsven, M. J. F., & Keyser, A. (1985). On parallelism between production and comprehension in agrammatism. In M.-L. Kean (Ed.), *Agrammatism. 165–206.* N.Y. etc.: Academic Press.

Kolk, H. & Heeschen, C. (1990). Adaptation symptoms and impairment symptoms in Broca's aphasia. *Aphasiology, 4,* 221–331.

Kolk, H. & Heeschen, C. (1992). Agrammatism, paragrammatism, and the management of language. *Language and Cognitive Processes, 7 (2),* 89–129.

Krauss, R. M. & Weinheimer, S. (1966). Concurrent feedback, confirmation, and the encoding of referents in verbal communication. *Journal of Personality and Social Psychology, 4:3,* 343–346.

Krauss, R. M. & Weinheimer, S. (1967). Effect of referent similarity and communication mode on verbal encoding. *Journal of Verbal Learning and Verbal Behavior, 6,* 359–363.

Labov, W. & Fanshell, D. (1977). *Therapeutic Discourse: Psychotherapy as Conversation.* N.Y.: Academic Press.

Lackner, J. R. (1980). Speech production: correction of semantic and grammatical errors during speech shadowing. In V. A. Fromkin (ed.), *Errors in Lingzistic Performance. 149–156.* N.Y. etc.: Academic Press.

Lerner, G. H. (1991). On the syntax of sentences-in-progress. *Language in Society, 20,* 441–458.

Levelt, W. J. M. (1983). Monitoring and self-repair in speech. *Cognition, 14,* 41–104.

Levelt, W. J. M. (1989). *Speaking. From Intention to Articulation.* Cambridge, MA: MIT Press.

Levelt, W. J. M. & Kelter, S. (1982). Surface form and memory in question answering. *Cognitive Psychology, 14,* 78–106.

Levinson, S. C. (1983). *Pragmatics.* Cambridge etc.: Cambridge University Press.

Lieberman, Ph. (1991). *Uniquely Human.* Cambridge, MA and London, England: Harvard University Press.

Ludwig, O. (1983). Writing systems and written language. In F. Coulmas & K. Ehlich (Eds.), *Writ-*

ing in Focus. 31–43. Berlin etc.: Mouton Publishers.

Lukatela, G., Gligorijevic, B., Kostic, A., & Turvey, M. T. (1980). Representation of inflected nouns in the internal lexicon. *Memory and Cognition*, 415–423.

McClelland, J. L., St. John, M., & Taraban, R. (1989). Sentence comprehension: a parallel distributed processing approach. *Language and Cognitive Processes, 4*, Special Issue, 287–335.

McNeill, D. (1987). *Psycholinguistics: A New Approach.* N.Y.: Harper and Row.

MacWhinney, B. & Bates, E. (Eds.) (1990). *The Cross-Linguistic Study of Sentence Processing.* Cambridge: Cambridge University Press.

Martin, R. C., Frederick Wetzel, W., Blossom-Stach, C., & Feher, E. (1989). Syntactic loss versus processing deficit: an assessment of two theories of agrammatism and syntactic comprehension deficits. *Cognition, 32*, 157–191.

Morais, J., Bertelson, P., Cary, L., & Alegria, J. (1986). Literacy training and speech segmentation. *Cognition, 24*, 157–191.

Mühlemann, T. & Foppa, K. (1989). Simultansprechen und Sprecherwechsel. *Sprache und Kognition, 1*, 1–8.

Nooteboom, S. G. (1980). Speaking and unspeaking: corections of phonological and lexical errors in spontaneous speech. In V. A. Fromkin (Ed.), *Errors in Linguistic Performance. 87–96.* N.Y. etc.: Academic Press.

Ochs, E. (1979). Planned and unplanned discourse. In T. Givon (Ed.), *Syntax and Semantics 12: Discourse and Syntax. 51–80.* N.Y. etc.: Academie Press.

Olson, D. R. & Hildyard, A. (1983). Literacy and the comprehension and expression of literal meaning. In F. Coulmas & K. Ehlich (Eds.), *Writing in Focus. 291–325.* Berlin etc.: Mouton Publishers.

Ong, W. J. (1982). *Orality and Literacy: The Technologizing of the Word.* London etc.: Methuen.

Pinker, S. (1991). Rules of language. *Science, 253*, 530–535.

Pylyshyn, Z. W. (1984). *Computation and Cognition.* Cambridge, MA: MIT Press.

Potter, M. C. & Lombardi, L. (1990). Regeneration in the short-term recall of sentences. *Journal of Memory and Language, 29*, 633–654.

Redeker, G. (1986). *Language Use in Informal Narratives.* Doctoral dissertation, UC Berkeley.

Ross, J. R. (1967). *Constraints on Variables in Syntax.* Ph.D. Thesis, MIT.

Ross, J. R. (1975). Where to do things with words. In P. Cole & J. L. Morgan (Eds.), *Syntax and Semantics 3: Speech Acts. 233–256.* N.Y. etc.: Academic Press.

Rumelhart, D. E. & McClelland, J. L. (1986). On learning the past tenses. In J. L. McClelland and D. E. Rumelhart (Eds.), *Parallel Distributed Processing, Vol. 2. 216–271.* Cambridge, MA: MIT Press.

Sacks, H., Schegloff, E. A., & Jefferson, G. (1974). A simplest systematics for the organization of turn-taking in conversation. *Language, 50*, 696–735.

Sadock, J. M. & Zwicky, A. M. (1985). Speech act distinctions in syntax. In T. Shopen (Ed.), *Language Typology and Syntactic Description, Vol. 1: Clause Structure. 155–196.* Cambridge etc.: Cambridge University Press.

Scheerer, E. (in press). Mündlichkeit und Schriftlichkeit: Implikationen für die Modellierung kognitiver Prozesse. In J .Baurmann, H. Günther und U. Knoop (Eds.), *HOMO SCRIBENS.* Tübingen: Niemeyer.

Schegloff, E. A. (1979). The relevance of repair to syntax-for-conversation. In T. Givon (Ed.), *Syntax and Semantics 12: Discourse and Syntax. 261–288.* N.Y. etc.: Academic Press.

Schegloff, E. A. (1984). On some questions and ambiguities in conversation. In J. M. Atkinson & J. Heritage (Eds.), *Structures of Social Action: Studies in Conversation Analysis. 28–52.* Cambridge etc.: Cambridge University Press.

Schegloff, E. A. & Sacks, H. (1973). Opening up closings. *Semiotica, 7*, 289–327.

Schenkein, J. (1980). A taxonomy for repeating action sequences in natural conversation. In B. Butterworth (Ed.), *Language Production, Vol. 1. 21–47.* London etc.: Academic Press.

Searle, J. R. (1969). *Speech Acts.* Cambridge: Cambridge University Press.

Searle, J. R. (1975). Indirect speech acts. In P. Cole & J. L. Morgan (Eds.), *Syntax and Semantics 3: Speech Acts. 59–82.* N.Y. etc: Academic Press.

Selkirk, E. (1982). *The Syntax of Words.* Cambridge, MA: MIT Press.

Seltz, O. (1922). *Über die Gesetze des geordneten Denkverlaufs. Zweiter Teil: Zur Psychologie des produktiven Denkens und des Irrtums.* Weimar: Dietsch und Brückner.

Senft, G. (1982). *Sprachliche Varietät und Variation im Sprachverhalten Kaiserslauterer Metallarbeiter.* Bern und Frankfurt a. M.: Peter Lang.

Shopen, T. (1972). *A Generative Theory of Ellipsis: A Consideration of the Linguistic Use of Silence.* Indiana University Linguistics Club.

Spencer, A. (1991). *Morphological Theory. An Introduction to Word Structure in Generative Grammar.* Oxford: Basil Blackwell Ltd.

Sperber, D. & Wilson, D. (1986). *Relevance: Communication and Cognition.* Oxford: Blackwell.

Stemberger, J. P. (1982). Syntactic errors in speech. *Journal of Psycholinguistic Research, 11*, 313–345.

Stemberger, J. P. & MacWhinney, B. (1986). Frequency and the lexical storage of regularly inflected forms. *Memory and Cognition, 14*, 17–26.

Tannen, D. (1982a). Oral and literate strategies in spoken and written narratives. *Language, 58*, 1–21.

Tannen, D. (1982b). The oral/literate continuum in discourse. In D. Tannen (Ed.), *Spoken and Written Language: Exploring Orality and Literacy. 1–16*. Norwood, NJ: Ablex Publishing Corporation.

Tannen, D. (Ed.) (1984). *Coherence in Spoken and Written Discourse*. Norwood: Ablex Publishing Corporation.

Tannen, D. (1987). Repetition in conversation: toward a poetics of talk. *Language, 63*, 574–605.

Wunderlich, D. (1976). *Studien zur Sprechakttheorie*. Frankfurt a. M.: Suhrkamp.

Claus Heeschen, Nijmegen (The Netherlands)

3. Phonological and Articulatory Characteristics of Spoken Language

1. Introduction

Speaking may be our most impressive motor skill. We speak rapidly, and production of each word involves intricate sequencing and temporal interleaving of gestures for the component, ordered consonants and vowels of the word. The problem of understanding speech production at this level is that of understanding how speakers accomplish the feat of fluent consonant and vowel production. Solving that problem involves solving another one, however. It is to understand what speaking is essentially. That is, it is to understand how a series of complicated actions of a vocal tract can serve to convey a message composed of rulefully-patterned symbols to members of a language community. In fact, the kind of solution an investigator seeks to the problem of understanding how vocal-tract actions are executed depends on how the investigator looks at the relation between vocal-tract action and the linguistic message itself.

Phonology is traditionally seen as the discipline that concerns itself with the building blocks of linguistic messages. It is the study of the structure of sound inventories of languages and of the participation of sounds in rules or processes. Phonetics, in contrast, concerns speech sounds as produced and perceived. Two extreme positions on the relationship between phonological messages and phonetic realizations are represented in the literature. One holds that the primary home for linguistic symbols, including phonological ones, is the human mind, itself housed in the human brain. The second holds that their primary home is the human vocal tract.

Consider the first position and the conceptualization of speech production to which it leads. For at least two reasons, the vocal tract is rejected as a natural home for phonological segments of the language. A philosophical reason is that phonemes are not the kinds of things that can occur or exist outside the mind. They are ideas or concepts without real-world actualization. Articulatory gestures or their acoustic consequences can serve as cues to phonological segments, but they cannot be phonological segments.

"[Segments] are abstractions. They are the end result of complex perceptual and cognitive processes in the listener's brain" (Repp 1981, 1462).

"Phonological representation is concerned with speakers' implicit knowledge, that is with information in the mind ... [Phonetic] representation ... is not cognitive because it concerns events in the world rather than events in the mind" (Pierrehumbert 1990).

A practical reason why phonological segments cannot occur in the vocal tract is that linguistic symbols have other properties, aside from being covert kinds of things, that preclude the vocal tract from representing them veridically or even analogically. In particular, a central and important fact about language is that its messages are composed of discrete symbols. Phonological segments are discrete in the sense that they do not overlap and blend. Moreover, until recently, they have been represented in linguistic theories as if they were composed of lists of coextensive (and by implication, cotemporal) features (cf.

Chomsky/Halle 1968). The features themselves described static postures of the vocal tract or their acoustic consequences; accordingly, the feature lists of a word described a succession of vocal-tract or acoustic snapshots. The vocal-tract actions that somehow convey a message to a listener have none of those properties. Actions associable with a given consonant or vowel do overlap and do appear to blend with actions of neighbors. Actions identifiable with the component features of a consonant or vowel are not cotemporal. Finally, fundamental units of articulation appear to be actions, not postures; accordingly, time is intrinsic to speech, rather than extrinsic as it is to the linguistic message. One interpretation of these mismatches is that they reflect the mismatch between the ideal of linguistic competence and the degraded physical reality of linguistic vocal performance; the latter necessarily is a considerable distortion of the former due to the limitations of mechanico-inertial systems. This way of looking at speech production promotes development of a kind of theory of the 'how' of speech production that have been termed 'translation theories' (Fowler/Rubin/Remez/Turvey 1980). The mismatch between the character of the planned message, presumably a sequence of linguistic symbols, and of its physical, phonetic, realization requires a translation over stages of processing out of the ideal, mental, domain of the plan into the real, physical-nonmental, domain of a vocal tract.

The other extreme perspective on the nature of speaking is that consonants and vowels are actions of the vocal tract that have linguistic, including phonological, significance in a language community. They are, certainly, psychological actions that require knowledge about them to be performed. However, the knowledge is not a superior 'ideal' that the actions cannot implement; rather, the knowledge is a b o u t the actions, derived from perceptual and articulatory experience with them. From this perspective, the mismatch between linguistic segments and articulation described above is apparent rather than real. It is the product of three kinds of error: 1. a mistaken ascription of primacy to linguistic knowledge (competence) over linguistic activity (performance); 2. an incorrect characterization of phonological segments in linguistic theory; 3. an incorrect characterization of the vocal tract actions of speech production. As to the first 'error', the argument is that we treat language differently from other human creations when we decide that its components exist only in the mind. Other human creations include, for example, automobiles, baseball games and musical pieces. Automobiles definitely exist in the world and so do baseball games and musical pieces when they are played. What is in the mind of those who know about automobiles, baseball and a musical piece, is only what they know about those things; it is not the things themselves. If linguistic concepts are like these other concepts, they are knowledge about real-world objects or events; the events have a psychological nature – in this case, they are actions of the vocal tract, identified as phonological segments. If the phonology in the mind of a language user is what the user knows about the actions that implement a linguistic message, then there need be no mismatch between knowledge and action. If a phonological theory ascribes properties to phonological segments as known that are impossible to realize in vocal-tract action, then the first hypothesis should be that the theory is wrong, not that vocal-tract action distorts components of linguistic competence. If descriptions of vocal-tract actions include properties, such as coarticulatory blending, that would distort the phonological message, then the first hypothesis should be that the descriptions are wrong. From this perspective, an important aim is to work on development of a phonology that does not ascribe properties to phonological segments that are unproduceable as vocal-tract action (cf. Browman/Goldstein 1986; Browman/Goldstein 1989). A second aim is to find a perspective on vocal-tract action from which macroscopic order is evident that conforms to the phonological structure of spoken utterances (e. g., Fowler/Rubin/Remez/Turvey 1980; Fowler 1990; Saltzman 1986; Saltzman/Munhall 1989).

This theoretical perspective promotes a theory of speech production different from a translation theory as outlined earlier. Speech production does not involve a translation out of an ideal, mental domain into a physical, nonmental, domain. Rather, the plan for a sequence of phonological segments, physically instantiated in the brain, replicates itself in a new physical medium, the moving vocal tract. A speech plan, in some way, brings about vocal-tract actions having linguistic significance.

In the remainder of this chapter, I pursue the different outlooks on a central aspect of speech production, coarticulation, that these different theoretical perspectives promote. I then consider the implications of our understanding of coarticulation for understanding another central aspect of speech production: the coordinated actions of the vocal tract that constitute token phonological segments.

2. Two Perspectives on Coarticulation

All sources of evidence regarding speech production, whether they are acoustic or articulatory, provide the same general picture of context-sensitivity in speech production. An acoustic signal displayed spectrographically or as a waveform, for example, can be divided into phonological-segment sized regions (e. g. Klatt 1973) by identifying acoustic properties that are more strongly associated with one particular segment of an utterance than with others. For example a stop burst can be assigned to a stop in a stop-vowel utterance, and the following voiced formants can be assigned to the vowel. Even so, however, the display has not thereby been partitioned into phonological segments or even into their acoustic consequences. This is so, in part, because there may be no obvious place to locate a boundary separating the acoustic consequences of one phoneme from those of another. For example, the voiceless formant transitions following a voiceless stop consonant in a consonant-vowel sequence belong with the stop, because they are voiceless, but they also belong with the vowel, because formants are characteristic of vowels and other sonorants (see, e. g. Peterson/Lehiste 1960). Indeed, generally, there are no boundaries between segments so that a partition leaves all and only the acoustic information for one segment on one side of the boundary and all and only that for another segment on the other side (cf. Fant/Lindblom 1961). Moreover, the overlap is not only in a potential boundary region. Spectral analysis of the signal well within a domain associated with a particular phonetic segment – well within the frication region for a fricative or within the steady-state formants, if any, of a vowel, for example – is likely to reveal influences of context. (I will use the term 'domain' to refer to the temporal region in which the features of a segment dominate in articulation or in the acoustic signal. The domain does not include the whole articulatory extent of a segment or the whole region in which it influences the acoustic signal, but only the region in which it is dominant; see also Löfqvist 1990.)

Examination of the articulatory behaviors that give rise to acoustic speech signals reveals a compatible picture. Articulatory movements can be found that are identifiable with one of the phonetic segments in an utterance – movement toward bilabial closure in a bV sequence, for example. In addition, boundaries can be located around that movement. In the example, a boundary may be located where closing is first detectable and another at the point of release of the closure. Once again, however, the boundaries are not boundaries between phonological segments or their articulatory consequences so that all and only movements associated with /b/ occur within the boundaries and movements associated with other segments fall outside the boundaries. During the closing and closure gestures, the tongue body will be conforming itself to the requirements of the following vowel (e. g. Öhman 1966), and once again, the movements within the boundaries are context-sensitive. For example, the jaw moves to a higher point of maximum closing for /b/ followed by a high than a low vowel (Keating/Lindblom/Lubker, cited in Keating 1990).

Sources of context sensitivity are bidirectional. Effects of earlier segments in the string extending beyond their domains of prominence are termed 'left-to-right', 'perseverative' or 'carryover' effects. Effects of later segments are called 'right-to-left' or 'anticipatory.' Estimates of the coarticulatory field – that is, the interval of time or the number of segmental domains affected by a segment in either direction – vary considerably, but may be quite large. For example, Magen (1989) reports anticipatory effects of V_3 on V_1 Cə C V_3 sequences in English. While some part of the carryover influences can bee ascribed to inertial properties of the vocal tract and to its inability instantaneously to adopt a characteristic posture for one phonological segment without exhibiting transitional movements between the postures, anticipatory coarticulation cannot have that explanation, and carryover effects are sometimes more extensive than can be realistically ascribed to these mechanical factors (Daniloff/Hammarberg 1973). These considerations have suggested to many investigators that coarticulation is planned. Generally accounts of coarticulation diverge along the theoretical lines distinguished in the introduction.

2.1. Coarticulation as Assimilation by Feature Spreading

In a translation theory, coarticulation serves an important function of, indeed, *translating* a planned symbol string into a form more compatible with the capabilities of vocal-tract action. (The role of phonetic rules generally, according to Keating (1990), is to make the linguistic representation "more physical.")

One example of a theory in which coarticulation serves that function is that of Daniloff/Hammarberg (1973). Daniloff/Hammarberg described the phonological segments that serve as "input" in a plan to speak as "canonical forms" – that is, "invariant, ideal, uncoarticulated forms" – the phonological types of a linguistic theory. These forms undergo "articulatory encoding" to tailor them to the vocal tract. The encoding processes include application of context-sensitive rules of feature spreading. An example they provide of such a rule is one that spreads a rounding feature from a vowel to a preceding /ʃ/: ʃ → $ʃ^{w}$ / _ [+ round, + V]. By this rule, the /ʃ/ in *shoe,* for example, acquires the feature [+ round] from its context, a following rounded vowel. Generally (following Henke 1966), rules cause a feature to spread in an anticipatory direction to any phonetic segment that is 'unspecified' for that feature. Feature values in phonological theory generally are binary, and a segment may be 'specified' for a feature by having either a '+' or a '–' value of that feature. (Accordingly, a rounded vowel is [+ round] while an unrounded vowel is [– round].) To count as an instance of a segment specified for some feature value, a token occurrence of the segment must have the appropriate feature value; changing the value may change one segment into another and hence, in a sequence of phonemes, may change one word into another. These feature values thereby serve a 'contrastive' function in the language. At least hypothetically, the contrastive feature values cannot be changed by a feature-spreading coarticulatory rule. However, some features are irrelevant to the identification of some segments. For example, in English, rounding is not contrastive for consonants; accordingly, making a consonant rounded does not change it from one consonant of English to another. Consonants are said to be 'unspecified' for rounding, and they are subject to coarticulatory rules of feature spreading.

Evidence compatible with the feature-spreading theory includes findings (or, perhaps, interpretations of findings; see 2.2) that lip rounding anticipates a rounded vowel across any number of preceding consonants (e. g. Daniloff/Moll 1968; Benguerel/Cowan 1974) and that nasality anticipates a nasal consonant across any number of vowels uninterrupted by oral consonants (Moll/Daniloff 1971).

The simple characterization of coarticulation fails in several ways. One is that the coarticulatory field very often does not respect boundaries drawn between segments. That is, the hypothesis of feature spreading as the sole source of coarticulation predicts that the spread feature should be uniformly present throughout the production of the segment – at least to the same extent that other features of the segment are present, but that is generally not the case (e. g., Benguerrel/Cowan 1974; Krakow 1989). Second, the magnitude of effects of ostensibly spread features is gradient rather than categorial. For example, Manuel/Krakow (1984) found that a following (front, high) vowel /e/, raises and fronts following (low, back) vowel /a/, but (front, high) /i/ raises it even more. Likewise, Marchal (1988) reported graded effects of one stop consonant on another in /kt/ sequences that suggested varying degrees of coarticulatory overlap between them. A third problem is that coarticulatory influences may affect realizations of specified features. In Marchal's findings, just cited, coarticulatory influences occur between stops specified for different places of articulation. A final problem relates to the idea of underspecification. The problem here is that segments considered to be unspecified for a feature involving some articulator – say, rounding and the lips (in English, consonants) or nasality and the velum (in English, vowels) – are not wholly neutral with respect to the demands they make on the articulator. Some consonants are associated with rounding movements of the lips (for example, /l/, /r/ and /s/ and /ʃ/ (Bell-Berti/Harris 1982; Delattre/Freeman 1968; Leidner 1973). Compatibly, vowels, ostensibly unspecified for nasality are associated with characteristic postures of the velum (Bell-Berti 1980; Moll 1962). Despite their not being wholly unspecified in terms of articulatory control, they are subject to coarticulatory influences from specified neighbors and they coarticulate with neighbors. For example, the different velum heights associated with vowels of different heights both influence velum height for neighboring consonants and they are recipients of coarticulatory influences from nasal consonants (Bell-Berti 1980). Accordingly, in contrast to the feature-spreading account of coarticulation, coarticulatory influences occur in the absence of any linguistic features to spread.

Recently, Keating (1988, 1990) has proposed an alternative account of specification and its role in coarticulation that preserves the idea of coarticulation as a participant in a translation from the mental to the physical domain of talking. She proposes that coarticulation includes processes at two levels at least, one phonological and one phonetic. At the phonological level, coarticulation is assimilatory feature spreading. Since Keating's focus has been on phonetic coarticulation, she simply alludes to this type of coarticulation without providing an example. However, a possible example is provided by Daniloff/Hammarberg (1973). They point out that in the word *width*, there is, apparently, a spreading of the interdental place of articulation of /θ/ to /d/ (which, by the way, is specified for a different place of articulation; however, in this case, the feature change does not yield a different phoneme of English). As for phonetic coarticulation, Keating proposes a "targets and connections" model. In the model, phonetic segments are associated with characteristic targets, and segments are sequenced by interpolating between successive targets. A novel aspect of Keating's idea of targets, however (but see Manuel 1987, for a similar idea), is that the targets are regions ("windows"), rather than fixed postures. Windows differ in their widths, and a target's instantiation within its window will depend on its neighbors in that the speaker will generally select the most efficient path from segment to segment that passes through each target region. The idea of target windows replaces the idea of underspecification as categorial with a gradient version. A segment with the narrowest possible window for some feature is "specified" for that feature value; one with the widest possible window for a feature is unspecified. However, most segments have intermediate target window sizes for their component features. Vowels have wider windows for velum height than do nasal and oral consonants, but the window is not as wide as possible. Accordingly, a vowel's window region does affect the articulatory path through the target window of neighboring segments.

This model handles the data of coarticulation considerably better than does the feature spreading model of Daniloff/Hammarberg (1973); yet it preserves the idea of coarticulation as among the processes that make the planned utterance 'more physical.' The targets and connections model is not obviously consistent with all of the data, however. In particular, one finding that the model does not seem to handle well is the ubiquity of coarticulatory fields that extend beyond immediate neighbors. The targets and connections idea explains how contiguous segments can be produced smoothly, but it does not readily predict strong coarticulatory influences of a segment C on A in an ABC sequence. Two other problems emerge below. They are that some coarticulation is difficult to characterize as anything other than overlap (for example, findings by Marchal 1988, cited above). A second is that a segment's 'aggressiveness' (here, having a narrow window) in its own domain appears always to be associated with a compatible degree of aggressiveness outside of its domain, frequently beyond any transitional region between target regions.

2.2. Coproduction Theories

A "coproduction" theory (Fowler 1977) explains coarticulation as the overlapping production of – to a first approximation – invariant sequences of consonants and vowels. The context sensitivity apparent in the acoustic signal and in articulation is not 'deep' context sensitivity in the sense that consonants or vowels have undergone assimilatory change (as in a feature spreading theory). Rather it is a more peripheral blending of consonants and vowels that are unchanged with respect to their essential, specified, properties.

Öhman's (1966; 1967) theory provides a seminal example of such a theory (but see also, however, (Kozhevnikov/Chistovich 1965). In a spectrographic analysis of $V_1 C V_2$ disyllables, Öhman noticed many instances in which the closing transitions into the consonant depended not only on V_1, but also on V_2. Likewise, transitions following consonant release depended on both vowels. X-ray tracings (see also Öhman 1967) showed clear evidence that the tongue body conformation during C closure was different in the context of different flanking vowels. Öhman (1966, 166) suggested that the stop gestures were "superimposed" on a diphthongal vowel-to-vowel gesture of the tongue body and that the "tongue is able to make a distorted vowel gesture, while it is executing the stop consonant". More speculatively, he proposed three neuromuscular systems for controlling the tongue. The systems, though distinct, would use overlapping muscles. One system, the apical system, is used to produce dental, alveolar and retroflex consonants; the dorsal system produces palatal and velar consonants, and the tongue body system produces vowels. During speech production, a consonant and vowel system may be controlling the tongue in overlapping time frames and the result is "a complex summation (neural, muscular and probably mechanical also) of the responses to each of the components of the instruction" (1966, 166). Öhman's observations have been replicated many times. For example, Perkell (1969) noticed that the /k/ constriction during /h∂kɛ/ consisted of a sliding movement of the tongue dorsum toward the front location for /ɛ/. Compatible evidence of vowel-to consonant anticipatory and carryover coarticulation and sometimes vowel-to-vowel coarticulation in V C Vs is provided by Barry/Kuenzel (1975), Butcher/Weiher (1976) and Carney/Moll (1971).

These findings are not captured naturally in a feature spreading account of coarticulation. The main reason is that they reveal the dynamic nature of changing articulatory parameter values during speech. Consider Perkell's finding just described. There is no change in a feature value for /k/'s place of articulation that would yield a sliding place value. The outcome is explained more naturally as a growing influence of /ɛ/'s articulatory demands during /k/.

Öhman (1967) developed a quantitative model of vowel-consonant-vowel coarticulation that did a satisfactory job of predicting the changing vocal-tract shapes (as indexed by X-ray tracings) during V C V production. Notably it includes a parameter value, k, and other parameters labeled q, to implement consonant and vowel production respectively over time. To implement the temporal articulatory domain of a consonant or vowel, the associated parameter increases over time and then decreases. That is, to generate coarticulatory influences of the vowel on the consonant, for example, the vowel's influence on the vocal tract gradually waxes and then wanes. Elsewhere, we have described this waxing and waning of a segment's implementation over time as a "prominence curve" (Fowler/Smith 1986); see Löfqvist's (1990) similar idea of "dominance").

In light of this evidence favoring coproduction, let us reconsider the data considered most supportive of feature spreading theory, evidence that lip rounding anticipates across consonant strings unspecified for rounding and that velum lowering anticipates across vowel strings unspecified for nasality. Difficulties with the idea of underspecification have already been cited. More than that, however, work by Bell-Berti and her colleagues show quite convincingly that the error of accepting underspecification has led to considerable overestimation of anticipation of velum lowering and lip rounding (see also Boyce/Krakow/Bell-Berti/Gelfer 1990).

2.2.1. Anticipatory Lowering of the Velum for Nasal Consonants

Consider the literature on nasalization first. Researchers typically examined C V_n N strings (where Ns are nasal consonants and the subscript on the vowel signifies that different numbers of vowels intervened between C and N). Velar lowering following C was taken as evidence for onset of anticipatory nasalization from N (Moll/Daniloff 1971). However, Bell-Berti (1980) points out that vowels are associated with lower velum heights than are oral consonants; accordingly the initial drop of the velum will be due at least to the vowel; it may or may not reflect an influence of N as well. That can be determined only by comparing C V_n N sequences with corresponding C V_n C sequences. Such a comparison indeed shows a lowering of the velum at the onset of a vowel string in C V_n C utterances that, of course, must be ascribed to the vowel rather than to coarticulatory effects of a nasal consonant (Bell-Berti/Krakow, submitted). When effects of the vowel are eliminated from velum movements in C V_n N utterances, findings are no longer consistent with feature spreading theories. Rather, they suggest an invariant onset of velum lowering relative to onset of nasal murmur in nasal consonant production. Bell-Berti/Harris (1981) interpret the findings as favoring a particular version of a coproduction theory, that they call "frame theory" in which the temporally-staggered onsets of component gestures of a phonetic segment are staggered in a time-invariant way.

The findings by Bell-Berti and her colleagues also help to explain an otherwise complicating finding by Bladon/Al-Bamerni (1982). Bladon/Al-Bamerni had found evidence for two patterns of anticipatory coarticulation of velum lowering – a one-step pattern of lowering, timed consistently with predictions of feature-spreading theory (that is, beginning at the onset of the first vowel in a string) and a two step pattern, the first step beginning at the onset of the first vowel and the second, as frame theory predicts, an invariant interval before the oral closing gesture for the nasal consonant. Bladon/Al-Bamerni were unable to find anything systematically different in the contexts in which each pattern was observed; therefore, they suggested that selection among the strategies was unsystematic. An alternative interpretation, however, is that sometimes the vocalic velum lowering movement (always beginning near vowel onset) overlaps completely with the lowering gesture for the nasal consonant, whereas at other times, it precedes velum lowering for the consonant. Bell-Berti/Krakow (submitted; see also Boyce/Krakow/Bell-Berti/Gelfer 1990) found increasing evidence of two- or multi-stage velum lowering as vocalic segments were added before the nasal consonant. Likewise, of their three talkers, one produced the target words at a considerably faster rate than the others and that subject showed a one-stage lowering pattern for all but the longest vowel segments. Finally, one talker who produced the words at two rates showed two- or multi-stage lowering only at the slower rate.

Overall, the findings on anticipatory velum lowering – originally considered to provide strong evidence in favor of a feature spreading theory of coarticulation – do not; rather, they provide better support for the view that coarticulation is coproduction. Notice, too, that Keating's targets and connections account must at least be modified to fit the data. In particular, the model does not predict that target windows for successive segments will overlap; however, the data just described shows convincingly that they do. That is, this model too must admit the possibility of coproduction. Coarticulation is not wholly finding the most efficient pathway from one target window to another; sometimes windows overlap.

2.2.2. Lip Rounding

The literature on lip rounding, like that on nasalization, has failed to support the feature spreading account. Generally, it supports frame theory. As Kent/Minifie (1977) pointed out, contradictory evidence was available even in one study commonly cited as supporting feature spreading, namely that of Benguerel/Cowan (1974). In their findings more than half the time, rounding spread not only through a preceding consonant string, but beyond it into a preconsonantal unrounded vowel. Bell-Berti/Harris (1979) obtained similar results for both of their speakers. The study by Bell-Berti/Harris (1979) and a later one (Bell-Berti/Harris 1982) showed a generally invariant relation between onset of EMG (orbicularis oris muscle of the lips) for a rounded vowel and measured acoustic onset of the rounded vowel over a variable number of prevocalic consonants.

The research by Bell-Berti/Harris tested for and found lip EMG activity for /l/, one of the consonants in the strings they used as stimuli. As noted earlier, other investigators have found rounding for other consonants. These consonantal influences on lip configuration are likely to have contaminated estimates of onset of lip rounding in the earlier research in the same way that the vocalic influences on velum height contaminated estimates of onset of velum lowering for nasal consonants. These contaminating influences can only be identified by examining control utterances that lack the specified segment (that is, V C_n V utterances in which both vowels are unrounded), and investigators have not done that generally. However, using appropriate control utterances, Boyce (1988) has shown that overlapping consonantal and vocalic lip movements approximately add so that effects of consonants on the lips in a utterance such as /kuktluk/ can be eliminated by subtracting the movement trace from /kiktlik/ from it. Whereas Boyce did not then test for the invariance of EMG onset relative to acoustic onset of the rounded vowel that Bell-Berti/Harris had reported earlier, she did find a clear intervocalic trough in lip movement activity and bimodal peaks of EMG activity in utterances with two rounded vowels. The pair of findings suggests that during the consonantal string /ktl/, rounding from the first vowel wanes while that for the second vowel increases. Hence there are two distinct rounding gestures that wax and wane in the consonantal string – just as Öhman's account of vowel-consonant production proposed. There is not a spreading of a rounding feature from vowel to consonant. Compatibly, Gelfer/Bell-Berti/Harris (1989) superimposed graphs of lip EMG activity (orbicularis oris) for utterances such as /ist # tu/ and

/ist # ti/ having varying numbers of intervocalic consonants and final /u/ or /i/. By eliminating the activity common to both utterances, and hence due to the consonant string, they were able to identify the onset time of EMG activity associated with the rounded vowel itself. Onset times bore a near-invariant relation to release of the occlusion of the final consonant in strings of two or more consonants.

2.2.3. Lingual Coarticulation

The literature on coarticulation involving the tongue supports and augments the idea of coarticulation as gestural overlap. Öhman's model suggests that demands on the articulators made by a segment increase gradually over time and decrease gradually. The serial ordering of segments in articulation is maintained not by preserving discreteness of segment production along the time axis, but, rather perhaps, by maintaining a serial ordering of their times of maximum control in the vocal tract. In addition, however, segments differ one from the other in the strengths of demands they place on different articulators (or on different articulatory systems; see below under 'coordination' and cf. Keating's idea of windows discussed above). The differences in strength have an observable consequence that is described differently (e. g. Farnetani 1990) depending on where it is observed. If discrete domains are identified for segments in an utterance by drawing boundaries at points where coarticulating segments shift in their relative dominance in the vocal tract, then one can say that in their own domain, segments that make strong demands on an articulator 'resist' coarticulatory influences from neighbors (Bladon/Al-Bamerni 1976); in the domains of near neighbors, they exert a strong coarticulatory influence. From the perspective of a coproduction theory, resistance to coarticulation and a strong coarticulatory influence covary because they are really the same thing – namely a segment's exerting a relatively strong influence on articulators throughout its temporal domain.

Recasens (1984; 1985; 1987; 1989) has conducted much of the work that has uncovered variation in coarticulation resistance in movements involving the tongue dorsum. In general, resistance to coarticulation of a consonant or vowel is associated with the amount of tongue dorsum-palatal contact associated with production of the segment (see also Farnetani 1990). Compatibly, using acoustic and electropalatographic measures, Recasens (1984; 1987) found a decrease in vowel-to-vowel coarticulation in VCV sequences in which C is produced with considerable contact between the tongue dorsum (an important articulator in vowel production) and the palate. For example, there is less V-to-C coarticulation across palatal /j/ than across dental /n/. Compatibly, the vowel /i/, which requires a constriction in the palatal region resists consonant-vowel coarticulatory influences moreso than do other vowels (Recasens 1985), and it resists vowel-to-vowel coarticulatory overlap as well (Recasens 1987; 1989). In addition, as noted earlier, segments such as /i/ that are resistant to coarticulation in their own coarticulatory domains themselves exert strong coarticulatory influences on neighbors (see Tables II-VI in Recasens 1987; see also Butcher/Weiher 1976; Farnetani/Vagges/Magno-Caldognetto 1985).

It may be tempting to conclude from this research that production of consonants and vowels is context sensitive after all in that coarticulatory anticipation of V2 in a VCV sequence must be delayed and reduced if V1 is /i/ as compared to /a/ or if C is /j/ as compared to /n/. However, possibly, the planned segment can be invariant, while its surface manifestations vary according to its neighbor's patterns of coarticulation resistance. Consider, by analogy, the different surface consequences of an invariant squeezing action of the hand depending on whether the hand is empty, or else holding a sponge or a rock. The outcome at the surface is different both in the extent to which the hand (metaphorically, the segment being produced) closes and in the extent that it deforms the sponge (a little coarticulation resistance) and the rock (a lot of resistance). Perhaps by the same token, an invariant plan for a segment can have different surface consequences if coarticulation resistance is implemented as a real physical variable in the vocal tract. There is one striking outcome reported by Recasens (1984) that suggests exactly that. He reported instances both of anticipatory and of carry-over coarticulation in which coarticulatory effects were discontinuous. That is, vowel-to-vowel effects were observed in VCV sequences even though, in consonants with considerable tongue dorsum/palatal contact, vowel-to-consonant coarticulation was absent. It is unlikely that talkers plan to begin production of V2 in V1, to stop production of V2 during C, and to recommence its production after C. An analogous plan for carryover coarticulation is even less likely.

2.3. Some Tentative Conclusions about Coarticulation

The findings just reviewed suggest the following summary. Each consonant or vowel of the language is implemented by one or more vocal-tract actions. Actions are of two varieties: gestures (Browman/Goldstein 1986) that are linguistically significant (and contrastive) and other, noncontrastive, ones that may occur because they are easier to produce than to suppress. Gestures for a segment may be timed or phased invariantly one with respect to another as frame theory proposes. Each vocal tract gesture has a prominence pattern of increasing then decreasing articulatory strength, where prominence refers to the extent to which the gesture exerts an influence on the character of movements in the vocal tract. Vocal tract actions differ one from the other in relative strength so that, for example, demands of /j/ or /i/ on the tongue dorsum-palate relation exceed those of /n/ and /a/. The extent to which a segment-specific action influences what is happening in the vocal tract at any point in time reflects the strength of that action and its strength relative to that of other ongoing actions affecting the same vocal-tract structures. 'Strength' appears to be implemented in such a way that its effects arise at the articulatory surface, not in differential planning for a segment depending on its context. The account is incomplete in a variety of ways, lacking detail in important areas, including a specification of how strength variations are realized. It is also too simple in some respects. In particular, patterns of relative timing of gestures for a segment are not invariant – they may vary over position in a syllable as Krakow (1989) has shown for the relative timing of velum lowering and lip closing actions for syllable-initial and -final /m/. They are likely to vary over stress and rate manipulations as well. In short, the state-of-the art in coarticulation research leaves investigators still with many problems to tackle.

3. Coordination

From the perspective of a coarticulating segment encroaching on the domain of a second segment, the second segment applies restrictions on where and to what extent encroachment can occur ('coarticulation resistance'). Accordingly, coarticulation by the same segment in the same (anticipatory, carryover) direction will be differentially manifested depending on the nature and strength of the restrictions applied in its coarticulatory field. Looked at from the perspective of the influenced segment, however, the restrictions are the segment's own identity; they are actions or postures the achievement of which counts as production of that segment. Somehow realization of the segment correspondingly prohibits contradictory actions. Here I examine implementation of those restrictions in speech production.

The vocal tract includes large numbers of muscles and structures that the muscles move or deform. Relative to the catalogue of movements that could occur were contractions of all possible combinations of vocal tract muscles used and contractions of all possible magnitudes, the movements that do occur in speech are limited in number and in kind. They are constrained, of course, to structure the air so that listeners can hear them. But more than that, they are low-dimensional movements – movements with order that spans groups of muscles and groups of vocal-tract structures. They are, indeed, coordinated actions.

Coordination achieves several things. Most importantly, structures of the vocal tract work together to achieve some end. For example, in production of /b/, the jaw and lips work together to achieve bilabial closure. The couplings among structures also preclude actions that violate the couplings; thereby they prohibit coarticulatory influences that would prevent the goal of the coordinative linkages. They do not completely eliminate variability or flexibility, however. For example, bilabial closure is realized with a variety of contributions by the jaw and lips. When /b/ is coarticulated with an open vowel, the jaw is lower during closure, and hence the lips do more of the closing work, than when /b/ coarticulates with /i/. Research using a perturbation procedure (e.g. Abbs/Gracco 1984; Kelso/Tuller/Vatikiotis-Bateson/Fowler 1984; Shaiman 1989) helps to expose couplings across structures of the vocal tract. In one of these experiments, Kelso/Tuller/Vatikiotis-Bateson/Fowler 1984) asked talkers to produce *It's a _ again,* with /baeb/ or /baez/ serving as target syllable. On a low proportion of trials, randomly selected, during the closing gesture for the second /b/ in /baeb/ or for the

/z/ in /baez/, the talker's jaw was unexpectedly braked, preventing its normal contribution to closure for the consonantal constriction. On perturbed relative to unperturbed trials, within 20 – 30 ms of the perturbation in /baeb/, the orbicularis oris muscle of the upper lip showed extra activation and by achievement of closure, the lip had moved farther down than on unperturbed trials. If the jaw was braked during closing for /z/, extra activation was observed in the genioglossus muscle of the tongue allowing the tongue to compensate for the unusually low position of the jaw. The upper lip did not show the same extra downward movement on /z/-perturbed trials that it showed on /b/-perturbed trials. Other research (Shaiman 1989) shows that when an articulator of the vocal tract is perturbed that is not involved in a consonantal closing gesture, closing on perturbed and unperturbed trials is alike. In short, the responses to perturbation are adaptive and they reveal a coupling among selective articulators of the vocal tract that jointly achieve some phonetic gestural end. Coupled structures and their neuromuscular underpinnings are know as 'synergies' or 'coordinative structures.' Whereas Löfqvist (1990) suggests that there are no dynamic perturbations in speech analogous to a jaw pull, perhaps there are. Coarticulatory encroachments from low vowels can perturb a talker's jaw, pulling it down during closure for /b/. Possibly, then, the couplings serve two functions; they bring about the coordinated action that constitutes a linguistic gesture of the vocal tract, and they permit only those coarticulatory encroachments that will not prevent the gesture from being realized.

The short-latency responses to the perturbations suggest that the couplings are low-level. That is, they are not cognitive couplings, but, rather neuromuscular ones. This may help to rationalize findings by Recasens summarized earlier of discontinuities in coarticulatory influences. Whereas it would be surprising for speakers to plan for V-to-V coarticulatory influences, yet plan for no V-to-C influences in a V C V sequence, the finding of discontinuities in coarticulation is less surprising if segments are planned to have an invariant coarticulatory field that then gets differentially suppressed by other synergies active in the vocal tract.

Following Browman/Goldstein (1986; 1989), we may call the vocal tract actions of a synergy a 'phonetic gesture' or, more simply, a 'gesture.' Phonetic gestures are, then, linguistically significant actions of the vocal tract. In the research using the perturbation technique just described, perturbations disrupted movements by one articulator among two or more that participated in a phonetic gesture. That is, perturbations and compensations were interarticulatory, but intragestural. However, some phonetic segments are defined by more than one gesture, and the timing or phasing between or among gestures may also be crucial to the identity of the segment. For example, the timing of an oral constriction gesture and a glottal devoicing gesture determines whether a consonant is preaspirated or aspirated (see, e. g., Löfqvist 1980; Löfqvist/Yoshioka 1984). Presumably, then, intrasegmental gestures must be coupled and one should see evidence of the coupling in perturbation experiments. To date, there is little evidence on the topic. However, Munhall/Löfqvist/Kelso (1988) have perturbed the lower lip during closing from a vowel to a /p/. The perturbation delayed achievement of closure, thereby lengthening the vowel. However, onset of glottal opening for /p/ was also delayed, giving rise to a perceptually adequate aspirated /p/. (Even so, there was disruption of the coordinative relation between the gestures such that the voice-onset times on perturbed trials were unusually long.)

Another index, perhaps, of a coupling relation between the gestures of a segment is provided by tests for invariant relative timing (as summarized in Löfqvist 1990). Coupling between gestures of a segment should give rise to invariance of relative timing between the gestures so that, as the segment is produced at various rates or with different levels of stress, temporal intervals between gesture onsets scale proportionately to changes in other intervals produced by the coupled actions. (The idea is that if the gestures are products of a common synergy, and rate changes are achieved by changes in a parameter that is common to the synergy, all temporal intervals produced by the gestures will scale proportionately.) Löfqvist (1990) applied a test for proportionality of intervals proposed by Gentner (1987) to several sets of data including measures of intrasegmental-intergestural intervals and intersegmental-intergestural intervals. Whereas 90% of tests for proportional changes in intervals over variation in rate and stress were rejected in tests of the latter intervals, just 33% were rejected in tests of the former intervals.

Löfqvist does not consider this particularly strong support for the proportional-durational test of coupling between gestures of a segment, because the reason why 67% of tests failed to reject the hypothesis of proportional durations for intrasegmental-intergestural intervals was not that intervals were relatively invariant, but rather because they were extremely noisy (see his Figures 11—15). Even so, his data do reveal marked differences in the temporal relations among gesture belonging to the same and to different phonological segments, with the latter relations showing systematic departures from the proportional-duration hypothesis and the former showing only unsystematic departures.

4. Speech Dynamics

There is a new development in the study of speech production that I will describe only briefly. It is as yet relatively untried; however, it promises to have a marked influence on research in the field. Although speech production is remarkable as a motor activity, it is not wholly unique. Some common issues arise in investigations of a variety of intentional motor skills. More fundamentally, however, some theorists suggest that intentional actions in general (Kugler/Turvey 1987; Kugler/Kelso/Turvey 1980) and speech production in particular (Saltzman 1986; Saltzman/Kelso 1987; Saltzman/Munhall 1989; Kelso/Tuller 1984) constitute a special instance of 'self-organization' in physical systems. Accordingly, they may be best understood by embedding their investigation in the larger context of the study of self-organizing physical systems. Complex physical systems that are open to the flow of energy from the environment, whether they are living systems or not, develop macroscopic, low dimensional patterned and stable activities that can be modeled as attractors of just a few sorts. Most simply, a physical system can be modeled as a 'point attractor' if, when perturbed, it tends to return to the same final target — much as the vocal tract does if it is perturbed during bilabial closure (e. g. Saltzman/Kelso 1987).

Saltzman and colleagues have shown that many central features of speech production, including adaptive responses to perturbations and consequences of coarticulatory overlap (see Saltzman/Munhall 1989), can be modeled if phonetic gestures are modeled as dynamical systems. On the other side, Tuller/Kelso (1990) have shown that speech production exhibits some of the central characteristic features of dynamical systems (cf. art. 37). Finally, Browman/Goldstein (1986) have developed an "articulatory phonology" whose primitive units, phonetic gestures, are defined by dynamical parameters of the vocal-tract point attractors of Saltzman's articulatory ("task-dynamic") model. Possibly, embedding the investigation of speech production in the context of studies of complex open physical systems generally will help to deepen our understanding of synergies and their achievement of low-dimensional, coordinated actions. In turn, understanding of these physical systems may literally add substance to the linguist's concepts of phonological segments and their features.

5. References

Abbs, J. & Gracco, V. (1984). Control of complex gestures: Orofacial muscle responses to load perturbations of the lip during speech. *Journal of Neurophysiology, 51,* 705—723.

Barry, W. & Kuenzel, H. (1975). Coarticulatory airflow characteristics of intervocalic voiceless plosives. *Journal of Phonetics, 3,* 263—282.

Bell-Berti, F. (1980). Velopharyngeal function: A spatio-temporal model. In N. Lass (Ed.), *Speech and language: Advances in basic research and practice. 291—316.* New York: Academic Press.

Bell-Berti, & F. Harris, K. (1979). Anticipatory coarticulation: Some implications from a study of lip rounding. *Journal of the Acoustical Society of America, 65,* 1268—1270.

Bell-Berti, F. & Harris, K. (1981). A temporal model of speech production. *Phonetica, 38,* 9—20.

Bell-Berti, F. & Harris, K. (1982). Temporal patterns of coarticulation: lip rounding. *Journal of the Acoustical Society of America, 71,* 449—454.

Bell-Berti, F. & Krakow, R. (1991). Anticipatory velar lowering: a coproduction account. *Journal of the Acoustical Society of America, 90,* 112—123.

Benguerel, A. & Cowan, H. (1974). Coarticulation of upper lip protrusion in French. *Phonetica, 30,* 41—55.

Bladon, A. & Al-Bamerni, A. (1976). Coarticulation resistance in English /l/. *Journal of Phonetics, 4,* 137—150.

Bladon, A. & Al-Bamerni, A. (1982). One-stage and two-stage temporal patterns of coarticulation. *Journal of the Acoustical Society of America, 72,* 104.

Boyce, S. (1988). *The influence of phonological structure on articulatory organization in Turkish and English: Vowel harmony and coarticulation.* PhD dissertation, Yale University.

Boyce, S., Krakow, R., Bell-Berti, F., & Gelfer, C. (1990). Converging sources of evidence for dissecting articulatory movements into gestures. *Journal of Phonetics, 18,* 173–188.

Browman, C. & Goldstein, L. (1986). Towards an articulatory phonology. In C. Ewan & J. Anderson (Eds.), *Phonology yearbook 3. 219–252.* Cambridge: Cambridge University Press.

Browman, C. & Goldstein, L. (1989). Articulatory gestures as phonological units. *Phonology, 6,* 201–252.

Butcher, A. & Weiher, E. (1976). An electropalatographic investigation of coarticulation in VCV sequences. *Journal of Phonetics, 4,* 59–74.

Carney, P. & Moll, K. (1971). A cinefluorographic investigation of fricative consonant-vowel coarticulation. *Phonetica, 23,* 192–202.

Chomsky, N. & Halle, M. (1968). *The sound pattern of English.* New York: Harper and Row.

Daniloff, R. Hammarberg, R. (1973). On defining coarticulation. *Journal of Phonetics, 1,* 239–248.

Daniloff, R. & Moll, K. (1968). Coarticulation of lip rounding. *Journal of Speech and Hearing Research, 11,* 707–721.

Delattre, P. & Freeman, D. (1968). A dialect study of American rs by X-ray motion picture. *Linguistics, 44,* 29–68.

Fant, G. & Lindblom, B. (1961). Studies of minimal speech and sound units. *Speech Transmission Laboratory: Quarterly Progress Report, 2,* 1–21.

Farnetani, E. (1990). V-C-V lingual coarticulation and its spatiotemporal domain. In W. J. Hardcastle & A. Marchal (Eds.), *Speech production and speech modeling. 93–130.* The Netherlands: Kluwer.

Farnetani, E., Vagges, K., & Magno-Caldognetto, E. (1985). Coarticulation in Italian /VtV/ sequences: A palatographic study. *Phonetica, 42,* 78–99.

Fowler, C., Rubin, P., Remez, R., & Turvey, M. (1980). Implications for speech production of a general theory of action. In B. Butterworth (Ed.), *Langage production I: Speech and talk. 373–420.* London: Academic Press.

Fowler, C. & Smith, M. (1986). Speech perception as "vector analysis": An approach to the problems of segmentation and invariance. In J. Perkell & D. Klatt (Eds.), *Invariance and variability of speech processes. 123–136.* Hillsdale, N. J.: Lawrence Erlbaum Associates.

Fowler, C. A. (1977). *Timing control in speech production.* Bloomington, Indiana: Indiana University Linguistics Club.

Fowler, C. A. (1990). Comments on the contributions by Pierrehumbert and Nearey. *Journal of Phonetics, 18,* 425–434.

Gelfer, C., Bell-Berti, F., & Harris, K. (1989). Determining the extent of coarticulation: Effects of experimental design. *Journal of the Acoustical Society of America, 86,* 2443–2445.

Gentner, D. (1987). Timing of skilled motor performance: Tests of the proportional duration model. *Psychological Review, 94,* 255–276.

Henke, W. (1966). *Dynamic articulatory models of speech production using computer simulation.* PhD dissertation, MIT.

Keating, P. (1988). Underspecification in phonetics. *Phonology, 5,* 275–292.

Keating, P. (1990). The window model of coarticulation: articulatory evidence. In J. Kingston & M. Beckman (Eds.), *Papers in laboratory phonology I. 451–470.* Cambridge: Cambridge University Press.

Kelso, J. A. S. & Tuller, B. (1984). Converging evidence in support of common dynamic principles for speech and movement control. *American Journal of Physiology, 246,* R982–R935.

Kelso, J. A. S., Tuller, B., Vatikiotis-Bateson, E., & Fowler, C. A. (1984). Functionally-specific articulatory cooperation following jaw perturbation during speech: Evidence for coordinative structures. *Journal of Experimental Psychology: Human Perception and Performance, 10,* 812–832.

Kent, R. & Minifie, F. (1977). Coarticulation in recent speech production models. *Journal of Phonetics, 5,* 115–144.

Klatt, D. (1973). Vowel-lengthening is syntactically determined. *Journal of Phonetics, 3,* 129–140.

Kozhevnikov, V. A. & Chistovich, L. A. (1965). *Speech: Articulation and Perception* (30, 543). Washington D. C.: Joint Publications Research Service.

Krakow, R. (1989). *The articulatory organization of syllables: A kinematic analysis of labial and velar gestures.* PhD, Yale University.

Kugler, P., Kelso, J. A. S., & Turvey, M. (1980). On the concept of coordinative structures as dissipative structures, I. Theoretical lines of convergence. In G. Stelmach & J. Requin (Eds.), *Tutorials in motor behavior. 3–47.* Amsterdam: North Holland.

Kugler, P. & Turvey, M. (1987). *Information, natural law and the self-assembly of rhythmic movement.* Hillsdale, N. J.: Lawrence Erlbaum Associates.

Leidner, D. (1973). *An electromyographic and acoustic study of American English liquids.* PhD, University of Connecticut.

Löfqvist, A. (1980). Interarticulator programming in stop production. *Journal of Phonetics, 8,* 475–490.

Löfqvist, A. (1990). Speech as audible gestures. In W. J. Hardcastle & A. Marchal (Eds.), *Speech production and speech modeling. 289–332.* The Netherlands: Kluwer.

Löfqvist, A. & Yoshioka, H. (1984). Intrasegmental timing: Laryngeal-oral coordination in vowel-consonant production. *Speech Communication, 3,* 279–289.

Magen, H. S. (1989). *An acoustic study of vowel-to-vowel coarticulation in English.* PhD dissertation, Yale University.

Manuel, S. (1987). *Acoustical and perceptual consequences of vowel-to-vowel coarticulation in three Bantu languages*. PhD dissertation, Yale University.

Manuel, S. & Krakow, R. (1984). Universal and language particular aspects of vowel-to-vowel coarticulation. *Haskins Laboratories Status Reports on Speech Research, SR-77/78*, 69–87.

Marchal, A. (1988). Coproduction: Evidence from EPG data. *Speech Communication, 7*, 287–295.

Moll, K. (1962). Velopharyngeal closure in vowels. *Journal of Speech and Hearing Research, 36*, 30–77.

Moll, K. & Daniloff, R. (1971). Investigation of the timing of velar movements during speech. *Journal of the Acoustical Society of America, 50*, 678–684.

Munhall, K., Löfqvist, A., & Kelso, J. A. S. (1988). Lip-larynx coordination in speech: A perturbation study. *Journal of the Acoustical Society of America, 80*, S109.

Öhman, S. (1966). Coarticulation in V C V utterances: Spectrographic measurements. *Journal of the Acoustical Society of America, 39*, 151–168.

Öhman, S. (1967). Peripheral motor commands in labial articulation. *Speech Transmission Laboratory: Quarterly Progress Report, 4*, 30–63.

Perkell, J. (1969). *Physiology of speech production: Results and implications of a quantitative cineradiographic study*. Cambridge, MA: MIT Press.

Peterson, G. & Lehiste, I. (1960). Duration of syllable nuclei. *Journal of the Acoustical Society of America, 32*, 693–703.

Pierrehumbert, J. (1990). Phonological and phonetic representations. *Journal of Phonetics, 18*, 315–394.

Recasens, D. (1984). V-to-C coarticulation in Catalan V C V sequences: An articulatory and acoustical study. *Journal of Phonetics, 12*, 61–73.

Recasens, D. (1985). Coarticulatory patterns and degrees of coarticulation resistance in Catalan C V sequences. *Language and Speech, 28*, 97–114.

Recasens, D. (1987). An acoustic analysis of V-to-C and V-to-V coarticulatory effects in Catalan and Spanish V C V sequences. *Journal of Phonetics, 15*, 299–312.

Recasens, D. (1989). Long range coarticulatory effects for tongue dorsum contact in V C V C V sequences. *Speech Communication, 8*, 293–301.

Repp, B. (1981). On levels of description is speech research. *Journal of the Acoustical Society of America, 69*, 1462–1464.

Saltzman, E. (1986). Task dynamic coordination of the speech articulators. In H. Heuer & C. Fromm (Eds.), *Generation and modeling of action patterns. 129–144.* New York: Springer-Verlag.

Saltzman, E. & Kelso, J. A. S. (1987). Skilled action: A task-dynamic approach. *Psychological Review, 94*, 84–106.

Saltzman, E. & Munhall, K. (1989). A dynamical approach to gestural patterning in speech production. *Ecological Psychology, 1*, 333–382.

Shaiman, S. (1989). Kinematic and electromyographic respones to perturbation of the jaw. *Journal of the Acoustical Society of America, 86*, 78–88.

Tuller, B. & Kelso, J. A. S. (1990). Phase transitions in speech production and their perceptual consequences. In M. Jeannerod (Ed.), *Attention and Performance VXII. 429–452.* Hillsdale, N. J.: Lawrence Erlbaum Associates.

Carol A. Fowler, Hanover, New Hampshire (USA)

4. Characteristics of Hesitation Phenomena

1. The Hesitant Nature of Speech

Normal spontaneous speech is not as smooth flowing as it might seem. Rather, it is characterized by hesitations which listeners filter out. These hesitations can take the form of silent pauses, filled pauses, such as *um* and *ah*, false starts, repetitions, or syllable lengthening. Excluding silent pauses that are so short that they could simply be a normal part of the articulation of certain sounds, it would be quite normal, for example, to find that in spontaneous speech a speaker produced a silent pause before 65% of the sentences uttered and a filled pause before 25%. Further, it would be quite normal for over 20% of clauses within the sentences to be preceded by a silent pause and for over 4% to be preceded by a filled pause. Pausing before words within clauses is less frequent, but is still perhaps more frequent than we realize – about 10% of words within clauses may be preceded by a silent pause and about 2% may be preceded by a filled pause. Apart from the frequency of pausing, the average length of the silent pauses that occur is probably surprising. Thus, the average length of the silent pauses before sentences within spontaneous speech may be over one and a half seconds. Before clauses within sentences the average length may be about one second and even before words within clauses the average length of the pauses that occur would be about 800 milliseconds. Along with all this pausing, there will be many false starts and repetitions, as well as syllable lengthening.

The degree of hesitation that characterizes normal spontaneous speech does not characterize reading or prepared speeches. This suggests that the marked degree of hesitation in spontaneous situations is probably due in large part to the major difference between the spontaneous situation and the prepared one. The difference is that what is said must be planned during the spontaneous speaking situation, but not in the prepared situations. It is thus usually assumed that hesitation in spontaneous speech is to a large extent a reflection of the mental processes of speech planning and that the analysis of hesitation phenomena will shed light on such processes. Since the early 50's, psycholinguists interested in production processes have sought to analyse the occurrence of hesitations in the hope of determining what mental processes are important in speech production and what unit or units of speech serve as planning units.

2. Planning Units

2.1. Transitional Probabilities

The earliest studies of hesitation phenomena in production were influenced greatly by the work of Lounsbury (1954), who was the first to discuss the possible use of hesitation pauses in testing hypotheses about encoding units. Drawing on Lounsbury's ideas, Goldman-Eisler (1958) investigated the status of the word as a possible encoding unit. She claimed from her data that words that were preceded by a pause had, on average, low transition probabilities, in that they were not very predictable. She concluded that pauses occur when speakers are selecting what word to say and, moreover, that once an utterance is begun only lexical decisions are made.

Maclay/Osgood (1959) also drew on Lounsbury's (1954) ideas. They compared pausing before content and function words, making the assumption that the former would have a lower transition probability and should therefore be preceded more often by pausing. The prediction was supported. Maclay/Osgood suggested that the results showed that the selection of a word is an important speech process. However, they also noted that when false starts in the speech were corrected, the correction typically involved not simply the unintended word, but also the function words associated with it. They thus suggested that the encoding unit is phrase-like, something like a key lexical item and its "tightly bound grammatical context" (Maclay/Osgood 1959, 41).

2.2. Sentences and Clauses

The works of Goldman-Eisler (1958) and Maclay/Osgood (1959) were somewhat naive methodologically and linguistically and have been strongly criticized (Boomer 1970; Rochester 1973). However, they were among the first studies relating hesitations and mental processing in speech production and they certainly were influential in sparking more research. Much of the subsequent work, though, is based on the conviction that the major planning unit of speech is likely to be larger than a word and probably one that can be defined linguistically. Boomer (1965) investigated the phonemic clause, which is a phonologically defined stretch of speech. Hawkins (1971) investigated the surface structure clause, a syntactically defined speech unit containing a finite (tensed) verb and its subject and predicate. Both Boomer and Hawkins found that the majority of pauses occurred either before or after the first word of the clause unit they studied, even though these clause units were defined on different bases. In fact, though, the phonological basis of the phonemic clause has been the subject of some dispute (Lieberman 1965; O'Connell/Slaymaker 1984) and many believe that the so-called phonemic clause often corresponds to the surface structure clause (Fodor/Bever/Garrett 1974). The work of Boomer and Hawkins does suggest that some unit larger than the word is important in speech planning. Unfortunately, though, in neither study do the initial boundaries of the clause units have an unambiguous interpretation, since the boundaries could have also been boundaries of other units, such as sentences. Goldman-Eisler (1972) appears to be the first of the production researchers to see that it might be important to characterize boundaries more carefully. In aiming to investigate the "psychological reality" of different linguistic units, Goldman-Eisler distinguished sentence boundaries from within-sentence clause boundaries. She found that there was more frequent and longer pausing at sentence boundaries than at within-sentence clause boundaries. Her primary conclusion from this was that speakers organize their messages in "highly cohesive sentence units" (Goldman-Eisler 1972, 110). However, she also found that the frequency and length of pausing were greater before the within-sentence clauses than before words within clauses. This suggests that the surface clause might indeed be an important unit in speech production, though Goldman-Eisler never noted this.

With even more care being taken to characterize boundaries unambiguously, later researchers have found that a unit often coextensive with the surface clause but sometimes smaller is of primary importance (Ford 1978; Ford 1982). Apart from surface structure clauses, one can identify clauses whose verb is non-finite or perhaps only implied. Thus, consider the sentence */(While we were on holidays)/(we liked/ to get up late/and take our time/ getting ready)/(before we went out/looking at the ruins/and all the other touristy things)/*. The sentence contains three finite (surface structure) clauses, indicated by parentheses, but it contains eight verbal units (basic clauses), indicated by slashes. Ford (1978; 1982) noted that since finite clause boundaries are always also basic clause boundaries, the findings from earlier research could result if it was in fact the basic clause that was important in speech production. Indeed, the work of Ford, examining silent and filled pausing in spontaneous speech, indicates that this is so. She found significant hesitation at basic clause boundaries regardless of whether or not the boundary was also a finite clause boundary. The two types of boundaries were indistinguishable in terms of pause rate and length. Moreover, it was found that the number of basic clauses within a finite clause had no effect on the amount of hesitation at the beginning of the finite clause. In short, no evidence of special status could be found for the finite clause. It is the basic clause boundaries that are of paramount importance for hesitations during sentences. Ford also examined sentence boundaries and found even more and longer hesitations there. Clearly, sentences have an important status, but for the production of these sentences it appears that it is the basic clause that is primary.

Holmes (1988) has observed the same pattern of hesitancy as Ford (1978; 1982) in spontaneous speech. Moreover, Holmes found that the same pattern does not hold for hesitations during reading aloud. For reading, she found very little pausing at basic clause boundaries that were not also finite clause boundaries. Pausing did occur at certain finite clause boundaries and these, she suggested, might have a listener and/or breathing function.

3. The Influence of Syntax

The basic clause is a syntactic unit, but it could also be considered a semantic unit, being essentially a simple propositional unit. One question that is of great interest is whether speakers make any syntactic decisions when they plan speech. The earliest studies attempted to see whether hesitations increased with syntactic complexity. Their methods of determining syntactic complexity were somewhat crude. Goldman-Eisler/Skarbek/Henderson (1965), Cook/Smith/Lalljee (1974), and Rochester/Gill (1973) used a global measure of the syntactic complexity of speech such as the Subordination Index, which is the percentage of all clauses which are subordinate clauses. In none of these studies was a relationship found between syntactic complexity and hesitations such as pausing, repetitions, stutters, and corrections. Taylor (1969), using measures of syntactic complexity based on Chomsky's (1957) transformational grammar and also on an immediate constituent analysis, failed to find a relationship between sentence initiation times and syntactic complexity. Goldman-Eisler/Skarbek/Henderson and Taylor concluded that the syntactic structure of sentences is automatically produced by speakers, the structuring being a matter of skill rather than of planning. Cook/Smith/Lalljee suggested that a global measure of complexity like the Subordination Index might not be appropriate to examine the possible effect of syntax on production. They suggested that a measure of individual clause complexity might be better. They did go on to find that pauses occurred more often before clauses that they considered syntactically more complex, but their measure of complexity was simply the number of words in a clause. Like Cook/Smith/Lalljee, Rochester/Gill also felt they should use a less global measure of complexity. They examined the degree of hesitation for sentences of different structure. They found that there were more hesitations at complement clause boundaries than at the boundaries of superficially similar relative clauses. The findings were seen as suggesting that syntactic structure influences the difficulty of speech production and thus that syntactic operations are an important part of speech processes. However, doubt is cast on this interpretation of the findings both by later studies and by Goldman-Eisler's (1972) findings. Goldman-Eisler found that relative clauses were preceded less often by pauses than were "other" subordinate clauses, but she also found that coordinate clauses were preceded even more often by pauses than were these subordinate clauses. Thus, it was coordinate clauses, which would be the simplest syntactically, that were the most likely to be preceded by a pause. Ford (1978) pointed out that the results suggest that pausing might not be a valid index of planning difficulty. She went on to examine pausing before and during clauses of different syntactic types. She found that all clause types had significant levels of pausing before and after the initial word, but that the pausing was the most frequent towards the beginning of coordinate clauses. She found, too, that the degree of pausing towards the beginning of the different clause types was influenced by the presence or absence of a conjunction, such as *but, which, that, to, while,* etcetera, with the patterning being different for each of the different structures studied. In a later study, Holmes (1988) found similar pausing patterns to Ford. Ford (1978) has suggested that the occurrence of hesitations might be dependent on the degree to which what has just been said is a complete linguistic unit, with longer and more frequent hesitations occurring before the least integrated clauses. The finding that hesitations do not increase with syntactic complexity does not mean, though, that speakers do not make syntactic decisions. In fact, studies that use secondary tasks such as 'click' perception and tracking to measure fluctuations in processing load (Ford/Holmes 1978; Ford 1978; Power 1986) have shown that processing is increased during syntactically more complex structures. The pattern of results found in the studies examining hesitations and different syntactic structures simply means that the level of hesitation that occurs cannot be attributable to complexity of syntactic planning, but must be attributable to something else, such as the degree of linguistic integration between clauses.

4. The Influence of Content

Like some of the researchers looking at hesitations and syntactic structure, the researchers interested in the influence of content on hesitations tend to assume that any increase in hesitation might be attributable to an increase in planning difficulty. Thus, the studies typically compare hesitation rates in speech which is assumed to be simple in content with rates in speech assumed to be more difficult in content. Goldman-Eisler (1961) compared pausing in speech for tasks requiring either cartoon description or interpretation. She found that proportionately more time was spent in pausing during interpretations, which she assumed would contain more difficult content than would descriptions. This result was also obtained by Goldman-Eisler/Skarbek/Henderson (1965). The findings were seen as supporting the idea that content decisions require some effort and thus some pausing. Several studies by other researchers have essentially replicated the findings (Levin/Silverman/Ford 1967; Reynolds/Paivio 1968; Taylor 1969; Siegman 1979), though at least one study obtained results which were the reverse of these studies (Rochester/Thurston/Rupp 1977). Unfortunately, the studies do not make a clear distinction between two potential causes of the pausing. It could be that speakers pause when they find it difficult to formulate very complex ideas into words (irrespective of the structures they might use). Alternatively, it could be that speakers have no views or knowledge about certain difficult topics and therefore pause because they have nothing substantial to say. Considering the emphasis Goldman-Eisler and her colleagues put on the generation of information during pausing, they seem to have had the first reason in mind. However, it is quite possible that the amount of pausing in the tasks was dependent on the second reason. In Taylor's (1969) study, for example, in which subjects were given words of different frequencies to use in sentences, it was found that some of the infrequent words were so infrequent that often subjects could not produce a sentence containing them. In the study by Levin/Silverman/Ford (1967), where comparisons were made of children's speech during descriptions and explanations, it was unexpectedly found that the children's spontaneous explanations of phenomena were less hesitant than explanations given on request. Ford (1978) has suggested that these findings add weight to the idea that pause rates in some of these studies might be dependent on whether or not speakers have anything to say. A similar suggestion has been made by Rosenberg (1977). He suggested that results might be contingent not on the difficulty of semantic planning but on the time taken to encode the input material. Remember, too, the finding from the studies of the influence of syntax on hesitations, that coordinated clauses are preceded by a pause the most often. Coordinated clauses are not only the simplest kind of clause, syntactically, but there is also no reason for believing that they are semantically complex. It seems that the rate of pausing may not be a valid index of the complexity of either the syntactic or semantic planning for the following clause.

5. Cognitive Rhythms

While much of the emphasis in investigations of hesitations has been at the clausal level, some research has focussed on larger, nonlinguistically defined units. Henderson/Goldman-Eisler/Skarbek (1966) reported that they found cycles, substantially longer than typical clauses or sentences, where periods of hesitant speech containing short utterances and long pauses alternated with periods of fluent speech containing long utterances and short pauses. They also found that the longer the total pause time during a hesitant period the longer the speech time during the succeeding fluent period. It was argued that the hesitant periods were for planning and that the fluent periods were the outcome of the planning, with each pair of hesitant and fluent periods being based on a cognitive rhythm – a rhythm of successive occurrence and decline of cognitive activity. The interpretation of the data was seriously criticized soon after it was reported. Schwartz/Jaffe (1968) and Jaffe/Breskin/Gerstman (1972) have shown that randomly generated sequences representing sound and silence durations show the same pattern as the reported hesitant/fluent cycles in speech. Butterworth (1975) aimed to show that the pattern of pausing is not random. He proposed that the cycles might correspond to "idea units". He presented subjects with transcripts of spontaneous speech containing hesitant/fluent cycles and asked them to divide the speech into "ideas". He claimed some success in showing a relationship between the cycles and idea units. Greene/Capella (1986) also claimed to find a relationship between cycles and ideational units. Beattie (1979; 1983) found that the incidence of gaze aversion during conversation, which is assumed to be related to increased cognitive planning (Nielsen 1962; Exline/Winters 1965; Kendon 1967), differed in the hesitant and fluent phases of cycles, with speakers averting their gaze at clause juncture pauses more often in hesitant phases than in fluent phases. Beattie (1983) suggested a model where speech is generated on a clause-by-clause basis during hesitant cycles whilst some suprasentential, probably semantic, plan is being generated for the next run of clauses, which will then be uttered relatively fluently. He suggested that considering the demands of conversation, the model would seem intuitively reasonable, with its flexibility allowing speakers to be coherent without losing the conversational floor. Butterworth/Goldman-Eisler (1979), in their study, found that speech related gestures are also differentially distributed during the hesitant and the fluent phases of cycles, again suggesting that the cycles might have some reality. Despite findings like these, though, the existence of cycles of cognitive rhythm is still controversial. Power (1983) claimed that in his studies of spontaneous speech there was no evidence of any cognitive rhythms. Further, he suggested that biased selections of speech were used in studies showing cognitive rhythm and that Butterworth/Goldman-Eisler's (1979) claim that rhythms are correlated with other variables should be treated with extreme caution since the rhythms are not typical of speech. Kowal/O'Connell (1985) argued that the empirical evidence for cognitive rhythms is based on an extremely small corpus, and, moreover, one that has not been described adequately. They also criticized the fact that the identification of phases of cognitive rhythm is subjective. Even Beattie (1984) admits that cognitive rhythms are nebulous and have depended on subjective judgement. Butterworth/Goldman-Eisler (1979), too, admit that their corpus was confined to samples clearly showing cognitive rhythm, suggesting that other samples do not show the rhythm. More research is required to settle the dispute. Speech may be planned at some level in idea units, but it is not certain whether such planning affects hesitation patterns in speech.

6. Implications for the Study of Language Pathology

It is obvious that much more work needs to be carried out on the pattern of hesitancy in speech. However, some progress has been made. First, it is clear that hesitations are quite typical in normal speech. Second, sentence boundaries are important locations of hesitations and, within sentences, basic clause boundaries are important. Third, while the incidence of hesitation does not increase with syntactic complexity, the incidence of hesitation is influenced by syntactic structure, with more pausing occurring before clauses that are less integrated with the preceding clause. It may be, too, that at least sometimes in speech, cycles of hesitancy alternating with fluency may be found and that these might relate to idea units. One challenge now is to use what is known about hesitancy patterns in normal speech as a background for the functional interpretation of language pathologies, since these pathologies may lead to pathological hesitations. Horner (1987) has noted that in studies of expressive language disorders, reference to fluency in normal speakers is absent, with a few exceptions (Buckingham/Kertesz 1974; Butterworth 1979; Golper/Thorpe/Tompkins et al. 1980; Yorkston/Beukelman 1980). She has also noted that a broad fluent versus nonfluent dichotomy is not always helpful to clinicians. It may be that by using what is known about hesitation patterns in normal speech as a background for the study of language pathologies, a greater understanding of these pathologies may be gained.

7. References

Beattie, G. W. (1979). Planning units in spontaneous speech: Some evidence from hesitation in speech and speaker gaze direction in conversation. *Linguistics, 17,* 61–78.

Beattie, G. W. (1983). *Talk: An analysis of speech and non-verbal behaviour in conversation.* Milton-Keyes: Open University Press.

Beattie, G. W. (1984). "Are there cognitive rhythms in speech?" – A reply to Power (1983). *Language and Speech, 27,* 193–195.

Boomer, D. S. (1965). Hesitation and grammatical encoding. *Language and Speech, 8,* 148–158.

Boomer, D. S. (1970). Review of F. Goldman-Eisler, Psycholinguistics: Experiments in spontaneous speech. *Lingua, 25,* 152–164.

Buckingham, H. W. & Kertesz, A. (1974). A linguistic analysis of fluent aphasia. *Brain and Language, 1,* 43–62.

Butterworth, B. (1975). Hesitation and semantic planning in speech. *Journal of Psycholinguistic Research, 4,* 75–87.

Butterworth, B. (1979). Hesitation and the production of verbal paraphasias and neologisms in jargon aphasia. *Brain and Language, 8,* 133–161.

Butterworth, B. & Goldman-Eisler, F. (1979). Recent studies on cognitive rhythm. In A. Siegman & S. Feldstein (Eds.), *Of speech and time: Temporal speech patterns in interpersonal contexts. 211–224.* Hillsdale, New Jersey: Lawrence Erlbaum Associates.

Chomsky, N. (1957). *Syntactic structures.* The Hague: Mouton.

Cook, M., Smith, J., & Lalljee, M. G. (1974). Filled pauses and syntactic complexity. *Language and Speech, 17,* 11–16.

Exline, R. V. & Winters, L. C. (1965). *Effects of cognitive difficulties and cognitive style upon eye contact in interviews.* Paper read at Eastern Psychological Association Meeting, 319–350.

Fodor, J. A., Bever, T. G., & Garrett, M. F. (1974). *The psychology of language: An introduction to psycholinguistics and generative grammar.* New York: McGraw-Hill.

Ford, M. (1978). *Planning units and syntax in sentence production.* Unpublished dissertation, University of Melbourne.

Ford, M. (1982). Sentence planning units: Implications for the speaker's representation of meaningful relations underlying sentences. In J. Bresnan (Ed.), *The mental representation of grammatical relations. 797–827.* Cambridge, Mass.: MIT Press.

Ford, M. & Holmes, V. M. (1978). Planning units and syntax in sentence production. *Cognition, 6,* 35–53.

Goldman-Eisler, F. (1958). Speech production and the predictability of words in context. *Quarterly Journal of Experimental Psychology, 10,* 96–106.

Goldman-Eisler, F. (1961). Hesitation and information in speech. In C. Cherry (Ed.), *Information theory. 162–174.* London: Butterworth.

Goldman-Eisler, F. (1972). Pauses, clauses, and sentences. *Language and Speech, 15,* 103–113.

Goldman-Eisler, F., Skarbek, A., & Henderson, A. (1965). Cognitive and neurochemical determination of sentence structure. *Language and Speech, 8,* 86–94.

Golper, L., Thorpe, P., Tompkins, C., Marshall, R., & Rau, M. (1980). Connected language sampling: An expanded index of aphasic behavior. In R. H. Brookshire (Ed.), *Clinical aphasiology: Conference proceedings, 10, 174–186.* Minneapolis, MN: BRK Publishers.

Greene, J. O. & Cappella, J. N. (1986). Cognition and talk: The relationship of semantic units to temporal patterns of fluency in spontaneous speech. *Language and Speech, 29,* 141–156.

Hawkins, P. R. (1971). The syntactic location of hesitation pauses. *Language and Speech, 14,* 277–288.

Henderson, A., Goldman-Eisler, F., & Skarbek, A. (1966). Sequential temporal patterns in spontaneous speech. *Language and Speech, 9,* 207–216.

Holmes, V. M. (1988). Hesitations and sentence planning. *Language and Cognitive Processes, 3,* 323–361.

Horner, J. (1987). Pause, planning, and paraphasia in expressive language disorders. *Topics in Language Disorders, 8,* 24–33.

Jaffe, J., Breskin, S., & Gerstman, L. J. (1972). Random generation of apparent speech rhythms. *Language and Speech, 15,* 68–71.

Kendon, A. (1967). Some functions of gaze direction in social interaction. *Acta Psychologica, 26,* 1–47.

Kowal, S. H. & O'Connell, D. C. (1985). Cognitive Rhythms reluctantly revisited. *Language and Speech, 28,* 93–95.

Levin, H., Silverman, I., & Ford, B. L. (1967). Hesitations in children's speech during explanation and description. *Journal of Verbal Learning and Verbal Behavior, 6,* 560–564.

Lieberman, P. (1965). On the acoustic basis of the perception of intonation by linguists. *Word, 21,* 40–54.

Lounsbury, F. G. (1954). Transitional probability, linguistic structure and systems of habit-family hierarchies. In C. E. Osgood & T. A. Sebeok (Eds.), *Psycholinguistics: A survey of theory and research problems. 93–101.* Bloomington: Indiana University Press.

Maclay, H. & Osgood, C. E. (1959). Hesitation phenomena in English speech. *Word, 15,* 19–44.

Nielsen, G. (1962). *Studies in self confrontation.* Copenhagen: Scandinavian University Books.

O'Connell, D. C. & Slaymaker, F. L. (1984). Evidence for the phonemic clause as an encoding unit. *Language and Communication, 4,* 273–283.

Power, M. J. (1983). Are there cognitive rhythms in speech? *Language and Speech, 26,* 253–261.

Power, M. J. (1986). A technique for measuring processing load during speech production. *Journal of Psycholinguistic Research, 15,* 371–382.

Reynolds, A. & Paivio, A. (1968). Cognitive and emotional determinants of speech. *Canadian Journal of Psychology, 22,* 164–175.

Rochester, S. R. (1973). The significance of pauses in spontaneous speech. *Journal of Psycholinguistic Research, 2,* 51–79.

Rochester, S. R. & Gill, J. (1973). Production of complex sentences in monologues and dialogues. *Journal of Verbal Learning and Verbal Behavior, 12,* 203–210.

Rochester, S. R., Thurston, S., & Rupp, J. (1977). Hesitations as clues to failures in coherence: A study of the thought-disordered speaker. In S. Rosenberg (Ed.), *Sentence production: Developments in research and theory. 65–87.* Hillsdale, New Jersey: Wiley.

Rosenberg, S. (1977). Semantic constraints on sentence production: An experimental approach. In S. Rosenberg (Ed.), *Sentence production: Developments in research and theory. 195–228.* Hillsdale, New Jersey: Wiley.

Schwartz, J. & Jaffe, J. (1968). Markovian prediction of sequential temporal patterns in spontaneous speech. *Language and Speech, 11,* 27–30.

Siegman, A. W. (1979). Cognition and hesitation in speech. In A. W. Siegman & S. Feldstein (Eds.), *Of speech and time: Temporal speech patterns in interpersonal contexts. 151–178.* Hillsdale, New Jersey: Lawrence Erlbaum Associates.

Taylor, I. (1969). Content and structure in sentence production. *Journal of Verbal Learning and Verbal Behavior, 8,* 170–175.

Yorkston, K. M. & Beukelman, D. R. (1980). An analysis of connected speech samples of aphasic and normal speakers. *Journal of Speech and Hearing Disorders, 45,* 27–36.

Marilyn Ford, Nathan, Brisbane, Queensland (Australia)

5. Spontaneous and Evoked Slips of the Tongue

1. Introduction

In the speech of any speaker of any language, regardless of health or age, errors occur at some (generally low) frequency. Such errors (or 'slips of the tongue') are frequently used as a tool to examine the organization of language in the speaker's cognitive system (cf. art. 7). In language pathology, the errors are used as a diagnostic tool to determine what is wrong and what type of treatment should be used. In order to do this, it is necessary to have a detailed classification system for errors, which includes knowledge of the factors that underlie the occurrence of errors.

There are several possible approaches to creating a classification system for errors. First, the exact description of an error is possible only within the context of a particular theory. Each theory categorizes and explains errors in different ways. It would thus be legitimate to take a single theory of language production and present the classification system entailed by that theory. However, a theory-bound classification system is inconvenient. When the theory changes, the classification system may also change, and the researcher must return to the data and reclassify many errors. Further, it is of limited use to researchers who use a different theory of language production which entails a different classification of the errors. A second approach would be to develop a theory-neutral classification system. An error's classification would be based on surface characteristics. Researchers using different models of language production could use the same classification system, but might assume different mechanisms underlying a particular type of error. A change in the theory need not entail a reanalysis of the data, but just a reinterpretation of mechanisms underlying the errors. A theory-neutral classification system is desirable, and I will attempt to present one here. Errors will be classifiable purely in terms of their surface characteristics, with as little contamination by particular theories of language production as possible. I will attempt to employ terminology that does not presuppose a particular underlying mechanism. For example, MacKay (1969) examined errors like in (1):

(1) ... *over training tia- — trials*

The consonant /r/ disappeared from the word *trials* under identity with the /r/ in *training*. MacKay termed the phenomenon motor masking, which presupposes a particular underlying mechanism. Shattuck-Hufnagel (1979) proposes a mechanism that has nothing in common with masking and renames it the trigger effect. Stemberger (1990) renames it repetition loss, which describes the error as the loss of a segment due to repetition of that segment elsewhere; this last term does not pre-judge how the error occurs. Wherever possible, such neutral terminology will be employed.

Where differences of opinion exist about the underlying system, a surface classification allows easy reanalysis. Suppose, for example, that a researcher believes that segment-sized units do not exist in language production, but instead believes that words are composed of syllable-sized units. In that case, the error in (1) would be a substitution of one syllable for another, motivated by sub-syllabic similarities with another syllable. But this is not a problem, since all errors classified as repetition loss errors can be re-categorized in the same way. Similarly, there are many factors that might facilitate the occurrence of an error in the speech of an individual; e.g., phoneme frequency, similarity of meaning or sound, etc. Not all researchers will agree that a particular putative contributing factor actually has any effect. But, if the researcher is aware of all the contributing factors that have been proposed, a decision can be made to ignore some of them.

Lastly, there is some problem with ambiguity. Often, a given surface error could come about for several different reasons. Consider the error in (2).

(2) *They main it the main store.* (*made*)

The error can be analyzed as the anticipation of the phoneme /n/ from the word *main* to replace the phoneme /d/ of the word *made*. However, the resulting mispronunciation makes the two words identical. It is possible that this is not a phoneme error, but rather the anticipation of the later word to replace the earlier word. How should such ambiguous errors be classified? In some sense, it would be best to classify them as ambiguous, and examine them from several possible analyses. In practice, however, researchers generally prefer to classify them in one specific way. That way is usually justified by considering the statistical characteristics of the different types of errors and deciding which would be more appropriate. For example, the two words in (2) belong to different parts of speech (verb vs. adjective); this is common for phoneme errors but rare for word errors (Garrett 1975), so most researchers would prefer to classify this as a sound error. However, such a decision will on occasion be wrong. How much the misclassification of errors affects the quality of an argument depends on what proportion of the data underlying it might be misclassified.

The classification system presented here is based on slips of the tongue by normal adult native speakers of a language. Errors also occur in other populations: adult native speakers with language pathologies, normal and disordered children, and nonnative speakers of a language. The system presented here may also be used with these populations.

2. Definitions and Typologies of Slips of the Tongue

There are a small number of dimensions that are needed to classify speech errors. The dimensions cross-classify almost perfectly; the same range of error types occurs in lexical errors as in phonological errors, though with large quantitative differences. Before discussing the categories, it is necessary to define some terms. (a) The target is what the speaker intended to say. (b) The error is what the speaker actually said. (c) The source is anything in the linguistic context or nonlinguistic environment that contributed whatever nontarget linguistic elements are found in the error; not all errors have sources.

The following dimensions are needed for the classification of speech errors. They characterize what the targets are, and how the errors differ from the targets. The last category (E) is meant to be exemplary only. The researcher can categorize an error as finely (e. g., target /b/ or passive) or as broadly as desired. No more will be said about this dimension.

Table 5.1: Classification Systems

A. Type of error
   1. substitution
   2. addition
   3. loss (deletion)
   4. blend
B. Linguistic Level
   1. semantic
   2. pragmatic
   3. lexical
   4. syntactic
   5. morphological
   6. phonological
   7. motor/phonetic
C. Source
   1. no source/noncontextual (paradigmatic)
   2. environmental (nonlinguistic)
   3. contextual (linguistic) (syntagmatic)
D. Directionality
   1. anticipation AB → BB
   2. perseveration AB → AA
   3. incomplete AB → A –
   4. anticipation/perseveration ABA → AAA
   5. complex
      a. exchange/shift AB → BA
      b. string ABC → AAA/CCC
      c. chain ABC → AAB/BCC
      d. blot-out ABC → BA/CB
      e. bumper-cars AB → CA/BC
      f. neologism
E. Linguistic Unit
   1. phonological unit
      a. phoneme
      b. phonological feature
      c. syllable
      d. stress/prosody
      e. etc.
   2. morpheme
      a. base
      b. prefix
      c. suffix
      d. regularization
      e. etc.
   3. word
      a. open class/closed class
      b. noun, verb, etc.
   4. syntactic unit
      a. phrase structure
      b. transformation
      c. etc.

A. Type of error

The number of things that could logically go wrong is fairly small: the speaker can use the wrong item (substitution, often termed 'replacement'), add extra items (addition), lose items (loss, often termed 'deletion'), or blend two items together (blend). The error item can have no source, or may be identical to an item in the context. All four types of errors can occur at all linguistic levels. A blend at the phonological level, for example, might be a feature error, where target /p/ and source /g/ are combined into error /b/.

There are some special terms that are used for particular subclasses of errors. When one morphological affix substitutes for another, they can belong to different morphological categories; e.g. progressive *-ing* for perfect *-ed*. However, it is often between two morphological patterns representing the same category. The most common error is a 'full' regularization, where the regular pattern substitutes for an irregular one, such as *falled* instead of *fell*. A less common error is a 'partial' regularization, where the regular pattern is added to the irregular one, such as *felled* instead of *fell*. Less common are irregularizations, where an irregular pattern is substituted for or added to a regular one, such as *glew* (or *glewed*) instead of *glowed*. Loss of an inflectional affix in languages where words have at most one affix, as in English, such as *walk* for *walks*, is called a base-form or no-marking error.

Word substitution errors can be of several types: they can resemble the target word (such as *rat*) semantically (e.g. *mouse*), phonologically (e.g. *mat*), or both (e.g. *cat*). Phonologically related substitutions are called malapropisms. If both semantic and phonological similarity is present, it is a mixed error. When one word substitutes for another, whether contextually or noncontextually, the error usually maintains the morphological markings of the target word rather than those of the source word; stranding is leaving behind the affixes of the source word, and accommodation is taking on the affixes of the target word, in the form appropriate for the error word (e.g. so target *decided to eat* becomes error *ate to decide*, not **eated to decide*). (Stranding and accommodation are also true of phonological errors; the error consonant takes on the allophonic characteristics appropriate to the error word, not those of the source word.) MacKay calls most semantically related word substitutions "synonymic intrusions". He notes that the related word can sometimes replace a word elsewhere in the sentence (e.g., *the lid for the top*, in place of *jar*). He terms these "displaced synonymic intrusions". It should be noted that the relationship is not always synonymic, however; the words may be antonyms or from the same semantic field. Two adjacent words in a sentence can be blended together, e.g. *shrig* for *shrimp and egg*. These are called haplology, telescoping, or sequence blend errors.

B. Linguistic level

In practice, an error can be identified as involving a syntactic element (e.g. a phrase structure or transformation), a morphological affix, a word (or base morpheme), a phonological element, or some aspect of motor performance. It is very difficult to spot purely semantic or pragmatic errors; these usually express themselves through incorrect words, morphemes, or syntax, and it is usually difficult to know whether the semantics and pragmatics were well-formed, but an error was made at a lower level, or if the semantics and pragmatics were in error, with appropriate flawless performance at lower levels.

C. Source

Many errors have a source, i.e. some element elsewhere in the linguistic context or nonlinguistic environment that inferes with the target element and in some way modifies what is produced. For example, when one phoneme substitutes for another, most often the error phoneme appears in a nearby word; or the plural suffix *-s* may appear not only on the target noun but also on a modifying adjective. If the element appears elsewhere in what the speaker is saying, whether in the same or a different clause, it is a contextual ('syntagmatic') error. If the error element appears external to the speaker (such as language that the speaker is hearing or reading, or an object or action that the speaker is observing), it is an environmental error. On occasion, the source may be in the speaker's cognitive system external to language, such as nonvocalized thoughts; this may be counted as an environmental error, or the researcher may choose to give it a separate classification (e.g. Freudian error).

Often, the researcher can find no apparent source for an error. In normals, this is most often true for word substitution errors, but is also often true of phonological errors. In aphasic speech, noncontextual ('paradigmatic') errors are relatively more common. Shattuck-Hufnagel (1979) emphasizes that this is a risky type of classification, as it is possible that there is a source that the researcher is overlooking, possibly interference from a related word or something in the environment where the relationship is not transparent enough to spot it with certainty. This category may thus serve as a garbage can in which to place errors with less transparent sources, and it is difficult to prove that errors ever truly lack a source.

D. Directionality

Directionality is a property only of contextual errors. It refers to the temporal relationship between the target and the source. Since spoken language consists of a single linear channel, the only simple relationships are that the source occurred before the target (and was perseverated) or after it (and was anticipated). In some cases, the source is ambiguous, since elements identical to the error both precede and follow the target (as /b/ both precedes and follows /r/ in the phrase *big red bugs*); it is impossible to determine whether the first /b/ is perseverated, or the second /b/ is anticipated, or both. These ambiguous errors are anticipation/perseverations; given the statistical properties of human speech, such ambiguities usually are found only with phonological and motor errors.

Complex errors also occur, in which there is an error at more than one point in the utterance. If the two errors are correlated, it is wrong to treat them as completely independent of each other. It should be stressed that I treat these as complex solely because there are errors at several points. It is possible that some complex error may be the most likely type of error, given the processing mechanisms used in speech production (as Shattuck-Hufnagel (1979), argues for exchanges). There are only two common types of complex error: exchanges and shifts. In exchanges, elements A and B are reversed, i. e. element A substitutes for element B, and vice versa. In shifts, an element is added at one place and lost from its target point. Exchanges and shifts can involve adjacent elements or distant ones; these may show different statistical properties. With adjacent elements, the error is ambiguous: in *atk* for *act*, do /k/ and /t/ substitute for one another, or was the /t/ added in front of the /k/ and lost from its original position? In word errors, it has been suggested that exchange errors involving adjacent words show normal syntactic stress patterns; in shifts, the word's syntactic stress moves with it (Cutler 1980; Stemberger 1985). In phonological errors, shifts may be more likely to violate phonotactic constraints.

Other complex errors are rare, and all may not yet be known. A string error is one in which an element is anticipated or perseverated to several words (e. g., *big bed bat* for *big red cat*). A chain is one in which element A displaces element B, which then displaces element C (e. g. *big bed rat* for *big red cat*). A string or chain can be both anticipatory and perseveratory; e. g. *caff* – *fat cat*, where /k/ is anticipated from *cat* to substitute for the /f/ of *fat*, which then perseverates to replace the /t/ of *fat*. In blot-out errors, an element disappears from its target position and substitutes for a nearby target item; it thus resembles a shift error. Similar errors may also occur combining noncontextual and contextual components. In bumper-cars errors, a noncontextual substitution on target A occurs, and the displaced element then is anticipated or perseverated to substitute for some target B.

Errors can sometimes be ambiguous between simple and complex errors. This happens when the speaker uses self-monitoring to detect that an error has occurred and then stops speaking and corrects the error. When that happens, we do not know what the rest of the utterance would have looked like. Most commonly, the ambiguity is between a simple anticipation and an exchange or shift, where the speaker stops talking before reaching the source; would the source have been correct (anticipation) or incorrect (exchange)? It is also possible that a perseveration might have been a perseveratory string or chain, but the speaker stopped so early that we cannot tell; but strings and chains are so uncommon that this is unlikely. These errors are best termed incompletes, without taking a stand on whether most are exchanges (Shattuck-Hufnagel 1979) or anticipations (Stemberger 1989).

The ultimate complex error has so many things going on that the target word is not even recognizable.

3. Conditioning Factors

There are a number of factors that potentially influence the occurrence of errors in speech. They can be divided into two broad classes: language-internal factors that relate primarily to linguistic representations and processes, and language-external factors that are due to other cognitive or biological factors.

3.1. Language-external Factors

There are a number of potential factors outside of language itself that might condition the occurrence of errors in language production, but few have been studied in any systematic fashion.

Cognitive load has been suggested as a likely factor: the number and difficulty of other tasks that the speaker is doing concurrently with speaking. If the speaker is distracted, few attentional resources can be spared for speech, and it is more likely that speech errors will occur. This is plausible, but has never been systematically studied. It is possible that the results of Warren (1986) that adults make speech errors more often than children could be a confound with this factor, as the adults in the study were teachers overseeing a large number of small children, who were themselves doing one thing at a time. Concurrent cognitive tasks certainly lead to errors. Harley (1984) examined environmental errors, in which something that is being perceived accidentally contaminates speech, suggesting that the functions being performed by different cognitive systems are not being kept apart sufficiently.

Internal thought in general has been suggested as a source of errors. Freud (1904) suggested that suppressed thoughts (often of a sexual nature) could intrude in the language production process and make errors of certain types more likely. Motley and Baars (1979) have shown experimentally that this is possible, and Motley (1985) provides a detailed discussion of the cognitive mechanisms that underlie it, treating it as a type of environmental error.

Rate of speaking affects the error rate: fast speech contains more errors than slow speech (Dell 1985). This may result from the stressing of processing resources, or it may be because the system does not always have enough time to do all the necessary processing, so that premature decisions must be made.

Tiredness, especially fatigue, may increase the rate of speech errors. This has not been studied systematically.

Drunkenness (and being under the influence of drugs) has been suggested as a factor that contributes to speech errors; comedians pretending to be drunk intentionally produce exchange 'errors'. Stemberger/Pisoni/Hathaway (1984) showed experimentally that this is the case, using the SLIPS task.

3.2. Language-internal Factors

Most of the research on factors that contribute to speech errors has been on language-internal factors. The factors relate especially to the way that linguistic elements are represented and to what size chunk is planned out at any given time. The bulk of the factors involve similarity between linguistic units.

With the Parallel Syllable Structure Constraint, errors tend to be between two phonological segments that are in parallel parts of the syllable: both in syllable onsets, both in syllable nuclei, or both in syllable codas. The tendencies for consonants to interact with consonants and for vowels to interact with vowels may derive partly from this factor. It is not an absolute. There can be errors between consonants in different parts of the syllable, and even between consonants and vowels, but they are relatively rare. The Parallel Syllable Structure Constraint holds most strongly in between-word errors; it holds less consistently in within-word errors, (Stemberger 1982 b).

Syllable structure also has an effect in terms of phonotactics, i. e. what constitutes a legal syllable in the language. Phonological errors generally obey the constraints of the language; i. e., violations account for only about 1% of normal errors (Stemberger 1984), and generally no more than 4% of aphasic errors (e. g. Dressler 1988). Errors like *dlorm* for *dorm* and *atk* for *act* occur only infrequently.

Syllable structure may affect how likely the speaker is to make an error on a given phonological element. If the element is closely integrated with another in syllable structure, it may be less likely to be replaced or deleted independently. MacKay (1970) argues that the lower error rate on vowels and syllable-final consonants relative to high-error syllable-initial consonants is due to differences in syllable structure. The vowel and the syllable-final consonant are joined together into the rime, and hence are part of the same unit, while syllable-initial consonants are separate; to have an error on just the vowel or just the syllable-final consonant, the rime would have to be broken apart, which may be less likely. Treiman (1988) suggests that the error rate within the rime (but not between the onset and vowel) may also be related to sonority: more sonorous syllable-final consonants cohere more strongly with the vowel, and that bond is less likely to be broken; most errors occur when the syllable-final consonant is an obstruent, fewer when it is a nasal, and least when it is a liquid or glide. The cohesiveness of subsyllabic units is also seen in blend errors (e. g. MacKay 1972): the switch point between the two target words is usually either at a syllable boundary or, if it is within the syllable, between the onset and rime, much less often between the vowel and coda.

Position in the word is important. Word-initial position is often special in perception (e. g. Cole/Jakimik/Cooper 1979; Stemberger/Elman/Haden 1986). Dell (1986) suggests that the greater error rate on word-initial consonants may come from an average greater activation level for word-initial consonants, which allows competing word-initial consonants to force their way in more efficiently in errors. Shattuck-Hufnagel (1987) also suggests that the effect derives from word position; since most syllable-initial errors are also word-initial and most syllable-final errors are also word-final, it is difficult to tease apart the separate effects of position in the syllable vs. position in the word, but the data suggest that position in the word may be the more important of the two.

There is also a segmental similarity effect: two segments are likely to be involved in an error together partly as a function of how similar they are in terms of phonological features. This has been found repeatedly for both normal and aphasic speech, regardless of the phonological feature system that has been used. For example, /p/ and /k/ differ by one feature (where /p/ has [labial], /k/ has [dorsal]), but /v/ and /k/ differ additionally by [continuant] and [voiced]. There are more errors between /p/ and /k/ than between /v/ and /k/, reflecting the difference in similarity. It has been noted that most errors on vowels involve vowels with similar stress: they are either both stressed or both unstressed.

Segmental similarity is also seen in the Repetition Effect: when a phonological element is repeated in two words in a sentence that are close to each other, that element is more likely to undergo a substitution or loss error. The effect is greatest when an entire phoneme is repeated, but can also been observed when there is a nearby phoneme that differs by only a single feature. The effect has been reported for both normal (MacKay 1969; Shattuck-Hufnagel 1979; Stemberger 1990; 1991a) and aphasic (Lecours/Lhermitte 1969) speech. Lexical similarities are also important in phonological errors, with the Repeated Phoneme Effect: when two words in a sentence contain the same phonemes, it is more likely that there will be substitution, addition, or loss errors elsewhere in the words. The effect seems to depend on an exact match of phonological elements in the two words (in parallel syllable positions); lesser degrees of similarity (such as having vowels that differ by a single feature) do not raise error rates at all (Stemberger 1990). Phonological similarity between two words has also been observed in lexical blend errors. The effect has yet to be reported in child speech errors (Stemberger 1989) or in aphasic speech (Kohn/Smith 1990). This may reflect some deep qualitative difference between these populations and normal adults, but may alternatively reflect a system in which all errors are more likely than in adult speech; if repeated phonemes have exactly the same degree of effect as in normal speech, it might be lost when the error rate increases greatly. Similarity between lexical items may also be important in lexical errors. Dell/Reich (1981) report that contextual word substitution errors involve words that are more similar to each other phonologically than would be expected by change. The interacting words also tend to be of the same part of speech.

Parallel morphological structure (prefix vs. base vs. suffix) has been suggested as a relevant factor conditioning morphological errors (Kean 1978; Stemberger 1983). Prefixes tend to interact with prefixes, suffixes with suffixes, infixes with infixes. Unfortunately, in most European languages, the types of things encoded by prefixes vs. suffixes are very different; data from languages with both prefixal and suffixal inflections would be useful.

Frequency has been implicated as an important factor affecting error rates: there tend to be more errors on low frequency elements than on high frequency elements. The frequency of a lexical item affects lexical errors (Hotopf 1983; Stemberger/MacWhinney 1986), as well as morphological and phonological errors (Stemberger/MacWhinney 1986; Bybee/Slobin 1982; Dell 1991). The frequency of a phonological element affects the rate of phonological errors (Motley/Baars 1975; Levitt/Healy 1985; Stemberger 1991a; 1991b; 1991d). Stemberger (1991d) argues that both type frequency and token frequency are important. Stemberger (1984) suggests that the token and type frequencies of syntactic elements such as phrase structures may play a role in syntactic errors, including telegraphic speech.

Markedness has been suggested as a relevant factor. Jakobson (1943/1968) proposed that marked segments tend to be replaced by unmarked segments in aphasia and child speech.

The Addition Bias also affects errors. In contextual errors, addition errors are far more common than loss errors (Stemberger 1989; 1990; 1991a; Stemberger/Treiman 1986). This holds for contextual phonological errors, involving both entire segments and individual features. In noncontextual errors (phonological, morphological, or lexical), it appears that loss is more prominent (Stemberger 1982b; 1984; 1990).

The distance between two interacting words, as well as whether the words are in the same syntactic phrase, has also been implicated. In phonological errors, the two consonants are usually less than seven words, and seven syllables, apart (Boomer/Laver 1968). Garrett (1980) reports that the two interacting words are usually in the same major syntactic phrase, especially for phonological errors. The two words involved in contextual lexical substitutions are usually within the same clause as well.

One last factor has been implicated for phonological errors: the Lexical Bias. Phonological errors tend to look like real words rather than nonwords (Motley/Baars 1975). This is true in both natural and experimental errors.

Factors that influence error rates may vary in magnitude depending on other things. Dell (1986; 1991) argues that factors are magnified in exchange errors, since the factor has an effect on each part of this complex error type. Berg (1988) and Stemberger (1991b) suggest that the relevant factor is error likelihood: factors have stronger effects on less common error types.

4. Experimental Procedures for Exploring Speech Errors

There are various experimental procedures that can be used for exploring speech errors. All involve setting up a situation in the laboratory where a speaker talks, and exploring the types of errors that occur and their frequencies. Most techniques address a single, highly specific type of error. Not all types of errors are easy to induce experimentally.

One of the major methodological drawbacks to using naturally occurring speech errors is the lack of control. The researcher may be interested in a highly specific aspect of language processing (say, the behavior of the English vowel /oy/ as in *boy*) which turns out to be very infrequent in natural speech. It is not uncommon to search a corpus of 7500 speech errors for errors relevant to a given hypothesis and to find only one or two (or even no) relevant errors. Further, there is no control over other factors that condition error phenomena, and one is forced to estimate how often a given factor would be present. These drawbacks often lead a researcher to conclude that finding any evidence for or against a given hypothesis is not feasible. Use of experimental situations to induce errors allows the researcher to exercise more control. Things which are infrequent in natural speech can be studied more easily. Other factors can be easily controlled. The methodological issues that the use of experimental procedures raise will be addressed below in section 5. The most widely used procedures with normals have focused on phonology and morphology, but a few studies have also examined syntax.

The simplest possible experimental task, and the most natural, would be to supply a speaker with a picture and ask them to describe it. This is standardly employed with disordered populations, where the error rate is so high that a fair number of errors occur even in short passages (e.g., the 'cookie jar picture'; cf. Goodglass/Kaplan 1983). In normals, however, the error rate is too low to be useful, and so something must be done to make the task more difficult and thereby raise the error rate. Levelt (1983) employed a task where words and letters (in different colors), laid out in a complex spatial array, were presented visually to the subject, who then describes the array. The complexity of the arrays leads to errors, primarily in the selection of lexical items. Another simple task would be confrontation naming, where a speaker must give the word for a picture; again, this is too simple for normals. A variation on this theme is to give speakers a definition of a word, and ask them to tell you what the word is; Brown/McNeill (1966) found that speakers sometimes go into a 'tip-of-the-tongue' state, in which partial information about the word is available to the speaker, and describe a set of questions for exploring what that partial information is. These are basically the only procedures used with normals that address primarily lexical errors.

There are several techniques for addressing phonological errors. The two most frequently employed tasks are the SLIPS task and the tongue-twister task.

The SLIPS task (an acronym for 'Spoonerisms from Laboratory-Induced Priming') makes use of priming to bias speakers to mispronounce words. A sample stimulus is provided in (3) (from Motely/Baars 1975).

(3) PRIME *dart board*
PRIME *dark born*
TARGET *barn door*

Pairs of words are presented to subjects, using a computer or tachistoscope. The first two pairs prime the speaker to produce phonemes in one order (here, /d/ in the first word, /b/ in the second order). The target pair reverses the order of the two phonemes (/b/ in the first word, /d/ in the second word). Subjects read these word pairs silently, one after the other, with only a single word pair visible at any given time. At certain points, a cue (either auditory or visual) is presented for the subject to say the last word pair that s/he read (from memory). This cue is used to increase uncertainty about what word pairs will be spoken aloud, so that the speaker may be unprepared to speak, which hopefully increases the error rate. The speaker usually says the word pair correctly, but on some proportion of trials (ranging from under 1% to over 20%, depending on the nature of the error that is being examined), the speaker makes an error, producing one or both consonants in the order in which they were primed, rather than in the actually presented order. Levitt/Healy (1985) found the prodecure to be effective with auditorily presented stimuli, and when the speaker spoke every pair of words. Dell (1984) provided clear evidence that the errors observed in this task are usually pronunciation errors in language production, and not reading errors.

The SLIPS task was originally developed using word-initial singleton consonants. It has also been used with word-initial consonant clusters (addition errors, loss errors, repetition loss errors), vowels, and post-vocalic consonants. It is likely to be effective with whatever type of error is of interest.

The errors in the SLIPS task are usually what is primed, but there are exceptions. First, exchanges are usually primed, but a majority of errors occur on just one of the two words. Second, nonprimed errors elsewhere in the word do occur, but at a much lower rate; Stemberger/Treiman's (1986) Experiment 4 shows that priming increases the error rate about 6 times. Third, priming can sometimes lead to errors of sorts other than those that are being primed. Stemberger and Treiman's Experiment 3 primed for reversal of two consonants, but many addition errors occurred (e. g. target *pump luck* yielded the primed substitution error *Lump luck* and the unprimed addition error *pLump luck* in about equal numbers). Stemberger's (1991d) Experiment 2 primed for reversal of a vowel and a syllabic /r/, but more often obtained addition errors (e. g., *shed curse* yielded *shRed curse*). Exploring the relative rates of several error types given the same priming is itself an interesting use of the task.

A tongue-twister task is also used to explore phonological errors. A subject repeats over and over a target phrase such as *unique New York*, in which several consonants and vowels repeat in different orders. Shattuck-Hufnagel (1983) has found that this technique deviates statistically from naturalistic speech errors in several ways, but that it works more like natural speech if the tongue-twister has normal syntax.

Phonological errors can also be explored using a task similar to the SLIPS task, in which subjects are instructed to say the target word pair aloud, either in the presented order or in the reverse order, depending on which cue is given. Subjects err by saying the words in the wrong order, or by mixing up the order of one or more phonemes. Error rates are generally around 2% – 3%.

Carter/Bradshaw (1984) and Fowler (1987) use a similar task as a language game. Subjects are given a word pair and instructed to reverse some phonological element(s) in the two words, e. g. the word-initial consonants. By seeing what subjects find difficult vs. easy, evidence is obtained about phonological representations.

Treiman (1983) used a blending task to explore phonological representations. She presented subjects with a syllable and a consonant, and instructed them to put them together. Error rates again reveal what is difficult vs. easy for the speaker to do.

Morphological errors have been explored using two tasks. The primary task is morphonaming (MacKay 1976; Bybee/Slobin 1982; Stemberger/MacWhinney 1986). It is a variant of the naming task (i. e. reading a single word aloud as quickly as possible) in which the speaker also manipulates the form of the word: one morphological category is replaced with another. Base forms of verbs have been replaced with past tense forms, progressive forms of verbs have been replaced with past tense or present tense forms, and definite forms of nouns have been replaced by indefinite forms. Subjects are usually correct, but on some trials produce base forms, full regularizations, partial regularizations, and irregularizations. Stemberger/Lewis (1986) combined morphonaming with SLIPS to study the interaction of phonological errors with morphological reduplication in Ewe.

Morphological errors of one type have also been explored using the embedding task (Stemberger, in progress). Speakers are given a sentence with the verb in a certain morphological form (e. g. past tense; *John ate it*), plus a verb in that same form (such as *didn't* or *decided to*). Subjects are instructed to take the second verb and add it to the sentence, making it the main verb of the sentence *(John didn't eat it)*. On some trials, subjects retain the original form of the verb *(John didn't ate it)*, but some verbs are more likely to be involved in such errors than others (esp. irregular verbs and verbs of low frequency).

Chen/Baars (1985) employed a similar task for studying syntactic errors. They presented subjects with two sentences, and cued them to produce one or the other. On some trials, subjects blended the two sentences together, producing errors that resemble naturally occurring syntactic errors. They were also able to cause the order of different nouns in the sentence to reverse, and this task is probably extendable to examine contextual word substitution errors in general.

There is one task that has been developed to examine lexical blend errors (Stemberger 1991c). Subjects are presented with two words visually, one above the other on a computer screen. The words are removed, and a row of arrows is then placed on the screen over the location of one of the words; if it is placed over the lower word, the arrows point up and the speaker must say the upper word; if it is placed over the upper word, the arrows point down and the speaker must say the lower word. On some trials (ca. 4.4%), the speaker says the wrong word. On other trials (ca. 1.5%), the speaker blends the two words together. This is useful for exploring factors that can affect blend errors.

5. Methodological Issues

There are methodological issues about the proper way to study speech error phenomena. These include whether the study is naturalistic or experimental, and how the data are gathered. The main issues for naturalistic error data are reliability and the estimation of chance. The main issue for experimental error data is ecological validity.

When gathering naturalistic error data, the most solid methodology is clearly one in which large amounts of speech are tape-recorded, and then analyzed for the occurrence of errors. This allows the researcher to spot errors under easy conditions (without the need for e. g. taking part in a conversation) and to back up and listen to a passage again to determine whether an error occurred. It also allows acoustic analysis of the error, if desired. Further, the correct speech can be examined to determine chance; for example, if the sample includes 5000 tokens of irregular past tense forms, along with 31 base form errors and regularizations, we know exactly what proportion of the time the speaker was successful when s/he intended to produce a past tense form. Tape-recording also allows a partial control for perceptual biases. By decreasing the processing load on the researcher, the researcher can devote more attention to the detection of errors. The researcher will notice a larger proportion of the errors than would otherwise be possible, and be more likely to notice errors that are less salient to human perceptual processing. Tape-recording speech in this way has drawbacks, however. First, the error rate is low (cf. art. 2). In a sample of ca. 200,000 words, Garnham/Shillcock/Brown et al. (1982) found only 191 errors; this is far too few to be useful in addressing most questions. To obtain the number of errors in many naturalistic corpora (ca. 7000), a sample of 7,000,000 words would be needed. This is too large to be feasible, so tape-recording is usually not done. Anne Cutler (personal communication 1987) did a small project in which she kept a tape-recorder going on a small tape with a one-minute loop of tape in it. Whenever she noticed an error, she would remove the tape and put in another one. This allows the recording of errors without the need to search through a large sample of speech, and allows a check on the researcher's categorization of the error and indeed on whether an error had really occurred, and allows the errors to be examined acoustically, but otherwise has none of the other advantages of tape-recording.

Most naturalistic work is done with pen and paper. The researcher listens to speech, being careful to distinguish normal speech from reading, detects an error just after it is made, and immediately writes it down in a notebook, along with whatever information is deemed appropriate (e. g. name, date, speaker's level of distraction, fatigue, or intoxication, if known). Some errors are missed. Errors that are hard to detect are presumably missed most often. Some people are better at detecting e. g. phonological errors than others. Some errors are detected, but the researcher forgets exactly what the speaker said before being able to write it down. Correct utterances are not recorded. The advantages of this approach are that anyone can do it, just about anywhere, with minimal equipment, and that it samples from a maximally large amount of speech without forcing the researcher to laboriously go through hundreds of hours of tape-recordings.

One drawback is that a lot of faith is being placed in the researcher's ability to detect and remember all types of errors equally. If some errors are easier to spot and remember long enough to record than others, statistical biases are introduced into the data that have more to say about perceptual processing and memory than language production. Although there is no way to directly assess the degree of bias present in any given corpus, there are ways to minimize its impact. First, a single highly trained and highly motivated person can collect all the errors; this at least insures that the same level of care is taken at all times, to the extent possible. Corpora that are collected by a large number of less highly motivated individuals (e. g., the corpus of Dell/Reich 1981) are more likely to contain perceptual biases. Second, when the data is analyzed, any difference between two categories of errors can be examined for whether it is likely to derive from a perceptual bias.

Consider two examples of possible perceptual biases (Cutler 1981; Stemberger 1982 a). (1) Naturalistic error corpora contain more errors on word-initial consonants than on word-final consonants, and perceptual studies have shown that untrained listeners detect errors more easily on word-initial consonants (Cole/Jakimik/Cooper 1979). The asymmetry in the naturalistic errors may be due to a perceptual bias. (2) Naturalistic error corpora find that most errors involve consonants differing by a single feature, and fewer involve consonants differing by two or more features. Error detection studies report that errors are easier to detect if the consonants differ by more than one feature. The observed asymmetry is in the direction o p p o s i t e what would be expected on the basis of perceptual biases, so it is probably a real property of speech production. With any asymmetry, if there is unlikely to be a perceptual bias that could produce the results, then the data may be taken at face value.

Another problem with naturalistic studies is how to determine chance. We cannot know the true error rate (i. e. the proportion of trials of a certain type that were in error) without knowing how many trials were correct. Different error types may differ in how many opportunities they have to occur in a given sample of speech. For example, if /t/ is twice as frequent as /k/, by chance /t/ should be mispronounced twice as often as /k/. Since true chance values are unknown, various imperfect means must be used to estimate chance. An incorrect estimation of chance can lead to spurious conclusions, suggesting that there is a difference where none truly exists, or that there is no difference where one in fact exists.

Another problem with naturalistic error data is that of determining reliability. A reliable study is one that can be replicated, and replication is usually considered to be required in experimental psychology. Naturalistic corpora require so much effort to collect that very few exist, and there are so few researchers that most analyses are done for only a single corpus.

There is a problem with controlling all the variables that might affect error rates. In naturalistic studies, there is no control. In analyses, there is usually little effort to tease out the effects of different variables. This would be very hard to do, in that even 3000 phonological errors is a small sample when separating out the effects of syllable position, similarity between segments, the Repeated Phoneme Effect, the Repetition Effect, phoneme and lexical frequency, distance between target and source (in words and syllables), etc. It is not surprising that no study has tried to control for all known important variables when examining the effects of a new one. Lastly, there is a problem with knowing what factors underlie a given error, especially hard-to-measure factors like those brought up in Freudian analyses. When looking at a given error made by a given subject, there may be so many possible causes that proving that e. g. repressed thoughts were an important component to the error may be next to impossible. At minimum, all other variables would have to be controlled, and a comparison with e. g. a case where repressed thoughts could not be a factor would have to be made, before a case could be made that a given factor is important. In natural speech, ambiguity is too rampant and too many complex variables are present to allow an easy decision about what factors are relevant.

For these reasons, many have turned to experimental studies of error phenomena. Experimental studies allow control of chance and of all variables other than the one of interest (except where natural confounds in the language prevent it from being controlled). They allow for the collection of a large number of relevant errors quickly. Studies can be replicated with different sets of stimuli and in different laboratories. Subjects' utterances are collected under low-noise conditions, analyzed without conflicting demands on attention (so that perceptual biases are less likely, and unclear utterances can be listened to repeatedly, at higher volume levels, with other listeners to judge what was wrong), and analyzed acoustically.

The major drawback to experimental studies is the question of ecological validity. First, there is the potential problem that the results do not reflect normal language production, but special strategies used only in the experimental situation. Significant results, however, will still reveal something about the speaker's language production system, as differences must reflect distinctions that the speaker has access to. However, no differences (null results) are hard to interpret; there may still be a difference, but the task-specific strategies adopted by the subjects obscure it. Note that these are general problems with the interpretation of experimental results, and are not peculiar to error studies. It has been suggested that the Lexical Bias, which is easier to find in experimental studies than in naturalistic studies, may be due to a special strategy used by subjects in e. g. the SLIPS task but not in natural speech. Stemberger (1991b) presents an overview of research with naturalistic and experimental data, and concludes that the results are largely the same with either approach; there are no clear cases of divergent results.

A second drawback is one of generalization. Experimental studies generally use a small sample of the possible relevant words of the language, and it is possible that some quirk of the words chosen might lead to results that would not have been observed if the full set of relevant words from the language had been used. That merely underscores the importance of replicating results.

Particular experimental tasks may have drawbacks of their own. One drawback is relatively low error rates. In the SLIPS task, some consonant contrasts may yield only a 2% error rate. Stemberger (1991b) presents one study where only four stimuli were possible and the error rate was only about 6%; he needed to run 250 subjects to get enough data to analyze. If the researcher has difficulty finding subjects to participate, experimental studies may be difficult to carry out.

Some experimental tasks are simple (such as reading a word pair from memory in SLIPS) and rely on skills that require no metalinguistic knowledge. Other tasks are more complex and may tap into a speaker's conscious knowledge or folk theories about linguistic representations (such as Carter/Bradshaw's (1984) task to reverse parts of the word pairs). The simpler and more ecological the task, the better.

Overall, no one methodology (experimental or naturalistic) is perfect. Interestingly, the strengths and weaknesses of the two approaches are almost complementary; when one has problems, the other does not. Several studies have combined the two approaches, investigating the same issues using both naturalistic and experimental data (e. g. Stemberger/Treiman 1986; Laubstein 1988). Such studies demonstrate replicability, control of extraneous variables, and ecological validity, and may be the most desirable way to proceed, if possible.

6. Conclusions

I have reviewed the types of errors that occur in speech production and presented a classification system for the analysis of such errors, which may be used for normal or disordered adults or children. The classification system is designed to be usable by all researchers regardless of the theory assumed. I have also reviewed the known factors that contribute to the occurrence of errors, both language-internal and language-external (including Freudian slips). I have discussed the methodological issues relative to the collection and interpretation of speech error data, both naturalistic and experimental, and described current experimental methods for investigating errors. It is hoped that this chapter will help to bring more standardization of error analyses to work on normal speech, and will also serve to bridge the gap with work on aphasic speech and language acquisition, by providing a common frame of reference.

7. References

Baars, B. J., Motley, M. T., & MacKay, D. G. (1975). Output editing for lexical status from artificially elicited slips of the tongue. *Journal of Verbal Learning and Verbal Behavior, 14,* 382–391.

Berg, T. (1988). *Die Abbildung des Sprachproduktionsprozesses in einem Aktivationsflussmodell: Untersuchungen an deutschen und englischen Versprechern.* Tübingen: Niemeyer.

Boomer, D. & Laver, J. (1968). Slips of the tongue. In V. Fromkin (Ed.), *Speech errors as linguistic evidence. 120–131.* The Hague: Mouton.

Brown, R. & McNeill, D. (1966). The "tip-of-the-tongue" phenomenon. *Journal of Verbal Learning and Verbal Behavior, 5,* 325–337.

Bybee, J. L. & Slobin, D. I. (1982). Rules and schemas in the development and use of the English past tense. *Language, 58,* 265–289.

Carter, R. & Bradshaw, J. (1984). Producing 'spoonerisms" on demand: Lexical, phonological, and orthographic factors in a new experimental paradigm. *Speech Communication, 3,* 347–360.

Chen, J.-Y. & Baars, B. J. (1985). The competing plans hypothesis as an alternative explanation of some "transformational errors". Presented at the meeting of the Eastern Psychological Association, Boston.

Cole, R. A., Jakimik, J., & Cooper, W. E. (1978). Perceptibility of phonetic features in fluent speech. *Journal of the Acoustical Society of America, 64,* 44–56.

Cutler, A. (1980). Errors of stress and intonation. In V. A. Fromkin (Ed.), *Errors in linguistic performance: Slips of the tongue, ear, Pen, and hand. 67–80.* New York: Academic Press.

Cutler, A. (1981). The reliability of speech error data. *Linguistics, 19,* 561–582.

Dell, G. S. (1984). The representation of serial order in speech: Evidence from the repeated phoneme effect in speech errors. *Journal of Experimental Psychology: Learning, Memory, & Cognition, 10,* 222–233.

Dell, G. S. (1985). Positive feedback in hierarchical connectionist models: Applications to language production. *Cognitive Science, 9,* 3–23.

Dell, G. S. (1986). A spreading activation theory of retrieval in sentence production. *Psychological Review, 93,* 283–321.

Dell, G. S. (1991). Effects of frequency and vocabulary type on phonological speech errors. *Language and Cognitive Processes, 5,* 313–349.

Dell, G. S., & Reich P. A. (1981). Stages in sentence production: An analysis of speech error data. *Journal of Verbal Learning and Verbal Behavior, 20,* 611–629.

Dressler, W. U. (1988). A linguistic classification of phonological paraphasias. In W. U. Dressler & J. Stark (Eds.), *Linguistic analyses of aphasic language. 1–23.* New York: Springer.

Fowler, C. (1987). Consonant-vowel cohesiveness in speech production as revealed by initial and final consonant exchanges. *Speech Communication, 6,* 231–244.

Freud, S. (1904). *Zur Psychopathologie des Alltagslebens.* Frankfurt am Main: Fischer, new ed. 1954.

Garnham, A., Shillcock, R. S., Brown, G. D. A., Mill, A. I. D., & Cutler, A. (1982). Slips of the tongue in the London-Lund corpus of spontaneous conversations. In A. Cutler (Ed.), *Slips of the tongue and language production. 251–264.* Berlin: Mouton.

Garrett, M. F. (1975). The analysis of sentence production. In G. Bower (Ed.), *Psychology of learning and motivation,* vol. 9. *133–177.* New York: Academic Press.

Garrett, M. F. (1980). The limits of accommodation. In V. Fromkin (Ed.), *Errors in linguistic performance: Slips of the tongue, ear, eye, and hand. 263–271.* New York: Academic Press.

Goodglass, H. & Kaplan, E. (1983). *The assessment of aphasia and related disorders. Stimulus cards.* Philadelphia: Lea & Febiger (2nd ed.).

Harley, T. A. (1984). A critique of top-down independent levels models of speech production: Evidence from non-plan internal speech errors. *Cognitive Science, 8,* 191–219.

Hotopf, W. H. N. (1983). Lexical slips of the tongue and pen: What they tell us about language production. In B. Butterworth (Ed.), *Language production, vol. 2. 147–199.* London: Academic Press.

Jakobson, R. (1941/1968). *Child language, aphasia, and phonological universals.* The Hague: Mouton.

Kean, M.-L. (1978). The linguistic interpretation of aphasic syndromes. In E. Walker (Ed.), *Explorations in the biology of language. 67–138.* Montgomery, VT: Bradford Books.

Kohn, S. E. & Smith, K. L. (1990). Between-word speech errors in conduction aphasia. *Cognitive Neuropsychology, 7,* 133–156.

Laubstein, A. S. (1988). Syllable structure: The speech error evidence. *Canadian Journal of Linguistics, 32,* 339–363.

Lecours, A. R. & Lhermitte, F. (1969). Phonemic paraphasias: linguistic structures and tentative hypotheses. *Cortex, 5,* 193–228.

Levelt, W. J. M. (1983). Monitoring and self-repair. *Cognition, 14,* 41–104.

Levitt, A. G. & Healy, A. F. (1985). The roles of phoneme frequency, similarity, and availability in the experimental elicitation of speech errors. *Journal of Memory and Language, 24,* 717–733.

MacKay, D. (1969). Forward and backward masking in motor systems. *Kybernetik, 2,* 57–64.

MacKay, D. G. (1970). Spoonerisms: The structure of errors in the serial order of speech. *Neuropsychologia, 8,* 323–350.

MacKay, D. (1972). The structure of words and syllables: evidence from errors in speech. *Cognitive Psychology, 3,* 210–227.

MacKay, D. G. (1976). On the retrieval and lexical structure of verbs. *Journal of Verbal Learning and Verbal Behavior, 15,* 169–182.

Motley, M. T. (1985). The production of verbal slips and double entendres as clues to the efficiency of normal speech production. *Journal of Language and Social Psychology, 4,* 275–293.

Motley, M. T. & Baars, B. J. (1975). Encoding sensitivities to phonological markedness and transition probability: Evidence from spoonerisms. *Human Communication Research, 2,* 351–361.

Motley, M. T. & Baars, B. J. (1979). Effects of cognitive set upon laboratory induced verbal (Freudian) slips. *Journal of Speech and Hearing Research, 22,* 421–432.

Shattuck-Hufnagel, S. (1979). Speech errors as evidence for a serial ordering mechanism in sentence production. In W. E. Cooper & E. C. T. Walker (Eds.), *Sentence processing. 295–342.* New York: Halsted Press.

Shattuck-Hufnagel, S. (1983). Sublexical units and suprasegmental structure in speech production planning. In P. F. MacNeilage (Ed.), *The production of speech. 109–136.* New York: Springer-Verlag.

Shattuck-Hufnagel, S. (1987). The role of word onset consonants in speech production planning: New evidence from speech error patterns. In E. Keller & M. Gopnik (Eds.), *Motor and sensory processing in language. 17–51.* Hillsdale, N. J.: Lawrence Erlbaum.

Stemberger, J. P. (1982 a). *The lexicon in a model of language production.* Doctoral Dissertation, UCSD. New York: Garland Publishing Inc. 1985.

Stemberger, J. P. (1982 b). The nature of segments in the lexicon: Evidence from speech errors. *Lingua, 56,* 43–67.

Stemberger, J. P. (1983). Inflectional malapropisms: Form-based errors in English morphology. *Linguistics, 21,* 573–602.

Stemberger, J. P. (1984). Structural errors in normal and agrammatic speech. *Cognitive Neuropsychology, 1,* 281–313.

Stemberger, J. P. (1985). An interactive activation model of language production. In: A. W. Ellis (Ed.), *Progress in the psychology of language, vol. 1. 143–186.* London: Lawrence Erlbaum.

Stemberger, J. P. (1989). Speech errors in early child language production. *Journal of Memory and Language, 28,* 164–188.

Stemberger, J. P. (1990). Wordshape errors in language production. *Cognition, 35,* 123–157.

Stemberger, J. P. (1991a). Apparent anti-frequency effects in language production: The Addition Bias and Phonological Underspecification. *Journal of Memory and Language, 30,* 161–185.

Stemberger, J. P. (1991b) Radical underspecification in language production. *Phonology, 8,* 73–112.

Stemberger, J. P. (1991c). Global similarity effects in phonological and morphological processing. Unpublished manuscript, University of Minnesota.

Stemberger, J. P. (1991d). Phonological frequency effects and superpositional memory. Unpublished manuscript, University of Minnesota.

Stemberger, J. P., Elman, J. L., & Haden, P. (1986). Interference between phonemes during phoneme monitoring: Evidence for an interactive activation model of speech perception. *JEP: HP & P, 11,* 475–489.

Stemberger, J. P. & Lewis, M. (1986). Reduplication in Ewe: Morphological accommodation to phonological errors. *Phonology Yearbook, 3,* 151–160.

Stemberger, J. P. & MacWhinney, B. (1986). Frequency and the lexical storage of regularly inflected forms. *Memory and Cognition, 14,* 17–26.

Stemberger, J. P., Pisoni, D. B., & Hathaway, S. N. (1985). Effects of alcohol intoxication on phonological errors in normal speech. *Research on Speech Perception Progress Reports, no. 11.* Bloomington, IN: Speech Research Laboratory, Department of Psychology, Indiana University.

Stemberger, J. P. & Treiman, R. (1986). The internal structure of word-initial consonant clusters. *Journal of Memory and Language, 25,* 163–180.

Treiman, R. (1983). The structure of spoken syllables: Evidence from novel word games. *Cognition, 15,* 49–74.

Treiman, R. (1988). The internal structure of the syllable. In G. Carlson & M. Tanenhaus (Eds.), *Linguistic structure in language processing. 27–52.* Dordrecht, Holland: Kluwer.

Warren, H. (1986). Slips of the tongue in very young children. *Journal of Psycholinguistic Research, 15,* 309–344.

Joseph Paul Stemberger, Minneapolis, Minnesota (USA)

6. Slips of the Pen, Tongue, and Typewriter: A Contrastive Analysis

This article reviews available data on spontaneous and evoked slips of the pen, tongue, and typewriter, and concludes that slips of the pen and typewriter exhibit different regularities from slips of the tongue and reflect different constraints on production. The comparison of these three classes of slips also clarifies some of the similarities and differences in the processes underlying speech, writing and typewriting.

1. Introduction

Speaking, writing, and typing are the main output modalities for expressing language among literate adults. However, speech has received far more scientific attention than typing and writing, and for good reasons. Typing and writing are relatively rare skills that have been recently acquired in our evolutionary history (Ellis 1988 b): No universal genetically-based processes have evolved specifically to represent writing and typing, unlike speech. If acquired at all, lexical and sublexical spelling processes are acquired after language, and are grafted onto semantic and syntactic processes for speech. As a result, patients with high level semantic or syntactic speech impairment invariably exhibit the same impairment in writing and typing (Ellis 1988 b). Finally, because different cultures have invented radically different systems for writing and typing, we cannot be sure *a priori* that orthographic processes do not differ for languages with fundamentally different graphic systems (Ellis 1986 b).

For studying some issues, however, typing offers major advantages over speech. The effect of skill on errors is one such issue: Degree of typing skill can be manipulated in ways not possible for speech. Input stimuli in studies of transcription typing can also be manipulated in ways not possible for speech. With typists instructed to type exactly what appears on a video display, a computer can replace an upcoming letter with another, different letter at some unpredictable time prior to typing. The time when such a change causes errors or disrupts timing indicates when control has passed from input transcription to keystroke execution (Salthouse 1984; 1985; 1986). Finally, typing errors offer technological advantages over speech errors for issues related to timing. Even the best techniques for inducing speech errors cannot measure time of output with the ease and precision routinely possible for computer analyzed keystrokes.

2. Errors: General Considerations

2.1. Units of Analysis in Writing and Typing

Three hierarchically related units of analysis have proven useful in studies of writing and typing: graphemes, allographs, and graphic motor patterns (Ellis 1979). 'Graphemes' correspond to letters of the alphabet, and can be expressed in three ways: as a keystroke in typing, as a letter in writing, or as a letter name in spelling words aloud (Ellis 1988 a). 'Allographs' are the various forms or variants of a grapheme that are accepted within a writing community, e. g., upper vs. lower case, and printed vs. cursive (Pulgram 1951; Gelb 1963). 'Graphic motor patterns' are particular sequences of muscle movements for expressing an allograph and may be unique to a given individual or context of use (van Galen 1980). The main focus of research has been whether graphic motor patterns succeed in depressing their key in typing and how they unfold in handwriting, i. e., the strokes composing a letter, their sequence, direction, relative size, position on a page, relative position on a line, and the muscles involved, e. g., finger muscles for horizontal surfaces and arm muscles for vertical surfaces (van Galen/Smyth/Meulenbroek/Hylkema 1989).

2.2. Errors: Definitional Issues

By general convention, errors are only recorded when the correct form is known and intended: The correct sequence of phonemic or graphemic components exists in memory, but the wrong components are inadvertently activated. This sine qua non aside, the definition of 'error' differs in subtle and largely unacknowledged ways in studies of tongue (cf. art. 5), pen and typing slips. By generally accepted definition, a typing error occurs when an inapproppriate key is depressed sufficiently to allow electrical contact. A key hit hard or long enough to cause repeated electrical contact therefore constitutes an error, and so does an accurate keystroke that is too weak to make electrical contact (Grudin 1983). However, analogous events have never been counted as pen or tongue slips. Collections of pen and tongue slips do not include locally faint, indistinct and awkward penstrokes, or faint, slurred and overly loud speech sounds.

The unique definition of typing error has contributed other, perhaps artificial differences between slips in the three output modalities. For example, most pen and tongue slips involve whole letters or speech sounds (Ellis 1979), but some can only be described as involving subcomponents of a speech sound (Fromkin 1973) or letter (Ellis 1979; 1988 a), e.g., the upstroke for *d* in the anticipatory pen slip, *made* → *mdde*. (Present examples are realistic, but invented, and the arrow in such formuli stands for 'could have been misproduced as'). Although all acts of speaking, writing, and typing can be described as involving a hierarchic organization of such components and subcomponents (MacKay 1987), typing slips can only involve whole letters or keystrokes by prior definition.

2.3. Organization of the Present Chapter

I first describe typing errors, then pen slips: their categories, temporal characteristics, and relation to variables such as experience, and graphemic, allographic, and motoric factors. Error detection and the role of different types of feedback are discussed next. Finally, I examine similarities, differences and gaps in existing research comparing errors in speech, writing and typing.

3. Typing Errors

3.1. Categories of Typing Errors

Studies of typing typically analyze errors into five main categories discussed below.

3.1.1. Substitution Errors in Typing

Videotapes of expert typists indicate that substitution errors (e.g., *type* → *typr*) usually involve adjacent keys, and result from a stroke with the wrong finger to the wrong key rather than from an inappropriate execution or movement trajectory with the correct finger (Grudin 1983). Whole word substitutions also occur (e.g., *perhaps* → *maybe*), but reflect misrepresentation of the input string rather than genuine errors.

The most interesting class of substitution errors, known as homologous intrusions (e.g., *type* → *tyqe*), involves substitution of the mirror-image or anatomically homologous finger and keyboard position on the opposite hand, a phenomenon that exceeds chance expectation (Book 1925; Grudin 1983 a; Munhall/Ostry 1983; Wells 1916). Under the usual interpretation, homologous intrusions result when a keystroke has been specified for the appropriate finger and key, but for the wrong hand (Salthouse 1986). However, studies of experimentally induced homologous intrusions in keying tasks that resemble typing suggest an alternative to this hand misspecification hypothesis. Under this priming hypothesis (MacKay 1971), units representing movements of anatomically homologous fingers are interconnected via the corpus callosum and prime one another prior to activation and actual movement. The priming hypothesis explains the built-in coordination of homologous fingers, and why tasks requiring simultaneous tapping with homologous fingers are performed especially rapidly and accurately. The priming hypothesis is also more general than the hand misspecification hypothesis, explaining additional phenomena such as why fewer homologous intrusions occur in the dominant hand (e.g., the right hand in right-handed subjects), and why instructions to 'pay attention to' one hand reduce the number of homologous intrusions in the attended relative to unattended hand (MacKay 1971). Finally, under the priming hypothesis, homologous intrusions represent a finger movement analog of speech errors known as blends (e.g., *sotally*, a blend of *solely* and *totally*; and *me together*, a blend of *me too*, and *we're together*; MacKay 1973).

3.1.2. Intrusion Errors in Typing

Extremely short interkey intervals follow intrusions (e.g., *type* → *tyupe*), which usually result from imprecise keystrokes: the appropriate finger strikes two keys together or hits a key in passing (Grudin 1983). Repetition intrusions (e.g., *type* → *tyype*) reflect either keyboard bounce or inadequate deactivation of a keystroke (Grudin 1983).

3.1.3. Omission Errors in Typing

Omission errors (e.g., *type* → *tpe*) usually result from strokes that are too weak to fully depress difficult-to-reach keys (e.g., q, b), and usually fall within keystroke intervals about twice the normal duration (Shaffer 1975). Medial letters of a word are more likely to be omitted than initial letters, a phenomenon observed originally in speech errors (MacKay 1969). Interestingly, some keystroke omissions seem to occur because the same letter or type of stroke was recently typed (e.g., *artificial* → *artifical*), as if an inhibitory process follows activation of underlying units, making repetition difficult (Grudin 1983; MacNeilage 1964). This too was observed originally in speech errors (MacKay 1987) and only very recently and elegantly in writing errors (van Galen 1990).

3.1.4. Transposition Errors in Typing

Most transpositions (e.g., *type* → *ytpe*) are cross-hand rather than within-hand, both absolutely and relative to chance, as if a preprogrammed letter upcoming on the other hand is ready to strike its key too early (Salthouse 1984; 1985; 1986). More than this is probably involved, however, because interstroke intervals are virtually identical for correctly sequenced vs. transposed letters: One of the transposed letters does not come especially early and the other especially late (Shaffer 1975; Grudin 1981; 1982). Rather, transposed keys change places in time and sequence, not unlike transposed sounds in speech errors such as *passification* → *fassipication* (MacKay, 1987).

3.1.5. Other Classes of Typing Errors

Four less frequent classes of typing error are migrations (e.g., *type* → *ptye*), anticipations (e.g., *type* → *etype*), misdoublings (e.g., *free* → *frre*), and alternations (e.g., *these* → *thses*). However, anticipations of nearby letters, as in *type* → *tpype*, are often counted as intrusions or transpositions, and indeed are indistinguishable from transpositions such as *type* → *tpye* if the typist has attempted to minimize the anticipation error (here, *tpype*) by not repeating *p* in its normal spot. Misdoublings such as *trre* (for *tree*) suggest that double letters are stored as a single letter together with a repeat tag that can become attached in error to the wrong letter (Lashley 1951). Alternations such as *thses* (for *these*) likewise suggest that alternating letters (here, the *e* in *ese*) are stored with an alternation tag that can become attached in error to the embedded letter (here, *s*).

3.2. Experience, Frequency and Typing Slips

Both experience (hours of typing over the course of a lifetime) and relative frequency (how often a given key is struck relative to all others) influence typing errors. Experience increases the proportion of across-hand vs. within-hand transpositions (Grudin 1983), perhaps because a single, hierarchically organized unit represents within-hand digrams (letter pairs) in expert typists. Experience also reduces the relative proportion of substitutions and homologous intrusions, which virtually disappear with high levels of typing skill (Grudin 1983). Finally, relative frequency also influences substitutions, which usually result in higher frequency digrams than correct or intended digrams (Grudin 1983).

3.3. Timing and Typing Errors

Because errors in typing, writing, speech, and other skills increase with speed or overall rate of output (MacKay 1982), it becomes an interesting question whether errors reflect 'local haste', a short-term burst in speed prior to the error. Timing characteristics of keystrokes before and after errors link some but not all types of error to local haste (Grudin 1981; 1983). Keystroke intervals immediately preceding omissions and transpositions are usually shorter than average, as if typists make these errors when attempting to perform faster than accuracy permits. However, interstroke intervals preceding substitutions and intrusions provide no corresponding evidence of local haste.

4. Classes of Pen Slips

Pen slips typically fall into four classes, discussed below, but over 10% allow dual classification, e.g., combined anticipation and perseveration (van Nes 1971). Transpositions (e.g., *results* → *resulst*) are a fifth, but quite infrequent type of writing error (van Nes 1971).

4.1. Anticipation Errors in Writing

Anticipations (e.g., *Writing* → *Triting*) represent the most frequent category of writing errors, comprising over 40% of most collections (van Nes 1971). As in speech, components within and between words are anticipated, often with contextual accommodation, as in *MacKay* → *MakcKay* and *Writing* → *Triting*, where the anticipated t becomes capitalized (T) to match the case of the W intended for that position (Ellis 1979; 1988 a; 1988 b). Such accommodations suggest that graphemes rather than allographs or graphic motor units are anticipated, followed by choice between upper vs. lower case at the allographic level (Ellis 1979). Also counted as anticipations are 'switches' where a writer starts to write one letter but switches at a point of similarity to an upcoming letter (e. g., *made* → *mdde*). Because switches always involve strokes or subcomponents of a letter, they can be said to occur during execution of graphic motor patterns (Ellis 1988 b).

4.2. Perseveration Errors in Writing

Perseveration errors are much less frequent than anticipations, comprising about 10% of most collections, and result from reactivation of a recently activated grapheme or graphic motor unit, as in stroke additions such as *n* → *m* (van Nes 1971).

4.3. Omission Errors in Writing

Dropping one or more strokes within a letter (e. g., *m* → *n*; *g* → *a*) is an interesting type of omission error. Another is letter masking (Ellis 1979), omission of a letter just written (e. g., *writing* → *writng*) or about to be written (e. g., *writing* → *wrting*). Letter masking may involve allographic units because masking followed by case accommodation (e. g., *Tutors* → *Tuors*) has never been observed (Ellis 1979).

5. Error Detection

Skilled typists normally detect from 50% to 70% of their typing errors, and as with speech errors, detect them very quickly: With instructions to stop typing after making an error, only one keystroke usually follows the error (Long 1976; Shaffer/Hardwick 1969). Indeed, typists detect some errors before they fully execute them because incorrect keys are often pressed more lightly than normal (Rabbitt 1978; Wells 1916). The interval following an error is longer than average, and exceeds intervals two or more keystrokes before or after the error, as if errors are registered at some level before normal typing is resumed (e. g., Salthouse 1984; 1985; 1986). Post-error pauses follow the second stroke of transpositions, as if both strokes are produced as a unit and detected as erroneous during the pause (Grudin 1983). Skilled typists also mistype words such as *the* without pausing or stopping (as instructed), as if these words represent multi-letter ballistic units (Grudin 1983).

6. Feedback in Handwriting and Typing

A visually based engram must play a role in detecting some typing errors because typists tend to detect about 30% fewer errors when prevented from seeing their typed copy (Long 1976; Rabbitt 1978; West 1967). However, only relatively unskilled typists exhibit this pattern: highly skilled touch typists generate comparable speed and accuracy whether they can see their copy or not (West 1967). Nonetheless, skilled typists occasionally glance at the keyboard to hit relatively unfamiliar keys (e. g.,], $, %, +, @, #, ^, &, *, {, <, 1–10), and to ensure that their fingers occupy home-row position (Cooper 1983). Visual feedback also plays a role in pen slips because eliminating visual feedback increases both errors (Smyth/Silvers 1987) and writing time, especially for repeated letters and strokes, as in *m*, *n*, *w* (van Galen/Smyth/Meulenbroek/Hylkema 1989).

The auditory feedback accompanying keystrokes is also related to typing errors because unskilled typists make more errors when this auditory feedback is delayed (Long 1976; 1976; Cooper 1983). Introducing an extraneous tone also disrupts subsequent taps in tasks resembling typing (Wing 1978).

7. Comparisons of Slips across Modalities

Because speech, typing and handwriting have been studied in virtual isolation in the past, comparisons of tongue, pen, and typing slips are virtually nonexistant. Even comparisons of errors involving tongue vs. ear in speech, and eye vs. hand in typing are rare, despite their importance for theories of error detection (MacKay 1987).

Preliminary comparisons suggest many differences between tongue, pen, and typing slips, despite the commonalities emphasized in preceding sections. Some of these skill-specific error characteristics reflect fundamental differences in how speech, typing and writing are coded and sequenced, while others are superficial, or follow from general principles.

7.1. Code and Processing Differences

Fundamental skill-specific differences in error patterns (for slips of the tongue cf. art. 5) arise from the fact that typing/writing employs a visual-spatial code (in addition to an initial phonological code; see van Nes 1985; van Galen 1990; and even Kao/Hoosain 1984) and this visual-spatial code is sequenced linearly rather than hierarchically. However, only a hierarchic rather than linear code is used in speech. For example, the *aba* in the word *abacus* is coded as two different syllables (a + ba) in speech, rather than as a linear string of phonemes. Other syllabic characteristics are also coded in speech, so that vowels can only substitute with other vowels, and syllable-initial consonants can only substitute with other syllable-initial consonants, and never with syllable-final consonants or vowels (MacKay 1987). As a result, analogs of typing errors such as alternations, e. g., *abacus* → *babcus*, do not occur in speech: Because of syllable structure constraints, a speech error involving the *b* or *a* in *abacus* might resemble *babacus* or *ubacas*, but not *babcus*, an output with fewer syllables and a fundamentally different syllable structure from *abacus* (MacKay 1973). In typing, however, vowels often substitute with consonants (e. g., *ramp* → *rmap*), and syllable-initial consonants often substitute with syllable-final consonants (e. g., *artful* → *arftul*).

Consonant clusters, another component of syllables, also differentiate tongue vs. typing slips. Although speech errors often involve consonant clusters, e. g., *slit throat* → *thrit sloat* (Fromkin 1973), analogous typing errors have never been reported, despite diligent search (Grudin 1983). Because touch typists are assumed to develop hierarchically organized graphemic units for frequent diads (letter pairs such as *th*), the absence of multiletter sustitutions in skilled typing is curious and suggests that typing units are sequenced in very different ways from the phonological units for speech.

Because graphemic and allographic representations with visual-spatial characteristics ultimately trigger keystrokes, typing errors often violate the phonological constraints seen in speech errors. Thus, phonological similarity plays only a minor role in writing and typing errors, but a major role in speech errors: For example, segment substitutions in speech tend to involve units that differ in only a single distinctive feature (MacKay 1969). In contrast, visual-spatial similarity is a more powerful factor in pen and typing slips, and represents the more likely explanation for the well-established effects of finger movement similarity and pen stroke similarity in pen (Ellis 1979), and typing slips (Grudin 1983). However, because speech production does not employ a visual-spatial code, at least for familiar words, visual similarity plays no role in tongue slips.

Differences between errors in speech vs. typing/writing can also arise from differences between orthography vs. phonology. For example, no basis for misdoublings exists in speech, unlike typing, because, unlike repeated letters, immediately repeated phonemes are virtually nonexistent in natural languages (MacKay 1970).

7.2. Superficial Cross-Modality Differences

The technology of typing, low level motoric factors, and language-specific graphic characteristics introduce superficial differences between tongue, pen and typing slips. Design of the standard Qwerty keyboard influences currently studied typing errors, and different types of errors may be observed in future studies with technologically more advanced keyboards (e. g., the Dvorjak keyboard, where the vowels occupy the left-hand home row; and chord keyboards, where simultaneously pressing several keys generates a single letter; Gopher/Karis/Koenig 1985). Low level motoric factors such as the cross-hand vs. within-hand factor in typing errors (Grudin 1983) contribute other superficial differences, and so do language specific graphic characteristics. Unlike English, for example, correspondence between graphemes and phonemes is almost perfect in Finnish (Ellis 1982), and it will come as no surprise if Finnish typing, lacking repeated graphemes, fails to exhibit misdoublings. Nor will it come as a surprise that grapheme repetition and grapheme-phoneme correspondence factors are irrelevant for Chinese, a language without graphemes (Pulgram 1951).

7.3. Differences Due to General Principles

Some skill-specific error characteristics follow from general principles that apply to all skills. For example, the principle of speed-accuracy trade-off (MacKay 1982) can account for the relative rareness of pen slips (Ellis 1982): Handwriting proceeds much more slowly than speech and typing, so that pen slips are infrequent by general principle. The relative predominance of anticipations over transpositions among pen slips may also follow from the slowness of handwriting: Because pen slips can be detected very rapidly relative to writing speed, writers can stop after detecting the first letter of transpositions, leaving on paper something indistinguishable from an anticipatory error (van Nes 1971). As a result, anticipations may be overreported, and potential transpositions underreported among slips of the pen. Finally, words are more often left incomplete following pen than tongue or typing slips (van Nes 1971), as if writing slowness allows writers to detect an error, stop, and begin the word anew.

8. References

Book, W. F. (1925). *Learning to Typewrite*. New York: Gregg.

Cooper, W. E. (1983). Introduction. In W. E. Cooper (Ed.), *Cognitive Aspects of Skilled Typewriting. 1–35*. New York: Springer-Verlag.

Ellis, A. W. (1979). Slips of the pen. *Visible Language, 13*, 265–282.

Ellis, A. W. (1982). Spelling and writing (and reading and speaking). In A. W. Ellis (Ed.), *Normality and Pathology in Cognitive Functions. 113–146*. London: Academic Press.

Ellis, A. W. (1988 a). Normal writing processes and peripheral acquired dysgraphias. *Language and Cognitive Processes, 3(2)*, 99–127.

Ellis, A. W. (1988 b). Modelling the writing process. In G. Denes, C. Semenza, P. Bisiacchi, & E. Andreewsky (Eds.), *Perspectives in Cognitive Neuropsychology. 189–211*. London: Lawrence Erlbaum.

Fromkin, V. A. (1973). *Speech Errors as Linguistic Evidence*. The Hague: Mouton.

Gelb, I. J. (1963). *A Study of Writing*. Chicago: Chicago University Press.

Gentner, D. R. (1983 a). The acquisition of typewriting skill. *Acta Psychologica, 54*, 233–248.

Gentner, D. R. (1983 b). Keystroke timing in transcription typing. In W. E. Cooper (Ed.), *Cognitive Aspects of Skilled Typewriting. 95–120*. New York: Springer-Verlag.

Gentner, D. R., Grudin, J. T., Larochelle, S., Norman, D. A., & Rumelhart, D. E. (1983). A glossary of terms including a classification of typing errors. In W. E. Cooper (Ed.), *Cognitive Aspects of Skilled Typewriting. 39–41*. New York: Springer-Verlag.

Gopher, D., Karis, D., & Koenig, W. (1985). The representation of movement schemas in long-term memory: Lessons from the acquisition of a transcription skill. *Acta Psychologica, 60*, 105–134.

Grudin, J. T. (1981). *The organization of serial order in typing*. Unpublished doctoral dissertation, University of California, San Diego.

Grudin, J. T. (1982). *Central control of timing in skilled typing* (Tech. Rep. No. ONR 8202). San Diego: University of California, Center for Human Information Processing.

Grudin, J. T. (1983). Error patterns in skilled and novice transcription typing. In W. E. Cooper (Ed.), *Cognitive Aspects of Skilled Typewriting. 121–144*. New York: Springer-Verlag.

Kao, H. S. R. & Hoosain, R. (Eds.) (1984). *Psychological Studies of the Chinese Language*. Hong Kong: The Chinese Language Society of Hong Kong.

Lashley, K. S. (1951). The problem of serial order in behavior. In L. A. Jeffress (Ed.), *Cerebral Mechanisms in Behavior. 112–136*. New York: Wiley.

Long, J. (1976). Visual feedback and skilled keying: Differential effects of masking the printed copy and the keyboard. *Ergonomics, 19*, 93–110.

MacKay, D. G. (1969). Forward and backward masking in motor systems. *Kybernetic, 6*, 57–64.

MacKay, D. G. (1970). Phoneme repetition in the structure of languages. *Language and Speech, 13*, 199–213.

MacKay, D. G. (1971). Stress pre-entry in motor systems. *American Journal of Psychology, 84*, 35–51.

MacKay, D. G. (1973). Complexity in output systems: Evidence from behavorial hybrids. *American Journal of Psychology, 86*, 4, 785–806.

MacKay, D. G. (1982). The problems of flexibility, fluency, and speed-accuracy trade-off in skilled behavior. *Psychological Review, 89*, 483–506.

MacKay, D. G. (1987). *The Organization of Perception and Action*. New York: Springer-Verlag.

MacNeilage, P. F. (1964). Typing errors as clues to serial ordering mechanisms in language behavior. *Language and Speech, 7*, 144–159.

Munhall, K. G. & Ostry, D. J. (1983). Mirror-Image movements in typing. In W. E. Cooper (Ed.), *Cognitive Aspects of Skilled Typewriting. 247–258*. New York: Springer-Verlag.

Pulgram, E. (1951). Phoneme and grapheme: a parallel. *Word, 7*, 15–20.

Rabbitt, P. (1978). Detection of errors by skilled typists. *Ergonomics, 21*, 945–958.

Salthouse, T. A. (1984). Effects of age and skill in typing. *Journal of Experimental Psychology: General, 113*, 345–371.

Salthouse, T. A. (1985). Anticipatory processing in transcription typing. *Journal of Applied Psychology, 70*, 264–271.

Salthouse, T. A. (1986). Perceptual, cognitive, and motoric aspects of transcription typing. *Journal of Applied Psychology*, *99*, 303–319.

Salthouse, T. A. & Saults, J. S. (1985). *The Multiple Spans of Transcription Typing*. Unpublished manuscript, University of Missouri, Department of Psychology, Columbia.

Shaffer, L. H. (1975). Control processes in typing. *Quarterly Journal of Experimental Psychology*, *27*, 419–432.

Shaffer, L. H. & Hardwick, J. (1969). Reading and typing. *Quarterly Journal of Experimental Psychology*, *21*, 381–383.

Smyth, M. M. & Silvers, G. (1987). Functions of vision in the control of handwriting, *Acta Psychologica*, *65*, 47–64.

Tenney, Y. T. (1980). Visual factors in spelling. In U. Frith (Ed.), *Cognitive Processes in Spelling*. *215–229*. London: Academic Press.

van Galen, G. P. (1980). Handwriting and drawing: A two-stage model of complex motor behaviour. In G. Stelmach & J. Requin (Eds.), *Tutorials in Motor Behavior*. Amsterdam: North Holland.

van Galen, G. P. (1990). Phonological and motoric demands in handwriting: Evidence for discrete transmission of information. *Acta Psychologica*, *74*, 259–276.

van Galen, G. P., Smyth, M. M., Meulenbroek, R. G. J., & Hylkema, H. (1989). The Role of Short-Term Memory and the Motor Buffer in Handwriting under visual and non-visual guidance. In R. Plamondon, C. Y. Suen & M. L. Simner (Eds.), *Computer Recognition and Human Production of Handwriting*. *253–271*. Singapore: World Scientific Publishing.

van Nes, F. L. (1971). Errors in the motor programme for handwriting. I.P.O. (Eindhoven), *Annual Progress Report*, *6*, 61–63.

van Nes, F. L. (1985). Verschrijvingen als informatiebron bij de studie van schrijfprocessen [Slips of the pen as a source of information processing in the study of handwriting processes]. In A. J. W. M. Thomassen, G. P. van Galen, & L. F. W. de Klerk (Eds.), *Studies over de schrijftmotoriek: Theorie en toepassing in het onderwijs* [Studies on handwriting movements: Theory and applications to education]. *87–110*. Lisse: Swets en Zeitlinger.

Wells, F. L. (1906). Linguistic lapses. In J. McK. Cattell & F. J. E. Woodbridge (Eds.), *Archives of Philosophy, Psychology and Scientific Methods No. 6*. *1–110*. New York: Science Press.

Wells, F. L. (1916). On the psychomotor mechanisms of typewriting. *American Journal of Psychology*, *27*, 47–70.

West, L. J. (1967). Vision and kinesthesis in the acquisition of typewriting skill. *Journal of Applied Psychology*, *51*, 161–166.

Wing, A. M. (1978). Response timing in handwriting. In G. Stelmach (Ed.), *Information Processing in Motor Control and Learning*. *469–485*. New York: Academic Press.

Donald G. MacKay, Los Angeles, California (USA)

7. Errors and their Relevance for Models of Language Production

1. Introduction

Research in language production must provide theories of systems for control of the real-time lexical, phonological, and phrasal organization of sentences that encode the communicative intentions of a speaker. Article 1 of this handbook outlines a family of hypotheses about the architecture of the language production process. The character of the system described there relies on a variety of evidence types. One of the most powerful is the patterning of diverse types of speech errors (cf. art. 5, for discussion of data issues and a typology of errors). We will consider how such data can be brought to bear on the analysis of language production and claims about how its component systems relate to each other.

I will use the term 'Message' (*M*) to refer to the proximal cause of sentence construction in the sense outlined in article 1: *M* is the real time representation that controls the integration of sentence form, and thus expresses the speaker's communicative intent at the time of utterance. The separation of production processes into a conceptual system for message construction and a language specific system for sentence construction is an empirical claim that the error data bears on, as does a range of related experimental findings. As a preliminary issue, we briefly consider the sense in which conceptual and sentence level processing are independent and some of the evidence that leads to such a hypothesis.

If 'sentence construction' were directly conceptual rather than linguistic, one would expect conceptual variables to affect it in the way that syntactic and phonological variables do. In particular, one might expect error processes in sentence construction to be dictated by conceptual variables of semantic class and relations as they are by syntactic class and syntactic relations. But, such is, in fact, not what the speech error data indicate. There, one finds powerful constraints of syntactic category and construction, and of phonological structure and prosody on error patterns, but one looks in vain for a similar impact of semantic variables. A proper summary remark is that the processes of sentence construction attested by speech error tolerate gross violations of semantic well-formedness in errors (e. g., lexical and sound movement errors); yet these same preserve basic syntactic and phonological structures. See Bierwisch (1982) for a direct and interesting discussion of this point. Other supporting observations are treated in subsequent sections of this paper. There are, of course, errors that violate syntactic and phonological structure – for example, morphological movement errors that are discussed in section 2.6 violate category restrictions on bound morpheme attachment – but these, in turn, strongly preserve lower levels of structural constraint. There is an apparent hierarchical principle at work – an error at the *i*th level of structure may violate strictures at the $i - 1$ level but not those at the $i + 1$ level.

There are, of course, a number of ways in which the semantic content of sentences must affect their form, and particular means for achieving this through message structure control of sentence formulation are outlined in article 1. We will consider aspects of this general question in section 4. The question, as always, is not whether, but how semantic constraints connect to the mechanisms that determine sentence form. And, for the sentence processing systems implicated in the speech errors to be discussed here, semantic control appears to be indirect. Aspects of the insulation of those systems from direct semantic control have also been tested in recent experimental efforts. These illustrate and amplify the point under discussion (see Bock 1990 for a provocative discussion of this issue). Studies by Bock/Loebell (1990) and by Bock/Loebell/Morey (1992) report assessments of how variations in the semantic roles associated with the noun phrases of a sentence may influence a speaker's formulation of surface constituency. The experimental technique relies on a syntactic persistence effect robustly established in earlier work by Bock and her colleagues. This work is part of a larger research program that has extensively studied the conditions and sensitivity of this methodology. In brief: Speakers are required to describe line drawings of simple scenes; the syntactic forms chosen for that performance have been shown to be affected by the syntactic form of an immediately prior (topically quite unrelated) sentence heard by a subject. Changes in the relative rates for generation of several different syntactic forms have been demonstrated in this syntactic 'priming' paradigm.

In Bock/Loebell (1990), two forms of PP datives were tested as priming forms; these expressed either benefactive or locative semantic relations. Variation in the phrasal constituency of the priming sentences did produce changes in the form of sentences chosen for picture descriptions, but differences in the semantic roles associated with the PP phrases did not: Locative constructions in the primes (e. g., *she drove her car to the church*) induced benefactive descriptions for transfer of possession pictures just as well as did benefactive constructions (e. g., *she gave her car to the church*). They report a similar result for passive sentences: locative by-phrases induced passive picture descriptions as readily as did passive by-phrases (i. e., those with agentive force).

In Bock/Loebell/Morey (1992), a contrast between actives and passives was tested by varying a semantic feature (animacy) of the NPs in subject position in the priming sentences. A priming sentence in active or passive voice could either match or not match a potential description for an experimental picture in the animacy feature associated with the NP chosen for its subject. The experimental pictures were designed such that only an active sentence could be used to describe them if an inanimate NP was used in subject position (viz., inanimate agents were depicted – as in an alarm clock waking a boy, or an ambulance hitting a policeman, etc). Strong form priming effects (more actives following active primes than passive primes) and animacy effects (more actives following inanimate subject primes than following animate subject primes) were observed, with no interaction. An animacy match was equally effective for inducing active sentence descriptions of the experimental pictures regardless of the thematic role (agent or patient) of the subject NP in the priming sentences: Inanimate subjects in passive priming sentences produced an increase in active sentence descriptions comparable to that for inanimate subjects in active primes.

A similar conclusion regarding conceptual control of phrasal structure has been suggested by Bock/Miller (1991). Rather than the priming paradigm, the focus here was on experimentally induced number agreement errors. Constructions in which the subject NP is separated from its verb by postnominal modifiers that differ in number (e. g., *a man with four children is/*are likely to be home evenings*) are prey to occasional failures of agreement that seem to reflect displaced control from the licit NP head to the more recent or adjacent NP. Bock/Miller tested for the influence of animacy and concreteness of the NP's assumed to trigger errors in these circumstances. And, again, control of this particular aspect of sentence form did not appear to be responsive to semantic features — features that are independently observed to be strongly correlated with assignment of subject status in natural and experimental sentence generation tasks.

On this general architectural point, therefore, speech error patterns and these recent experimental outcomes are in concord: There is a significant processing boundary between conceptual and sentence representation. Exploring the relation of representations in *M* to sentence formulation processes provides a way to address that boundary. Some aspects of this that will arise in upcoming discussion include:

(a) The elaboration of both message level structures and sentence level structures is deployed in time, but not to the same scale — see the discussion of incremental planning for *M*, article 1. The computational window for *M* is not the same as that for various *S* levels, and this reflects the fact that the objects being manipulated are not the same. Aspects of error patterns bear directly on this.

(b) The relation of *M* to sentence processes is feed forward only (i. e., no decision about a feature of *M* is contingent on a feature developed by sentence level processes). W h a t a speaker decides to say is not affected by the processing that encodes *M* into sentences — and, on the face of it, should not. This is merely to say that if the syntactic, lexical, and phonological encoding mechanisms directly changed *M*, it would yield bizarre results (e. g., language with the appearance of schizophrenic speech, perhaps (cf. art. 53). Note: this is emphatically not to say that events at sentence level do not have any impact on processes at *M*. See section 4.

In the error analysis, we will discuss three classes of systems: Phrasal construction, phonological coding and lexical selection. Primary focus is on the data from spontaneous speech errors, augmented by observation of other natural features of production and by some experimental findings. The general interpretive formula we follow assumes that errors result from misassignments of elements to locations in the target utterance. What are the functional 'elements', what defines 'location' and what triggers error? These are central questions about the mental representations and processes at issue. We assume that error interactions arise from elements being part of the 'same' process/representation. Constraints on error interactions, therefore, may plausibly be taken to indicate what structure is present at the point of error, and that is the target of our analysis.

The error data has two broad classes we will attend to in outlining an initial case for the major architectural features of the language production system. These are m u l t i p l e s i t e e r r o r s — e. g., movement errors, and s i n g l e s i t e e r r o r s — e. g., substitutions and deletions (cf. also art. 5). In speaking of multiple sites, I refer to sites in the intended target sentence — i. e., 'plan internal errors' in the sense discussed by Butterworth (1982). Errors that involve two identifiable error loci (i. e., exchanges, shifts, anticipations, and perseverations) are of particular relevance to the analysis of phrasal level processes. They display differences in patterning characteristic of the grammatical type of the elements involved, and from these an organization of processing structures may be inferred. Exchanges are of particular import because of their unambiguous indication of domains of interaction in planning. This discussion will be amplified and refined in terms of single site errors, and of cases for which the error description may implicate multiple message or sentence representations. This latter entails parallelism in the formulation processes that map from *M* to articulation. There is, as we will see in the error data, evidence that encoding processes may diverge into more than a single stream.

We begin our examination of error patterns with those that suggest planning structures for phrasal organization. Subsequently we will turn to error data relevant to lexical retrieval. In the process, we will examine some aspects of phonological processing and note some of the experimental findings that extend and modulate our understanding of speech error patterns.

2. Phrasal Processing

At the outset, we should recall Levelt's discussion of sentence construction (cf. also art. 1). He describes it as a lexically driven, incremental process. To say that it is lexically driven means that encoding operations are controlled by the semantic and grammatical properties of words ('lemmas' in his usage). To say that it is incremental means that sub-parts of *M* are translated into sentence format as they become available during message construction – subject, of course, to the constraints of grammatical form that are expressed in the syntax of the language. The information derived from lemma entries drives sentence construction, with lemma recovery under initial control of *M*. In complementary fashion, an established sentence environment (i. e., initial utterance, or projection from early decisions to structurally linked later utterance positions) constrains lexical recovery – e. g., in the grammatical category that will instantiate a conceptual structure in a lemma. This way of talking suggests not only a mutual dependence of the processes of lexical recovery and sentence formulation, but also a certain separation of the processes. Precisely this latter point is immediately attested in speech error patterns that move words and morphemes separately from their structural frames. And, as we will later see in section 3, the joint import of the patterns for movement errors and those for substitution errors links lexical selection processes to phrasal construction processes quite systematically. Our first target then, is the evidence for organization of the subsystems in sentence construction.

2.1. Accommodations to Error

Several features of speech error distributions indicate the existence of more than one level of processing that implicates phrasal structure, and thus begins to outline the general architecture of the production system. One clear indication that multiple levels of representation intervene between *M* and articulatory control derives from the phenomenon of accommodation in speech errors (Fromkin 1971; Bierwisch 1982). The systems that account for regular morphological and phonological processes must apply after the processing stage(s) that gives rise to errors that mislocate words, morphemes and sound elements (e. g., 1–3), thus dictating a separation of the processing level that fixes detailed phonetic representations from that for abstract segmental and morphological structures.

(1) "... a meating arathon ..." [an eating marathon] (a/an alternation; Fromkin 1971)
(2) "... even the best team losts." [... even the best teams lost.] (/z/ changes to /s/)
(3) "drei Wochen im Tag gearbeitet." [... drei Tage in der Woche gearbeitet] (number marking; Bierwisch 1982)

Accommodatory effects are quite general and robustly represented in data from a number of different investigators (see, e. g., Stemberger (1984) re length accommodation in German errors; see Garcia-Albea/del Viso/Igoa (1988) for a general treatment re Spanish errors). We note that observations of some accommodatory effects (e. g., changes in word final inflectional affixes) may be influenced to a greater extent than other error classes by perceptual normalization of the error products (Cutler 1982). However, the generality of such effects for cases in which perceptual error is a less plausible contributor make its existence not open to serious question. Precise measurement of the acoustic and articulatory character of error elements in these and other error types will be required to determine the full and detailed extent of accommodatory effects. See Shattuck-Hufnagel (1985) for some confirmatory observation; see Mowrey/MacKay (1990) for evidence that non-standard articulatory configurations may result from experimental inductions of error that use 'tongue twister' techniques.

2.2. Sound Movement Errors

Given the reasons cited in 2.1. to distinguish the processing of abstract phonological forms from that which fixes their specific phonetic realizations, we are led to ask what speech error can tell us about the nature of the higher ordered levels of sound structure processing. Several aspects of sound errors suggest basic features of that speech planning system. Some examples of sound errors are given in 4–6.

(4) "but, I was in stuch a state of anxiety that I didn't notice." [such a state]

(5) "You have clatic ..., clatic sting?" [static cling]

(6) "... like a lilting willy." [wilting lilly; Cutler 1983]

These errors have been widely remarked to show the following characteristics (Meringer 1908; Boomer/Laver 1968; MacKay 1970; Nooteboom 1969; Fromkin 1971; Caldognetto/Tonelli/Vagges/Cosi 1987; del Viso/Igoa/Garcia-Albea 1990):

- The majority of such errors occur within phrases,
- the source syllables are metrically similar (re strong/weak distinction),
- the word with primary phrasal stress is more often involved than chance would predict,
- there are strong phonological similarities between the interacting elements themselves and also between their immediate segmental environments (see also Dell 1984).

These regularities are reported for Dutch, English, German, Italian and Spanish on the basis of substantial error corpora. Other reports based smaller samples from other languages (e. g., Arabic, Swedish) are in general accord. There are language specific effects, some of which we note later, but the overall generalizations concerning phonological similarity effects seem secure. From facts of this kind, we may infer that the level at which these processing errors occur is constrained by phrasal boundaries, and that sufficient phrasal detail is present to represent major phrasal stress features. Both syntactic and prosodic characterization of the relevant phrasal structure has been suggested (see section 2.6.). We may, in short, hypothesize a syntactic and/or phonological planning structure incorporating the distinctions reflected in these errors; that structure mediates the segmental interpretation of lexical targets.

There are several additional error features that concern structure building at this level of processing. Systematic features of sound errors implicate subanalyses of words in terms of phonemes, syllables, and features. So, for example, the modal sublexical error, particularly for exchanges, is a single segment slot; errors unambiguously identifiable as single feature multisite errors are observed, though they are not common (Fromkin 1971). Combining these observations with that concerning the strong similarities of interacting segments in sound errors – most segments in exchange errors, for example, differ only by a feature or two – suggests that sound errors are plausibly characterized in terms of processes that associate feature bundles with abstract segmental slots in a lexical and/or syllabic framework. Target segment similarity defined in terms of featural overlap is a determining factor, as is environmental similarity.

The relevant similarities, however, extend beyond the featural analysis of target and environment segments. In particular, a variety of observations have been interpreted as a reflection of the role of syllable structure in the production processes that give rise to systematic error. Segmental speech errors correspond in syllable position (Fromkin 1971; Shattuck-Hufnagel 1975; Caldognetto/Tonelli 1985; del Viso/Igoa/Garcia-Albea 1990; see also Crompton 1982). The positional constraint appears to govern interactions of segments: Initial segments interact with other initial segments, and similarly for medial and final segments. Note that movement errors do not generally involve syllable sized chunks – if one sets aside those errors that are ambiguous as to their classification, as is the case for monosyllablic morphemes, or cases with ambiguous segment boundaries (Shattuck-Hufnagel 1983; del Viso/Igoa/Garica-Albea 1990). Their lack of independent movement and the evidence for a constraining effect on segment movement errors suggests that syllabic structure is part of the planning framework; this contrasts with a hypothesis that syllables are individually controlled units of a processing vocabulary that must be recovered for assignment to a structural frame in a way analogous to the retrieval and assignment processes that do seem to be at work for sound segments or words. This general construal of segmental and syllabic processes seems quite in keeping with the tenor of contemporary phonological theory, and is all the more cogent given the evidence for an independent representation of stress as part of the processing framework that segments are attached to. For a related discussion that stresses the separation of segmental slots and their phonetic content, see Stemberger (1990).

He discusses several features of 'word shape' errors (i. e., those that substitute, add, or delete segment slots in a word) and argues for incorporating a coarse coding in lexical representations for production processing models.

Shattuck-Hufnagel (1987) has suggested a somewhat different perspective with interesting implications for the role of syllable structure. She has argued that word onset consonants should be considered a processing class. Two observations in particular warrant close study:

(a) In error corpora, word initial consonants predominate in sound error processes. This bias is found primarily in multisite errors (i. e., those with a source in the intended utterance – as contrasted with simple substitutions). Further, Shattuck-Hufnagel notes that much of the evidence usually taken for strong syllable structure constraint on sound errors can be accounted for by the word onset effect. That is, the position correspondence would be stated as a word position effect rather than a syllable position effect.

(b) Experimentally induced errors indicate that such a bias may depend on phrasal structure. In a memory/repetition task (using phonetically balanced 'tongue twisters'), Shattuck-Hufnagel found a word initial bias, as is typical of natural error corpora. That bias was linked to phrasal structure in the test strings: Word lists did not show a consistent word initial error bias, but the same test words in phrasally organized strings showed a strong and consistent position asymmetry.

We note that a word onset position effect appears for German (Bierwisch 1982), and has been reported for Italian (Caldognetto/Tonelli/Vagges/Cosi 1987); its relation to the syllable onset bias is not established for these cases. By contrast, the evidence from Spanish does not reveal a word onset bias. Syllable initial errors in non-onset positions in words were reported to be about twice as frequent as syllable initial errors in word onset positions (del Viso/Igoa/Garcia-Albea 1990). These language specific differences do not have a well developed account at present. One suggestion made by del Viso/Igoa/Garcia/Albea is that syllable initial error bias might reflect the statistical distribution of syllable types in Spanish, and tests controlling for this are compatible with that view. One other difference between Spanish and English sound errors that might play a role is that a much larger percentage of movement errors in Spanish were word internal than in English – word internal sound errors in English are substantially less common than errors between words. This suggests possible differences in the relevant sound planning domains and this might be associated with differences in word onset effects. As present, this is a speculation. We will reconsider the word onset position bias in the context of some more detailed suggestions concerning sound planning structures.

As an account of the normal production planning mechanisms underlying sound errors, Shattuck-Hufnagel (1979) proposed a segment to slot association process (a "scan-copier") for serial assignment of the phonetic content of lexical items; sound segment descriptions are sequentially copied from the lexical source set to marked sites in a planning framework for the target sentence and a monitor mechanism checks off elements as they are assigned to frame slots. Types of errors that involve interaction between different sites in the target (exchanges, anticipations, perseverations) arise from different patterns of monitor failure. The likelihood of failures is a function of segmental similarity, parallel frame positions, and phonetic similarity of frame environments. This descriptive mechanism readily encompasses the principal classes of sound movement errors.

Dell (1986), Harley (1984), Berg (1985), Stemberger (1985), and others have discussed network models of sound errors (as well as for morphological and lexical errors that we will turn to shortly). Though there are differences of detail, the general interactive nature of the accounts is similar. We describe aspects of Dell's model here as an illustration of the approach applied to sound errors. Network proposals for relations between lexical and phrasal processing will be taken up in later sections. The model uses spreading activation in a network to account for natural and experimentally induced sound errors and for network simulation results. In Dell's system, a network lexicon feeds independently constructed representations of sentence structure; the sentence structures provide controlling activation for the network, in which established connectivity reflects the stable relations among levels of lexical structure (lexical, morphological, syllabic, segmental and featural). The network integrates word forms and these are assigned to their structurally determined position in the sentence. Because of the network organization, varying degrees of interaction among the different levels of structural representation may be reconstructed by adjustment of the connections, their strengths, and time course.

Sound errors in this system, as in Shattuck-Hufnagel's, are driven by similarities between processing elements. Dell's treatment introduces the additional factor of a "confusion of levels" – processing activity at levels other than the phonological can interfere with sound planning processes. To illustrate briefly: Processing of lexical items is underway at several levels of the network simultaneously, and lexical focus will differ across levels. For an anticipation error, the sequence goes as follows: the phonetic elements of the lexical node that is the focus of processing at the semantic and/or syntactic level will receive activation from that planning activity; this activation is, strictly speaking, not relevant to the processing objectives of the higher level, but because of network connectivity, it will occur. And, since higher levels are on average ahead of lower levels, the activation motivated by the higher order processes will boost activation for phones scheduled for output later than the phones that are the focus of phonological processing for the most immediate pronunciation target. Such a later ordered phone may, thus, occasionally exceed activation levels for a correct phone and intrude in its place. Note the importance of phonetic similarity in this process. Similarities between target and potentially intruding phones permit the latter to share activation from the legitimate phonological nodes, thereby increasing the likelihood of intrusion. Perseverations are caused by 'rebound activation'. In Dell's model, correct assignment of a word to its position in a structure sets its activation to zero. But, because it is highly activated just prior to this selection, its immediate net neighbors are excited; their heightened activation can send a delayed activation boost to an already selected word. Exchanges arise by the continuation of these processes: The phone that has been displaced in an anticipation error retains its relatively high level of activation – this will not have been dissipated by the selection process, and thus it may occur in the position intended for the intruding phone.

The network account of errors describes them as jointly influenced by different structural levels. How does this fit the earlier observation about distinctions between message and sentence level processes and between whatever different levels of sentence production processing activity may be motivated by error analysis or other argument? Dell's model includes several distinct types of sentence representation, but a single lexical net. The lexical net permits 'leakage' between the processing components in such a system. Several types of findings have been advanced as demonstrations of processing interactions between levels of sentence structure mediated in this way. One that we will consider here concerns evidence for lexical biases in sound errors; others will be examined in later sections.

The core issue regarding lexical bias in sound level processing is the question whether sound errors create words (e. g., see elements in 4–6). The answer is: sometimes. It is clear for all current error corpora that a majority of error products for sound errors are nonwords (55–65 percent: Fromkin 1971; Garrett 1976; del Viso/Igoa/Garica-Albea 1990; figures vary depending on the error classes and error positions included). So a basic separation of segmental interpretation processes from lexical processes is not in doubt. But the theoretically salient issue posed by Dell needs a more finely tuned answer, for the incidence of created words in error corpora, even though a minority, has been reported to exceed chance estimates (Dell/Reich 1981). Errors involving initial consonants in exchanges, and in anticipatory or perseveratory substitutions showed significant elevation in lexical outcomes. Moreover, a lexical bias has also been reported for experimentally induced errors (Baars/Motley/MacKay 1975; Dell 1986). A network model of the processes that integrate the sound structure of words, suitably tuned, would readily accommodate such influences (see, e. g., Dell 1986, for a network simulation of sound errors), while a processing model with autonomous levels in which the integration of sound structure follows lexical access for word form would require an alternative account of interactive effects between sound error products and lexical representations.

It should be noted that del Viso/Igoa/Garcia-Albea did not find a lexical bias effect for sound errors in their Spanish corpus. Two differences of procedure are instructive. They did not restrict their analysis to just initial segments and did not restrict it to just consonant errors; they tested vowels and non-initial errors. Twenty-seven percent of their sound errors were vowel errors; moreover, no word initial error position bias holds in Spanish. So, maintaining these features of Dell/Reich's analysis was infeasible – it would have restricted the Spanish analysis to a minority of their corpus. However, in determining their estimates of chance for lexical and non-lexical error outcomes, they did retain Dell and Reich's restriction to sound movements that yielded phonologically acceptable sequences in the language. The differences in analysis are plausible as an account of the contrasting outcomes for the lexical bias effect in Spanish and English and should be systematically examined for their consequence in other error corpora.

Whatever the resolution of lexical bias effects in natural error corpora, there are still good grounds to pursue the issue based on experimental evidence for lexical effects. Three possibilities to be entertained include:

- A network interaction between lexical nodes and the nodes that create phonological structures – phonemes, syllables, and features (Dell 1986).
- An editorial bias introduced by interpretive monitoring via the comprehension system. There is evidence in favor of such editorial processes as a factor in the experimental effects of Baars/Motley/MacKay. In their study, a lexical bias appeared only when the error induction materials were real lexical items.
- An error checking routine internal to the processes that create phonological phrases. The late contact with the lexicon would be represented not as a factor controlling sound level processing, but as a check on the accuracy of sound processing. This suggestion remains to be developed, but on one line of thought, it might connect to Shattuck-Hufnagel's word onset bias. She has suggested that the susceptibility of word onset segments to error may arise because word initial and non-initial segmental information are transferred from lexical source to planning frame at different times. The late transfer of onset information might be linked to its role in coordinating lexical retrieval targets and frame insertion sites (see Garrett 1988).

No strong basis for a choice between these alternatives is presently available. The possibility that the bias is not generally displayed in natural error corpora when more inclusive treatments of error classes are made suggests a problem with the standard network treatment. It ought to work for all classes of sound errors and in all word positions unless, of course, arguments motivated by the network architecture can be offered for elements and environments tested in the Spanish results. A comprehension based editorial monitor account, as discussed by Levelt (cf. art. 1), is perhaps least problematic on current evidence, though internal 'editorial' effects of the error checking sort are an interesting possibility for future development.

2.3. Word Exchanges

The preceding observations about sound errors implicate kinds of process and representation that control planning for detailed pronunciation of the intended output. The structures so implicated, however, are not sufficient to account for the full range of error data. In particular, though a phrasally bounded structure is involved and lexical structure is relevant, it is sublexical structure that is salient, with clearly syntactic matters not prominent. By contrast, properties of word and morpheme exchanges and of shifts (e. g., Fromkin 1971; Bierwisch 1982; Garrett 1975; 1980) clearly indicate a syntactically constrained processing level distinct from that at which sound movement errors occur. Initially, we examine exchanges, turning later to other word movement errors. Examples appear in 7–9.

(7) "Bensinger takes to that left field wall like water takes to a duck ..., er, like a duck takes to water, I guess."

(8) "... see if your week's clear in an eye." [... your eye's clear in a week.]

(9) "... she sings everything she writes". [... writes every thing she sings]

Word exchanges and sound movement errors, particularly sound exchanges sharply contrast in their typical character:

- Word exchanges are predominantly between phrases, and in a significant number of cases, between adjacent clauses. Moreover, and most importantly, they occur almost exclusively for words of corresponding grammatical category, and frequently span several intervening words (Bierwisch 1982; Garrett 1975).
- Sound exchanges rarely cross clause boundaries, and are predominantly phrase internal, usually spanning only a word or two; they do not show a grammatical category constraint like that for word ex-

changes (Garrett 1975; 1980; del Viso/Igoa/Garcia-Albea 1990).

In addition to these points, there are two further significant contrasts, both 'negative' features. The first lies in the very different involvement of phonological variables as constraining or contributing factors in the two error classes: Word exchanges show limited evidence of such properties (see section 4 for more detailed discussion of this issue), whereas, as just noted, the sound errors show manifold phonological similarities for both the error elements themselves and their environments. The second contrast is between semantically based word substitutions (to be discussed in section 3) and word exchanges. Using the target/intrusion pairs from word substitution errors to index the relevant semantic relations between word exchange elements again reveals sharp differences: word exchanges are not semantically similar in the ways characteristic of word substitutions. These contrasts, and others to be discussed momentarily, indicate a processing stage, prior to the sound structure level, but distinct from the message level, at which the syntactic relations among words, but not their surface phonological representation, are determined. It must be a multiphrasal level (as opposed to the single phrasal domain implicated in sound errors); the limiting domain is arguably two clauses – word exchanges rarely implicate elements of non-adjacent clauses.

2.4. Stranding Exchanges

At this point, we focus the error analysis on a third class of exchanges. These move morphemes, and they have features in common with word and sound exchanges, but they also display important additional properties. Such errors move stem morphemes; affixal morphemes, predominantly from inflectional classes, are 'stranded' (Garrett 1975; Garcia-Albea/del Viso/Igoa 1988).

(10) "That's why they sell the *cheap*s drink." [drinks cheap]

(11) "I'm not in the *read* for *mood*ing." [mood for reading]

(12) "You *order*ed up *end*ing some fish dish ..." [ended up ordering]

Based on the diagnostic variables used to analyze the sound exchanges and word exchanges, morpheme exchanges appear to arise in two ways – either at the multiphrasal planning stage that gives rise to word exchanges, or at the single phrase stage that gives rise to sound exchanges (Garrett 1980). The key observation is that when morpheme stranding errors involve elements of distinct phrases, the categorial constraint typical of word exchanges holds strongly, otherwise not. By test comparison, there is no such change in the evidence for a grammatical category constraint when one focuses on those sound exchange errors (relatively few) that do cross phrase boundaries.

There is another more general grammatical category effect that emerges here and is of considerable moment. The separation of stem and affix in stranding errors is but one manifestation of a broad contrast between major and minor category words. When words exchange – as discussed in 2.4. – they are from lexical classes that have phrasal projections: N, V, Adj, P. Minor grammatical category free forms, as well as bound affixal elements, are rarely found in word exchanges. Moreover, this general category distinction also applies to source words for sound exchanges. Those sound elements that participate in exchanges are parts of major category items; minor category words are rarely found to be unambiguously the source of a segment involved in a simple two locus sound exchange. These observations have been combined in a hypothesis about all exchange errors (Garrett 1975; 1980): exchanges arise from misassignment of a lexical form, or segments of a lexical form, to a structural frame. These latter may be planning structures appropriate either to syntactic or to phonological phrasing (Garrett 1982). In both instances, the lexical content of the planning structures is assumed to be independently retrieved under the control of higher ordered structures (i. e., *M* structure in the case of lemma retrieval, and syntactic structure in the case of word form retrieval; see section 3). On this hypothesis, non-lexical formatives are incorporated as features of planning frames, and are, therefore, not subject to exchange processes. This provides an account of stranding errors, and predicts that stranded elements should not themselves be observed to exchange in other error cases. This prediction seems to be generally well supported in error corpora (Garrett 1975; Stemberger 1985; Garcia-Albea/del Viso/Igoa 1988). Similarly, this hypothesis accounts for the restriction of word exchanges and the source words for sound exchanges to major categories. The error outcomes may be seen as a consequence of the assignment of particular classes of processing elements to direct access via *M* substructures (or inheritance from that access stage – see section 3.1.), as opposed to an indirect access via the recruitment of planning structures. The former are candidates for exchange processes, the latter are not. We will return to this point.

Further to these matters, we note that the construal of error mechanism just outlined fits an aspect of error structure not yet introduced. This concerns stress assignments for elements in movement errors. The generalization is that phrasal stress is preserved in exchanges, i.e. the moved elements do not take their stress with them, but are stressed according to their error induced environment (Fromkin 1971). Phrasal stress is not, on this observation, a feature of the elements undergoing insertion into planning structures. If stress is conceived of as a feature of the planning frames (or computed from it), stress should be, as it is, 'stranded' in word and morpheme exchanges.

2.5. Shift Errors

To the patterns so far reviewed, we add those for another major category of movement errors. These are morpheme 'shift errors' (e.g., 13–15). The elements typical of these errors are minor category words and inflectional affixes (Garrett 1975; Garcia-Albea/del Viso/Igoa 1988):

(13) "mermaid_ move*s* their legs together." [mermaids move their legs together]

(14) "... doing the studies, then come_ up*ing* with the analysis" [doing the studies, then coming up with the analysis]

(15) "If you can't figure_ what that out is, ..." [figure out what that is]

The complementarity with exchanges is quite striking. With minor exception, the most frequently observed elements in unambiguous shift errors are not found either as elements of word or morpheme exchanges or as sources for sound exchange errors. One descriptive hypothesis that accommodates this is that morpheme shifts, bound or free, occur posterior to all exchanges. They arise as a consequence of operations that interpret the non-lexical features of planning frames for insertion into the terminal string of their phrasal configuration. A further observation about stress errors reinforces the distinctiveness of shifts. As noted in 2.4., exchange errors preserve phrasal stress. But, word shifts often distort it (Cutler 1980). A shifted element, most often a minor category word, and bearing some stress for contrastive or emphasis reasons, will appear with stress in its new, error induced location. These facts indicate a significant processing difference between the error elements involved in word shifts and those characteristic of word exchanges, extending the case for a distinction between syntactically and phonologically organized processing representations.

There is a strong grammatical category effect 'nested' within the preceding characterization of movement error processes that deserves more explicit notice. As noted, major and minor grammatical category words behave quite differently. The contrasts between these two classes of elements have been expressed as a hypothesis about computational vocabularies in the production system: 'Open class' (OC) elements (viz., major category items that participate in exchanges) are recruited by direct retrieval processes – i.e., under message structure control. Some properties of the direct access process are inferable from word substitution errors (see section 3). The 'closed class' (CC) elements (minor category elements that rarely appear in exchanges, but commonly appear in shifts) are, on this account, recruited as parts of structural frames, most particularly planning frames associated with phonological phrasing (Garrett 1975; 1980). This hypothesis has variant forms – the one just stated is the most general. Lapointe/Dell (1989; see also Bock 1989) have suggested a more restricted version in which only bound morphemes are treated as frame elements, and an alternative account of error constraints on minor category free forms is given based on frequency and stress factors. Resolution of the appropriateness of a categorical analysis versus one in terms of correlated variables like length, stress, and frequency in closed class elements is difficult and is a matter of current research. Dell (1991), for example, has reported recent results showing that frequency is inversely related to error likelihood for experimentally induced sound errors and that this applies to both open and closed class elements. The relation of this finding to the full range of CC vocabulary effects in error data remains to be worked out.

2.6. A Summary Description of Speech Error Patterns

The several aspects of error patterning so far discussed may be incorporated in the form of a proposal for the successive assignment of lexical content to two levels of phrasally organized processing structures. By way of a summary description here, we may relate these distinctions to the structure discussed in article 1 and outlined in figure 1.1 there. Note that the processes designated for sentence formulation in that treatment include an initial syntactic mapping under *M* level control; this requires lemma retrieval and subsequent incorporation into syntactic representations. This process is followed by the construction of phonological phrases, which involve the recovery of the word forms that are associated with lemmas and (with appropriate morphological processing) the integration of phonological phrasing for the sentence. The error processes we have reviewed to this point are based entirely on error cases displaying an interaction between two sites in the target utterance, and their patterns indicate multiple processing levels in sentence formulation that readily correspond to the major distinctions outlined in Levelt's figure 1.1 (cf. art. 1). The errors provide evidence for:

(a) a multiphrasal level of planning, possibly with a two clause limiting domain; these are processes that build abstract logical and syntactic representations (i. e., phonologically uninterpreted);

(b) a single phrase level that provides for abstract phonological interpretation of phrasal structures, with a subsequent dependent process that determines the phonetic detail; the domain is perhaps best captured in terms of phonological phrasing;

(c) a significant restriction on information flow between processing levels, and in particular, a significant autonomy of the indicated sentence level processes with respect to the semantic variables represented at *M*;

(d) a dissociation of lexical content and phonetic segment content from their respective phrasal environments in the processes that build sentence form.

As a final note, we cite the relation between interpretations of movement error data and that for hesitation distributions (e. g. Ford 1982; Holmes 1988) and repair processes (e. g., Levelt 1983). Such evidence is not reviewed here, but the implications for the types of major planning structures are broadly compatible with those for speech errors. In section 4, we consider some other experimental findings that can be used to evaluate and modulate aspects of the error interpretations so far considered. Those matters will be taken up after discussion of major aspects of lexical retrieval and their relation to phrasal processes.

3. Lexical Retrieval and Phrasal Construction

We earlier remarked the mutual dependence of lexical selection and phrasal construction. Hypotheses about phrasal processing systems can indicate what lexical structures must be available at given points in the sentence construction process. And, conversely, independently generated hypotheses about lexical retrieval can suggest ways in which phrasal integration may be controlled by the availability of lexical structure. This issue emerges quite clearly in analysis of the patterns in lexical errors: there is a natural fit between the independently motivated lexical retrieval hypotheses discussed in this section and the distinction between syntactic and phonological levels of phrasal integration motivated on the basis of the sound, morpheme, and word movement errors.

Lexical retrieval can go wrong in two ways: failure to generate an output, and generation of the wrong output. The 'wrong' output can be defective in several ways. These two general modes of failure are expressed respectively in 'tip of the tongue' (T.O.T.) observations and in word substitution errors. In T.O.T. cases, the semantic force of the word in question is available to the speaker, but the word form fails to be generated at the scheduled moment for its use, and the speaker is aware of this failure. Such failures may vary in their duration and our disposition to label any given such incident as a 'T.O.T. state' will depend in part on whether and when it resolves. The potential linkages to hesitation phenomena are obvious (cf. art. 4). In word substitutions, failure manifests itself when an unintended word replaces the intended word. We focus on word substitutions here. The processing implications of the two kinds of lexical failures are, however, similar in respects that we will note.

3.1. Word Substitutions

An essential consideration in the study of word substitutions for purposes of developing a retrieval theory is that the errors identified for analysis must plausibly be lexical substitutions – quite obviously, we wish to exclude cases that result from sublexical error – e. g., sound errors that make words. Somewhat less obviously, word errors may also result from other aspects of the production process not straightforwardly based on retrieval mechanisms. Word substitutions are, in fact, diverse in their superficial properties and apparent causes: anticipatory and perseveratory copying (e. g., 16), discourse (17) and environmental (18) intrusions, and those with no apparent discourse or environmental source (e. g., 19–24). These latter are the focus of current interest. Errors like those in 16–18 are ambiguous as to their source or multiply determined, and there is good indication that some at least include attentional factors (i. e., the environmental intrusions). Environmental errors in particular seem responsive to several distinct influences, form, meaning and situational, where the situational information is as often topic irrelevant as relevant.

(16) anticipations or perseverations: "the crazy *idea* who has a good idea, but doesn't have a grant, ..." [guy]

(17) conversational intrusions; immediate prior mention: [remark follows a series of temperature reports] "... it's been hot and muggy – the kind of weather that shortens *temperatures*." [tempers]

(18) environmental intrusions: "You found your *pen*?" [bag] [addressee was waving a pen in speaker's face while cleaning it; the question actually concerned a misplaced briefcase.]

(19) "I've got whipped cream on my *mushroom*." [mustache]

(20) "People don't know – people who've never sat on an *envelope*." [elephant]

(21) "Does it make *tradition* ..., uh, transition at the appropriate point?"

(22) "He rode his bike to school *tomorrow*." [yesterday]

(23) "The picture on the front was the *whale* from Jaws." [shark]

(24) "*Ask* me whether you think it'll do the job." [tell]

The substitution type with the least problematic interpretation for retrieval claims is that for which there is no identifiable topical relevance and for which there has been no mention in prior discourse, either topic relevant or irrelevant. Separating errors into subtypes can be difficult or impossible given limited information about the discourse or the environment of the errors – as is sometimes the case in the diary method of error collection (cf. art. 5). Broad decisions about the likelihood of topical relevance for a given lexical target may be made based on the conversational setting, but detailed recording of prior remarks in a discourse or, more difficult still, of unrelated collateral discussions or events is necessary for a secure assignment to the environmental errors category. It is essential to attempt the separation, however, for the structural properties of the clear cases of lexical retrieval error do differ from those of environmental and discourse errors, and this is particularly so for the analysis of meaning related cases (see Harley 1984; Garrett 1992 a; 1992 b).

When one restricts, insofar as feasible, the error cases to be analyzed in the ways discussed above, the remaining substitutions are, by and large, those that have a relation of form (e. g., 19–21) or meaning (e. g., 22–24) to the intended target word. Fay/Cutler's (1977) discussion of such word substitutions laid out the basic contrasts that have engaged much of subsequent enquiry. They evaluated relations between target and intrusion words by contrasting meaning related and form related substitution pairs. They reasoned that when a meaning relation was absent, the form parameters of potential relevance to storage and retrieval could be identified. Accordingly, they analyzed form similarity for cases showing no plausible meaning link; these they labeled 'malapropism' errors. Errors with a readily identifiable meaning relation were used as a comparison set. The differences in form similarities for the two sets are, in fact, quite striking: For the malapropisms, Fay and Cutler found a significant correspondence for phonological segments, stress placement, and length in syllables, with the most marked segmental similarity at word onset. Later work (Hurford 1981; Cutler/Fay 1982) showed that although greatest similarity is indeed for word initial segments, there is also strong overall similarity. The major regularities are robust, appearing in several independent corpora. These findings suggest a special status for the parameters of word form that link target and error words. Initial sounds, length in syllables and stress location are arguably principal factors in the organization of the inventory of lexical forms, and hence constitute the normally effective descriptions for word form retrieval.

Fay and Cutler interpreted the patterns in word substitutions as supporting two processing claims: (a) initial word selection is based on a direct mapping from meaning representations to words, and when defective, the selection process yields semantically related word substitutions; (b) word forms are stored in an inventory organized on the basis of phonological resemblance, and an error in retrieval of a word form yields a nearby, hence similar, item in this space. Notice that this account does not require a lemma/word form distinction – though not incompatible with it. Two further features of word substitutions suggest a more detailed account that distinguishes lemma and word form representations: First, there is a powerful constraint of grammatical category for both meaning and form related substitutions: target and intrusion correspond – nouns intrude for nouns, verbs for verbs and adjectives for adjectives. Second, there is a dissociation between meaning and form relations: target and intrusion words that are clearly related in form do not often show a strong meaning relation, and, conversely, substitutions with a strong meaning relation do not have readily discerned relations of form. This latter dissociation might seem foregone, given that the relation between word form and word meaning is conventional. But, processing representations may exploit, or at least reflect, adventitious correlations of form and meaning. In network formulations of process, this condition is likely. Thus, this error pattern has import for our analysis of the way in which the stored representations of words are organized for retrieval during sentence construction and for our evaluation of the kinds of mechanism that may implement that organization.

Assuming for the moment an uncomplicated account, the dissociation indicates that meaning and form based retrieval are separate operations. Both such processes are syntactically constrained, and hence part of language specific processes, not of those that determine *M*. This has been described as a two-step retrieval process (Fromkin 1971; Butterworth 1980; Garrett 1976; 1978) that is integrated with systems for phrasal construction in sentence production. On this account, information about word form is not available at the stage of initial lexical selection, and a separate retrieval operation is required at the point when segmental structure is specified. Following Levelt (1989) and others, the first of these two retrieval stages is referred to as 'lemma activation', by which one means the identification of a specific lexical item with its semantic and syntactic specification, but without the specification of its phonological form. The second stage corresponds to his 'word form' retrieval (cf. also art. 1).

Here we note specifically, that the two levels of sentence processing indicated by the movement errors discussed in 2.1.–2.6. correlate directly with the two major types of lexical processing implied in the patterns of lexical substitution errors. The two levels of sentence structure motivated by several types of movement errors may plausibly be associated, respectively, with a message driven process that provides lexical content for abstract syntactic structures, and with a form-driven process that associates the phonological descriptions of words with their phrasal environments. There is, therefore, good empirical reason based on specifically sentence level processes to assign a two stage structure to the systems that account for lexical retrieval in language production. Movement error interpretation complements and reinforces the interpretation of patterns independently identified in the word substitution errors.

One plausible construal of the grammatical category correspondence between target and intrusion in word substitutions is that it too reflects the dependence of lexical recovery on grammatical frames: the grammatical category constraint is imposed in the phrasal integration process. We might also recall in this connection the strong constraint of grammatical category on word exchanges. The picture that emerges concerning word exchange errors at the initial stages of sentence formulation is that these must arise after the conceptual nomination of lexical content for target sentences, and before their phonological interpretation – witness the simultaneous lack of apparent semantic or phonological constraint word exchanges. We will return to this picture in section 4.

An alternative account of the category constraint would interpret it as a fact about the organization of lemma and word form inventories – i.e., the inventories are cross-classified by grammatical category. Such an interpretation has little independent support and is not readily assessed. One observation that tells against it is Cutler's (1980) analysis of apparent lexical stress errors – e.g. '*psyCHOlogy*' pronounced as '*psychoLOgy*'. These appear only for morphologically complex forms and she argues that such errors are, therefore, not stress shift errors per se, but confusions between derivationally related word forms, thus suggesting a common storage site for derived variants.

Many other findings suggest a similar view of lexical retrieval processes. First, tip of the tongue states in both natural speech situations and in experiment match word substitution structures in essential respects. T.O.T. states are a canonical demonstration of conceptual and word-form dissociation. And, for word form variables, T.O.T. data indicate greater than chance ability to guess the initial sounds of words, and significant, though weaker, knowledge of word length and stress (Brown/McNeill 1966; Browman 1978). The speech error patterns may also be compared to studies of lexical retrieval failures in aphasia and related disorders: see Buckingham (1979); see Garrett (1992 b) for an account of some semantic error patterns in language disorders that indicate a lemma/word form distinction; see Butterworth (1979) for a discussion linking this view of lexical retrieval to hesitation and neologistic speech in jargon aphasia. Bock (1987 b) notes the correspondence of the two-step retrieval hypothesis in sentence production to stages offered in accounts of experimental studies of object naming. Kempen/Huijbers (1983) report experimental effects supporting a lexically specific but phonologically uninterpreted stage of processing in picture descriptions.

3.2. Form and Meaning Interactions

The differences between meaning and form based word substitution errors that motivate the two-step retrieval theory are strongly marked in the data. Nevertheless, the boundary between the error types may be less absolute than it seems. Despite the appearance of dissociation, joint form and meaning similarities for target and intrusion pairs have been reported to exceed probabilities of random convergence (Dell/Reich 1981; Stemberger 1984; Harley 1984). The strength and detailed character of such effects are important in determining their theoretical interpretation. If such effects are negligible, a two stage system integrated with phrasal and phonological processes as outlined in 3.1. is preferred. Indeed, a network system of the sort introduced in section 2.2. might even be used to model such a two step process, and if so, the patterns of connectivity would necessarily be set so as not to support significant levels of form and meaning interaction, although other types of interaction between levels might be incorporated (e. g., a relation between lexical and sound structure integration). Alternatively, one might seek to model the two processes in a network representation of the lexicon so that form and meaning descriptions could interact more extensively in the processes that govern the insertion of lexical items into phrasal environments. We will consider this latter possibility.

The general claim (Dell/Reich 1981; Harley 1984; Stemberger 1984) is for a phonological influence on semantic errors, and the principal evidence for this focuses on the overlap of initial consonants in target and intrusion words. Dell and Reich's report showed a significant elevation in segment overlap for word onset positions in semantic substitutions in their error corpus. A related claim (Stemberger 1985; Aitchison/Straf 1982; Harley 1984) is that word substitutions showing both strong semantic and strong phonological similarity, while infrequent, are still more likely than chance (e. g.: '*lobster*' for '*oyster*'; '*amnesia*' for '*anaesthesia*'). In sharp contrast, a recent similar study of semantic errors in Spanish (del Viso/Igoa/Garcia-Albea 1990) found no indication of a segmental overlap for semantic errors in their corpus. However, they supplemented the segmental analysis with tests for stress and length and did find greater than chance correspondences for these variables. While the result of the Spanish error analysis significantly complicates the claim for segmental similarity effects in semantic word substitutions, the length and stress effects are nevertheless relevant to the general question of evidence for form and meaning interactions. The apparent form relations between target and error words in semantic errors have been interpreted as support for an interactive activation account of lexical selection.

Dell's (1986) account of these effects emphasizes the general nature of the segmental overlap effects across the set of lexical representations. That is, strong overlap cases are taken to be just the most noticeable instances of a quite general increase in the likelihood of semantic error when a semantic target shares phonetic segments with a potential (on semantic grounds) intruding item, particularly when the shared segments are word initial. Such a position bias makes sense in light of the heightened salience of that factor in word form retrieval as evidenced by the malapropism errors. The magnitude of effects for semantic errors reported by Dell and Reich is not comparable to that for form based errors; but, arguably, they need not be, given that in the mixed cases, form similarities do not have to carry the burden of error generation alone. The network formulation permits a trading relation between form and meaning similarity.

What is the import of the evidences of meaning and form interactions? Do they compromise a basic processing contrast between meaning related and form related word substitutions? Assuming future research shows that current estimates of the level of effect are representative, that does not appear to be the case: phonological similarities for form based word substitutions are qualitatively as well as quantitatively different from those for meaning based substitutions. While segmental overlap in word initial positions is a well motivated and relevant comparison, it does underestimate the strength of the contrast between form and meaning based word substitutions. Not only is the level of effect very different in magnitude at the first four segment positions, the form related errors, unlike semantic errors, also show strong overall similarities. Fay and Cutler also report a subtler point: the featural differences at the initial mismatch points between target and intrusion in form based errors are less than for semantic errors. The point to take from this is that, even if a network were in fact the indicated mechanism to adopt because of its capacity to accommodate evidence for form and meaning interaction, it would likely be one in which the tuning for separation of the two information classes would be more significant than that for their joint effects. This point is made more salient by the experimental results we review next.

Two recent experiments have addressed the relation of form and meaning representations in lexical retrieval for production. They yield conflicting results. Schriefers/Meyer/Levelt (1990) used a picture naming task with simultaneous lexical probes (subjects were to ignore the word and name the picture). On the basis of established norms for the naming targets for their pictures, they chose probe words either semantically or phonetically similar to the target name for the picture. The temporal relation between probe word and picture presentation was varied in order to explore the time course of activation for the picture naming response, with facilitatory and inhibitory effects on naming times as dependent measures. They found evidence for two nonoverlapping stages: an initial stage in which only semantic effects were observed and an end stage with only phonological effects. Such a pattern poses difficulties for a network implementation that preserves significant semantic and phonetic connectivity, though straightforwardly compatible with a two stage retrieval model of lexical processing. By contrast, Martin/Weissberg/Saffran (1989) report a result showing an interaction of meaning and form. They also used picture naming, but their pictures were used in sets designed to test for degrees of phonological and semantic similarity. Subjects were required to trace a pattern through an array of pictures, successively naming the pictured objects, and substitution errors were tabulated. The picture sets contained (a) items semantically distinct, but phonologically similar, or (b) with the complementary relation, or (c) with joint similarities (e. g., *parrot*, *pigeon*, *penguin* – all birds and all with the same initial phone). Semantic and phonological similarities were independently conducive to error, and their joint presence produced a significant interaction. This result seems to favor a model in which both types of description are simultaneously active in lexical retrieval.

The differences between these two experimental outcomes may be less problematic than their opposed interpretation would suggest. It seems likely that the procedural differences between the two studies resulted in their tapping different aspects of lexical naming performances. In particular, the Martin et al. method provides a good opportunity for the effects of working memory representations and attentional focus to contribute to performance in addition to immediate retrieval operations that are predominantly under internal semantic control. This seems particularly likely given that subjects repeated the naming response for a given pictured stimulus several times in a test session. These conditions are similar in many respects to those we noted in our discussion of the role of environmental contaminants in the analysis of word substitution errors. Words that intrude into the intended stream of speech and that can be linked to immediately prior utterance, or identified as intrusions from an irrelevant written word, picture or object in the speaker's view, are normally excluded from the error analysis aimed at identifying the nature of lexical retrieval systems on the grounds that these errors incorporate additional mechanisms whose interaction with basic retrieval devices remains to be established. Of course, it is always open to question the separation between environmental intrusion errors and the semantic or form based errors that motivate the two-step retrieval account. For example, Stemberger (1985) and Harley (1984) both treat all these lexical errors in terms of a common network mechanism that does not sharply distinguish adventitious extralinguistic influences on encoding from those intrinsic features of the meassage and sentence structures underlying the intended speech act. The general problem of how to approach the treatment of the error data in a way that does not affect its utility for deciding between competing theoretical treatments is extremely difficult and beset with metatheoretic thorns of the most troublesome sort. In the present case, the convergence of the Schriefers et al. experimental study with the word substitution distinctions drawn in section 3.1. encourages a continued investigation of the possibility that a form of the two-stage lexical retrieval model, perhaps in a network instantiation that preserves limited interactive potential, is a useful line to explore.

4. Relations of Phrasal and Lexical Processes: Error Data and Experimental Evidence

4.1. Interactions of Syntax and Word Form

In their analysis of error data, Dell/Reich (1981) also report evidence of a phonological similarity for word exchanges (where, by working hypothesis outlined in section 2.3., word form is not specified). Their objective was to test the role of phonological factors for lexical insertion processes at the functional syntactic level. Lexical assignments to structure at that level are the hypothesized locus of most word exchanges. The similarity factor assessed here, as for the meaning related word substitutions, was initial segment overlap. They reported a significant correspondence at word onset sites for the words in between phrase exchanges with matching grammatical category. Moreover, the similarity for the word and morpheme exchanges presumed to be characteristic of the initial stages of sentence formulation did not differ in degree from the similarity observed for other word and morpheme exchanges that did not satisfy the disjoint phrase and matching grammatical category criteria – i.e., exchanges that would be assigned to a later level of processing at which phonological interpretations of the lexical content items would be more likely to be available. Several observations are relevant to our evaluation of the implications of these findings.

First, we must consider some contrasting results in the analysis of the Spanish error corpus by del Viso/Igoa/Garcia-Albea. They examined the same question Dell and Reich raised about relations between word exchange elements but detected no evidence of segmental similarity for the two words at all – not even a trend. Nor was there any effect observed for the variables they used to supplement their analysis – stress and length variables. These latter, it will be recalled showed an elevated incidence in semantic word substitutions. In brief, no hint of form similarity was detected. The reason for the language difference is unclear at present. The phonological similarity effects at issue are not large and the observation base still somewhat limited, especially given the variability inherent in the data being relied on, so the possibility of sampling error cannot be dismissed for any of the analyses. Neither can we ignore the possibility of actual differences in the processing systems that reflect the structural differences in the languages. This matter must be left open.

A finding of phonological influences on exchange errors requires explanation, and may indicate that networklike processes are at work. Note, however, that such an effect does not compromise the original points of contrast between the word and sound exchange errors. The segmental similarity effects under discussion are not of the same order as those observable for the processes in which phonological form is clearly the target of the processing operations. Moreover, the distributional evidence that indicates a distinction between syntactic and phonological processing systems remains. It is a correlated claim for absence of phonological representations at the early syntactic processing level that is at question. In addressing this kind of issue, there is an important distinction to be borne in mind. That distinction is between performance effects that reflect the structural organization of a processing system and those that may reflect detailed features of the mechanisms that implement its structural organization and associated computations. Dell's (1986) modeling of the phonological effects on meaning based and syntactic errors preserves this distinction in its identification of interactive effects with connectivity in a network processor for lexical structure that feeds independent systems responsible for integration of sentence form.

4.2. Lexical and Syntactic Integration

Several additional experimental findings need consideration at this point. These provide another perspective on the relation of lexical retrieval processes to phrasal construction, and thereby on the interpretation we have considered for the data from speech errors.

Consider first some additional work by Bock. She has addressed these issues in a number of experiments. For example, she used the picture description task described in section 1 to compare the influence of conceptual and phonological variables on sentence form (Bock 1986 a). The pictures that are the targets for description were preceded by a prime word that was either phonologically related or semantically related to one of the nouns required to label objects or participants in the depicted events. The two classes of primes produced different effects: Semantically primed nouns were more likely to surface as sentence subjects than unprimed nouns, and there were corresponding shifts between active and passive voice as a function of roles for pictured objects that the prime words referred to; phonological primes did not produce a similar effect. Two questions suggest themselves: first, what produces the semantic priming effects, and second, why were the phonological primes not effective?

Bock related the semantic priming result to the way in which phrasal schemata are recruited by relevant semantic functions. On her account, conceptual factors associated with thematic roles (e. g., agent, patient) effect the ultimate assignment of lexical items to surface grammatical roles (e. g., subject, direct object). Conceptual accessibility can thus determine which (appropriate) argument is assigned to the subject role – the more highly activated an item, the quicker it is linked to a surface role in the structure. This view is also supported in a report by Bock/Warren (1985) of canges in grammatical role assignments for NP's differing in conceptual accessibility – in this case, indexed by their imagery value. In a recall task, more accessible nouns shifted to subject roles. Similar findings – with prototypicality as the test vehicle – were reported by Kelly/Bock/Keil (1986). See Bock (1987 a) for further discussion.

A way to look at the question about phonological primes is in terms of differences between the availability of representations for picture contents when conceptually driven and when driven by lexical form. The availability of word forms affects sentence processes at a point when the factors that determine phrasal configuration have already been determined. Thus, a significant impact of semantic primes on alternations of sentence form in the absence of similar consequence for phonological primes may be understood in terms of the point in sentence formulation at which the two types of description are relevant. This account fits the general picture suggested by speech error analysis.

There are, however, circumstances in which the availability of word forms does have an impact on sentence form, and these effects must connect to those just cited. Levelt/Maassen (1981) used a task in which speakers described two moving figures in simple visual arrays. Restrictions were imposed on the type of syntactic construction permitted for descriptions; time to initiate utterance was measured. By independent pre-test, they determined response latencies for naming the figures used in the arrays, and compared these to utterance order for nouns in the array descriptions to determine if variations in the availability of the lexical items affected order of mention. Though there was an effect of lexical accessibility (in onset time to utterance), there was no consequence for order of mention of the terms in the various conjuncts tested. Levelt and Maassen interpreted this to show that the ordering of sentence contents at *M* occurs independently of lexical search. However, there was evidence that lexical accessibility affected choice of syntactic frames. In a follow on experiment, subjects were permitted alternative syntactic forms for their descriptions, and shifts from NP conjuncts to sentence conjuncts occurred when less accessible forms were used, suggesting that lexical accessibility may affect the choice of surface syntactic form. Bock (1987 a) reports a similar effect in another phonological priming experiment. Similarities between prime and target words were much stronger than in the previously cited experiment; here, priming effects were inhibitory – a primed word tended to come later in the picture descriptions, and there were concomitant shifts in active/passive use. For both the Levelt and Maassen and the Bock experiment, effects on fluency were observed: more nonfluencies and longer time to utterance initiation when a less accessible target word was about to be used. These syntactic variations seem most naturally characterized as 'failure triggered' switches in form, rather than effects of word form retrieval on syntactic planning. Such a construal fits both the nonfluency effects and the form switches. When a first ordered form is unavailable, and phonological integration of its constituent phrase accordingly delayed, there is a switch to an expression that uses an available lexical form. On this point, note that Levelt/Maassen (1981) found an increase in utterance duration just prior to switches between alternate sentence forms.

The preceding discussion assumes that when variations in sentence form observed in these experiments are direct, they are based on conceptual accessibility, and that when such variation is observed in response to lexical accessibility, the impact on sentence formulation is indirect – i.e., a late switch to an alternative formulation. Two observations follow. First, this analysis is compatible with the kind of architecture derivable from the speech error analysis, and more specifically, with the model outlined in art. 1. Second, an implication of this interpretation is that some form of parallelism may be part of the processing scheme. The non-fluency observed in connection with switches in form raises the possibility that it may not be true parallel processing in which more than a single full form is routinely readied, but more a 'fast recovery' that repairs difficulty by reassembly of already developed substructures. Is a significant parallelism representative of normal production processes? Evidence that we consider next indicates that it is, and we will conclude our review of interpretations of the speech error data with a short discussion of that evidence.

4.3. Parallel Processes in Sentence Construction: Blend Errors

Parallelism requires simultaneous, multiple representations at one or more of the processes intervening between conceptual activity and articulation. In one respect, this condition clearly obtains. If we accept the reality of more than a single train of thought, the stage is set for two *M* level representations to coexist, only one of which is meant for expression. Further, our ability to adjust expression, in apparent real time, to accommodate stylistic variation suggests coexistence of multiple sentence level representations. Such editorial work could be a pseudo-parallelism, of course, with alternatives computed serially. However, a particular error phenomenon – blending – argues for a parallelism internal to the sentence construction system.

Blends come in both lexical (e.g., 25, 26) and phrasal (e.g. 27, 28) varieties. Word blends differ from word substitutions in an essential feature. They hold between items that are equally acceptable as candidates for a given phrasal slot (i.e., they preserve intended truth value; word substitutions do not). Phrasal blends show the same meaning constraint as word blends: They reflect competition between two ways to say the same thing.

(25) "You'll never evoid that ..." [evade/avoid]

(26) "Ich muss meine Liste noch verweitern." [vergrössern/erweitern; Bierwisch 1971]

(27) "It doesn't care ..., no ..., I don't matter." Successive blends: [I don't care] and [It doesn't matter]

(28) "Für mich kommt es ähnlich vor." [Für mich ist das ähnlich/Mir kommt das ähnlich vor]

Butterworth's discussion of blend errors (1982) distinguishes 'plan internal' errors, 'alternative plan' errors (those with equivalent meanings), and 'competing plan' errors (those with different meanings). He observes that theories of error processes focused on plan internal errors do not provide a satisfactory account of alternative plan errors; some form of parallelism is required. Blends do seem to be alternative plan errors – an interaction between distinct encodings of a given message rather than an interaction between distinct elements in a single encoding of a message. To describe them, two or more higher order representations must be assumed. Another important feature of blends is that they show influences from distinct levels of processing activity. Both word (MacKay 1972; Dell/Reich 1981) and phrasal (Fay 1982) blends show effects of syntactic and phonological similarity as well as semantic equivalence. This has sometimes been taken as an indication of interactive processing. Such a conclusion is not forced. The presence of different types of constraint can readily be explained by assuming that meaning equivalence is required to initiate parallel encodings, but form similarity is a condition on path blending (rather than pruning).

Blends are alternative plan errors in Butterworth's terminology and they make the primary point for current purposes. But the competing plans case must also be mentioned – those errors that represent a train of thought not intended for utterance. The processing implication is different for alternative and competing plans since alternative plans do not require distinct representations at *M*; competing plans do. There are certainly instances in which error seems to be linked to thought trains outside the intended message – Freud's (1904) accounts of error are the most obvious example. Harley (1984) discusses other relevant cases that he terms 'cognitive intrusions' and the error category of 'environmental contaminants' mentioned in section 3 is also representative.

Cognitive and environmental intrusions demonstrate that some aspect of the message system can be engaged by more than one conceptual input, and the blends demonstrate a capacity to entertain more than a single phrasal or lexical encoding for a given message. Sophisticated editorial functions will be required to control competing lines of processing activity thereby attested. Baars (1980) has argued that failure to control such competition accounts for most speech errors. Whatever the merits of that general perspective, it is worth noting that the devices in question are relevant to more than the phenomena of speech error. Ultimately, they may also provide an account of our capability to control the stylistic and functional conventions of our language and to adjust our expression in real time to the changing demands of natural communicative settings.

5. References

Aitchison, J. & Straf, M. (1982). Lexical storage and retrieval: A developing skill? In A. Cutler (Ed.), *Slips of the Tongue. 197–241.* Amsterdam: Mouton.

Baars, B. J. (1980). The competing plans hypothesis. A heuristic viewpoint on the causes of errors in speech. In H. Dechert & M. Raupach (Eds.), *Temporal Variables in Speech. 39–49.* The Hague/Paris/New York: Mouton.

Baars, B., Motley, M., & MacKay, D. (1975). Output editing for lexical status from artificially elicited slips of the tongue. *Journal of Verbal Learning and Verbal Behavior, 14*, 382–391.

Berg, Th. (1985). Is voice de suprasegmental? *Linguistics, 23*, 883–915.

Bierwisch, M. (1982). Linguistics and language error. In A. Cutler (Ed.), *Slips of the Tongue. 29–72.* Amsterdam: Mouton.

Bock, J. K. (1986 a). Meaning, sound and syntax: Lexical priming in language production. *Journal of Experimental Psychology: Learning, Memory, and Cognition, 12*, 575–586.

Bock, J. K. (1986 b). Syntactic persistence in language production. *Cognitive Psychology, 18*, 355–387.

Bock, J. K. (1987 a). An effect of the accessibilty of word forms on sentence structures. *Journal of Memory and Language, 26*, 119–137.

Bock, J. K. (1987 b). Coordinating words and syntax in speech plans. In A. Ellis (Ed.), *Progress in the Psychology of Language. Vol. 3. 337–390.* London: Erlbaum.

Bock, J. K. (1989). Closed class immanence in sentence production. *Cognition, 31*, 163–186.

Bock, J. K. (1990). Structure in language: Creating form in talk. *American Psychologist, 45,* 1221–1236.

Bock, J. K. & Loebell, H. (1990) Framing sentences. *Cognition, 35*, 1–39.

Bock, J. K., Loebell, H., & Morey, R. (1992). From conceptual roles to syntactic relations: Bridging the syntactic cleft: *Psychological Review, 99*, 150–171.

Bock, J. K. & Miller, C. (1991). Broken agreement. *Cognitive Psychology, 23*, 45–93.

Bock, J. K. & Warren, R. K. (1985). Conceptual accessibility and syntactic structure in sentence formulation. *Cognition*, 21, 47–67.

Boomer, D. & Laver J. (1968). Slips of the tongue. *British J. of Disorders of Communication, 3*, 2–12.

Brown R. & McNeill, D. (1966). The tip of the tongue phenomenon. *Journal of Verbal Learning and Verbal Behavior, 5*, 325–337.

Browman, C. (1978). Tip of the tongue and slip of the ear: Implications for. language processing. *UCLS Working Papers in Phonetic, No. 42.*

Buckingham, H. (1979). Linguistic aspects of lexical retrieval disturbances in the posterior fluent aphasias. In H. Whitaker & H. A. Whitaker (Eds.), *Studies in Neurolinguistics, Vol. 4. 269–291.* New Nork: Academic Press.

Butterworth, B. (1979). Hesitation and the production of verbal paraphasias and neologisms in jargon aphasia. *Brain and Language, 8*, 133–61.

Butterworth, B. (1980). Some constraints on models of language production. In B. Butterworth (Ed.), *Language Production: Vol 1. Speech and Talk* 423–459. London: Academic Press.

Butterworth, B. (1982). Speech errors: Old data in search of new theories. In A. Cutler (Ed.), *Slips of the Tongue and Language Production. 73–108.* Amsterdam: Mouton.

Caldognetto, E., Tonelli, L. (1985). Syllabic constraints on phonological speech errors in Italian.

In W. Dressler & L. Tonelli (Eds.), *Natural Phonology from Eisenstadt. 73–88.* Padova: CSLEP.

Caldognetto, E., Tonelli, L., K. Vagges & P. Cosi (1987). The organization of constraints on phonological speech errors. *In Proceedings of the XIth International Congress of Phonetic Sciences, Tallinn, U.S.S.R. Vol. 3. 50.4.1–50.4.4.*

Crompton, A. (1982). Syllables and segments in speech production. In A. Cutler (Ed.), *Slips of the Tongue and Language Production. 663–716.* Amsterdam: Mouton.

Cutler, A. (1980). Errors of stress and intonation. In V. Fromkin (Ed.), *Errors in Linguistic Performance. 67–80.* New York: Academic Press.

Cutler, A. (1982). The reliability of speech error data. In A. Cutler (Ed.), *Slips of the Tongue and Language Production. 7–28.* Amsterdam: Mouton.

Cutler, A. (1983). Lexical complexity and sentence processing. In G. B. Flores d'Arcais & J. R. Jarvella (Eds.), *The Process of Language Understanding. 43–79.* Chichester: Wiley.

Cutler, A. & Fay, D. (1982). One mental lexicon, Phonologically arranged: Comments on Hurford's comments. *Linguistc Inquiry, 13, 1,* 107–113.

del Viso, S., Igoa, J. & Garcia-Albea, J. (1990). Mechanisms of phonological encoding: Evidence from slips of the tongue in Spanish. Paper presented at the 3rd Annual CUNY Conference Human Sentence Processing, New York, NY.

Dell, G. (1984). Representation of serial order in speech: Evidence from the repeated phoneme effect in speech errors. *Journal of Experimental Psychology: Learning, Memory, and Cognition, 10,* 222–233.

Dell, G. (1986). A spreading activation theory of retrieval in sentence production. *Psychological Review, 93,* 283–321.

Dell, G. (1991). Effects of frequency and vocabulary type on phonological speech errors. *Language and Cognitive Processes, 5,* 313–349.

Dell, G. & Reich, P. (1981). Stages in sentence production: An analysis of speech error data. *Journal of Verbal Learning and Verbal Behavior, 20,* 611–629.

Fay, D. (1982). Substitutions and splices: A study of sentence blends. In A. Cutler (Ed.), *Slips of the Tongue and Language Production. 163–195.* Amsterdam: Mouton.

Fay, D. & Cutler, A. (1977). Malapropisms and the structure of the mental lexicon. *Linguistic Inquiry, 8,* 505–520.

Ford, M. (1982). Sentence planning units: Implications for the speaker's representation of meaningful relations underlyind sentences. In J. Bresnan (Ed.), *The Mental Representation of Grammatical Relations. 785–851.* Cambridge, MA: MIT Press.

Freud, S. (1904). *Zur Psychopathologie des Alltagslebens.* Frankfurt/M.: Fischer, new ed. 1954.

Fromkin, V. (1971). The non-anomalous nature of anomalous utterances. *Language, 47,* 27–52.

Garica-Albea, J., del Viso, S. & Igoa, J. (1988). Movement errors and levels of processing in sentence processing. Paper presented at 1st Annual CUNY Conference on Human Sentence Processing, New York, NY.

Garrett, M. F. (1975). The analysis of sentence production. In: G. Bower (Ed.), *The Psychology of Learning and Motivation: Advances in Research and Theory,* vol. 9. *133–177.* New York: Academic Press.

Garrett, M. F. (1976). Syntactic processes in sentence production. In R. Wales & E. Walker (Eds.), *New Approaches to Language Mechanisms. 231–256.* Amsterdam: North Holland Press.

Garrett, M. F. (1978). Word and sentence perception. In R. Held, H.-L. Teuber & H. Leibowicz (Eds.), *Handbook of Sensory Physiology, Vol. VIII: Perception. 611–625.* New York/Heidelberg: Springer.

Garrett, M. F. (1980). Levels of processing in sentence production. In B. Butterworth (Ed.), *Language Production: Vol. 1. Speech and Talk. 177–220.* London: Academic Press.

Garrett, M. F. (1982). Production of speech: Observations from normal and pathological language use. In A. Ellis (Ed.), *Normality and Pathology in Cognitive Functions. 19–76.* London: Academic Press.

Garrett, M. F. (1988). Processes in Language Production. In F. Newmeyer (Ed.), *Linguistics: The Cambridge Survey. Vol. III Language: Psychological and Biological Aspects. 69–96.* New York: Cambridge University Press.

Garrett, M. F. (1992 a). Lexical retrieval processes: Semantic field effects. In E. Kittay & A. Leherer (Eds.), *Frames, Fields and Contrasts.* Hillsdale, NJ: Erlbaum.

Garrett, M. F. (1992 b). Disorders of lexical selection. In. W. J. M. Levelt (Ed.), *Lexical Access in Speech Production: Special issue of Cognition, 42,* 143–180.

Harley, T. (1984). A critique of top-down independent levels models of speech production. Evidence from non-plan-internal speech errors. *Cognitive Science, 8,* 191–219.

Holmes, V. M. (1988). Hesitation and sentence planning. *Language and Cognitive Processes, 3,* 323–361.

Hurford, J. R. (1981). Malapropisms, left-to-right listing, and lexicalism. *Linguistic Inquiry, 12,* 419–423.

Kelly, M., Bock, K. & Keil, F. (1986). Prototypicality in a linguistic context: Effects on sentence structure. *Journal of Memory and Language, 25,* 59–74.

Kempen, G., Huijbers, P. (1983). The lexicalization process in lexicalization and naming: Indirect election of words. *Cognition, 14*, 185–209.

LaPointe, S. & Dell, G. (1989). A synthesis of some recent work in language production. In G. Carlson & M. Tannenhaus (Eds.), *Linguistic Structure and Language Processing. 107–156.* Dordrecht: Kluwer.

Levelt, W. J. M. (1983). Monitoring and self-repair in speech. *Cognition, 14*, 41–104.

Levelt, W. J. M. (1989). *Speaking: From Intention to Articulation.* Cambridge, MA: MIT Press.

Levelt, W. J. M. & Maassen, B. (1981). Lexical search and order of mention in sentence production. In W. Klein & W. J. M. Levelt (Eds.), *Crossing the Boundaries in Linguistics: Studies Presented to Manfred Bierwisch. 221–252.* Dordrecht: Reidel.

Martin, N., Weissberg, R. & Saffran, E. (1989). Variables influencing the occurrence of naming errors: Implications for models of lexical retrieval. *Journal of Memory and Language, 28*, 462–485.

MacKay, D. G. (1970). Spoonerisms: The structure of error in the serial order of speech. *Neuropsychologia, 8*, 323–350.

MacKay, D. G. (1972). The structure of words and syllables: Evidence from errors in speech. *Cognitive Psychology, 3*, 210–227.

Mowrey, R. A. & MacKay, I. R. A. (1990). Phonological primitives: electro-myographic speech error evidence. *The Journal of the Acoustical Society of America, 88 (3)*, 1299–1313.

Nooteboom, S. (1969). The tongue slips into patterns. In A. Sciarone, A. van Essen & A. Van Raad (Eds.), *Leyden Studies in Linguistics and Phonetics. 114–132.* The Hague: Morton.

Meringer, R. (1908). *Aus dem Leben der Sprache.* Berlin: Behr's.

Schriefers, H., Meyer, A. & Levelt, W. (1990). Exploring the time course of lexical access in language production: Picture-word interference studies. *Journal of Memory and Language, 29*, 86–102.

Shattuck-Hufnagel, S. (1979). Speech errors as evidence for a serial order mechanism in sentence production. In W. Cooper & E. Walker (Eds.), *Sentence Processing. 295–342.* Hillsdale, NJ: Erlbaum.

Shattuck-Hufnagel, S. (1983). Sublexical units and suprasegmental structure in speech production planning. In P. MacNeilage (Ed.), *The Production of Speech. 109–136.* New York: Springer.

Shattuck-Hufnagel, S. (1985). Context similarity constraints on segmental speech errors: An experimental investigation of the role of word position and lexical stress. In J. Lauter (Ed.), *On the Planning and Production of Speech in Normal and Hearing Impaired Individuals: A Seminar in Honor of S. Richard Silverman. ASHA Reports, 15.*

Shattuck-Hufnagel, S. (1987). The role of word-onset consonants in speech production planning: New evidence from speech error patterns. In E. Kellar & M. Gopnik (Eds.), *Motor and Sensory Processing in Language. 17–51.* Hillsdale, NJ: Erlbaum.

Shattuck-Hufnagel, S. & Klatt, D. H. (1979). The limited use of distinctive features and markedness in speech production. *Journal of Verbal Learning and Verbal Behavior, 18*, 41–55.

Stemberger, J. (1984). Length as a suprasegmental: Evidence from speech errors. *Language, 60*, 895–913.

Stemberger, J. (1985). An interactive activation model of language production. In A. Ellis (Ed.), *Progress in the Psychology of Language, Vol 1. 143–186.* London: Erlbaum.

Stemberger, J. (1990). Wordshape errors in language production. *Cognition, 35*, 123–157.

Merrill F. Garrett, Tucson, Arizona (USA)

8. Disordered Language in Creative Writing

1. Introduction

In his 'Reflections on Language', Chomsky (1976) writes:

"Creativity is predicated on a system of rules and forms, in part determined by intrinsic human capacities. Without such constraints, we have arbitrary and random behavior, not creative acts."

As Chomsky has always emphasized, there is one sense of the term 'creative' in which all normal use of language is creative. The attack on behaviourist analyses of language performance (Chomsky 1959) was predicated upon the observation that (almost) no instance of normal langunge-use is a 'stimulus-occasioned' act in the technical sense of that expression. Each sentence is, as it were, freshly coined to express a thought appropriate to, but not determined by, the context of situation. The Cartesian tradition and German romanticism converged in placing the utmost stress upon this distinction between human language and the restricted, stimulus-bound repertoires of both the 'speaking machines' of the automata makers and the 'communicative signs' employed by animals other than ourselves (Chomsky 1966).

In this sense, to speak in clichés is itself a pathology of language. To command only a small repertoire of 'verbal responses', each evoked by a well-defined class of stimuli is a sign of either developmental or acquired language disorder. Broca's patient Lelong, who replied "Tois" (trois) to all questions that demanded a numerical answer illustrates the point in extreme form (Broca 1861).

'Formulaic' speech (from conventional greetings to swearing) constitutes a minute fraction of any normal user's repertoire. Such "ready made" (Jackson 1874) speech may even have a right hemisphere source (van Lancker 1987). That is, it may be programmed from a biological substrate that is not specialized for the normal, free, 'creative' use of language. The point was initially made by Jackson (1874) who noted the (unintended) humour that can arise from the combination of 'propositional' and 'automatic' speech. His most famous example concerns "the Communist orator" who "began his oration 'Thank God, I am an Atheist'."

Had Jackson's speaker intended to make an argument (about theological predeterminism, for example) from his choice of words, the discussion would have moved to a second sense of 'creativity': rule-breaking creativity. This notion, which ranges all the way from simple-minded puns (a newspaper article on fashions in child-rearing entitled "Spock the difference") to the linguistic plurabelleties of 'Finnegans Wake', is the topic of the following sections.

2. Rule-Breaking

Although normal rule-governed creativity draws upon 'rules' that are 'automatically' obeyed, rule-breaking creativity must meet three (related) criteria that go considerably beyond the mere malfunctioning of a rule-system: The 'error' must be produced by intent on the part of the writer; both writer and reader should recognize the 'error' and know the 'correct' form; the writer (and preferably the reader also) must recognize the point of the 'error'. In short, such 'errors' made in full 'conscious' awareness of their deviance are not errors.

Consider, for example, the selection restriction on the lexical items that can appear in the slot A __ AGO. Those items must be either specific temporal nouns (minute, month, century etc.) or noun phrases (very long time, short while, etc.). Our corpus of aphasic language in which we attempted to elicit these expressions includes such errors as: "a big ... ago", "a long ago", and "a message ago". The full eliciting context was HE LEFT A __ AGO, and the patients' task was to fill in the blank (either orally or in writing).

No patient produced a response as deviant as "a grief ago", an example from Dylan Thomas, discussed in Chomsky (1961). But Thomas' semi-grammatical phrase depends for its effect precisely upon using "grief" as if it were an ordinary temporal noun. The expression derives its power from the brevity attendant upon this particular way of forcing the reader to reclassify the lexical features of "grief" to make the word compatible with the selection restrictions of the frame. The same poetic force does not reside in the (prosaic but fully grammatical) expressions that would convey Thomas' meaning: 'In a state of grief, subjective time can appear to pass very slowly', or 'Although she died a year ago, it seems like only yesterday.' "A grief ago" is compatible with either interpretation (or both); only the rest of the poem can specify.

Not all examples of intentional rule-breaking have the depth of true poetry; on occasion catchy cleverness will suffice. Some years ago, the advertising hoardings displayed the ungrammatical sentence:

"The birds is coming."

Fans of Alfred Hitchcock had no difficulty in interpreting the message as its well-formed variant:

"'The Birds' is coming".

But the ungrammatical form was no doubt more eye-catching and memorable. Superficially equivalent examples of failure of number agreement in aphasia ("The children is playing") may be equally striking to the examiner but express no communicative intent specific to the form of error.

By contrast, the finest examples of deviance are those that achieve a perfect match of form and meaning. When Arthur Rimbaud wanted to convey that his multiple potentialities and personalities had destroyed the Cartesian unity of his 'self', he wrote:

"Je est un autre."

It is difficult to imagine a more succinct expression of alienation. Rimbaud as artist retains full control of the language whatever fragmentation of personality Rimbaud the man may suffer (or 'pretend' to suffer in his poetic persona).

Creative rule-breaking in the above sense can extend all the way from spelling to narrative structure. The one word (or nonword) title of Samuel Beckett's poem on the life and times of René Descartes manages to incorporate three of the work's themes: Descartes' argument with William Harvey ("dear blood-swirling Harvey"); his opinion of his employer, Christina, Queen of Sweden, who demanded tutorials in bed at five a. m.; his unwillingness to divulge his date of birth lest some astrologer attempt to predict his fate. The title is, of course, WHOROSCOPE.

The closest approximation we can find in our records of aphasic subjects is a woman with a mild dysgraphia who we asked to write "horoscope" to dictation. She wrote HORRORSCOPE, looked intently at her response for a few seconds and then remarked: "I hope it's not going to be that bad." (We will return to this pattern of recognized error later).

At the level of text, convention demands that anaphoric reference be clear, a condition that can usually be met by introducing the full referring phrase (e. g. "Joseph K") before the corresponding anaphoric pronoun ("he"). Although there are within-sentence conditions under which the order can be reversed ("After he had shaved, Joseph dressed"), this order is either incomprehensible or misleading when the context is expressed in two sentences ("He shaved. Then Joseph left").

Here is an anomic patient recounting the story of *Cinderella*.

"They all wanted to marry him. She couldn't go to the ... go dancing. They were ugly but she was beautiful and he was very handsome. It turned into a pear ... no ...."

Although the disorganization extends considerably beyond a lack of specific noun phrases, the reader is not exactly helped by all the antecedentless pronouns.

A superficially similar pattern is seen in the opening paragraphs of John Le Carré's 'A Small Town of Germany'. The text is littered with *he's* and *they's* that have no priorly-introduced full noun phrases. The point, however (as befits a good spy novel), is that the characters do not know at this point who is following whom. Since the traditional narrator, the unseen but omniscient author, has removed himself from the text, the reader is left as confused as the characters. The reader accordingly e x p e r i e n c e s the character's disorientation in consequence of a stylistic device that is rather more subtle than being overtly informed of that dislocation. When, some pages later, the reader is given the relevant information, it must be integrated with the opening passages by the puzzle-solving faculty, and not by linguistic rule.

3. Chance and Choice

'Modernism', that is, the literary experimentation of the late nineteenth and early twentieth century, was in part an exploration of how far language could be pushed before a complete breakdown of linguistic communication would occur.

The poets could initially rely upon closed-class items to mark the syntactic structure of neologisms (Bratley/Dakin 1967):

"Twas brillig, and the slithy toves
Did gyre and gimble in the wabe."

And even when those cues were removed, metre and rhyme still sufficed to impose strict form on what might otherwise appear to be jargon aphasia. Christian Morgenstern's 'The Great Lalula' must be read aloud before its very traditional beauty can be appreciated:

"Kroklokwafzi? Semememi!
Seiokrontro – prafriplo:
Bifzi, bafzi; hulalemi:
Quasti basti bo ...
Lalu lalu lalu lalu la! [...]"

By contrast, the protest poets who recited the following line in Zurich cafés in 1915 did so in a monotone:

"bevordadadawarwardadada."

But they could rely upon the literacy of their audience to provide the correct parsing:

"Bevor Dada da war, war Dada da."
(Before Dada was there, was Dada there).

The real problems arose when prose (or 'free' verse) was subjected to a drastic removal of normal syntactic and/or semantic constraints. Consider the following seven passages:

1: This long time when he did this best time, and he could thus have been bound, and in this long time, when he could be this to first use of this long time ...

2: We all know the significance of the issue in respect of payment we respectfully speak to them for ten bottles of brown ale ...
3: There is coagulation in cold and there is none in prudence ...
4: When dogs cross the air in a diamond like ideas and the appendix of the meninx tells the time of the alarm programme ...
5: The gun – don't know what's the matter with him, dreadfully dreadfully done on drum ...
6: Yellow which but honest milk the showed years the cheezes markets scant complexity all the odour not of gold on soft to believes ...
7: It being, you know, there all for all insurance policies being, insurance policies being, insurance policies being, a very good investment, death being inevitable ... .

One of these passages is a fifth order statistical approximation to English, contained in Morton (1964); one is from a novel by Gertrude Stein ('Tender Buttons'); one is a piece of 'automatic writing', produced in a 'quasi-trance' state by Miss Stein, reported in Solomons/Stein (1896) and discussed by Skinner (1961); one is a Dadaist poem by Tristan Tzara (1977) that he claims to have constructed by taking a newspaper article, cutting out the words, shaking them in a bag, and then transcribing them one at a time. One passage was actually constructed in this fashion (by us). One passage is an example of jargon aphasia after left hemisphere stroke (Rochford 1974), and one was produced by a schizophrenic patient with auditory hallucinations and paranoid delusions (Hoffman/Sledge 1984).

Critiques of 'modernism' have usually claimed that 'advanced' writing, once described as 'experimental', has gone a step (or more) too far. Writing by 'free association' has tilted the creative balance between chance and choice too far in the direction of chance. In consequence, the claim unfolds, the distinction between genuine creative writing and the quasi-random productions of (some) aphasics and madmen has been obliterated; the reader is presented with the verbal equivalent of a Rorschach ink-blot and left to make of it what he or she will.

The purported upshot is that the reader will be unable to distinguish the sources of the seven texts we have quoted. We are accordingly inclined to leave this as an exercise for the reader, but will provide some hints. The passage that was truly constructed by random choice of words from a newspaper article is (rather obviously) number six. Tzara *must* have been cheating when he claimed to be making Dada poems by this method and this method *alone*. All the remaining passages contain far too much structure (albeit of varying natures) to reflect the operation of chance without choice.

In matters of aesthetic evaluation the issue is not how texts are generated; it is rather how the final (published) version is selected. As the old story goes, granted unlimited time, typewriters, and monkeys, the complete works of Shakespeare could be produced by random processes. Whether anyone other than William Shakespeare could have selected 'The Tempest' from the morass is the real question. We observe likewise that examples of jargon aphasia or schizophrenic language that resemble modernist texts are *selected* for that resemblance.

It is told that Rav Shimshon of Ostropol wrote a *complete* kabbalistic commentary on the Talmud. Upon consulting the spirits in his dreams for their evaluation of his work he was informed that it was too long. Rav Shimshon pruned the work, reconsulted the spirits and was told it was too obscure. After many more recursive procedures of this nature, the good Rabbi ended up with the text of 'Perush Rashi', the standard commentary on the Talmud written some centuries earlier. Who knows but that Rashi did not write his commentary by the same method? Jorge Luis Borges tells an illuminating variant of this parable in his short story 'Pierre Menard, author of the Quixote'.

When Skinner (1961) writes: "The mere generation of the effects of repetition and surprise is not in itself a literary achievement", he is undoubtely correct. But as we have indicated, the issue is which surprises and repetitions an author chooses to leave in the final text. With respect to repetition, consider the following three brief passages:

1: A rose is a rose is a rose.
2: My sister, my sister, my sister had a holiday in Sweden.
3: We bought a ca, ca, car (laughs). Car. Just one!

The first sentence is Gertrude Stein's most famous line. We have no idea how she produced it, but in the context of her other writings the line bears a very explicit meaning. It is part of her attack upon what she regarded as overblown 'patriarchal poetry'. The tendency of male poets to produce such lines as "O, my Luve's like a red red rose", "A rose-red city half as old as time" or "Each Morn a thousand Roses brings" was regarded by Miss Stein as sheer sentimental indulgence. And who is to say that she is wrong? We do, however, note that the 'quotation' is wrong. Just as 'Casablanca' does not contain the immortal line "Play it again, Sam", so Gertrude Stein never wrote the sentence everyone knows. What she did write (in 'Sacred Emily') was:

"Rose is a rose is a rose is a rose."

And this line enables her not only to state the tautology but also to parody the recipients of her attack.

The second line is an example of palilalia in a patient with Parkinson's disease (Marshall 1977). No communicative intent underlies the repetition. The third example was produced by a patient with mild Wernicke's aphasia. Although the 'stuttering' was unintentional, the joke arises from the fact that the patient herself could recognize the inappropriateness of her repetitions, and comment upon them in a highly appropriate fashion.

Some forms of creative writing show a similar interplay between accident and design. To describe 'Finnegans Wake' as an example of 'stream of consciousness' writing may contain a (small) measure of truth, as the "gossipaceous Anna Livia" would no doubt admit. But a five-hundred page novel in which the last sentence ("A way a lone a last a loved a long the") is the beginning of the first ("riverrun, past Eve and Adam's, from swerve of shore to bend of bay ...") surely reflects a larger measure of conscious artistic control.

It is an accident of English that a patient with deep dyslexia can read *slovenly* as "hot" (via *oven*), but the patient can make nothing from the accident. It is likewise an accident of French that "taire" is contained in "commentaire", but it is Edmond Jabès (in 'Le Livre des Questions') who notices that:

"In the night of 'commentary' (commentaire), there shines the proud verb 'to be silent' (taire)."

4. Form and Meaning

Bilingual and multilingual patients with language disorder are frequently observed to switch and mix languages; the classic sourcebook of cases is Paradis (1983). The cause is often a word-finding difficulty in one language where the expression is available in another. Here is a German/Czech bilingual who himself provides the correct explanation:

'Es fahlen mit die výrazý" (Paradis 1983, 685)

(I can't think of expressions).

In poets who can think of words in either language, the challenge of combining them has sometimes proved hard to resist. Here the young Rainer Maria Rilke (writing from "Mütterchen Prag") demonstrates his prowess in 'Der kleine Dratenik' (The little tinker):

" 'Nur einen Krajcar, nur einen
für ein Stück Brot, milost panku!' "
Da! – Und er stammelt mit Dank zu,
doch läßt nicht Ruh er den Beinen."

(" 'Just a penny, just one, for a bit of bread, Sir!' There! And he stammers his thanks as his legs jump up and down.")

Rilke continues to maintain rhyme and metre across the two languages for a few more verses, seemingly without effort (and therein lies the art.) Nonetheless, the poem remains an exercise in virtuosity; the linguistic mix per se adds little depth of feeling.

From another bilingual city (Montréal), Abraham Klein can control the equivalent technical skills (in free verse) and express thereby his joy in linguistic duplexity:

"Grand port of navigations, multiple
The lexicons uncargo'd at your quays,
Sonnant though strange to me; but chiefest, I,
Auditor of your music, cherish the
Jointed double-melodied vocabulaire
Where English vocable and roll Ecossic,
Mollified by the parle of French
Bilinguefact your air!"

Here form and meaning conspire to celebrate bilingualism.

Above all, it is James Joyce who, in 'Finnegans Wake', celebrates the language of Europe, from Dublin to Trieste (and beyond). The title does indeed refer to the wake held on the death of Finnegan, and marks his demise in (French) 'fin' and (Italian) 'fine'. But the title (and the book) also demand that the Finnegans awake (again). "Shem the Penman" points the way:

"Nomad may roam with Nabuch but let naaman laugh at Jordan! For we, we have taken our sheet upon her stones where we have hanged our hearts in her trees; and we list, as she bibs us by the waters of babalong."

Just as Joyce is an intrinsically polyglott writer, so Jabès, in a comparable passage, is dependent upon a specific language.

"Nomadism. The Name justifies the nomad."

Yes, but only in the French original, where 'The Name' is 'Le Nom'. But both writers are 'Freudians' in that their work seems to deny the very existence of accident in language and language-use. It is this Freudian turn that accounts, in part, for the (only seemingly) 'disordered' nature of much creative writing in the twentieth century:

"Out of the fog of the word 'to know' (savoir) looms the word 'to see' (voir), he said.
Knowing is essentially seeing" ('Le Livre des Questions').

5. References

Bratley, P. & Dakin, D. J. (1967). A limited dictionary for syntactic analysis. In D. Michie (Ed.), *Machine Intelligence 2*. Edinburgh: Oliver and Boyd.

Broca, P. (1861). Remarques sur le siège de la faculté de langage suivies d'une observation d'aphémie. *Bulletin de la Societé d'Anatomie, 6*, 330–357.

Chomsky, N. (1959). A review of B. F. Skinner's *Verbal Behavior. Language, 35*, 26–58.

Chomsky, N. (1961). Some methodological remarks on generative grammar. *Word, 17*, 219–239.

Chomsky, N. (1966). *Cartesian Linguistics*. New York: Harper and Row.

Chomsky, N. (1976). *Reflections on Language*. London: Temple Smith.

Hoffman, R. & Sledge, W. (1984). A microgenetic model of paragrammatisms produced by a schizophrenic speaker. *Brain and Language, 21*, 147–173.

Jackson, J. H. (1874). On the nature of the duality of the brain. *Medical Press and Circular, 1*, 19–63.

Marshall, J. C. (1977). Disorders in the expression of language. In J. Morton & J. C. Marshall (Eds.), *Psycholinguistics Series, Volume 1*. London: Elek.

Morton, J. (1964). A model for continuous language behavior. *Language and Speech, 7*, 40–70.

Paradis, M. (Ed.) (1983). *Readings on Aphasia in Bilinguals and Polyglots*. Montreal: Didier.

Rochford, G. (1974). Are jargon dysphasics dysphasic? *British Journal of Disorders of Communication, 9*, 35–44.

Skinner, B. F. (1961). *Cumulative Record*. London: Methuen.

Solomons, L. M. & Stein, G. (1896). Normal motor automatisms. *Psychological Review, 3*, 492–512.

Tzara, T. (1977). *Seven Dada Manifestos and Lampisteries*. London: John Calder.

Van Lancker, D. (1987). Nonpropositional speech: Neurolinguistic studies. In A. W. Ellis (Ed.), *Progress in the Psychology of Language*, Volume 3. 49–118. London: Lawrence Erlbaum.

John C. Marshall/Jennifer M. Gurd, Oxford (UK)

II. Acquired Organic Pathologies of Language Behavior: Neurolinguistic Disorders

9. Clinical Symptoms and Syndromes of Aphasia

1. Definition

The term *aphasia* denotes acquired disturbances of language processing resulting from brain damage. This attempt at a definition contains four crucial aspects, namely:
– aphasia is acquired,
– aphasia affects linguistic processes,
– other cognitive functions are relatively spared,
– aphasia is a consequence of brain damage.

The fact that aphasia is acquired distinguishes it from developmental language deficits, which occasionally have been termed "childhood aphasia" (e. g. Eisenson 1972). According to the above definition, the term "childhood aphasia" is restricted to those cases, in which brain damage resulted in aphasia after language had been acquired to some extent.

2. Epidemiology and Etiology

Aphasia is a common symptom of cerebral disease. Brust/Shafer/Richter/Bruun (1976) estimated 84000 new cases per year in the US. Only a minority of patients recover completely from their language deficit (21% – Kertesz/McCabe 1977; 25% – Brust/Shafer/Richter/Bruun 1976). The most frequent cause of aphasia is ischemic infarction in the territory of supply of the left middle cerebral artery, occurring in about 75% of aphasic patients (The figures vary because of differing criteria for case admission). Other causes, such as hemorrhages, tumor, trauma, cerebral infection, and circumscribed atrophic pathology account for the rest of the cases. Regardless of etiology, left hemisphere pathology is a far more frequent cause of aphasia than brain damage to the right hemisphere.

The reason for this imbalance between the cerebral hemispheres is the lateralization of higher mental functions in the brain. In almost all right handed people, the left hemisphere is dominant for language functions. A review of the neurophysiological aspects of lateralization in the human brain is given by Nass/Gazzaniga (1987).

3. Symptoms of Aphasia

The description of an aphasic patient's language performance is based on two types of observations. These are the analysis of the patients linguistic and communicative performance in a conversational situation, and a comparison of performance in the various modalities, such as repetition, writing to dictation, reading aloud, speech and script comprehension, oral and written naming.

3.1. Spontaneous Speech

Both in spontaneous productions and elicited utterances, symptoms of aphasia can be described and categorized according to the linguistic levels that are involved. The following discussion will focus upon the lexical/semantic, phonological, and syntactic levels and upon automatized speech elements. In addition, the fluency of speech production (Benson 1967; Kertesz 1979), the accuracy and speed of articulation, and prosodic features are usually included in the description of aphasic patients' productions.

3.1.1. Lexical/Semantic/Structure

This level includes word finding, word selection, word combination, and the differentiation of word meanings. Word finding difficulties are a feature of central importance in all types of aphasia, but also occur in normal speakers under conditions of fatigue and distraction and more often in more diffuse conditions such as dementia and disorders of consciousness. These difficulties may manifest themselves in hesitations and interruptions of speech flow, in the use of circumlocutory phrases or in the discontinuation of the phrase and subsequent pursuit of the topic in a different form.

The term 'semantic paraphasia' describes the incorrect use of a word. The proximity to the presumably intended target may be more or less close, and the term 'close semantic paraphasia' may be used to denote semantic relatedness (e. g. *wheels* for *bicycle*). In the course of speech, it may be difficult to decide which words are paraphasic, as in "It's kind of empty to mark these customers, too" (from Buckingham/Kertesz 1976). Productions containing semantic paraphasias to the extent that they are rendered incomprehensible are termed 'semantic jargon'.

Semantic violations may occur in compound words, e. g. the paraphasia *hair phone* for *comb*. For this type of error, the term 'semantic neologism' may be used. This terminology lends itself to confusion, as the unspecified terms 'neologism' and 'neologistic jargon' are frequently used synonymously for 'phonemic neologism' and 'phonemic jargon'.

3.1.2. Phonological Structure

This level describes the selection of phonemes and their sequencing in order to form the sound structures of words, but not their articulatory or phonatory realisation. In practice, a distinction between phonological and articulatory disturbances is sometimes difficult, especially with the frequent combination of Broca's aphasia, speech apraxia and dysarthria. The segmental sound structure of a word may be altered by the following types of errors: omission, substitution, the addition of individual phonemes and errors of sequence. These alterations are termed phonological or phonemic paraphasias. Apart from disturbances of phoneme selection, errors of sequence may occur as perseverations and anticipations. These latter types, which also occur in slips of the tongue of normal speakers, suggest that the phonemic structure or of a word or even a phrase is available as a whole during its realisation.

As phonemes are defined as those elements that distinguish between sound structures of different lexical meaning, phonological and lexical errors cannot always be distinguished in the single event.

In some types of aphasia, most notably conduction aphasia, the patient does attempt to correct his/her output, be it phonologically acceptable or not. Both the production of phonemic paraphasias and disturbances of output monitoring and correction may result in the behaviors of 'conduite d'approche' and 'conduite d'ecart' that denote the step by step approximation or digression from the intended target phonological structure: *a bursh ... bish ... b-rush ... bush ... bursh ... brush* (naming a brush).

Words that are phonemically so distorted that they do not resemble known word forms are termed "phonemic neologisms", and when the speech output is incomprehensible because of such neologisms, it is termed 'neologistic' or 'phonemic jargon". In phonemic jargon, function words may be preserved, although almost every content word is distorted (Buckingham/Kertesz 1976).

3.1.3. Syntactic Structure

Following Pick (1913) and Kleist (1934), syntactic errors in aphasia have been classified as 'agrammatic' and 'paragrammatic'. As stereotypies and speech automatisms may consist of well-formed phrases, only propositional utterances should be considered for the evaluation of syntactic impairment. Both types of errors, agrammatic and paragrammatic, denote deviations from the standard grammatical form required in syntactically connected productions. Unfortunately, little is known about grammatical norms in common colloquial speech. Therefore the diagnosis of agrammatic and paragrammatic errors in clinical practice depends on their frequency and their deviation from the subjective norm of the assesser.

In general, an error is agrammatic, when a necessary grammatical element is missing. The missing element could be an inflectional morpheme, a function word or an auxiliary or modal verb in a complex verb phrase. Tissot/Mounin/Lhermitte (1973) cite the following features of agrammatism:

- the deletion of function words in discourse,
- the predominance of nouns,
- the loss of verb inflection with substitution of infinite for finite forms,
- loss of agreement between person, number, and gender.

In mild cases, the patient may be able to apply grammar with some effort, but reduce this effort by using simple and/or stereotyped sentence frames, frequently consisting of SPO main clauses. In severe cases of agrammatism, the aphasic only has access to major grammatical categories – nouns, verbs, adjectives, and adverbs. Function words – prepositions, conjunctions, and pronouns – are strikingly rare in agrammatic language productions. However, not all function words and not all flection morphemes are affected. The conjunction *and* may be used abundantly, and – in English-speaking agrammatics – the present participle is frequently used in place of the conjugated verb.

In contrast to agrammatics, paragrammatics are able to apply grammatical rules. They inflect nouns and verbs and use function words, but their speech deviates from the grammatical norm. Paragrammatic patients also violate rules governing the sequential organization of the sentence structure and sentence termination. Typically, sentence structures are long and complex, with many subordinate and parenthetical clauses, but also with overlapping or blending of sentence structures (... *when I went to the doctor gave me an injection* ...). Also frequent is the multiple occurrence of the same constituent in different positions in a phrase (*not even in hospital they could not help* ...), but this type of violation is not unusual among normal speakers, too. Another type of paragrammatic error is the incorrect use of inflections and function words, which led to the interpretation of paragrammatism as "extended paraphasia" (Goodglass/Kaplan 1972).

It has been argued that agrammatism and paragrammatism are not mutually exclusive, i. e. the same patient may produce both agrammatic and paragrammatic errors, and that agrammatic speakers, when forced to inflect and use function words tend to produce paragrammatic errors (Heeschen 1985).

3.1.4. Automatic Speech Elements

This level focusses on utterances that frequently recur in a stereotypical manner and are produced by the patient contrary to his or her communicative intention (as assumed by the communication partner, Huber/Poeck/Weniger (1982). In aphasic patients, such utterances may be produced in the form of automatisms, echolalia, perseverations, and stereotypies (for definitions, see Table 9.1.). In conditions other than aphasia, palilalia and tics are repetitive speech phenomena that occur mainly in extrapyramidal disease.

From a clinical point of view, it is important to note that automatisms (with extremely rare exceptions, Leischner 1951) only occur in aphasia, whereas echolalia, perseveration, and stereotypy may also be characteristic of brain damage that does not result in aphasia (Kleist 1934; Wallesch 1990; 1991). A number of authors, most notably Luria (1970), viewed both perseveration and echolalia as characteristic of frontal lobe pathology and indicative of a pathological level of stimulus-boundness.

Haag/Huber/Hündgen/et al. (1985) drew attention to the presence of two different modes of production of perseveration and automatism. In the 'mode of disinhibition' the stereotyped utterance is produced instantly, thus possibly blocking access to target related productions, whereas in the 'mode of failure' the perseverate is uttered only after search for appropriate material has failed.

Alajouanine (1956) and Code (1982) identified two basic types of automatisms, those with an actual linguistic meaning ("real word recurrent utterances", Code 1982) and those without one ("non-meaningful recurrent utterances", Code 1982). In line with Hughlings Jackson (1879), Code (1989) views the former as holistically produced, non-propositional productions of right hemisphere speech mechanisms, and the latter as the product of a severely compromised left hemisphere phonological system.

3.2. Performance in Language Modalities

The Wernicke (1874) – Lichtheim (1885) model has influenced aphasiology ever since its construction (Fig. 9.1.), since it forms one of the foundations of early as well as modern aphasia tests. In this model, (spoken) language processing is performed by three interconnected components: a sensory speech center, a motor speech center, and a concept center. Other than the motor and sensory centers that have been equated by some autors (e. g. Lichtheim 1885; Geschwind 1984) with Broca's and Wernicke's areas, respectively, the concept center was not thought to be localized in a delimited brain area (Lichtheim 1885). Only the latter was supposed to be linked to other, e. g. visual, association centers.

In the Wernicke – Lichtheim model, the connection between the sensory and the motor speech center is used for repetition without semantic analysis, the one between sensory and concept center for language comprehension, and that between concept and motor speech center for productions that do not necessarily rely on the act of language comprehension, e.g. visual object naming. Consequently, the integrity of the three sides of the triangle can be investigated separately by the three tasks of repetition, naming, and comprehension. Vice versa, if the model corresponded to anatomical reality as was assumed for all its parts with the exception of the concept center, it should predict the existence of aphasia types with prominent dysfunction of the motor or sensory speech center, the pathways between the two and those from sensory to concept and from concept to motor center. The pathway lesions were of special interest, because for them the model would forecast dissociations between repetition and the other language modalities:

1) a type of aphasia with impaired repetition, but intact comprehension and naming (Fig. 9.1, lesion 1),
2) a type of aphasia with intact repetition and comprehension, but impaired naming (Fig. 9.1, lesion 2), and
3) a type of aphasia with intact repetition and naming, but impaired comprehension (Fig. 9.1, lesion 3).

Aphasia syndromes resembling the predicted types were in fact discovered and termed according to the model as
1) conduction aphasia,
2) transcortical motor aphasia, and
3) transcortical sensory aphasia.

In the Wernicke–Lichtheim and most other aphasia classification systems, the diagnosis of an aphasia syndrome is made on the basis

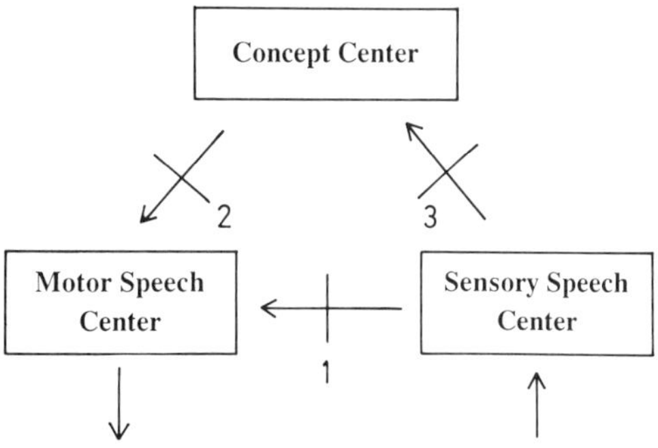

Fig. 9.1: The Wernicke-Lichtheim model. Hypothetical lesions:
1) resulting in conduction aphasia
2) resulting in transcortical motor aphasia
3) resulting in transcortical sensory aphasia

of associations and dissociations between symptoms. Whereas in this and related models, performances in naming, repetition, and comprehension are explained as two-stage cognitive processes, modern linguistic research has demonstrated that these are complex and multi-stage processes (see e.g. Caplan 1987).

The classic tasks included in aphasia tests: repetition, naming, auditory and script comprehension, writing to dictation, and sometimes written naming and script copying frequently allow more detailed observations of aphasic symptoms than conversational speech.

3.2.1. Naming

Table 9.2. summarizes error types and mechanisms in visual confrontation naming.

Echolalia:

"the automatic and compulsive repetition of words by the patient in the absence of the understanding of their meaning" (Brain 1965, 105); "repetition of the investigator's utterances with or without mild changes in position and choice of words" (Huber/Poeck/Weniger 1982)

Perseveration:

"the recurrence, out of context and in the absence of the original stimulus, of some behavioral act" (Buckingham/Whitaker/Whitaker 1979, 329)

Speech automatism:

"a constantly recurring utterance which is formally rigid, consists of neologistic sequences of syllables, interchangeable words or phrases, does not fit into the linguistic context either lexically or syntactically, and which the patient produces in contrast to the intention expected by his interlocutor" (Huber/Poeck/Weniger 1982, 81).

Table 9.1: Definitions of types repetitive verbal behavior occurring in aphasia

Type	Mechanism
delayed naming	slowed activation/selection of target lexical entry
self-correction	recognition of error; retrieval of target lexical entry
circumlocution	failure to retrieve specific lexical entry; conveys semantic information
phonemic paraphasia	error in phoneme selection and sequencing
semantic paraphasia	retrieval of lexical entry semantically related to target
malapropism	retrieval of lexical entry word-form related to target (Blanken 1990)
unrelated word	failure to gain access to appropriate semantic category/error in visual analysis (visually related paraphasia)
lexical neologism	combination of two lexical entries
phonemic neologism	extreme phoneme selection and sequencing error
perseveration	failure to inhibit a previous response
automatism	inhibition of response by production of automatism
gesture	compensation for failure to retrieve target
no response	

Table 9.2: Error types and error mechanisms in naming (based on Linebaugh 1990)

In comparison to the analysis of spontaneous speech, naming has the obvious advantage, that the lexical target is known to the investigator. Therefore, errors can be more easily classified and analyzed linguistically (see e. g. Morton 1985). Naming contains fewer degrees of freedom than conversational speech. Therefore, many aphasics may find naming a relatively easy task. Conversely, naming may expose impairments of lexical access and word form production in those patients, who are circumlocutory in spontaneous speech. Naming tasks are frequently employed for research purposes, e. g. when performance in the oral and written modality or across separate categories of the lexicon are investigated.

Visual confrontation naming is focally impaired in the conditions of visual agnosia and the so-called "optic aphasia" (Coslett/Saffran 1989). Briefly, in visual agnosia, the patient is unable to recognize an object seen or a picture of an object because of a disturbance of higher visual or visual-semantic functions. These patients would also be unable to indicate the use of an object seen by pantomime, but would be able to respond with the correct name to a specific noise or to a question. The term optic aphasia is used to describe a disconnection between the anatomically quite distinct respresentations of visuognostic and language functions. Consequently, patients suffering from this condition are unable to name an object but would be able to describe it by pantomime. This behaviour is also frequent in aphasics, but unlike other aphasics, a patient with pure 'optic aphasia' would flawlessly answer questions such as *What do you call the liquid you make cheese from?* As the lesion in the brain that results in optic aphasia is situated in the temporo-parieto-occipital border zone of the left hemisphere, this visuo-verbal disconnection syndrome may be combined with anomic or Wernicke's aphasia, thus leading to a combination of aphasic and visual access word retrieval deficits. Consequently, it is worthwhile to include naming of prototypical sounds or in response to questions in routine aphasia assessment.

3.2.2. Repetition

With respect to linguistic levels, repetition is best suited for investigating articulatory and phonological disturbances. Usually, the patient is not required to perform semantic and lexical search processes in order to repeat. Some patients, however, may have to rely on a semantic route in this task (Katz/Goodglass 1990). Increasing word or phrase length in a repetition task imposes increasing demands on the patient's phonological short term memory. In a detailed analysis of a single case of conduction aphasia, Caramazza/Basili/Koller/Berndt (1981) compared various theories accounting for repetition deficits and showed that in their case an auditory-verbal short-term memory deficit gave the best explanation for the observed behavior. In their view, their case provided strong evidence for a relationship between a nonlinguistic processing component and particular aphasic symptoms. Other explanatory theories for repetition deficits include 1) a disconnection between receptive and expressive speech areas (Geschwind 1965), 2) a limitation of information transmission between these areas (Kinsbourne 1972), 3) an impairment of memory for sequence (Tzortzis/Albert 1974), and 4) an impairment of the transformation of a phonological representation into a phonetic string (Kohn 1984).

A detailed analysis of repetition should consist of:
- lexical and nonlexical stimuli
- stimuli of varying length
- as well as other language modalities

such as phonemic and lexical comprehension, reading and writing to dictation.

3.2.3. Comprehension

Intactness or only mild impairment of spoken language comprehension is often wrongly assumed in aphasic patients. Clinicians often overlook the fact that in conversation or informal assessment, the patient may make use of situational cues. In formal assessment, forced choice decision tasks are often easier for the patient than those that demand production, both with respect to linguistic and neuropsychological processing demands. Only when norms derived from aphasic patients are employed, such as in the Boston Diagnostic Aphasia Examination (Goodglass/Kaplan 1972), the Western Aphasia Battery (Kertesz 1979), or the Aachen Aphasia Test (Huber/Poeck/Weniger/Willmes 1983; Huber/Poeck/Willmes 1984), valid statements can be made concerning comprehension deficits.

Obviously, this implies the demand to assess all linguistic levels in auditory comprehension: the phonological, lexical, and sentence, and even the text level (for a review, see Riedel 1981). However, the investigation of comprehension is hampered by the fact, that the analysis of errors is much more difficult than in expression and must be accomplished by linguistically refined sets of distractors and variations (e. g., Baker/Blumstein/Goodglass 1981; Caramazza/Zurif 1976; Parisi/Pizzamiglio 1970; Goodglass/Gleason/Hyde 1970).

Besides linguistic deficits at various stages, a number of nonlinguistic dysfunctions may affect comprehension in the communication and the assessment situation:
- auditory impairment, including auditory agnosia (Spreen/Benton/Fincham 1965)
- attentional deficits, including hemineglect. With hemineglect, the patient may not attend to an auditory stimulus from the neglected side and, in a multiple choice response task, may not react to those stimuli that are presented contralaterally to the lesion (Heilman/Valenstein 1972).
- impairments of prelinguistic processing, such as phonological short term memory deficits and verbal agnosia (Albert/Bear 1974).
- deficits affecting the required action, which in most instances involves pointing to one of a set of items. Especially patients with a lesion in the parietal lobe may suffer from a distortion of their extrapersonal coordinate system which may result in systematic or unsystematic deviations in directed, visually guided pointing and reaching movements (Ratcliff/Davies-Jones 1972).

4. Syndromes of Aphasia

Even in the early days of aphasia research did investigators note variations in linguistic performance among patients. These variations were assigned heuristic value in terms of explanation of the respective pathologies and in terms of models of normal language processing, both with respect to the brain structures involved in completing language tasks (e. g. Wernicke 1874) as well as denoting cognitive components in linguistic performance (e. g. Jackson 1879/80; Pick 1913).

This position has repeatedly been disputed. Among others, Pierre Marie (1906) and Bay (1962) claimed that there is but one aphasia and that differences in clinical symptomatology resulted from additional, e. g. speech motor, symptoms that were peripheral to central language processes. More recently, Poeck (1983), Caramazza (1984) and Marshall (1986) questioned the significance of aphasic syndromes for the examination of linguistic theories.

In medicine, the term 'syndrome' denotes a cooccurrence of symptomes at a greater than chance frequency. This set of symptoms constitutes the syndrome. It is not imperative that all symptoms of the syndrome are present in a given patient. The statistical cluster is supposed to reflect an underlying common pathophysiological source of the various symptoms. In line with this medical approach, Poeck (1983) suggested that indeed the common pathophysiological basis of the aphasia syndromes was rather one reflecting vascular territories than linguistic regularities.

Application of the medical use of the term to patterns of aphasic symptoms and of adequate statistical methods clearly demonstrates that there are syndromes of aphasia (Kertesz 1979, 83ff; Huber/Poeck/Weniger/Willmes 1983). These statistical methods, mainly cluster and nearest neighbour network analyses, group patients according to similarities in degree and patterns of deficits. As some patient subgroups are more similar than others, this approach must produce ambiguous results because certain parameters must be preset:

– the level at which similarities are to be considered. If this is set high, the cluster analysis produces a large number of mainly small groups. A low level, on the other hand, leads to few, large, inhomogenous clusters.
– the minimal number of members in a cluster that is required if clinical significance is to be assumed. This is also an awkward problem, because on the one hand, some syndromes considered meaningful (e. g. "isolation of the speech area", (Geschwind/Quadfasel/Segarra 1968; "surface dyslexia", Patterson/Marshall/Coltheart 1985) are in fact exceedingly rare. On the other hand, some patients with additional pathology or unusal lesion configurations can be expected to be nonclassifiable.

These two problems – how similar members of a cluster should be and how small meaningful groups may be – are central not only for statistical grouping but also for the more intuitive clinical classification. Here, the second problem is usually dealt with on the basis of patholinguistic and/or pathophysiological theory. Small groups that are considered meaningful are interpreted, those that are not, discarded. Differences in the theoretical approaches of various researchers are therefore reflected in a great number of classifications systems. These are also influenced by the patient population, upon which the clinician's experience is based. Relevant differences relate to whether vascular or nonvascular (e. g. war trauma: Luria 1970) etiologies and whether acute or chronic patients predominate.

As has already been pointed out, ischemic vascular lesions predominate the etiologies of aphasia in peace-time. The lesions fall into certain patterns that depend upon which branch of the middle cerebral artery (or, occasionally, the anterior or posterior cerebral artery) or which region between areas of supply of such branches is affected. Most patients with ischemic infarction are over 50 years of age and many suffer form diffuse or multifocal pathology. Their ability to compensate for their deficits may therefore be reduced.

Patient series from neurological teaching hospitals usually comprise acutely aphasic patients in whom diffuse effects of the focal lesion contribute to the clinical picture, whereas those from rehabilitation hospitals are more chronic with less widespread effects of pathology, their symptomatology reflecting compensatory processes and strategies to a greater extent.

Three approaches have been advanced for the classification of aphasic patients. One, originally proposed by Wernicke (1874) distinguishes syndromes on the basis of assumed dissociations across modalities, resulting in terms such as 'motor' and 'sensory' or 'expressive' and 'receptive' aphasia (e. g. Weisenburg/McBride 1935). More recently, this approach has been employed by Goodglass/Kaplan (1972) and Kertesz (1979). A second class of attempts at a taxonomy focused on anatomical distinctions, e. g. "anterior" and "posterior" aphasia (Benson 1967). In fact, a wide range of classification systems is a combination of these two, using both dissociations between modalities and anatomical models for syndrome interpretation (e. g. Nielsen 1938; Geschwind 1965; Goodglass/Kaplan 1972; Kertesz/Phipps 1977; Benson 1979). The third approach that is most interesting in the present context focuses on linguistic symptomatology, mainly in spontaneous language production.

Both speed of production and phrase length vary greatly in aphasic patients. Accordingly, Benson (1967) suggested that this was a feature distinguishing enough to separate different types of aphasia under the headings of 'nonfluent' and 'fluent' disorders. Head (1926) and Wepman/Jones (1961) proposed that linguistic categories be used, resulting in terms such as "semantic" or "syntactic" aphasia. In line with Jackson's (1866) distinction between "positive" and "negative" symptoms Wallesch (1991) based his classification system on the dominant impairment in language production and distinguishes aphasia syndromes with predominant deficit (Broca's, global, anomic, and transcortical motor aphasia) from those, in which the patients production is characterized by linguistic errors (Wernicke's and conduction aphasia).

In reaction to the theoretical confusion manifested in the multitude of classification systems (for an overview, see McNeil 1988), a number of aphasiologists deliberately used historic terms to denote clinical syndromes, but explicitly or implicitly rejected the theoretical connotations linked to these.

In the following, the classification originally developed by researchers in Aachen and currently used by the German neurolinguistic school will be described (Huber/Stachowiak/Poeck/Kerschensteiner 1975; Huber/Poeck/Weniger 1982; 1989; Huber/Poeck/Weniger/Willmes 1983; Kerschensteiner/Poeck/Huber et al. 1978; Poeck/Kerschensteiner/Stachowiak/Huber 1974; Stachowiak/Huber/Kerschensteiner et al. 1977). At the time of its construction, it was assumed that the syndromes of Broca's, Wernicke's, global, and amnestic/anomic aphasia were linguistically meaningful, and also, that a development from one syndrome to the other ("Syndromwandel", Leischner 1979) was not possible without alterations in the underlying pathology. Both positions have since been rejected by the Aachen group (Poeck 1983; Willmes/Poeck 1984).

The syndrome descriptions consist of an overview of the neurolinguistic features, a description of the typical underlying pathology and common accompanying symptoms and differential diagnostic considerations. The following syndromes are to be presented: Global aphasia, Broca's aphasia, anomic aphasia, Wernicke's aphasia, conduction aphasia, and the transcortical aphasias.

4.1. Global Aphasia

4.1.1. Synonymous or Related Terms

Total aphasia (Dejerine 1906; Leischner 1979); grande aphasie de Broca (Marie 1906), expressive-receptive aphasia (Weisenburg/McBride 1935).

4.1.2. Neurolinguistic Description

The term 'global' denotes that all language functions are severely affected in this syndrome. Propositional language is either almost absent, or reduced to single words or fragmented phrases produced with great effort. However, even maximally impaired patients have been reported to produce adequate single word utterances or short phrases under extreme stress (Jackson 1866). Some stereotypical expressions may be preserved and used adequately in some situations (Andresen 1985). A subgroup of patients are able to produce highly overlearned sequences such as prayers, popular songs or series (Brunner/Kornhuber/Seemüller et al. 1982; Blanken/Dittmann/Haas/Wallesch 1988).

Huber/Poeck/Weniger (1989) suggest a distinction between four types of global aphasia, namely 1) 'standard global aphasia' with hardly any spontaneous language production, 2) an iterative type with prominent recurring utterances that are fluently produced in most cases, 3) a neologistic type with fluent or nonfluent neologistic jargon that contains stereotyped elements, and 4) one subgroup with predominant production of stereotyped phrases and fragments thereof. Poeck/de Bleser/von Keyserlingk (1984a) considered patients with fluent production of consonant-vocal recurring utterances to represent a special form of global aphasia and, in the absence of detectable differences in lesion anatomy between these and nonfluent standard global aphasics, speculated that these patients were characterized by an abnormal premorbid organization of the cerebral language system.

Brunner/Kornhuber/Seemüller et al. (1982) emphasized the presence or at least elicibility of speech automatisms in global aphasia and used them as the leading symptom in the diagnosis of this syndrome. This position has been challenged by a recent paper by Blanken/Wallesch/Papagno (1990) which cited the presence of automatisms in patients suffering from aphasia of a lesser degree.

As all language processes are severely affected in global aphasia, these patients are greatly impaired in all modalities and in all subtests used for aphasia assessment, with two possible exceptions. First, echolalia may be present in global aphasia, frequently causing repetition scores to exceed the bottom region. Second, the patient's intelligence and social performance being less affected from the effects of the brain lesion than his/her language abilities, comprehension especially in an informal situation may appear to be, or in fact be, quite adequate.

Linguistically controlled comprehension tests or the Token Test (De Renzi/Vignolo 1962) are able to disclose severe impairment in such patients.

When propositional utterances are produced by global aphasics at all, they are laborious, phonologically distorted, highly dysprosodic and asyntactical. A systematic simplification such as is present in the agrammatic phrases of Broca's aphasics does not occur. Those propositional utterances, that are produced consist of syntactically unconnected single words. Stereotypical utterances, on the other hand, are frequently produced fluently, with little effort, and with marked prosodical contour. In a large proportion of patients, closer analysis of prosody reveals that it may also be stereotypical (De Bleser/Poeck 1984). An analysis of utterance lengths in response to different forms of questions led Blanken/Dittmann/Haas/Wallesch (1988) to the conclusion that the format of stereotypical productions was not stereotyped but showed significant effects of the question type.

4.1.3. Lesion Localization and Etiology

In right-handed people and most left-handed ones, global aphasia is the result of severe damage to the cerebral representation of language functions in the core of the region of supply of the left middle cerebral artery (Fig.9.2). The critical area includes Broca's and Wernicke's areas, the insula, the left basal ganglia, and their fibre connections. As all these parts of the brain are supplied by the same artery, the middle cerebral, the most common cause of global aphasia is large ischemic infarction in this artery's territory. Large hemorrhages in the left basal ganglia, which occur with vascular malformations or with severe hypertension, may cut off the language cortex from its subcortical connections and may thus result in a functionally equivalent extent of damage.

However, whether or not a patient will develop global aphasia cannot be predicted on the basis of the anatomical lesion as shown, e. g., by computer tomography (CT) alone. Lesion size and localization seem to interact with age (Eslinger/Damasio 1981; Habib/Ali-Cherif/Poncet 1987), intelligence, motivation, intensity and adequacy of therapy, psychosocial variables, duration of illness (Willmes/Poeck 1984), and even sex (Pizzamiglio/Mammucari/Razzano 1985). Even with lesions of extreme size (complete infarctions of the middle cerebral artery territory), younger patients will ultimately develop Broca's aphasia in most instances (Haas/Blanken/Mezger/Wallesch 1988). In a series of patients globally aphasic more than 3 weeks post stroke, Vignolo/Boccardi/Caverni (1986) were able to demonstrate a great variation in lesion localization.

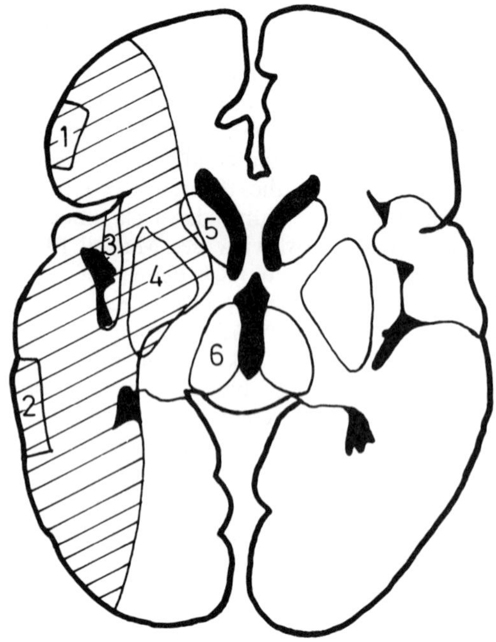

Fig. 9.2: Schematic horizontal cut through the brain demonstrating anatomical regions assumed to be involved in language processing:
Broca's area (1), Wernicke's area (2), insula (3), basal ganglia: nucleus lenticularis (4), head of caudate nucleus (5), thalamus (6).
The hatched region corresponds to the area of supply of the middle cerebral artery.

4.1.4. Accompanying Symptoms

In most instances, globally aphasic patients have suffered large left hemisphere lesions including both cortical and subcortical structures. With few exceptions, when the perirolandic cortex, the anterior limb of the internal capsule and the anterior parts of the basal ganglia are spared, a right hemiparesis affecting the right upper limb most prominently is common. Other frequent symptoms include dysarthria, speech apraxia, ideomotor apraxia (Wallesch/Haas/Blanken 1988) constructional apraxia (Leischner 1979), a right visual field defect, and especially in the early stages right hemineglect and localization-unspecific deficits such as psychomotor slowing, fatigue and verbal and nonverbal perseveration (Allison/Hurwitz 1967).

4.1.5. Differential Diagnosis

The differential diagnosis of global aphasia includes other disorders that may lead to severely compromised communication, such as clouded consciousness, advanced dementia, psychotic, psychogenic and traumatic mutism, anarthria and severe dysarthria, the combination of milder forms of aphasia with speech apraxia, and Broca's aphasia.

A diagnosis of global aphasia should be made with caution in the acute stage, i. e., not before the first four weeks post onset. The acute disruption of brain function in acute stroke may lead to severe language deficits even in such patients that may eventually recover completely (Wallesch/Bak/Schulte-Mönting 1992). Also, clouding of consciousness is frequent in these patients and increases the communication impairment (Wallesch/Bak/Schulte-Mönting 1992). Therefore, a diagnosis of global aphasia should only be considered in patients appearing alert, responsive, and cooperative. This precondition is justified on the basis of the definition given in the introduction and thus rules out most cases of clouding of consciousness, psychosis, and advanced dementia.

Linguistic analysis and therefore aphasia assessment proves difficult, when a patient does not speak. If speechlessness is due to a disorder affecting articulation only, such as anarthria or severe dysarthria, both comprehension and written expression are intact. The same would hold for pure cases of speech apraxia, but they are excessively rare. Mutism, both of psychotic/psychogenic and of neurogenic origin is characterized by the lack of a perceptible attempt to articulate (for a review, see Lebrun 1989). Comprehension and writing are intact or largely preserved in most, but not in all mute patients.

The combination of Broca's aphasia and speech apraxia is frequent and may lead to severely restricted and largely incomprehensible speech production. In most cases, the assessment of written language and of comprehension will allow a differentiation from global aphasia. It has to be kept in mind, that a transition from global to Broca's aphasia is not uncommon (about 20% according to Willmes/Poeck 1984), therefore a clear-cut dichotomy between the two syndromes cannot be expected.

4.2. Broca's Aphasia

4.2.1. Synonymous or Related Terms

Aphemia (Broca 1865), cortical motor aphasia (Wernicke 1874; Lichtheim 1885), central motor aphasia (Goldstein 1948), motor aphasia (Leischner 1979), expressive aphasia (Weisenburg/McBride 1935), verbal aphasia (Head 1926), word muteness (Kleist 1934), syntactic aphasia (Wepman/Jones 1961), efferent motor aphasia (Luria 1970), anterior aphasia (Benson 1967), agrammatic aphasia (Brown 1972).

4.2.2. Neurolinguistic Description

Our present-day conception of Broca's aphasia is quite different both from Broca's original case and his interpretation (Berker/Berker/Smith 1986). The patient, Leborgne or "Monsieur Tan", was globally aphasic with no speech except for a cv-recurring utterance ("tan"). Broca interpreted his deficit quite similar to modern concepts of speech apraxia.

The principal feature of Broca's aphasia is a reduction of linguistic proficiency. This is quite specific at the syntactic level, resulting in agrammatism, which has been proposed to be an axial symptom of this syndrome (Kerschensteiner/Poeck/Huber et al. 1978).

Whereas the total lack of functors in telegraphic style is easily detected even by the untrained observer, mild degrees of agrammatism may escape notice. In mild Broca's aphasia, the patient's productions may be characterized only by a reduction of the use of subordinate clauses, multiple objects, or the genitive, and time relations between verb forms may be simplified. These symptoms are pathognomonic only when a more elaborate premorbid use of language can be established.

In the vast majority of Broca's aphasics, the deficit in linguistic proficiency affects phonological and lexical processes as well as the generation of syntactic structure. However, occasionally patients with 'pure' or 'fluent' agrammatism are described (Miceli/Mazzucchi/Menn/Goodglass 1983). It is a question of definition, whether these are included in the syndrome of Broca's aphasia. In any case, these patients demonstrate the dissociability of grammatic impairment from the other features of Broca's aphasia. Case reports of patients with rather specific morphological (Kolk/van Grunsven/Keyser 1985) or syntactical deficits (Nadeau 1988) contribute not only to the dissolution of the syndrome concept of Broca's aphasia but also of a unitary view of agrammatism (for a review, see Goodglass/Menn 1985).

Patients suffering from standard Broca's aphasia exhibit a deficit of lexical retrieval resulting in time-consuming, laborious and frequently unsuccessful attempts at word-finding. Semantic paraphasia, in most cases of semantically related words, and production of less-specified superordinates or filler words may occur. Both phonological assembly and articulation are slowed down and laborious. The patients tend to simplify consonant clusters by elision or interposition of 'schwas' (short, unstressed and phonologically underspecified vowels). It is often impossible to decide to what extent the laborious articulation is due to phonological, apractic and dysarthric disturbances which co-occur in many patients. Whether or not a distinction between these levels of speech production is artificial, has been discussed (Buckingham 1983; Rosenbek 1984).

In short, Broca aphasics need effort to produce a proposition despite their agrammatism, retrieve the required words or comprehensible substitutes, assemble the phonological string as well as possible and produce acceptable articulation. All these impairments add up to the prominent impression of nonfluency, and indeed Broca's aphasia is paradigmatic for the non-fluent group of aphasias (Benson 1967).

4.2.3. Lesion Localization and Etiology

Broca's aphasia is usually the result of a large infarction in the territory of supply of the left middle cerebral artery. The anterior branches of this vessel seem to be involved in all infarction cases. The anterior insula has been described as the core lesion area (Blunk/de Bleser/Willmes/Zeumer 1981; Poeck/de Bleser/von Keyserlingk 1984b). The infarction of Broca's area in the foot of the second and third frontal convolution alone causes mutism in the acute stage with rapidly improving articulation and no persisting language deficit (Mohr/Pessin/Finkelstein et al. 1978). Broca's aphasia is not confined to infarct cases, but may occur with any pathology that damages the left hemisphere language representation extensively but locally and allows ample time for compensation, such as herpes encephalitis, hemorrhage, and circumscribed trauma. It does not occur with rapidly growing tumors. Aphasia in this condition rather resembles the syndromes of acute aphasia.

4.2.4. Accompanying Symptoms

As Broca's aphasia arises in conjunction with rather large lesions of the cerebral language region focussing on its anterior aspect, parts of the brain that are involved in motor functions such as the motor and premotor cortex, the anterior limb of the internal capsule and parts of the basal ganglia are usually affected. Consequently, right hemiparesis, mostly affecting the arm and the lower face (brachiofacial paresis), as well as cortical dysarthria are frequent accompanying symptoms. Due to the large cortical representation of the hand, its paresis is usually most marked and most disabling. A right visual field defect and right hemineglect are less common than in Wernicke's and global aphasia. Depression has been reported to occur more frequently in Broca's and global aphasia than in the other syndromes (Starkstein/Robinson/Price 1987). The extension of the lesion into the left frontal lobe has been speculated to cause this mood disorder.

4.2.5. Differential Diagnosis

Broca's aphasia has to be distinguished from other aphasic and nonaphasic causes on nonfluency. Nonaphasic causes include speech motor impairment such as anarthria, dysarthria and speech apraxia that are frequently combined with Broca's aphasia, but in their pure forms can easily be distinguished by preserved writing and comprehension abilities, reduced speech output with clouded consciousness and dementia, and psychiatric conditions such as mutism in schizophrenia and severe depression. Whereas aphasics clearly show that they are motivated to communicate, this is not the case with reduced consciousness, dementia, and psychosis.

Aphasic syndromes sharing the feature of nonfluency include global aphasia, severe anomic aphasia, transcortical motor aphasia, acute nonfluent aphasia, and severe conduction aphasia. As has already been pointed out, the distinction between global and Broca's aphasia is a matter of degree at times and the former may evolve into the latter (Willmes/Poeck 1984). Severe cases of anomic aphasia may be unable to complete a statement because of word retrieval failure. These patients, however, exhibit their major deficit with respect to content words and have little if any problems in generating functors, whereas Broca's aphasics show a dissociation in the opposite direction. The primary deficit in transcortical motor aphasia is not linguistic but involves the generation of speech in situations containing many degrees of freedom (see below). These patients are severely impaired and highly nonfluent in conversation, but increase their level of performance the more constraints are imposed upon their production (repetition > reading aloud > confrontation naming > response to pronoun question). Agrammatism is not prominent in this syndrome, therefore repetition of sentences is usually grammatical. Acute nonfluent aphasia does not exhibit the features of compensation that are characteristic for Broca's aphasia, i. e. the production of propositional phrases despite agrammatism and nonfluency. Finally, nonfluency in conduction aphasia is characterized by the sequence of phonological approaches known as conduite d'approche that again affects content words more than functors.

4.3. Wernicke's Aphasia

4.3.1. Synonymous or Related Terms

Sensory aphasia (Wernicke 1874, Goldstein 1948), receptive aphasia (Weisenburg/McBride 1935), syntactic aphasia (Head 1926), pragmatic aphasia (Wepman/Jones 1961), posterior aphasia (Benson 1967), semantic aphasia (Brown 1972).

4.3.2. Neurolinguistic Description

Wernicke's aphasia is characterized by its "para"-symptomatology (paraphasia, paragrammatism), which has been interpreted as a deficit of choosing between elements of one linguistic class, a disorder of similarity (Jakobson 1968).

Phonemic paraphasias in the spontaneous speech of Wernicke's aphasics are produced without hesitation, fluently and usually without subsequent attempts at correction. Attempts at a phonemic approach towards the target may be present, most frequently in naming, but these are more characteristic for conduction aphasia. With increasing frequency of phonemic paraphasia, phonemic neologisms and neologistic jargon occur. In Wernicke's patients whose spontaneous speech is free from phonemic paraphasia, neologisms may be revealed with forced word production such as in confrontation naming or when the interlocutor insists on a specific information in conversation. A significant but incomplete correlation between expressive and receptive phonological disorder has been reported (Miceli/Gainotti/Caltagirone/Masullo 1980).

Although most lexical retrieval problems in Wernicke's aphasia may lead to rather adequate circumscriptions, the use of filler words and phrases or related semantic paraphasias, wild paraphasic misnaming, in which the production has no perceptible relation to the assumed target, is the diagnostically salient symptom on the lexical level. The patients may also violate rules of composite generation, thus producing nonexistent and inappropriate semantic neologisms.

Both the phonological and semantic disturbances may be so severe that they result in jargon. With phonemic jargon the adequacy of the syntactic structure cannot be judged, although the presence of such structure can often be easily detected, as undistorted function words frequently stand out and segment the utterances (Buckingham/Kertesz 1976; Brown 1981) and syntactic morphology may be used correctly with neologisms. If the lexical content is sufficiently comprehensible, violations of syntactic format, sentence blendings frequently to an extent that sentence boundaries cannot be determined, doubling of constituents, choice of inadequate functors and inappropriate or nonexistent inflections can be detected.

Spontaneous speech is usually fluent, occasionally exceeding the norm, the patient obviously attempting to overcome communication problems by verbose explanations and circumlocutions, which themselves are affected by the language disorder.

Huber/Stachowiak/Poeck/Kerschensteiner (1975) and Huber/Poeck/Weniger (1989) in line with Kertesz/Benson (1970) distinguish two types of Wernicke's aphasia, one with predominant semantic paraphasia with the extreme of semantic jargon, the other with predominant phonological disturbance and neologistic jargon.

As a rule, language comprehension is more severely impaired in Wernicke's than in Broca's aphasia. This assumed dichotomy is of central importance for a number of classification systems (Wernicke 1874; Lichtheim 1885; Geschwind 1965; Goodglass/Kaplan 1972; Kertesz 1979; Benson 1979). As outlined above, the decision whether a classification is being based on the comparison between modalities or supramodal linguistic characteristics is crucial for the inherent logic of taxonomical systems. Patients suffering from Wernicke's aphasia as described here with only mildly impaired comprehension are not infrequent. Especially in patients with acute aphasia with predominant phonemic paraphasia, even to the extent of phonemic jargon, the comprehension deficit may only be mild. In some of these patients, also writing may be much better preserved than oral production. These patients seem to suffer from a disorder at a quite peripheral level of word form assembly.

4.3.3. Lesion Localization and Etiology

Error intrusion – the critical feature of Wernicke's aphasia as described here – is more common in the acute stage, whereas chronic aphasics frequently regain output control that allows for error suppression. Whereas processes of functional compensation lead to the evolution of Broca's aphasia from a more global impairment, such processes result in the development from aphasia characterized by para-symptoms to anomic or unspecific residual aphasia (Willmes/Poeck 1984). Consequently, fluent, paraphasic aphasia is frequent in the first few weeks post onset (20% Wernicke's aphasia after 4 to 6 weeks in a collective of 96 vascular aphasics, Willmes/Poeck 1984), but is rare among chronic aphasics (3% in the series of Willmes/Poeck 1984).

As the intrusion of errors can be overcome especially by those patients who learn to regain output control, chronic Wernicke's aphasia is most common in patients suffering from diffuse or multifocal brain pathology in addition to their aphasia-inducing lesion and among the elderly (Eslinger/Damasio 1981).

The most common cause of Wernicke's aphasia is posterior left middle cerebral artery infarction including Wernicke's area in the posterior third of the left superior temporal gyrus. Other etiologies such as hemorrhage, tumor, and especially trauma are more common than with Broca's aphasia. A detailed study of the effects of lesions of Wernicke's area upon language comprehension has been conducted by Naeser/Helm-Estabrooks/Haas et al. (1987).

Occasionally, paraphasic speech and comprehension deficit result from lesions to the deep nuclei of the forebrain (thalamus and basal ganglia) or the white matter of the anterior limb of the internal capsule (Wallesch 1985; Wallesch/Papagno 1989).

4.3.4. Accompanying Symptoms

In most cases of Wernicke's aphasia, the obvious neurological symptomatology is scarce. Because of the posterior temporal lobe lesion, the motor system is usually not affected (Benson 1979). A right sided visual field defect is common but may be difficult to establish in a noncooperating patient. In patients suffering from acute Wernicke's aphasia, a lack of insight into their condition is common (Gainotti 1972). They seem to attribute the communication impairment to their communication partners and may get impatient, loud, aggressive and even paranoid. Lack of concern and psychiatric symptoms have been attributed to the connections of the temporal lobe with the limbic system.

4.3.5. Differential Diagnosis

Paraphasic or neologistic productions may also occur in conduction aphasia, dementia, confusional states and schizophrenia. The latter three conditions can usually be discriminated by behavioral observation and neurological examination. However, it is not uncommon that an acutely aphasic patient of the Wernicke type without hemiparesis, without insight into his or her impairment and consequently with seemingly inappropriate behavior is misdiagnosed as confused or acutely psychotic and admitted to a psychiatric ward. Psychotic and aphasic neologistic jargon are not always easily distinguished (Lecours 1982). In confused patients, the cognitive content is deranged rather than the linguistic content. A patient interviewer will be able to establish formally appropriate communication with a confused patient and thus obtain information about misperceptions, delusions, anxiety and disorientation. Spontaneous speech in mild dementia is quite free from linguistic errors and mainly characterized by word finding deficit (Blanken/Dittmann/Haas/Wallesch 1987). In more severe cases, perseveration, echolalia, neologism, and finally mutism are the most prominent symptoms (Leischner 1951; Appell/Kertesz/Fishman 1982; Obler/Albert 1982), most of them being not characteristic of Wernicke's aphasia.

Conduction aphasia has frequently been viewed as a variant of Wernicke's aphasia (Lhermitte/Gautier 1969). The differential diagnosis will be discussed, after this syndrome has been described.

4.4. Anomic Aphasia

4.4.1. Synonymous or Related Terms

Anomia (Goodglass/Kaplan 1972), amnesic/amnestic aphasia (Weisenburg/McBride 1935; Huber/Poeck/Weniger/Willmes 1983), nominal aphasia (Head 1926; Brain 1965), semantic aphasia (Wepman/Jones 1961; Luria 1970).

4.4.2. Neurolinguistic Description

The key symptom of anomic aphasia is a disturbance of lexical access and/or retrieval. Phonology and syntax are only mildly affected. The prominent feature of this syndrome is a word-finding deficit. The word finding disorder manifests itself in pauses, circumlocutions, real word paraphasias that are in most instances semantically related to the target, evasion of the target word by use of empty phrases (*well, you know*), substitutes without specific meaning (*thing*), circumscription by verbal or nonverbal means, or abandonment of the ongoing phrase and continuation of the statement in different form.

Most of these strategies are communicatively adequate. Therefore the patients' communication impairment may appear quite mild. The spontaneous speech is usually fluent except for the word-finding pauses but is characterized by a lack of content density. The deficit becomes quite striking, when one and only one word is demanded and cannot be evaded, such as in naming.

4.4.3. Lesion Localization and Etiology

The lesion is usually situated in the posterior border regions of the core language area in the left hemisphere and spares Broca's and Wernicke's areas and the insula. In most instances the temporoparietal junction or the inferior parietal lobe is affected. Anomic aphasia is relatively frequent with non-ischemic causes of aphasia such as hemorrhages, trauma and tumors.

4.4.4. Accompanying Symptoms

The typical localization of the lesion in anomic aphasia behind and above Wernicke's area accounts for the frequency of symptoms of visuo-verbal disconnection in patients suffering from anomic aphasia. If the lesion extends into the subcortical pathways that connect the visual association cortex with the cortical language region, as is frequently the case with infarctions of the border zone between the territories of the posterior and middle cerebral arteries, then the patient may suffer from so-called "optic aphasia" (Coslett/Saffran 1989 see above).

Due to the usually posterior lesion, right visual field defects are common and motor symptoms such as hemiparesis and dysarthria are rare with anomic aphasia.

4.4.5. Differential Diagnosis

A number of other neurolinguistic pathologies resemble anomic aphasia in that word-finding deficits are their prominent feature. Fatigue, intoxication, distraction and depression may lead to this symptom in otherwise healthy subjects. Diffuse brain diseases such as dementia or states of clouded consciousness result in a weakening of the cognitive processes of word concept generation that are prior to lexical access (Blanken/Dittmann/Haas/Wallesch 1987). Furthermore, word-finding impairment is a core symptom of the other aphasia syndromes as well. In well-recovered patients who had originally suffered from one of the other aphasia types, it frequently is the most prominent residual impairment. Finally, modality-specific naming deficits (e. g., 'optic aphasia') may resemble anomic aphasia, when only one modality is assessed.

The easiest way to rule out diffuse brain diseases as the cause of a lexical access impairment is an assessment of cognitive functions that are not closely linked to language abilities. There are, however, aspects of behaviour even in a visual confrontation naming task that allow differentiation between aphasic and diffuse impairment. Naming errors that are related to the visual structure of the target but that are semantically unrelated are exceptionally rare in aphasic patients but frequent in subjects suffering from dementia, clouding of consciousness (Bayles/Tomoeda 1983) and visual impairment. Also, whereas the symptoms of perseveration and echolalia are frequent and quite disinhibited in dementia, they are rare in aphasics, who mainly show them after effort and subsequent failure to produce a target (for a review, see Wallesch 1990).

Especially patients who had recovered well from Wernicke's aphasia frequently have quite isolated word finding impairment. It has been debated whether this development indicates a pattern of syndrome evolution ("Syndromwandel", Leischner 1979; Willmes/Poeck 1984), these patients being truly anomic aphasics, or whether they retain a mild form of Wernicke's aphasia. Mainly two features allow a discrimination between improved Wernicke's and anomic aphasia:

- the occurrence of phonemic or wild semantic paraphasia or paragrammatism with fatigue
- the production of phonemic neologisms when naming of the target proves impossible.

4.6. Conduction Aphasia

4.6.1. Synonymous or Related Terms

Repetition aphasia (Weisenburg/McBride, 1935), Central Aphasia (Goldstein 1948), Phonemic Aphasia (Brown 1972).

4.6.2. Neurolinguistic Description

Conduction aphasia was predicted by Wernicke's (1874) model as a disconnection between the sensory and motor language centers. Even Wernicke himself focussed less on the disorder of repetition (Lichtheim 1885 drew attention to this aspect), and more on these patients' failing attempts at self-correction resulting from lack of control of the motor center:

"Vieles gelingt ihm geläufig, besonders leicht hingeworfene Redensarten; dann kommt er an ein Wort des Anstosses, bleibt daran hängen; müht sich, ärgert sich, und fast jedes Wort, das er dann stockend vorbringt, ist unsinnig; er verbessert sich immer wieder, und je mehr er sich müht, desto schlimmer wird der Zustand" (Wernicke 1874, 47–48).

("Many productions succeed, especially small talk; but then a critical word comes up and he gets stuck; he struggles, gets angry, and almost every word that is now haltingly produced is meaningless; he continues to correct himself, but the more he tries, the worse it gets").

There is no general agreement as to the frequency of conduction aphasia. Benson/Sheramatta/Bouchard/et al. (1973) report that 5 to 10% of their aphasia admissions suffered from this syndrome. In a recent study by one of the present authors (Wallesch/Bak 1991), 19 out of 112 acutely aphasic patients exhibited a focal deficit of repetition, but only 1 out of 74 was diagnosed as conduction aphasic at the chronic stage.

Benson/Sheramatta/Bouchard et al. (1973) advance the following criteria for diagnosis: 1) fluent, paraphasic conversational speech; 2) absence of significant difficulty in comprehension; 3) repetition disturbance of a significant degree. The last symptom is regarded as critical. However, "significance" is a statistical term and can only be evaluated if aphasia assessment is based on psychometric criteria, as in the Aachen Aphasia Test (Huber/Poeck/Willmes 1984) or the Western Aphasia Battery (Kertesz, 1982).

Most patients suffering from conduction aphasia are focally impaired not only in repetition, but also in reading aloud and writing to dictation. Their performance is quite characteristic: either they succeed instantly, or they perform a series of attempts at self correction, mainly aiming at the phonological structure, that fail more often than not ('conduite d'approche' and 'conduite d'ecart'). The word of onset of the sequence is sometimes even accurate, and in many instances it is the best approach at the target.

As already observed by Wernicke (1874), these patients' speech production is fluent in stereotypes, but laborious and phonologically distorted in propositional productions where they get stuck and the sequence of correction attempts is initiated.

An analysis of phonological picture naming errors in conduction aphasics conducted by Joanette/Keller/Lecours (1980) revealed that these patients seem to have a quite clear notion of the target structure. Similar data obtained by Kohn (1984) indicate that in conduction aphasia the phonological representation of a word cannot immediately be translated into a phonemic string. Errors in these translations, and probably also deficient output monitoring as demonstrated by the non-acceptance of correct productions, are able to account for the long sequences of 'conduite d'approche' and 'conduite d'ecart' in these patients.

4.6.3. Lesion Localization and Etiology

In accordance with Wernicke's model, conduction aphasia has traditionally been correlated with a lesion of the arcuate fasciculus that is thought to constitute an anatomical link between Wernicke's and Broca's areas (Geschwind 1965; Benson/Sheramatta/Bouchard et al. 1973; Damasio/Damasio 1980; Tanabe/Sawade/Inoue et al. 1987). However, there are cases in the literature, where this structure was spared (Green/Howes 1977).

4.6.4. Differential Diagnosis

Conduction aphasia resembles the phonemic subtype of Wernicke's aphasia in the prominent production of phonemic paraphasia, and speech apraxia in the cumbersome attempts at output correction.

Conduction aphasia may be a transitional stage in the evolution of Wernicke's aphasia (Pashek/Holland 1989). A distinction between the two syndromes may be based on the patient's behavior in connection with phonemic paraphasia. A conduction aphasic will recognize almost all paraphasias and start a sequence of correction attempts, whereas most paraphasias will be produced without notice in Wernicke's aphasia. Clinically, performance in comprehension and repetition tasks may contribute to the differential diagnosis. In this author's opinion, a diagnosis should not be founded on these observations, unless a classification system based on comparisons across modalities such as that proposed by Kertesz (1979) is generally applied.

Conduction aphasia may co-occur with facial (Benson/Sheramatta/Bouchard et al. 1973) and speech apraxia (Blumstein/Cooper/Goodglass et al. 1980). A distinction between apraxic (articulatory) and conduction aphasic (phonemic) errors can usually be made on the basis of observations or measurements of articulatory movements. Parapraxia (frequently erroneous, searching movements in order to establish correct place and mode or articulation) is not a feature of conduction aphasia.

4.7. The Transcortical Aphasias

Whereas conduction aphasia was predicted by the Wernicke-Lichtheim model as a focal disconnection of the direct pathway between Wernicke's and Broca's areas, the transcortical aphasias were defined as syndromes in which these areas and their direct connection was intact and more central parts of the language system disconnected (see Fig. 1). Consequently, patients suffering from these syndromes were defined by their rather intact ability to repeat.

Three transcortical syndromes are distinguished: transcortical motor aphasia, transcortical sensory aphasia, and mixed transcortical aphasis (= "isolation of the speech area", Geschwind/Quadfasel/Segarra 1968).

4.7.1. Transcortical Motor Aphasia

The key features of transcortical motor aphasia are paucity of spontaneous speech and largely preserved language comprehension and repetition. The Wernicke–Lichtheim model explains this syndrome as a disconnection between the concept center and the motor speech area. The syndrome is common with acute aphasia, usually following a period of complete mutism, and rare with chronic aphasia. During improvement, naming recovers while the patient continues to suffer from very restricted language production in conversation, leaving the patient with "aphasia sine aphasia" (von Stockert 1975). This development clearly contradicts the Wernicke–Lichtheim model.

The deficit has been explained on the basis of a heightened excitability threshold of the cerebral speech production apparatus, which performs well in restricted settings with available cues that may trigger output, and badly in open situations with many degrees of freedom (Goldstein 1948; Rubens 1976).

Transcortical motor aphasia is usually the consequence of a lesion outside the anterior parts of the classical language area. It is frequently observed for very short periods of time (hours or few days) following neurosurgical manipulations of the left frontal lobe. Transcortical motor aphasia of longer duration is usually seen after vascular or nonvascular lesions of the left frontal lobe outside Broca's area, especially of the left supplementary motor area at the medial aspect of the lobe (Rubens 1976) or with lesions in the depth of the left hemisphere (Wallesch/Papagno 1989). The supplementary motor area has been speculated to mediate internally generated intentions as opposed to external response demands that are conveyed through the lateral parts of the frontal lobe (Goldberg 1985). Linguistic functions as such are considered intact. Therefore, the status of transcortical motor aphasia as an aphasia as defined above remains doubtful.

4.7.2. Transcortical Sensory and Mixed Transcortical Aphasia

Both syndromes are rare and most patients are characterized by disinhibited echolalia. This disinhibition results in a high level of performance in repetition tasks. However, as Goldstein (1948) pointed out, there are patients suffering from transcortical sensory or mixed aphasia, in whom repetition is not disinhibited but performed only voluntarily. For the latter type of patients, a number of linguistic routes have been described that may account for the sparing of repetition (for a review, see Gonzales Rothi 1990).

In transcortical sensory aphasia, language production is fluent and characterized by mainly semantic paraphasia. In mixed transcortical aphasia the output is scarce except for echolalia. Naming and comprehension are severly impaired in both syndromes.

Mixed transcortical aphasia has also been termed "isolation of the speech area" syndrome (Geschwind/Quadfasel/Segerra 1968), because intact syntactic and morphological operations can be demonstrated in these patients' repetitions.

Mixed transcortical and transcortical sensory aphasia with preserved control of repetition may occur as acute syndromes and are compatible with partial recovery (Kertesz/McCabe 1977; Kertesz/Sheppard/MacKenzie 1982), and transcortical sensory aphasia may also be encountered as an intermediate stage in the resolution of Wernicke's aphasia (Kertesz/Harlock/Coates 1979). The latter syndrome has also been described as a transitional stage in the dissolution of language in dementia (Albert/Goodglass/Helm et al. 1981).

Vascular, degenerative, and traumatic lesions may give rise to transcortical sensory and mixed aphasia. Most studies agree that the pathology is situated either in the posterior temporal lobe or in the temporal isthmus that connects this lobe with other areas of the brain (Geschwind/Quadfasel/Segerra 1968; Kertesz/Sheppard/MacKenzie 1982; Alexander/Hiltbrunner/Fischer 1989).

4.8. Patterns of Evolution

In the description of the aphasia sydromes, it has repeatedly been stated that a syndrome may be the result of evolution or unstable over time. The temporal dynamics of patterns of aphasia have traditionally been given only little consideration, and this neglect is a major cause of the confusion that exists in the taxonomy of aphasia.

Patients suffering from acute aphasia not only present symptoms of acute focal dysfunction. For a number of weeks, their language and behavioral performance is also determined by the effects of diffuse cerebral impairment, as is manifested by the high incidence of symptoms of clouded consciousness, attentional impairment and rapid fluctuations in performance (Wallesch/Bak 1991). These deficits preclude detailed linguistic assessment. Kertesz (1979) and Wallesch/Bak (1991) analysed 64 and 66 patients respectively that were investigated in the third to sixth week post onset by means of cluster analysis. Both studies produced similar results with respect to syndromes of acute aphasia. They found:

1) a cluster of mild aphasia with prominent word finding difficulty
2) a cluster of mild aphasia with prominent comprehension deficit
3) a cluster of moderate aphasia with low repetition
4) a cluster of severe aphasia with preserved comprehension
5) a cluster of severe aphasia with deficitis in all modalities.

According to his classification system, Kertesz terms these clusters anomic, Wernicke, conduction, Broca, and global aphasia, respectively. Wallesch/Bak do not go this far, as the clusters obtained in their study proved to be quite heterogeneous with respect to outcome. In their series, an evolution to chronic Wernicke's aphasia occurred in clusters 3) and 4), but not in 2). Patients included in cluster 4) did not conform in their language production to Broca's aphasia as defined above, but produced almost no output except for stereotypes.

In a series published by Kertesz (1984), 12 out of 21 initially globally aphasic patients evolved to Broca's aphasia. In addition, 15 out of 17 Broca's and 6 out of 9 conduction aphasics became anomic. Only 4 out of 9 Wernicke aphasics remained in this category, and 19 out of 29 anomic aphasics recovered completely.

Willmes/Poeck (1984) investigated the evolution of 95 vascular aphasics from 4 to 6 weeks until 7 months post stroke. The patients were classified by discriminant analysis on the basis of the Aachen Aphasia test (Huber/Poeck/Weniger/Willmes 1983) into the categories of global, Broca, Wernicke, and anomic aphasia. Out of 21 global aphasics, 11 remained in this class and 5 developed Broca's aphasia. Only 3 out of 19 Wernicke's aphasics remained; 10 became anomic and 4 recovered completely. Five out of 13 Broca's aphasics recovered, 5 retained this syndrome. Sixteen out of 33 anomic aphasics recovered completely, and another 5 exhibited only minimal symptoms after 7 months. All these findings indicate that a massive change of syndrome assignment ("Syndromwandel", Leischner 1979) takes place within the first months of aphasia. In our experience, transition from global to Broca's aphasia may occur even years post onset.

4.9. Alternative Classification Systems

A classification system has been presented that was based on neurolinguistic symptomatology. The major disadvantage of this approach is that it does not provide a clear discrimination in every single case, e. g. a patient may exhibit features both of Broca's and conduction or Broca's and transcortical motor aphasia.

The most frequently advanced alternative type of classification system is one that com-

Aphasia type	Fluency	Comprehension	Repetition	Naming
global	0–4	0–3.9	0–4.9	0–6
Broca's	0–4	4–10	0–7.9	0–8
Isolation	0–4	0–3.9	5–10	0–6
Transcortical motor	0–4	4–10	8–10	0–8
Wernicke's	5–10	0–6.9	0–7.9	0–9
Transcortical sensory	5–10	0–6.9	8–10	0–9
Conduction	5–10	7–10	0–6.9	0–9
Anomic	5–10	7–10	7–10	0–9

Table 9.3: Criteria for Classification (Kertesz 1979, 58)

pares performance across modalities (e. g., Goodglass/Kaplan 1972, Benson 1979; Kertesz 1979). As the most elaborated and best documented system, Kertesz' will be presented.

Based on the standardization sample of his Western Aphasia Battery and a scoring system from 0 (maximal impairment) to 10 (normal performance), Kertesz (1979) advanced the following criteria for classification (Table 9.3.).

This system obviously allows unequivocal syndrome diagnosis. On the other hand, it negates qualitative distinctions between syndromes. Mild changes in performance may result in seemingly qualitative transitions. Furthermore, one must suspect that syndromes thus defined may contain quite heterogenic patient populations. Consequently, Kertesz' (1979) own cluster analyses only imperfectly reflected his syndrome assignments. However, as the status of syndromes becomes more and more questioned (Caramazza 1984; Marshall 1986), this operational approach may be the clinically most justified.

Another approach to aphasia classification is based on pathophysiological considerations. The first system of this sort was, of course, Wernicke's (1874). The most notable modern taxonomy is Luria's (1970; 1974; Luria/Hutton 1977). Luria's neuropsychological and neurophysiological theories led to the identification of a frontal 'dynamic' aphasia, a condition in which the drive to produce statements is mainly affected. Luria's approach also encouraged a separation of Broca's aphasia into an efferent and an afferent motor subtype. The afferent/efferent dichotomy was also used by Kertesz/Phipps (1977) for the subdivision of conduction aphasia.

Luria's taxonomy implicitly assumes that the interactions between afferents and efferents and the functions of the frontal lobe are clarified well enough to allow them to form the basis for aphasia interpretation. The last ten years of neurophysiological research, however, have been characterized by the growing insight that our theories of brain function have been too simplistic (e. g. Evarts/Shinoda/Wise 1984; Phillips/Zeki/Barlow 1984). At the present time, a note of caution must be expressed not to attempt to solve linguistic problems by employing neurophysiological theories. Incidentally, this warning was already advanced by Freud (1891).

5. References

Alajouanine, T. (1956). Verbal realization in aphasia. *Brain*, *79*, 1–28.

Albert, M. L., Bear, D. (1974). Time to understand. A case study of word deafness with reference to the role of time in auditory comprehension. *Brain*, *97*, 373–384.

Albert, M. L., Goodglass, H., Helm, N. A., Rubens, A. B., & Alexander, M. P. (1981). *Clinical aspects of dysphasia.* Wien: Springer.

Alexander, M. P., Hiltbrunner, B., & Fischer, R. S. (1989). Distributed anatomy of transcortical sensory aphasia. *Archives of Neurology*, *46*, 885–892.

Allison, R. S. & Hurwitz, L. J. (1967). On perseveration in aphasics. *Brain*, *90*, 429–448.

Andresen, H. (1985). Selektiv erhaltene sprachliche Fähigkeiten bei schwerer Aphasie. *Osnabrücker Beiträge zur Sprachtheorie*, *32*, 43–72.

Appell, J., Kertesz, A., & Fishman, M. (1982). A study of language functions in Alzheimer patients. *Brain and Language*, *17*, 73–91.

Baker, E., Blumstein, S., & Goodglass, H. (1981). Interaction between phonological and semantic factors in auditory discrimination. *Neuropsychologia*, *19*, 1–15.

Bay, E. (1962). Aphasia and nonverbal disorders of language. *Brain*, *85*, 411–426.

Bayles, K. A. & Tomoeda, C. K. (1983). Confrontation naming impairment in dementia. *Brain and Language, 19,* 98–114.

Benson, D. F. (1967). Fluency in aphasia. Correlations with radioactive scan localization. *Cortex, 3,* 373–394.

Benson, D. F. (1979). *Aphasia, alexia, and agraphia.* New York: Churchill Livingstone.

Benson, D. F., Sherematta, W. A., Bouchard, R., Segarra, J. M., Prince, D., & Geschwind, N. (1973). Conduction aphasia: a clinicopathological study. *Archives of Neurology, 30,* 307–310.

Berker, E. A., Berker, A. H., & Smith, A. (1986). Translation of Broca's 1865 report. *Archives of Neurology, 43,* 1065–1072.

Blanken, G. (1990). Formal paraphasias: A single case study. *Brain and Language, 38,* 534–554.

Blanken, G., de Langen, E., Dittmann, J., & Wallesch, C. W. (1989). Implications of preserved written language abilities for the functional basis of speech automatisms (recurring utterances): a single case study. *Cognitive Neuropsychology, 6,* 211–249.

Blanken, G., Dittmann, J., Haas, J. C., & Wallesch, C. W. (1987). Spontaneous speech in senile dementia and aphasia. Implications for a neurolinguistic model of language production. *Cognition, 27,* 47–74.

Blanken, G., Dittmann, J., Haas, J. C., & Wallesch, C. W. (1988). Producing speech automatisms (recurring utterances): Looking for what is left. *Aphasiology, 2,* 545–566.

Blanken, G., Wallesch, C. W., & Papagno, C. (1990). Dissociations of language functions in aphasics with speech automatisms (recurring utterances). *Cortex, 26,* 41–63.

Blumstein, S., Cooper, W., Goodglass, H., Statlender, S., & Gottlieb, J. (1980). Production deficits in aphasia: A voice onset time analysis. *Brain and Language, 9,* 153–170.

Blunk, R., De Bleser, R., Willmes, K., & Zeumer, H. (1981): A refined method to relate morphological and functional aspects of aphasia. *European Neurology, 20,* 69–79.

Brain, W. R. (1965). *Speech disorders.* London: Butterworth.

Broca, P. (1865). Sur la siege de la faculte du langage articule. *Bulletin de la Societe Anthropologique du Paris, 6,* 337–393.

Brown, J. W. (1972). *Aphasia, apraxia and agnosia.* Springfield: Thomas.

Brown, J. W. (1981). *Jargonaphasia.* New York: Academic Press.

Brunner, R. J., Kornhuber, H. H., Seemüller, E., Suger, G., & Wallesch, C. W. (1982). Basal ganglia participation in language pathology. *Brain and Language, 16,* 281–299.

Brust, J., Shafer, S., Richter, R., & Bruun, B. (1976). Aphasia in acute stroke. *Stroke, 7,* 167–174.

Buckingham, H. W. (1983). Apraxia of language vs. apraxia of speech. In R. A. Magill (Ed.), *Memory and control of action. 275–320.* Amsterdam: North Holland.

Buckingham, H. W., Kertesz, A. (1976). *Neologistic jargon aphasia.* Amsterdam: Swets & Zeitlinger.

Buckingham, H. W., Whitaker, H., & Whitaker, H. A. (1979). On linguistic perseveration. In H. & H. A. Whitaker (Eds.), *Studies in neurolinguistics, vol. 4. 329–352.* New York: Academic Press.

Caplan, D. (1987). *Neurolinguistics and linguistic aphasiology.* Cambridge: Cambridge University Press.

Caramazza, A. (1984). The logic of neuropsychological research and the problem of patient classification in aphasia. *Brain and Language, 21,* 9–20.

Caramazza, A., Basili, A. G., Koller, J. J., & Berndt, R. S. (1981). An investigation of repetition and language processing in a case of conduction aphasia. *Brain and Language, 14,* 235–271.

Caramazza, A. & Zurif, E. (1976). Dissociations of algorithmic and heuristic processes in comprehension: evidence from aphasia. *Brain and Language, 3,* 572–582.

Code, C. (1982). Neurolinguistic analysis of recurrent utterances in aphasia. *Cortex, 18,* 141–152.

Code, C. (1989). Recurrent utterances and automatisms in aphasia. In C. Code (Ed.), *The characteristics of aphasia. 155–177.* London: Taylor & Francis.

Coslett, H. B. & Saffran, E. M. (1989). Preserved object recognition and reading comprehension in optic aphasia. *Brain, 112,* 1091–1110.

Damasio, H. & Damasio, A. R. (1980). The anatomical basis of conduction aphasia. *Brain, 103,* 337–350.

De Bleser, R. & Poeck, K. (1984). Aphasia with exclusively consonant-vowel recurring utterances; Tan-tan revisited. In F. C. Rose (Ed.), *Progress in aphasiology. 51–57.* New York: Raven.

Dejerine, J. (1906). L'aphasie motrice. Sa localisation et sa physiologie pathologique. *Presse medicale, 55,* 453–457.

De Renzi, E. & Vignolo, L. A. (1962). The Token Test. A sensitive test to detect receptive disturbances in aphasics. *Brain, 85,* 665–678.

Eisenson, J. (1972). *Aphasia in children.* New York: Harper & Row.

Eslinger, P. J. & Damasio, A. R. (1981). Age and type of aphasia in patients with stroke. *Journal of Neurology, Neurosurgery and Psychiatry, 44,* 377–381.

Evarts, E. V., Shinoda, Y., & Wise, S. P. (1984). *Neurophysiological approaches to higher brain functions.* New York: Wiley.

Freud, S. (1891). *Zur Auffassung der Aphasien.* Leipzig: Deuticke.

Gainotti, G. (1972). Emotional behaviour and hemispheric side of the lesion. *Cortex, 8,* 41–55.

Geschwind, N. (1965). Disconnection syndromes in animals and man. Part II. *Brain, 103,* 337–350.

Geschwind, N. (1984). Neural mechanisms, aphasia, and theories of language. In D. Caplan, A. R. Lecours, & A. Smith (Eds.), *Biological perspectives on language. 31–39.* Cambridge, Mass.: MIT Press.

Geschwind, N., Quadfasel, F., & Segarra, J. (1968). Isolation of the speech area. *Neuropsychologia, 6,* 327–340.

Goldberg, G. (1985): Supplementary motor area structure and function: Review and hypothesis. *Behav. Brain. Res., 8,* 567–616.

Goldstein, K. (1948). *Aftereffects of brain injuries in war.* New York: Grune & Stratton.

Gonzales Rothi, L. J. (1990). Transcortical aphasias. In L. L. LaPointe (Ed.), *Aphasia and acquired neurogenic language disorders. 78–95.* New York: Thieme.

Goodglass, H., Gleason, J. B., & Hyde, M. (1970). Some dimensions of auditory language comprehension in aphasia. *Journal of Speech and Hearing Research, 13,* 595–606.

Goodglass, H. & Kaplan, E. (1972). *The assessment of aphasia and related disorders.* Philadelphia: Lea & Febiger.

Goodglass, H. & Menn, L. (1985). Is agrammatism a unitary phenomenon? In M. L. Kean (Ed.), *Agrammatism. 1–26.* Orlando: Academic Press.

Green, E. & Howes, D. (1977). The nature of conduction aphasia: A study of anatomical and clinical features and of underlying mechanisms. In H. & H. A. Whitaker (Eds.), *Studies in Neurolinguistics, vol. 3. 123–155.* New York: Academic Press.

Haag, E., Huber, W., Hündgen, R., Stiller, U., & Willmes, K. (1985). Repetitives sprachliches Verhalten bei schwerer Aphasie. *Nervenarzt, 56,* 543–552.

Haas, J. C., Blanken, G., Mezger, G., & Wallesch, C. W. (1988). Is there an anatomical basis for the production of speech automatisms. *Aphasiology, 3,* 557–565.

Habib, M., Ali-Cherif, A., & Poncet, M. (1987). Age-related changes in aphasia type and stroke location. *Brain and Language, 31,* 245–251.

Head, H. (1926). *Aphasia and kindred disorders of speech.* New York: Macmillan.

Heeschen, C. (1985). Agrammatism vs. Paragrammatism: A fictitious opposition. In M. L. Kean (Ed.), *Agrammatism.* Orlando: Academic Press.

Heilman, K. M., Valenstein, E. (1972). Auditory neglect in man. *Archives of Neurology, 26,* 32–35.

Huber, W., Poeck, K., & Weniger, D. (1982). Aphasie. In K. Poeck (Ed.), *Klinische Neuropsychologie 1ed. 66–107.* Stuttgart: Thieme.

Huber, W., Poeck, K., & Weniger, D. (1989). Aphasie. In K. Poeck (Ed.), *Klinische Neuropsychologie 2ed. 89–137.* Stuttgart: Thieme.

Huber, W., Poeck, K., Weniger, D., & Willmes, K. (1983). *Der Aachener Aphasie Test.* Göttingen: Hogrefe.

Huber, W., Poeck, K., & Willmes, K. (1984). The Aachen Aphasia Test. In F. C. Rose (Ed.), *Progress in aphasiology. 291–303.* New York: Raven.

Huber, W., Stachowiak, F. J., Poeck, K., & Kerschensteiner, M. (1975). Die Wernicke-Aphasie. Klinisches Bild und Überlegungen zur neurolinguistischen Struktur. *Journal of Neurology, 210,* 77–97.

Jackson, J. H. (1866). On a case of loss of power of expression: inability to talk, to write and to read correctly after convulsive attacks. *British Medical Journal, 92,* 326–330.

Jackson, J. H. (1879/80). On affections of speech from disease of the brain. *Brain, 2,* 323–356.

Jakobson, R. (1968). Child language, aphasia and phonological universals. The Hague: Mouton.

Joanette, Y., Keller, E., & Lecours, A. R. (1980). Sequences of phonemic approximations in aphasia. *Brain and Language, 11,* 30–44.

Jones, L. V., Wepman, J. M. (1961). Dimensions of language performance in aphasia. *Journal of Speech Research, 4,* 220–232.

Katz, R. B. & Goodglass, H. (1990). Deep dysphasia: analysis of a rare form of repetition disorder. *Brain and Language, 39,* 153–185.

Kerschensteiner, M., Poeck, K., Huber, W., Stachowiak, F. J., & Weniger, D. (1978). Die Broca-Aphasie. Klinisches Bild und Überlegungen zur neurolinguistischen Struktur. *Journal of Neurology, 217,* 223–242.

Kertesz, A. (1979). *Aphasia and associated disorders.* New York: Grune & Stratton.

Kertesz, A. (1984). Recovery from aphasia. In F. C. Rose (Ed.), *Progress in aphasiology. 23–39.* New York: Raven.

Kertesz, A. & Benson, D. F. (1970). Neologistic jargon – a clinico-pathological study. *Cortex, 6,* 362–386.

Kertesz, A., Harlock, W., & Coates, R. (1979). Computer tomographic localization, lesion size, and prognosis in aphasia and nonverbal impairment. *Brain and Language, 8,* 34–50.

Kertesz, A. & McCabe, P. (1977). Recovery patterns and prognosis in aphasia. *Brain, 100,* 1–18.

Kertesz, A. & Phipps, J. B. (1977). Numerical taxonomy of aphasia. *Brain and Language, 4,* 1–10.

Kertesz, A., Sheppard, A., & MacKenzie, R. (1982). Localization in transcortical sensory aphasia. *Archives of Neurology, 39,* 475–478.

Kinsbourne, M. (1972). Behavioral analysis of the repetition deficit in conduction aphasia. *Neurology, 22*, 1126–1132.

Kleist, K. (1934). *Gehirnpathologie*. Leipzig: Barth.

Kohn, S. E. (1984). The nature of the phonological disorder in conduction aphasia. *Brain and Language, 23*, 97–115.

Kolk, H. H. J., van Grunsven, M. J. F., & Keyser, A. (1985). On parallelism between production and comprehension in agrammatism. In M. L. Kean (Ed.), *Agrammatism*. Orlando: Academic Press.

Lebrun, Y. (1989). *Mutism*. London: Taylor & Francis.

Lecours, A. R. (1982). Simulation of speech production without a computer. In M. A. Arbib, D. Caplan, & J. C. Marshall (Eds.), *Neural models of language processes. 345–370*. New York: Academic Press.

Leischner, A. (1951). Über den Verfall der menschlichen Sprache. *Archiv für Psychiatrie und Zeitschrift Neurologie, 187*, 250–267.

Leischner, A. (1979). *Aphasien und Sprachentwicklungsstörungen 1ed.* Stuttgart: Thieme.

Lhermitte, F. & Gautier, J. C. (1969). Aphasia. In P. J. Vinken & G. W. Bruyn (Eds.), *Handbook of Clinical Neurology, vol. 4. 84–104*. Amsterdam: North Holland.

Lichtheim, L. (1885). On aphasia. *Brain, 7*, 433–484.

Linebaugh, C. W. (1990). Lexical retrieval problems: anomia. In L. L. LaPointe (Ed.), *Aphasia and related neurogenic language disorders. 96–112*. New York: Thieme.

Luria, A. R. (1970). *Traumatic aphasia*. Paris: Mouton.

Luria, A. R. (1974). Language and the brain. Towards the basic problems of neurolinguistics. *Brain and Language, 1*, 1–14.

Luria, A. R. & Hutton, J. T. (1977). A modern assessment of the basic forms of aphasia. *Brain and Language, 4*, 129–151.

Marie, P. (1906). Revision de la question de l'aphasia. I. La troisieme circonvolution frontale gauche ne joue aucun role dans la fonction de langage. *Semaine medicale (Paris), 26*, 241–247.

Marshall, J. C. (1986). The description and interpretation of aphasic language disorder. *Neuropsychologia, 24*, 5–24.

McNeil, M. R. (1988). Aphasia in the adult. In N. J. Laas, L. V. McReynolds, J. L. Northern, & D. E. Yoder (Eds.), *Handbook of Speech-Language Pathology and Audiology. 738–786*. Toronto: B. C. Decker.

Miceli, G., Gainotti, G., Caltagirone, C., & Masullo, C. (1980). Some aspects of phonological impairment in aphasia. *Brain and Language, 11*, 159–169.

Miceli, G., Mazzucchi, A., Menn, L., & Goodglass, H. (1983). Contrasting cases of Italian agrammatic aphasia without comprehension disorder. *Brain and Language, 18*, 65–97.

Mohr, J. P., Pessin, M. S., Finkelstein, S., Funkenstein, H. H., Duncan, G. W., & Davis, K. R. (1978). Broca aphasia: Pathologic and clinical. *Neurology, 28*, 311–324.

Morton, J. (1985). Naming. In S. Newman & R. Epstein (Eds.), *Current perspectives in dysphasia. 217–230*. London: Churchill Livingstone.

Nadeau, S. E. (1988). Impaired grammar with normal fluency and phonology. Implications for Broca's aphasia. *Brain, 111*, 1111–1137.

Naeser, M. A., Helm-Estabrooks, N., Haas, G., Auerbach, S., & Srinivasan, M. (1987). Relationship between lesion extent in Wernicke's area on computed tomographic scan and predicting recovery of comprehension in Wernicke's aphasia. *Archives of Neurology, 44*, 73–82.

Nass, R. D., Gazzaniga, M. S. (1987). Cerebral lateralization and specialization in human central nervous system. In V. B. Mountcastle (Ed.), *Handbook of Physiology, sec. 1: The Nervous System, vol. V, part 2. 701–761*. Bethesda: American Physiological Society.

Nielsen, J. M. (1938). The unsolved problem in aphasia. I. Alexia in "motor" aphasia. *Bulletin of the Los Angeles Neurological Society, 4*, 114–122.

Obler, L. K. & Albert, M. L. (1982). Language in the elderly aphasic and in the dementing patient. In M. L. Taylor Sarno (Ed.), *Acquired aphasia. 385–398*. New York: Academic Press.

Parisi, D. & Pizzamiglio, L. (1970). Syntactic comprehension in aphasia. *Cortex, 2*, 204–215.

Pashek, G. V. & Holland, A. L. (1989). Evolution of aphasia in the first year post onset. *Cortex, 24*, 411–424.

Patterson, K. E., Marshall, J. C., & Coltheart, M. (1985). *Surface dyslexia*. London: Erlbaum.

Phillips, C. G., Zeki, S., & Barlow, H. B. (1984). Localization of function in the cerebral cortex. *Brain, 107*, 327–362.

Pick, A. (1913). *Die agrammatischen Sprachstörungen*. Berlin: Spinger.

Pizzamiglio, L., Mammucari, A., & Razzano, C. (1985). Evidence for sex differences in brain organization in recovery in aphasia. *Brain and Language, 25*, 213–223.

Poeck, K. (1983). What do we mean by "aphasic syndromes"? A neurologist's view. *Brain and Language, 20*, 79–89.

Poeck, K., de Bleser, R., & von Keyserlingk, D. G. (1984 a). Neurolinguistic status and localization of lesion in aphasic patients with exclusively consonant-vowel recurring utterances. *Brain, 107*, 199–217.

Poeck, K., de Bleser, R., & von Keyserlingk, D. G. (1984b). Computed tomography localization of standard aphasic syndromes. In F. C. Rose (Ed.), *Progress in aphasiology. 71–89*. New York: Raven.

Poeck, K., Huber, W., & Willmes, K. (1989). Outcome of intensive language treatment in aphasia. *Journal of Speech and Hearing Disorders, 54*, 471–479.

Poeck, K., Kerschensteiner, M., Stachowiak, F. J., & Huber, W. (1974). Die amnestische Aphasie. Klinisches Bild und Überlegungen zur neurolinguistischen Struktur. *Journal of Neurology, 207*, 1–17.

Ratcliff, G. & Davies-Jones, G. A. (1972). Defective visual localization in focal brain wounds. *Brain, 95*, 46–60.

Riedel, K. (1981). Auditory comprehension in aphasia. In M. T. Sarno (Ed.), *Acquired aphasia. 215–269*. New York: Academic Press.

Rosenbek, J. C. (1984). Advances in the evaluation and treatment of speech apraxia. In F. C. Rose (Ed.), *Progress in aphasiology. 327–336*. New York: Raven.

Rubens, A. B. (1976). Transcortical motor aphasia. In H. & H. A. Whitaker (Eds.), *Studies in neurolinguistics, vol. 1. 293–303*. New York: Academic Press.

Spreen, O., Benton, A. L., & Fincham, R. W. (1965). Auditory agnosia without aphasia. *Archives of Neurology, 13*, 84–92.

Stachowiak, F. J., Huber, W., Kerschensteiner, M., Poeck, K., & Weniger, D. (1977). Die globale Aphasie. Klinisches Bild und Überlegungen zur neurolinguistischen Struktur. *Journal of Neurology, 214*, 75–84.

Starkstein, S. E., Robinson, R. G., & Price, T. R. (1987): Comparison of cortical and subcortical lesions in the production of poststroke mood disorders. *Brain, 110*, 1045–1059.

Tanabe, H., Sawade, T., Inoue, N., Ogawa, M., Kuriyama, Y., & Shiraishi, J. (1987). Conduction aphasia and the arcuate fasciculus. *Acta Neurologica Scandinavica, 76*, 422–427.

Tissot, R. J., Mounin, G., & Lhermitte, F. (1973). *L'agrammatisme*. Brussels: Dessart.

Tzortzis, C., Albert, M. (1974). Impairment of memory for sequences in conduction aphasia. *Neuropsychologia, 12*. 355–366.

Vignolo, L. A., Boccardi, E., & Caverni, E. (1986). Unexpected CT-scan findings in global aphasia. *Cortex, 22*, 55–70.

von Stockert, T. R. (1975). Aphasia sine aphasia. *Brain and Language, 1*, 277–282.

Wallesch, C. W. (1985). Two syndromes of aphasia occurring with ischemic lesions involving the left basal ganglia. *Brain and Language, 25*, 357–361.

Wallesch, C. W. (1990). Repetitive verbal behaviour: neurological and functional considerations. *Aphasiology, 4*, 133–154.

Wallesch, C. W. (1991). Aphasia. In M. Swash & J. Oxbury (Eds.), *Clinical Neurology, vol. 1. 10–29*. Edinburgh: Churchill Livingstone.

Wallesch, C. W. & Bak, T. (1991): Acute aphasia. In A. Hartmann, W. Kuschinsky & S. Hoyer (Eds.), *Cerebral ischemia and dementia*. Berlin: Springer.

Wallesch, C. W., Bak, T., & Schulte-Mönting, J. (1992). Acute aphasia – patterns and prognosis. Aphasiology, *6*, 273–285.

Wallesch, C. W., Haas, J. C., & Blanken, G. (1988). On the neurological status of speech automatisms and its implications for neurolinguistic models. *Aphasiology, 3*, 435–447.

Wallesch, C. W. & Papagno, C. (1989). Subcortical aphasia. In F. C. Rose, R. Whurr, & M. A. Wyke (Eds.), *Aphasia. 256–287* London: Cole & Whurr.

Weisenburg, T. & McBride, K. (1935). *Aphasia, a clinical and psychological study*. New York. Commonwealth Fund.

Wepman, J. M. & Jones, L. V. (1961). *The language modalities test for aphasia*. Chicago: Education Industries Service.

Wernicke, C. (1874). *Der aphasische Symptomencomplex*. Breslau: Cohn & Weigert.

Willmes, K. & Poeck, K. (1984). Ergebnisse einer multizentrischen Untersuchung über die Spontanprognose von Aphasien vaskulärer Ätiologie. *Nervenarzt, 55*, 62–71.

Claus-W. Wallesch, Freiburg (Germany)/
Andrew Kertesz, London, Ontario (Canada)

10. Cerebral Organization of Language

1. Introduction

Current theories of cortical mechanisms of cognition are related to the development of anatomical techniques to trace cortical connections and long tracts, and to stain neurons. Anatomists, such as Gall/Spurzheim (1810) began to assign functions to cortical regions, elevating them to the status of cortical organs for every conceivable mental activity. They originated phrenology, the study of skull landmarks reflecting cerebral function, and this was carried to absurdity by charlatans. Scientific support for the localization of function came from the physiologists of the second half of the 19th century who observed the close relationship of stimulated cortical points and movements in animals (Fritsch/Hitzig 1870), extirpation of occipital cortex and loss of vision (Munk 1881), and from clinicians who correlated language impairment with the left perisylvian brain lesions (Broca 1861; Wernicke 1874). Associationist psychology, reflex physiology, the neuronal theory, and improved anatomical methods, such as myelin staining and cytoarchitectonics, contributed the anatomically based concepts of language function. Cortical lesions in dogs led Goltz (1881) to conclude that the cerebral cortex is the organ of intelligence, which is permanently impaired by large lesions, but smaller lesions cannot cause permanent or selective deficits. A similar conclusion was reached by Lashley (1933) who promoted the idea of equipotentiality of brain regions on the basis of rat experiments. Further sophistication in the clinical, psychological and experimental investigations contributed evidence both for localized cerebral function, as well as for widespread and integrated activity. Extremely localizationist or equipotentialist views are no longer tenable, in view of the available information.

2. Anatomical Issues

The hemispheres are divided anatomically into frontal, parietal, temporal, and occipital lobes. The Sylvian fissure separates the temporal lobe from the frontal and parietal lobes, and the Rolandic fissure separates the frontal from the parietal lobe. The separation of the occipital lobe from the temporal and the parietal lobes is less obvious on the lateral surface, but medially, the parieto-occipital fissure is distinctive and reaches the calcarine sulcus. On the lateral surface an arbitrary line is drawn between the parieto-occipital fissure and the pre-occipital notch. Further gyral and sulcal subdivisions are more variable, but the superior, middle, and inferior frontal and temporal gyri, the precentral and post-central gyri, the supramarginal, angular and superior parietal gyri on the convexities are usually identifiable. From the medial surface above the corpus callosum, which connects the two hemispheres, the cingulate gyrus and posteriorly the paracentral lobule, the precuneus and the cuneus and inferiorly the lingual and fusiform gyri are quite consistent. These gyral subdivisions do not always correspond to cyto-architectonic boundaries very accurately, but they are important anatomical landmarks for functional studies as well.

The basal ganglia are essential relay systems between subcortical and cortical structures. Recent evidence links them closely to cortical mechanisms of language. Therefore, it is important to have a brief description and to emphasize the connections between the subcortical region and language cortex. The most important basal ganglia from the point of view of cognition are the striatum, the globus pallidus, and the thalamus. The striatum consists of the putamen and the caudate which are separated by the anterior internal capsule but they are considered to be a unit functionally. The globus pallidus is medial to the putamen and forms the lenticular nucleus with it. The thalamus is the most medial of the nuclei of the basal ganglia, and occupies the two sides of the third ventricle. The thalamus is an important relay station for the ascending sensory and extra-pyramidal motor systems up to the cortex. It receives important input from the cerebellum, the striatum and the globus pallidus. All this input is integrated into the thalamocortical projections that reach every aspect of the cortex. The thalamocortical connections for language are not yet agreed upon, except some, for example the projections from the pulvinar to Wernicke's area are well recognized on the basis of physiological studies.

Cortical areas are usually defined by various histological techniques used. Classical cytoarchitectonics has been based on staining the Nissl substance in neurones. Myeloarchitectonics, angio-architectonics, pigment architectonics, chemoarchitectonics and transmitter architectonics provide further information about cortical regions. The following summary is based on traditional cytoarchitectonics with some recent evidence mainly from pigment architectonics (Sanides 1970).

Heterotypical cortex, such as the hippocampal formation and the olfactory cortex (paleocortex), usually contains a few, poorly distinguished bands of neurons. Mesocortex refers to areas between allocortex and isocortex and is characterized by greater lamination. It includes the paralimbic areas of the caudal orbitofrontal cortex, the insula, the parahippocampal gyrus, the temporal pole and the cingulate.

Isocortex or homotypical cortex occupies the greatest surface in the human brain and has six layers. Starting from surface these are: 1) molecular layer (10% of cortical thickness). This is relatively acellular consisting mostly of tangential axons from horizontal cells and ascending collaterals. II) The outer granular layer (9%) contains small cells that is ill-defined from the next layer. III) Pyramidal layer represents about 30% of the cortex and contains lower cell density but greater average cell size. IV) Inner granular layer (10%) high density, small cells. This is the least consistent layer and at times it is missing ('agranular' cortex). V) Ganglionic layer (20%). This layer provides major cortical efferent tracts, such as the pyramidal tract and callosal commissural fibers. VI) The fusiform layer (21%).

Isocortex is further subdivided to unimodal (modality specific) and multimodal cortex by functional considerations (Mesulam 1985). Heteromodal (multimodal) cortex is closer in structure to paralimbic cortex and it is considered developmentally and functionally between paralimbic and unimodal areas (Mesulam 1985). Ideotypic cortex is the highly specialized unimodal cortex of the primary areas with characteristic cytoarchitectonic features, such as the striate cortex for vision, the koniocortex for audition (Heschl's gyrus) and somatic sensation (post-central cortex), and the macro-pyramidal cortex of the motor strip.

The cytoarchitectonic specificity of language cortex is controversial. Brodmann (1909) claimed such specificity for Broca's area 44 and also for the superior temporal (area 22) and the inferior parietal (area 40) region, but this was rejected by Mayendorf (1930), and Bailey/von Bonin (1951). Nevertheless, recent studies show distinct pigment architectonics in area 44 and in the superior temporal region (Galaburda/Sanides 1980).

Cerebral connections follow a certain pattern that distinguishes between primary and other cortical areas according to Flechsig (1901), who specifically established, on the basis of myelogenetic studies, that primary areas are interconnected only through secondary and tertiary association areas. Although recently there has been some evidence that modifies Flechsig's rule, it remains an important principle of cortical organization.

3. Physiological Issues

Cortico-cortical connections were explored physiologically by Dusser de Barenne/McCulloch (1938), who applied strychnine locally and detected increased electrical activity at distant sites of the brain. Since then, electrical recordings and tracer techniques (see below) confirmed these early anatomical and physiological studies. The importance of cortical connections and the mechanisms of disconnections in the production of the neurobehavioral syndromes was recently placed in modern perspective by Geschwind (1965). More recently the term connectionism has been used in an entirely different sense in brain modelling and artificial intelligence (McClelland/Rumelhart 1986).

The extent to which functions can be localized in the brain is variable. There are functions about which there is less argument concerning localization to a certain cortical region. These are the primary sensory and motor areas including the cortical areas for special senses, such as hearing and vision, that are clearly responsible for perceiving the environment and initiating further cerebral processes. On the other hand, the greatest volume of cortex is concerned with cognition that is less obviously localizable. Freud (1891) conceived the language substrate as a continuous cortical area in the left hemisphere extending between "the primary acoustic and optic areas, and the origin of the motor tracts". The lesions of the "necessarily ill defined parts of the speech region" border on receptive and motor cortical fields and "cut off one of the elements of speech association from its connexions with the others". Head (1926) emphasized the distinction between the localizable functions of motion, sensation and vision, which have a clear relationship to body parts, muscles, sensory inputs and stimuli, and "disorders of speech or similar higher grade functions ... in that there is no such relation to parts of the body or their projection in space".

Even the localization of primary motor functions in the prerolandic cortex has been the subject of argument, especially concerning to what extent a part of a movement, or whole actions are cortically represented. Stimulation and ablation studies indicated that fairly complex movements seem to be affected together. Primary areas have distinctive cytoarchitecture but recent investigations indicated that they are not uniform in function (Zeki 1983). Cerebral maps of even the primary areas do not appear to be fixed, passive representations, as some recent work showed a great deal of plasticity of function, for example, in the somatosensory cortex (Merzenich/Kaas/Wall et al. 1983). Sensory representation or motor function in the cortex is dynamic, changing with time and antecedent activity, and attentional mechanisms of the moment.

Cortical areas that could be modular in their function have been established, despite the changeability and plasticity of physiological maps. The anatomy of a cortical module as a piece of neural tissue subserving a function is conceptualized by some to be similar to the printed circuits in a computer (Szentagothai 1978). The reality of such cortical modules has been established to some extent in the sensory 'barrels' or cylindrically organized anatomical units in lamina 4 of the somesthetic cortex of rats (Woolsey/Van Der Loos 1970). On the other hand the 'orientation' columns in the visual cortex do not have an obvious anatomical demarcation and they are only defined by electrophysiological response to functional stimuli (Hubel/Wiesel 1968).

The selectivity of certain cortical columnar organizations are not always reflected in lesion analysis. Large lesions of the cortex that are known to have certain physiological response properties produced only a slight deficit of that function. In other words, behavioural studies do not always replicate physiological ones, partly because physiological function in the intact brain may be different from reorganized function after a lesion. There are numerous methodological differences between physiological and behavioural studies that account for the discrepancies. Much of the actual matching of cortical physiology with behavioural functions remains controversial (Phillips/Zeki/Barlow 1984).

Functional representation in the brain is demonstrated by the response of discrete groupings of cells in the somatosensory cortex to particular sensory stimuli (Mountcastle 1957). However, the correlation between neural events and subjective experience is difficult to establish. Arguments for the so-called 'grandmother cell' that would respond exclusively to one type of stimulus (Barlow 1972) have been replaced by the concept of modifiable networks responding to different stimulation at different times. These consist of a variable number of neurons and show a great deal of plasticity. Recent considerations of cortical function suggest that there is more information about a stimulus in an assembly of cells than in any one of them because of the possible patterns of covariations among the cells (MacKay 1978). From the perceptual network, the association areas receive information which is at some stage assigned a psychological percept, such as a colour, shape, or a lexical item according to what memories or precepts are available to match the perception. The influencing of the perceptual process by memories, the so-called 'top down' processing, seems to be an important function of the secondary and perhaps tertiary association areas. Language may serve a special integrative function by mediating or facilitating multi-modality associations (Geschwind 1965).

Secondary association regions adjacent to the primary cortical areas are less closely tied to specific function, and large areas of the brain commonly called tertiary association areas seem even less clearly identified with any particular function, showing a great deal of plasticity and versatility. Some of these tertiary association areas, however, have a definite hemispheric specialization. For example, the unique role of the left hemisphere association areas in language is well-established since Broca, notwithstanding the recent interest in right hemispheric contributions to language. There is some evidence for oral and visual comprehension of concrete nouns by the right hemisphere from callosotomies (Zaidel 1976). The fact that the right hemisphere produced automatic or emotional utterances has been suspected since Jackson (1878) and left hemispherectomies in adults also suggested that the right hemisphere is not as speechless, or devoid of language as was formerly thought (Smith 1966) (see Code 1987 for review) of right hemisphere contributions to language.

The temporal lobe tertiary association areas integrate auditory, visual, and even tactile sensory, information. Anatomical evidence indicates that the sensory system projects through a series of cortical fields from primary sensory areas to the insular region of the temporal lobe, which is closely connected with the limbic areas important in the consolidation of memory (Turner/Mishkin/Knapp 1980). The dominant (usually) left temporal lobe is crucial for comprehension of syntax and phonology. Single word lexical comprehension may be shared with the right hemisphere.

The frontal cortex has been divided into the precentral motor association area that in the inferior region includes Broca's area. The area in front of these precentral areas is collectively called the prefrontal cortex. The extensive connections of this complex association cortex have been reviewed by Goldman-Rakic (1987) and the functional studies in man by Stuss/Benson, (1984). First Bianchi (1895) and then Nauta (1971) suggested that the prefrontal cortex had a unique role of synthesizing inner and outer sensory worlds. The prefrontal cortex appears to be the ultimate target of several sensory cascades as shown by the cortico-cortical connections using the Nauta method (Pandya/Kuypers 1979; Jones/Powell 1970). Various synthetic functions, such as 'response inhibition,' 'short-term memory,' 'polymodal integration,' 'planning,' 'the temporal structuring of behaviour,' were allocated to various regions of the prefrontal cortex (Fuster 1980; Jacobsen 1936; Mishkin 1964). Goldman-Rakic (1987) argued that the prefrontal cortex is necessary for regulating behaviour guided by representations or internalized models of reality but not for behaviour directly guided by external stimuli. The two most directly involved areas of the frontal cortex with language are the left inferior posterior frontal lobe, with an important role in articulation, and the medial supplementary motor area on the left, which plays a role in the initiation of speech.

The parietal lobes are important polysensory areas bilaterally. The simultaneous injections of distinguishable anterograde tracers revealed that these areas are mutually interconnected with as many as 15 other cortical areas in the monkey (Selemon/Goldman-Rakic 1988). The left parietal polymodal tertiary association area is considered to have a specific integrative function between visual and auditory language processes (Wernicke 1874; Geschwind 1965).

4. Functional Issues

Clinicians, physiologists and psychologists have different concepts about what brain functions are. Psychological formulations may not be appropriate to describe actual brain connectivity. On the other hand, anatomy and physiology may not be sufficient, even if it were known to the finest detail to answer all questions about behaviour. Recent advances in cognitive modelling are important in the interpretation of functional deficits (Ellis/Young 1988). These models are based on the principles of information processing and the computer metaphor. Fractionation or staging of function however present many methodological and conceptual problems. Reduction of a complex behaviour to its components is fraught with the hazard of losing the meaning and biological significance of the behaviour to the organism. From the point of view of localization, more complex behaviours, such as comprehension, are likely to have widespread input and will be affected by lesions in many areas. Fractionated functions, such as the "phonological input lexicon", are often the component of other complex behaviours and are even less likely to be localizable than a clinically tangible and often examined behaviour, such as auditory verbal comprehension.

Functional modeling in the past often assumed a serial activation. However, recent physiological studies and computer modelling has emphasized that mental processes operate in parallel, as well as serially (Hinton/Anderson 1981; McClelland/Rumelhart 1986; Van Essen 1985). Discrete units of cognition presumably have some counterparts in a neural organization, but so far there is little evidence that much of the fractionation of function through cognitive modelling has a corresponding physiological organization. Attempts to segregate perception from central processing have often proved to be unsuccessful (Dreyfus 1979). Previous knowledge, in other words the precept, has considerable influence on how stimuli are perceived and this is called, 'top down' processing.

Many language functions, such as naming, seem to be distributed in a diffuse fashion through the language area, as they are affected by lesions from many locations. The widespread distribution of certain cognitive functions, such as directed attention, and memory is biologically predictable, considering their connection to many other processes. Other integrative functions, such as problem solving, intelligence or judgement have so many components, that it has been impossible to localize them. Some of these cognitive functions still require definitions. Complex cognitive tasks are not likely to be restricted to gyri or even lobar structures.

5. Biological Issues

The time elapsed from the onset of the deficit is a major factor to be considered with localization. The early deficit that may be related to edema, cellular function, transient ischemia, etc., is followed by a great deal of early spontaneous recovery in trauma or stroke. The chronic deficit is related not only to a loss of function, but to compensatory changes by functionally connected structures, such as homologous contralateral areas or neighbouring areas during subsequent stages of recovery. The deficit with acute lesion is usually more severe than in the recovered state, although the lesion is the same. Failure to consider this variable may lead to conflicting conclusions about localization (Kertesz 1979).

It is often argued that the performance observed should not be attributed to the damaged area that functions without some of its components, but to other functionally related or even unrelated structures, which take over from the damaged one. At times after a lesion, not only deficits or negative symptoms are observed but also new behaviour or positive symptoms may appear. Positive symptoms may represent elements of neural activity that had been controlled or suppressed by the structure destroyed by the lesion. It has been suggested that sometimes a second lesion even promotes recovery by eliminating this mechanism (Irle 1987).

A performance observed after electrical stimulation of the brain, the local application of neurotransmitters or recording from single units is the function of other connected structures as well (Glassman 1978). To a certain extent, this consideration remains important in the interpretation of any method, but it does not justify the elimination of the search for an anatomical substrate for function.

The sudden removal of large areas of functioning brain in stroke or experimental lesions may produce distant effects in functionally connected neural structures. This is also known as diaschisis since von Monakow (1914) introduced the idea. Slowly growing tumors, on the other hand, often displace tissues with relatively little functional deficit. Rapidly expanding tumors produce distant effects by edema, hemorrhage and vascular occlusion. Therefore, in many instances, lesions of the same size or location will not produce the same deficit unless the study is strictly controlled for etiology. This principle is often violated in many studies of functional localization in neuropsychology.

Behaviour in a complex nervous system may be disturbed because the whole system or only a component of it is affected with similar results, provided that the impaired component is crucial enough in the performance of a function. This, however, could also mean that the same phenomenon is observed from lesions at different locations. The concept of the organism using alternate structures for a function implies "redundancy" and could also account for some of the recovery of complex cognitive function (Stein/Rosen/Butters 1974). That the same function is represented at various levels of the nervous system is the well known principle of "hierarchical" representation, and it is somewhat different from the reduplication implied in redundancy. There is a third possibility, namely, the 'taking over' by completely unrelated structures or 'vicarious functioning'.

Age has always been considered a major factor in recovery. When a child sustains brain damage, the plasticity of the brain allows for compensation, as long as the lesion is not a progressive one. Hemispherectomy in a young child or damage to the prepubertal brain results in almost complete recovery from aphasia (Basser 1962), just like a prepubertal child can acquire a second language without an accent, indicating the possibility of hormonal influence on limiting plasticity. Certain aphasic syndromes, such as fluent or Wernicke's aphasia, appear to be more frequent in older age. Whether this is related to anatomical differences in the vasculature affected or continuing functional lateralization

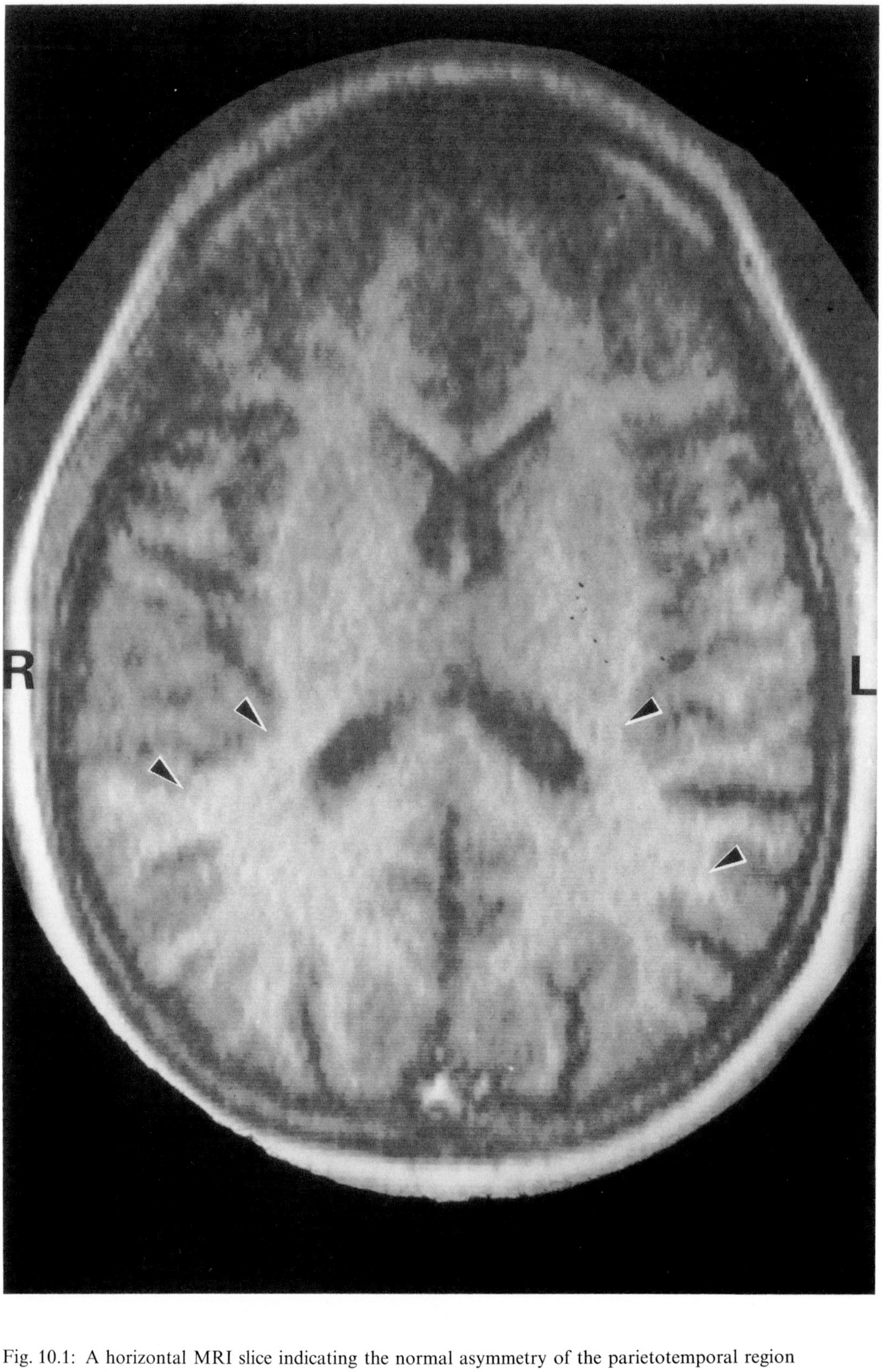

Fig. 10.1: A horizontal MRI slice indicating the normal asymmetry of the parietotemporal region

remains controversial (Brown/Jaffe 1975; Kertesz/Sheppard 1981; Code/Rowley 1987).

Sex differences in cerebral organization are considered to be significant by some studies. It is assumed that language may be more bilaterally distributed in women, therefore lesions may have different effects in different sexes (McGlone 1977; Kimura 1983). Recent epidemiological and clinicoanatomical studies of aphasia did not support inter – and intrahemispheric sex differences (Kertesz/Sheppard 1981; Kertesz/Benke 1989). This is not to deny that there may be important sex differences in other abilities or in psychological deficits.

Handedness is considered an important factor in cerebral dominance for certain functions. Left handers may have somewhat different cerebral organization, not just mirroring right handers but also important qualitative differences which may result in certain lesions producing different deficits in left and in right handers. Gloning/Gloning/Haub/Quatember (1969) suspected that left handers are likely to become aphasic regardless of which hemisphere is damaged, but others found less left handers among aphasics than expected from the general population even in the acute stage (Kertesz 1979; Code/Rowley 1987). This is also compatible with more bilaterally distributed language in left handedness. In the chronic stage, one would expect to see less left handed aphasics because of the suggested better recovery from the deficit (Gloning/Gloning/Haub/Quatember 1969), but this was challenged subsequently (Borod/Carper/Naeser 1990).

Anatomical asymmetries and individual differences in brain structure may be associated with functional differences as well. Anatomical differences between individuals are often observable but they are difficult to quantitate. Hemispheric asymmetries of the cerebral cortex suggest a structural basis for language dominance. Heschl originally noted two transverse gyri in the temporal operculum on the right, and usually one on the left. The length of Heschl's gyrus is usually greater on the left side. The central portion of Heschl's gyrus appears to be larger in the left hemisphere. It has been postulated that this area corresponds to the representation of the frequency range of the human voice. Cunningham (1892) observed Sylvian fissures curving up more sharply on the right and lying horizontally on the left. This was confirmed quantitatively by Rubens/ Mahowald/Hutton (1976). Pfeifer (1936) called attention to the larger planum temporale, the area behind Heschl's gyrus on the left. Geschwind/Levitsky (1968) found this in 65% of brains. This may account for the variable extent to which superior temporal lobe lesions affect language. This asymmetry has been confirmed in newborns (Witelson 1973; Wada/Clarke/Hamm 1975), indicating that there may be a 'prewired' structural feature of our brain allowing the development of language dominance on the left. The cytoarchitectonic asymmetry of the planum temporale, mentioned before, accompanies the gross anatomical asymmetry (Galaburda/Sanides 1980).

One of the most obvious asymmetries on magnetic resonance imaging (MRI) is at the posterior opercular regions. The larger left planum or opercular sulci continue at a larger angle posteriorly (Fig. 10.1). A sharper demarcation of the opercular region from the parietal sulci is seen on the right. Hand preference, hand performance, dichotic listening, and visual field preference measures were correlated with several measures of anatomical asymmetries seen on MRI (Kertesz/Polk/Black/Howell 1990). The sulcal demarcation, anterior frontal width and parietal width correlated best with hand performance, as measured on a dot tapping task (Kertesz/Black/Polk/Howell 1986).

6. Language Function and Lesion Localization

The observation that lesions in the same location were associated with the same deficit or the same behaviour encouraged clinicians and anatomists to draw conclusions from lesions about how the brain functions from clinicoanatomical correlation. This principle received further support from modern neuroscience, the combination of lesion experiments with histochemical and physiological techniques (Mishkin 1978; Goldman-Rakic 1988) and recent imaging techniques that actually display functional changes on line with cognitive processing, such as PET, SPECT or electrophysiology.

Clinicoanatomical correlation in the past suffered from the variability of the deficit descriptions and lack of availability of in vivo localization. Patients who came to autopsy in the past often had poorly explored deficits and a large interval between the clinical and anatomical findings. Modern methods of in vivo localization allowed the application of standardized language testing of a group of similar patients at a well defined stage of stroke, with simultaneous in vivo localization (Kertesz/Harlock/Coates 1979). An example of this method is illustrated in Fig. 10.2, summarizing our CT studies of aphasia (Kertesz/Harlock/Coates 1979).

6.1. Language Production

Spoken language incorporates many subfunctions, which have been categorized by linguists as articulation, fluency, syntax utilization, phonology, lexicon, linguistic prosody, pragmatics, etc. The function of articulated language has been much studied since Broca by neuropsychologists, linguists, neurologists, physiologists, and speech pathologists. Speech output differs substantially, whether it is in response to questions (responsive speech), extemporaneous expression of ideas (descriptive speech) or repetition. The clinical syndrome of Broca's aphasia affects speech output with certain characteristics. Patients with this syndrome speak effortfully with hesitations, pauses, word finding difficulty, phonemic errors (substitutions, deletions, transpositions, anticipations), unintelligible utterances (or stereotypies), and impaired syntax (agrammatism), but comprehension is relatively preserved. Broca's aphasia can be reliably defined by standardized test scores (Kertesz 1979) or by careful clinical description. Many identifiable, even dissociable, central processes contribute to the syndrome, but none of these have so far a reliable localization, only the syndrome as a whole.

Severe persisting Broca's aphasia is associated with large lesions that include not only Broca's area (posterior third of F 3 and the frontal operculum), but also the inferior parietal and often the anterior temporal region

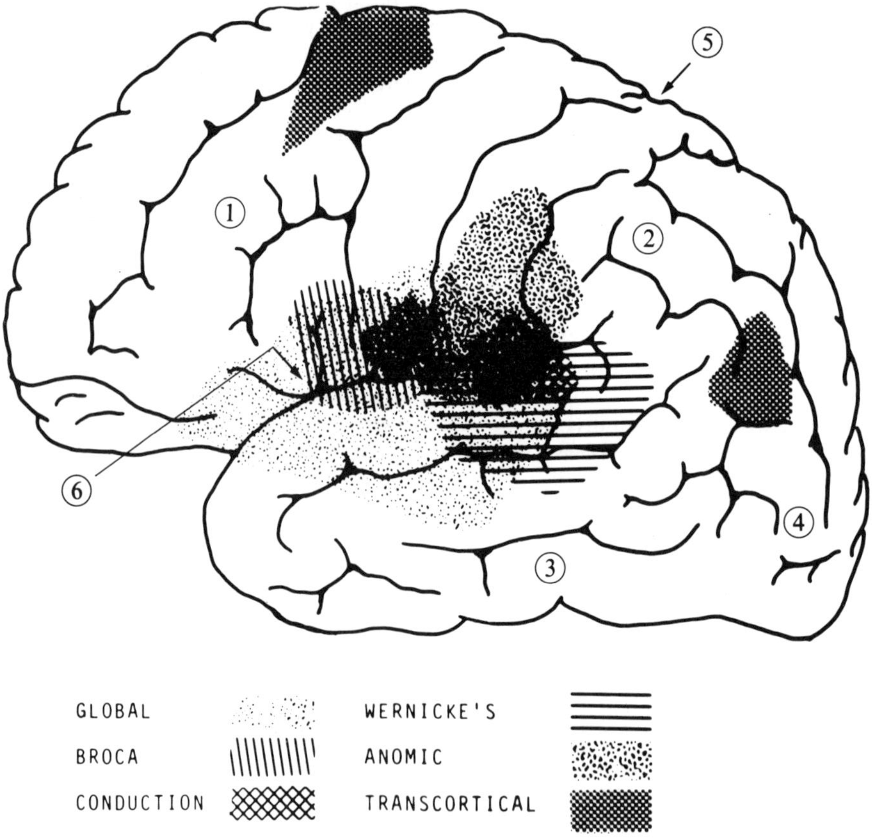

Fig. 10.2: The lateral surface of the brain and its major anatomical landmarks, with a summary of CT lesions of various aphasia types.

① Frontal lobe — ② parietal lobe — ③ temporal lobe — ④ occipital lobe — ⑤ Rolandic fissure — ⑥ Sylvian fissure

(Mohr 1976; Kertesz/Harlock/Coates 1979). Small lesions involving only Broca's area are compatible with good recovery. Pure Broca's area lesions produce a transient motor aphasia (also called 'cortical motor aphasia', 'pure motor aphasia'). Pure motor aphasia has been associated with anterior subcortical, as well as opercular, inferior rolandic, and insular cortical lesions (Kertesz 1984; Lecours/Lhermitte 1976; Suguishita/Konno/Kabe et al. 1987; Tonkonogy/Goodglass 1981).

The role of language cortex in articulation has been studied through experimental psychology, neurophysiology and behavioural neurology. Liberman/Cooper/Shankweiler/Studdert-Kennedy (1967) made important contributions to show the close relationship between phoneme articulation and phonological perception. Anterior language cortex lesions produce impairment of the isolated individual lip movement, and posterior lesions of sequential articulatory movement (Mateer/Kimura 1977). The manual signing systems in the deaf are also disrupted by a left hemisphere damage which is distributed similarly to damage in case of verbal disorders. This is evidence that language cortex is specified for language per se, regardless of the expressive modality, and gestural mechanisms of expression in manual signers are equivalent to articulatory mechanisms in hearing speakers (Poizner/Klima/Bellugi 1987).

Persistent non-fluency was associated with lesions extending to the rolandic cortical region and underlying white matter in previous studies (Mayendorf 1926; Levine/Sweet 1983; Knopman/Selnes/Niccum et al. 1983). The involvement of the central white matter was also important for the fluency deficit in the head injured population of Russell/Espir (1961) and Ludlow/Rosenberg/Fair et al. (1986), and in stroke (Naeser/Palumbo/Helm-Estabrooks et al. 1989). The centrum semiovale or periventricular white matter, that is involved in persistent cases of global or Broca's aphasia, often includes the pyramidal tract, thalamocortical somatosensory fibers, the body of the caudate nucleus, striatocortical connections, callosal radiations, the subcallosal fasciculus, thalamocortical projections from the dorsomedial and ventrolateral nuclei, and the occipitofrontal fasciculus. Motor and premotor phonemic assembly mechanisms are elaborated by a cortical/subcortical network that can be damaged partially, and followed by good recovery. However, if both cortical and subcortical components of the network are impaired, the deficit is more severe (Brunner/Kornhuber/Seemüller et al. 1982) and recovery is much less likely.

Global aphasia is defined by the loss of speech output, as well as comprehension, usually associated with destruction of both the anterior and posterior language areas (Kertesz/Lesk/McCabe 1977). However, Mazzocchi/Vignolo (1979) and Vignolo/Boccardi/Caverni (1986) found that occasionally Wernicke's area is spared. Even 'Broca's area' cortex may not be destroyed, although it is usually disconnected from the rest of the language cortex by white matter involvement (Naeser/Palumbo/Helm-Estabrooks et al. 1989). There are also case reports of patients with initial global aphasia without hemiplegia who recover dramatically when they have posterior-frontal and posterior-temporal lesions but sparing of the central structures (Van Horn/Hawes 1982; Ferro 1983).

Transcortical motor aphasia also is characterized by poor spontaneous speech but very good repetition and comprehension. There is a variable naming deficit and the writing output is also poor. The localization of lesions is characteristically the mesial frontal region or the supplementary speech area in the dominant hemisphere (Goldstein 1948; Chushid/de Gutierrez-Mahoney/Margules-Lavergne 1954; Arseni/Botez 1961; Kornyey 1975; Rubens 1975). The importance of the supplementary motor area on the left was recognized by Penfield/Roberts (1959), who renamed it the 'supplementary speech area' because of the frequent speech arrest that was found during stimulation of this region. Lesions anterior and superior to Broca's area were also described in transcortical motor aphasia, although some of these descriptions stretched the definition of this syndrome with only a relative preservation of repetition over speech output. Lesion localization in this syndrome as in others will depend on the strictness of its definition. It is generally agreed that the supplementary motor area and its connections to Broca's area are important in initiating speech. The lack of speech initiation is often considered to be a part of a general hypokinetic syndrome associated with frontal lobe lesions.

6.2. Comprehension

The motor-sensory dichotomy of language originated from Meynert (1866) who, among others, recognized that the frontal part of the brain is concerned with motor mechanisms and the posterior part of the brain with sensory processing. Wernicke (1874) developed this further, publishing 12 cases of sensory aphasia (two autopsied) in his historic article. Subsequent autopsy and CT studies confirmed that Heschl's gyrus, the planum temporale and the superior temporal gyrus are involved as a rule in sensory aphasia and extensions into the posterior insula, temporal isthmus, the middle and inferior temporal gyri, and the supramarginal and angular gyri add to the variety of clinical features. In the spectrum of Wernicke's aphasia, some of the clinical entities have different localization. 'Pure word deafness' should be restricted to the relatively rare condition when the patient complains of not understanding speech, but hearing, reading, and speech output remain undisturbed. Auditory agnosia for nonverbal sounds and amusia is often associated, although these symptoms may be seen with right sided lesions without the verbal component. In cortical deafness which is the result of bilateral temporal lesions, the patient appears clinically deaf, with preserved primary hearing, but impaired central auditory processes (Kertesz 1983). Neologistic jargon output is distinctive and is associated with lesions of both the superior temporal and inferior parietal regions (Kertesz/Benson 1970). Wernicke's aphasia with semantic jargon is correlated with lesions that are somewhat smaller and more temporal and inferior than those with neologisms or phonemic paraphasias (Kertesz 1983). Other CT studies indicated that patients with semantic substitutions have lesions posterior to those with phonemic paraphasias (Cappa/Cavallotti/Vignolo 1981). However, these studies included a mixture of aphasic types. Patients with transcortical sensory aphasia who have semantic jargon have far more posterior lesions, usually in the watershed area between the middle cerebral and posterior cerebral circulation (Kertesz/Sheppard/MacKenzie 1982). Persisting comprehension deficit was associated with lesion extension inferiorly and anteriorly from Wernicke's area in a mixed group of aphasics that also included global and Broca's type patients (Selnes/Knopman/Niccum et al. 1983). In a recent study of lesion extent in Wernicke's aphasia by Naeser/Helm-Estabrooks/Haas et al. (1987), the extent of involvement of *Wernicke's area* appeared to differentiate good recovery from poor. Our studies of lesion location and size in Wernicke's aphasia suggest that ipsilateral connected structures, especially in the inferior parietal lobule, are the most likely to substitute after damage. The supramarginal and angular gyrus appear as the most likely compensating structures (Kertesz 1988).

Language comprehension is a complex process that involves analysis of acoustic and phonological properties of input, as well as the recognition of syntactic and lexical elements (Liberman/Cooper/Shankweiler/Studdert-Kennedy 1967). This rapid parallel processing of input and matching it to linguistic precepts is an analytical left hemisphere function. The most likely candidate to perform this is the auditory association cortex, localized to the superior temporal gyrus region and the planum temporale, located behind Heschl's gyrus (Wernicke's area). Wernicke already postulated that the auditory association area plays a monitoring role in language output (presaging modern concepts of feedback and parallel processing), and that its damage results in paraphasic, faulty speech. The left hemisphere mediates sequencing and temporal order which are important to language comprehension and output alike (Bradshaw/Nettleton 1981). Conduction aphasia is associated with lesions in the arcuate fasciculus, (so named by Burdach 1819), as well as in the insula (Damasio/Damasio 1983). Usually both structures are involved, although one may predominate over the other. The arcuate fasciculus carries massive temporofrontal connections considered essential for the elaboration of language (Wernicke 1874; Dejerine/Dejerine-Klumpke 1895; Polyak 1927; Geschwind 1965). The language cortex is anatomically contiguous from Wernicke's to Broca's area through the temporal operculum, insula and the frontal operculum. Pierre Marie emphasized the significance of the region of the 'quadrilateral' area that included the insula and the underlying subcortical region. He was criticized by Dejerine and Klumpke for excluding the frontal operculum and inferior frontal lobe from his concept of language cortex (Lecours/Caplan 1984). Subsequent anatomists have also pointed out the contiguity of language cortex which becomes evident when the Sylvian fissure is unfolded (Krieg 1963).

Syntax

Complex functions, such as syntactical processing, are much more difficult to correlate with specific lesion sites, although they can be fractionated linguistically. Extension of the lesions to the inferior parietal lobule and the central region of the rolandic cortex, above the Sylvian fissure, are the prerequisites of persistent agrammatic aphasia. Complex syntactic manipulations may be impaired without typical agrammatic speech in parietal (Luria 1970) and in frontal lesions (Nadeau 1988). Paragrammatism or faulty use of grammar is seen in Wernicke's aphasia, usually with impaired posterior temporal and inferior parietal language cortex. Agrammatism, and telegraphic speech is associated with Broca's aphasia due to fairly extensive frontal and central perisylvian lesions.

6.3. Lexicon and Lexical Access

Naming disturbances are elicited from all patients with aphasia and the lesions are distributed in the anterior, central and posterior portions of the brain, therefore it has not been considered a function with consistent clinical localization (Kertesz 1979). Various types of anomia however have been distinguished, and certain differences in brain damage associated with these types have been described (Benson 1979). Lexical retrieval and semantic analysis are left hemisphere functions, but they are likely related to a wide, overlapping network of cortical mechanisms, rather than consistently identifiable single cortical areas. Yet anterior and central lesions are more likely to produce lexical retrieval deficit without a loss of semantic representation. Posterior temporoparietal lesions often produce naming difficulty that is associated with some comprehension deficit for the same lexical item or a loss of meaning of words, even though they may be used in a correct grammatical sentence. Head (1926) called these cases 'semantic aphasia'. Some category specific anomias have been described as a consequence of temporal lobe encephalitis, such as the inability to name fruits while preserving the names of flowers (McKenna/Warrington 1988).

6.4. Subcortical-Cortical Mechanism

The role of subcortical structures in language is not fully understood. Motor impairments dominate the deficit in lesions of the basal ganglia. This is ranging from dysarthria and hypophonia (which has been known to occur commonly after thalamotomies) to severe global aphasia. Anomic aphasia is often observed, presenting as a disturbance of word retrieval and rather hesitant speech. The often preserved repetition is called a "transcortical feature" (Selby 1967; Cappa/Vignolo 1979). Bell (1968) considered the deficit to be similar to the aphasias of the frontal regions. Lesions in the putamen and the anterior internal capsule produce slow, anomic, dysarthric speech, and with posterior extension, comprehension is also impaired and paraphasic speech and jargon appear (Barat/Mazaux/Bioulac et al. 1981; Naeser/Alexander/Helm-Estabrooks et al. 1982; Damasio/Damasio/Rizzo et al. 1982).

Isolated lesions of the caudate or putamen are rare, but both have been described as causing transient speech deficits. Thalamic lesions produce fluctuating jargon aphasia alternating with relatively non-fluent speech (Mohr/Walters/Duncan 1975). Repetition is often preserved (Cappa/Vignolo 1979). Although subcortical lesions are often said to produce atypical syndromes, (Damasio/Damasio/Rizzo et al. 1982) when an attempt is made to compare the scores of patients with subcortical lesions with equivalent sized cortical lesions, the differences are not significant (Kertesz 1984). Distant cortical hypometabolism or lesions are considered as a possible reason for the deficit, in addition to whatever intrinsic coordinating or processing may take place in the basal ganglia (Metter/Wasterlain/Kuhl et al. 1981; Baron/D'Antona/Serdaru et al. 1986).

6.5. Alexia and Agraphia

Disturbances of reading and writing occur with lesions of distinct cortical localization, but also in various combinations with aphasia. These language functions are also subserved by networks and therefore more than one lesion site will account for the same syndrome. Dejerine (1892) made the classical distinction between pure alexia with left occipital lesions that usually involve the splenium or its radiation, and alexia with agraphia that are associated with parietal, at times specifically angular gyrus lesions on the left side. Dejerine postulated that the lesion in pure alexia disconnects the callosal input for letters and colours from the intract right hemisphere to the left parietal language area, in addition to destroying the left occipital area. This was the prime model for the disconnection theories that postulated the existence of white matter lesions disconnecting various cortical language processors (Geschwind 1965). The recent linguistic distinction of deep and surface dyslexia (deep and surface refers to linguistic, not anatomical structures) is based on error analysis of the reading on non-words and orthographically irregular words. Deep dyslexia seems to be related to large perisylvian infarcts and corresponds to what other authors describe as aphasic alexia (or the third alexia). Surface dyslexia or reading without comprehension is seen with temporal damage mainly (Bub/Kertesz 1982). Other varieties of lesions that disconnect primary visual input from the angular gyrus were termed "preangular" or "subangular" alexias by Greenblatt (1983).

Agraphia is also associated with parietal lobe lesions on the dominant side but agraphia is common with any lesion producing aphasia, although dissociations have also been observed. Frontal lobe lesions can also produce agraphia, although the existence of Exner's center in the second frontal convolution in front of the hand area of the precentral gyrus has not been generally supported. Recent studies showed a considerable amount of agraphia with purely subcortical lesions, which is somewhat different from agraphia due to cortical lesions because it seems that mostly the graphomotor aspects rather than grammatical and semantic aspects are involved (Kertesz 1984). This type of agraphia used to be designated apraxic agraphia.

Ideographic (Kanji) and syllabic (Kana) writing disorders in Japanese have been reported to be associated with different lesion localization, suggesting different neuronal processing. Kanji processing is semantic and context dependent. Kana, on the other hand, can be read aloud without semantic processing. Iwata (1984) suggested that semantic processing takes place through inferior occipitotemporal connections, because lesions in this area interfere with Kanji selectively (Kawahata/Nagata/Shishido 1988; Kawamura/Hirayama/Hasegawa et al. 1987). Dorsal connections through the angular gyrus are involved in Kana (or phonological) processing, similar to Indo-European languages. Pure agraphia for Kanji has also been reported with subcortical damage under-cutting the left inferior temporal gyrus (Mochizuki/Ohtomo 1988).

7. Language Function and Cortical Stimulation

Cortical stimulation, excision and direct recording developed for epilepsy surgery are important contributions to cortical localization. Initially it was used by physiologists to map the function of the cerebral cortex in animals, and subsequently neurosurgeons, such as Foerster and Penfield, tried to identify cortical areas using stimulation in preparation for their excisions. Sensory, motor and language functions can be spared using this technique. Penfield/Roberts (1959) mapped the language areas extensively and Van Buren/Fedio/Frederick (1978), Ojemann/Whitaker (1978), Ojemann/Mateer (1979), Lüders/Lesser/Dinner et al. (1988), and Creutzfeldt/Ojemann/Lettich (1989) have added further information concerning cortical localization. The studies of Ojemann and his collaborators have shown that stimulation of Broca's area produces the most consistent naming difficulty. They also found a rather peculiar mosaic of language function where a couple of millimetres made a great deal of difference in determining what functional alterations were obtained on stimulation. For instance, one site would interfere with language but not the site next to it, and a very small change in the location of the electrodes would change the results. Language appeared to be concentrically organized around the Sylvian fissure rather than following the anteroposterior dichotomy of the lesion studies. The anterior and central system was concerned with articulatory organization of speech and stimulation of this region impaired facial movement and arrested speech. The second system involved the inferior frontal, superior temporal and parietal peri-Sylvian cortex, and stimulation disrupted the sequence of movements as well as phonemic perception. Outside this zone, stimulation site disrupted naming, reading, syntax, and next to it the outermost system involved shortterm verbal memory.

Recording from neurons in the superior temporal gyrus showed activation on listening to verbal material, particularly to phonological distinctions. Differences in meaning or inflection were associated with changes in the pattern of neuronal discharge from the middle and inferior temporal gyrus (Creutzfeldt/Ojemann/Lettich 1989). Medial temporal lobe recording produced stimulus specific firing on sight of a particular word or face during epilepsy surgery. This region seemed to encode distinct stimuli in a given context, with a remarkable degree of specificity (Heit/Smith/Halgren 1988). Implanted subdural electrodes were also used to record and to stimulate ambulant patients. In addition to the perisylvian language cortex, stimulation of the inferior basal region also produced speech arrest more on the left than the right (Lüders/Lesser/Dinner et al. 1988).

Transcranial magnetic stimulation of human brain has been recently reported for eliciting motor function (Barker/Jalinous/Freeston 1985). The threshold for excitation of motor cortex is markedly reduced by slight voluntary contraction of the target muscle. The mechanism of facilitation is neural activity at the spinal and cortical level. It is assumed that dendrites and presynaptic terminals, or even cell bodies and efferent axons will be stimulated by increasing strength magnetic stimuli (Mills/Murray/Hess 1987). Magnetic stimulation of language cortex has also been tried, but so far only negative phenomenon, such as anomia has been obtained.

7.1. Cortical Electrophysiology

Electroencephalography (*EEG*) and Event-Related Potentials (*ERP*) are physiological methods of localizing cortical activity and function. EEG represents a summation of remote physiological events. The original observations of suppression of alpha rhythm in the dominant hemisphere during verbal tasks and in the non-dominant side during spatial tasks (Galin/Ornstein 1972) have been further elaborated. Intercortical connections were assessed by measuring the degree of correlation between pairs of electrodes, called cortical coupling (Callaway/Harris 1974). Computerized statistical treatment of EEG data is used to display functional alterations and their locations in colour coded images that is often called 'brain mapping'. ERP uses averaging computers to link brain potentials to certain stimuli and averaging out the rest of the background activity. Differences in ERP lateralization were observed by using verbal and nonverbal stimuli (Buchsbaum/Fedio 1970), words vs. nonsense syllables (Shelburne 1972), and contextual meaning (Brown/Marsh/Smith 1973; Teyler/Roemer/Harrison et al. 1973). Long latency ERPs are sensitive to task relevance and expectancy. The 300 msec. positive component is called 'P 300' which is considered endogenous and less dependent on stimulus characteristics. Another example of ERPs associated with language processing is the 'N 400 potential' which is related to the occurrence of context incongruity in serial semantic tasks (Kutas/Hillyard 1980; Neville/Kutas/Schmidt 1982). ERP studies are technically difficult because of the many artefacts that interfere with the study. The stimulation has to be very short and have a definite onset, duration and offset, in order to be connected with the cerebral event. Although the technique reflects a physiological event connected with actual cerebral processing, the resolution of localization is poor and the potentials are usually distributed over a large area of the scalp and the brain.

7.2. Functional Activation

Positron Emission Tomographic (*PET*) studies of activity related changes in cerebral blood flow, and cerebral oxygen metabolism, using short half-life oxygen-15 and a technique of subtraction of flow during control tasks confirmed certain notions of cortical localization. They also provided evidence for localization of certain functions that has not been possible on the basis of clinicopathological lesion analysis (Petersen/Fox/Posner et al. 1988). Areas related to motor output and articulation were the sensory-motor cortex at the lower end of the rolandic fissure and near Broca's area which is by itself not surprising. Bilateral Sylvian activation during speech was confirmed, but the lack of specificity for language was also pointed out because activation occurred when subjects moved their mouth and tongue without speaking. The left inferior frontal area was considered to participate in processing semantic associations (a verb with a noun). The anterior cingulate gyrus appeared to be part of an anterior attentional system indicated by its activation while monitoring lists of words for a semantic category. Auditory processing activated the primary auditory cortex bilaterally, but the activation was specific for words on the left temporoparietal cortex and in the anterior-superior temporal region. These studies also showed that Wernicke's area was not necessarily activated in reading, and suggested that visual verbal information appears to have access to 'output coding' without phonological recoding in the posterior temporal cortex. They found simple repetition was independent from semantic association confirming in a sense the original Wernicke–Lichtheim model (Lichtheim 1885). Activation for semantic association did not appear to be modality specific and it appeared to be coupled with output activation, especially in the median frontal and anterior cingulate regions.

In another report (Posner/Petersen/Fox/Raichle 1988) the ventral occipital lobe was the processor of the visual word form, as it was activated by passively looking at visually presented nouns. The left lateral frontal lobe is involved in semantics used in coding word associations but not requiring motor or verbal output (e. g., attending to, but not speaking, words in a specific class from a presented list). The supramarginal gyrus appears to process phonological tasks (e. g. determining whether words rhyme), whereas the anterior cingulate region is activated when the brain selects language or other information for action (e. g., naming presented words). The data suggest that a posterior system processes early visual images and anterior attention systems select information for output.

8. Conclusion

The concepts of cortical fields and flexible cortical networks have replaced the rigid mosaicism of cortical centres. The evidence for widespread cerebral activation in cortical functions has been substantial. The reticular activating system, the ubiquitous thalamocortical projections, as well as the multiplicity of limbic and cortical connections indicated that central nervous system activity is complex and much of the brain may be activated even for simpler acts of cognition. These physiological notions have been confirmed lately by the multiple areas that are shown to be activated on the cerebral blood flow (CBF) and positron emission tomography (PET) technique in reasonably well-defined stages of mental activity. Indirect measures of function, such as EEG, event-related averaged potentials, or the distribution of neurotransmitters also support the widespread and interactive nature of cerebral activity. Nevertheless, local components of many forms of cognition can be distinguished functionally, physiologically, and anatomically, even though their plasticity, overlap, and interdependence is recognized.

Hughlings Jackson's statement remains, as paraphrased here, axiomatic: One can only localize lesions (and accompanying physiological and metabolic changes) associated with certain behavioural alterations but not function. Does this mean that the study of lesion-behaviour correlation is useless? The answer is an emphatic no, because as Phillips/Zeki/Barlow (1984) stated, "the original method, that of studying and trying to explain the deficits of function associated with specific lesions, is still capable of yielding interesting results, and is in a sense the final arbiter; if you cannot show the expected deficits of function after a local lesion, you probably have not got the right answer about what function that local region performs". Evidence from physiological studies and deficit analysis indicates that the concepts of modularity of language function are useful, provided it is realized that these functions are integrated and participate in more diffusely distributed processes. The lesion evidence has an important role in determining the structural constraints of functional networks. Evidence from clinicopathological localization has a great deal to offer in steering cognitive modelling towards biological reality and providing the structural guidance for the interpretation of further physiological and psychological data. Lesion localization, quite apart from the theoretical considerations, has an important clinical use in interpreting syndromes and in determining prognosis.

9. References

Arseni, C. & Botez, M. I (1961). Speech disturbances caused by tumors of the supplementary motor area. *Acta Psychiatrica Scandinavica*, 36, 279–299.

Bailey, P. & von Bonin, G. V. (1951). *The isocortex of man*. Urbana: University Of Illinois Press.

Barat, M., Mazaux, J. M., Bioulac, B., Giroire, J. M., Vital, C., & Arne, L. (1981). Troubles du langage de type aphasique et lesions putaminocaudees: observation anatomoclinique. *Revue Neurologique*, *137*, 343–356.

Barker, A. T., Jalinous, R., & Freeston, I. L. (1985). Non-invasive magnetic stimulation of the human motor cortex. *Lancet*, *2*, 1106–1107.

Barlow, H. B. (1972). Single units and sensation: a neuron doctrine for perceptual psychology? *Perception*, *1*, 371–394.

Baron, J. C., D'Antona, R., Serdaru, M., Pantano, P., Bousser, M. G., & Samson, Y. (1986). Hypometabolisme cortical apres lesion thalamique chez l'homme: etude par la tomographie a positrons. *Revue Neurologique*, *142*, 465–474.

Basser, L. S. (1962). Hemiplegia of early onset and the faculty of speech with special reference to the effects of hemispherectomy. *Brain*, *85*, 427–460.

Bell, D. S. (1968). Speech functions of the thalamus inferred from the effects of thalamotomy. *Brain*, *91*, 619–638.

Benson, D. F. (1979). *Aphasia, alexia and agraphia*. Edinburgh & London: Churchill-Livingstone.

Bianchi, L. (1895). The functions of the frontal lobes. *Brain*, *18*, 497–522.

Borod, J. C., Carper, J. M., & Naeser, M. (1990). Long-term language recovery in left-handed aphasic patients. *Aphasiology*, *4*, 561–572.

Bradshaw, J. L. & Nettleton, N. C. (1981). The nature of hemispheric specialization. *Behavioural and Brain Sciences*, *4*, 51–63.

Broca, P (1861). Remarques sur le siege de la faculte du langage articule suivies d'une observation d'amphemie (perte de la parole). *Bulletin et Memoires de la Societe Anatomique de Paris*, *36*, 330–357.

Brodmann, K. (1909). *Vergleichende Lokalisationslehre der Grosshirnrinde*. Leipzig: Barth.

Brown, W. S. & Jaffe, J. (1975). Hypothesis on cerebral dominance. *Neuropsychologia*, *13*, 107–110.

Brown, W. S., Marsh, J. T., & Smith, J. C. (1973). Contextual meaning effects on speech-evoked potentials. *Behavioral Biology*, *9*, 755–761.

Brunner, R. J., Kornhuber, H. H., Seemüller, E., Suger, G., & Wallesch, C. W. (1982). Basal ganglia participation in language pathology. *Brain and Language*, *16*, 281–299.

Bub, D. & Kertesz, A. (1982). Deep agraphia. *Brain and Language*, *17*, 146–165.

Buchsbaum, M. & Fedio, P. (1970). Hemispheric differences in evoked potentials to verbal and nonverbal stimuli in the left and right visual fields. *Physiology and Behaviour*, *5*, 207–210.

Burdach, K. F. (1819–1826). *Vom Baue und Leben des Gehirns*. Leipzig: Dyk'sche Buchhandlung.

Callaway, E. & Harris, P. R. (1974). Coupling between cortical potentials from different areas. *Science*, *183*, 873–875.

Cappa, S. F., Cavallotti, G., & Vignolo, L. A. (1981). Phonemic and lexical errors in fluent aphasia; correlation with lesion site. *Neuropsychologia*, *19*, 171–179.

Cappa, S. F. & Vignolo, L. A. (1979). "Transcortical" features of aphasia following left thalamic hemorrhage. *Cortex*, *15*, 121–130.

Chusid, J., de Gutierrez-Mahoney, C., & Margules-Lavergne, M. (1954). Speech disturbances in association with parasagittal frontal lesions. *Journal of Neurosurgery*, *11*, 193–204.

Code, C. (1987). *Language, aphasia, and the right hemisphere*. New York: Wiley and Sons.

Code, C. & Rowley, D. (1987). Age and aphasia type: the interaction of sex time since onset and handedness. *Aphasiology*, *1*, 339–345.

Creutzfeldt, O., Ojemann, G., & Lettich, E. (1989). Neuronal activity in the human lateral temporal lobe. I. Responses to speech. *Experimental Brain Research*, *77*, 451–475.

Cunningham, D. J. (1892). *Contribution to the surface anatomy of the cerebral hemispheres*. Dublin: Royal Irish Academy.

Damasio, A. R. & Damasio, H. (1983). Localization of lesions in achromatopsia and prosopagnosia. In A. Kertesz (Ed.), *Localization in neuropsychology*. New York: Academic Press.

Damasio, A. R., Damasio, H., Rizzo, M., Varney, N., & Gersh, F. (1982). Aphasia with nonhemorrhagic lesions in the basal ganglia and internal capsule. *Archives of Neurology*, *39*, 15–20.

Dejerine, J. (1892). Contribution a l'etude anatomo-pathologique et clinique des differentes varietes de cecite verbale. *Comptes Rendus des Seances de la Societe de Biologie et de Ses Filiales*, *4*, 61–90.

Dejerine, J. & Dejerine-Klumpke, A. (1895). *Anatomie des centres nerveux*. Paris: Ruef et Cie, 1895.

Dreyfus, H. L. (1979). *What computers can't do: The limits of artificial intelligence*. 2nd edition. New York: Harper & Row.

Dusser de Barenne, J. G. & McCulloch, W. S. (1938). The direct functional interrelation of sensory cortex and optic thalamus. *Journal of Neurophysiology*, *1*, 176–186.

Ellis, A. W. & Young, A. W. (1988). *Human cognitive neuropsychology*. Hove, U. K.: Lawrence Erlbaum Associates.

Ferro, J. M. (1983). Global aphasia without hemiparesis. *Neurology*, *33*, 1106.

Flechsig, P. (1901). Developmental (myelogenetic) localisation of the cerebral cortex in the human subject. *Lancet*, ii, 1027–1029.

Freud, S. (1891). *Zur Auffassung der Aphasien, eine Kritische Studie*. Leipzig: Deuticke. (Translated by E. Stengel, London: Imago, 1953).

Fritsch, G. T. & Hitzig, E. (1870). Über die elektrische Erregbarkeit des Grosshirns. *Archiv für Anatomie und Physiologie*, Leipzig, 300–322.

Fuster, J. M. (1980). *The prefrontal cortex*. New York: Raven Press.

Galaburda, A. M. & Sanides, F. (1980). Cytoarchitectonic organization of the human auditory cortex. *Journal of Comparative Neurology*, *190*, 597–610.

Galin, D. & Ornstein, R. (1972). Lateral specialization of cognitive mode: an EEG study. *Psychophysiology*, *9*, 412–418.

Gall, F. J. & Spurzheim, J. C. (1810). *Anatomie et Physiologie due Systeme Nerveux en General, et du Cerveau en Particulier*. Paris: Schoell and Co.

Geschwind, N. (1965). Disconnexion syndromes in animals and man. *Brain*, *88*, 237–294, 585–644.

Geschwind, N. & Levitsky, W. (1968). Human brain: Left-right asymmetries in temporal speech regions. *Science*, *161*, 186–187.

Glassmann, R. B. (1978). The logic of the lesion experiment and its role in the neural sciences. In S. Finger (Ed.), *Recovery from brain damage*. New York: Plenum Press.

Gloning, I., Gloning, K., Haub, G., & Quatember, R. (1969). Comparison of verbal behaviour in right-handed and non-right-handed patients with anatomically verified lesions of one hemisphere. *Cortex*, *5*, 43–52.

Goldman-Rakic, P. S. (1987). Circuitry of the prefrontal cortex and the regulation of behavior by representational memory. *Handbook of Physiology*, *5* (Part 1, Ch. 9), 373–417.

Goldman-Rakic, P. S. (1988). Topography of cognition: Parallel distributed networks in primate association cortex. *Annual Review of Neuroscience*, *11*, 137–156.

Goldstein, K. (1948). *Language and language disturbances*. New York: Grune & Stratton.

Goltz, F. (1881). *Transactions of the 7th International Medical Congress*, Vol. 1, W. MacCormac (Ed.). London: J. W. Kolkmann, 1881.

Greenblatt, S. H. (1983). Localization of lesions in alexia. In A. Kertesz (Ed.), *Localization in neuropsychology*. New York: Academic Press.

Head, H. (1926). *Aphasia and kindred disorders of speech*. Cambridge: Cambridge University Press.

Heit, G., Smith, M. E., & Halgren, E. (1988). Neural encoding of individual words and faces by the human hippocampus and amygdala. *Nature*, *333*, 773–775.

Hinton, G. E. & Anderson, J. A. (1981). *Parallel models of associative memory*. Hillsdale, N. J.: Lawrence Erlbaum Assoc. Inc.

Hubel, D. & Wiesel, T. (1968). Receptive fields and functional architecture of monkey striate cortex. *Journal of Physiology*, *195*, 215–243.

Irle, E. (1987). Lesion size and recovery of function: some new perspectives. *Brain Research Reviews*, *12*, 307–320.

Iwata, M. (1984). Kanji versus Kana: Neuropsychological correlations of the Japanese writing system. *Trends in Neuroscience*, *7*, 290–293.

Jackson, J. H. (1878). On affections of speech from disease of the brain. *Brain*, *1*, 304–330.

Jacobsen, C. C. (1936). Studies of cerebral function in primates. *Comparative Psychology and Monographs*, *13*, 1–68.

Jones, E. G. & Powell, T. P. (1970). An anatomical study of converging sensory pathways within the cerebral cortex of the monkey. *Brain*, *93*, 793–820.

Kawahata, N., Nagata, K., & Shishido, F. (1988). Alexia with agraphia due to the left posterior inferior temporal lobe lesions – Neuropsychological analysis and its pathogenic mechanisms. *Brain and Language*, *33*, 296–310.

Kawamura, M., Hirayama, K., Hasegawa, K., Takahashi, N., & Yamaura, A. (1987). Alexia with agraphia of kanji (Japanese morphograms). *Journal of Neurology, Neurosurgery & Psychiatry*, *5*, 1125–1129.

Kertesz, A. (1979). *Aphasia and associated disorders: Taxonomy, localization and recovery*. New York: Grune & Stratton.

Kertesz, A. (1983). Localization of lesions in Wernicke's aphasia. In A. Kertesz (Ed.), *Localization in neuropsychology*. New York: Academic Press.

Kertesz, A. (1984). Apraxia of speech. In J. C. Rosenbek, M. R. McNeil & A. E. Aronson (Eds.), *Apraxia of Speech: Physiology, Acoustics. Linguistics. Management*. San Diego, CA.: College-Hill Press.

Kertesz, A. (1988). What do we learn from recovery from aphasia? In S. G. Waxman (Ed.), *Advances of Neurology, Vol. 47: Functional recovery in neurological disease*. 277–292. New York: Raven Press.

Kertesz, A. & Benke, T. (1989). Sex equality in intrahemispheric language organization. *Brain and Language*, *37*, 401–408.

Kertesz, A. & Benson, D. F. (1970). Neologistic jargon – a clinico-pathological study. *Cortex*, *6*, 362–386.

Kertesz, A., Black, S. E., Polk, M., & Howell, J. (1986). Cerebral asymmetries on magnetic resonance imaging. *Cortex*, *22*, 117–127.

Kertesz, A., Harlock, W., & Coates, R. (1979). Computer tomographic localization, lesion size and prognosis in aphasia. *Brain and Language*, *8*, 34–50.

Kertesz, A., Lesk, D., & McCabe, P. (1977). Isotope localization of infarcts in aphasia. *Archives of Neurology*, *34*, 590–601.

Kertesz, A., Polk, M., Black, S. E., & Howell, J. (1990). Sex handedness and the morphometry of cerebral asymmetries on magnetic resonance imaging. *Brain Research*, *530*, 40–48.

Kertesz, A. & Sheppard, A. (1981). The epidemiology of aphasic and cognitive impairment in stroke – age, sex, aphasia type and laterality differences. *Brain*, *104*, 117–128.

Kertesz, A., Sheppard, A., & MacKenzie, R. A. (1982). Localization in transcortical sensory aphasia. *Archives of Neurology*, *39*, 475–478.

Kimura, D. (1983). Sex differences in cerebral organization for speech and praxic functions. *Canadian Journal of Psychology*, *37*, 19–35.

Knopman, D. S., Selnes, O. A., Niccum, N., Rubens, A. B., Yock, D., & Larson, D. (1983). A longitudinal study of speech fluency in aphasia: CT correlates of recovery and persistent nonfluency. *Neurology*, *33*, 1170–1178.

Kornyey, E. (1975). Aphasie transcorticale et echolalie: Le probleme de l'initiative de la parole. *Revue Neurologique*, *131*, 347–363.

Krieg, W. J. S. (1963). *Connections of the cerebral cortex*. Evanston, Il.: Brain Books.

Kutas, M. & Hillyard, S. A. (1980). Reading senseless sentences: Brain potentials reflect semantic incongruity. *Science*, *207*, 203–205.

Lashley, K. S. (1933). Integrative functions of the cerebral cortex. *Physiological Review*, *13*, 1–42.

Lecours, A. R. & Caplan, D. (1984). Augusta Dejerine-Klumpke or "the lesion in anatomy". *Brain & Cognition*, *3*, 166–197.

Lecours, A. R. & Lhermitte, F. (1976). The 'pure form' of the phonetic disintegration syndrome (pure anarthria): anatomo-clinical report of a historical case. *Brain and Language*, *3*, 88–113.

Levine, D. N. & Sweet, E. (1983). Localization of lesions in Broca's motor aphasia. In A. Kertesz (Ed.), *Localization in Neuropsychology*, New York: Academic Press.

Liberman, A. M., Cooper, F. S., Shankweiler, D. R., & Studdert-Kennedy, M. (1967). Perception of the speech code. *Psychological Review*, *74*, 431–461.

Lichtheim, L. (1885). On aphasia. *Brain*, *7*, 443.

Lüders, H., Lesser, R. P., Dinner, D. S., Morris, H. H., Wyllie, E., & Godoy, J. (1988). Localization of cortical function: New information from extraoperative monitoring of patients with epilepsy. *Epilepsia*, *29*, S 56–S 65.

Ludlow, C. L., Rosenberg, J., Fair, C., Buck, D., Schesselman, S., & Salazar, A. (1986). Brain lesions associated with nonfluent aphasia fifteen years following penetrating head injury. *Brain*, *109*, 55–80.

Luria, A. (1970). *Traumatic Aphasia*. Hague: Mouton.

MacKay, D. M. (1978). The dynamics of perception. In P. A. Buser & A. Rougeul-Buser (Eds.), *Cerebral correlates of conscious experience*, Amsterdam: Elsevier.

Mateer, C. & Kimura, D. (1977). Impairment of nonverbal oral movements in aphasia. *Brain and Language*, *4*, 262–276.

Maydendorf, E. Niessl von (1926). Über die sog. Brocaische Windung und ihre angebliche Bedeutung für den motorischen Sprachakt. *Monatsschrift für Psychiatrie und Neurologie*, *61*, 129–146.

Mayendorf, E. Niessl von (1930). *Vom Lokalisationsproblem der artikulierten Sprache*. Leipzig: Barth.

Mazzocchi, F. & Vignolo, L. A. (1979). Localisation of lesions in aphasia: Clinical CT scan correlation in stroke patients. *Cortex*, *15*, 627–654.

McGlone, J. (1977). Sex differences in the cerebral organization of verbal functions in patients with unilateral brain lesions. *Brain*, *100*, 775–793.

McKenna, R. A. & Warrington, E. K. (1988). Category specific naming preservation: a single case study. *Journal of Neurology, Neurosurgery and Psychiatry*, *41*, 571–574.

McClelland, J. L. & Rumelhart, D. E. (1986). *Parallel distributed processing: Explorations in the microstructure of cognition, Vol. 2: Psychological and biological models*, London: MIT Press.

Merzenich, M. M., Kaas, J. H., Wall, J., Nelson, R. J., Sur, M., & Felleman, D. (1983). Topographic reorganisation of somatosensory cortical areas 3 b and 1 in adult monkeys following restricted deafferentation. *Neuroscience*, *8*, 33–55.

Mesulam, M. M. (1985). *Principles of behavioural neurology*. Philadelphia: FA Davis.

Metter, E. J., Wasterlain, C. G., Kuhl, D. E., Hanson, W. R., & Phelps, M. E. (1981). ^{18}FDG positron emission computed tomography in a study of aphasia. *Annals of Neurology*, *10*, 173–183.

Meynert, T. (1866). Ein Fall von Sprachstörung anatomisch begründet. *Medizinisches Jahrbuch und Zeitschrift für die Gesamte Ärzteschaft*, *12*, 152–187.

Mills, K. R., Murray, N. M., & Hess, C. W. (1987). Magnetic and electrical transcranial brain stimulation: Physiological mechanisms and clinical applications. *Neurosurgery*, *20*, 164–168.

Mishkin, M. (19649. Perseveration of central sets after frontal lesions in monkeys. In J. M. Warren, K. Akert (Eds.), *The Frontal Granular Cortex and Behavior*, New York: McGraw-Hill.

Mishkin, M. (1978). Memory in monkeys severely impaired by combined but not by separate removal of amygdala and hippocampus. *Nature*, *272*, 297–298.

Mochizuki, H. & Ohtomo, R. (1988). Pure alexia in Japanese and agraphia without alexia in kanji. *Archives of Neurology*, *45*, 1157–1159.

Mohr, J. P. (1976). Broca's area and Broca's aphasia. In H. Whitaker & H. A. Whitaker (Eds.), *Studies in neurolinguistics* (Vol. 1). New York: Academic Press.

Mohr, J. P., Walters, W. C. & Duncan, G. W. (1975). Thalamic hemorrhage and aphasia. *Brain and Language*, *2*, 3–17.

Mountcastle, V. B. (1957). Modality and topographic properties of single neurons of cat's somatic sensory cortex. *Journal of Neurophysiology*, *20*, 408–434.

Munk, H. (1881). *Über die Funktionen der Grosshirnrinde. Gesammelte Mitteilungen aus den Jahren 1877–1880*. Berlin: Hirschwald.

Nadeau, S. E. (1988). Impaired grammar with normal fluency and phonology. Implications for Broca's aphasia. *Brain*, *111*, 1111–1137.

Naeser, M. A., Alexander, M. P., Helm-Estabrooks, N., Levine, H. L., Laughlin, S. A., & Geschwind, N. (1982). Aphasia with predominantly subcortical lesion sites: Description of three capsular/putaminal aphasia syndromes. *Archives of Neurology*, *39*, 2–14.

Naeser, M. A., Helm-Estabrooks, N., Haas, G., Auerbach, S., & Scrinivasan, M. (1987). Relationship between lesion extent in Wernicke's area on computed tomographic scan and predicting recovery of comprehension in Wernicke's aphasia. *Archives of Neurology, 44*, 73–82.

Naeser, M. A., Palumbo, C. L., Helm-Estabrooks, N., Stiassny-Eder, D., & Albert, M. L. (1989). Severe nonfluency in aphasia. Role of the medial subcallosal fasiculus and other white matter pathways in recovery of spontaneous speech. *Brain, 112*, 1–38.

Nauta, W. J. H. (1971). The problem of the frontal lobe: A reinterpretation. *Journal of Psychiatric Research, 8*, 167–187.

Neville, H. J., Kutas, M., & Schmidt, A. (1982). Event-related potential studies of cerebral specialization during reading. I. Studies of normal adults. *Brain and Language, 16*, 300–315.

Ojemann, G. A. & Mateer, C. (1979). Human language cortex: Localization of memory, syntax and sequential motor-phoneme identification systems. *Science, 250*, 1401–1403.

Ojemann, G. A. & Whitaker, H. A. (1978). Language localization and variability. *Brain and Language, 6*, 239–260.

Pandya, D. N. & Kuypers, H. G. J. M. (1979). Cortico-cortical connections in the rhesus monkey. *Brain Research, 13*, 13–36.

Penfield, W. & Roberts, L. (1959). *Speech and Brain Mechanisms*. Princeton, N. J.: Princeton University Press.

Petersen, S. E., Fox, P. T., Posner, M. I., Mintun, M., & Raichle, M. E. (1988). Positron emission tomographic studies of the cortical anatomy of singleword processing. *Nature, 331*, 585–589.

Pfeifer, R. A. (1936). Pathologie der Hörstrahlung und der cortikalen Hörspäre. In O. Bumke and O. Foerster (Eds.), *Handbuch der Neurologie* Bd. VI. 533–626. Berlin: Springer-Verlag.

Phillips, C. G., Zeki, S., & Barlow, H. B. (1984). Localization of function in the cerebral cortex. *Brain, 107*, 327–361.

Poizner, H., Klima, E. S., & Bellugi, U. (1987). *What the hands reveal about the brain*. Cambridge, Mass.: The MIT Press.

Polyak, S. (1927). An experimental study of the association callosal and projection fibers of the cerebral cortex of the cat. *Journal of Comparative Neurology, 44*, 197–258.

Posner, M. I., Petersen, S. E., Fox, P. T., & Raichle, M. E. (1988). Localization of cognitive operations in the human brain. *Science, 240*, 1627–1631.

Rubens, A. B. (1975). Aphasia with infarction in the territory of the anterior cerebral artery. *Cortex, 11*, 239–250.

Rubens, A. B., Mahowald, M. W., & Hutton, J. T. (1976). Asymmetry of the lateral (sylvian) fissures in man. *Neurology, 26*, 620–624.

Russell, W. R. & Espir, M. L. E. (1961). *Traumatic aphasia*. London: Oxford University Press.

Sanides, F. (1970). Functional architecture of motor and sensory cortices in primates in the light of a new concept of neocortex evolution. In C. R. Noback & W. Montagna (Eds.), *The primate brain*. New York: Appleton.

Selby, G. (1967). Stereotaxic surgery for the relief of Parkinson's disease. II. An analysis of the results of a series of 303 patients (413 operations). *Journal of the Neurological Sciences, 5*, 343–375.

Selemon, L. D. & Goldman-Rakic, P. S. (1988). Common cortical and subcortical targets of the dorsolateral, prefrontal and posterior parietal cortices in the rhesus monkey: evidence for a distributed neural network subserving spatially guided behaviour. *Journal of Neuroscience, 8*, 4049–4068.

Selnes, O. A., Knopman, D. S., Niccum, N., Rubens, A. B., & Larson, D. (1983). Computed tomographic scan correlates of auditory comprehension deficits in aphasia: a prospective recovery study. *Annals of Neurology, 13*, 558–566.

Shelburne, S. A. (1972). Visual evoked responses to word and nonsense syllable stimuli. *Cortex, 12*, 325–336.

Smith, A. (1966). Speech and other functions after left (dominant) hemispherectomy. *Journal of Neurology, Neurosurgery and Psychiatry, 29*, 467–471, 1966.

Stein, D. G., Rosen, J. J., & Butters, N. (1974). *Plasticity and Recovery of Function in the Central Nervous System*. New York: Academic Press.

Stuss, D. T. & Benson, D. F. (1984). Neuropsychological studies of the frontal lobes. *Psychological Bulletin, 95*, 3–28.

Sugishita, M., Konno, K., Kabe, S., Yunoki, K., Togashi, O., & Kawamura, M. (1987). Electropalatographic analysis of apraxia of speech in a left hander and in a right hander. *Brain, 110*, 1393–1417.

Szentagothai, J. (1978). The neuron network of the cerebral cortex: a functional interpretation. *Proceedings of the Royal Society, B, 201*, 219–248.

Teyler, T. J., Roemer, R. A., Harrison, T., et al. (1973). Human scalp-recorded evoked-potential correlates of linguistic stimuli. *Bulletin of the Psychonomic Society, 1*, 333–324.

Tonkonogy, J. & Goodglass, H. (1981). Language function, foot of the third frontal gyrus, and rolandic operculum. *Archives of Neurology, 38*, 486–490.

Turner, B. H., Mishkin, M., & Knapp, M. (1980). Organization of the amygdalo petal projections from modality-specific cortical association areas in the monkey. *Journal of Comparative Neurology, 191*, 515–543.

Van Buren, J., Fedio, P., & Frederick, G. (1978). Mechanism and localization of speech in the parietotemporal cortex. *Neurosurgery, 2*, 233–239.

Van Essen, D. C. (1985). Functional organization of primate visual cortex. In A. Peters & F. G. Jones (Eds.), *Cerebral Cortex* (Vol. 3). New York: Plenum Press.

Van Horn, G. & Hawes, A. (1982). Global aphasia without hemiparesis: a sign of embolic encephalopathy. *Neurology, 32*, 403–406.

Vignolo, L. A., Boccardi, E., & Caverni, L. (1986). Unexpected CT-scan findings in global aphasia. *Cortex, 22*, 55–69.

von Monakow, C. (1914). *Die Lokalisation im Grosshirn und der Abbau der Funktionen durch cortikale Herde*. Wiesbaden: Bergmann.

Wada, J. A., Clarke, R., & Hamm, A. (1975). Cerebral hemispheric asymmetry in humans. Cortical speech zones in 100 adult and 100 infant brains. *Archives of Neurology*, 32, 239–246.

Wernicke, C. (1874). *Der aphasische Symptomencomplex*. Breslau: Cohn & Weigart, in Boston Studies on the Philosophy of Science, vol. IV. Dordrecht, Reidel.

Witelson, S. F. (1973). Left hemisphere specialization for language in the newborn. Neuroanatomical evidence of asymmetry. *Brain, 96*, 641–646.

Woolsey, T. & Van der Loos, H. (1970). The structural organization of layer IV in the somatosensory region (S 1) of mouse cerebral cortex. *Brain Research, Amsterdam, 17*, 205–242.

Zaidel, E. (1976). Auditory vocabulary of the right hemisphere following brain bisection or hemidecortication. *Cortex, 12*, 187–211.

Zeki, S. M. (1983). The distribution of wavelength and orientation selective cells in different areas of monkey visual cortex. *Proceedings of the Royal Society, B, 217*, 449–470.

Andrew Kertesz, London, Ontario (Canada)/
Claus-W. Wallesch, Freiburg (Germany)

11. Diagnostic Methods in Aphasiology

1. Introduction

Descriptions of more or less detailed clinical examination procedures for acquired language disorders in individual patients are as old as aphasiology itself. Case reports from the second half of the nineteenth century were often quite detailed. They concentrated on the specific impairments of the patient under study rather than on characteristics of the examination procedures themselves. This state of affairs was not specific to the examination of language disorders. In accord with the development of general psychology at the beginning of the 20th century, objective and standardized assessment procedures were constructed for the measurement of the comparatively complex concept of intelligence. Whereas there was a rapid development of intelligence tests according to Benton's review (1967, 35), the assessment of aphasia progressed slowly. The well known detailed and systematic examination by Head (1926) lacked standardized administration, scoring and normative data. The first extensive standardized test battery in English by Weisenburg/McBride (1935), as well as other batteries developed in the 1950s by Wepman (1951), Eisenson (*Examination for Aphasia*, EFA; 1954), Wepman/Jones (*Language Modalities Test for Aphasia*, LMTA; 1961) and Schuell (1955) still fall under Benton's criticism, namely, that there is little evidence in published form that the batteries are well standardized, objective and useful. For more details concerning the underlying theory and composition of individual tasks, the reader is referred to reviews such as those by Kertesz (1986), Lang (1981) and Spreen/Risser (1981).

Since the 1960s as the need for diagnostic assessment, planning of language therapeutic interventions and comparability of patients in experimental research on aphasia increased, several comprehensive aphasia test batteries have been developed and published. Among the tests in widespread use for the English language are the *Minnesota Test for Differential Diagnosis of Aphasia* (MTDDA; Schuell 1973), the *Porch Index of Communicative*

Ability (PICA; Porch 1967; 1973), the *Neurosensory Center Comprehensive Examination for Aphasia* (NCCEA; Spreen/Benton 1977), the *Boston Diagnostic Aphasia Examination* (BDAE; Goodglass/Kaplan 1972; 1983), and the *Western Aphasia Battery* (WAB; Kertesz 1982). Several other batteries, screening tests, and tests of specific aspects of language behavior are reviewed by Kertesz (1986), Lang (1981), Skenes/McCauley (1985) as well as Spreen/Risser (1981). Although based on different and even controversial theoretical conceptualizations of aphasia, all batteries assess or rate various aspects of oral expression or spontaneous speech as well as its information content. Furthermore they comprise one or more (sub)tests calling for repetition, confrontation naming, reading and writing (to dictation) and auditory and written comprehension tasks. The test batteries are language modality based, providing a pattern of type and severity of impairments (Kertesz 1986; 1988). Almost all of the batteries also contain additional or supplementary arithmetic, memory, praxis, visual recognition, drawing or spatial orientation subtests making the examination more comprehensive clinically.

Test authors became increasingly concerned with the requirements for standardized psychological tests as summarized in the Standards for Educational and Psychological Testing (AERA/APA/NCME 1985). It is these requirements which distinguish the relatively informal though frequently well-structured and systematically executed clinical examination for aphasia from a formal test. The review paper by Skenes/McCauley (1985) is explicitly devoted to checking whether criteria listed by the AERA/APA/NCME (1985) as essential standards were met. These criteria include information about test development, tester qualification, appropriate interpretations of test scores and subscores, test instructions and scoring, normative data, and the fundamental psychometric properties of validity and reliability. Kertesz (1988) lists 10 properties an ideal aphasia test should have. Regrettably, none of the aphasia tests evaluated met all of the seven criteria cited by Skenes/McCauley. Comprehensive diagnostic assessment of type and severity of language disorders is only one of several functions formal assessments fulfill. Screening, assessment for counseling and rehabilitation and progress evaluation are discussed by Spreen/Risser (1981). More recently, David (1990, 103) has summarized additional reasons for testing. She includes monitoring recovery, predicting outcome, consistent sampling for a database of precise descriptions, comparison of affected versus unaffected skills with well-known syndromes and over time, and assistance of communication with other professionals. The reviews by Kertesz, Lang, Skenes/McCauley and Spreen/Risser also provide state of the art information on tests focussing on specific aspects of language behavior and screening tests such as the *Token Test* (De Renzi/Vignolo 1962) and the *Boston Naming Test* (BNT; Kaplan/Goodglass/Weintraub 1983). The papers also evaluate functional communication, including the *Functional Communication Profile* (FCP; Sarno 1969) and the *Communicative Abilities in Daily Living* (CADL; Holland 1980). As has been claimed repeatedly, obviously none of the existing tests can meet all of the stated functions. But at the same time, during the process of testing itself the experienced clinician can gain insight into a wealth of information needed for preliminary hypotheses about the sources of the overt features of language disorders. It is also obvious that whenever a test in the field of aphasia has passed the laborious and time consuming process of test development, validation and standardization, it is already outdated to some extent. This is particularly true for the last decade, which has witnessed many advances from experimental studies and theoretical developments in psycholinguistics, neurolinguistic aphasiology (Caplan 1987) and cognitive neuropsychology in general (Shallice 1988).

In recent years, acquired language disorders have come to be approached from the perspective of information processing models with the aim of identifying neurally realized computational subsystems supporting language processing. Consequently, the classical aphasia syndrome categories – characterized as polytypic (Schwartz 1984) or psychologically weak (Caramazza 1984) – and test batteries using these categories have been challenged for not supplying explanatory evidence concerning the nature of a patient's underlying language processing disorders. Inquiries into and controversial discussions about the adequate methodology of drawing inferences from impaired performance to normal cognitive (language) processing (Caramazza/McCloskey 1988; Caramazza/Badecker 1989; Zurif/Gardner/Brownell 1989; Shallice 1988) have led many researchers to conclude that only by means of in-depth single case studies one can validly relate overt impaired performance and the processing structure of normal cognitive systems. Such an approach clearly leads one to challenge the adequacy of aphasia test batteries in current use (Byng/Kay/Edmundson/Scott 1990) both with respect to diagnostic purposes and to providing adequate information for a language therapeutic approach that is geared at the underlying language processing deficit in a given patient.

In the following, no detailed and comprehensive description and evaluation of existing aphasia test instruments will be given. Readers seeking more information may turn to the references given above as well as to a recent book edited by LaPointe (1990). Also beyond the scope of this article is a thorough discussion of particular models of normal language processing and their implications for the assessment of aphasia. Rather, the different approaches and tests will be evaluated from a psychometric perspective. In the last three decades, measurement models in psychology have advanced considerably (Jones/Appelbaum 1989). Neuropsychology and aphasiology in particular have not yet succeeded in incorporating these psychometric accomplishments into their body of assessment procedures to a sufficiently large extent. — First, the test battery approach and the single case approach will be treated in turn; then suggestions for bridging the gap between both will be made. Finally specific diagnostic assessment problems in comparative aphasiology (Bates/Wulfeck 1989), in the study of bilingual or polyglot aphasia (Paradis 1989) and in the early acute phase will be touched on.

2. The Test Battery Approach

2.1. Concepts

As with any other complex (psychological) construct, there have been various conceptions of language and of aphasia, which in turn have an influence on the collection and composition of tasks comprising an aphasia test battery. (1) For instance, some researchers view aphasic disorders as reflecting a unitary reduction or loss of language capabilities across all language modalities. The MTDDA is an example for this approach systematically examining a variety of language behaviors in different modalities at different levels of task difficulty. (2) Other investigators believe that aphasic disorders affect the information flow in an input to complex central integrative processing to output language model. Consistent with this opproach, the subtests of the PICA are arranged into three groups of subtests according to whether a verbal, gestural or graphic output is required. (3) An approach linked more directly to the neurological substrate considers aphasic disorders to be of different types (syndromes) characterized by a typical pattern of (selectively) impaired components of language functioning caused by the locus (and extent) of the patient's brain lesion. The BDAE and the WAB are taken to be the most explicit examples of the 'neo-localization' approach. Both tests provide more or less explicit and strict criteria for how to assign a patient's performance profile across a variety of conversational speech and language modality based subtests to one of a fixed set of classical aphasia syndromes. (4) Some researchers feel that one can do away with a particular language model and diagnostic types of aphasia. Based on clinical experience one can choose tasks of varying complexity in order to assess a patient's ability to speak or understand spoken and written language as well as to read and write. The NCCEA, providing a 20-subtest profile of percentile scores is a good example of such a pragmatic approach. (5) With a more psycholinguistically oriented approach — viewing aphasic language disorders as impairments in the instrumental use of language — one can go beyond the exclusive assessment of verbal input and output skills. With careful selection of items according to basic structural characteristics of the language system in a particular language, it is hoped that these items can reveal something about underlying linguistic impairments (Weniger 1990, 110). The Aachen Aphasia Test (AAT; Huber/Poeck/Weniger/Willmes 1983; Huber/Poeck/Willmes 1984), for example, attempts to reconcile the clinical approach often centering around aphasic syndromes and the psycholinguistic approach as much as possible in a standard assessment procedure of clinically acceptable length and detail. In a frequently cited article Poeck (1983) argues that vascular aphasic syndromes are no natural combinations of symptoms (no strong syndromes). Instead, they are mainly artifacts produced by the vascularization of the language areas in the brain. Yet he considers them to be useful artifacts in that they allow for a probabilistically-based formation of sufficiently well-separated, sufficiently homogeneous subgroups with respect to linguistically well-controlled predominantly expressive language tasks in a sufficiently large percentage of cerebrovascular cases. In a psycholinguistic approach, components of language processing that are modality specific as well as those that are language dependent can be discerned descriptively. The former are generally subdivided into primary ones directly related to the sound structure of language (acoustic perception and articulatory performance), and secondary ones related to the graphemic structure of language (reading and writing). On the other hand, linguistic components comprise phonologic, syntactic, lexical and semantic levels of processing. For each level, specific linguistic units like phonemes, morphemes, sentences can be discerned with particular regularities for their selection and combination. This characterization will be exemplified in more detail in section 2.2.1. on construct validity.

2.2. Psychometric Properties

In the introduction it was claimed that aphasia test batteries have not been examined adequately with more recent models and methods from psychometrics. In some instances, however, the aphasia tests were constructed prior to the publication or easy availability of these methods. Many textbooks and review articles on psychometric methods extensively treat objectivity, reliability, and validity of psychological tests (Messick 1980; AERA/APA/NCME 1985; Jones/Appelbaum 1989). There is a growing tendency to consider construct validity to be the most fundamental type of validity (Wainer/Braun 1988).

2.2.1. Construct Validity

The construct validity of aphasia tests has commonly been evaluated by means of factor-analytic procedures and principle components analysis. If different subtests had been conceptualized to assess the same or a similar type of language skills they should be correlated substantially, being reducable to a few 'underlying dimensions' or even to just one general language factor (Schuell/Jenkins/Carroll 1962). It has gone unnoticed, however, that there is a longstanding discussion about the theoretical problems inherent in the common factor model, factorial underdeterminacy in particular (Steiger/Schönemann 1978). It is generally assumed that the strong first factor, reported for almost all aphasia test batteries reflects the general, pervasive influence of aphasic language impairment. A more cautious interpretation must take into account the large interindividual variability in level of impairment usually present in larger samples of aphasic patients with the individual subject's performance often located at a similar level of impairment across subtests. This fact almost inevitably leads to high intercorrelations on the average, giving rise to a strong first factor. The high mean intercorrelation overrides the pattern of relations among the correlation coefficients, which itself could be a stable property across different samples as well as across various aphasia tests. Although this phenomenon has been known for some time, it seems to have been recognized only rather recently with regard to the PICA (Clark/Crockett/Klonoff 1979). — Willmes/Poeck/Weniger/Huber (1983) have introduced the approach of facet theory (Canter 1985; Shye 1978) together with nonmetric multidimensional scaling procedures (Guttman 1967; Schlesinger/Guttman 1969) to the evaluation of the construct validity of the AAT. Facet theory provides a rich conceptual framework within which the domain of language tasks used in the assessment of aphasia can be structured. The linguistic tasks included in any aphasia test battery can be characterized by the following definition: An item belongs to the universe/domain of language items if its domain asks about a language regularity of a linguistic unit and asks for a response in a language modality towards that linguistic unit and its range is ordered from very right to very wrong with respect to that linguistic regularity. Regularity and unit are dependent facets since the regularities of individual languages are always tied to particular units. Similarity relations among phonetic features, classificatory relations within semantic fields and recursive hierarchical relations among syntactic structures are to be found for phonemes, lexemes, and sentences, respectively. Regularities and units are modality independent. Lexemes and sentences exhibiting the same regularities can be selected for all modalities. In Huber/Poeck/Willmes (1984) items in the different subtests of the AAT are characterized in this way with a more detailed elaboration of the regularity facet, which has not been paid much explicit attention in many other test batteries. To give an example, in the AAT auditory and written comprehension are examined using a word-to-picture multiple choice matching task also containing line drawings of semantically related lexical items (Weniger 1990). The facet theoretic definition can be directly related to predictions about the solution of a nonmetric multidimensional scaling procedure (e. g. Smallest Space Analysis; Lingoes 1973) applied to the matrix of monotonicity coefficients (Raveh 1978) or other correlation coefficients. Ordinal rather than metric relationships among correlation coefficients – as in factor analysis – are mapped into a space of as few dimensions as possible in such a way that the relations among distances between subtests in the space are in close agreement with the orderings among the similarity coefficients. Taking into account only the ordinal aspects of similarities among linguistic tasks within aphasia tests is more appropriate to the psycholinguistic framework for an aphasia test. Figure 11.1 depicts the 2-dimensional Smallest Space Analysis representation for the original PICA correlation matrix (Clark/Crockett/Klonoff 1979).

A radex-like structure, postulated by Willmes/Poeck/Weniger/Huber (1983) to be present for any aphasia test constructed according to language modalities with subtests incorporating different degrees or types of linguistic complexity, can clearly be discerned. The modality facet plays a polar, unordered role with similar subtests located in a sector emanating from some center. A modular(ordered) linguistic complexity facet induces concentric ellipses about that origin according to whether more or less central language processing is required for carrying out the respective task. The representation makes it obvious that the original grouping of tasks into a verbal, a graphic, and a gestural subtotal score must be qualified. Effects of the linguistic units facet cannot be observed, because total scores across the same ten common objects/nouns entered the correlation matrix and the prototypicality, semantic similarity as well as phonotactic properties of the items have not been controlled for. – The consistently high positive correlations found among linguistic tasks in seemingly all aphasia tests, which is a problem for the interpretation of factor analytic results, can easily be related to a first law of language items (cf. Shye 1978) which postulates nonnegative correlations among any two items from the domain of language tasks whenever

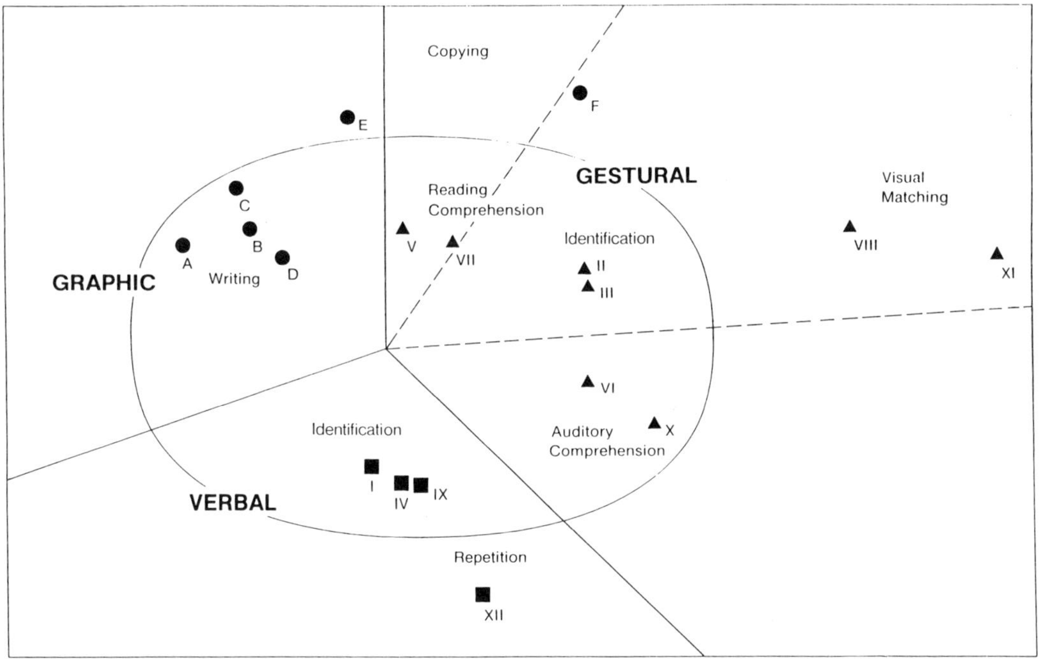

Fig. 11.1: Reanalysis of the original standardization sample subtest intercorrelation matrix for the PICA (Clark/Crockett/Klonoff 1979; n = 150) with a nonmetric multidimensional scaling procedure: Smallest Space Analysis (SSA-I, Lingoes 1973): 2-dimensional solution, alienation coefficient = 0.118; original labeling of subtests

the sample of aphasic patients is not selected artificially. – Other aspects of construct validity are related to predictions about the level of difficulties of particular items. If the linguistic regularity examined is expected to induce varying item difficulty, appropriate (mostly nonparametric) statistical tests should be applied to empirically verify gradation levels of complexity.

2.2.2. Criterion Validity

In aphasiology, the criterion usually is a set of syndrome categories. High correlation with a categorical criterion is equivalent to a good distinction between syndrome groups of patients based on the multivariate profile of test scores. Not all aphasia tests were designed to allow for a syndrome classification. Nevertheless, most of them try to distinguish several subtypes of aphasia by giving a description of their respective test-profile characteristics. The first edition of the BDAE (Goodglass/Kaplan 1972) provides ranges of profile ratings for six spontaneous speech characteristics, an auditory comprehension score as well as the Z-score profile of severity ratings, fluency variables and subtest performances of a typical case for a particular syndrome. – Syndrome groups have also been differenciated by means of a purely statistically based approach. A prototypical example of such a classification method is the WAB which uses techniques from numerical taxonomy, particularly cluster analyses. Although the hierarchical cluster analyses carried out for the profile of fluency, comprehension, repetition, naming and information content of spontaneous speech (Kertesz/Phipps 1977) yielded a larger number of clusters (cf. Risser/Spreen 1985), a classification table with 8 aphasic syndromes was set up giving score intervals for all 8 syndromes in such a way that every profile can unambiguously be assigned to one category. This classification system has been criticized for not containing a category 'non-classifiable'. Poeck (1983) among others has claimed that only probability statements from an adequate statistical model should be used for classification purposes. In keeping with this criticism, a multivariate nonparametric discriminant analysis procedure was applied to the AAT. In this way it could be examined whether the clinical, neurolinguistic classification of aphasic patients according to a list of key symptoms had empirical support from the AAT spontaneous speech ratings and subtest performances. More than 80% were reclassified in accordance with the clinical expert judgement. Based on the standardization sample of about 400 patients each new patient examined with the AAT can be assigned a syndrome classification probability. Operationally, each patient with a posterior probability of more than 70% is considered to be classifiable. From a technical point of view, it is important to note that only multivariate classification procedures not assuming multivariate normality and identical scatter of scores in all groups seem to be adequate, since distributions of scores from aphasic patients' samples tend to be highly skewed, of very different scatter or bi- or multimodal. – Of course, against any discriminant analysis procedure a circularity argument can be raised, since the apriori grouping of cases is not based on strictly independent information. But it is hard to conceive, just where such information should be obtained. Therefore the tentative classification of a new case – as everybody will agree – should never be based on an automatic allocation procedure alone. Objections to the usefulness of syndrome categories have been given in the introduction. For a recent summary of arguments against syndrome categories see Byng/Kay/Edmundson/Scott (1990). – Although considered to be of less importance, a comprehensive aphasia test should also discriminate well between aphasic patients, non-aphasic brain damaged patients and healthy controls. Mild aphasic impairments should also be discerned reliably. Spreen/Risser (1981) among others have pointed out, that no aphasia test can be expected to perfectly discriminate between mild aphasia and normal language functioning. – Another approach to the latter problem would be to use short screening batteries like the Sklar Aphasia Scale (SAS; Sklar 1973) or specific tests like the Token Test (DeRenzi/Vignolo 1962). Although the Token Test was originally designed to tap mild impairments of auditory comprehension, the original version as well as many modified or shortened versions have proven to show high discriminatory power (for an overview see Boller/Dennis 1979). As it turned out, the written language subtest of the AAT slightly outperformed the Token Test. The combination of both subtests yielded a correct selection of 91% of the aphasic and 95% of the non-aphasic patients. Contrary to the opinion expressed earlier by Orgass/Poeck (1969), the AAT thus manages to combine good selection properties with a reliable differentiation of ability levels, a goal which is hard to accomplish for purely psychometric reasons.

2.3. Reliability

The psychometric property of reliability is concerned with how precise a psychological test is as a measurement instrument, since the total score of a (sub-)test only estimates the unknown true ability/impairment level. High reliability is thus required for diagnostic statements about individual patients' performances. A second aspect of reliability, namely retest-reliability, is related to the stability of performances across two (or more) assessments with the same test instrument.

2.3.1. Internal Consistency

A consistency coefficient like Cronbach's alpha coefficient (1951) indicates, how homogeneous a set of items is in grading subjects according to level of performance. Only when there is high internal consistency of no less than about 0.90, can a subtest total score be assumed to express the performances for the individual items. Only then is the confidence interval for the true score (Guilford 1965; Lord/Novick 1968) small enough to allow for a reliable distinction between different levels of performance. In any case, this requirement can only be met if the number of items contained in a subtest is large enough.

2.3.2. Generalizability Theory

Generalizability theory, an elaboration of the internal consistency approach (Brennan 1983), based on estimates of variance components known from analysis of variance, makes it possible to decompose the total variability in a batch of test items into several specific components, each of which is associated with a different facet of the test. Applied to the AAT, generalizability studies showed that the items within the various parts comprising one subtest were more homogeneous than across parts within one subtest.

2.3.3. Test-Retest Reliability

The most problematic aspect of reliability with respect to the assessment of aphasia is so-called test-retest reliability. Since quantitative and even qualitative changes in the level and pattern of performances must be expected, particularly in the course of early recovery, it is not interesting to examine long-term stability. What one does want to know, however, is whether changes in performance before and after some period of language treatment can reliably be attributed to the treatment and not to unspecific practice effects. Rigorous verification of retest reliability for aphasia tests would therefore require both stability in level of performance and high correlation between test scores from two test administrations within a short time interval. Both properties could be demonstrated for the AAT for a time interval of only two days both for patients with short and long duration of the aphasia.

2.3.4. Intra- and Interrater Agreement

Whenever a subject's responses cannot simply be categorized as correct or false without losing away too much information in the process, ratings are required. In line with this reasoning, the BDAE, WAB or AAT use spontaneous speech ratings to judge the severity of a given symptom as well as those aspects of responses that cannot readily be measured otherwise. Usually, rating scales only have ordinal properties. In the linguistic subtests of the AAT, the item responses are scored on 4-point scales, the scale points being defined by descriptions of possible aphasic symptoms, which are assumed to express similar degrees of impairment across all items within a subtest. – With rating scales of about 5 levels or more, interrater agreement can be studied also with methods from generalizability theory or by Krippendorff's model (1970). This model also allows for the distinction of systematic discrepancies between raters in terms of scale mean and scale units (cf. Weniger/Willmes/Huber/Poeck 1981 for an application to the AAT). Correlational methods computing pairwise agreement between judges are not adequate because they are insensitive to differences in scale means. In order to analyze pairwise agreement for categorical scales, the kappa-coefficient (Cohen 1968) or versions correcting for rater biases (Krauth 1984) should be used. Schouten (1980) developped a coefficient for more than two raters. – For the assessment of intra-rater stability across two or several ratings of the same behaviors basically the same methods can be used. It is considered mandatory, to conduct such interrater studies with a sizeable number of potential test users on a sizeable number of patients to be judged.

2.4. Interpretation of Test Results

In his review paper, Lang (1981) regrets that for none of the test batteries a statistically based evaluation of the test profile is provided. Test authors only made suggestions for a descriptive comparison of strengths and weaknesses of a patient's subtest performances. Performances might also be evaluated by relating the individual test profile to typical profiles for a particular syndrome group. H. P. Huber (1973) has introduced a comprehensive approach to the inferential statistical evaluation of an individual test profile. The methods are based on the classical test theory model (Lord/Novick 1968). The prerequisites to be fulfilled by an aphasia test are the availability of standard norms from a large sample of no less than 400 and sufficiently high subtest reliability coefficients computed from a sizeable sample as well. Willmes (1985) has demonstrated the application of these procedures to the analysis of one and the comparison of two AAT-subtest profiles of one patient obtained before and after a period of intensive language therapy. First, subtest performances within one profile can be examined for significant differences, i. e. for differences which cannot be attributed to measurement errors alone. Second, the so-called diagnostic validity for a significant (reliable) difference can be computed, i. e. the probability of obtaining a still larger difference in the aphasic population. For an in-depth study of an aphasic patient with a particular repetition (or reading) disorder, for example, one could require as a strict prerequisite screening criterion that the repetition (or reading) performance in the baseline test is diagnostically validly worse than those in the other subtests (or written language tasks). Third, two profiles of one patient can be compared with respect to level and shape of the profiles. In case of differences in shape, detailed analyses of differential changes in subtest performances can be carried out. A particularly interesting kind of profile pattern is that of a unimodal deficit or peak in performance. To evaluate the efficacy of a particular treatment approach, it is helpful to demonstrate differential changes with the subtest(s) assessing the trained functions improving more. From this perspective Risser/Spreen's (1985, 466) claim that the AAT has diagnostic classification as its primary goal, must certainly be qualified.

2.5. Alternative Models for Test Construction and Scoring

For the vast majority of assessment procedures in neuropsychology only the classical test theory model (Lord/Novick 1968) has been employed, although it is a weak model in terms of its measurement properties. Item parameters, like item difficulty, are dependent on the distribution of ability, levels in the sample used to estimate them, i. e. no specifically objective comparisons of both, item parameters and subject abilities are possible. If a probabilistic test model (latent trait model; Jones/Appelbaum 1989) is shown to hold, these latter properties can be assumed to hold as well (Rasch 1961; Wright/Masters 1982). Consequently, item difficulties and person abilities can be measured on the same latent dimension with interval scale properties. For a test with dichotomous item scoring, the number of correct responses (irrespective of their pattern) is directly related to an ability level on an interval scale. In the classical test theory approach the total scores are only assumed to show such scale properties, i. e. one assumes without testing that identical differences between test raw scores at different levels of performance represent the same amount of difference in ability. — Willmes (1981) has successfully applied the simple Rasch model for dichotomous item scoring to the German version of the Token Test. It turned out that parts I to IV together fulfilled the Rasch model well, i. e. they measured one latent trait. The same was true for the fifth part containing various syntactic constructions. But the latent ability was different from that of the first four parts despite the high intercorrelations observed between all five parts. In addition, a variant of the model, the linear logistic model (Fischer 1983) allows for testing more specific hypotheses about the item parameters. This analysis for the Token Test revealed among other things that all three structural parameters as well as the different syntactic constructions and the difference in memory load play a crucial role in determining the item difficulties. — One drawback for the applicability of latent trait models in aphasiology is that they require large sample sizes of no less than 100—200 subjects in order to provide sufficiently precise parameter estimates. — More recent latent trait models (Wright/Masters 1982) can also handle items with more than two ordered response categories. In case of model fit, they also yield ability estimates on a unidimensional latent continuum. The partial credit model relates the probability of scoring x rather than x — 1 on a scale ranging from 0 to m to an ability parameter and a set of m so called step parameters. They indicate the points on the latent continuum at which the probability for the next higher item score becomes more likely than the actual score. An example is given in Figure 11.2. The partial credit model was applied to the reading aloud section of the AAT-subtest Written Language. The ten items have a 0 – 3 scoring. A large random sample of n = 378 aphasic patients was chosen from the AAT-database (Willmes/Ratajczak 1987) representing a wide range of severity levels. For each item the location of the step points on the latent continuum is depicted. Items are ordered according to the step points for the highest score 3. The figure 11.2. clearly demonstrates that distances between step values for one item as well as among different items may vary considerably although the scoring criteria are identical for all items. For the most difficult item 10 ('Why does she want to give it to me'), it is plausible that it only requires a medium ability level to read correctly more than two thirds of the simple words, yielding a score of 2. It requires, however, much more ability to get all of the 'little words' correct in the correct sequence. These results clearly indicate that the simple sum of item scores is only a crude estimate of the patient's ability. – Along a similar line of argument, the collapsing of the multidimensional scoring scheme for the PICA into a presumably unidimensional 16-point scale is highly questionable (cf. Martin 1977). Not even the ordinal properties of that scale let alone its unidimensionality have been demonstrated convincingly.

3. The Single Case Study Approach in Cognitive Neuropsychology

Although models of cognitive neuropsychology have become rather elaborate and the methodology of drawing inferences from impaired performance to normal cognitive processing have been extensively discussed (Caramazza/McCloskey 1988; Caramazza/Badecker 1989; Zurif/Gardner/Brownell 1989; Shallice 1988) related problems pertaining to psychometric methods and statistical procedures for evaluation have not been followed up with similar interest and rigor. – A wealth of single subject designs has been described in several publications (Hersen/Barlow 1976; Kratochwill 1978; Kazdin 1982; Barlow/Hersen 1985). A recent book edited by Valsiner (1986) addresses the single case approach from a broader perspective. The volume by McReynolds/Kearns (1983) is particularly concerned with communication disorders. These designs are mostly centered around the evaluation of one treatment or the compari-

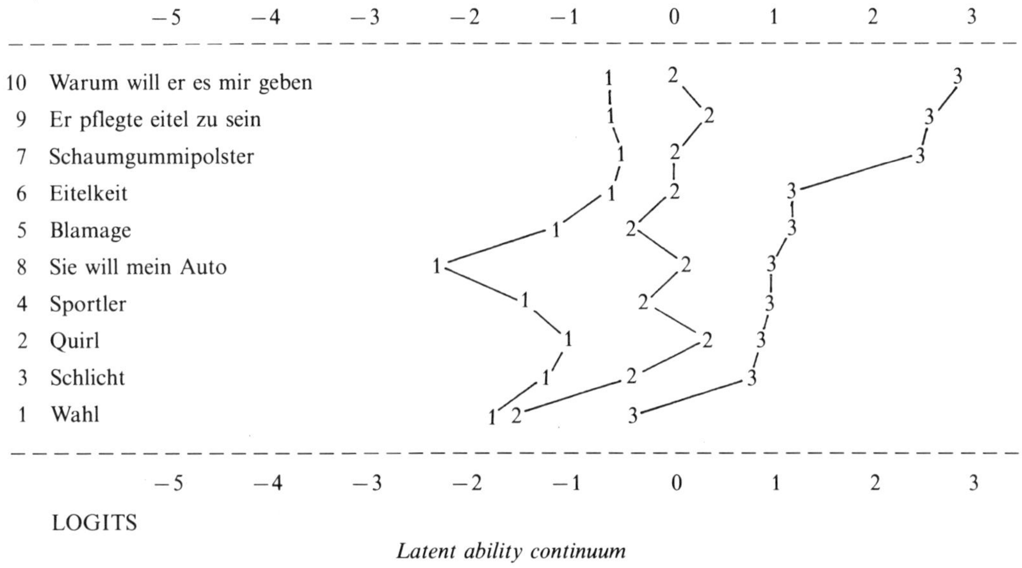

Fig. 11.2: Analysis of the AAT-subtest section 'Reading Aloud' with the partial credit probabilistic test model (CREDIT, Wright/Masters 1982); n = 378 aphasic subjects from the AAT-database (Willmes/Ratajczak 1987): depicted are the item step values for the item scores 0 (left) to 3 (right)

son of two or more treatments. Pring (1986) and Wilson (1987) present recent overviews. Single case designs are, however, particularly suited to research areas, for which changes in behavior are quite rapid and effects of treatments can be reversed. Coltheart (1983) and Howard (1986) have treated methodologically adequate single case experimental designs for scientific studies concerned with the treatment of aphasia. They describe the crossover treatment design, which is well suited for the demonstration of specific treatment effects. This situation is quite different from behavior modification studies. In-depth analysis of an individual patient aimed at tapping the source of some processing deficit within some model of normal cognitive functioning, comprises assessments of at least two sets of items. These test procedures are, in general, specifically tailored to the requirements of the particular investigation. The methodological approach chosen leads to a theory driven, sometimes ad hoc collection of items. Obviously, no sound empirical evidence concerning the particular reliability and (construct) validity properties of the items comprising a specific task, as well as the various tasks themselves, are available. Even if some tasks have been employed repeatedly in several single-case studies, the adequacy of the items, without arguing their theoretical appropriateness, remains a matter of observational impression.

3.1. Criterion-Referenced Assessment and Content Validity

In exemplary applications of the cognitive neuropsychological approach, content validity is implicitly taken to be the major criterion for item generation and selection. A test is called content valid (Berk 1980; Klauer 1987), when it contains or represents a universe of items (behavioral domain), e. g. the universe of legal neologisms for a particular language or the universe of temporal prepositions. A domain can be defined by exhaustive enumeration of its members or, more often, by stating the properties which any item from the particular domain has to fulfil. In both cases, the test actually used is composed of a representative sample from that domain. – Every item is completely characterized by a stimulus and a response component, yielding a specific item format. This general framework, tacitly employed in rudimentary form in cognitive neuropsychology, is well established in educational and occupational testing (Jones/Appelbaum 1989). It is associated with criterion-referenced measurement or mastery testing (Hambleton/Novick 1973; De Gruijter/van der Kamp 1984). Two important aspects are the stratification of a domain into subsets and the formation of representative samples from each of them in order to be able to draw inferences from the item sample to the whole domain. Representativeness can often be obtained by drawing a random sample of prespecified size from the subset. Distinct representative samples constitute data independent content valid parallel tests. A one-to-one relationship between a task domain and one component or route in some processing model does not hold in general. Several types of tasks or subdomains may be relevant and informative. – The degree of competence (ability) of a given subject for some domain is defined as the probability of solving items from a particular domain correctly (Klauer 1987). In this way a stochastic relationship is established between some latent competence and the observable behavior. Empirically, the level of competence is estimated from a representative sample from that domain. The properties of the ability estimate depend on the particular model used. – A second important aspect is the (dichotomous) classification according to mastery/non-mastery with respect to some domain. The individual competence is at the mastery level when it is larger than some criterion probability of say 0.90 or above. In criterion-referenced testing, the individual test performance is related to a certain level of competence, not to a distribution of scores within some reference population.

3.2. Statistical Assessment of (double) Dissociations

The relative merits of associations and dissociations for theory discovery and model falsification are discussed by Shallice (1988, Chapter 10). In this chapter, he distinguishes between three types of dissociations between two tasks, A and B, performance on B assumed to be better than on A: classical, trend, and robust dissociation. The distinction is based on whether B is performed in the normal range or below it, A being performed significantly worse than B. A robust dissociation is a strong dissociation for which a subject's competence with respect to both tasks can be expressed by means of standardized scores obtained for non brain-damaged subjects. Willmes (1990) has delineated statistical procedures based on the binomial model

(Lord/Novick 1968; Klauer 1987) for pass/fail-scored items. By means of these tests, operational definitions for the above types of dissociations are feasible. The sampling model variant of the binomial model, not requiring identical item difficulty but random sampling of items from a domain for each new subject, seems to be particularly adequate for concurrent types of language tasks. Statistical procedures are considered necessary because in many instances dissociations of the all or none type, i. e. (almost) perfect performance for one type of task as opposed to (almost) zero performance for another type, are not easily found. The journal '*Cognitive Neuropsychology*' but also other leading journals in the field of neuropsychology or aphasiology in particular, contain many examples of the weaker type of dissociation. The statistical procedures described in Willmes (1990) are mostly based on Fisher's exact test for fourfold tables and an exact version of the McNemar test with explicit consideration of the power of the statistical tests. This approach gives rise to a rational decision on the number of items required for a particular task. Regrettably, this number usually tends to be larger than those numbers often encountered in actual single-case studies. A related argument pertains to demonstrating how stable differences in an individual's ability for the theoretically most relevant discrepancies between performances according to some processing model actually are. Shallice (1988, 234) has pointed out that for a valid demonstration of a double dissociation it is not sufficient to find two complementary dissociations for two patients. Rather one has to show, that both patients exhibit complementary and significant differences between both tasks. Details are explained by Willmes (1990). – Whenever items are scored on an ordinal scale or the responses have metric properties like reaction times, different statistical methods have to be used. If the same language items are used under two (or several) different conditions, exact versions of the Wilcoxon test (Friedman test) are appropriate as are dependent two-sample (several samples) permutation tests (Edgington 1987). The set of items now plays the role of the sample of subjects in experimental research. Efficient algorithms are available to carry out the necessary computations. For the comparison of two (several) different sets of items, exact versions of the Mann–Whitney U test (Kruskal–Wallis test) or independent two-(several) sample permutation tests can be used. – Inherent differences in task difficulty pose a crucial problem for the valid interpretation of a dissociation (Blanken 1988; Shallice 1988; Sergent 1988). This objection is particularly important in those instances, in which performance is poorer on the (presumably) more demanding task, and normal subjects show ceiling performance on both tasks. It has been suggested and demonstrated by Huber/Willmes/Göddenhenrich (1988), that normative data from the general aphasic population, if available, can also provide relevant information concerning the gradation of performance on the different tasks. (See Willmes (1990) for an example.) This last argument will be taken up in section 3.3.

3.3. Bridging the Gap between Standard Assessments and Single Case Studies

In the introduction to his book on cognitive neuropsychology, Shallice (1988, 30) argues that a prerequisite for an in-depth (experimental) study of an individual patient is the availability of results from standard clinical 'baseline' tests. A pragmatic reason is that others should be enabled to gain a global impression of a patient's condition. Similarly important is the argument that the particular experimental tasks might provide pseudo-support for a theoretical claim, the effect being produced by some concomitant or different impairment which had gone unnoticed without more comprehensive clinical testing. To the contrary, Byng/Kay/Edmundson/Scott (1990) maintain that existing aphasia test batteries should no longer be central to the assessment of aphasic language impairment. The main reason is that psycholinguistic factors are poorly controlled. Byng and coauthors presented examples from the test batteries under scrutiny for which this claim is true, often simply because too few items were used. Instead, they propose the cognitive neuropsychological approach as an adequate theoretical framework. Adequate test procedures are thought to be of the following type: a large collection of tasks, all designed to assess a particular aspect of language processing, serves as a test reservoir from which the tasks assumed to be relevant for a particular patient have to be selected by the investigator. Implicitly, these tasks have been designed according to the conceptual framework of criterion-referenced testing as described in 3.1. The examiner's choice and sequencing of tasks is guided by the quantitative and qualitative performance of the individual patient. The first comprehensive collection of such tasks is the *Psycholinguistic Assessments of Language Processing in Aphasia* (PALPA, Kay/Lesser/Coltheart 1992) made up of six sections devoted to phonological and auditory lexical input processing, semantics (words and pictures) and picture naming, syntactic-semantic factors and morphological processing, orthographic and visual input processing, phonological and lexical output processing in oral reading and inner speech, and finally processes in written spelling. Each section in turn is composed of 7 to 11 sets of items, selected with respect to psycholinguistically relevant factors. All in all there are several thousand items, particular sets of words and non-words included in several processing tasks. – The authors of the PALPA acknowledge that standardization of such content valid sets of tasks both for aphasic and nonaphasic subjects would be very useful, in order to have empirical evidence for the gradation of item difficulties and patterns of responses. A methodological problem is however invoked when different parts of such a huge battery are standardized for different samples. – Since examination of a single patient with the whole battery is not feasible, guidelines for where to start and – depending on the performance observed – which task(s) to chose next are required. This problem is well known from educational psychology as the determination of psychometric hierarchies using order analysis (Dayton/Macready 1976). The concept of mastery and the related inverse concept of failure can also be employed to operationally define progression to another task. The authors of the PALPA admit that the psycholinguistic approach to assessment is still in its infancy. The relation between a particular model and a particular task is not always clearcut, nor is the validity of the model; yet the approach to assessment is hypothesis driven. Although very large, the battery is in no way complete. The analysis of spontaneous or elicited speech or of functional communication are definitely lacking. A recent development in assessing the latter type of verbal behavior is the *Amsterdam Nijmegen Everyday Language Test* (ANELT; Blomert/Koster/van Mier/Kean 1987). – Poeck/Göddenhenrich (1988) have described a collection of standard assessment procedures, which, based on psycholinguistic research results, are geared at the identification of dissociations in several areas of interest. With respect to the lexical discrimination supplement, Huber/Willmes/Göddenhenrich (1988) were able to demonstrate two crucial problems for the psycholinguistic approach. In this test, selective or predominant impairment of the phonological versus the semantic lexicon is assessed. It contains items requiring discrimination between semantically (phonemically) similar words as well as line drawings of objects representing the same words, and in another set discrimination between neologisms is required. Within a sample of 61 aphasic patients, application of the binomial model for the detection of trend dissociations resulted in the following: 20 out of 35 trend dissociations revealed poorer performance for neologisms. The legal neologisms were never processed significantly better. But only one of them was a strong dissociation. When taking into account the percentile ranks instead of the raw scores, even the number of trend dissociations, defined as a difference of at least 20 percentile ranks (also suggested by Reinvang 1985) dropped to two, one patient now showing a markedly better performance for neologisms. Another patient exhibited a seemingly better preserved ability for the processing of phonologically similar words both for raw scores and percentiles. Taking into account the huge left-hemispheric lesion covering the entire territory of the middle cerebral artery, makes the above pattern of performance implausible. It could rather be argued that phonemic similarity of the distractors in the multiple-choice set, which were dissimilar semantically, did not pose a problem for the intact capacities of the right hemisphere to process the high frequency nouns.

4. Two Specific Assessment Problems

4.1. Comparative Aphasiology

There is growing interest in cross-linguistic studies of aphasic patients. Comparative aphasiology addresses the question: Which are the qualitative and quantitative similarities and differences in aphasic symptoms in various languages affected in mono- and bilingual aphasic patients (Bates/Wulfeck 1989; Paradis 1989). Basically, there are two approaches to this kind of problem: In-depth studies of a large corpus of language in a small number of patients such as the CLAS-project (Cross Language Agrammatism Study, Menn/Obler 1990) or investigations of a very large number of patients by means of a standard test battery, the best known being the *Bilingual Aphasia Test* (BAT, Paradis 1987). With the first approach it is hard to ascertain comparability of the patient's aphasias. The second approach might not satisfactorily consider specific linguistic and sociocultural aspects of the languages under study. In any case, a standardized assessment is helpful for two purposes: Selection of patients from different language communities, who show a very similar level and pattern of performance, and baseline assessment of a bi- or multilingual patient. Merely counting the number of tasks for which a certain percentage of items was solved correctly for the different languages studied is not sufficient evidence (Nilipour/Ashayeri 1989). – The test versions in the different languages cannot be simple translations of each other. The task is to reconcile the constructional principles of the test with the structural properties of the languages of interest. But assumed equivalence of linguistic complexity in different languages must also be demonstrated empirically. For the AAT, the Italian version (De Bleser/Denes/Luzzatti et al. 1986) and the Dutch version (Graetz/De Bleser/Willmes/Heeschen 1991) have been shown to exhibit similar validity and reliability properties (Luzzatti/Willmes/Bisiacchi et al. 1987; De Bleser/Willmes/Graetz/Hagoort 1991), although interesting differences are present in detail. For instance, compound nouns in the third part of the repetition subtest must have a different structure in German/Dutch and Italian. While the German language is very productive in their formation, in Italian increasing difficulty can be accomplished only by introducing syntagmatic sequences. Only for Italian Broca's aphasics, items with a relatively large number of bound morphemes were disproportionately difficult. In German compound nouns, even if they are composed of bound morphemes, seem to be processed as coherent lexical entries. – In order to obtain comparable norms, the patient recruitment process must be very similar for the different test versions. With the psychometric single case analysis procedures outlined in 2.3., patients can be selected who show very similar levels and patterns of performance. The same procedures can be applied for baseline assessment of a bilingual patient. Also the various courses of recovery across languages, as classified by Paradis (1989, 11) can be tested with these statistical procedures for the individual patient.

4.2. Assessment of Acute Aphasia

Standardized assessment in the very early stages of aphasia has gained interest only recently. It is used to screen for the presence of aphasia in order to substantiate the clinical examination. In addition, the early course of recovery should be documented so that the best time to start speech therapeutic stimulation can be determined. The type of test suggested so far was just a shortened and more easy version of a standard assessment procedure (Acute Aphasia Screening Protocol, AASP, Crary/Haak/Malinsky 1989; The Frenchay Aphasia Screening Test, FAST, Enderby/Wood/Wade/Hewer 1987). In this way, test authors wanted to account for the general and neurological state of the aphasic patients on the ward. But in the first weeks post onset, no clearcut distinction can be made between persistent structural brain damage and transient functional disorders. Biniek/Huber/Willmes et al. (1991) have suggested an assessment procedure which systematically exploits stimulation of expressive language functions. In several subtests of ten items each, four levels of stimulation are discerned: verbal request e. g. to identify a common real object by pointing to and raising it; repeated verbal request; demonstration of the pointing movement by the examiner; repeated demonstration together with additional tactile stimulation by guiding the non-paretic hand of the patient to carry out the movement. Even 3 days post stroke the Aachen Aphasia Bedside Test (AABT) showed satisfactory psychometric properties (Biniek 1991).

5. Conclusion

Compared to the reviews by Benton (1967) and Spreen/Risser (1981) the assessment of aphasia has witnessed considerable progress. A variety of new test batteries have been published with an increasing concern for constructional and psychometric quality. The approach of cognitive neuropsychology has led to an ongoing debate about the adequacy of standard batteries for an in-depth analysis of the nature of an individual patient's language impairments. It has also led to the proliferation of a new type of content valid tasks which allow for a more direct assignment of observed performances to underlying language processing deficits. It has been argued that these collections of tasks also have to be subjected to the arduous examination of their psychometric properties. Modern psychometric models and methods have been discussed which enable the examiner to base diagnostic decisions on firmer grounds. Yet, it must be kept in mind that the availability of new theoretical developments and empirical results will again challenge the adequacy of any existing battery or set of tasks.

6. References

American Educational Research Association, American Psychological Association & National Council on Measurement in Education (1985). *Standards for educational and psychological testing.* Washington, DC: American Psychological Association.

Barlow, D. H. & Hersen, M. (1985). *Single case experimental studies.* London: Pergamon Press.

Bates, E. & Wulfeck, B. (1989). Comparative aphasiology: a cross-linguistic approach to language breakdown. *Aphasiology, 3,* 111–142.

Benton, A. L. (1967). Problems of test construction in the field of aphasia. *Cortex, 3,* 32–58.

Berk, R. A. (Ed.) (1980). *Criterion-referenced measurement: the state of the art.* Baltimore: Johns Hopkins University Press.

Biniek, R. (1991). Akute Aphasien. Habilitation thesis. Medical Faculty, RWTH Aachen, Aachen.

Biniek, R., Huber, W., Willmes, K., Glindemann, R., Brand, H., Fiedler, A., & Annen, C. (1991). Ein Test zur Erfassung von Sprach- und Sprechstörungen in der Akutphase nach Schlaganfällen. *Nervenarzt, 62,* 108–115.

Blanken, G. (1988). Anmerkungen zur Methodologie der kognitiven Neurolinguistik. *Neurolinguistik, 2,* 127–147.

Blomert, L., Koster, Ch., van Mier, H., & Kean, M. L. (1987). Verbal communication abilities of aphasic patients: The Everyday Language Test. *Aphasiology, 1,* 463–474.

Boller, F. & Dennis, M. (Eds.) (1979). *Auditory comprehension: clinical and experimental studies with the Token Test.* New York: Academic Press.

Brennan, R. L. (1983). *Elements of generalizability theory.* Iowa City: ACT Publications.

Byng, S., Kay, J., Edmundson, A., & Scott, C. (1990). Aphasia tests reconsidered. *Aphasiology, 4,* 67–91.

Canter, D. (Ed.) (1985). *Facet theory: approaches to social research.* New York: Springer.

Caplan, D. (1987). *Neurolinguistics and linguistic aphasiology: an introduction.* Cambridge, Mass.: Cambridge University Press.

Caramazza, A. (1984). The logic of neuropsychological research and the problem of patient classification in aphasia. *Brain and Language, 21,* 9–20.

Caramazza, A. & Badecker, W. (1989). Patient classification in neuropsychological research. *Brain and Cognition, 10,* 256–295.

Caramazza, A. & McCloskey, M. (1988). The case for single-patient studies. *Cognitive Neuropsychology, 5,* 517–528.

Clark, C., Crockett, D. J., & Klonoff, H. (1979). Factor analysis of the Porch Index of Communication Ability. *Brain and Language, 7,* 1–7.

Cohen, J. (1968). Weighted Kappa: nominal scale agreement with provision for scaled disagreement or partial credit. *Psychological Bulletin, 70,* 213–220.

Coltheart, M. (1983). Aphasia therapy research: a single case study approach. In C. Code & D. J. Muller (Eds.), *Aphasia therapy.* 194–202. London: Edward Arnold.

Crary, M. A., Haak, N. J., & Malinsky, A. E. (1989). Preliminary psychometric evaluation of an acute aphasia screening protocol. *Aphasiology, 3,* 611–618.

Cronbach, L. J. (1951). Coefficient alpha and the internal structure of tests. *Psychometrika, 16,* 297–334.

David, R. M. (1990). Aphasia assessment: the acid tests. *Aphasiology, 4,* 103–107.

Dayton, C. M. & Macready, G. B. (1976). A probabilistic model for validation of behavioral hierarchies. *Psychometrika, 41,* 189–204.

De Bleser, R., Denes, G. F., Luzzatti, C., Mazzucchi, A., Poeck, K., Spinnler, H., & Willmes, K. (1986). L'Aachener Aphasie Test (AAT) I. Problemi e soluzioni per una versione italiana del test e per uno studio crosslinguistico dei disturbi afasici. *Archivio di Psicologia, Neurologia e Psichiatria, 47,* 209–237.

De Bleser, R., Willmes, K., Graetz, P., & Hagoort, P. (1991). De Akense Afasie Test II: psychometrische kenmerken van de nederlandstalige versie. *Logopedie en foniatrie, 63,* 207–217.

De Gruijter, D. N. M. & van der Kamp L. J. T. (1984). *Statistical methods in psychological and educational testing.* Lisse: Swets and Zeitlinger.

De Renzi, E. & Vignolo, L. (1962). The Token Test: a sensitive test to detect receptive disturbances in aphasia. *Brain, 85,* 665–678.

Edgington, E. S. (1987). *Randomization Tests.* (2nd ed.). New York: Marcel Dekker.

Eisenson, J. (1954). *Examining for aphasia: a manual for the examination of aphasia and related disturbances.* New York: The Psychological Corporation.

Enderby, P. M., Wood, V. A., Wade, D. T., & Hewer, R. L. (1987). The Frenchay Aphasia Screening Test: a short, simple test for aphasia appropriate for nonspecialists. *International Journal of Rehabilitation Medicine, 8,* 166–170.

Fischer, G. H. (1983). Logistic latent trait models with linear constraints. *Psychometrika, 48,* 3–26.

Goodglass, H. & Kaplan, E. (1972, 2nd ed. 1983). *The assessment of aphasia and related disorders.* Philadelphia: Lea and Febiger.

Graetz, P., De Bleser, R., Willmes, K., & Heeschen C. (1991). De Akense Afasie Test: constructie van de nederlandstalige versie van de AAT. *Logopedie en foniatrie, 63,* 58–68.

Guilford, J. P. (1965). *Psychometric methods* (4th ed.). New York: McGraw-Hill.

Guttman, L. (1967). The development of nonmetric space analysis. A letter to Professor John Ross. *Multivariate Behavioral Research, 2,* 71–82.

Hambleton, R. K. & Novick, M. R. (1973). Toward an integration of theory and method for criterion referenced tests. *Journal of Educational Measurement, 10,* 159–170.

Head, H. (1926). *Aphasia and kindred disorders of speech.* New York: Macmillan.

Hersen, M. & Barlow, D. H. (1976). *Single case experimental designs: strategies for studying behavior change.* New York: Pergamon Press.

Holland, A. L. (1980). *Communicative Abilities in Daily Living; Manual.* Baltimore: University Park Press.

Howard, D. (1986). Beyond randomized controlled trials: the case for effective case studies of the effects of treatment in aphasia. *British Journal of Disorders of Communication, 21,* 89–102.

Huber, H. P. (1973). *Psychometrische Einzelfalldiagnostik.* Weinheim: Beltz.

Huber, W., Poeck, K., Weniger, D., & Willmes, K. (1983). Der Aachener Aphasie Test (AAT). Göttingen: Hogrefe.

Huber, W., Poeck, K., & Willmes, K. (1984). The Aachen Aphasia Test. In F. C. Rose (Ed.), *Advances in neurology, vol. 42: Progress in aphasiology. 291–303.* New York: Raven Press.

Huber, W., Willmes, K., & Göddenhenrich, S. (1988). Die Diagnose von aphasischen Leistungsdissoziationen beim lexikalischen Diskriminieren. In K.-B. Günther (Ed.), *Sprachstörungen: Probleme ihrer Diagnostik bei mentalen Retardierungen, Entwicklungsdysphasien und Aphasien. 306–329.* Heidelberg: Edition Schindele.

Jones, L. V. & Appelbaum, M. I. (1989). Psychometric methods. *Annual Review of Psychology, 40,* 23–43.

Kaplan, E., Goodglass, H., & Weintraub, S. (1983). *The Boston Naming Test.* Philadelphia: Lea and Febiger.

Kay, J., Lesser, R., & Coltheart, M. (1992) *Psycholinguistic Assessments of Language Processing in Aphasia.* London: Lawrence Erlbaum.

Kazdin, A. E. (1982). *Single case research designs: methods for clinical and applied settings.* New York: Oxford University Press.

Kertesz, A. (1982). *Western Aphasia Battery.* New York: Grune and Stratton.

Kertesz, A. (1986). Assessment of aphasia. In T. Incagnoli, G. Goldstein, & C. J. Golden (Eds.), *Clinical application of neuropsychological test batteries.* 329–360. New York: Plenum Press.

Kertesz, A. (1988). Is there a need for standardized aphasia tests? Why, how, what and when to test aphasics. *Aphasiology, 2,* 313–318.

Kertesz, A. & Phipps, J. (1977). Numerical taxonomy of aphasia. *Brain and Language, 4,* 1–10.

Klauer, K.-J. (1987). *Kriteriumsorientierte Tests.* Göttingen: Hogrefe.

Kratochwill, T. R. (1978). *Single subject research: strategies for evaluating change.* New York: Academic Press.

Krauth, J. (1984). A modification of kappa for interobserver bias. *Biometrical Journal, 26,* 435–445.

Krippendorff, K. (1970). Estimating the reliability, systematic error, and random error of interval data. *Educational and Psychological Measurement, 30,* 61–70.

Lang, C. (1981). Aphasietestung mit psychometrischen Verfahren. *Fortschritte Neurologie Psychiatrie, 49,* 164–178.

LaPointe, L. L. (Ed.) (1990). *Aphasia and related neurogenic language disorders.* New York: Thieme.

Lingoes, J. C. (1973). *The Guttman-Lingoes nonmetric program series.* Ann Arbor: Mathesis Press.

Lord, F. M. & Novick, M. R. (1968). *Statistical theories of mental test scores.* Reading, MA: Addison-Wesley.

Luzzatti, C., Willmes, K., Bisiacchi, P., De Bleser, R., Faglia, L., Mazzucchi, A., Posteraro, L., & Taricco, M. (1987). L'Aachener Aphasie Test (AAT) II. Proprietà psicometriche della versione italiana. *Archivio di Psicologia, Neurologia e Psichiatria, 48,* 480–519.

Martin, A. D. (1977). Aphasia testing: a second look at the Porch Index of Communicative Ability. *Journal of Speech and Hearing Disorders, 42,* 547–562.

McReynolds, L. J. & Kearns, K. P. (1983). *Single subject experimental designs in communicative disorders.* Baltimore: University Park Press.

Menn, L. & Obler, L. K. (1990). *Agrammatic aphasia: a cross-language narrative sourcebook, vol. 1–3.* Amsterdam/Philadelphia: John Benjamins.

Messick, S. (1980). The validity and ethics of assessment. *American Psychologist, 35,* 1012–1027.

Nilipour, R. & Ashayeri, H. (1989). Alternating antagonism between two languages with successive recovery of a third in a bilingual aphasic patient. *Brain and Language, 36,* 23–48.

Orgass, B. & Poeck, K. (1969). Assessment of aphasia by psychometric methods. *Cortex, 5,* 317–330.

Paradis, M. (1987). *The assessment of bilingual aphasia.* Hillsdale, NJ: Lawrence Erlbaum Associates.

Paradis, M. (1989). Bilingual and polyglot aphasia. In F. Boller & J. Grafman (Eds.), *Handbook of neuropsychology, vol. 2.* 117–140. Amsterdam: Elsevier.

Poeck, K. (1983). What do we mean by aphasic syndromes? A neurologist's view. *Brain and Language, 20,* 79–89.

Poeck, K. & Göddenhenrich, S. (1988). Standardized tests for the detection of dissociations in aphasic language performance. *Aphasiology, 2,* 375–380.

Porch, B. E. (1967). *Porch Index of Communicative Ability: theory and development (vol. 1).* Palo Alto: Consulting Psychologists Press.

Porch, B. E. (1973). *Porch Index of Communicative Ability: administration, scoring, and interpretation (vol. 2).* Palo Alto: Consulting Psychologists Press.

Pring, T. R. (1986). Evaluating the effects of speech therapy for aphasics: developing the single case methodology. *British Journal of Disorders of Communication, 21,* 103–115.

Rasch, G. (1961). On general laws and the meaning of measurement in psychology. In *Proceedings of the 4th Berkeley Symposion on Mathematical Statistics and Probability. 321–333.* Berkeley: University of California Press.

Raveh, A. (1978). Finding periodical patterns in time series with monotone trend: a new technique. In S. Shye (Ed.), *Theory construction and data analysis in the behavioral sciences. 371–390.* San Francisco: Jossey-Bass.

Reinvang, I. (1985). *Aphasia and brain organization.* New York: Plenum Press.

Risser, A. & Spreen, O. (1985). Test review: The Western Aphasia Battery. *Journal of Clinical and Experimental Neuropsychology, 7,* 463–470.

Sarno, M. T. (1969). *The Functional Communication Profile: Manual of directions.* New York: New York University Medical Center – The Institute of Rehabilitation Medicine.

Schlesinger, I. M. & Guttman, L. (1969). Smallest space analysis of intelligence and achievement tests. *Psychological Bulletin, 71,* 95–100.

Schouten, H. J. A. (1980). Measuring pairwise agreement among many observers. *Biometrical Journal, 22,* 497–504.

Schuell, H. (1955). *Minnesota Test for Differential Diagnosis of Aphasia (research ed.).* Minneapolis: University of Minnesota.

Schuell, H. (1973). *Differential diagnosis of aphasia with the Minnesota Test (2nd ed.).* Minneapolis: University of Minnesota Press.

Schuell, H., Jenkins, J. J., & Carroll, J. B. (1962). A factor analysis of the Minnesota Test for Differential Diagnosis of Aphasia. *Journal of Speech and Hearing Research, 5,* 350–369.

Schwartz, M. F. (1984). What the classical aphasia categories can't do for us, and why. *Brain and Language, 21,* 3–8.

Sergent, J. (1988). Some theoretical and methodological issues in neuropsychological research. In F. Boller & J. Grafman (Eds.), *Handbook of Neuropsychology, vol. 1. 69–81.* Amsterdam: Elsevier.

Shallice, T. (1988). *From neuropsychology to mental structure.* Cambridge: Cambridge University Press.

Shye, S. (Ed.) (1978). *Theory construction and data analysis in the behavioral sciences.* San Francisco: Jossey-Bass.

Skenes, L. L. & McCauley, R. J. (1985). Psychometric review of nine aphasia tests. *Journal of Communication Disorders, 18,* 461–474.

Sklar, M. (1973). *Sklar Aphasia Scale (rev. ed.).* Los Angeles: Western Psychological Services.

Spreen, O. & Benton, A. L. (1977). *Neurosensory Center Comprehensive Examination for Aphasia (1977 revision).* Victoria, BC: Neuropsychology Laboratory, University of Victoria.

Spreen, O. & Risser, A. (1981). Assessment of aphasia. In M. T. Sarno (Ed.) *Aquired aphasia. 67–127.* New York: Academic Press.

Steiger, J. H. & Schönemann, P. H. (1978). A history of factor indeterminacy. In S. Shye (Ed.), *Theory construction and data analysis in the behavioral Sciences.* San Francisco: Jossey-Bass.

Valsiner, J. (Ed.) (1986). *The individual subject and scientific psychology.* New York: Plenum Press.

Wainer, H. & Braun H. I. (Eds.) (1988). *Test Validity.* Hillsdale, NJ: Lawrence Erlbaum Associates.

Weisenburg, T. H. & McBride, K. E. (1935). *Aphasia.* New York: Commonwealth Fund.

Weniger, D. (1990). Diagnostic tests as tools of assessment and models of information procession: a gap to bridge. *Aphasiology, 4,* 109–113.

Weniger, D., Willmes, K., Huber, W., & Poeck, K. (1981). Der Aachener Aphasie Test; Reliabilität und Auswertungsobjektivität. *Nervenarzt, 52,* 269–277.

Wepman, J. M. (1951). *Recovery from aphasia.* New York: Ronald.

Wepman, J. M. & Jones, L. V. (1961). *Studies in aphasia: an approach to testing.* Chicago: Educational Industry Service.

Willmes, K. (1981). A new look at the Token Test using probabilistic test models. *Neuropsychologia, 19,* 631–645.

Willmes, K. (1985). An approach to analyzing a single subject's scores obtained in a standardized test with application to the Aachen Aphasia Test (AAT). *Journal of Clinical and Experimental Neuropsychology, 7,* 331–352.

Willmes, K. (1990). Statistical methods for a single-case study approach to aphasia therapy research. *Aphasiology*, *4*, 415–436.

Willmes, K. Poeck, K., Weniger, D., & Huber, W. (1983). Facet theory applied to the construction and validation of the Aachen Aphasia Test. *Brain and Language*, *18*, 259–276.

Willmes, K. & Ratajczak. H. (1987). The design and application of a data- and methodbase system for the Aachen Aphasia Test. *Neuropsychologia*, *25*, 725–733.

Wilson, B. (1987). Single case experimental designs in neuropsychological rehabilitation. *Journal of Clinical and Experimental Neuropsychology*, *9*, 527–544.

Wright, B. D. & Masters, G. N. (1982). *Rating scale analysis*. Chicago: Mesa Press.

Zurif, E. B., Gardner, H., & Brownell, H. H. (1989). The case against the case against group studies. *Brain and Cognition*, *10*, 237–255.

Klaus Willmes, Aachen (Germany)

12. Semantic Disorders in Aphasia

1. Introduction

A normal mature speaker of a language should be able to recognize that some expressions in that language are 'meaningful' while other expressions are 'meaningless' (except under very special circumstances). The distinction can be drawn at the level of individual lexical items and at the combinational level of the grammar. – Thus at the word-level (in English) there is, for example, a contrast between *blink* (with the meaning "to rapidly close and open one's eyes involuntarily") and *blick* (a pseudo-word that is phonologically well-formed but is without denotation or clear connotation in the language). At the sentence-level, there is a similar contrast between the meaningful sentence "Healthy young babies sleep soundly" and the semantically-anomalous sentence "Colourless green ideas sleep furiously." The former sentence in turn contrasts with "Sleep young soundly babies healthy" in which lexical meaningfulness is maintained in the absence of appropriate syntactic constrains; the other sentence contrasts with "Bleenless grune floops sneded rudly" in which morphological markers give the impression of a well-formed Adjective + Adjective + Noun + Verb + Adverb sequence despite the lack of recognizable lexical items.

The lexicon itself is not a mere listing of individual words but is rather organized in semantic fields. Thus *red*, *green*, *blue* (etc.) are all colour terms, while *mother*, *father*, *cousin* (etc.) are kinship terms. Relationships such as synonymy (*small* and *little*) or antonymy (*small* and *large*) hold between some terms in some fields, whilst in many fields hierarchical structures are found; the sequence *terrier*, *dog*, *mammal*, *animal*, *thing* is ordered by class-inclusion. At the sentence-level, such lexical relationships lead to semantic entailments: "If John is thinner than Fred, then Fred must be fatter than John"; "if Rover is a terrier, then Rover must be a dog." – These, then, are just a few of the linguistic phenomena that might be regarded (pre-theoretically) as falling within the domain of the semantic component of the grammar. A considerably fuller discussion can be found in such sources as Fodor (1977) and Ladusaw (1988).

Within theoretical linguistics, many foundational issues remain controversial. Thus the distinction between 'concepts' (that are not necessarily linguistic entities) and 'semantic primitives' (that fall within the domain of linguistics per se) is still unclear; similarly, the distinction between semantic and 'encyclopedic' knowledge is problematic (Katz/Fodor 1963). The entire notion of semantic decomposition (with a defined level of semantic representation within the grammar) has been attacked. It was originally argued (Katz/Fodor 1963) that 'complex' words (e. g. *kill*) should be psychologically recoded by sequences of semantic 'primitives' (e. g. 'CAUSE TO DIE') for the process of comprehension to take place. Fodor/Fodor/Garrett (1975), however, have provided evidence that no such 'automatic' decomposition takes place, and that it is rather the case that semantic entailments are mediated by inference rules or meaning postulates. Thus the entailment from "Fred killed Bill" to "Bill died" would depend upon activation of the meaning postulates "For any x and any y, if x killed y, then x caused y to die. If x caused y to die, then y died." Such meaning postulates are stored in long-term memory and are retrieved when the relevant inferential processes are demanded; they are not part of the 'on-line' representations that are automatically computed within the language module. Similarly, Chomsky (1981) has argued that many of the traditional concerns of "real semantics" (e. g. considerations of truth and reference) do not strictly-speaking fall within the domain of the grammar. The study of "the relation between language or language use and the world" (Chomsky 1981) is extra-linguistic; the rules of logical form (LF) that determine quantifier binding and coreferentiality (for example) constitute the 'semantic' boundary of universal grammar.

For the most part, investigations of 'semantic disorder' in aphasia (and other acquired neurological pathologies) have taken a fairly traditional view of 'semantics'. At the lexical level, mistakes in spontaneous speech (and in reading aloud and writing) that bear some similarity in meaning to the target have been categorized as 'semantic errors.' Likewise, in studies of single-word comprehension, such tests as word-picture matching often provoke errors that appear semantically-related to the target. Disorders of logical form and the integration of semantic information into a 'mental model' (Johnson-Laird 1983) of situations described in language have received somewhat less attention.

2. Lexical Semantics

Semantic paraphasias in spontaneous speech (and in naming to visual confrontation) are common in almost all types of aphasia and in many patients whose primary diagnosis is neurodegenerative disease (Alzheimer's disease or Pick's disease, for example). The patient will say *wife* (for *husband*), *north* (for *south*), *cold* (for *hot*) and so forth across a wide range of semantic fields (Buckingham/Rekart 1979). These lexical selection deficits seem closely analogous to the slips-of-the-tongue that can be observed (albeit at a much lower rate) in normal speakers (Fromkin 1973; Buckingham 1980).

Although such errors as the substitution of *see* for *hear* are descriptively 'semantic', they do not necessarily implicate an impairment at that level (Ellis/Kay/Franklin 1992). It is, for example, possible that substitutions of this nature arise when the phonological (or graphemic) form of the 'intended' word is unavailable. In circumstances where an entry in the phonological lexicon is 'blocked' (either momentarily or permanently), the patient may access a semantic entry that is close in meaning to the intended word and then access the phonological form that is appropriate to that entry.

This account presupposes, of course, some kind of 'spreading activation' (Stemberger 1985) along the links in a semantic network (Miller/Fellbaum 1991), combined with a 'threshold' model (Morton 1979) that determines the final response outcome. In cases where 'phonological blocking' has given rise to (apparently) 'semantic' errors, phonological cueing (Myers/Goodglass 1978) should facilitate word retrieval, while semantic cueing should have no effect, or even a deleterious effect (Podroza/Darley 1977). On this analysis, some semantic 'errors' (e. g. *table* – "chair") would actually be reduced circumlocutions whereby the patient is attempting to express (e. g.) "I know it's a piece of furniture, similar to a chair, but I can't find the exact word." In cases where other evidence is indicative of good comprehension, or where the patients can show that they are aware that their 'semantic' errors are indeed mistakes, a phonological blocking hypothesis has high priority in the explanation of errors on confrontation naming tests, reading aloud, or word repetition (Morton/Patterson 1980; Newcombe/Marshall 1980; Howard/Franklin 1988). The ubiquitous presence of word-frequency effects (McKenna/Warrington 1980) may have their primary locus within the phonological lexicon.

There are, however, many aphasic patients who show semantic errors on 'output' (or expressive) tasks in conjunction with a disorder of lexical comprehension (Gainotti/Silveri/Villa/Miceli 1986). In such cases, the simplest hypothesis is clearly that an impairment within the semantic system is responsible for the conjoint occurrence of semantic errors in both (e. g.) overt naming and in verbal comprehension, as assessed by forced-choice picture pointing in response to a spoken (or written) word (Butterworth/Howard/McLoughlin 1984; Howard/Orchard-Lisle 1984; Hillis/Rapp/Romani/Caramazza 1990). In some cases of this nature, it may be possible to argue that conceptual (as opposed to strictly semantic) knowledge is intact. – Thus the patient of Howard/Orchard-Lisle (1984), was a 'global' aphasic who made frequent semantic errors on object-naming; she also accepted many semantic co-ordinates as correct names for objects (e. g. *needle* as the name of a thimble, or *lion* as the name of a tiger). Nonetheless, she performed within the normal control range on a test of 'picture association'; she could for example, correctly match a picture of an eskimo to an igloo rather than a house (the semantic distractor). If such 'pictorial associations' are regarded as 'conceptual', the patient's poor performance on the other tasks would seem intrinsic to a lexical semantic system.

Testing for a semantic deficit should include picture-naming (with both oral and written responses), picture-pointing (to the pictorial referents of spoken and written words) with semantic distractors among the pictures, miming (to both spoken and written stimuli), and producing 'names' to spoken or written definitions. In the 'ideal' case, the evidence will all converge upon a semantic locus.

Disorders of the semantic system could result from impaired access to semantic memory or from degraded representations within semantic memory (Warrington 1981). Degradation could in turn be total (i. e. loss of a semantic item), partial (e. g. superordinate information is preserved, subordinate information lost), or distorted (e. g. erroneous specification of a semantic item). Excellent discussions of how to distinguish between such possibilities can be found in Caramazza/Hillis/Rapp/Romani (1990), and Caplan (1992). Item-by-item consistency of performance over different verbal semantic tasks is clearly the best indicant that damage to a central semantic store is implicated (Shallice 1988). Likewise, the existence of semantic priming effects in many aphasic patients with poor lexical comprehension shows that items cannot have been totally lost from semantic memory (Blumstein/Milberg/Shrier 1982).

Many of the most interesting studies of semantic impairment have been conducted with patients whose primary neurological diagnosis is non-specific degenerative disease (Warrington 1975), Alzheimer's disease (Schwartz 1990), or Pick's disease (Marin/Glenn/Rafal 1983). In these conditions (as in many aphasias) semantic superordinate information is typically preserved with loss of subordinate features (Chertkow/Bub 1990). In the latter two (degenerative) conditions, there is often a particular pattern of semantic dissolution in which the hierarchy of semantic features (from most specific to most general) is lost. This pattern is not, however, seen in all patients with degenerative language disorder. Thus Funnell (1992) has reported a case of Alzheimer's disease in which comprehension of general categorical knowledge declined together with knowledge of specific distinguishing semantic features.

3. Category- and Modality-Specific Deficits

Whatever the form of semantic representations turns out to be (ordered feature sets, network associations, meaning postulates etc.), it is obvious that the human mind draws functional semantic distinctions and hence that the structure of the human brain (on pain of Cartesian dualism) must honour those distinctions. It has nonetheless seemed remarkable to many recent investigators that brain damage, either focal or (more surprisingly) diffuse can selectively impair (or leave preserved against a background of more general semantic impairment) specific semantic categories. – For example: Yamadori/Albert (1973) reported a patient, with trauma of the left posterior temporo-parietal region, who could neither name nor understand the names of "room objects and body parts" despite reasonable performance on other semantic classes. The most commonly reported dissociation, however, is between living and nonliving objects. Warrington/Shallice (1984) and Silveri/Gainotti (1988) have shown that in patients with herpes simplex encephalitis, naming and word-picture matching for nonliving things can be considerably better than for living things (and foods). Sartori /Job (1988) report a similarly selective deficit for animals, fruit, and vegetables; the impairment was seen on both picture-naming and naming to verbal definition. Likewise, Silveri/Daniele/Giustolisi/Gainotti (1991) found a severe impairment on confrontation naming of living things (flowers, fruits and animals) with relative preservation of naming non-living objects in patients with dementia of Alzheimer's type. A similar case of progressive selective deficit in naming and auditory verbal comprehension of animals, fruits and vegetables was reported by Basso/Capitani/Laiacona (1988) in a case of degenerative disease with progressive aphasia but without generalized dementia.

It would seem unlikely that all of the above dissociation can be 'explained away' on the basis of the confounding effects of such variables as word frequency, age of acquisition, or general familiarity, although Funnell/Sheridan (1992) have drawn attention to some possible confounds with familiarity. The most convincing evidence that the 'categorial' effect is truly categorial would be a demonstration that in other patients there is relative preservation of knowledge of living things compared to non-living things (as assessed by a variety of verbal-visual matching tasks). Two such patients have been reported by Warrington/McCarthy (1983; 1987). – The performance of the latter patient (Warrington/McCarthy 1987) did not, however, show a clean, clear-cut distinction between the two (general) categories. For example, within the (overall) well-preserved category of living things, there was a selective deficit in the comprehension of names of body parts; likewise, within the (overall) impaired category of non-living things, knowledge of large objects (e. g. buildings) was well-preserved. – It remains, then, an open question whether the evidence truly supports the categorical dichotomy between living and non-living, or whether some other set of distinctions is required. Warrington/McCarthy (1987) suggest that the relative importance of 'physical' versus 'functional' properties involved in the definitions of different objects may be implicated (see also Farah/McMullen/Meyer 1991; and Damasio 1990). The notion that visually-based versus language-based knowledge representations are involved in some selective naming disorders is also supported by the case of 'animal name' anomia reported by Hart/Gordon (1992).

The counterintuitive claim that knowledge representations can be intact even in cases of category-specific anomia seems to follow from a pattern of results reported by Hart/Berndt/Caramazza (1985). Their patient, with a lesion of left frontal cortex and the basal ganglia, had a residual anomia that was particularly severe for the categories of fruit and vegetables. He could name to visual confrontation such rare items as an abacus and a sphinx, yet was unable to name correctly common fruits. The same dissociation was found on naming to palpation and from verbal definitions. Sorting pictures into different conceptual classes was also especially difficult with fruits and vegetables. Initially, this pattern seems to indicate a loss of the knowledge base for these classes. Yet when the patient was given the names of fruits and vegetables he could perform word-picture matching well. He could likewise classify the words into appropriate semantic categories, and correctly judge and describe the size, colour, texture and shape of the fruits and vegetables that the words refer to. The names of fruits and vegetables seem then to be the key that unlocks intact conceptual knowledge that cannot be accessed from visual or tactile experience or from verbal definitions. – The case of Hart/Berndt/Caramazza (1985) contrasts with and complements a case of modality-specific semantic disorder reported by McCarthy/Warrington (1988). Their patient had sustained relatively focal damage to the left temporal lobe. He appeared to show a category-specific impairment in that his ability to define the characteristics of animals or plants in response to their spoken names was selectively impaired by contrast with his definitions of inanimate objects. For example: In response to *pig* the patient could only volunteer that it was an animal, whereas *wheelbarrow* elicited the response "the item we have here in the gardens for carrying bits and pieces; wheelbarrows are used by people doing maintenance here on your buildings. They can put their cement and all sorts of things in it to carry it around"! – However, the patient has not lost the knowledge-base pertaining to animals and plants. Although, for example, in response to the word *rhinoceros* the patient could only say "Animal, can't give you any functions", he can access a wide range of information from a picture of a rhinoceros: "Enormous, weighs over one ton, lives in Africa." A similar case is reported by Bub/Black/Hampson/Kertesz (1988).

The general issue at stake here is whether there is a single, central semantic (or conceptual) system that can be accessed from different sensory modalities and that drives different output modes. By contrast, are there distinct (multiple) semantic systems, each linked to its own input and output channels? McCarthy/Warrington (1988) and Shallice (1988) draw the conclusion that semantic information is multiply represented in the normal brain and that this duplication is intrinsically linked to the input modalities (including language) whereby we gain knowledge of the world. If this were so, one would expect to see, after brain damage, the kind of dissociations between different access modes to semantic information reported by Hart/Berndt/Caramazza (1985) and McCarthy/Warrington (1988). – The notion of modality-specific semantic systems would also help to explain how in some aphasic patients, semantic errors can occur in naming to one modality of stimulus presentation but not another. For example, Lhermitte/Chedru/Chain (1973) reported a patient with normal object- naming to palpation (for both hands) but who made substantial numbers of semantic errors when naming to visual confrontation. Many of these errors (e. g. *knife* – "plate") could not be 'explained away' as high-level perceptual deficits. The converse dissociation was reported by Beauvois/Saillant/Meininger/Lhermitte (1978). Their patient has essentially intact naming to visual confrontation, but made substantial numbers of semantic errors when naming to palpation (with either hand). Again, the majority of these errors (e. g. *cork* – "bottle") could not be interpreted as due to sensory or perceptual deficits.

It remains to be seen whether theorists who support the notion of a unitary, modality-neutral semantic system (Riddoch/Humphreys/Coltheart/Funnell 1988) can convincingly interpret the full range of apparently modality-specific semantic disorders.

4. Sentence Semantics and Logical Form

Much (if not all) of what might be thought of as 'sentential semantics' is conjointly determined by lexical structure and the syntax. Thus the standard interpretation of why many aphasic patients cannot, for example, understand 'reversible' passives (Caplan/Hildebrandt 1988) is syntactic. In a sentence such as *The boy was helped by the girl*, the assignment of the thematic role 'AGENT' to *the girl* is determined by the syntax (e. g., by the fact that the prepositional phrase *by the girl* is immediately dominated by the label Verb Phrase). Failure to assign the correct hierarchical syntactic structures to sentences will accordingly leave the patient with no option but to interpret thematic roles on the basis of linear (non-linguistic) strategies (e. g. the first noun phrase is the AGENT) and/or pragmatic considerations of plausibility. With respect to these cases, it is implausible (or impossible) that *the flowers* could be the AGENT of the sentence (*The flowers were watered by Jill.*

Similar considerations apply to many phenomena of coreference. To borrow an example from Caplan (1992), there is a clear contrast between the interpretation of the two sentences: *Susan said that a friend of Mary's washed herself* and *Susan said that a friend of Mary's washed her*. In the former sentence, *herself* must refer to *friend* (and cannot refer to either *Susan* or *Mary*); in the latter sentence, *her* can refer to either *Susan* or *Mary* (but cannot refer to *friend*). These (semantic) facts are, however, determined by the 'syntactic' positions in which reflexives (*herself*) and pronouns (*her*) can occur.

In an important discussion, Caplan (1992) considers whether any patients exist who have (reasonably) intact lexical semantics but who nonetheless are unable to assign any thematic roles (or other sentential semantic features) to phrases in sentences. His conclusion is that no such patient has been reported (but cf. Schwartz/Saffran/Marin 1980); in all known patients with a cognitive disorder of sentence comprehension, the problem can be traced back to either a lexical impairment or a syntactic impairment. Caplan's claim does, however, depend upon a view of lexical semantics in which it is possible to state that the full lexical meaning of (e. g.) *woman* does not involve knowing that a woman is a (potential) agent. The theoretical problem, of course, is how to distinguish between a patient who assigns thematic roles to the noun phrases in sentences at random and one who simply assigns no thematic roles at all. In the former case, the disorder can always be interpreted as a major loss of syntactic processing; only an impairment of the latter type would be specific to sentential semantics.

The fullest discussion of sentential semantics and logical form in the context of aphasic breakdown is provided by Saddy (1991). The patient that Saddy reprots shows a 'standard' impairment in the comprehension of reversible passives with definite and indefinite noun phrases (*a man, the woman*). However, when the universal quantifier (every) is used in otherwise equivalent sentences, the patient's performance is essentially normal. He is even aware of 'scope' differences in such sentences; that is, he recognizes that for *A child was photographed by every woman*, there are two permissable readings, one in which the same child is photographed and one in which different children are photographed. – Saddy's study throws an entirely new light on the whole range of impairments in sentence comprehension in aphasia; the comprehension disorder in his own patient (and perhaps many others with 'agrammatic' comprehension) is due, Saddy suggests, to an inability to distinguish different event-types; the patient treats all event-arguments as nominal. If indefinates have no intrinsic quantificational force, reversible passives such as *A man was filmed by a woman* will be interpreted by the patient as referring to a man, a woman, and an act of filming. Nonetheless, the correct thematic roles of the two noun phrases will not be known to the patient since the verbal predicate binders are not available in a representation in which the verb phrase is treated as nominal. – By contrast, at the level of logical form, a quantifier (such as *every*) can act as a proxy binder for the predicate argument of the verb. In this case, a truth value can be assigned to the representation, with the consequent improvement in comprehension.

5. Conclusions

Further advances in the study of semantic disorders in aphasia will depend crucially upon better specification of the nature of semantic representations. At the level of lexical semantics many controversies remain to be resolved concerning the plausibility of lexical decomposition (Fodor/Garrett/Walker/Parkes 1980; Jackendoff 1991). Similarly, psychological studies of 'meaning' have provided no firm distinction between 'dictionary' knowledge and 'encyclopedic' knowledge. The theoretical construct 'semantic memory' (as employed in both psycho- and neurolinguistics) incorporates the knowledge that 'lions are wild animals' (for example). Yet it remains inclear whether such information lies within the domain of the lexical component of the grammar.

Hillert (1992) proposes that lexical semantics should be taken to refer solely to "grammatical constraints" on lexical items. If this suggestion is correct, category-specific deficits (involving the living/non-living distinction, for example) would need to be interpreted as consequent upon syntactic distinctions between the two classes of nouns. Whether this proposal can be carried out in a principled fashion is not obvious. There are, however, clear cases of category-specific deficits where a syntactic characterization would be plausible. Examples include cases with specific impairment of verb comprehension and retrieval (McCarthy/Warrington 1985), and cases where proper nouns are differentially impaired (Semenza/Zettin 1988; Lucchelli/De Renzi 1992). Proper names are "pure referring expressions" (Semenza/Zettin 1989) that have distinctive syntactic properties.

The finding that some patients with Wernicke's aphasia appear to have relatively good comprehension when tested with 'on-line' measures raises further problems (Tyler 1992). It seems that such techniques as phoneme- and word-monitoring, speeded naming, and lexical decision (all in sentential or discrete contexts) can reveal processing profiles that are close to normal in patients who show severe comprehension deficits on traditional 'off-line' testing. Tyler (1992) takes these findings to imply a distinction between 'automatic' processes of structure-building (internal to the language-faculty?) and what might be called processes of meta-comprehension that manipulate and act upon the output of unconsciously-computed representations.

If this way of looking at Tyler's results is correct (see also Hillert 1992), many current ways of interpreting the notion of semantic (or 'conceptual') disorder in aphasia may need to be dramatically revised.

6. References

Basso, A., Capitani, E., & Laiacona, M. (1988). Progressive language impairment without dementia: a case with isolated category specific semantic defect. *Journal of Neurology, Neurosurgery, and Psychiatry*, *51*, 1201–1207.

Beauvois, M. F., Saillant, B., Meininger, V., & Lhermitte, F. (1978). Bilateral tactile aphasia: A tacto-verbal dysfunction. *Brain*, *101*, 381–401.

Blumstein, S. E., Milberg, W., & Shrier, R. (1982). Semantic processing in aphasia: Evidence from an auditory lexical decision task. *Brain and Language*, *17*, 301–315.

Bub, D. N., Black, S., Hampson, E., & Kertesz, A. (1988). Semantic encoding of pictures and words: Some neuropsychological observations. *Cognitive Neuropsychology*, *5*, 27–66.

Buckingham, H. (1980). On correlating aphasic errors with slips of the tongue. *Applied Psycholinguistics*, *1*, 199–220.

Buckingham, H. & Rekart, D. M. (1979). Semantic paraphasias. *Journal of Communication Disorders, 12*, 197–209.

Butterworth, B., Howard, D., & McLoughlin, P. (1984). The semantic deficit in aphasia: The relationship between semantic errors in auditory comprehension and picture naming. *Neuropsychologia, 22*, 409–426.

Caplan, D. (1992). *Language: Structure, Processing, and Disorders*. Cambridge, Mass.: MIT Press.

Caplan, D. & Hildebrandt, N. (1988). *Disorders of Syntactic Comprehension*. Cambridge, Mass.: MIT Press.

Caramazza, A., Hillis, A. E., Rapp, B. C., & Romani, C. (1990). The multiple semantics hypothesis: Multiple confusions? *Cognitive Neuropsychology, 7*, 161–189.

Chertkow, H. & Bub, D. (1990). Semantic memory loss in Alzheimer's disease: What do indirect measures measure? *Brain, 113*, 397–417.

Chomsky, N. (1981). *Lectures on Government and Binding*. Dordrecht: Foris.

Damasio, A. R. (1990). Category-related recognition defects as a clue to the neural substrates of knowledge. *Trends in the Neurosciences, 13*, 95–98.

Ellis, A. W., Kay, J., & Franklin, S. (1992). Anomia: Differentiating between semantic and phonological deficits. In D. I. Margolin (Ed.), *Cognitive Neuropsychology in Clinical Practice. 207–228*. New York: Oxford University Press.

Farah, M. J., McMullen, P. A., & Meyer, M. M. (1991). Can recognition of living things be selectively impaired? *Neuropsychologia, 29*, 185–193.

Fodor, J. D. (1977). *Semantics: Theories of Meaning in Generative Grammar*. Hassocks, Sussex: Harvester Press.

Fodor, J. A., Garrett, M., Walker, E., & Parkes, C. (1980). Against definitions. *Cognition, 8*, 263–367.

Fodor, J. D., Fodor, J. A., & Garrett, M. (1975). The psychological unreality of semantic representations. *Linguistic Inquiry, 6*, 515–532.

Fromkin, V. (Ed.) (1973). *Speech Errors as Linguistic Evidence*. The Hague: Mouton.

Funnell, E. (1992). Progressive loss of semantic memory in a case of Alzheimer's disease. *Proceedings of the Royal Society, London. B 249*, 287–291.

Funnell, E. & Sheridan, J. (1992). Categories of knowledge? Unfamiliar aspects of living and nonliving things. *Cognitive Neuropsychology, 9*, 135–153.

Gainotti, G., Silveri, M. C., Villa, G., & Miceli, G. (1986). Anomia with and without lexical comprehension disorders. *Brain and Language, 29*, 18–33.

Hart, J., Berndt, R. S., & Caramazza, A. (1985). Category-specific naming deficit following cerebral infarction. *Nature, 316*, 439–440.

Hart, J. & Gordon, B. (1992). Neural subsystems for object knowledge. *Nature, 359*, 60–64.

Hillert, D. (1992). Lexical semantics and aphasia: A state-of-the-art review. *Journal of Neurolinguistics, 7*, 1–43.

Hillis, A., Rapp, B., Romani, C., & Caramazza, A. (1990). Selective impairment of semantics in lexical processing. *Cognitive Neuropsychology, 7*, 191–243.

Howard, D. & Franklin, S. (1988). *Missing the Meaning?* Cambridge, Mass.: MIT Press.

Howard, D. & Orchard-Lisle, V. (1984). On the origin of semantic errors in naming: Evidence from a case of a global aphasic. *Cognitive Neuropsychology, 1*, 163–190.

Jackendoff, R. (1991). Parts and boundaries. *Cognition, 41*, 9–45.

Johnson-Laird, P. N. (1983). *Mental Models*. Cambridge: Cambridge University Press.

Katz, J. J. & Fodor, J. A. (1963). The structure of a semantic theory. *Language, 39*, 170–210.

Ladusaw, W. A. (1988). Semantic theory. In F. J. Newmeyer (Ed.), *Linguistics: The Cambridge Survey (Volume 1). 89–112*. Cambridge: Cambridge University Press.

Lucchelli, F. & De Renzi, E. (1992). Proper name anomia. *Cortex, 28*, 221–230.

Lhermitte, F., Chedru, F., & Chain, F. (1973). A propos d'un cas d'agnosie visuelle. *Revue Neurologique, 128*, 301–322.

McCarthy, R. A. & Warrington, E. K. (1985). Category specificity in an agrammatic patient: The relative impairment of verb retrieval and comprehension. *Neuropsychologia, 23*, 709–727.

McCarthy, R. A. & Warrington, E. K. (1988). Evidence for modality-specific meaning systems in the brain. *Nature, 334*, 428–430.

McKenna, P. & Warrington, E. K. (1980). Testing for nominal aphasia. *Journal of Neurology, Neurosurgery, and Psychiatry, 43*, 781–788.

Marin, O. S. M., Glenn, C. G., & Rafal, R. D. (1983). Visual problem solving in the absence of lexical semantics: Evidence from dementia. *Brain and Cognition, 2*, 285–311.

Miller, G. A. & Fellbaum, C. (1991). Semantic networks of English. *Cognition, 41*, 197–229.

Morton, J. (1979). Word recognition. In J. Morton & J. C. Marshall (Eds.), *Psycholinguistics Series, Volume 2. 109–156*. London: Elek.

Morton, J. & Patterson, K. E. (1980). A new attempt at an interpretation, or, an attempt at a new interpretation. In M. Coltheart, K. E. Patterson & J. C. Marshall (Eds.), *Deep Dyslexia. 91–118*. London: Routledge.

Myers, D. & Goodglass, H. (1978). The effects of cuing on picture naming in aphasia. *Cortex, 14*, 178–189.

Newcombe, F. & Marshall, J. C. (1980). Response monitoring and response blocking in deep dyslexia. In M. Coltheart, K. E. Patterson & J. C. Marshall (Eds.), *Deep Dyslexia. 160–175*. London: Routledge.

Podraza, B. L. & Darley, F. L. (1977). Effect of auditory prestimulation on naming in aphasia. *Journal of Speech and Hearing Research, 20*, 669–683.

Riddoch, M. J., Humphreys, G. W., Coltheart, M., & Funnell, E. (1988). Semantic system or systems? Neuropsychological evidence reexamined. *Cognitive Neuropsychology, 5*, 3–25.

Saddy, J. D. (1991). *Investigations into Grammatical Knowledge*. Ph. D. Thesis: Massachusetts Institute of Technology.

Sartori, G. & Job, R. (1988). The oyster with four legs: A neuropsychological study of the interaction of visual and semantic information. *Cognitive Neuropsychology, 5*, 105–132.

Schwartz, M. F. (Ed.) (1990). *Modular Deficits in Alzheimer-Type Dementia*. Cambridge, Mass.: MIT Press.

Schwartz, M. F., Saffran, E., & Marin, O. (1980). The word order problem in agrammatism I: Comprehension. *Brain and Language, 10*, 249–262.

Semenza, C. & Zettin, M. (1988). Generating proper names: a case of selective inability. *Cognitive Neuropsychology, 5*, 711–721.

Semenza, C. & Zettin, M. (1989). Evidence from aphasia for the role of proper names as pure referring expressions. *Nature, 342*, 678–679.

Shallice, T. (1988). Specialization within the semantic system. *Cognitive Neuropsychology, 5*, 133–142.

Silveri, M. C. & Gainotti, G. (1988). Interaction between vision and language in category-specific semantic impairment. *Cognitive Neuropsychology, 5*, 677–709.

Silveri, M. C., Daniele, A., Giustolisi, L., & Gainotti, G. (1991). Dissociation between knowledge of living and nonliving things in dementia of the Alzheimer type. *Neurology, 41*, 545–546.

Stemberger, J. P. (1985). An interactive activation model of language production. In A. W. Ellis (Ed.), *Progress in the Psychology of Language, Volume 1. 143–186*. London: Erlbaum.

Tyler, L. K. (1992). *Spoken Language Comprehension*. Cambridge, Mass.: MIT Press.

Warrington, E. K. (1975). The selective impairment of semantic memory. *Quarterly Journal of Experimental Psychology, 27*, 635–657.

Warrington, E. K. (1981). Neuropsychological studies of verbal semantic systems. *Philosophical Transactions of the Royal Society, London. B 295*, 411–423.

Warrington, E. K. & McCarthy, R. (1983). Category specific access dysphasia. *Brain, 106*, 859–878.

Warrington, E. K. & McCarthy, R. (1987). Categories of knowledge: Further fractionation and an attempted integration. *Brain, 110*, 1273–1296.

Warrington, E. K. & Shallice, T. (1984). Category specific semantic impairments. *Brain, 107*, 829–853.

Yamadori, A. & Albert, M. L. (1973). Word category aphasia. *Cortex, 9*, 112–125.

Jennifer M. Gurd/John C. Marshall
Oxford (UK)

13. Syntactic Disorders in Aphasia

1. Introduction

Aphasia, an organic disorder of the language system due to brain damage, may take many different forms, from a near-total destruction of the linguistic system in global aphasia to a loss of low-frequency name retrieval in anomic aphasia. Syntactic disorders are generally associated with the symptoms of agrammatic or paragrammatic speech production, which are usually present in Broca's and Wernicke's aphasia, respectively. Agrammatic production is typically characterized by slow, effortful speech which consists of syntactically simplified utterances. The lexical categories are used in their citation form rather than in the forms required for syntactically connected speech. In contrast to agrammatic production, paragrammatic production is generally fluent retaining the syntactic complexity of normal speech. However, the syntactic plan of the utterance is frequently disturbed by blends and other syntactic contaminations, symptoms which may occasionally also occur in normal speech (Fay 1980). Furthermore, the associated phenomena are very heterogeneous, ranging from extreme phonological to extreme semantic deviations.

The sophistication of knowledge and research about these two disorders has turned out to be very asymmetrical. Whereas agrammatism has given rise to numerous theoretical speculations about the underlying mechanisms of the deficit, there is only a small number of studies on paragrammatism and these have not reached a comparable depth. One reason may be that it is not clear whether the paragrammatic symptom is rooted in a specifiable linguistic principle, or whether it is more likely a breakdown of general monitoring mechanisms. Consequently, the ascription of paragrammatism to a competence disorder has always been extremely shaky, in contrast to agrammatism, where the issue of a competence versus performance deficit remains controversial.

For these reasons, the survey on syntactic disorders in aphasia will almost exclusively be confined to a discussion of the phenomenon of agrammatism.

2. Major Historical Forerunners

The study of syntactic disorders in aphasia started at the turn of the century in German aphasiology (Pick 1898; 1913) with the introduction of syntax as an object of research in linguistics and psycholinguistics (Wundt 1900; Bühler 1918). Until then, the psychology of language and its disorders had focused on the isolated word.

From the linguistic perspective, this word-centered analysis can be explained by the emphasis in linguistic research on reconstructing proto-Indoeuropean, which basically meant the reconstruction of phonology and morphology. Due to the free word order, the syntax per se of the classical languages was felt to be trivial.

From the psychological point of view, the dominant paradigm in the 19th century was an associationist model, according to which a word was mentally represented by different interconnected memory systems ('engrams') for each peripheral sensory input and output channel (motor, auditory, tactile, visual, etc.) (Charcot 1883; Wernicke 1886).

In the first quarter of this century, language disturbances were studied with more syntactic scrutiny in selected single cases. However, the paradigm of classical associationism was carried on by some authors like Kleist (1914), who postulated motor engrams for sentences in analogy to the earlier ideas about motor and acoustic word engrams. In his theory, a loss of motor sentence engrams would lead to agrammatic speech production, while a lesion in the sensory area would entail the loss of coordination of preserved motor engrams, leading to paragrammatic speech production.

It is important to see that in subsequent work a rather strict separation was assumed between syntax and morphology. Word order, a property of syntax, was considered to be a natural result of the language of thought, which had to be distinguished from grammaticalisation with function words and morphological devices. Frequently comparisons were made between inflecting languages such as German and isolating languages such as Chinese or developing languages such as child or pidgin language. This separation of morphology and syntax played a role in the conceptualisation of linguistic processing. The levels of word order formation, of lexical insertion, and of grammaticalisation were considered distinct stages in language production. According to this conception, a disturbance occuring at any one level would thus lead to a specific corresponding subtype of grammatical disorder. Pick (1913) subsumed such disorders under the heading of "expressive agrammatism". Disturbances of the language of thought were termed "pseudo-agrammatism". Similar proposals were also made with respect to different stages in language comprehension (Bühler 1909; Pick 1909). These ideas are reminiscent of modern theories of sentence processing like Garrett's (1980).

Goldstein (1913) argued in favor of a central grammatical deficit ("zentrale Aphasie"), although this would mostly be associated with either a motor or a sensory deficit. Agrammatic and paragrammatic output was the result of a combination of the central grammatical disorder plus additional motor or sensory disorders, respectively. A revival of this theory has been proposed in Heeschen (1985).

In an influential case study, Salomon (1914) was able to demonstrate the existence of what was then called 'impressive' or 'sensory' agrammatism, i. e. a disturbance of grammatical elements in comprehension, in a patient with agrammatic speech production. He argued that these two disorders should always co-occur because of a lack of control of motor images (including grammatical elements) on comprehension in patients with agrammatic expression. A modern version of this hypothesis is that agrammatism results from a disorder in the central syntactic parser (Berndt/Caramazza 1980).

Isserlin (1922) reported three patients with different subtypes of grammatical production disorders (agrammatism, paragrammatism). Whereas expressive agrammatism could occur with or without impressive agrammatism, patients with paragrammatic production would invariably have severe grammatical comprehension problems as well. He suggested that agrammatic speech could be the result of an adaptation to the general motor deficit. This explanation has found a recent revival in Kolk/van Grunsven (1985).

This short survey of the history shows that there have been different theoretical explanations of morphosyntactic disorders and different characterizations of agrammatism affecting either speech alone or in conjunction with comprehension. Some of these explanations have found a revival in more recent work. Yet, knowledge of grammatical disorders has advanced considerably for at least two reasons. First, there is a better understanding of the nature of syntax due to the post-war increase in theoretical linguistic research and second, models of normal sentence processing have been developed in the new science of experimental psycholinguistics. Apart from these aspects, however, the German aphasiological tradition had already laid most of the important foundations for the study of morphosyntactic disorders as it is pursued today.

3. Agrammatism as a Central Syntactic Deficit

In the transition from European to American-dominated aphasiology, Roman Jakobson's integrative work emphasized the role of linguistics in the study of language disorders. Jakobson, a linguist of the Prague school, was influenced by the work of the Russian neurologist A. R. Luria and after his emigration to America by Geschwind and other contemporaries. His most influential aphasiological work is Jakobson (1941). Although the main emphasis was on phonological issues, Jakobson's proposals on contiguity and similarity were generalized to morpho-syntactic issues as well. He suggested that the two fundamental axes in language, the syntagmatic and the paradigmatic, were selectively vulnerable in aphasia. 'Efferent' (motor) aphasia was seen as a contiguity disorder affecting the combination of words and other morphemes to higher units as well as the retrieval of bound morphemes and syntactically relevant forms, whereas the selection process was relatively preserved. The reverse pattern was proposed for sensory aphasia. Patients with this disorder would retain relative stability in the syntagmatic organization of speech while showing serious selection deficits. (See Jakobson 1956; 1963). In evaluating Jakobson's contribution to the field, one has to keep in mind that his perspective was exclusively theoretical, and that it was up to other researchers to validate his classifications empirically (See Osgood/Miron 1963).

Modern American work on linguistic aspects of aphasia was initially strongly influenced by Jakobson's ideas. They gave rise to a large number of group studies showing double dissociations between 'anterior' aphasics (with disturbed syntax but preserved semantics) and 'posterior' aphasics (with preserved syntax but impaired semantics). (See Caramazza/Berndt 1978 for a review.)

Another major source of influence on psycho- and neurolinguistics in the late fifties and sixties was the Chomskyan model of generative transformational grammar (Chomsky 1957). This initiated a cognitive revolution leading to the final rejection of behaviorist psychology. Inspired by experimental psycholinguistic results, the linguistic grammar was thought to be quite directly implemented into a processing model. The syntax consisted of a set of context-free rewrite rules such as S → NP VP, NP → DET N etc., and a number of transformations which relate (semantically interpreted) deep structures or 'kernel sentences' generated by the rewrite system to various surface forms. Syntactic complexity could then be seen as the number of transformations which must operate on a kernel to derive a certain surface form. This has become known as the 'derivational theory of complexity'. (See Fodor/Bever/Garrett 1974 for a detailed evaluation and Berwick/Weinberg 1984).

As a natural consequence of the choice of this model as a quasi-processing model, aphasiological work in this tradition shifted away from questions of linguistic modality as had been suggested in most of the classical work. Aphasia was now taken to be a central linguistic deficit which affects all aspects of language processing.

As dictated by the derivational grammar of Chomsky (1957; 1965), the emphasis was naturally on linguistic production. Myerson/Goodglass (1972), for example, wrote the grammar of three agrammatic patients in terms of phrase structure rules which would account for their spontaneous speech.

On the other hand, since aphasia was taken to be a central linguistic deficit, comprehension should equally be affected in aphasics. Marshall (1977), for example, explicitly rejected the assumption that agrammatism would be a mere output problem, a disorder of the 'pronunciation' side of otherwise fully specified structures. Prominent studies of aphasic – mainly agrammatic – comprehension appeared in the seventies. Shewan/Canter (1971) found a syntactic complexity effect for aphasics in general in a sentence picture matching task. The variables in this task were untransformed ('kernel') sentences versus passive, negated and negative passive sentences.

Heilman/Scholes (1976) investigated Broca's aphasics for their comprehension of sentences which were disambiguated by the placement of the definite article such as *They fed her dog the biscuits* versus *They fed her the dog biscuits*. The patients performed at chance level in this task, although they did not show lexical problems.

Caramazza/Zurif (1976) found evidence that Broca's and conduction aphasics had a specific syntactic parsing problem which they could often circumvent by making use of semantic cues such as animacy. The patients examined showed good comprehension of sentences with 'irreversible' participants such as *The bicycle that the boy is holding is broken*, while their performance became unreliable with semantically 'reversible' sentences such as *The man that the woman is hugging is happy*. In the latter case, a heuristic strategy (see Bever 1970) cannot be employed, and comprehension requires a thorough syntactic analysis. In a similar vein, Goodglass/Blumstein/Gleason et al. (1979) found that subject relatives like *The man greeted by the woman was smoking a pipe* were more difficult for Broca's aphasics to comprehend than synonymous coordinated constructions like *The woman greeted the man and he was smoking a pipe*. The authors concluded that the patients' problems could not rest in the linguistic memory load but specifically in the processing of syntactically complex structures. Schwartz/Saffran/Marin (1980) and Saffran/Schwartz/Marin (1980) examined whether word order (as generated by the base component of a generative grammar) can be appreciated by agrammatics in comprehension and in production. This would, for instance, be predicted by a phonological or morpholexical deficit explanation (discussed in the next paragraph). Their data indicated that certain patients are entirely unable to use order information, not only in (reversible) passive sentences but also in simple English SVO sentences and locative constructions such as *The circle is in the square*. (See, however, the criticism concerning certain theoretical issues in Caplan 1983).

Evidence for a central syntactic deficit in agrammatics with Broca's aphasia was not only found in comprehension tasks but also in experiments that rely on metalinguistic abilities. Following a paradigm invented by Levelt (1970), Zurif/Caramazza/Myerson (1972) asked Broca's aphasics to rank the relatedness of words that occurred in a sentence. The results of such a relatedness ranking procedure in normals has a fairly close resemblance to syntactic surface structures. However, the result achieved by the aphasic patients suggested that constituents will be syntactically integrated only as long as they make a referential semantic contribution, e. g., a possessive pronoun but not an article would be properly attached to a noun, a verb but not a copula would be attached to an object noun (phrase) etc. (See also Zurif/Caramazza 1976.) Using the same technique, Zurif/Green/Caramazza/Goodenough (1976) focused more on the processing of the function word vocabulary.

Most of the studies which fall in this period of research dealt with the English language. One notable exception was the influential study of German aphasics by von Stockert and Bader (1976). These authors used a task in which the patient had to put three cards with constituents in an order which resulted in a sentence. The materials used normal sentences such as *Die Milch/läuft/aus der Kanne* ('The milk runs out of the pitcher'), semantically deviant sentences such as *Das Klavier/spielt/auf dem Karl* ('The piano plays on Charles'), as well as properly inflected nonwords like *Das Wampel/wird/gewampelt*. Von

Stockert and Bader found that in solving this task Broca's aphasics followed a semantic strategy, while Wernicke's aphasics followed a morphosyntactic strategy. Both strategies lead to the correct result in normal sentences, but there were differences with respect to semantically deviant sentences. Whereas Broca's used a semantic solution, thus ignoring morphological mismatches, Wernicke's were sensitive to the morphosyntax, thus ignoring the semantic deviance. This study strongly established the double dissociation between morphosyntax and semantics with respect to the two major clinical groups of Broca's and Wernicke's aphasics. De Bleser/Dronsek/Bayer (1988), however, could not replicate these results with a different group of subjects.

The studies reported above are just a suggestive sample of work in this period. What they have in common is the assumption of a central syntactic deficit that embraces each aspect of linguistic processing. It then becomes difficult to distinguish such a deficit from a loss of syntactic competence. In fact, Whitaker (1969) assumed explicitly that aphasia proper is a loss of linguistic competence but he revised this later on (see Whitaker 1970) and abandoned the competence-performance distinction for the neuropsychological enterprise altogether. (See the discussion in Schnitzer 1978.) Similarly, Weigl/Bierwisch (1970) argued against aphasia as a deficit of linguistic (or syntactic) competence. They reported a patient who, once 'deblocked' for a given sentence S, showed access to a class of transformationally related sentences {S 1, S 2, ..., Sn} which were inaccessible to the patient before. Thus, it seemed plausible to distinguish a central syntactic processing deficit from disordered competence, on the one hand, and from a modality specific deficit, on the other hand. While there is no conclusive evidence in the entire neuropsychological literature in favor of a competence deficit, a number of cases have been reported which point to the possibility of a modality specific disruption of morpho-syntactic processing. We will return to such cases below.

4. Agrammatism as a Morpholexical Deficit

Although agrammatism appeared to be a syntactic disorder, there were attempts to reduce it to a morphological or phonological (processing or central) disorder. The basic claim was that agrammatics cannot access or process the elements of the so-called 'closed class' vocabulary like normal subjects. Closed class elements are function words such as determiners, auxiliaries, pronouns etc., perhaps also prepositions and certain adverbs, but also bound morphemes (in this research mainly with emphasis on syntax-relevant inflectional morphemes). Items of the open class are the lexical elements of the noun, verb, and adjective class. Bradley (1978) showed in experiments with normal subjects that the recognition speed for items of the open class is a function of the frequency of the individual item, while there is no such effect for items of the closed class. Bradley/Garrett/Zurif (1980) showed that agrammatics require the same recognition time for both vocabulary types. (See also Friederici 1985 for German.) As suggested by the investigation of speech errors (see Fromkin 1980; Meringer/Mayer 1895; Cutler 1981), there is evidence that the closed class items are inserted into the syntactic (production) frame (see Garrett 1975; 1980) before the open class items are inserted. In this case, one could interpret the processing results of agrammatics as an inability to establish in real time the syntactic frame (Garrett's "positional level") necessary for the insertion of open class items. The idea of abnormal access to the closed class vocabulary had a strong impact on research in the late seventies and early eighties. Kean (1977) tried to give a more precise characterization of the deficit in terms of classical generative phonology. Given a theory of distinct word- and morpheme-boundaries in the phonological representation, Kean's central claim was that agrammatics strip a sentence down to its minimal phonological words. This procedure would then eliminate what is traditionally considered to be the functional elements ('grammatical morphemes') of speech. As long as a language like English with relatively poor morphology and rather rigid word order is considered, the predictions may be borne out, but it has been shown that it fails to characterize agrammatic speech in morphologically richer languages like German (see Heeschen 1985, Bayer/De Bleser/Dronsek 1987), Hebrew and Russian (Grodzinsky 1984) and many others (see Menn/Obler 1989). In addition, it has been observed that agrammatic patients tend to leave out verbs in general and not only auxiliary verbs (see Miceli/Silveri/Villa/Caramazza 1984). Of course, this does not conform easily to the established vocabulary type explanations. (With respect to the verb forms predominantly used by agrammatics, see also the account in terms of markedness theory by Lapointe (1985)). We will return to the role of functional categories below. What can be established, however, is that the deficit can neither be reduced to a purely morphophonological disorder nor to a pure production problem that leaves language comprehension intact.

5. Modality Specificity and Performance Disorders

The studies reported so far have in common that they mostly assume an invariant core of the deficit which enables us to assign individual patients to a group such as agrammatic and paragrammatic aphasics. According to this view, variability within such a homogeneous group would stem from different degrees of severity of the disorder. However, such a syndrome interpretation has been challenged in modern cognitive neuropsychology. With respect to the notion 'agrammatism', Badecker and Caramazza (1985) have argued that it is not a unitary phenomenon at all but rather a conglomeration of a set of quite heterogeneous clinical symptoms which may or may not co-occur in a single patient. Indeed, it has repeatedly been observed that there are patients with agrammatic speech but a much better preserved comprehension system. For example, Miceli/Mazzucchi/Menn/Goodglass (1983) described two Italian patients with a clinical picture of agrammatism in their spontaneous speech, although their comprehension did not show the features of a syntactic deficit. Furthermore, Linebarger/Schwartz/Saffran (1983) presented evidence that four English speaking patients with agrammatic production and a clear comprehension disorder (as verified by sentence picture matching tasks) showed a surprisingly good performance in grammaticality judgement tasks. The authors explained their results as a pure performance disorder in which the abstract knowledge of grammar (in the sense of Chomskyan competence) is retained but cannot be put to use. The reason for this was sought in the inability of these patients to map syntactic representation onto semantic representations, although both syntax and semantics must be preserved on a more abstract level.

Studies like these undermine the symptom-based classification of patients according to spontaneous speech phenomena and explanations in terms of a common linguistic deficit. Badecker/Caramazza (1985) argued that notions like 'agrammatism' or 'paragrammatism' should be banned from a scientific enterprise until the nature of the deficit is clarified by in-depth studies of single cases. Methodologically, this would disqualify group studies because averaging across clinically defined patients could conceal the underlyingly non-uniform functional deficits. On the one hand, it seems rather uncontroversial that group studies of agrammatic (or seemingly agrammatic) patients are unacceptable as long as the clinical criteria are not sufficiently articulated (as in terms like "Broca's aphasia with agrammatic speech production"). On the other hand, it has persistently been argued that there is a common functional deficit among certain patients which does allow for a unitary explanation in terms of linguistic and psycholinguistic theory (see Grodzinsky 1991a for a recent defense). Researchers such as David Caplan have suggested a different solution to the controversy about single case versus group studies. They propose a multiple case approach which adopts the depth and methodology of single case studies, but still expects generalizability across individual cases. This methodological approach is often used in modern linguistically oriented studies.

6. Current Syntactic Accounts

As pointed out in some detail in Berwick/Weinberg (1984), the theory of Government and Binding (GB) (Chomsky 1981; 1982 and subsequent work) has provided a new perspective on the relation between grammar and parser and also about linguistic theory and its relevance for psycholinguistics. In a nutshell, GB has minimized rule systems as well as transformations in favor of generalized phrase structure (X-bar syntax) and a number of 'modules' which are thought to hold universally. Among these are principles of case- and thematic-relations, binding, control etc. Language specific differences are attributed to a finite set of so-called 'parameters' which are induced by experience (lexical learning). In parsing models making use of GB-type grammars, the principles and parameters of

Universal Grammar are thought to work on-line as filtering devices keeping track of the local well-formedness of syntactic projections that are induced by access to lexical items and functional categories (cf. Kolb/Thiersch 1991) for a computer implementation of English and German). Various proposals exist as to the characterization of syntactic deficits in terms of the GB-framework, in particular those deficits affecting comprehension. Grodzinsky (1990; 1991 b) interprets agrammatic comprehension as an impaired access to a properly annotated syntactic (surface) structure. Consider English sentences such as *The girl was pushed by the boy* (passive) or *It was the girl who the boy pushed* (object cleft). In order to assign the proper thematic relations, it is necessary to associate the NP *the girl* or *who* with an empty element *e* (a kind of placeholder) in the underlying argument position. [*The girl$_i$ was pushed e_i by the boy; It was the girl$_i$ who$_i$ the boy pushed e_i*]. According to Grodzinsky, agrammatic patients do not have access to these empty categories and therefore fail to assign proper thematic relations to sentences of this kind. The chance level performance on such sentences which has repeatedly been observed is neither found in active sentences nor with adjectival passives such as *The soldier was enraged at the boy*, in which there is no empty element to be associated. In other cases such as *It was the girl who pushed the boy*, an 'Agent-First' strategy (see Bever 1970) would lead to the correct thematic assignment (although perhaps for the wrong reason). According to Grodzinky, one can go so far as to use aphasiological data as an evaluation metric for different syntactic theories such as Lexical Functional Grammar (see Bresnan 1982) and Generalized Phrase Structure Grammar (see Gazdar/Klein/Pullum/Sag 1985). (For an overview see Sells 1985.) Since LFG and GPSG do not treat passive and other constructions as instantiations of syntactic movement, as GB does, Grodzinsky claims that they are not 'breakdown compatible' and therefore inferior to the GB account. In a similar vein, Caplan/Hildebrandt (1988) argue that the patterns of comprehension breakdown in aphasics would favor a GB-type grammar as the basis of the syntactic processor, although their motivation is somewhat different. These authors found patients with double dissociations in their comprehension of sentences involving different kinds of empty categories (such as Wh-traces, NP-traces and PRO, which have a completely different status in GB). Work of this kind can be seen as a further development of the classical syntactic deficit theory of agrammatism.

There are also newer attempts at a characterization in terms of the vocabulary type morpholexical approach mentioned above, but these are now recast into a new model of syntax that has started with Chomsky (1986; 1989) and Pollock (1989). This further development takes functional elements like complementizers and various inflectional elements as syntactic (not morphological) heads which project in (X-bar) syntax, like the lexical categories N, V, A and P. One could then assume that the nature of the agrammatic deficit can by and large be characterized as a loss of the functional heads that give rise to the frame into which lexical projections have to be inserted in order to derive full representations. In this sense, this explanation looks like a revival of the vocabulary approach. However, it is in fact quite different because the deficit is not ascribed to the morpholexical or phonological level, but rather to syntax proper.

Bayer/De Bleser/Dronsek (1987) and De Bleser/Bayer (1988) also presented evidence from production experiments which reveal far more inflectional abilities in agrammatics than usually assumed.

Ouhalla (1990) attempted to derive the so-called 'word order problem' (see Schwartz/Saffran/Marin 1980) from the idea that lexical projections such as VP are pure representations of a thematic grid which does not reveal anything about the order of constituents. Functional projections are thought to be needed in order to assign arguments to their ultimate position in a phrase marker. According to this hypothesis, English speaking agrammatics should not be in a position to distinguish between reversible sentences such as *The boy sees the girl* and *The girl sees the boy* because for them the bracketing may equally be [*boy* [*see girl*] or [[*girl see*] *boy*]. Unfortunately, this claim has not yet been established on the basis of experiment data.

7. Conclusion

The conclusion to be drawn from this overview is that our thinking about agrammatic disturbances has never abandoned the idea that they may best be characterized as a syntactic deficit. Especially the transition from the earlier work in the Chomsky tradition to the latest developments in this theory has suggested that this is the invariant core of most of the work in linguistic aphasiology. However, a central counterpoint has been that even the most severely agrammatic aphasics were found to be sensitive to some structure which has to be characterized as syntactic by all means. This has lead to the idea that linguistic knowledge may be so abstract that one cannot really expect it to be affected by a focal brain lesion. Consequently, most of the cases cannot be explained by a central syntactic deficit but rather by some kind of processing disorder. Seen from this perspective, one would hope that further research on the relation between the grammar and the parser will shed light on the nature of the syntactic disorder in aphasics. On the other hand, one can consider aphasia research as one branch of linguistics and cognitive science which plays an essential role in finding a solution to these problems.

8. References

Badecker, W. & Caramazza, A. (1985). On considerations of method and theory governing the use of clinical categories in neurolinguistics and cognitive neuropsychology: The case against agrammatism. *Cognition, 20*, 97–125.

Bayer, J., De Bleser, R., & Dronsek, C. (1987). Form und Funktion von Kasus bei Agrammatismus. *Linguistische Berichte. Sonderheft 1*, 81–117.

Berndt, R. & Caramazza, A. (1980). A redefinition of the syndrome of Broca's aphasia: Implications for a neuropsychological model of language. *Applied Psycholinguistics, 1*, 225–278.

Berwick, R. & Weinberg, A. (1984). Parsing efficiency, computational complexity, and the evaluation of grammatical theories. *Linguistic Inquiry, 13*, 165–191.

Bever, T. (1970). The cognitive basis for linguistic structures. In J. R. Hayes (Ed.), *Cognition and the Development of Language. 297–352.* New York: Wiley.

Bradley, D. C. (1978). *Computational Distinctions of Vocabulary Type.* Unpublished Ph. D. dissertation. MIT Cambridge, Mass.

Bradley, D., Garrett, M. & Zurif, E. B. (1980). Syntactic deficits in Broca's aphasia. In D. Caplan (Ed.), *Biological Studies of Mental Processes. 269–286.* Cambridge, Mass.: MIT Press.

Bresnan, J. (Ed.) (1982). *The Mental Representation of Grammatical Relations.* Cambridge, Mass.: MIT Press.

Bühler, K. (1909). Über das Sprachverständnis vom Standpunkt der Normalpsychologie. In *Bericht über den III. Kongress für experimentelle Psychologie.* Frankfurt/M. 22.–25. 04. 1908. Leipzig, *94–130.*

Bühler, K. (1918). Kritische Musterung der neueren Theorien des Satzes. *Indogermanisches Jahrbuch, 6*, 1–20.

Caplan, D. (1983). A note on the word order problem in agrammatism. *Brain and Language, 20.* 155–165.

Caplan, D. & Hildebrandt, N. (1988). *Disorders of Syntactic Comprehension.* Cambridge, Mass.: MIT Press.

Caramazza, A. & Berndt, R. (1978). Semantic and syntactic processes in aphasia: a review of the literature. *Psychological Bulletin, 85*, 898–918.

Caramazza, A. & Zurif, E. B. (1976). Dissociation of algorhithmic and heuristic processes in language comprehension: Evidence from aphasia. *Brain and Language, 3*, 572–582.

Charcot, J. M. (1883). Des differentes formes de l'aphasie. *Progres Medical, 11*, 441.

Chomsky, N. (1957). *Syntactic Structures.* The Hague: Mouton.

Chomsky, N. (1965). *Aspects of the Theory of Syntax.* Cambridge, Mass.: MIT Press.

Chomsky, N. (1981). *Lectures on Government and Binding.* Studies in Generative Grammar 9. Dordrecht: Foris.

Chomsky, N. (1982). *Some Concepts and Consequences of the Theory of Government and Binding.* Linguistic Inquiry Monographs. Cambridge, Mass.: MIT Press.

Chomsky, N. (1986). *Barriers.* Linguistic Inquiry Monographs. Cambridge, Mass.: MIT Press.

Chomsky, N. (1989). Some notes on economy of derivation and representation. In I. Laka & A. Majahan (Eds.), *MIT Working Papers in Linguistics 10, Functional Heads and Clause Structure, 43–74.*

Cutler, A. (Ed.) (1981). The reliability of speech error data. (Special issue on errors in spontaneous speech). *Linguistics, 19*, 7–8.

De Bleser, R. & Bayer, J. (1988). On the role of inflectional morphology in agrammatism. In M. Hammond & M. Noonan (Eds.), *Theoretical Morphology. 45–69.* New York: Academic Press.

De Bleser, R., Dronsek, C., & Bayer, J. (1988). Morphosyntactic processing in German agrammatism: A replication and revision of Von Stockert/Bader (1976). *Cortex, 24*, 53–76.

Fay, D. (1980). Transformational errors. In V. Fromkin (Ed.), *Errors in Linguistic Performance: Slips of the Tongue, Ear, Pen, and Hand. 111–122.* New York: Academic Press.

Fodor, J. A., Bever, T., & Garrett, M. F. (1974). *The Psychology of Language.* New York: Mc Graw-Hill.

Friederici, A. (1985). Levels of processing and vocabulary types: Evidence from on-line comprehension in normals and agrammatics. *Cognition, 19*, 2, 133–162.

Fromkin, V. L. (Ed.) (1980). *Errors in Linguistic Performance: Slips of the Tongue, Ear, Pen, and Hand.* New York: Academic Press.

Garrett, M. F. (1975). The analysis of sentence production. In G. Bower (Ed.), *The Psychology of Learning and Motivation: Advances in Research and Theory 9. 133–177.* New York: Academic Press.

Garrett, M. F. (1980). Levels of processing in sentence production. In B. Butterworth (Ed.), *Language Production 1. 177–220.* London: Academic Press.

Gazdar, G., Klein, E., Pullum, G., & Sag, I. (1985). *Generalized Phrase Structure Grammar.* Cambridge, Mass: Harvard University Press.

Goldstein, K. (1913). Die Störungen der Grammatik bei Hirnkranken. *Monatsschrift für Psychiatrie und Neurologie, 36*, 540–568.

Goodglass, H., Blumstein, S. E., Berko Gleason, J., Hyde, M., Green, E., & Statlender, S. (1979). The effect of syntactic encoding on sentence comprehension in aphasia. *Brain and Language, 7*, 201–209.

Grodzinsky, Y. (1984). The syntactic characterization of agrammatism. *Cognition, 16*, 99–120.

Grodzinsky, Y. (1990). *Theoretical Perspectives on Language Deficits.* Cambridge, Mass.: MIT Press.

Grodzinsky, Y. (1991 a). There is an entity called agrammatic aphasia. *Brain and Language, 41*, 555–564.

Grodzinsky, Y. (1991 b). Neuropsychological reasons for a transformational analysis of verbal passive. *Natural Language and Linguistic Theory*, 9, 1–23.

Heeschen, C. (1985). Agrammatism versus paragrammatism: A fictious opposition. In M. L. Kean (Ed.), *Agrammatism.* 207–248. New York: Academic Press.

Heilman, K. & Scholes, R. J. (1976). The Nature of comprehension errors in Broca's, conduction and Wernicke's aphasics. *Cortex, 12*, 258–265.

Isserlin, M. (1922). Über Agrammatismus. *Zeitschrift für die Gesamte Neurologie und Psychiatrie, 75*, 322–410.

Jakobson, R. (1941). *Kindersprache, Aphasie und allgemeine Lautgesetze.* Uppsala: Universitets Arsskrift. Translated as *Child Language, Aphasia and Phonological Universals.* The Hague: Mouton, 1968.

Jakobson, R. (1956). Two aspects of language and two types of aphasic disturbances. In R. Jakobson & M. Halle (Eds.), *Fundamentals of Language. 55–82.* The Hague: Mouton.

Jakobson, R. (1963). Toward a linguistic classification of aphasic impairments. Reprint in R. Jakobson (1971), *Selected Writings, vol. II, Word and Language. 289–306.* The Hague: Mouton.

Kean, M. L. (1977). The linguistic interpretation of aphasic syndromes. *Cognition, 5*, 9–46.

Kleist, K. (1914). Aphasie und Geisteskrankheit. *Münchener medizinische Wochenschrift, 61*, 8–12.

Kolb, H. P. & Thiersch, C. (1991). Levels and empty categories in a principles and parameters approach to parsing. In K. Netter & H. Haider (Eds.), *Representational and Derivational Approaches to Generative Grammar. 251–301.* Dordrecht: Reidel.

Kolk, H. & van Grunsven, M. (1985). On parallelism in agrammatism. In M.-L. Kean (Ed.), *Agrammatism. 165–208.* New York: Academic Press.

Lapointe, S. (1983). Some issues in the linguistic description of agrammatism. *Cognition, 14*, 1–41.

Lapointe, S. (1985). A theory of verb form use in the speech of agrammatic aphasics. *Brain and Language, 24*, 100–155.

Levelt, W. J. M. (1970). A scaling approach to the study of syntactic relations. In G. B. Flores d'Arcais & W. J. M. Levelt (Eds.), *Advances in Psycholinguistics. 109–121.* Amsterdam: North Holland.

Linebarger, M., Schwartz, M., & Saffran, E. (1983). Sensitivity to grammatical structure in so-called agrammatic aphasics. *Cognition, 13*, 361–392.

Marshall, J. C. (1977). Disorders in the expression of language. In J. Morton & J. C. Marshall (Eds.), *Development and Pathology.* Psycholinguistics Series 1, 125–160. London: Elek Science.

Menn, L. & Obler, L. K. (1989). *Agrammatic Aphasia. A Cross-Language Narrative Sourcebook.* Amsterdam: John Benjamins.

Meringer, R. & Mayer, K. (1895). *Versprechen und Verlesen.* Stuttgart: Göschen'sche Verlagsbuchhandlung.

Miceli, G., Mazzucchi, A., Menn, L., & Goodglass, H. (1983). Contrasting cases of Italian agrammatic aphasia without comprehension disorder. *Brain and Language, 19*, 65–97.

Miceli, M., Silveri, C., Villa, G., & Caramazza, A. (1984). On the basis for the agrammatic's difficulty in producing main verbs. *Cortex, 20*, 207–220.

Myerson, R. & Goodglass, H. (1972). Transformational grammars of three agrammatic patients. *Language and Speech, 15*, 40–50.

Osgood, C. E. & Miron, M. S. (Eds.) (1963). *Approaches to the Study of Aphasia.* Urbana: University of Illinois Press.

Ouhalla, J. (1990). *Functional Categories, Agrammatism and Language Aquisition.* (Unpublished Manuscript.) Queen Mary and Westfield College, London University.

Pick, A. (1898). Über Agrammatismus als Folge cerebraler Herderkrankungen. In A. Pick, *Beiträge zur Pathologie und pathologischen Anatomie des Zentralnervensystems. 123–133.* Berlin: Karger.

Pick, A. (1909). *Über Sprachverständnis.* Leipzig: Barth.

Pick, A., (1913). *Die agrammatischen Sprachstörungen. Studien zur psychologischen Grundlegung der Aphasielehre.* Teil I (part II never appeared). Berlin: Springer.

Pollock, J.-Y. (1989). Verb movement, universal grammar, and the structure of IP. *Linguistic Inquiry, 20,* 365–424.

Saffran, E., Schwartz, M., & Marin, O. (1980). The word order problem in agrammatism II. Production. *Brain and Language, 10,* 132–144.

Salomon, E. (1914). Motorische Aphasie mit Agrammatismus und sensorisch-agrammatische Störungen. *Monatsschrift für Psychiatrie und Neurologie, 35,* 181–208, 216–175.

Shewan, C. M. & Canter, C. J. (1971). Effects of vocabulary, syntax, and sentence length on auditory comprehension in aphasic patients. *Cortex, 7,* 209–226.

Schnitzer, M. L. (1978). Toward a neurolinguistic theory of language. *Brain and Language, 6,* 342–361.

Schwartz, M., Saffran, E., & Marin, O. (1980). The Word Order Problem in Agrammatism I. Comprehension. *Brain and Language, 10,* 263–280.

Sells, P. (1985). *Lectures on Contemporary Syntactic Theories.* Stanford: CSLI.

Von Stockert, Th. & Bader, L. (1976). Some relations of grammar and lexicon in aphasia. *Cortex, 12,* 49–60.

Weigl, E. & Bierwisch, M. (1970). Neuropsychology and linguistics: Topics of common research. *Foundations of Language, 6,* 1–18.

Wernicke, C. (1886). Nervenheilkunde. Die neueren Arbeiten über Aphasie. *Fortschritte der Medicin, 4,* 371–377, 463–482.

Whitaker, H. A. (1969). On the representation of language in the human brain. *Working Papers in Phonetics, 12,* UCLA.

Whitaker, H. A. (1970). Linguistic competence: Evidence from aphasia. *Glossa, 4,* 1, 46–54.

Wundt, W. (1900). *Völkerpsychologie. Eine Untersuchung der Entwicklungsgesetze von Sprache, Mythos und Sitte.* Leipzig: Engelmann.

Zurif, E. B. & Caramazza, A. (1976). Psycholinguistic structures in aphasia: Studies in syntax and semantics. In H. Whitaker & H. A. Whitaker (Eds.), *Studies in Neurolinguistics, Vol. 1. 261–292.* New York: Academic Press.

Zurif, E. B., Caramazza, A., & Myerson, R. (1972). Grammatical judgments of agrammatic aphasics. *Neuropsychologia, 10,* 405–417.

Zurif, E. B., Green, E., Caramazza, A., & Goodenough, C. (1976). Grammatical intuitions of aphasic patients: Sensitivity to functors. *Cortex, 12,* 183–186.

Ria De Bleser, Aachen (Germany)/
Josef Bayer, Düsseldorf (Germany)

14. Disorders of Word Class Processing in Aphasia

1. Syntactic Categories

It is a basic assumption of any investigation into the nature of language that a given word of a language can be assigned to one or another syntactic category or word class. Two taxonomies of words are common; the open-closed class distinction, which divides the lexical inventory in terms of productivity, and syntactic categorization, which divides the lexical inventory in terms of grammatical role. This chapter will outline the basic concept of categorization and present an overview of the literature from aphasia that bears on the role of syntactic categorization in language processing. The first section of the chapter is concerned with the linguistic notions underlying the concept of syntactic categories. A theory of categorization is developed and related to the open-closed class description. The second section presents an overview of the literature pertaining to category effects. The third section offers a sketch of the various theoretic approaches which bear on processes sensitive to category distinctions and offers an alternative approach to category sensitivity.

1.1. Grammatical Word Classes: The Open Class – Closed Class Distinction in Linguistic Terms

The expression 'open and closed' class vocabulary reflects the observation that the lexical inventory of a language can be divided along the lines of productivity. The open class members of the inventory are those grammatical classes of the language which it is possible to expand. Languages employ a variety of devices to achieve this end; new coinage (xerox), borrowing from other languages (le weekend), blending two or more existing items (photo-copy), acronyms (Scuba) and back formation (xeroxing) are representative. Most new vocabulary comes into a language as either nouns or verbs. The productive rules of the grammar may then serve to generate adjectives and even adverbs from these sources. The closed class members are those which belong to a class which is not generally possible to expand; determiners, demonstratives, quantifiers, modals, auxiliaries. Prepositions fall under the closed class definition. However, this word type has proven to behave anomalously with respect to other closed class items in psycholinguistics investigations (see 2.2.1.).

A partial explanation for this anomalous behavior may be found in a linguistically based characterization of categories. The linguistic characterization of the 'major' or 'lexical' and 'minor' or 'functional' syntactic categories makes almost the same division of the word inventory as the open-closed distinction, however, under this characterization pronouns and prepositions are patterned with the 'open' class set.

In general, the notion of category is used pretheoretically in psycholinguistic investigations. Making the notion of a category specific and providing a vocabulary of primitive terms allows for a clearer understanding of the questions raised and the evidence revealed. The syntactic feature approach to categorization outlined below is based upon an approach common in the generative linguistics tradition. It was suggested in Chomsky (1965) and developed in Chomsky (1975; 1986; 1988), Emmonds (1985) and Jackendoff (1977). Akmajian/Demers/Harnish (1984); O'Grady/Dobrolovsky/Aronoff (1989) and Sells (1985) provide accessible introductions to contemporary linguistic ideas. A comprehensive introduction to the semantic notions relevant to the discussion can be found in Chierchia/McConnell-Ginet (1990).

1.1.1. Determining the Open Class Vocabulary

The productivity partition in the lexical inventory of languages corresponds quite closely to the linguistic distinction between 'functional' and 'lexical' grammatical classes. This gross distinction in category types follows from a feature system that takes noun and verb status as being featural primitives of lexical item (cf. Chomsky 1965; 1975; Emmonds 1985; Jackendoff 1977). The major categories are characterized as [±noun], henceforth [±N], and [±verb], henceforth [±V]. On the basis of this basic feature system four categories of lexical elements are predicted; [+N, −V], [−N, +V], [+N, +V] and [−N, −V]. Since the noun-verb distinction is taken as primitive, these two grammatical classes are captured as the two maximally contrasting feature sets; thus a noun is a lexical item that is marked as being [+N, −V], a verb is a lexical item that is marked as being [−N, +V]. Two other grammatical classes are also determined by this system, a grammatical class that has properties of both nouns and verbs, [+N, +V] and a grammatical class that has the properties of neither, [−N, −V].

1.1.2. Noun−Verb Distinction

These two feature sets are taken to determine the class of prepositions and the class of adjectives and adverbs respectively. To understand this assertion we must consider what the feature sets imply. We understand nouns to be labels for sets of properties that characterize objects, concrete or abstract, e. g., *dogs, trees, handbook articles* etc. As such, nouns are canonical examples of the kind of things that can be arguments of predication. Verbs, on the other hand, are labels for actions or states, e. g., *to read, to stand, to laugh* etc. They are canonical examples of predicates. A verbal predicate combines with its arguments to generate a complex proposition.

(1) [dogs] + [laugh] → [dogs laugh]

1.1.3. [+N, +V]

For a grammatical class to have both verbal and nominal properties means that members of this class will both be predicates and arguments of predicates. This would seem to be a good characterization of prepositions. Prepositions can be considered to exhibit [+verb] properties since they are predicates that combine with noun phrase complements to form prepositional phrases.

(2) [$_{\text{p}}$ Under] + [$_{\text{NP}}$ the tree] → [$_{\text{pp}}$[$_{\text{p}}$ Under] [$_{\text{NP}}$ the tree]]

Prepositions can be considered to exhibit [+noun] properties too, since prepositional phrases may also be arguments to predicates.

(3) [$_{\text{VP}}$[$_{\text{V}}$ put] [$_{\text{NP}}$ the book] [$_{\text{PP}}$[$_{\text{P}}$ Under] [$_{\text{NP}}$ the tree]]

1.1.4. [−N, −V]

The grammatical class determined by the features [−N, −V] will neither be a potential argument for some predicate nor will it take arguments. This feature combination is taken to characterize modifiers like adjectives. In most cases an adjective does not take arguments nor can it stand as the argument of a predicate.

(4) *[pitiful the boy]
*Bill [fixed pitiful]

The members of the class of adjectives do not always conform to this characterization. For instance, the adjective *proud* may be used like other adjectives as in (5):

(5) Bill is proud
Sue is a proud woman

however, *proud* also has verb-like properties in that it may take an argument as in (6):

(6) Bill is [proud [of Sue]]

In fact in many languages adjectives behave like verbs (see Dixon 1977).

Adverbs may also fall into this classification. They too can neither be arguments of predicates (7a) nor take arguments as predicates (7b).

(7a) *[quickly the boy]
(7b) *Bill [fixed quickly]

These two types of modifiers can be thought of as grammatical classes that correspond to the subtraction of a +value from either a nominal or verbal specification. Adjectives are nominal modifiers and can be taken to be the result of subtracting the +value from the [+N, −V] nominal specification. Adverbs, on the other hand, are verbal modifiers and can be taken to be the result of subtracting the +value from the [−N, +V] verbal specification. In both cases the resulting feature specification is [−N, −V]. Thus, for English, the taxonomy of grammatical classes outlined here does not distinguish between adjectives and adverbs. However, the partition does effectively capture the set of grammatical classes that correspond to the open class vocabulary. We leave a discussion of prepositions for later.

The characterization of prepositions as [+N, +V] and adjectives as [−N, −V] is the reverse of the traditional view. In Chomsky (1965; 1970) the fact that adjectives commonly pattern with nouns is taken as evidence that adjectives should be treated as being [+N]. Thus prepositions are treated as [−N, −V] and adjectives as [+N, +V]. Our treatment of prepositions as [+N, +V] and adjectives as [−N, −V] captures the fact that prepositions behave as hybrids with respect to language disorders and processing. They are sometimes retained like [+N] elements and sometimes impaired like [+V] elements.

We see then that the major lexical categories noun, verb, preposition and ad-positions can be characterized in terms of the two binary features [±noun] and [±verb]. This of course leaves unaccounted quite an important portion of the lexical inventory. What remains is the 'minor categories' determiners, demonstratives, quantifiers, comparatives, complementizers, auxiliaries, modals, aspect and tense markers, logical operators, negation and inflectional morphology. This heterogeneous set is referred to as members of the 'functional' vocabulary and correspond to the closed class. Note that the lexical–functional split is not identical to the open-closed split. Prepositions, pronouns and reflexives are members of the closed class vocabulary but fall into the 'lexical' class. There are no open class members that would be characterized as 'functional'.

1.2. Closed Class Elements – Functional Vocabulary

The closed class or functional vocabulary is not quite so easy to define. It is not entirely closed. While it is true that new closed class words are rarely introduced into a language, some of the operations applying to the open class can also be used to generate an infinite number of complex closed class constructions, i.e., [*more than seven but less than twelve*] ...

It is also not adequate to treat the functional vocabulary as the complement set of the 'lexical' vocabulary, that is, to suggest that anything that is not captured by the ±N, ±V features is 'functional'. The reason this approach fails is that most of the functional vocabulary could be characterized as [−N, −V] and differentiation within the set would not be possible.

One potential route to follow is to introduce a third feature to the category feature inventory, ±functional. However, for this to be a reasonable approach we must be convinced that there could be something very basic about the notion 'functional'. So basic that it could be treated as a featural primitive.

This approach is not implausible. There is an important distinction between those words that are members of the 'lexical' or open classes and those that are members of the 'functional' or closed classes. The difference lies in their role in the linguistic act of referring. Members of the 'lexical' vocabulary are used as general labels describing objects, events and states while the members of the 'functional' vocabulary are used, usually but not necessarily, in combination with 'lexical' elements, to pick out particular objects, events and states and to assert propositions.

In isolation we understand the 'lexical' word /dog/ to refer to an 'animal that has four legs, fur and barks', but the use of /dog/ in isolation can not be used to convey reference to a particular dog. In English, if the noun *dog* is used in a sentence without the accompaniment of an appropriate 'functional' element it can only be interpreted as either a proper name or a mass term. Consider the sentence in (8)

(8) Bill likes dog.

This sentence asserts either that Bill likes someone or something named *dog* or Bill is partial to dog meat. It cannot mean *Bill likes that dog over there*, or *Bill likes some dog or other*. Such a meaning is conveyed only through the appearance of an appropriate 'functional' element. In this case one of the determiners.

(9) Bill likes {a, the, this, that, some, every ...} dog

The reason that (8) has the interpretation it does is due to the fact that in English there is no determiner possible with proper names (*John likes (*the) Tom*) or necessary with mass terms (*John likes (the) sand*). Thus either of these interpretations is available for /dog/ in (8). In other languages such conditions will be different.

So, in English, /dog/ without a 'functional' element means 'animal that has four legs, fur and barks'. The ability to use /dog/ to refer to some individual animal or set of animals depends upon some member of the 'functional' vocabulary.

The same is true for verbs. A verb in isolation is a label for a kind of event or state. It is only through cooccurrence with tense and auxiliary elements, 'functional' elements, that a verb can be understood to refer to instances of events or states.

(10) *Bill [to like] the dog
Bill [has liked] the dog

Because of this special role played by the 'functional' vocabulary in reference to instances of objects, events or states, the ability to determine that an expression is a description of a particular situation and then to determine whether it is a true description or not depends crucially on the 'functional' vocabulary.

There does seem then to be a principled distinction that can be drawn between the referential properties of the 'lexical' or open class vocabulary and the 'functional' or closed class vocabulary. On this basis we can feel more comfortable about the introduction of [±functional], henceforth [±F], as a class feature (Saddy 1991).

This addition now expands the category inventory from four to eight. The 'major' syntactic categories are those picked out by the feature [−F]. The addition of the [−F] feature to the ±noun, ±verb feature set adds no new information. It simply makes explicit the non-referential property of the members of the 'major' categories. The four 'major' categories are still distinguished by virture of association with predicate or argument properties.

(11) [−F, +N, −V] = (Noun)
[−F, −N, +V] = (Verb)
[−F, +N, +V] = (Preposition)
[−F, −N, −V] = (Ad-Position)

The four 'new' categories, corresponding to the so called 'minor' categories, are characterized by the feature [+F].

(12) [+F, +N, −V]
[+F, −N, +V]
[+F, +N, +V]
[+F, −N, −V]

The correlation between the [−F] feature sets and their [+F] counterparts is not as straightforward as might be hoped. This is due to the fact that functional elements serve to do more than determine the referential properties of either arguments or predicates.

It is clear that [+F, +N, −V] will pick out those functional elements that contribute to the referential properties of nouns, i.e., determiners, quantifiers, numerals, and [+F, −N, +V] will pick out those functional elements that contribute to the referential properties of verbs, i.e., auxiliaries, tense.

In the case of [+F, +N, +V], however, there are no functional elements that contribute to the referential properties of prepositions in the same way as determiners contribute to nominal reference or tense contributes to event reference. We simply do not pick out particular instantiations of 'under-ness' or 'on-ness'. The feature set picks out functional elements that apply to combinations of arguments and predicates. In functional or referential terms a combination of arguments and predicates is a proposition. We do have functional elements such as voice or mood, and negation, which determine the nature of propositions as a whole. These are the functional elements that are determined by the features [+F, +N, +V].

(13) Bill will kiss the horse (active voice)
The horse will be kissed by Bill (passive voice)
Kiss the horse! (imperative voice)
Bill did not kiss the horse (negated proposition)

Similarly, elements of the feature set [+F, −N, −V] do not pick out functional elements that contribute to the referential properties of adpositions since we do not refer to particular instances of 'pretty-ness' or 'quickly-ness'. Rather, this feature set picks out those functional elements that are indifferent to predicate or argument status. These will be elements such as intensifiers, comparatives and logical operators which can serve to modify any referential domain.

(14) [[more than six but less than 24] eggs]
[a [more green than blue] parrot]
[[more in than out] of the box]

The preceding discussion provided an argument in favor of principled categorial distinctions internal to the closed class or functional vocabulary. The distinctions offered correspond, more or less, to our intuitive notions; determiners should be different than auxiliaries. Intuitive notions, however, can not be relied upon and indeed the distinctions determined by the featural approach outlined above are not entirely transparent. For instance, should tense and voice belong to distinct categories as predicted? The featural approach does have the advantage of making fairly clear distinctions on the basis of a linguistic analysis. If the distinctions are valid we would expect to find psycholinguistic evidence in support of the contrasts. The literature does provide examples of special sensitivity to the functional vocabulary in general (2.1., 2.2.6.) as well as to distinctions within the functional domain (2.2., 2.2.1., 2.2.2., 2.2.3., 2.2.4., 2.2.5.).

2. Disorders of Language Processing in Aphasia

2.1. Open Versus Closed Class

Over the last decade a considerable amount of attention in the aphasiological literature has been focussed on the distinction between the processing of open and closed class elements. It was in particular with the work of Bradley (1978; Bradley/Garrett/Zurif 1980) that this issue became central to the discussion of agrammatic Broca's behavior. Early descriptions of agrammatism had focussed on the analysis of these patients' production behavior, later studies centered around these patients' behavior in language perception. This shift of research interest towards the domain of language comprehension in Broca's aphasics was initiated by a study conducted by Caramazza/Zurif (1976). These authors had shown that Broca patients used heuristic strategies and not structural analyses when understanding sentences. In their study they had used sentences which necessarily required a structural analysis in order to be understood correctly. From their results they concluded that Broca's aphasia should not be described as a production deficit, but that an adequate definition of the deficit seen in these patients was that of a central syntactic impairment.

The early descriptions of Broca's aphasics' production behavior had stressed these patients' inability to produce function words and bound morphemes in spontaneous speech. Bradley/Garrett/Zurif (1980) reasoned that if Broca's aphasics suffer from a central deficit rather than from a selective deficit in production, similar aspects might be affected in production and in comprehension. Thus they investigated the aphasics' ability to process open and closed class words in a visual lexical decision paradigm. They found that normal subjects recognized these two word classes differently. While lexical decision times for open class words were a function of the words' frequency, lexical decision times for the function words were not. Moreover, open and closed class words behaved differently when they were part of a nonword constructed out of an open or closed class word and an independently occurring suffix (e.g., *thinage, thanage*). Bradley found an interference effect in the lexical decision times for the nonwords containing an open class element but no such effect for the nonwords containing a closed class element. The interpretation of this interference effect was that in order to determine that an item such as *thinage* as a nonword requires the listener to identify *thin* as an adjective, and then to check whether the word formation rule used correctly applies to the category of adjectives. For closed class elements lexical decision times could be much shorter as in this case the subject only has to identify the word class in order to know that productive rules do not apply. These results led Bradley and her colleagues to hypothesize that there is a specialized lexical access system that is responsible for retrieving closed class items. This specialized system's function is to provide fast access to those elements that carry the structural information which would allow the early structuring of the incoming input.

The agrammatic Broca patients who were tested with the same paradigm did not show a similar processing difference for the two word classes. Lexical decision times for both open and closed class words were a function of the words' frequency, and moreover they did not show an interference effect for the open class nonwords. Bradley and colleagues therefore suggested that agrammatism could be characterized by the loss of the specialized retrieval system for the closed class elements.

Given the importance of this result a number of investigators tried to replicate the findings. But the difference in the frequency sensitivity of the two word classes for normal subjects was not replicated (e. g., Kolk/Blomert 1985; Gordon/Caramazza 1982; 1983; 1985; Friederici/Heeschen 1983; Matthei/Kean 1989; Segui/Mehler/Frauenfelder/Morton 1982). The nonword interference effect for the open class nonwords, however, was replicated (e. g., Kolk/Bloomert 1985; Matthei/Kean 1989).

Gordon/Caramazza (1982) took the nonreplication as a basis to reject the hypothesis put forward by Bradley Garrett/Zurif (1980). Matthei/Kean (1989) viewed the difference in processing the two types of nonwords to indicate that normals first identify syntactic category and then look up the particular morphological rules that may apply. The absence of a similar nonword interference effect in Broca's aphasics as shown by Bradley was interpreted as an insensitivity to syntactic class information. This interpretation, however, seems to be too strong given other findings concerning these patient's sensitivity to syntactic class (e. g., Andreewsky/Seron 1975; Rosenthal/Goldblum 1989, see below).

Friederici (1983; 1985) argued that the inability to find a processing difference between open and closed class words in a lexical decision task does not necessarily call into question the hypothesis that there are two different processing devices involved. When words are presented in isolation – as it is done in a lexical decision task – function words may not be processed differently from open class words as in this situation function words do not serve their structural function. The latter is only relevant when these elements appear in sentential context. When presented in isolation in a lexical decision task they may simply be processed according to their form and not with respect to their grammatical function. Therefore, Friederici (1983; 1985) investigated the aphasics' ability to process open and closed class words in sentential context. She used a word monitoring paradigm in which the subjects had to detect a word which was specified before each trial. Each trial consisted of a pair of sentences, the first sentence being a context sentence which was either semantically related or unrelated to the second sentence which contained the target word. Target words were members of the open class (nouns) or members of the closed class (determiners, demonstratives, conjunctions). Normal subjects showed two effects, first, monitoring reaction times were faster for function words than for content words, and second, semantic context had an effect on the recognition of open class words but not on the recognition of closed class words. Agrammatic Broca patients also demonstrated a context effect for open class words and not for closed class words, but in contrast to normal subjects and non-agrammatic aphasic controls agrammatic aphasics' monitoring reaction times were much longer for closed class words than for open class words.

These results demonstrate a general processing distinction between the open and closed class in normals and a selective processing deficiency for one word class in the agrammatics.

2.2. Processing Contrasts for "Minor" Category Items

2.2.1. Prepositions

In the experiment reported above, Friederici (1985) also tested whether a potential difference in the processing of open and closed class words is a function of class membership or of the functional role a given element plays in the sentence. To investigate this question prepositional forms were used as targets. These elements appeared in different functional roles in the sentence (e. g., (1) lexical preposition, (2) obligatory preposition and (3) verb particle).

(15) Peter steht auf dem Stuhl.
Peter stands on the chair.

(16) Peter hofft auf den Sommer.
Peter hopes for the summer.

(17) Peter steht auf.
Peter stands up.

Agrammatic aphasics displayed a different pattern of monitoring times for the three different sentence types. Prepositional forms in sentences of type (17) were processed like open class items showing a clear semantic relatedness effect. As verb particles are part of the lexical entry of the verb this pattern is not unexpected. Prepositions in sentences of type (16) were processed similar to other closed class words, very slow but independent of semantic variables. The use of these obligatory prepositions is primarily structurally guided, namely in as far as the primary decision that has to be made when this word is used, is whether the verb should be used with a prepositional phrase or with another complement *(Peter hopes that the summer will come soon.)*. Once this decision is taken the particular preposition is chosen indirectly by the verb. Prepositions in sentences of type (15) show a behavior which lies between the two other types. This may be a reflection of the fact that lexical prepositions carry referential information (location) as well as structural information (head of PP). These results suggest that processing of a given element is not a function of class membership, but rather dependent on the functional role this element plays in the sentence. Moreover, with respect to agrammatism this result implies that agrammatic Broca patients are sensitive to the functional role a particular element plays in the sentence. The long reaction times to those elements which carry structural information were interpreted as being due to a slowed access to the structural information closed class words encode. An alternative interpretation of these data may be tried within the framework of lexical hypothesis as proposed by Levelt (1989) for production. According to this theory closed class elements are accessed partly indirectly through the lexical entry (lemma) of major category items (e. g., articles requiring gender information, inflections encoding tense or obligatory prepositions as in (16)), other closed class elements are conceptually activated and accessed directly (e. g., modals or lexical prepositions as in (15)). Under the hypothesis that agrammatic Broca's aphasics suffer from a selective impairment of fast access to those closed class elements that are indirectly activated via the lemma, the performance observed could be a reflection of such a deficit (we will turn to this proposal below).

2.2.2. Auxiliaries

There is evidence from another study that agrammatic Broca patients are able to retrieve the structural information encoded in closed class elements, but that access to this type of information is slowed down. Friederici/Kilborn (1989), for example, have shown that in a cross-modal syntactic priming paradigm Broca patients just like normal controls demonstrate a syntactic priming effect. Contrary to normal controls, however, their overall lexical decision times on a visually presented letter string increase dramatically when the visual target is preceded by sentential context as compared to when presented in isolation. Interestingly the authors found a difference between the subjects' sensitivity to two types of auxiliaries. Subjects showed larger syntactic priming effects for auxiliaries encoding mood (18) and (18*) than for those encoding tense (19) and (19*).

(18) Der Mann hat gelacht.
The man has laughed.

(18*) Der Mann ist gelacht.
The man is laughed.

(19) Der Mann ist geblieben.
The man has stayed.

(19*) Der Mann wurde geblieben.
The man was (passive marker) stayed.

Within the framework proposed above these two types of auxiliaries differ with respect to the type of information they encode and therefore the degree to which they are accessed directly. Closed class elements encoding mood may be accessed more directly than those encoding tense. The hypothesis that Broca aphasics' impairment in accessing closed class words may cut along the lines of direct versus indirect access also provides a possible explanation for these data.

2.2.3. Determiners

Numerous studies have stressed the agrammatics' inability to phrasally integrate articles and nouns in production and in metalinguistic tasks (e. g., Gleason/Goodglass/Green et al. 1975; Zurif/Caramazza/Myerson 1972). A similar inability has also been claimed to be present in comprehension. Heilman/Scholes (1976) presented Broca's aphasics with pairs of sentences that differed in the placement of the article indicating a noun phrase (e. g., *She showed her baby the pictures* versus *She showed her the baby pictures*). Agrammatic Broca aphasics had considerable problems in a sentence picture matching task when required to indicate which picture depicted each sentence. The correct understanding of the difference between these two sentences depends on the ability to construct and interpret a phrasal node – an ability which these patients seem to miss.

Caplan/Matthei/Giglev (1981) suggested that agrammatic aphasics might be able to process the article enough to make a decision at the lexical node level. They had shown that Broca patients were able to distinguish sentences like *Can you show Bill walking the dog*, where *walking* is the verb, from sentences like *Can you show Bill the walking dog*, where *walking* is an adjective.

Grossman/Carey/Zurif/Diller (1986) showed that Broca aphasics were able to distinguish between common nouns (e. g., *a rose*) and proper nouns (e. g., *Rose*). This grammatical form class distinction is marked by the presence or absence of an article. The agrammatic Broca patients they tested were clearly sensitive to the presence and absence of an article as a marker of lexical category. They suggested that this indicated that these patients can make grammatical decisions at the lexical node level.

It seems that agrammatic Broca's aphasics are sensitive to determiners as syntactic markers in comprehension. This type of patient, moreover, seems to be able to process the article's gender information, at least in off-line comprehension tasks (e. g., Rosenthal/Goldblum 1989).

2.2.4. Bound Morphology

There are a number of reports of aphasic patients who have problems in producing morphologically complex words (e. g., Goodglass/Berko 1960; Goodglass/Gleason/Ackerman/Hyde 1972). Systematic studies on the aphasic comprehension performance on morphologically complex words are less numerous.

Comprehension studies using off-line as well as on-line techniques have shown that agrammatic Broca's aphasics are sensitive to inflectional morphology (Friederici/Wessels/Emmorey/Bellugi in press; Lukatela/Crain/Shankweiler 1988; Tyler/Cobb 1987). Tyler/Cobb (1987) testing one agrammatic patient in an on-line task report that this patient is sensitive to derivational, but not to inflectional morphology.

Tyler/Behrens/Cobb/Marslen-Wilson (1990) reported a processing distinction between stems and affixes in a non-fluent patient with agrammatic output (patient BN). This patient unlike the agrammatic patient DE (Tyler/Cobb 1987) showed no difference in processing derivational and inflectional morphology, he appeared to be insensitive to both inflectional and derivational morphology in a word monitoring and a grammaticality judgment task. In evaluating this patient's problem further, they conducted a number of experiments in which they tested BN's sensitivity to violations of the stems and to violations of inflections. This patient demonstrated sensitivity to violations of the relation between verb stem and noun stem in a sentence, (a) with respect to pragmatic aspects, (b) with respect to semantic selectional restrictions and (c) with respect to subcategorization rules. When violations occurred in inflectional suffixes (a) encoding syntactic aspects, such as transitivity or (b) anaphoric aspects, such as tense marking he showed no sensitivity to violations.

Friederici/Wessels/Emmorey/Bellugi (in press) also using an on-line technique found that agrammatic patients are sensitive to inflectional morphology as marker of syntactic category (noun vs verb), but do not respect the particular information (tense, person, number) a given verb inflection carries. Lukatela/Crain/Shankweiler (1988) report that in an off-line task this type of patient is sensitive to inflectional morphology. Thus it seems that in off-line tasks agrammatic patients are able to retrieve the syntactic information encoded in closed class elements, but that on-line only part of the information can be retrieved. What seems to be accessible online is syntactic category information.

Evidence for differential on-line sensitivity with respect to the inflection – derivation distinction has been offered (Tyler/Behrens/

Cobb/Marslen-Wilson 1990). Differential on-line sensitivity with respect to different subsets within inflectional morphology has not been investigated in aphasia. Data from studies with normal sign language learners, however, suggest a processing distinction between inflectional elements marking tense and aspect (Emmorey/Bellugi/Friederici/Horn in press).

2.2.5. Determiners and Auxiliaries

Off-line evidence that agrammatic Broca's show sensitivity to different members of the functional domain is also available. Saddy (1990) reports on an agrammatic individual's performance on an insertion paradigm. In this off-line task the subject is presented with a well formed sentence and is given a word or phrase and is asked to show where that word or phrase could be included in the initial sentence. For instance, the subject may be presented with a sentence such as

(20) A man watched the children playing

and given the word *six* to insert. The subject's task is to indicate by pointing and/or speaking where the word *six* could be included in the sentence. The ability to give the correct response

(21) A man watched the six children playing

indicates that the subject has recognized the syntactic properties of the item to be inserted and has been able to evaluate those properties with respect to the stimulus sentence. Saddy's subject was able to perform insertions of functional items associated with the nominal paradigm, determiners, numerals, quantifiers, nominal negation and complementizers, but was unable to perform any insertions of functional elements associated with the verbal paradigm; auxiliaries, do support, verbal negation. This sensitivity to contrasts internal to the functional paradigm is parallel in some respects to the pattern of impairment found with respect to the processing of nouns versus verbs (see 2.3.1.).

2.2.6. Category Ambiguous Elements

The syntactic information encoded in closed class elements is part of what Rosenthal/Goldblum (1989) call 'the grammatical prerequisites for agrammatic behavior in comprehension'. They put forward the argument that the behavior of agrammatic subjects reported in the literature (e. g., Linebarger/Schwartz/Saffran 1983; Saddy 1990; Shankweiler/Crain/Correll/Tuller 1989; Wulfeck 1987) can not be explained without the assumption of such prerequisites. These studies had shown that agrammatic patients are able to judge a sentence's grammaticality.

The argument was further supported on logical grounds by claiming that a subject who shows a selective deficit for a given syntactic class must be sensitive to syntactic class information. Rosenthal/Goldblum (1989) exemplify this argument referring to data reported by Andreewsky/Seron (1975). These authors report the reading performance of a patient whose comprehension was severely agrammatic. When asked to read a sentence like (22) which contained the same word form *car* twice, but in different word class roles (noun vs conjunction),

(22) Le *car* ralentit *car* le moteur chauffe.
The *bus* slows down *because* the engine overheats.

the patient read (22')

(22') car ralentit moteur chauffe.

This behavior, i. e., the selective omission of all closed class elements, requires the ability to distinguish between different grammatical classes as a prerequisite.

This fact has been neglected in particular by those who took the telegraphic language output in agrammatic Broca's aphasics' production as an indication of a syntactic deficit (for an overview see Berndt/Caramazza 1980). But it seems that in production agrammatic subjects respect syntactic category not only by omitting closed class elements selectively. Also when required to produce in a sentence as much closed class morphology as possible, agrammatic Broca patients respect syntactic category. Kolk (personal communication) found that agrammatics produce within-class substitution errors in a forced production task. Bates/Friederici/Wulfeck (1987) reported that German and Italian agrammatics demonstrated a considerable amount of within-category substitution errors for closed class words in a picture description task.

Additional evidence that those patients who seem to show a selective deficit for closed class elements indeed respect syntactic category information comes from a number of studies focussing on the distinction between nouns and verbs. Most interestingly these patients are able to disambiguate noun-verb ambiguities on the basis of sentential-structural information (Hagoort 1990) (see 2.3.2.)

2.3. Processing Contrast for Major Category Items

2.3.1. Nouns and Verbs

There are a number of studies which demonstrate a contrast in the processing of nouns and verbs (Miceli/Silveri/Villa/Caramazza 1984; Zingeser/Berndt 1990) and the aphasics' ability to retrieve verbs as compared to other word categories (McCarthy/Warrington 1985).

Miceli/Silveri/Villa/Caramazza (1984) tested agrammatic and anomic patients in an object and an action naming task. Agrammatics showed a marked impairment in naming actions, in contrast to anomics and normal controls who named actions better than objects. The action naming impairment in agrammatics was interpreted as a lexical deficit. McCarthy/Warrington (1985) discuss a case of an agrammatic patient who also showed a selective impairment of verb retrieval and attributed this to a lexical deficit as well. Zingeser/Berndt (1990) demonstrated a dissociation between nouns and verbs in a variety of production tasks with different aphasic groups. Agrammatics produced fewer verbs than nouns, whereas anomics produced more verbs than nouns in the same tasks. They offer different interpretations for these data, one which goes beyond the lexical level. They discuss that the selective impairment for verbs within the open class may be due to the fact that the lexical representation of the verbs is syntactically richer than that of nouns (e. g., the lexical entry of the verb includes information about the verb argument structure). If the full syntactic information is retrieved every time the subject accesses the verb, even when the verb is produced in isolation as in an action naming task, than this may explain why verb retrieval is much harder than noun retrieval for agrammatics.

2.3.2. Noun-Verb Ambiguity Resolution

The finding that agrammatic aphasics show a selective difficulty with verbs compared to nouns must mean that these subjects are able to distinguish between these two syntactic categories. The work by Hagoort (1990) shows that agrammatic patients are indeed able to do so. In a word priming task with two priming words and one target he used words that were ambiguous with respect to word category (e. g., noun-verb ambiguity, *sail-sail*) and those which were not (e. g., noun-noun ambiguity, *bank-bank*). The critical question for such a priming situation is whether both meanings of the ambiguous word are activated or not. This is usually shown by an equally strong priming effect for a target word under a condition which semantically primes one of the readings (e. g., *table-bank-chair* for the noun-noun ambiguities and *sea-sail-ship* for the noun-verb ambiguities) and one which does not (e. g., *robbery-bank-chair* and *plant-sail-harbour*). With an interstimulus interval between the members of the triplet of 500 msec he found for normal controls that both the contextually biased and the non-biased meaning were activated and that Broca patients demonstrated the same tendency for the two types of ambiguities as the normal controls. With an interstimulus interval of 100 msec, however, Broca patients behaved differently from normal controls. While normal controls still showed activation of multiple meanings for the noun-noun ambiguities and for the noun-verb ambiguities, Broca patients showed multiple activation only for the noun-noun ambiguity, but not for the noun-verb ambiguity. This suggests that at the interstimulus interval of 100 msec Broca's aphasics benefit less or not at all from the form class difference between both readings of the ambiguities. These data are compatible with the view that agrammatic Broca's aphasics have access to the syntactic category information, but that access is dramatically slowed down. It may not be available within the time window of the 100 msec interval.

3. Theories of Agrammatism Connected to Category Distinction

There are a number of theories of agrammatism which directly bear on the distinction between different categories. First there is the lexical hypothesis put forward by Bradley and colleagues (1978; Bradley/Garrett/Zurif 1980) mentioned above. The hypothesis is based on the distinction between open and closed class elements. The claim is that agrammatic Broca's aphasics have lost a special retrieval system for the closed class elements, a retrieval device which guarantees the fast access to this class of items in normal processing. The authors define the difference between the open and the closed class on the basis of the class's productivity. The open class can be enlarged by the application of word formation rules while the closed class can not.

Another aspect, however, is the functional role these elements play in sentences. Garrett (1975) proposed that in language production elements of the open class are selected by semantic features whereas elements of the closed class are part of the sentence frame and selected at a different level of representation. Evidence supporting the processing distinction between the major category items and the minor category items came from normal speech errors. Garrett (1975) had shown that elements of the open class behave differently from elements of the closed class in speech errors. However, it became obvious that certain members of the closed class did not behave according to the set. Prepositions behaved like open class elements when they were heads of phrases, but like closed class elements when they were not.

Kean (1979) proposed to base the distinction between major and minor category items on phonological grounds. Within this framework major category items were defined as phonological words or non-clitic elements and minor category items as clitics. The distinction being that phonological words have a phonological word boundary to each side whereas clitic elements only have a boundary to one side and are clitisized to a major category item. Since agrammatics omit primarily phonological clitics, agrammatism was characterized as a phonological deficit.

Friederici (1985; 1988) defined the agrammatic deficit in computational terms. Her claim is that agrammatic patients have selectively slow access to the syntactic information given by the closed class elements as compared to open class elements. As a consequence the syntactic information is not available when needed to parse the incoming information. According to this view some of the syntactic information encoded in closed class elements is available, however, not within the time window necessary for normal parsing.

3.1. An Alternative Approach

An alternative approach to distinctions internal to the functional domain is offered in Levelt (1989). Levelt's account is concerned with production mechanisms but can be considered as a general approach to potential distinctions. Levelt distinguishes between those members of the functional domain that are partially determined indirectly in response to particular requirements of a major class item and those that are 'conceptually' determined. For example, a determiner that shows gender concord will have its shape determined by the gender of the nominal that it 'determines' while a marker for sentential negation would be accessed directly. Garrett (1992) refers to this distinction as 'direct' versus 'indirect' election. An immediately appealing result is that this approach will distinguish between different types of prepositions; those that head prepositional phrase but are entirely determined by the verb they occur with, i. e., *give x TO y,* and, those that occur as verbal particles, i. e., *pick the book UP*, are 'indirectly' elected. While those that occur as heads of independent adjuncts are 'directly' elected. Such a distinction is in accord with the psycholinguistic results concerning prepositions (2.2.1.).

Levelt's approach clearly makes different delineations within the functional domain. This theory's appeal lies in its reflection of processing loads. The functional domain is partitioned in accord with the complexity of computation involved in determining (or decoding) a given form. Within this theory it is possible that functional elements that are members of distinct groups, under the featural approach will be members of the same 'election' grouping. Furthermore, the cross-linguistic predictions made by the two approaches are distinct. The featural approach would predict that members of the same featural category should pattern together regardless of their 'election' status, while Levelt's approach would predict that the difficulty of a given category could vary from language to language on the basis of its 'election' status. While Levelt's approach does appeal to syntactic or semantically based category distinctions within the functional domain, the relative difficulty of processing these elements should be independent of their syntactic/semantic class.

The literature does not speak directly to the election-category contrast. The relevant data, however, should not be hard to generate. We suggest that this avenue of investigation should prove to be a fruitful one as it addresses the distinction between formal knowledge and procedural mechanisms in a fairly straightforward manner.

Acknowledgement: A. D. Friederici was supported by the Alfried-Krupp-Prize. While the article was written, D. Saddy was a Guest-Researcher to the Cognitive Science Lab Berlin with the support of the Alfried-Krupp von Bohlen und Halbach-Stiftung.

4. References

Akmajian, A., Demers, R. & Harnish, R. (1984). *Linguistics: An Introduction to Language and Communication.* Cambridge, MA: MIT Press.

Andreewsky, E. & Seron, X. (1975). Implicit processing of grammatical rules in a classical case of agrammatism. *Cortex, 9,* 379–390.

Bates, E., Friederici, A., & Wulfeck, B. (1987). Grammatical morphology in aphasia: Evidence from three languages. *Cortex, 23,* 545–574.

Berndt, R. S. & Caramazza, A. (1980). A redefinition of the syndrome of Broca's aphasia: Implications for a neuropsychological model of language: *Applied Psycholinguistics, 1,* 225–278.

Bradley, D. C. (1978). *Computational distinction of vocabulary type.* Unpublished doctoral dissertation, Massachusetts Institute of Technology.

Bradley, D. C., Garrett, M. F., & Zurif, E. B. (1980). Syntactic deficits in Broca's aphasia. In D. Caplan (Ed.), *Biological Studies of Mental Processes. 269–286.* Cambridge, MA: MIT Press.

Caplan, D., Matthei, B., & Gigley, S. (1981). Comprehension of gerundive constructions by Broca's aphasics. *Brain and Language, 13,* 145–160.

Caramazza, A. & Zurif, E. B. (1976). Dissociation of algorithmic and heuristic processes in language comprehension: Evidence from aphasia. *Brain and Language, 3,* 572–582.

Chierchia, G. & McConnell-Ginet, S. (1990). *An Introduction to Semantics.* Cambridge, MA: MIT Press.

Chomsky, N. (1965). *Aspects of the Theory of Syntax.* Cambridge, MA: MIT Press.

Chomsky, N. (1970). Remarks on nominalization. In R. Jacobs & P. Rosenbaum (Eds.) *Readings in English Transformational Grammar.* 184–221. Waltham, Mass.

Chomsky, N. (1975). *Reflections on Language.* New York: Pantheon Books.

Chomsky, N. (1986). *Knowledge of Language.* New York: Praeger.

Chomsky, N. (1988). *Language and Problems of Knowledge: The Managua Lectures.* Cambridge, MA: MIT Press.

Dixon, R. M. W. (1977). Where have all the adjectives gone? *Studies in Language, 1,* 19–80.

Emmonds, J. (1985). *A Unified Theory of Syntactic Categories.* Dordrecht: Foris Publications.

Emmorey, K., Bellugi, U., Friederici, A. D., & Horn, P. (in press). Effects of age of acquisition on grammatical sensitivity: Evidence from on-line and off-line tasks. *Journal of Memory and Language.*

Friederici, A. D. (1983). Aphasics' perception of words in sentential context: Some real-time processing evidence. *Neuropsychologia, 21,* 351–358.

Friederici, A. D. (1985). Levels of processing and vocabulary types: Evidence from on-line comprehension in normals and agrammatics. *Cognition, 19,* 133–167.

Friederici, A. D. (1988). Agrammatic comprehension: Picture of a computational mismatch. *Aphasiology, 2,* 279–284.

Friederici, A. D. & Heeschen, C. (1983). Lexical decision of inflected open class items and inflected closed class words. Paper presented at the 21st Annual Meeting of the Academy of Aphasia, Minneapolis, MN, October, 1983.

Friederici, A. D. & Kilborn, K. (1989). Temporal constraints on language processing: Syntactic priming in Broca's aphasia. *Journal of Cognitive Neuroscience, 1,* 262–272.

Friederici, A. D., Wessels, J., Emmorey, K., & Bellugi, U. (in press). Sensitivity to inflectional morphology in aphasia: A real-time processing perspective. *Brain and Language.*

Garrett, M. F. (1975). The analysis of sentence production. In G. Bower (Ed.), *The Psychology of Learning and Motivation: Advances in Research and Theory. 133–177.* New York: Academic Press.

Garrett M. F. (1992). Disorders of lexical selection. *Cognition, 42,* 143–180.

Gleason, J. B., Goodglass, H., Green E., Ackerman, N., & Hyde, M. (1975). The retrieval of syntax in Broca's aphasia. *Brain and Language, 2,* 451–471.

Goodglass, H. & Berko, J. (1960). Agrammatism and inflectional morphology in English. *Journal of Speech and Hearing Research, 3,* 257–267.

Goodglass, H., Gleason, J., Ackerman, N., & Hyde, M. (1972). Some linguistic structures in the speech of a Broca's aphasic. *Cortex, 8,* 191–212.

Gordon, B. & Caramazza, A. (1982). Lexical decision for open- and closed-class words: Failure to replicate differential frequency sensitivity. *Brain and Language, 15,* 143–160.

Gordon, B. & Caramazza, A. (1983). Closed- and open-class lexical access in agrammatic and fluent aphasics. *Brain and Language, 19,* 335–345.

Gordon, B. & Caramazza, A. (1985). Lexical access and frequency sensitivity: Frequency saturation and open/closed class equivalence. *Cognition, 21,* 95–115.

Grossman, M., Carey, S., Zurif, E., & Diller, L. (1986). Proper and common nouns: Form class judgements in Broca's aphasia. *Brain and Language, 28,* 114–125.

Hagoort, P. (1990). Tracking the time course of Language Understanding in Aphasia. Doctoral Dissertation, Katholic University of Nijmegen.

Heilman, K. & Scholes, R. (1976). The nature of comprehension errors in Broca's conduction, and Wernicke's aphasics. *Cortex, 12,* 258–265.

Jackendoff, R. (1977). *X-bar Syntax: A Study of Phrase Structure.* Cambridge, MA: MIT Press.

Kean, M.-L. (1979). Agrammatism: A phonological deficit? *Cognition, 7,* 69–83.

Kolk, H. & Blomert, L. (1985). On the Bradley hypothesis concerning agrammatism: The non-word-interference effect. *Brain and Language, 26,* 94–105.

Levelt, W. J. M. (1989). *Speaking: From Intention to Articulation.* Cambridge, MA: MIT Press.

Linebarger, M. C., Schwartz, M. F., & Saffran, E. M. (1983). Sensitivity to grammatical structure in so-called agrammatic aphasics. *Cognition, 13,* 361–392.

Lukatela, K., Crain, S., & Shankweiler, D. (1988). Sensitivity to inflectional morphology in agrammatism: Investigation of a highly inflected language. *Brain and Language, 33,* 1–15.

Matthei, E. H. & Kean, M.-L. (1989). Postaccess Processes in the Open vs. Closed Class Distinction. *Brain and Language, 36,* 163–180.

McCarthy, R. & Warrington, E. K. (1985). Category-specificity in an agrammatic patient: The relative impairment of verb retrieval and comprehension. *Neuropsychologia, 23,* 709–727.

Miceli, G., Silveri, M. C., Villa, G., & Caramazza, A. (1984). On the basis for the agrammatics' difficulty in producing main verbs. *Cortex, 20,* 207–220.

O'Grady, W., Dobrovolsky, M., & Aronoff, M. (1989). *Contemporary Linguistics. An Introduction.* New York: St. Martins's Press.

Rosenthal, V. & Goldblum, M.-C. (1989). On certain grammatical prerequisites for agrammatic behaviour in comprehension. *Journal of Neurolinguistics, 4,* 179–211.

Saddy, J. D. (1990). Investigations into Grammatical Knowledge. Doctoral Dissertation, MIT, Cambridge, MA.

Saddy, J. D. (1991). A feature classification system for syntactic categories. Cognitive Science Lab Berlin, Free University of Berlin, June 1991.

Segui, J., Mehler, J., Frauenfelder, U., & Morton, J. (1982). The word frequency effect and lexical access. *Neuropsychologia, 20,* 615–627.

Sells, P. (1985). Lectures on Contemporara Syntactic Theories. CSLI Lecture Notes. Stanford: Ventura Hall.

Shankweiler, D., Crain, S. Correll, P., & Tuller, B. (1989). Reception of language in Broca's aphasia. *Language and Cognitive Processes, 4,* 1–33.

Tyler, L. K., Behrens, S., Cobb, H., & Marslen-Wilson, W. (1990). Processing distinctions between stems and affixes: Evidence from a non-fluent aphasic patient. *Cognition, 36,* 129–153.

Tyler, L. K. & Cobb, H. (1987). Processing bound grammatical morphemes in context: The case of an aphasic patient. *Language and Cognitive Processes, 2,* 245–262.

Wulfeck, B. (1987). Grammaticality judgments and sentence comprehension in agrammatic aphasia. *Journal of Speech and Hearing Research, 31,* 72–81.

Zingeser, L. B. & Berndt, R. S. (1990). Retrieval of Nouns and Verbs in Agrammatism and Anomia. *Brain and Language, 39,* 14–32.

Zurif, E. B., Caramazza, A., & Myerson, R. (1972). Grammatical judgments of agrammatic aphasics. *Neuropsychologia, 10,* 405–417.

Angela D. Friederici, Berlin (Germany)/ Douglas Saddy, Brisbane, Queensland (Australia)

15. Disorders of Lexical Morphology in Aphasia

1. Introduction

Morphological paraphasias – e. g., producing *walking* for *walked* – are an often observed feature of language impairment. Errors of this type are prominent in the major, clinically-defined disorders of sentence production – agrammatism and paragrammatism (see Butterworth/Howard 1987; Kean 1978; Miceli/Silveri/Romani/Caramazza 1989; and Tissot/Mounin/Lhermitte 1973, for recent discussions; see also papers in Nespoulous/Villiard 1990), and in various disorders of single-word production in reading, writing, and naming (e. g., De Bleser/Bayer 1990; see also papers in Coltheart/Patterson/Marshall 1980). In addition, failure to differentiate among morphologically related forms has been implicated in comprehension impairments (e. g., Tyler/Behrens/Cobb/Marslen-Wilson 1990; Tyler/Cobb 1987).

2. Morphological Errors and their Interpretation

A central problem in the analysis of lexical deficits is whether the production of morphological paraphasias reflects – in some cases at least – a deficit to mechanisms that are strictly devoted to processing affixed forms. To make such a case, one must show that paraphasias like *darkness* → *darkly* do not result from whole-word substitutions (analogous to *index* → *insect*, or *center* → *cent*) or from sub-lexical, non-morphological substitutions (as seen in word and non-word paraphasias like *belt* [bɛlt] → *bell* [bɛl] and *index* [ɪndɛks] → [ɪndɛk]). If morphological errors were the only variety of lexical error that a patient produced, the argument for a 'true' deficit to lexical morphology would be relatively straightforward (although not entirely unproblematic since even in this case we would not be able to assert with complete confidence that these errors arise from a morphological processing deficit). As it is, there is a notable absence of such pure cases. Even when morphological lapses are the predominant type of lexical paraphasia, they do not appear to occur as the only variety of lexical error in any reported case. In an ongoing project involving the study of nearly 100 patients who produce morphological paraphasias in reading and repetition tasks, none presented with a 'pure' morphological deficit (in the sense that no other type of lexical error occurs). This may not be a matter of coincidence. Given that lexical morphology embodies the capacity to relate (in a rule-governed fashion) an extended set of lexical meanings to an extended stock of lexical forms, a deficit affecting this capacity may invariably induce semantic and/or phonological and/or orthographic errors as well.

The two most common patterns of performance in reading tasks include the production of morphological errors in conjunction with visual errors (e. g., Job/Sartori 1984; Patterson 1982) or visual and semantic errors (Badecker/Caramazza 1987; Coltheart 1980; Patterson 1980). Two recent cases have been described whose paraphasias are limited to morphological and semantic paraphasias (Caramazza/Hillis 1990). Similar cases of acquired dysgraphia present written morphological errors cooccurring with phonological paragraphias (Bub/Kertesz 1982; Shallice 1981) and with semantic errors (Patterson/Shewell 1987).

Setting aside those cases where segmental errors can result in the production of forms that coincidentally are related morphologically to the target (as when consonant cluster simplification at a peripheral stage of lexical processing derives *weld* [wɛld] from the intended *welds* [wɛldz]), morphological paraphasias must be contrasted with whole-word substitutions in order to assess the possible involvement of disrupted mechanisms of morpheme composition or parsing. For example, Badecker/Caramazza (1987), Funnell (1987) and Pillon/de Partz/Raison/Seron (1991) argue that factors such as the relative frequency of an affixed word and its stem, abstractness, and the visual similarity of lexically related forms can account for some patients' tendency to produce morphological errors on affixed words. If this were true in every patient, there would be little evidence in the neuropsychological literature for morphological composition as a normal (and disruptable) component of lexical production. There are cases, though, where it is possible to implicate the operation of mechanisms that are specifically devoted to the production (and/or comprehension) of morphologically complex words. For example, evidence for deficit to mechanisms of morphological composition, and for lexical deficits that selectively disrupt inflectional morphology can be found from case studies of acquired aphasia. Below, we briefly discuss serval illustrative cases.

2.1. Errors of Morphological Composition: Retrieval Versus Composition

Patient SJD is an English speaking patient who presents with an acquired lexical output impairment affecting spontaneous speech and a variety of single-word processing tasks such as reading and repetition (Badecker/Caramazza 1991). Morphological errors are the predominant error type in SJD's reading performance: SJD also produced whole-word substitutions (e. g., reading *summit* for *summon*); and phonemic paraphasias (e. g., *shrilly* [šrɪli] → [šruli]. The fact that SJD produced relatively few non-word phonemic paraphasias in comparison to the proportion of morphological errors (13% versus 65% of her reading errors, respectively) speaks strongly against the possibility that her morphological errors were merely the product of sub-morphemic, phonological errors. This possibility is also ruled out by the fact that SJD produced morphological errors (affix omissions and substitutions) in reading words like *bowled* [bold] and *links* [lɪŋks], but no comparable errors for their monomorphemic homophones *bold* [bold] and *lynx* [lɪŋks]. Had errors like *bowled* → *bowling* [bolɪŋ] arisen as the product of segmental substitutions (as opposed to morpheme substitutions), one should observe similar errors (e. g., *bold* → *bowls* [bolz] for the monomorphemic items as well. Similarly, one can show that it was the morpho-phonological structure of affixed words (and not their morpho-semantic or morpho-syntactic complexity) that affected her performance: SJD produced errors on regularly inflected verbs (e. g., *helped*), but not for irregular inflections (as in *swept*).

Several phenomena indicated that SJD's morphological output errors could not be reduced to whole-word substitutions, the most striking of which was the production of illegal combinations of morphemes (e. g., *poorest* → *'poorless, the most poorless indians have very little money'*). If SJD's morphological paraphasias were simply a special case of whole-word misselection (analogous to the substitution of monomorphemic forms in her error *fluid* → *fluent*), then one would expect all of her affix insertion and substitution errors to consist of grammatically well-formed combinations. Instead, morphologically illegal forms like *youthful* → **youthly* were evident in SJD's reading, repetition, writing to dictation and spontaneous speech. Furthermore, both the legal and illegal combinations of morphemes in her insertion and substitution errors tended to involve inflectional and productive derivational affixes. A preference for inflection and productive derivation over non-productive derivation would not be expected if mechanisms of word formation were not directly implicated in the generation of the morphological paraphasias. Hence, one conclusion that can be drawn from this case is that, in some patients, the production of morphological errors reflects an impairment to mechanisms that are devoted to morphological composition (and/or decomposition) in normal performance.

2.2. Inflection versus Derivation

A case of acquired impairment which provides some indication of the morphological distinctions that are made in the language processing system is that of patient FS, an Italian speaking patient who presented with a lexical impairment that resulted in morphological paraphasias in spontaneous speech and in single word processing tasks such as repetition (Miceli/Caramazza 1988). FS produced a substantial number of morphological substitution errors in a variety of tasks, but these errors predominantly affected the inflectional specification of a word (gender and number markers for nouns and adjectives; and tense, aspect, person and number specifications of verbs). Derivational morphology was virtually unaffected. FS's errors also included phonological paraphasias, but these can be distinguished from his inflectional substitutions in a relatively straightforward manner. For example, FS's morphological paraphasias tended to result in the production of 'citation forms' – i. e., the minimally marked members of a paradigm (infinitival forms of verbs, singular forms for nouns, masculine singular forms for adjectives) that regularly serves as the base for word formation – regardless of whether the particular inflected forms were among the least frequent items of an inflectional paradigm. (For a discussion of the grammatical role of citation forms, see Burzio (1989).) Furthermore, the tendency to produce citation forms could not be reduced to a tendency to produce particular phonological shapes, since the preference for citation forms held constant even when the phonological form of the citation-form suffix varied. For instance, when FS repeated adjective forms, he exhibited a strong tendency to use the masculine singular form for those adjectives that allow a four-way inflectional contrast (masc. sg., masc. pl., fem. sg., fem. pl.), and the singular form for those adjectives which only allow a two-way contrast (sg. vs pl.). Notably, the maximally disfavored inflection for the former adjective type (fem. pl., as in *car-e*) was phonologically identical to the favored inflection for the adjectives showing a two way contrast (sg., as in *fort-e*). Indications that these inflectional errors do not arise as simple whole-word substitutions derives from the fact that the misselected inflections that occurred in FS's performance would occasionally result in the production of a morphologically illegal combination of stem and affix – as in the spontaneous speech error *studi-o* ('office,' masc. sg.) → **studi-a* (*fem. sg.), where the noun is inflected with the gender inappropriate ending; or the repetition error *mor-issimo* ('die,' third conjugation inflection) → **mor-este* (second conjugation ending) (Badecker/Caramazza 1989). Hence, FS's performance is significant both for the evidence it provides for morphological composition and for the motivation it provides for the lexical distinction between inflectional and derivational morphology.

3. Jargonaphasia and Word-Formation Mechanisms

Studies of preserved inflectional capacity in patients who present with severe semantic and syntactic deficits have been proposed as evidence that mechanisms for inflectional morphology are functionally independent of the sentence-level mechanisms they must interact with (De Bleser/Bayer 1986), a claim that runs counter to the split morphology model advanced by Anderson (1982). The classic cases of preserved inflection that motivate compositional mechanisms of inflection involve aphasic patients whose speech includes neologistic jargon. Several studies have reported patients whose neologisms cannot all be described as phonological deformations of a target word (e. g., Buckingham 1981; Butterworth/Howard 1987; Caplan/Keller/Locke 1972). One reason for holding this position is that in many instances, the neologisms bear no phonological similarity to their target. In addition to being segmentally dissimilar, they may differ from a target form in the number of syllables and in stress pattern (Buckingham 1981). Nevertheless, the production of neologistic jargon often cooccurs with a preserved capacity to inflect words, and this capacity extends to neologisms as well. In some case, patients' use of inflections (on neologisms and on actual stems) will, on occasion, be grammatically inappropriate. However, of the five patients described by Butterworth/Howard (1987, 24), two never made inflectional errors on neologisms, and for the remaining patients, the number of inflections occurring in obligatory contexts (as well as the number of uninflected neologisms in syntactic contexts that excluded inflections) far outweighed the few cases where they failed to occur in contexts that required them, or where they intruded ungrammatically. Regardless of their syntactic appropriateness, though, the very presence of the inflection on the non-lexical base forms indicates that the lexical system distinguishes stem and affix representations. In particular, inflected neologisms provide an additional form of evidence for the existence of mechanisms for morphological composition in the phonological output lexicon. See also Semenza/Butterworth/Panzeri/Ferreri (1990) for a related case involving derivational morphology.

4. Morphological Deficits in Sentence Comprehension and Production

Several studies have documented cases of sentence comprehension impairment that strongly implicate morphological deficits (Tyler/Behrens/Cobb/Marslen-Wilson 1990; Tyler/Cobb 1988). For example, patient DE was found to be selectively impaired in processing inflections in normal speech comprehension (Tyler/Cobb 1988). In a word monitoring task, DE was sensitive to the contextual appropriateness of a word when the wrong derived form was used (as in *He was the most wasteful/*wastage/*wastely cook she had ever met*), but not when an inappropriate inflection intruded (as in *It often causes/*causing/*causely pain in my loose filling*). In a similar study (Tyler/Behrens/Cobb/Marslen-Wilson 1990), patient BN exhibited a more pervasive morphological impairment in that his monitoring performance indicated an insensitivity to both syntactic ill-formedness – based on the use of inappropriate inflected or derived forms (the examples with *wastage* and *causing*) – and to lexical ill-formedness (the examples with **wastely* and **causely*).

Current theories of sentence production (e. g., Garrett 1982; Lapointe 1985) predict that morphological paraphasias (e. g., agreement errors) can result from deficits to sentence processing mechanisms while single-word processing remains unimpaired. Two recent studies (Caramazza/Hillis 1989; Nespoulous/Dordain/Perron et al. 1988) describe patients who are intact in single word processing tasks, but who exhibit selective deficits in processing grammatical morphemes in sentence processing tasks. In the case of patient 'Clermont' (Nespoulous/Dordain/Perron et al. 1988), only free-standing grammatical morphemes were affected. Patient ML (Caramazza/Hillis 1989) produced some inflectional (morpho-lexical) substitutions in addition to omitting and substituting free-standing grammatical morphemes, although the proportion of such morphological agreement errors is small in comparison to the number of function word errors. While the presence of agreement errors in ML's speech supports the hypothesis that "morphological deficits" can arise from damage to syntactic (non-lexical) processing components, a stronger case for this position can be envisioned. Studies which document contrasting patterns of inflectional impairment (e. g., Miceli/Silveri/Romani/Caramazza 1989) have provided some indications that grammatical agreement may be differentially affected (resulting, for example, in divergent error rates for subject-verb, noun-adjective, and determiner-noun agreement), although the relative contribution of lexical and syntactic deficits in most of the reported cases has not been established. Clearly this is one distinction that deserves greater attention.

5. Morphological Representation and Processing

Evidence from disorders of lexical morphology indicates that lexical processing does not rely solely on retrieving precompiled affixed forms — as suggested in certain current linguistic and psycholinguistic theories (e. g., Bybee 1985; Halle 1973; Lukatela/Gligorijevic/Kostic/Turvey 1980) — and that, instead, lexical composition does play a role (as supposed by Stemberger (1982) and others). Of course, this position does not rule out that some precompilation for regularly affixed forms does play a role in lexical processing — see, for example, Stemberger/MacWhinney (1986). Similarly, there is good evidence for processing distinctions among morphological types — e. g., the inflection/derivation distinction exhibited by FS (Miceli/Caramazza 1988) and DE (Tyler/Cobb 1988) — that also find support in linguistic frameworks (e. g., Anderson 1982). Further contact between linguistic theory and neurolinguistic research is desirable as many aspects of the normal processing system remain unclear. For example, what is the basis for the association between morphological and phonological processing deficits? The theory of 'Lexical Phonology' (Kaisse/Shaw 1985; Kiparsky 1982; 1985) provides one formal linguistic model that could be consistent with this association, but a compelling case for this account has not as yet been made based on neurolinguistic or other processing evidence. Another issue concerns the apparent asymmetry of sparing of stem processing in patients like SJD (Badecker/Caramazza 1991) in the presence of impaired affix processing. One possibility is that this pattern reflects a distinction between stored phonological forms for words, on the one hand, and word-formation rules, on the other (as proposed in word-based theories of morphology — e. g., Anderson 1988; 1992; Aronoff 1976). Alternatively, it may be that a morpheme-based lexicon is organized so as to differentiate bound and free-standing morphemes in a dissociable fashion (as some versions of Lexical Phonology would have it). These are but a few of the many issues that must be resolved in order to complete our understanding of acquired deficits in lexical morphology.

Acknowledgement: The preparation of this material was supported by NIH grant DC00366 to The Johns Hopkins University.

6. References

Anderson, S. (1982). Where's Morphology? *Linguistic Inquiry, 13,* 571—612.

Anderson, S. (1988). Morphological theory. In F. Newmeyer (Ed.), *Linguistics: The Cambridge Survey,* Vol. 1. *146—191.* Cambridge: Cambridge University Press.

Anderson, S. (1992). *A-Morphous Morphology.* Cambridge: Cambridge University Press.

Aronoff, M. (1976). *Word Formation in Generative Grammar.* Cambridge, MA: MIT Press.

Badecker, W. & Caramazza, A. (1987). The analysis of morphological errors in a case of acquired dyslexia. *Brain and Language, 32,* 278—305.

Badecker, W. & Caramazza, A. (1989). A lexical distinction between inflection and derivation. *Linguistic Inquiry, 20,* 108—116.

Badecker, W. & Caramazza, A. (1991). Morphological composition in the lexical output system. *Cognitive Neuropsychology, 8,* 335—367.

Bub, D. & Kertesz, A. (1982). Evidence for lexicographic processing in a patient with preserved written over single word naming. *Brain, 105,* 697—717.

Buckingham, H. (1981). Where do neologisms come from? In J. Brown (Ed.) *Jargonaphasia. 39—62.* New York: Academic Press.

Burzio, L. (1989). Prosodic reduction. In C. Kirschner & J. DeCesaris (Eds.), *Studies in Romance Linguistics. 51—68.* Amsterdam: Benjamins.

Butterworth, B. & Howard, D. (1987). Paragrammatisms. *Cognition, 26,* 1—37.

Bybee, J. (1985). *Morphology: A Study of the Relation between Meaning and Form.* Amsterdam: Benjamins.

Caplan, D., Keller, L., & Locke S. (1972). Inflection of neologisms in aphasia. *Brain, 95,* 169—172.

Caramazza, A. & Hillis, A. (1989). The disruption of sentence production: Some dissociations. *Brain and Language, 36,* 625–650.

Caramazza, A. & Hillis, A. (1990). Where do semantic errors come from? *Cortex, 26,* 95–122.

Coltheart, M. (1980). Deep dyslexia: A review of the syndrome. In M. Coltheart, K. Patterson & J. Marshall (Eds.), *Deep Dyslexia. 22–47.* London: Routledge & Kegan Paul.

Coltheart, M. Patterson, K., & Marshall, J. (Eds.) (1980). *Deep Dyslexia.* London: Routledge and Kegan Paul.

De Bleser, R. & Bayer, J. (1986). German word formation and aphasia. *The Linguistic Review, 5,* 1–40.

De Bleser, R. & Bayer, J. (1990). Morphological reading errors in a German case of deep dyslexia. In J.-L. Nespoulous & P. Villard (Eds.), *Morphology, Phonology and Aphasia. 32–59.* Berlin: Springer-Verlag.

Funnell, E. (1987). Morphological errors in acquired dyslexia: A case of mistaken identity. *The Quarterly Journal of Experimental Psychology, 39A,* 497–539.

Garrett, M. (1982). Production of speech: Observations from normal and pathological language use. In A. Ellis (Ed.), *Normality and Pathology in Language Cognitive Functions. 19–76.* London: Academic Press.

Halle, M. (1973). Prolegomena to a theory of word formation. *Linguistic Inquiry, 4,* 3–16.

Job, R. & Sartori, G. (1984). Morphological decomposition: Evidence from crossed phonological dyslexia. *The Quarterly Journal of Experimental Psychology, 36A,* 435–458.

Kaisse, E. & Shaw, P. (1985). On the theory of lexical phonology. *Phonology Yearbook, 2,* 1–30.

Kean, M.-L. (1978). The linguistic interpretation of aphasic syndromes: Agrammatism in Broca's aphasia, an example. *Cognition, 5,* 9–46.

Kiparsky, P. (1982). Lexical morphology and phonology. In I.-S. Yang (Ed.), *Linguistics in the Morning Calm. 3–91.* Seoul: Hanshin.

Kiparski, P. (1985). Some consequences of lexical phonology. *Phonology Yearbook, 2,* 85–134.

Lapointe, S. (1985). A theory of verb form use in the speech of agrammatic aphasia. *Brain and Language, 24* 100–155.

Lukatela, G., Gligorijevic, B., Kostic, A., & Turvey, M. (1980). Representation of inflected nouns in the lexicon. *Memory and Cognition, 8,* 415–423.

Miceli, G., & Caramazza, A. (1988). Dissociation of inflectional and derivational morphology. *Brain and Language, 35,* 24–65.

Miceli, G., Silveri, M., Romani, C., & Caramazza, A. (1989). Variation in the pattern of omissions and substitutions of grammatical morphemes in the spontaneous speech of so-called agrammatic patients. *Brain and Language, 36,* 447–492.

Nespoulous, J.-L., Dordain, M., Perron, C., Ska, B. Bub, D., Caplan, D., Mehler, J., & Lecours, A. (1988). Agrammatism in sentence production without comprehension deficits: Reduced availability of syntactic structures and/or grammatical morphemes? A case study. *Brain and Language, 33,* 273–295.

Nespoulous, J.-L. & Villard, P. (Eds.). (1990). *Morphology, Phonology and Aphasia.* Berlin: Springer-Verlag.

Patterson, K. (1980). Derivational errors. In M. Coltheart, K. Patterson & J. Marshall (Eds.), *Deep Dyslexia. 286–306* London: Routledge & Kegan Paul.

Patterson, K. (1982). The relation between reading and phonological coding: Further neuropsychological observations. In A. Ellis (Ed.), *Normality and Pathology in Cognitive Functions. 77–111.* London: Academic Press.

Patterson, K. & Shewell, C. (1987). Speak and spell: Dissociations and word-class effects. In M. Coltheart, R. Job & G. Sartori (Eds.), *Cognitive Neuropsychology of Language. 273–294.* London: Erlbaum.

Pillon, A., de Partz, M.-P., Raison, A.-M., & Seron, X. (1991). *L'orange, c'est le frutier de l'orangine:* A case of morphological impairment? *Language and Cognitive Processes, 6,* 137–167.

Semenza, C., Butterworth, B., Panzeri, M., & Ferreri, T. (1990). Word formation: New evidence from aphasia. *Neuropsychologia, 28,* 499–502.

Shallice, T. (1981). Phonological agraphia and the lexical route in writing. *Brain, 104,* 413–429.

Stemberger, J. (1982). *The lexicon in a model of language production.* PhD thesis, University of California at San Diego.

Stemberger, J. & MacWhinney, B. (1986). Frequency and the lexical storage of regularly inflected forms. *Memory and Cognition, 14,* 17–26.

Tissot, R., Mounin, G., & Lhermitte, F. (1973). *L'agrammatisme.* Paris: Dessart.

Tyler, A., Behrens, S., Cobb, H., & Marslen-Wilson, W. (1990). Processing distinctions between stems and affixes: Evidence from a non-fluent aphasic patient. *Cognition, 36,* 129–153.

Tyler, L. & Cobb, H. (1987). Processing bound grammatical morphemes in context: The case of an aphasic patient. *Language and Cognitive Processes, 2,* 245–262.

William Badecker/Alfonso Caramazza, Baltimore, Maryland (USA)

16. Disorders of Word-Form Processing in Aphasia

1. Introduction

1.1. Neologistic Jargon Aphasia – A Syndrome

Neologistic jargon aphasia is one form of Wernicke's aphasia and represents but one type of jargon aphasia, the others comprising phonemic jargon aphasia and semantic jargon aphasia (Brown 1977). Neologisms, on the other hand, may be produced by patients who have other forms of aphasia and their appearance need not be restricted to the productions of patients with Neologistic jargon aphasia.

1.2. Neologism – The Term

1.2.1. Dictionary Definition of Neologism

A neologism is defined as "a new word, usage, or expression" or "a meaningless word coined by a psychotic" (Webster's Seventh New Collegiate Dictionary 1963; cf. art 55). Novelty, meaningless, and unrecognizability are most often key descriptors of neology in most accepted definitions of the term.

1.2.2. The Term Neologism in the Aphasia Literature

A survey of the treatment of the neologism in the aphasia literature over the past 100 or so years reveals a certain degree of disparity. Most investigators at least agree that the neologism is a bizarre and unrecognizable form for which meaning cannot be gleaned. Critchley (1970, 61), for example, writes that there are literal (phonemic) and verbal paraphasias as well as other word form errors that "... need not necessarily be a dictionary word but may be a fragment of nonsense or gibberish: in other words a 'neologism'." Alajouanine (1972, 33) described neologisms as "... new terms devoid of any linguistic meaning ..." Moreover, other aphasiologists (Lecours/Lhermitte 1972; Eisenson 1973) have included as neologisms various types of blended words or incorrect combinations of roots and affixes, where the form is novel but where the blended units are for the most part discernable. The objective of the present chapter will be to establish the range of sources for the generation of various types of neologistic word forms.

2. Productive Sources for Neologisms

2.1. Phonemic Paraphasia

The phonemic, or literal, paraphasia has been observed at least since the work of Wernicke (1874; also see Eggert 1977 and Buckingham 1989a) [cf. Chapter 17 of this Handbook] Substitutions, omissions, additions and transpositions of phonemes, when kept to a minimum, will not in general obliterate the recognizability of a target word; a plethora of these types of derailments will. Therefore, it is perfectly reasonable to suggest that severe phonemic paraphasia could produce a bizarre and unrecognizable form. This account is most often an article of faith, since the very unrecognizability prevents certainty – a perennial problem with most studies of neology in aphasia. Nevertheless, many aphasiologists have explained certain neologisms in this way. Wernicke (1906, trans. in Eggert 1977, 227), in a updating of Wernicke (1874), characterizes the jargon aphasia in the general syndrome of sensory aphasia where, "... the distortion words (phonemic paraphasia – HWB) in spontaneous speech may degenerate into complete unintelligibility commonly referred to as jargon aphasia." Kertesz/Benson (1970, 385) characterizing the neology in neologistic jargon write, "Linguistically, neologistic jargon appears to consist of phonemic (literal) substitutions which distort the original word to the degree that it becomes a neologism." Similarly, Brown (1977, 42) feels that, "... the neologism at times appears as a phonemic error severe enough to render the word unintelligible." The Boston Diagnostic Aphasia Examination (Goodglass/Kaplan 1983, 36) tells the scorer that neologisms are distinguished from phonemic paraphasias based on whether or not less than half of the intended word is discernable as an intact unit. This wording indicates that there is a continuum of phonemic paraphasic severity. The Boston Diagnostic Aphasia Examination also allows a neologistic distortion to be comprised of the "introduction of extraneous phonemes." They do not, however, instruct the scorer to consider the source of those extraneous phonemes. Investigators such as Butterworth (1979, 147) have even used the term "target related neologism" to describe mild phonemic paraphasic errors that do not destroy the target's recognizability. Only a strict adherence to the novel aspect of a neologism would justify calling the phonemic paraphasia a type of neologism (target related).

2.2. The Two-Stage Error Neologism

2.2.1. Initial Semantic Substitution

Certain investigators (Pick 1931; Brown 1972; 1977) have suggested that unrecognizable jargon forms could arise from "... the not infrequent mixture of verbal and literal paraphasia" (Pick 1931, 57). Verbal paraphasias are substitutions of full word forms, where the substitution is based either on meaning or form. Most who have discussed the two-stage source for the neologism have focused on the semantic substitution. For example, when characterizing neologistic jargon aphasia, Brown (1977, 43) hypothesizes that the neologism may arise through the production of "... semantic paraphasias ... that would not achieve correct phonemic realization, the result being a phonemic distortion superimposed on a semantic paraphasia." No doubt, Brown was influenced by Pick, whose work Brown translated from German into English (Brown 1972). Lecours/Lhermitte (1972, 304–5) in similar fashion write, "... on peut suggerer que ces neologismes sont des paraphasies monemiques dont la composante lexicale est secondairement le siege d'une transformation phonemique."

2.2.2. Initial Formal Substitution

As we shall see later in this chapter, most models of lexical selection include a form-based access as well as a meaning-based access to the lexicon. On-line formal malapropisms in speech errors (Fay/Cutler 1977) as well the classical malapropisms (Zwicky 1982) provide evidence that lexical substitutions may be produced on the basis of phonological (formal) similarity. Recently, Blanken (1990) reported on an aphasic patient who exhibited frequent phonologically related verbal paraphasias (a sort of 'aphasic malapropism') on different sorts of tasks. To fill out the picture on the two-stage error neologism, therefore, formal as well as semantic verbal paraphasias should be allowed to serve as the input to the subsequent phonological disruption component.

2.3. Incorrect Morphological Affixation

Recognizable roots and morphological affixes may be combined in unconventional and inappropriate ways by certain types of aphasics (and various kinds of psychotic patients) [cf. Chapter 15 of this Handbook]. These forms have often been referred to as neologisms. In the French literature these forms are termed 'monemic' paraphasias, the moneme resting at the level of the morpheme in the linguistics of André Martinet (1960). For example, Lecours (1975, 85) writes that, "There is ... a type of aphasic neologism ... in which segments of words corresponding for the most part to monemes are the involved units. ... Nearly all of the 317 neologisms are constituted of two easily identified monemes, a lexical one and an affix ..."

2.4. The Blend as a Neologism

2.4.1. Two Semantically Related Forms Blended

The simultaneous selection of two meaning related lexical items that are fused in the process produce forms that have been referred to as neologisms. For example, Lecours/Lhermitte (1972, 97) describe the "production of such neologisms" as the error mammimal from a blend ('telescopage' in their terms) of mammal and animal. Similarly, Eisenson (1973, 16) demonstrates, "Other neologisms (which) may comprise combinations of words or of morphemes which do indicate intent and meaning." His examples are *spoon* + *fork* yielding *spork; flower* + *rose* yielding *flose; scent* + *smell* yielding *sment*. These neologisms for Eisenson are referred to as 'contaminations.' Obviously, their componente are neither bizarre nor unrecognizable.

2.4.2. Target Word and Perseverated Word Blends

Buckingham/Whitaker/Whitaker (1979) and Buckingham (1985) have documented blends of target words with words perseverated from previous productions. These reports analyzed the perseverate *drink* as it blended with the production of subsequent words in a repetition task. When asked to repeat words such as *cross* and *crack*, the patient produced *draw* and *drack*.

2.5. Random Generator Produced Neologism

It has been suggested that the very bizarre and nonsensical form of neologism (referred to as "abstruse" in Lecours (1982)) could stem from segmental and/or syllabic constructional processes that somehow go into operation when a patient experiences a complete lexical access block. The neologism so generated would be a surrogate word for the unaccesed target and would be produced under the conditions of anomia. This sort of neologism has been viewed as "masking" what would otherwise have been an unfilled pause in the speech output. The notion of the "random generator" was first suggested in the literature in Butterworth (1979), but previous work such as Buckingham/Kertesz (1976) and Lecours/Rouillon (1976) had indicated that segmental material could be formed to 'fill in' otherwise anomic gaps, the results being the bizarre looking neology of jargonaphasia. In addition, if one looks closely at Case # 4 in Wernicke (1874, trans. in Eggert 1977, 128–9) one can find something very close to the surrogate neologism compensating for unaccessed words. Case # 4 dealt with a conduction aphasic with jargon, where Wernicke wrote that the patient often, "... produced meaningless combinations of words and syllables, a jargon which was difficult to record." Wernicke further noted that when the patient would block during a sentence, he would, "... compensate for his errors by the use of meaningless words or new combinations or (sic) syllables. In this way he was able to complete the sentence." Thus, the neologisms of Wernicke's patient (Case # 4) appeared to be producted at word block junctures. In recent publications, Buckingham (1990b) has garnered evidence to argue that the notion of a mechanism like the random generator is fully justified, and that in fact it is part and parcel of the normal cognitive machinery underlying phonological knowledge for all speaker/hearers.

2.6. Syllable and Segment Structure Constraints on Neologisms

Practically all studies of neologistic production have indicated that neologisms are formed from the stock of segments in the native language of the speaker, but typically phoneme frequency counts may not be abided by (e. g. Butterworth 1979). Further, although there is at least one recent report that some neologisms exhibit motor abnormalities in the acute stages (Dogil 1989), most studies of neologisms have demonstrated that they are more or less fluently articulated and that they obey the language specific phonotactic constraints of the aphasic's premorbid native language. As far as the random generator mechanism is concerned, it has been argued that it is a segment generator (Butterworth 1979) or that perhaps it is a syllable generator (Buckingham 1981). The random generating mechanism must, in any event, 'know' the phonotactics of the language, since as mentioned neologisms follow those patterns. Were the mechanism to generate syllabic units, the phonotactic constraints would be built in so to speak. The question remains an open one, however. On Butterworth's (1979) view, the random generator produces only the bizarre, "abstruse", and non-target related neologism and only after approximately 400 msecs have transpired, presumably indicating failed lexical access. Butterworth did not observe this several millisecond pause before semantic paraphasias, nor before simple phonemic paraphasias (what Butterworth called "target related neologisms"). This, to Butterworth, of course indicated that the abstruse neologism is not scaffolded off of some target word that has been obliterated by phonemic paraphasia, but rather that its segmental makeup stems from productions of segments that are not the result of distortions of underlying words but rather are surrogate forms created de novo by the random production mechanism. The word 'random' should obviously not be taken to imply that any haphazzard stringing together of phonemes would be permitted. Rather, Butterworth chose the word 'random' to indicate that his phoneme count from the stock of neologisms in his corpus did not accord with the frequency counts for phonemes in English.

3. Production Models for Neologisms

3.1. The Merrill Garrett Model

The model constructed by Merrill Garrett (1982; 1984; 1988; 1990) [cf. Chapter 7 of this Handbook] can serve to locate and characterize various sorts of aphasic derailments in the aphasiological literature (Buckingham 1980; 1985; 1986; 1987; 1989b; Kohn 1984; 1985; and Schwartz 1987, among others). Garrett's original work dealt exclusively with slips-of-the-tongue, but more recently he has shown how his model does, indeed, provide the basic architecture for characterizing aphasic errors of one sort or another. In some of my recent work (1985; 1986; 1989b), I have tried to show that the random generator proposed by Butterworth (1979) and the scan-copier and checkoff monitor proposed by Shattuck-Hufnagel (1979) need to be incorporated into the overall model of Garrett in order to achieve a fuller account of neologisms and phonemic paraphasias.

3.1.1. The Functional Level in the Garrett Model

At the Functional Level, case role relations for the content words are established under direct control of the Message Level, and the words themselves are selected purely on the basis of their meaning. At this point, there is no phonological appreciation of lexical items. Word access at this level is often referred to as the first lexical lookup. Therefore, lexical paraphasic substitutions based upon meaning similarity (along some metric – either paradigmatic or syntagmatic) would be the result of a computational derailment at this point, and therefore the computations here are pre-phonological. In addition, most theorists posit something like a "linking address" or a "pointer" that ultimately connects the semantic lexical object with the lexical object that bears the phonological form. Prior research going back at least to the original work of Jakobson (1941) has demonstrated that at least some degree of network-type linkages exist among words with similar meaning and words with similar form. At the Functional Level, therefore, access may fail, and some semantic associate may be selected, linked to some other form. On the other hand, the linking address of some semantic lexical object may point to the appropriate form needed, but that pointer may very likely be directed to a form embedded somehow in the network of phonologically related forms that do not share meaning. The form-related substitution would not, in any event, take place at the Functional Level during the first lexical lookup. Furthermore, two forms, later to be blended, may be accessed at the Functional Level. It has most often been observed that blended forms share at least some meaning parameters.

3.1.2. The Positional Level in the Garrett Model

The Positional Level is the location of very important computations, derailments of which lead to typical sorts of aphasic errors. It is at this level where syntactic matrices are established and the slots in those matrices filled appropriately with content and function morphemes. The slotting computations for the contentives and for the functors operate separately, and breakdowns with each may be dissociated. Since neology affects contentives almost exclusively, my focus will be on the contentives – especially nouns. Lexical selection at this level (the second lexical lookup) will be computed on the basis of phonological form, aided of course by the fact that the previously semantically accessed form will for the most part point to the appropriate phonological representation. Lexical paraphasic substitutions at the Positional Level will necessarily be formal verbal paraphasias, such as those reported in Blanken (1990). An operating buffer working memory component must be established among the Positional Level computations so that the representative segments of the contentives may be readied for utterance order and ultimately articulated. I have argued elsewhere (e. g. Buckingham 1986) that serial ordering mechanisms such as those suggested by Shattuck-Hufnagel (1979) are needed at Garrett's Positional Level in order to facilitate the mapping of underlying phonological segmental representations onto utterance order syllabic templates. The operations of the mechanism largely scan the representative form and copy the segments onto the syllable template matrices. Furthermore, I have suggested (Buckingham 1986) that the scan-copying is computed as the contentives are being slotted into their phrasal matrix positions. That, of course, is when the language output requires normal phrasing, such as with message level driven spontaneous speech. When one repeats, names objects, or reads isolated words aloud for an examiner, where something like message level control is much less involved, the units into which words are slotted will obviously be much smaller, but the serial ordering mechanism will still be copying representative segments onto syllabic templates. Interestingly, some studies (e. g. Pate/Saffran/Martin 1987) have shown more segmental manipulation derailments for single word production than for full phrase production. When the serial ordering mechanisms such as the scan-copier misfire, segmental disorders (phonemic paraphasia) appear [cf. Chapter 17 of this Handbook]. The theory alluded to above that accounts for neologisms in terms of severe phonemic paraphasia must implicate the phonemic manipulation computations at the Positional Level. Practically all phonemic errors obey syllable constraints. Segmental substitutions never result in an unpermitted sequence of sounds. A /t/ will never be substituted for a /p/ in a word such as *please*. An omission will rarely, if ever, set up an unpermitted or heavily marked sequence of sounds. Beland/Caplan/Nespoulous (1990) demonstrated that intervocalic consonants do not in general delete, since that would leave the highly marked situation of two contiguous vowels. Additions of segments do not set up unpermitted sequences, and transpositions of phonemes are constrained in at least two manners. A linear transposition of a phoneme will not set up an unpermitted sequence, nor will it in general move to a syllabic position other than the type in which it originated, unless it is transposed within the confiness of one syllable. In that case, for instance, a coda consonant can move to onset position – providing, of course, that the phoneme in question may in fact occur in the onset position. That is, the /f/ in *after*, may move to the onset position (the slot for which is unfilled in the underlying representation) in the error *fafter*, but the velar nasal in the coda cluster of *ink* would not move to onset position, since velar nasals are phonotactically ruled out there in English. Neologisms generated by the random generator would initially be placed into the operating buffer and scan copied onto the syllable templates in similar fashion to normally accessed words. Subsequent phonemic alterations of the original abstruse neologism would be brought about by scan copying misfirings, the neologism failing to be erased from the buffer. Note that perseveration may be characterized as a failure to be deleted from the buffer for some reason. The heavy involvement of alliteration and assonance in neologistic production implies that the repeated segments are not cleared from the buffer in normal fashion and become available for repeated production. In Shattuck-Hufnagel's (1979) model, there is what she calls a "checkoff monitor," whose responsibility is to erase or clear from the buffer an element once it is copied onto its productive template. If there is a failure of the checkoff monitor, the segment will remain available to be copied again. In this way, the so called "doublet" (Buckingham 1990a) will appear.

In sum, the various types of neologisms can be characterized in terms of the levels and mechanisms we have just discussed. Target related neologisms (simple phonemic paraphasia) result from derailments of the scan copier at the Positional Level. Abstruse neologisms could result from exascerbated involvement of this mechanism at this level, or they may result from the production of a surrogate form produced by the random generator when no word form can be accessed from the lexicon. Note that this does not mean that the first lexical lookup was necessarily unsuccessful, only that the second lexical lookup was. The two-stage neologism would arise from an initial first lexical lookup error. That semantic substitution would be placed into the buffer, where the scan copier would derail as well. If the linking address mistakenly points to a form similar in its phonological makeup to the target, then this may lead the second lexical lookup to select the formally similar word. This word be placed into the buffer, where again the scan copier could malfunction. Blended neologisms would stem from the splicing of simultaneously selected words at the Functional Level during the first lexical lookup. It is not clear as yet exactly how the phonological splicing takes place, but from the examples in the literature it appears as if the splicing is done such that the result meets the phonotactic constraints of the language. For example, the blend of *spork* for *spoon* and *fork* splices between the onset and the peak of *fork*, while the blend of *flose* for *flower* and *rose* splices between the onset and the peak for *rose*. The root/affixal morpheme neologistic blends would be a bit more difficult to account for, owing to the fact that inflectional morphemes are inserted at the Positional Level of matrix building. Derivational morphemes, however, may be initially affixed to their roots at the Functional Level and may therefore be accessed as part of the derived lexical form as it is stored in the lexicon. If that is the case, neologisms involving inappropriate derivational affixation may be produced at a level distinct from inflectional morpheme affixation errors. (See Badecker/Caramazza (1989) and Chapt. 15 in this Handbook for further remarks on derivational vs. inflectional morphology and how they dissociate in aphasia) – The problem of incorporating a model such as Garrett's for the characterization of aphasic errors is that Garrett's model was originally set up to handle normal spontaneous speech. In fact, it was originally constructed from slips-of-the-tongue, which for the most part are on-line computational derailments that occur during spontaneous speech that is under message level control. However, much of the data derived from studies of aphasia is garnered in experimental settings, under tighter controls, and with specific stimuli that are presented to subjects, who are then to respond in certain ways. This is not spontaneous speech, and the ensuing responses are not under the message level control of spontaneous speech. We must, then, condider the production of neologisms when experimental stimuli intervene.

3.2. When Experimental Stimuli Intervene

3.2.1. Visual

3.2.1.1. Object Naming

The drive, or control, for single word productions on confrontation examination eminates from the will to respond in some way to a presented stimulus. The semantic system, rather than being accessed under message level control through the above mentioned first lexical lookup, is now approached subsequent to visual recognition. Once the necessary semantic units are accessed through the visual modality, the pointers will be invoked for accessing either the phonological output lexicon (the form representations that directly feed into the articulatory system) for the spoken label or the orthographic output lexicon (the graphemic forms that directly feed into the written system) for the written label (see Rapp/Caramazza 1991 for this sort of architecture). The manipulations of the segmental material from, say, the phonological output lexicon for oral naming should be quantitatively similar to those operations under message level control. For single word production on confrontation naming an underlying phonological form must be accessed and the segments scan copied for sequential ordering. Errors could occur here as well, and the result would be phonemic paraphasia on naming. The paraphasia could be severe enough to produce a bizarre label. There is no reason why there could not be a block upon accessing the phonological output lexicon, in which case any segments produced could have stemmed from other sources. The basic point here, however, is that the same scan copying mechanism and phonological output component are invoked in the tasks of naming and spontaneous speech, although the level of control will be different. Furthermore, neologistic responses to naming will have a similar range of possible sources except that the operating buffer size will be more restricted when only a single word is being readied for production.

3.2.1.2. Oral Reading

Neologisms have been described in oral reading (e. g. Buckingham 1985). Subjects may be requested to read words in the language (with differing frequency counts), or they may be asked to read non-existing words aloud (cf. Chapter 22 in this Handbook). Presumably, at least, the non-words will be graphotactically (and accordingly, therefore, phonotactically) permissible. The semantic system would be activated for words, the grapheme-phoneme conversion system for non-words. For oral reading, obviously, a phonological response is needed, and only in the case of real word reading will the phonological output lexicon be accessed. Again, the architecture of Rapp/Caramazza (1991) is useful. For oral reading, material gets to the buffer either from the phonological output lexicon (again, related to the second lexical lookup in spontaneous speech models like Garrett's) or from the phoneme-grapheme conversion system. Neologistic oral reading could have several possible sources. Scan copying derailments in the phonological buffer may be severe enough to render the spoken word neologistic. What is more likely to happen is a differential breakdown depending upon word frequency or some type of word saliency. The oral reading of non-words is notorious for inducing paraphasic responses, as is the oral reading of very low frequency words. Also involved is the recent observation from interactive activation models that if a nonword bears a good deal of phonological similarity to a real word, then that fact alone would predict better oral reading response. This argues that at times the phoneme-grapheme conversion system will work better if a non-word bears some resemblance to a real word. The oral reading neology reported for real words (non-words were not tested in the patient) in Buckingham (1985) did not appear to involve the orthographic input lexicon or the semantic system. There was evidence that the patient understood the word she was reading neologistically, and so the neologisms minimally involved either the phonological output lexicon or the segmental manipulations in the phonological buffer. Had non-words been read normally (which is doubtful, but it was not tested), then that would have implicated the phonological output lexicon. The patient named and repeated neologistically as well, but she nevertheless appeared to understand the target words involved (i. e. “lemma” access (Levelt 1989) had been successful). In each case, it could very well have been a dysfunction in the phonological output lexicon (i. e. something at or during the second lexical lookup).

3.2.2. Auditory Input (repetition)

Auditory input for repetition, as opposed to some form of passive word recognition, must ultimately pass through a phonological output system, aided or not by the semantic system. That is, word frequency, saliency, operativity, and grammatical class are factors that often influence repeatability, but these issues are not necessarily involved in the repetition of non-words. Furthermore, the syndrome of transcortical sensory aphasia (Berndt 1988) would indicate that there is some sort of shunt between what Caramazza calls the phonological input lexicon and the phonological output system bypassing the semantic component. Other forms of Isolation of the speech area (e. g. Geschwind/Quadfasel/Segarra 1968; Whitaker 1976) would again support the possibility of short-circuiting (in a reflex and automatistic fashion) the semantic system while repeating. However, it must be pointed out that the ‘echolalic’ nature of these sorts of reflex-like repetitions is most likely under different control systems than are the repetitions of other types of aphasic patients, such as conductions. These types of transcortical or isolation syndrome patients rarely, if ever, produce neologisms when repeating. Theirs does not appear to be a problem with the buffer manipulations of phonemic segments. However, there is often a great deal of phonemic paraphasia on repetition items in Wernicke’s and in conduction aphasics, which seems to involve the same selection and ordering mechanisms we have postulated for other stimulus settings. Obviously, what puts the pressure on these sequential selection and ordering processes is the relative low ‘strength’ level of the stored phonological lexical representations or the evanescent quality of the acoustic input stimulus itself. That is, when analyzing phonemic paraphasias and neology on repetition tasks, we must not only consider the possibility of a specific disruption with the phoneme manipulating mechanisms themselves, but we must also consider the nature of representative shapes or the nature of the acoustic trace. One recently discovered and innovative way to investigate these questions has centered around behaviors whereby patients produce sequences of phonemic approximations as they attempt to produce the required response – the ‘conduite d’approche’ or ‘d’ecart.’

3.2.3. Conduite d’Approche or d’Ecart

Sequences of productive attempts to produce some target can be collected from spontaneous speech, repetition, object naming, oral reading and can serve as a rich data base for the analysis of segmental paraphasic processes as the patient gets closer (d’approche) or further away (d’ecart) from the target. The pioneering study of conduite d’approche is found in Joanette/Keller/Lecours (1980). Comparing Broca’s, conductions and Wernicke’s aphasics over several types of tasks, they found that the conductions generally showed a continuous progression toward to target in terms of both vowels and consonants, while the Broca’s aphasics showed a progressive improvement for vowels, but in terms of features, they did not get as close to vowel targets as did the conductions. The Broca’s consonantal sequences did not appear to approach target consonants with any regularity. Wernicke’s patients exhibited neither consonantal nor vowel approximations, and thus performed worse than the other two groups. Interestingly enough, when the task was repetition, the conductions (predictably) did not approach the targets as successfully. In addition, when the sequence of attempts was lengthy, the sequences showed less approximation to targets. Short sequences generally approached the target better. Important factors for performance appeared to involve the initial ‘strength’ of the target item and its permanence. The conduction patients’ monitoring system was intact, and they were able to ‘hold on’ to the representation better than the Wernicke’s, being able to profit more successfully from each attempted production as they compared it with the target being approached and self-corrected accordingly. On the other hand, Wernicke’s aphasics likely have some impairment in the monitoring system (which seems to correlate with their low comprehension abilities), which in turn prohibits successful self-correction. Therefore, for these authors, it seemed reasonable to suppose that phonemic paraphasias may stem from not only phoneme manipulating mechanisms but also from an inpaired input to these mechanisms. In all, the conductions were superior to the Wernicke's. The Broca's aphasics, on the other hand, had more serious motoric problems, which was most likely at the root of their problems with consonantal approximations. In a more recent publication, Valdois/Joanette/Nespoulous (1989) also found that a conduction aphasic exhibited constant progression towards targets, while two Wernicke's aphasics only demonstrated irregular progressions. In this study, regardless of the length of sequences, the conduction patient approximated successfully. On the other hand, for the Wernicke's patients, length of approximation determined approximation success. Only short sequences resulted in any successful approximations, and those successes seemed to depend exclusively on the success rate performed on the l a s t approximation, i. e. a very irregular sequence. Furthermore, the conductions's attempts typically included all the phonemes in the target segment, whereas the attempts of the Wernicke's subject often lacked certain segments of the target. Finally, Wernicke's patients often lost some of the segmental information along the way, owing to segmental complexity, length of material, or syllabic constituency. These factors did not seem to hinder the maintenence of segmental information for the conduction aphasic. In sum, the Montreal studies demonstrate that conduction aphasics are better than their Wernicke counterparts in approaching targets, and that in so doing they are much more able to hold on to the form they are after and to continuously compare what they produce with their ultimate goal — uttering the target correctly.

Not everyone, however, has found conductions to be so successful on the conduite d'approche. Kohn (1989) found in a case study that her conduction aphasic's series of approximations were not particularly effective in leading to correct responses. Such stark contrasts as Kohn's and the Montreal studies need explanation. It may simply come down to differences in severity of involvement for the different conduction aphasics, but the final word is not in quite yet on clearcut and qualitative distinctions on successive approximation investigations. As concerns neologisms, it would be interesting to find patients whose initial attempts are bizarrely neologistic and then to follow closely the conduite d'approache patterns in them. It would be predicted that the abstruse type of neologism in patients with impaired comprehension, highly disrupted representative lexical shapes, and depressed monitoring skills would not show any necessary progression towards targets and many even show the conduite d'ecart. On the other hand, it would be predicted that the patient with an initial neologism stemming from phonemic paraphasia with otherwise intact monitoring and relatively mild impairment with the scan copier may very well produce subsequent attempts that successively rid themselves of phonemic error, ultimately yielding the target, or at least something very close to it.

3.2.4. Specific Sensory Deficits

3.2.4.1. Altered Phonological Representations

The notion of altered phonological representations is a notorious difficult one to track, and in fact it is highly unlikely that brain damage would selectively disrupt some discrete aspect in phonological representation. Rather, what seems more plausible is that in some fashion sensory nervous system damage gives rise to some sort of overall 'weakness' or instability in phonological forms, under the assumption that those forms must be 'strong' and stable in order for their segments to be manipulated by selection and ordering mechanisms. One would imagine that to keep representative segments stable, there would have to be a proper balance between excitation and inhibition mechanisms to keep the needed items in sharp focus, while simultaneously inhibiting the arousal of similar but unwanted items. The claim, then, is that sensory damage may disturb these normal excitatory-inhibitory mechanisms, which in turn will destablize phonological segments, thus preventing the symbol manipulating operations from gaining access to items with the proper amount of resolution. Luria (1973) has suggested that if, for instance, all semantically or phonologically similar words are evoked to equal threshold levels with no proper inhibition of all but the desired item, then all the items will present simultaneously and with equal strength, thereby blocking access to a n y of them. This would be the point in the output of the jargonaphasic where, as argued above, the random generator could produce a string of syllables that would look unrecognizable but that would serve as a surrogate word.

In another sense, damage to acoustic images for word representations would disrupt any ability to auditorily guide the production mechanism, thus leaving the motor articulatory system to 'run on' without sensory control. Certainly, Wernicke felt that this situation could lead to neology. Ultimately, we must get a better handle on how sensory deficits of one sort or another could serve as the pathophysiological underpinnings of neologistic production.

3.2.4.2. Rapidly Vanishing Acoustic-Verbal Traces

In the most obvious sense, a sensory disorder that involves short-term acoustic verbal memory will be devastating for patients who are asked to repeat acoustic-verbal stimuli. The ability to subvocally rehearse the item or to hold on to the item while its segments are being operated upon by sequencing mechanisms will disrupt repetition as well as writing to dictation. Quite often, in these situations, patients will produce what they can manage, and the result will often be phonologically incorrect in one way or another and to varying degrees of severity. Furthermore, as the acoustic trace fades from a pathologically shortened short-term memory store, the segments of that form will be increasingly weakened or decayed such that the selecting and ordering mechanisms – even if they are perfectly intact – will have little or nothing to work on.

In addition, serial ordering capabilities themselves may be compromised by the brain damage, as is often the case with left, posterior temporal/parietal lesions (Kimura 1982). These capacities would be related to the proper functioning of the scan copier mechanism, and so a sensory deficit could lead to disruption of the sequential ordering mechanisms without necessarily involving the representative forms themselves.

3.2.4.3. Self-Monitoring Abilities

It has often been observed that comprehension disorders and self-monitoring deficits go hand in hand, and as comprehension improves, so does the ability of the patient to monitor his/her own speech output. Note that an ability to monitor one's own output does not automatically insure that, once caught, the error can be self-corrected. It is a well-known fact that there are patients who produce errors and immediately monitor them as being incorrect, but who do not necessarily produce the correct form subsequent to the recognition of the error. Patients with self-monitoring deficits produce errors but proceed as if they had not done so. The typical neologistic jargonaphasic behaves most often in this manner – producing bizarre forms with apparent disregard. Consequently, a sensory deficit that leads to a disruption of self-monitoring could easily exacerbate neologistic production. Obviously, however, there would have to be a concurrent problem with one or another production mechanism that would produce the neologism in the first place. Lack of self-monitoring would simply allow the productions to continue unchecked.

4. Conclusion

Suffice it to say that there are numerous ways for the language production system to breakdown such that words will be compromised. Representative systems/levels as characterized by available production models may be affected as well as the operations that manipulate the segments from those systems. Error production is greatly exacerbated as well in those cases where the overall operating tone of the organism is disturbed. Abnormalities in short-term verbal memory, in disinhibition, and in self-monitoring will all play one role or another in disorders of word form processing in aphasia.

5. References

Alajouanine, T. (1956). Verbal realization in aphasia. *Brain, 79,* 1–28. Reprinted in M. T. Sarno (Ed.), *Aphasia: Selected readings. 19–36.* New York: Appleton-Century-Crofts. 1972.

Badecker, W. & Caramazza, A. (1989). A lexical distinction between inflection and derivation. *Linguistic Inquiry, 20,* 108–116.

Beland, R., Caplan, D., & Nespoulous, J. L. (1990). The role of abstract phonological representations in word production: Evidence from phonemic paraphasias. In R. Beland, J. Ryalls, & A. R. Lecours (Eds.), "Phonological and phonetic aspects of aphasia," in special issue of the *Journal of Neurolinguistics, 5,* 125–164.

Berndt, R. S. (1988). Repetition in aphasia: Implications for models of language processing. In F. Boller & J. Grafman (Eds.), *Handbook of neuropsychology,* vol. 1, *329–348.* Amsterdam: Elsevier.

Blanken, G. (1990). Formal paraphasias: A single case study. *Brain and Language, 38,* 534–554.

Brown, J. W. (1972). *Aphasia, apraxia, and agnosia.* Springfield, Il: C. C. Thomas.

Brown, J. W. (1977). *Mind, brain, and consciousness: The neuropsychology of cognition.* New York: Academic Press.

Buckingham, H. W. (1980). On correlating aphasic errors with slips-of-the-tongue. *Applied Psycholinguistics, 1,* 199–200.

Buckingham, H. W. (1981). Where do neologisms come from? In J. W. Brown (Ed.), *Jargonaphasia. 39–62.* New York: Academic Press.

Buckingham, H. W. (1985). Perseveration in aphasia. In S. Newman & R. Epstein (Eds.), *Current perspectives in aphasia. 113–154.* Edinburgh: Churchill Livingstone.

Buckingham, H. W. (1986). The scan-copier mechanism and the positional level of language production: Evidence from phonemic paraphasia. *Cognitive Science, 10,* 195–217.

Buckingham, H. W. (1987). Phonemic paraphasias and psycholinguistic production models for neologistic jargon. *Aphasiology, 1,* 381–400.

Buckingham, H. W. (1989a). Phonological paraphasia. In C. Code (Ed.), *The characteristics of aphasia. 89–110.* London: Taylor & Francis.

Buckingham, H. W. (1989b). Mechanisms underlying aphasic transformations. In A. Ardila & P. Ostrosky-Solis (Eds.), *Brain organization of language and cognitive processes. 123–145.* New York: Plenum.

Buckingham, H. W. (1990a). Principle of sonority, doublet creation, and the checkoff monitor. In J. L. Nespoulous & P. Villiard (Eds.), *Morphology, phonology, and aphasia. 193–205.* New York: Springer-Verlag.

Buckingham, H. W. (1990b). Abstruse neologisms, retrieval deficits and the random generator. In R. Beland, J. Ryalls, & A. R. Lecours (Eds.), "Phonological and phonetic aspects of aphasia," in special issue of the *Journal of Neurolinguistics, 5,* 215–235..

Buckingham, H. W. & Kertesz, A. (1976). *Neologistic jargon aphasia.* Amsterdam: Swets & Zeitlinger.

Buckingham, H. W., Whitaker, H., & Whitaker, H. A. (1979). On linguistic perseveration. In H. Whitaker & H. A. Whitaker (Eds.), *Studies in neurolinguistics, Vol. 4. 329–352.* New York: Academic Press.

Butterworth, B. (1979). Hesitation and the production of verbal paraphasias and neologisms in jargon aphasia. *Brain and Language, 18,* 133–161.

Critchley, M. (1970). *Aphasiology.* London: Edward Arnold. Chapter on "Articulatory defects in aphasia: The problem of Broca's aphemia" reprinted in H. Goodglass & S. Blumstein (Eds.), *Psycholinguistics and aphasia. 51–68.* Baltimore: Johns Hopkins. 1973.

Dogil, G. (1989). The phonological and acoustic form of neologistic jargon aphasia. *Clinical Linguistics and Phonetics, 3,* 265–279.

Eggert, G. (Ed.) (1977). *Wernicke's works on aphasia: A sourcebook and review.* The Hague: Mouton.

Eisenson, J. (1973). *Adult aphasia: Assessment and treatment.* Englewood Cliffs, NJ: Prentice-Hall.

Fay, D. & Cutler, A. (1977). Malapropisms and the structure of the mental lexicon. *Linguistic Inquiry, 8,* 505–520.

Garrett, M. F. (1982). Production of speech: Observations from normal and pathological language use. In A. Ellis (Ed.), *Normality and pathology in cognitive functions. 19–76,* London: Academic Press.

Garrett, M. F. (1984). The organization of processing structure for language production: Applications to aphasic speech. In D. Caplan, A. Lecours, & A. Smith (Eds.), *Biological perspectives on language. 172–193.* Cambridge, MA: The MIT Press.

Garrett, M. F. (1988). Processes in language production. In F. Newmeyer (Ed.), *Linguistics: The Cambridge survey. III language: Psychological and biological aspects. 69–96.* Cambridge, England: Cambridge University Press.

Garrett, M. F. (1990). Sentence processing. In D. N. Osherson & Lasnik (Eds.), *An invitation to cognitive science: Language.* Vol. 3. *133–175.* Cambridge, MA: The MIT Press.

Geschwind, N., Quadfasel, F. A., & Segarra, J. M. (1968). Isolation of the speech area. *Neuropsychologia, 6,* 327–340.

Goodglass, H. & Kaplan, E. (1983). *The assessment of aphasia and related disorders.* (2nd ed.). Philadelphia: Lea & Febiger.

Jakobson, R. (1941). *Aphasie. Kindersprache und allgemeine Lautgesetze.* Uppsala: Almquist u. Wilsells.

Joanette, Y, Keller, E., & Lecours, A. R. (1980). Sequences of phonemic approximations in aphasia. *Brain and Language, 11,* 30–40.

Kertesz, A. & Benson, D. F. (1970). Neologistic jargon: A clinicopathological study. *Cortex, 6,* 362–386.

Kimura, D. (1982). Left-hemisphere control of oral and brachial movements and their relation to comprehension. *Philosophical Transactions of the Royal Society of London, B298,* 135–149.

Kohn, S. E. (1984). The nature of the phonological disorder in conduction aphasia. *Brain and Language, 23,* 97–115.

Kohn, S. E. (1985). *Phonological breakdown in aphasia.* PhD Dissertation, Tuffs University, Department of Psychology.

Kohn, S. E. (1989). The nature of the phonemic string deficit in conduction aphasia. *Aphasiology, 3,* 209–239.

Lecours, A. R. (1975). Methods for the description of aphasic transformations of language. In E. H. Lenneberg & E. Lenneberg (Eds.), *Founda-*

tions of language development: A multidisciplinary approach. 75–94. New York: Academic Press.

Lecours, A. R. (1982). On neologisms. In J. Mehler, E. C. T. Walker, & M. F. Garrett (Eds.), *Perspectives on mental representation. 217–247.* Hillsdale, NJ: Erlbaum.

Lecours, A. R. & Lhermitte, F. (1972). Recherches sur le language des aphasiques: 4. Analyse d'un corpus de neologismes; Notion de paraphasie monemique. *L'encephale, 61,* 295–315.

Lecours, A. R. & Rouillon, F. (1976). Neurolinguistic analysis of jargonaphasia and jargonagraphia. In H. Whitaker & H. A. Whitaker (Eds.), *Studies in neurolinguistics.* Vol. 2. *95–144.* New York: Academic Press.

Levelt, W. J. M. (1989). *Speaking. From intention to articulation.* Cambridge, MA: MIT Press.

Luria, A. R. (1973). *The working brain: An introduction to neuropsychology.* New York: Basic Books.

Martinet, A. (1960). *Eléments de linguistique générale.* Paris: A. Colin.

Pate, D. S., Saffran, E. M., & Martin, N. (1987) Specifying the nature of the production impairment in a conduction aphasic: A case study. *Language and Cognitive Processes, 2,* 43–84.

Pick, A. (1931) *Aphasia.* Translated by J. W. Brown, 1973. Springfield, Il: C. C. Thomas.

Rapp, B. & Caramazza, A. (1991). Lexical deficits. In M. T. Sarno (Ed.), *Acquired aphasia* (2nd ed.). 181–222. Orlando, FL: Academic Press.

Schwartz, M. F. (1987) Patterns of speech production deficit within and across aphasia syndromes: Application of a psycholinguistic model. In M. Coltheart, G. Sartori, & R. Job (Eds.), *The cognitive neuropsychology of language. 163–199.* London: Erlbaum.

Shattuck-Hufnagel, S. (1979). Speech errors as evidence for a serial-ordering mechanism in sentence production. In W. E. Cooper & E. C. T. Walker (Eds.), *Sentence processing: Psycholinguistic studies presented to Merrill Garrett. 295–342.* Hillsdale, NJ: Erlbaum.

Valdois, S., Joanette, Y., & Nespoulous, J. L. (1989). Intrinsic organization of sequences of phonemic approximations: A preliminary study. *Aphasiology, 3,* 55–73.

Wernicke, C. (1874). *The aphasic symptom complex: A psychological study on an anatomic basis.* Breslau: Cohn & Weigert. [Translated and reprinted in Eggert (1977) Op. Cit., 91–145.]

Wernicke, C. (1906). *The aphasia symptom complex.* Die Deutsche Klinik. [Translated and reprinted in Eggert (1977), Op. Cit., 219–283].

Whitaker, H. (1976). A case of the isolation of the language function. In H. Whitaker & H. A. Whitaker (Eds.), *Studies in neurolinguistics.* Vol. 2. *1–58.* New York: Academic Press.

Zwicky, A. M. (1982). Classical malapropisms and the creation of a mental lexicon. In L. K. Obler & L. Menn (Eds.), *Exceptional language and linguistics. 115–132.* New York: Academic Press.

Hugh W. Buckingham, Baton Rouge, Louisiana (USA)

17. Segmental Disorders in Aphasia

1. Introduction

This chapter evaluates segmental, or phonemic, output errors in aphasia within the context of a cognitive model of single-word production. Given the prevalence of phonemic paraphasias across different classes of aphasia, the examination of segmental errors involves a broad range of patients (Kohn/Goodglass 1985).

There are a limited number of ways in which speech output can be disrupted at the segmental level. Phonemes can either be substituted, omitted, added, misordered, or distorted. The surrounding phonemic context can influence the production of some of these errors, such as the addition or substitution of a phoneme that is elsewhere in the target (*apple* → *papple*). Substitution errors vary with respect to the type of distinctive feature (e. g. place, manner, voicing) and number of distinctive features that are incorrect. Another layer of complexity involves the distribution of segmental errors with respect to syllabic structure (e. g. effects of number of syllables, consonant-vowel [C-V] structure).

At first pass, one can be struck by a degree of similarity among different types of aphasics with respect to their segmental errors. As Blumstein (1973) documented, the spontaneous speech of Broca's, Wernicke's, and conduction aphasics is similar in terms of, for example, the type of error (e. g. substitutions were most prevalent for all three groups) and the degree of phonological distortion (e. g. most substitutions differed from their targets by one distinctive feature for all three groups).

Differences among aphasic types emerge when the effects of different methods of data elicitation and experimental analysis are considered (Kohn 1985; 1988). For example, in spontaneous speech, where targets are not always identifiable, more utterances are likely to be classified as neologisms and not submitted to phonological analysis, than in picture naming, oral reading, and repetition. It is not surprising, then, that results of picture naming and repetition only partially agree with Blumstein's findings based on spontaneous speech: While the phonemic substitutions made by Broca's aphasics during picture naming and repetition are consistent with Blumstein's original results (e. g. Monoi/Fukusako/Itoh/Sasanuma 1983), those made by conduction and Wernickes's aphasics tend to alter two or more subphonemic components (e. g. Burns/Canter 1977). Consequently, it is possible to distinguish the phonological output behavior of different aphasia syndromes by carefully examining phonemic errors.

In the current climate of debate about aphasia diagnosis, serious questions have been raised about the use of the traditional aphasia syndromes for examining experimental data (e. g. Caramazza/Badecker 1989). However, as an independent means for comparing results across studies, the traditional aphasia diagnoses still provide a valid framework (Kohn/Smith 1992a), especially given that most of the relevant literature involves patients with such diagnoses. Accordingly, the data presented here will be organized in terms of patterns of behaviors that point to different levels of breakdown in word production (i. e., distinct neurolinguistic deficits). The aphasia syndrome most often identified with each neurolinguistic deficit will serve as the focus of discussion for each deficit.

This chapter begins by identifying the relevant clinical populations, in order to raise diagnostic issues that affect data interpretation (2.). Then, the theoretical orientation for evaluating the data is presented via a brief exposition of a word-production model and expected symptoms of breakdown at each level of processing (3.). The final major section (4.) focuses on the experimental data that distinguish functional deficits responsible for segmental errors. Most of these data were elicited by tests of noun production that vary according to the modality of input (i. e., picture naming, oral reading, repetition). A separate subsection is devoted to breakdown at each of the three levels in the production model.

2. The Clinical Population under Examination

Experimental investigations of segmental errors in aphasia typically involve one or more of the following syndromes: Broca's aphasia, conduction aphasia, and Wernicke's aphasia (cf. art. 9 for clinical details). In addition, relevant work has been done involving patients with 'apraxia of speech' (cf. art. 40 for clinical details).

It is important to note that in discussing experimental data on phonological production, a distinction is rarely drawn between Broca's aphasia and apraxia of speech; these terms are often used as synonyms (e. g. Blumstein/Baum 1987; Ryalls 1987; Canter/Trost/Burns 1985). Consequently, this chapter will be unable to determine whether different articulatory-based deficits are associated with these two diagnostic categories.

Apraxia of speech has also been associated with conduction aphasia (e. g. Kent/McNeil 1987; McNeil/Liss/Tseng/Kent 1990). However, rather than cloud issues concerning the speech production deficits commonly associated with conduction aphasia, the results of such studies encourage one to consider that, in addition to more abstract phonological disturbances, some conduction aphasics may also possess "speech abnormalities at the phonetic-motoric level" (Kent/McNeil 1987, 213). In a similar vein, some researchers have suggested that conduction aphasia entails two subtypes – one with high speech fluency and impaired auditory comprehension, and the other with reduced speech fluency and relatively intact auditory comprehension (Kertesz/Phipps 1977). The former subtype can involve a secondary diagnosis given to a resolving Wernicke's aphasia (Kohn 1988).

Because of a lack of clinical information, not all of the aforementioned complexities in diagnosis will be addressed. Nonetheless, these diagnostic issues should be remembered when considering possible conflicts or weaknesses in the data.

3. An approach to the Interpretation of Segmental Output Errors in Aphasia

As stated in the Introduction, the aphasia data on segmental output errors is examined here with respect to a model of single-word production. In order to clarify this process, the model used is described first (3.1.), and then the expected behavioral manifestations of major types of disruption to the model are identified (3.2.).

3.1. A Model of Phonological Word Production

The model that guides this chapter identifies only basic distinctions needed for a discussion of segmental errors in aphasic word production. This model incorporates many aspects of other models (e.g., Caramazza/Miceli/Villa 1986; Patterson 1988; Butterworth 1985), but does not include routes that bypass the lexicon for the oral reading and repetition of novel stimuli, in accordance with an analogy approach to these processes (cf. Friedman/Kohn 1990; see Figure 17.1).

As displayed in Figure 17.1, the current state of our knowledge about segmental errors in aphasia suggests the existence of the following three stages in the phonological process of single-word production: (1) phonological – the accessing of a stored representation from the phonological lexicon; (2) phonemic – the construction of a segmental representation on the basis of the stored lexical form; (3) phonetic – development of a phonetic-articulatory representation by integrating context-sensitive phonological information into the phonemic representation. This model remains neutral with respect to whether there are separate lexicons for input and output, because this controversial issue is not relevant to the current discussion (cf. Patterson 1988)

Following Ellis (1985), entries in the phonological lexicon represent root morphemes, and are susceptible to partial activation. These entries are hierarchically coded with basic phonological information that cannot be realized from context, such as consonant-vowel (CV) structure and nonredundant segmental features (e.g. three-place onsets in English begin with /s/ [*spr*ay], so that the features of the first consonant need not be specified; Crompton 1982; Kohn 1985; Caplan/Vanier/Baker 1986).

Once the appropriate representation has been activated in the phonological lexicon (i.e., stage one), segmental information not stored permanently is integrated at the next stage (e.g. the /s/ is now specified in three-place onsets). This process is basically linear (cf. Kohn/Smith 1992b; Nespoulous/Joanette/Ska et al. 1987), with the end result being a phonemic-level representation that retains syllabic structure (Kohn/Smith 1990a). To align this stage with most current box and arrow models, which contain some sort of output buffer and consider phonological production to involve a single lexical stage of phonological access, construction of the phonemic representation is located within the phonemic buffer (Figure 17.1) and will be referred to as post-lexical. This depiction is consistent with Caplan/Vanier/Baker's (1986) distinction between "underlying phonological representations" and "superficial phonological representations." The former can be related to representations in the phonological lexicon and the latter to phonemic representations at the level of the phonemic buffer.

The procedures associated with the first two stages of the production model may apply only to content words. Given the rarity of segmental errors with functors in both the aphasic and normal speech error corpora, it has been suggested that functors "are accessed in a different manner (i.e., as whole units rather than as conglomerations of separable segments) from content words" (Christman/Buckingham 1989, 114). Alternatively, the rarity of segmental distortions in the aphasic production of functors has been attributed to a frequency effect. Miller/Ellis (1987) argue that such errors are rare in all high frequency words, functors included. Given the ambiguity surrounding this issue, and the relative paucity of data on this topic, we will restrict our attention to the production of content words.

At the third stage of word production, phonemes undergo phonetic variation that is described clearly by the two categories of allophones distinguished by Ladefoged (1971; 1972): (1) extrinsic allophones, where a consonant is modified according to its immediate context (e.g. aspiration of word-initial stop consonants in English); and (2) intrinsic allophones, which result from the partial over-

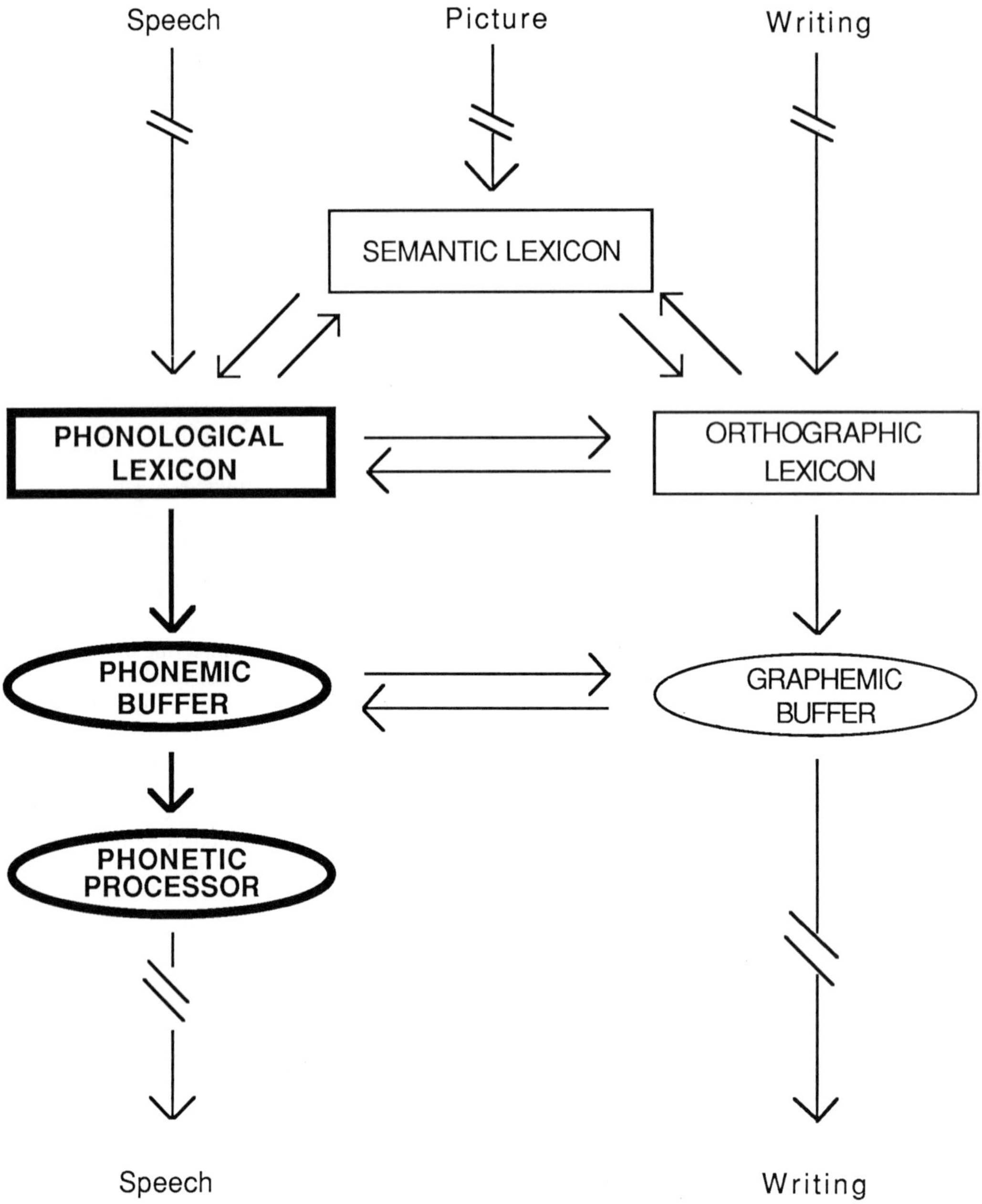

Fig. 17.1: A schematic model of single-word production (Components discussed are in bold)

lapping of the articulation of neighboring phonemes, i. e., coarticulation (e. g. lip rounding for /s/ in *spew*; Ladefoged 1972). Given the occurrence of coarticulatory effects of up to seven segments in both directions (MacNeilage 1982), phonetic representations must be highly integrated, with the boundaries of segments being obscured (Katz 1988). This contrasts with the more linear nature of representations at the previous stage.

It is likely that vowels are central to the coarticulatory process, so that the features of consonants are adjusted according to the vowel context (Kohn 1988; Ryalls 1987). This notion follows from the fact that the articulatory gestures for vowels are less complicated than those for consonants (Monoi/Fukusako/Itoh/Sasanuma 1983; Niemi/Koivuselka-Sallinen/Hanninen 1985), and it is consistent with the observation that in varied CV configurations, the acoustic cues that distinguish place, manner and voicing are more systematic for vowels than for consonants (Pisoni 1975). Thus, vowel formants entail "a more-or-less steady state or static acoustic property" (Ryalls 1986, 65). From the standpoint of coarticulation, then, basic CV patterns can be ordered in terms of increasing phonetic difficulty as follows: vowels, single consonants, consonant clusters (Burns/Canter 1977).

3.2. Symptoms of Breakdown in Phonological Production

On the basis of the current model, predictions can be made about the segmental speech errors that should arise with disruption at each stage. As will be seen, some symptoms can occur at more than one level (e. g. word-length effect), so that the identification of a functional deficit will depend upon a set of behaviors (i. e., a symptom-complex).

Disruption within the phonological lexicon (stage 1) leads to segmental errors when access difficulties involve partial activation and/or conflation of representations. If one follows an analogy model, in which unfamiliar words and nonwords are processed lexically (via the construction of abstract phonological representations from a synthesis of information from stored representations), a lexical-level phonological disturbance should impair the production of nonwords as well as real words.

The products of impaired lexical phonological processing can be articulated, because the subsequent, phonemic, stage can build a representation from incomplete or confused lexical information following rules of canonical phonological structure. This claim is consistent with the fact that even abstruse neologisms (i. e., phonological productions with no recognizable lexical source; cf. art. 16) abide by phonotactic constraints (Christman/Buckingham 1989).

It follows from this characterization of breakdown that utterances based on disrupted access to lexical phonological representations can contain information that is unrelated to the target at both the syllabic and segmental level (e. g. extra syllables [Kohn 1985; Valdois/Joanette/Nespoulous 1989], random phonemic substitutions [Miller/Ellis 1987]). There should be increased difficulty as words increase in length, given the greater probability of deficient access as the amount of representational information increases (Friedman/Kohn 1990). Note that there is no direct means for error correction with breakdown at this lexical stage because the first step in the phonological production system is disrupted (Kohn 1985).

A deficit at the phonemic level (stage 2) leads to phonological distortions that preserve the basic structure of the target, because utterances are based on accurate lexical phonological information. Thus, full attempts should maintain basic CV structure and a majority of target phonemes. Simplified CV structures may be used generally to reduce the programming load, but should not surface at a rate that suggests particular difficulty with certain syllabic structures, as expected with a phonetic deficit (see 4.3.). Performance with real words and nonwords should be comparable, because the deficit is post-lexical (i. e., occurs after the level at which words and nonwords are inherently different).

Given the linear nature of this stage, processing difficulty should be affected by length, both in terms of an increase in errors as words increase in length, and in the frequent production of word fragments (i. e., partial productions of targets that create dysfluencies). The distance of substitutions from their targets depends, in part, on the amount of information that must be integrated; substitutions that differ by more than one distinctive feature can occur when the stored information about features is minimal. If featural information is integrated in parallel across segments, errors can involve the misordering of phonemes (e. g. copies, transpositions; Kohn 1985; but see Kohn/Smith 1992b).

The distribution of segmental errors following a disturbance at the phonetic level (stage 3) should be systematically related to the target CV structure, according to the degree of articulatory difficulty of different CV configurations. Thus, vowels should be least susceptible to error with breakdown at this stage because of their relatively static acoustic nature and their likely central role in coarticulation (3.1.). Consonant substitutions should occur when the phonetic distortion of an articulatory dimension (e. g. place, manner, voicing) results in a segment crossing the perceptual boundary into another phonetic category (MacNeilage 1982; Buckingham 1983); these errors should be related to motor difficulty (e. g. consonant devoicing). MacNeilage (1982) posits that a misarticulation involving more than one dimension is less likely to be perceived as an acceptable example of a phonetic category, and, thus will be labeled as a distortion. Taken together, a phonetic deficit should result in a high proportion of perceived consonant substitutions involving only one dimension, plus frequent distortions. Because of the far reaching effects of coarticulation, and in contrast to the two previous stages, segmental errors due to a phonetic deficit should not necessarily increase incrementally as words increase in length.

4. Segmental Error Patterns in Aphasia that Reflect Different Phonological Deficits

On the basis of the theoretical framework presented in the previous section, experimental evidence for breakdown at each of the three levels in the word-production model are now considered. This is accomplished by identifying the aphasia syndrome that most typically exhibits the set of symptoms of breakdown at each processing level. In this way, the dominant phonological deficit associated with each of the major aphasia syndromes is explored.

4.1. Segmental Error Patterns that Reflect Impaired Access to Representations in the Phonological Lexicon

Wernicke's aphasia is the syndrome that has been most consistently associated with impaired access to entries in the phonological lexicon. The segmental output errors of these aphasics points to the disruption of information at two basic levels within a phonological representation — syllabic and segmental.

One symptom of incompletely accessed syllabic information is the production of paraphasias that complicate the target structure via syllable addition (3.2.). Valdois/Joanette/Nespoulous (1989) found, in comparing sequences of "phonemic approximations" in the spontaneous speech of Wernicke's and conduction aphasics, that the former produced a larger proportion of error sequences with extra syllables (15 vs. 1 %). Because syllable additions can be motivated by (accurate) phonological information, such as the simplification of CV structure via vowel epenthesis (e. g. *pretzel* → /prɛtəsl̩/), Kohn (1985) distinguished syllable addition errors that were "motivated" vs. unmotivated by the target word in the picture naming of Broca's (BA), Wernicke's (WA) and conduction aphasics (CA; see 4.3.). In contrast to the other two groups, a majority of the syllable additions produced by the Wernicke's aphasics were unmotivated by the target structure, and, thus, seemed due to a breakdown in lexical access (e. g., *rhinoceros* → *disseragerus*; WA = .74, BA = .19, CA = .47).

Kohn (1985) identified two other types of segmental errors that reflect disruption of the basic syllabic structure of words. These errors were most strongly associated with the Wernicke's aphasics: (a) attempts with randomly scrambled, as opposed to misordered, target phonemes (*candelabra* → *calenbranda*; WA = .12 vs. CA = .03 and BA = .02 of incorrect attempts with correct number of syllables); (b) errors that changed the syllabic status of a sonorant (*pretzel* → *pestler*; WA = .11 vs. BA = .005 and CA = .05 for targets containing sonorants).

Phoneme additions also complicate target structures, and have been particularly associated with Wernicke's aphasics. In examining picture naming and repetition, Burns/Canter (1977) found that their Wernicke's aphasics produced more phoneme additions than their conduction aphasics. Using the same test materials, Trost/Canter (1974) found Broca's aphasics to produce fewer consonant additions than either group (but see Kohn 1985).

Consistent with the evidence that Wernicke's aphasics are particularly prone to making errors that complicate the phonological structure of targets, there is evidence that they tend not to simplify the structure. In an examination of speech across several linguistic contexts, Keller (1984) found no tendency for a group of French-speaking Wernicke's aphasics to simplify consonant clusters.

When deficient lexical access creates segmental errors that do not affect syllabic structure, incomplete information about individual target phonemes is the source. Such segmental errors should surface frequently as phonemic substitutions that are remotely related to their targets. Several studies report the prevalence of such segmental errors in Wernicke's aphasics.

Burns/Canter (1977) found that a majority of the substitutions of conduction and Wernicke's aphasics involved errors along two or more subphonemic components (e. g. place and manner). They state that this pattern was more marked for Wernicke's than for conduction aphasics, but do not present separate data for each group (see 4.2. for discussion of distant substitutions in conduction aphasia).

Miller/Ellis (1987) evaluated the substitutions of a Wernicke's aphasic by comparing them to experimentally generated "pseudosubstitutions". The "pseudoerrors" were constructed by extracting the incorrect phonemes from the patient's attempts and randomly reassigning them to the empty slots created by the phoneme extractions. They found no significant difference between the phonetic distance between actual phoneme substitutions and their targets vs. between the "pseudosubstitutions" and their targets, suggesting that the real substitutions were unrelated to the target phonemes that they replaced.

Inadequate lexical access to segmental information in Wernicke's aphasia has also been suggested by the low proportion of target phonemes contained in their utterances. Valdois/Joanette/Nespoulous (1989) examined sequences of phonemic approximations, and found that only 53 % of those produced by Wernicke's aphasics represented all target phonemes, and that 26 % of them never contained several target phonemes. This contrasted with the performance of their conduction aphasics, who produced all target phonemes in 63 % of the sequences, with the remaining sequences missing only one segment. Similarly, Kohn (1985) found that during picture naming, Wernicke's aphasics produced the most "phonologically oriented sequences" with not more than 50 % of the target phonemes (WA = .16 vs. BA = .08 and CA = .05).

An increase in segmental errors as words increase in length is also indicative of phonological disruption at the lexical stage. Burns/Canter (1977) claim that their Wernicke's aphasics produced more phonological errors during the repetition of multisyllabic vs. monosyllabic words, but the details are not clear. In a longitudinal examination of a Wernicke's aphasic, Kohn/Smith (1990 b) found the number of pictures named correctly after phonological errors (i. e., with some indication of activation difficulty) decreased as targets increased in length. Interestingly, there was no effect of length for targets that were immediately named correctly (i. e., where no overt signs of impaired phonological access were displayed). This dual pattern spanned the four testing sessions that were administered between 3 days and 5 months post onset.

A final way in which segmental errors have been linked to a lexical problem is in terms of an inability to correct these errors. Kohn (1985) found in examining picture naming sequences of phonologically-oriented errors, that Wernicke's aphasics, in comparison to conduction and Broca's aphasics, produced the most sequences where the first and last attempts contained the same number of target phonemes and the fewest sequences in which the proportion of target phonemes increased from the first to the last attempt. Similar results have been reported more recently by Valdois/Joanette/Nespoulous (1989). Studies by Joanette/Keller/Lecours (1980) and Miller/Ellis (1987) have found the error sequences of Wernicke's aphasics to actually deteriorate, so that the final attempt is phonologically more distant from the target than the initial attempt.

It was argued earlier that a breakdown in lexical phonological processing will affect the production of nonwords. This association is illustrated by a case presented by Friedman/Kohn (1990). Here, the production of nonwords was far more impaired than the production of real words. The authors argue that this is predicted by an analogy model of nonword production that involves the activation of neighbor words to synthesize a novel representation.

Such a model would also seem to predict that the processing involved in activating whole representations can be dissociated from that involved in constructing representations from components of stored representations (i. e. via analogy). This dissociation would help account for other aspects of the longitudinal case of Wernicke's aphasia described above (Kohn/Smith 1990 b). This patient's output problems are also best described as the result of impaired activation of entries in the phonological lexicon, but, in contrast to the previous case, the production of nonwords and real words was comparable. The same model can account for both cases if one assumes that the previous case (Friedman/Kohn 1990) represents breakdown that results in greater damage to the analogy mode and the other case (Kohn/Smith 1990 b) represents breakdown that results in greater damage to the whole-representation mode of lexical access.

4.2. Segmental Error Patterns that Reflect Impaired Construction of the Phonemic Representation

A phonemic-level output deficit has frequently been associated with conduction aphasia. This deficit affects the length as well as the segments of target words.

One way in which word length is affected is through the production of word fragments (i. e. truncated phonemic representations). In an examination of picture naming performance, Kohn (1984) found that conduction aphasics produced significantly more of such responses than either Broca's or Wernicke's aphasics. Valdois/Joanette/Nespoulous (1989) found similar results in examining sequences of phonemic approximations in the spontaneous speech of Wernicke's and conduction aphasics: 28 % of the conduction aphasics' sequences contained one-syllable attempts to multisyllabic targets, as compared to only 19 % for the Wernicke's aphasics'.

Another way that a phonemic output deficit is sensitive to target length is through an increased number of segmental errors as targets increase in the number of syllables. The association of such a length effect in conduction aphasia is robust. In examining the oral reading and repetition of one- to four-syllable words, Nespoulous/Joanette/Ska et al. (1987) observed the greatest number of errors on the longest targets. Kohn (Kohn 1989; Kohn/Smith 1991) has reported two cases of conduction aphasia in which correct performance across picture naming, repetition and oral reading declined as targets increased in length. Across a similar range of tests, Caplan/Vanier/Baker (1986) found a marked effect of word length in another case of conduction aphasia.

Because of the post-lexical nature of a phonemic deficit, there should be comparable performance between nonword and real word production, both in terms of the effect of target length and overall level of success. Such findings have been reported in three case studies of conduction aphasia (Caplan/Vanier/Baker 1986; Kohn 1989; Kohn/Smith 1991).

One way to lessen the impact of a phonemic output disorder is to reduce the complexity of phonemic representations by relying on unmarked CV forms. There is equivocal data on this subject with respect to conduction aphasia. Nespoulous/Joanette/Beland et al. (1984) found no clear preference for either creating or destroying consonant sequences, while Keller (1984) found a preference in some conduction aphasics for producing single phonemes instead of sequences of consonants and vowels.

It was argued earlier that phonemic breakdown can distort target phonemes in two ways: phoneme substitutions, which can be distant from their targets, and phoneme misorderings. A prevalence of phoneme substitutions in conduction aphasia that differ from their targets by more than one distinctive feature has been reported in a number of studies. In examining the picture naming and noun repetition of conduction aphasics, Burns/Canter (1977) found that substitutions involving two or more subphonemic component alterations were more frequent than those involving a single component. Similar findings have been reported by Monoi/Fukusako/Itoh/Sasanuma (1983) for Japanese speaking conduction aphasics. In examining French-speaking conduction aphasics, Nespoulous/Joanette/Ska et al. (1987) found that 57 % of their substitutions during repetition differed by two or more features and 56 % of their substitutions during oral reading differed by two or more features.

While distant phonemic substitutions are also associated with lexical level breakdown, the other type of phonemic-level distortion, namely misordered phonemes, are essentially unique to this level. Nespoulous/Joanette/Ska et al. (1987) found that in contrast to Broca's aphasics, conduction aphasics produced more "contextually-determined" errors, or errors involving the "serial ordering" of phonemes, during single-word repetition and oral reading. Once again Monoi/Fukusako/Itoh/Sasanuma (1983) present similar findings for Japanese-speaking aphasics (but see Kohn 1985).

Errors involving misordered phonemes in conduction aphasics have recently received attention because of their apparent resemblance to normal slips of the tongue (Nespoulous/Joanette/Ska et al. 1987; Buckingham 1987). This association is particularly appealing, because the normal data have also been associated with disruption at a stage of phonemic planning (Shattuck-Hufnagel 1979; 1983). However, comparisons between the speech errors of conduction aphasics and normal speakers are questionable, because the conduction aphasic errors typically examined arise on tests of single-word production, while the normal speech errors typically examined involve the interaction between the phonemes of words during connected speech.

In an effort to present a more valid comparison, Kohn (1989; Kohn/Smith 1990 a) examined the sentence repetition of a conduction aphasic for the distribution of errors that resulted from an interaction between the phonemes of two words. Results indicated similarities, as well as differences, between the aphasic and normal speech errors. For example, both sets of errors usually involve the interaction of single segments of words from major lexical categories. However, while the normal errors typically involve word-onsets and occur within phrases, those of the conduction aphasic typically involved vowels and syllable-final consonants, and crossed phrase boundaries. These and other differences indicated that the word-interaction errors of the conduction aphasic resulted from the perseveration of segments from one planning phrase to another, as opposed to the mislocation of segments during the construction of a phonemic representation, which has been emphasized with normal speech errors (Shattuck-Hufnagel 1979; 1983). In terms of a production model, the aphasic data were interpreted as reflecting an inability to clear information from the phonemic output buffer. More research in aphasia on segmental misorderings that span words is needed.

4.3. Segmental Error Patterns that Reflect Impaired Phonetic Processing

The syndrome most often associated with a phonetic-level output deficit is Broca's aphasia. The segmental errors of these aphasics reflect misarticulation or impaired coarticulatory programming in a variety of ways.

In contrast to breakdown at the prior two stages, errors should not necessarily increase as targets increase in length. Indeed, the segmental errors of Broca's aphasics appear to be concentrated in monosyllabic words (Nespoulous/Joanette/Ska et al. 1987).

The segmental errors of Broca's aphasics that affect syllabic structure are related to coarticulatory complexity, as opposed to inadequate lexical access. Both Nespoulous/Joanette/Beland et al. (1984) and Keller (1984) found that their Broca's aphasics tended to simplify, as opposed to create, consonant sequences. Keller found the same pattern for vowels. On both repetition and picture naming, Canter/Trost/Burns (1985) found a prevalence of errors involving consonant clusters as opposed to consonant singletons for their Broca's, but not fluent, aphasics.

Other types of errors that reduce the complexity of CV structure were reported by Kohn (1985), who found that in comparison to conduction and Wernicke's aphasics, Broca's aphasics produced the most errors involving vowel epenthesis/consonant reduplication (*pretzel* ⟶ /prɛs/alr̩/), and involving consonant additions before word-initial vowels during picture naming. Finally, the prevalence of errors of "transitionalization" in the Broca's, but not in conduction and Wernicke's, aphasics is also consistent with a simplification of the coarticulatory program in these aphasics (Canter/Trost/Burns 1985). This error type involves a variety of processes that disturb the normal flow of articulation (e. g. articulatory hiatus, intrusive vowel, prolongation).

Consistent with the proposed importance of vowels to phonetic programming, a number of studies have reported the relative preservation of vowels vs. consonants for Broca's, in contrast to conduction and Wernicke's, aphasics. Niemi/Koivuselka-Sallinen/Hanninen (1985) report this pattern for Finnish-speaking Broca's aphasics. With respect to Japanese aphasics, Monoi/Fukusako/Itoh/Sasanuma (1983) found that their Broca's aphasics produced a mean of 92.1 % of their errors on picture naming and 97.3 % on repetition involved consonants, while their conduction aphasics displayed almost equal susceptibility to consonant and vowel errors during picture naming and repetition. On picture naming, Kohn (1985) found significantly fewer vowel omissions for her Broca's, than conduction and Wernicke's, aphasics. Trost/Canter's (1974) examination of vowel errors in Broca's aphasia revealed no instances where a vowel error constituted the only error in a monosyllabic word. This led them to conclude "that vowels were misarticulated in relation to articulatory difficulty on contiguous consonants" (Trost/Canter 1974, 69–70).

A concentration of segmental errors in word-initial vs. word-final position in Broca's aphasia has been identified as another sign of articulatory difficulty. Canter/Trost/Burns (1985) report this pattern to hold strongly for consonant clusters, but weakly for singletons (but see Niemi/Koivuselka-Sallinen/Hanninen 1985, for possible cross-language differences).

When types of segmental errors are considered, distortions, predicted to occur with a phonetic disorder, have been reported in Broca's aphasics, but not in conduction or Wernicke's aphasics (Canter/Trost/Burns 1985; Burns/Canter 1977). Identifiable substitutions should be the closest to their targets following damage at this stage. Therefore, it is not surprising that Nespoulous/Joanette/Beland et al. (1984) found that during repetition, their French-speaking Broca's aphasics produced more consonant substitutions that changed one distinctive feature than did their conduction aphasics, that Monoi/Fukusako/Itoh/Sasanuma (1983) report similar results for Japanese-speaking aphasics, and that Canter/Trost/Burns (1985) report similar findings when comparing Broca's with fluent (i. e. conduction and Wernicke's) aphasics. The latter two studies examined picture naming, as well as repetition.

Further details about phonemic substitutions in Broca's aphasia support the interpretation of these errors as phonetic in nature. In contrast to those of conduction and Wernicke's aphasics, MacNeilage (1982) found that the likelihood of a phoneme being substituted by a Broca's aphasic was inversely related to its frequency in babbling and adult language. This inverse relationship was taken as reflecting the influence of an articulatory deficit. Errors involving place of articulation in Broca's aphasia tend to be close approximations. Trost/Canter (1974) found that slightly more than half of such errors produced by Broca's aphasics were off by only one place (e. g. the substitutions of dental for bilabial phonemes). MacNeilage (1982) identified two types of voicing errors that suggest the presence of motor difficulty: the devoicing of fricatives and final stop consonants. Such voicing errors were prevalent in Broca's aphasics, but not in conduction and Wernicke's aphasics. Similar results have been reported by Nespoulous/Joanette/Beland et al. (1984) with respect to the repetition performance of Broca's and conduction aphasics.

Another method that has documented phonetic deficiencies affecting segmental production in Broca's aphasia involves asking normal listeners to judge recorded aphasics productions. Katz (1988) asked normal speakers to determine which of two possible vowels occurred in aphasic CV productions in which he had removed the aperiodic portion corresponding to the consonant. In relation to productions by normal speakers and posterior aphasics, those by Broca's aphasics were judged less accurately by normal speakers. Katz (1988, p. 362) suggests that the "lower perceptual scores for the anterior aphasics' productions are presumably due to there being less coarticulatory information present in these subjects' stimuli." However, he notes that such a coarticulatory disturbance is not across the board, in that it seems to be in evidence when the coordination of two or more independent articulators or two regions of the same articulator are involved. This notion is supported by detailed acoustic analyses that go beyond the scope of this chapter (e. g. Shinn/Blumstein 1983).

Finally, we have been viewing breakdown at each level as though it were fairly uniform across patients. This approach is dictated by the lack of detailed information about individual subjects. However, with respect to phonetic processing, a recent case study allows us to speculate about how types of phonetic processing can be differentially affected by brain damage. Marshall/Gandour/Windsor (1988) describe a patient who was initially diagnosed as having Broca's aphasia with apraxia of speech. What is remarkable about this patient is that with the use of an electrolarynx his speech was essentially normal. The authors use this case to argue that the programming of oral and laryngeal gestures can be dissociated (i. e., apraxia of speech vs. apraxia of phonation).

4.4. Aspects of Segmental Errors that Span Deficits/Syndromes

This chapter has focused on data that differentiate phonological deficits and corresponding syndromes. However, as indicated by Blumstein's (1973) findings (see 1.), some aspects of the aphasia data reveal similarities in the behavioral manifestations of different deficits and/or syndromes. For example, the relative distribution of types of segmental errors involving single consonants during picture naming and repetition is similar for Broca's, Wernicke's, and conduction aphasics: Substitutions are the most prevalent, followed by additions, and then omissions (Trost/Canter 1974; Burns/Canter 1977; but see Monoi/Fukusako/Itoh/Sasanuma 1983). The distinctive features involved in the substitution errors are similar across the three diagnostic groups: Errors involving place of articulation are most prevalent, followed by manner, voicing, and then nasality (Burns/Canter 1977).

There are some similarities across syndromes in terms of the relative difficulty of certain production tests. In particular, if a disparity is shown between test scores, picture naming is usually more impaired than repetition. This pattern suggests that the more that word production depends on lexical phonological access, the more difficult it is (Kohn 1988). Trost/Canter (1974) report this pattern for Broca's aphasics, Burns/Canter (1977) report this pattern for both conduction and Wernicke's aphasics, Kohn (1989; Kohn/Smith 1990a; 1990b; 1991) reports this in two separate cases of conduction aphasia and one case of Wernicke's aphasia (in one case of conduction aphasia this did not reach significance). With respect to conduction aphasia, these findings conflict with the notion that repetition is particularly impaired in conduction aphasia, which some still support (Albert/Goodglass/Helm et al. 1981), but can be aligned with the notion of a general phonemic output deficit, as being argued here (Kohn/Smith 1991).

Finally, it should be noted that the current chapter's association of a syndrome with a single level of phonological breakdown does not necessarily exclude the co-occurence of other, less prominent, sources of phonological breakdown. For example, it has been suggested that Broca's aphasics also produce phonemic errors, and that both Wernicke's and conduction aphasics produce phonetic errors (e. g. Blumstein/Cooper/Goodglass et al. 1980). The association of conduction aphasia with some degree of articulatory disturbance has received some attention in the literature (Valdois/Joanette/Nespoulous/Poncet 1988; Keller 1984).

5. Summary

Difficulties in segmental production associated with the major aphasia syndromes have been examined in order to broadly characterize the deficit that distinguishes each syndrome. It was argued that Wernicke's aphasics primarily suffer the most basic deficit, in that a majority of their errors reflect impaired access to representations stored in the phonological lexicon. Conduction aphasia was seen primarily as involving a breakdown at a subsequent stage of phonological production, in which the stored representation is transformed into a complete phonemic representation. Finally, our evaluation of Broca's aphasia is perhaps the best documented and most widely held. The phonological disturbance of these aphasics primarily involves a phonetic-level disturbance.

6. References

Albert, M. L., Goodglass, H., Helm, N. A., Rubens, A. B., & Alexander, M. P. (1981). *Clinical aspects of dysphasia.* New York: Springer-Verlag.

Blumstein, S. E. (1973). *A phonological investigation of aphasic speech.* The Hague: Mouton.

Blumstein, S. E. & Baum, S. (1987). Consonant production deficits in aphasia. In J. H. Ryalls (Ed.), *Phonetic approaches to speech production in aphasia and related disorders.* 3–21. Boston: Little, Brown and Co.

Blumstein, S. E., Cooper, W. E., Goodglass, H., Statlender, S., & Gottlieb, J. (1980). Production deficits in aphasia: A voice-onset time analysis. *Brain and Language, 9,* 153–170.

Buckingham, H. W. (1983). Apraxia of language vs. apraxia of speech. In R. A. Magill (Ed.), *Memory and control of action.* 275–292. Amsterdam: North-Holland.

Buckingham, H. W. (1987). Phonemic paraphasias and psycholinguistic production models for neologistic jargon. *Aphasiology, 1,* 381–400.

Buckingham, H. W. (1989). Phonological paraphasia. In C. Code (Ed.), *The characteristics of aphasia.* 89–110. London: Taylor & Francis.

Burns, M. S. & Canter, G. J. (1977). Phonemic behavior of aphasic patients with posterior cerebral lesions. *Brain and Language, 4,* 492–507.

Butterworth, B. (1985). Jargon aphasia: Processes and strategies. In S. K. Newman & R. Epstein (Eds.), *Current perspectives in dysphasia.* 61–96. Edinburgh: Churchill Livinstone.

Canter, G. J., Trost, J. E., & Burns, M. S. (1985). Contrasting speech patterns in apraxia of speech and phonemic paraphasia. *Brain and Language, 24,* 204–222.

Caplan, D., Vanier, M., & Baker, C. (1986). A case study of reproduction conduction aphasia I: Word production. *Cognitive Neuropsychology, 3,* 99–128.

Caramazza, A. & Badecker, W. (1989). Patient classification in neuropsychological research. *Brain and Language, 10,* 256–295.

Caramazza, A., Miceli, G., & Villa, G. (1986). The role of the (output) phonological buffer in reading, writing, and repetition. *Cognitive Neuropsychology, 3,* 37–76.

Christman, S. S. & Buckingham, H. W. (1989). Jargonaphasia. In C. Code (Ed.), *The characteristics of aphasia.* 111–130. London: Taylor & Francis.

Crompton, A. (1982). Syllables and segments in speech production. In A. Cutler (Ed.), *Slips of the tongue and language production.* 663–716. New York: Mouton.

Ellis, A. W. (1985). The production of spoken words: A cognitive neuropsychology perspective.

In A. W. Ellis (Ed.), *Progress in the psychology of language*. Vol. 2. 107–146. London: Lawrence Erlbaum.

Friedman, R. B. & Kohn, S. E. (1990). Impaired activation of the phonological lexicon: Effects upon oral reading. *Brain and Language, 38,* 278–297.

Joanette, Y., Keller, E., & Lecours, A. R. (1980). Sequences of phonemic approximations in aphasia. *Brain and Language, 11,* 30–44.

Katz, W. F. (1988). Anticipatory coarticulation in aphasia: Acoustic and perceptual data. *Brain and Language, 35,* 340–368.

Keller, E. (1984). Simplification and gesture reduction in phonological disorders of apraxia and aphasia. In J. C. Rosenbek, M. McNeil, & A. E. Aronson (Eds.), *Apraxia of speech: Physiology, acoustics, linguistics, management*. 221–256. San Diego: College-Hill Press.

Kent, R. D. & McNeil, M. R. (1987). Relative timing of sentence repetition in apraxia of speech and conduction aphasia. In J. H. Ryalls (Ed.), *Phonetic approaches to speech production in aphasia and related disorders*. 181–220. Boston: Little, Brown and Co.

Kertesz, A. & Phipps, J. B. (1977). Numerical taxonomy of aphasia. *Brain and Language, 4,* 1–10.

Kohn, S. E. (1984). The nature of the phonological disorder in conduction aphasia. *Brain and Language. 23,* 97–115.

Kohn, S. E. (1985). Phonological breakdown in aphasia. Ph. D. dissertation, Tufts University, Department of Psychology.

Kohn, S. E. (1988). Phonological production deficits in aphasia. In H. A. Whitaker (Ed.), *Phonological processes and brain mechanisms*. 93–117. New York: Springer-Verlag.

Kohn, S. E. (1989). The nature of the phonemic string deficit in conduction aphasia. *Aphasiology, 3,* 209–239.

Kohn, S. E. & Goodglass, H. (1985). Picture-naming in aphasia. *Brain and Language, 24,* 266–283.

Kohn, S. E. & Smith, K. L. (1990a). Between-word speech errors in conduction aphasia. *Cognitive Neuropsychology, 7,* 133–156.

Kohn, S. E. & Smith, K. L. (1990 b). Evolution of impaired access to the phonological lexicon. Presented at the Academy of Aphasia, Baltimore, MD.

Kohn, S. E. & Smith, K. L. (1991). The relationship between oral spelling and phonological breakdown in a conduction aphasic. *Cortex, 27,* 631–639.

Kohn, S. E. & Smith, K. L. (1992 a). Introduction: On the notion of 'aphasia syndrome'. In S. E. Kohn (Ed.) *Conduction aphasia*. 1–21. New York: Lawrence Erlbaum.

Kohn, S. E. & Smith, K. L. (1992 b). Distinguishing two phonological output deficits: Activation of stored phonological representations vs. construction of phonemic representations. Unpublished manuscript, Braintree Hospital.

Ladefoged, P. (1971). The limits of phonology. In B. Spang-Thomson (Ed.), *Form and substance*. 47–56. Copenhagen: Akademisk Forlag.

Ladefoged, P. (1972). Phonetic prerequisites for a distinctive feature theory. In A. Valdman (Ed.), *Papers in linguistics and phonetics to the memory of Pierre Delattre*. 273–285. The Hague: Mouton.

MacNeilage, P. F. (1982). Speech production mechanisms in aphasia. In S. Grillner & B. Lindblom (Eds.), *Proceedings of the international symposium on speech motor control*. 43–60. New York: Pergamon.

Marshall, J. C. (1986). The description and interpretation of aphasic language disorder. *Neuropsychologia, 24,* 5–24.

Marshall, R. C., Gandour, J., & Windsor, J. (1988). Selective impairment of phonation: A case study. *Brain and Language, 35,* 313–339.

McNeil, M. R., Liss, J. M., Tseng, C.-H., & Kent, R. D. (1990). Effects of speech rate on the absolute and relative timing of apraxic and conduction aphasic sentence production. *Brain and Language, 38,* 135–158.

Miller, D. & Ellis, A. W. (1987). Speech and writing errors in "neologistic jargonaphasia": A lexical activation hypothesis. In M. Coltheart, G. Sartori, & R. Job (Eds.), *The cognitive neuropsychology of language*. 253–272. London: Lawrence Erlbaum.

Monoi, H., Fukusako, Y., Itoh, M., & Sasanuma, S. (1983). Speech sound errors in patients with conduction and Broca's aphasia. *Brain and Language, 20,* 175–194.

Nespoulous, J.-L., Joanette, Y., Beland, R., Caplan, D., & Lecours, A. R. (1984). Phonologic disturbances in aphasia: Is there a "markedness effect" in aphasic phonemic errors? In F. C. Rose (Ed.), *Advances in Neurology, vol. 42, Progress in aphasiology*. 203–214. London: Raven Press.

Nespoulous, J.-L., Joanette, Y., Ska, B., Caplan, D., & Lecours, A. R. (1987). Production deficits in Broca's and conduction aphasia: Repetition versus reading. In E. Keller & M. Gopnik (Eds.), *Motor and sensory processes in language*. 53–82. New Jersey: Lawrence Erlbaum.

Niemi, J., Koivuselka-Sallinen, P., & Hanninen, R. (1985). Phoneme errors in Broca's aphasia: Three Finnish cases. *Brain and Language, 26,* 28–48.

Patterson, K. (1988). Acquired disorders of spelling. In G. Denes, C. Semenza, & P. Bisiacchi (Eds.), *Perspectives on cognitive neuropsychology*. 213–230. New Jersey: Lawrence Erlbaum.

Pisoni, D. B. (1975). Mechanisms of auditory discrimination and coding of linguistic information. *Acta Symbolica, 6,* 65–111.

Ryalls, J. H. (1986). A study of vowel production in aphasia. *Brain and Language, 29,* 48–67.

Ryalls, J. H. (1987). Vowel production in aphasia: Towards an account of the consonant-vowel dissociation. In J. H. Ryalls (Ed.), *Phonetic approaches to speech production in aphasia and related disorders*. 23–43. Boston: Little, Brown and Co.

Shattuck-Hufnagel, S. (1979). Speech errors as evidence for a serial-ordering mechanism in sentence production. In W. E. Cooper & E. C. T. Walker (Eds.), *Sentence processing: Psycholinguistic studies presented to Merrill Garrett*. 295–342. New Jersey: Lawrence Erlbaum.

Shattuck-Hufnagel, S. (1983). Sublexical units and suprasegmental structure in speech production planning. In P. F. MacNeilage (Ed.), *The production of speech*. 109–136. New York: Springer.

Shinn, P. & Blumstein, S. E. (1983). Phonetic disintegration in aphasia: Acoustic analysis of spectral characteristics for place of articulation. *Brain and Language, 20*, 90–114.

Trost, J. E. & Canter, G. J. (1974). Apraxia of speech in patients with Broca's aphasia: A study of phoneme production accuracy and error patterns. *Brain and Language, 1*, 63–79.

Valdois, S., Joanette, Y., & Nespoulous, J.-L. (1989). Intrinsic organization of sequences of phonemic approximations: A preliminary study. *Aphasiology, 3*, 55–73.

Valdois, S., Joanette, Y., Nespoulous, J.-L., & Poncet, M. (1988). Afferent motor aphasia and conduction aphasia. In H. A. Whitaker (Ed.), *Phonological processes and brain mechanism*. 59–92. New York: Springer-Verlag.

Susan E. Kohn, Boston, Massachusetts (USA)

18. Disorders of Prosody in Aphasia

1. Characteristics of Prosody

Prosody is a feature of spoken language and refers to variations in three acoustic properties of the speech wave: duration, amplitude, and fundamental frequency (F_0). The perceptual correlates of these properties are speech rate and timing, loudness, and pitch (Lehiste 1970; Fromkin 1978). A further prosodic phenomenon is stress. As a sign of prominence it does not correspond to a single acoustic property of the speech wave. Prosodic phenomena are generally classed as being suprasegmental: They are not an inherent feature of the linguistic sound structure of an utterance but rather 'built on' the acoustic variables which define the phonetic realization of speech sounds. Furthermore, they cannot be established without comparing the phonetic quality of adjacent sounds; the amount of articulatory effort required to stress a sound depends on the effort with which other sounds are produced.

A characteristic of prosodic phenomena such as pitch and stress is that they display varying degrees of linguistic involvement. Stress can have a phonemic function when differentiating between a compound noun and a noun phrase. When the position of stress in a given morpheme is fixed the assigned stress pattern provides for a morphological distinction between compound words. Stress may also be used to mark the focus of attention in a sentence, the word selected for primary stress being a matter of communicative intent and not linguistic rules. In the literature on the processing of stress in brain-damaged patients a distinction is made between lexical and emphatic stress.

Like stress, pitch has functions at word and sentence levels; on the former the vibration of the vocal folds during voice production (the physiological correlate of pitch/fundamental frequency F_0) are referred to as tone, on the latter as intonation. In many languages tone is used to mark differences in the meaning of roots and stems, with the number of tone levels being distinguished varying from one language to the other. Tone also serves as a marker for grammatical distinctions. Not all sentential variations of F_0 are arbitrary; they are governed by grammatical properties of the utterance, including its mode, stress pattern, and syntactic structure (cf. Cooper/Sorensen 1981). Declarative utterances are frequently characterized by a gradually declining pattern of F_0; a rise in F_0 at the end of an utterance is typical for questions – irrespective of its syntactic structure. Depending on the attitude or emotional state to be conveyed intonation becomes a means for expressing contextual aspects of the intended message.

2. The Perception of Prosodic Features in Aphasia

2.1. The Influence of Linguistic Function

Disorders in the receptive processing of prosody have been approached from two angles: the pertinent acoustic properties are either examined as semiotic cues to the linguistic structure and the affective intent of an utterance or as psycho-physical entities. The extent to which stress and pitch contribute to the linguistic structuring of an utterance has been associated with hemispheric asymmetries in the processing of prosody. Two hypotheses have been advanced as to the perceptual processing of prosodic features. The functionalist hypothesis posits that the function of a prosodic feature rather than its perceptual attributes determines the lateralization of processing and that a continuum may be discerned between the two hemispheres. A number of dichotic listening studies have shown that both hemispheres may be engaged independently and simultaneously in the processing of the tonal and the phonetic components of a verbal stimulus. Within this conceptual framework asymmetries in the processing of prosody are discussed in terms of a parallel processing hypothesis.

The functionalist hypothesis predominates in the literature. Focussing on the linguistic functions of pitch contours Van Lancker (1980) has proposed a scale of hemispheric specialization, the range of which is determined by the domain taken as frame of reference (sound, syllable, word, phrase, sentence). Right hemisphere (RH) specialization is assumed to increase as one moves up in the hierarchy from sound to utterance. Supportive evidence has come from some dichotic listening studies. Van Lancker/Fromkin (1973) found a right ear advantage (REA) when native speakers of Thai were required to identify pairs of words differing only in tone. The same tones presented as hums yielded no significant differences between the two ears. Behrens (1985) had English-speaking subjects decide whether the right or left ear had received the stimulus item with stress on the first syllable. The stimuli were pairs of compound nouns and noun phrases, distinguished phonemically by placement of stress. A REA was found; the same task performed with filtered stimulus pairs led to a reversal of ear advantage.

The results of studies on the processing of intonation are less straightforward. Zurif/Mendelsohn (1972) examined the effect of linguistic structure on hemispheric preferences in the processing of intonation. Using sequences of nonsense words, spoken with a monotone voice or a syntactically meaningful variation of pitch, they obtained a REA in the structured condition. This result is at variance with that of a study by Blumstein/Cooper (1974) in which the stimuli were sentences of a (syntactically) different mode. Irrespective of task demands (matching, identification of sentence mode or contour pattern) the filtered sentences tended to yield a left ear advantage (LEA). Filtering (elimination of phonemic cues) appears to diminish the effect of syntactic structure on a potential REA. Although speech stimuli were not filtered, Shipley-Brown/Dingwall/Berlin et al. (1988) failed to find a dissociation between the perception of linguistic and affective intonation. For both types of intonation judgment a LEA was obtained, possibly due to the blocked order of stimulus presentation.

According to the functionalist hypothesis receptive abilities in the processing of prosodic features are more likely to be impaired in aphasia when these subserve linguistic functions. Perception of tonal contrasts have been reported to be impaired in aphasia (Gandour/Dardarananda 1983); sample size and task demands (visual identification of aurally perceived words) make further studies necessary. Blumstein/Goodglass (1972) examined the ability of aphasic patients to use stress cues in discriminating lexically between stress-contrasted minimal pairs. Both the Broca's and the Wernicke's aphasics made more overall errors than the normal controls, but the pattern of errors was the same in all three groups, indicating that the ability to perceive phonemic differences as signalled by stress placement is preserved in aphasia. Replicating the study with some modifications Emmorey (1987) found fluent and nonfluent aphasics to perform less well than normal controls and RH-damaged patients. In a German study (cf. Weniger 1984) aphasic patients also exhibited impaired performance when required to differentiate a change in meaning as marked by a shift in stress placement. The linguistic structure of some of these stimuli placed increased demands on parsing skills, exacerbating deficits in stress perception.

There is some experimental evidence suggesting that the ability to use stress as a cue in disambiguating phonemically similar strings of sounds could be tied up with the parsing skills demanded by the stimulus materials. Baum/Daniloff/Daniloff/Lewis (1982) probed the effects which different types of changes in sentential stress placement have upon the comprehension of agrammatic aphasic patients. Contrast items in which stress either signalled a lexical distinction or a shift in morpheme boundary elicited more errors than the items in which stress marked the major point of attention. There was a strong positive correlation between error scores on the three contrast sets and severity of the overall language impairment.

Agrammatic patients have been shown to be rather sensitive to violations of syntactic structure when making grammaticality judgments despite their poor ability to make use of syntactic devices in comprehension tasks. Two potential prosodic cues to syntactic structure are segmental lengthening and pause placement (Cooper/Paccia-Cooper 1980). The F_0 pattern may contribute to the detection of features of syntactic organization. Longer syntactic units are initiated with higher frequencies than shorter ones and a calibration of F_0 contour is found at major syntactic boundaries. Such prosodic cues could be affecting the grammaticality judgments of agrammatic patients. The possible influence of such cues on patients' sensitivity to grammaticality has been examined by Berndt/Salosoo/Mitchum/Blumstein (1988). Grammatical well-formedness had to be judged under three listening conditions: In the first, all sentences were spoken with an appropriate intonation contour, the contours of the ungrammatical sentences being modeled on grammatical ones of comparable structure. The same sentence stimuli were subsequently presented after possible prosodic cues had been removed by a flattening of F_0. To control for the loss of signal clarity a set of vocoded stimuli with normal intonation was used as a baseline. The normal listening condition replicated previous findings. Contrary to normal controls and RH damaged patients the aphasic patients did somewhat less well in the two signal-processed conditions; but the observed effects do not reveal intonational cues as a prime source of information for aphasic patients in judging grammatical well-formedness.

Numerous studies have been devoted to the dissociable processing of the verbal and tonal components of an utterance. The assumption underlying most of these studies is that the left hemisphere (LH) is more engaged in processing linguistic-propositional aspects of an utterance while the RH appears to be more adept at processing affective-tonal ones (Schlanger/Schlanger/Gerstman 1976; Ross/Mesulam 1981; Ross/Harney/de Lacoste-Utamsing/Purdy 1981; Speedie/Branch Coslett/Heilman 1984). In accordance with the functionalist hypothesis patients with LH lesions have been reported to be impaired in their abilities to identify intonation contours as commands, questions, and statements (Heilman/Bowers/Speedie/Branch Coslett 1984). One way of tapping dissociations in the perceptual processing of the verbal and tonal components of an utterance is to use stimulus sentences which on half of the trials are intonated with the affective tone conveyed by the meaning of the sentence; on the other half of the trials the affective intonation is incongruent with the verbal content of the sentence. The performance of patients with RH lesions has been found to be more disrupted by inconsistencies between tone and content than that of patients with LH lesions when instructed to judge the affective tone of the sentences (Bowers/Branch Coslett/Bauer et al. 1987). In the congruent condition RH-damaged patients could benefit from attending to the verbal content in making their judgements, in the incongruent condition such a compensatory strategy was less successful. Such compensatory performance was also manifested in a study by Gensior (cf. Weniger 1984). Right brain-damaged patients had no difficulty identifying the emotional attitude of sentences intonated with a neutral tone of voice (as it could be inferred from the verbal content); the same patients displayed impaired performance when required to use intonation as a cue in distinguishing between the two propositionally possible meanings of a stimulus sentence. Aphasic patients showed the reverse pattern of behaviour (for mood judgments with/without prior exposure to a verbally conveyed affective context cf. Tomkins/Flowers 1987). As such manipulations of stimulus materials and task demands show, caution is warranted in the interpretation of findings which point to a hemisphere specialization for linguistic and affective aspects of intonation.

Only few studies have thus far explored the possibility that the two hemispheres may simultaneously participate in processing that component of a verbal stimulus for which it is specialized, the linguistic medium not being viewed as merely a carrier of tonal information (Goodglass/Calderon 1977; Ley/Bryden 1982; with monaural stimulus presentation cf. Safer/Leventhal 1977). In a study by Hartje/Willmes/Weniger (1985) emotionally intonated sets of consonant-vowel (CV) syllables were presented dichotically to patients with unilateral left or right brain damage, together with a group of controls; the task was to identify both the two intonation contours and the two syllable sequences. The two groups of brain-damaged patients performed as well as normals in identifying that stimulus component for which their intact hemisphere is taken to be functionally dominant; if performance of the intact hemisphere is considered on that stimulus component for which it is functionally non-dominant (syllables in the RH of LH-damaged patients, intonation in the LH of RH-damaged patients) brain-damaged patients do less well than normals, the difference reaching significance only for the identification of syllable sequences.

2.2. The Influence of Acoustic Attributes

In recent years some attempts have been made to determine the properties of the speech sound which could be responsible for the receptive disorders of prosody. The superiority of the LH for linguistic processing appears to reside strongly on the ability to perceive (and produce) rapid temporal changes. Temporal alterations in formant transition have been found to influence the magnitude of the REA in normals required to identify perceived CV-syllables (Schwartz/Tallal 1980). As shown by Robin/Tranel/Damasio (1990) aphasic patients need longer interstimulus intervals (ISI) than normals to detect the presence of a gap between two tones. The size of the ISI also affects their ability to discern the two closest tones in a sequence of six; compared to RH-damaged patients aphasic patients do less well in such temporal sequencing tasks. Conversely, patients with RH lesions require larger frequency differences between tones in order to match or discriminate consecutive tones (cf. Sidtis/Volpe 1988). In a study concerned with the differential processing of linguistic and affective intonation the performance of patients with RH lesions was found to be connected with a deficient extraction of pitch information; duration cues appeared to guide the matching decisions more than variations in the pattern of F_0 (Van Lancker/Sidtis in press).

3. The Production of Stress and Pitch in Aphasia

3.1. Prosodic Structuring

Disorders in the expressive use of prosody have also been studied from two angles: focus of attention is either on the articulatory-acoustic features which provide for a prosodic structuring of the utterance or on the physiological mechanisms which mediate the prosodic modulation of an utterance. To capture the characteristics of disorders in suprasegmental output an acoustic analysis of the speech wave is usually performed. Besides providing for a systematic evaluation of recorded speech samples such analyses have contributed to the view that dysprosody may be a perceptual phenomenon, not actually present in the acoustic speech signal.

The results of the few studies on the ability of aphasic patients to signal phonemic differences by means of stress placement or tone variation are rather inconclusive. In a word repetition task Chinese-speaking nonfluent aphasic patients displayed equally high error scores in producing syllable-initial consonants as in producing tone contrasts (Packard 1986). However, the aphasic patients in a study by Gandour/Petty/Dardaranada (1988) were able to produce tone contrasts in a reading task at a rather high level of proficiency (as measured by the distinctiveness of the produced contrasts). Whether tone production at the phonological level has a favorable recovery (as argued) or is a matter of spared pitch remains uncertain.

As stress cannot be associated with a single acoustic property, Emmorey (1987) used both pitch and duration measurements in analizing how successfully nonfluent aphasic patients are able to produce stress contrasts in a naming task. These patients made no use of pitch in distinguishing between noun compounds and noun phrases but signalled distinctions by means of duration cues. The two fluent aphasic patients produced the distinctions as well as normals, supporting the view that the ability to access and output suprasegmental information is largely spared in left posterior damaged patients.

At the sentential level the use of duration may not be intact in (nonfluent) patients described as having a Broca's aphasia. Instead of showing a lengthening of words in final position, these patients have been reported to have an increased mean duration of words in nonfinal position, as evidenced in reading tasks (Danly/Shapiro 1982). Whether such abberant lengthenings are the outcome of deficient syntactic planning or the result of difficulties in maintaining the flow of speech is not easily resolved, given that these patients are able to produce normal F_0 declination slopes in short sentences. Breaking sentences into smaller units than normals by more frequent use of F_0 resetting (initiation of a new intonation contour after a major syntactic boundary) may be indicative of a deficit in long-range programming of linguistic units but do not exclude a certain loss of phonatory control (cf. Ryalls 1982). The finding that the speech production of patients with a Broca's aphasia contains more continuation rises (localized increase in F_0 just prior to a syntactic boundary) may be interpreted along the same line of argumentation. Noteworthy is that the frequency of the continuation rises correlates positively with the severity of the language disorder. Of relevance with respect to the ability to maintain a normal F_0 pattern is a case study by Gandour/Petty/Dardarananda (1989), indicating that the critical variable is the temporal domain over which F_0 must be controlled. Although patients with a Wernicke's aphasia do not exhibit any observable deficits in the pattern of F_0 when producing neologisms and semantic and phonemic paraphasias, their F_0 configurations reveal shorter-than-normal domains of speech planning (cf. Danly/Cooper/Shapiro 1983).

Ever since Jackson's (1879–80) elaborations on the loss of speech as a disruption in the ability to use words propositionally, intonation has been viewed as a device for assigning recurring utterances (real words or non-meaningful strings of speech sounds) some propositional value. As disturbances of speech prosody have been associated primarily with RH brain damage, the prosodic production of non-propositional forms of speech by aphasic patients is commonly attributed to processing mechanisms of the intact RH. There is some evidence suggesting that linguistic and affective prosody may be dissociable in patients with RH lesions (Shapiro/Danly 1985; Emmorey 1987; Behrens 1988; 1989); however, as some researchers have pointed out, the amelodic speech of RH-damaged patients may not be specifically tied to disturbances in the emotional realm but rather the outcome of deficits in laryngeal tuning (cf. Ryalls/Behrens 1988). The question whether aphasic patients with extremely reduced speech production make variable use of pitch changes in order to mark different intents has thus far received little attention (cf. Poeck/De Bleser/Graf von Keyserlingk 1984).

3.2. Prosodic Modulation

Computer-implemented techniques of signal processing have made acoustic descriptions of prosodic characteristics of speech more accessible; however, they have not yet led to an increase in studies aimed at providing acoustic measures of prosodic disturbances. Prosodic anomalies may be expected in the speech of brain-damaged patients with motor speech problems. It is the speech of patients described as being dysarthric and/or apractic that has been examined in some detail (cf. Kent/Rosenbeck 1982). The dysfluency observed in these patients has been attributed to deteriorations in the coordination and sequencing of articulatory movements: articulatory prolongation (lengthening of transitional as well as steady-state segments in the speech pattern) and syllable segregation or dissociation, depending on the amount of prosodic cohesion maintained across syllables (in the presence of intersyllabic intervals). Aberrancies in the patterning of F_0 are linked to deficiencies in the temporal programming of laryngeal movements, monotone speech also being a possible outcome of failures in complete oral clozure for stop consonants.

Deficits in the motor control of prosody have been associated with neural structures of the language dominant LH. But since patients with RH lesions also exhibit restricted F_0 variation more interactive models of speech modulation are needed to account for the differential contributions of the two hemispheres in mediating prosody. Attentional mechanisms are likely to be just as crucial as temporal organization in the regulation of speech prosody (cf. Branch Coslett/Bowers/Heilman 1987).

4. The Foreign Accent Syndrome

The emergence of a foreign accent in speech subsequent to a lateralized brain lesion is rare and usually accompanied by aphasic symptoms. Speech output is described as being affected by changes in the production of specific segmental features of vowels (length and tenseness) and consonants (voicing) as well as in the patterning of F_0 (cf. Blumstein/Alexander/Ryalls et al. 1987). Characteristic for the articulatory and prosodic disruptions observed in a speaker with a foreign accent is that these exemplify features of attested natural languages (cf. Gurd/Bessell/Bladon/Bamford 1988).

5. References

Baum, S. R., Daniloff, J. K., Daniloff, R., & Lewis, J. (1982). Sentence comprehension by Broca's aphasics: Effects of some suprasegmental variables. *Brain and Language, 17*, 261–271.

Behrens, S. J. (1985). The perception of stress and lateralization of prosody. *Brain and Language, 26*, 332–348.

Behrens, S. J. (1988). The role of the right hemisphere in the production of linguistic stress. *Brain and Language, 33*, 104–127.

Behrens, S. J. (1989). Characterizing sentence intonation in a right hemisphere damaged population. *Brain and Language, 37*, 181–200.

Berndt, R. S., Salasoo, A., Mitchum, C., & Blumstein, S. (1988). The role of intonation cues in aphasic patients' performance of the grammaticality judgement task. *Brain and Language, 34*, 65–97.

Blumstein, S., Alexander, M. P., Ryalls, J., Katz, W., & Dworetzky, B. (1987). On the nature of the foreign accent syndrome: a case study. *Brain and Language, 31*, 215–244.

Blumstein, S. & Cooper, W. E. (1974). Hemispheric processing of intonation contours. *Cortex, 10*, 154–168.

Blumstein, S. & Goodglass, H. (1972). The perception of stress as a semantic cue in aphasia. *Journal of Speech and Hearing Research, 15*, 800–906.

Bowers, D., Branch Coslett, H. B., Bauer, R. M., Speedie, L. J., & Heilman, K. M. (1987). Comprehension of emotional prosody following unilateral hemispheric lesions: processing defect versus distraction defect. *Neuropsychologia, 25*, 317–328.

Branch Coslett, H., Bowers, D., & Heilman, K. (1987). Reduction in cerebral activation after right hemisphere stroke. *Neurology, 37*, 957–962.

Cooper, W. E. & Paccia-Cooper, J. (1980). *Syntax and speech.* Cambridge, Mass.: Harvard University Press.

Cooper, W. E. & Sorensen, J. M. (1981). *Fundamental frequency in sentence production.* New York: Springer Verlag.

Danly, M., Cooper, W. E., & Shapiro, B. (1983). Fundamental frequency, language processing, and linguistic structure in Wernicke's aphasia. *Brain and Language, 19*, 1–24.

Danly, M. & Shapiro, B. (1982). Speech prosody in Broca's aphasia. *Brain and Language, 16*, 171–190.

Emmorey, K. D. (1987). The neurological substrates for prosodic aspects of speech. *Brain and Language, 30*, 305–320.

Fromkin, V. A. (Ed.) (1978). *Tone. A linguistic survey.* New York: Academic Press.

Gandour, J. & Dardarananda, R. (1983). Identification of tonal contrasts in Thai aphasic patients. *Brain and Language, 18*, 98–114.

Gandour, J., Petty, S. H., & Dardarananda, R. (1988). Perception and production of tone in aphasia. *Brain and Language, 35*, 201–240.

Gandour, J., Petty, S. H., & Dardarananda, R. (1989). Dysprosody in Broca's aphasia: a case study. *Brain and Language, 37*, 232–257.

Goodglass, H. & Calderon, M. (1977). Parallel processing of verbal and musical stimuli in right and left hemispheres. *Neuropsychologia, 15*, 397–407.

Gurd, J. M., Bessell, N. J., Bladon, R. A., & Bamford, J. M. (1988). A case of the foreign accent syndrome, with follow-up clinical, neuropsychological and phonetic descriptions. *Neuropsychologia, 26*, 237–251.

Hartje, W., Willmes, K., & Weniger, D. (1985). Is there parallel and independent hemisphere processing of intonational and phonetic components of dichotic speech stimuli? *Brain and Language, 24*, 83–99.

Heilman, K. M., Bowers, D., Speedie, L., & Branch Coslett, H. (1984). Comprehension of affective and nonaffective prosody. *Neurology, 34*, 917–921.

Jackson, H. (1879–80). On affections of speech from disease of the brain. *Brain, 2*, 203–222.

Kent, R. D. & Rosenbek, J. C. (1982). Prosodic disturbance and neurologic lesion. *Brain and Language, 15*, 259–291.

Lehiste, I. (1970). *Suprasegmentals.* Cambridge, Mass.: MIT Press.

Ley, R. G. & Bryden, M. P. (1982). A dissociation of right and left hemispheric effects for recognizing emotional tone and verbal content. *Brain and Cognition, 1*, 3–9.

Packard, J. J. (1986). Tone production deficits in nonfluent aphasic Chinese speech. *Brain and Language, 29*, 212–223.

Poeck, K., De Bleser, R., & Graf von Keyserlingk, D. (1984). Neurolinguistic status and localization of lesion in aphasic patients with exclusivley consonant-vowel recurring utterances. *Brain, 107*, 199–217.

Robin, D. A., Tranel, D., & Damasio, H. (1990). Auditory perception of temporal and spectral events in patients with focal left and right cerebral lesions. *Brain and Language, 39*, 539–555.

Ross, E. D., Harney, J. H., de Lacoste-Utamsing, C., & Purdy, P. D. (1981). How the brain integrates affective and propositional language into a unified behavioral function. *Archives of Neurology, 38*, 745–748.

Ross, E. D. & Mesulam, M. M. (1979). Dominant language functions of the right hemisphere? *Archives of Neurology, 36*, 144–148.

Ryalls, J. H. (1982). Intonation in Broca's aphasia. *Neuropsychologia, 20*, 355–360.

Ryalls, J. H. & Behrens, S. J. (1988). An overview of changes in fundamental frequency associated with cortical insult. *Aphasiology, 2*, 107–115.

Safer, M. A. & Leventhal, H. (1977). Ear differences in evaluating emotional tones of voice and verbal content. *Journal of Experimental Psychology: Human Perception and Performance, 3*, 75–82.

Schlanger, B. B., Schlanger, P., & Gerstman, L. J. (1976). The perception of emotionally toned sentences by right hemisphere damaged and aphasic subjects. *Brain and Language, 3*, 396–403.

Schwartz, J. & Tallal, P. (1989). Rate of acoustic change may underlie hemispheric specialization of speech production. *Science, 207*, 1380–1381.

Shapiro, B. E. & Danly, M. (1985). The role of the right hemisphere in the control of speech prosody in propositional and affective contexts. *Brain and Language, 25*, 19–36.

Shipley-Brown, F., Dingwall, W. D., Berlin, C.I., Yeni-Komshian, G., & Gordon-Salant, S. (1988). Hemispheric processing of affective and linguistic intonation contours in normal subjects. *Brain and Language, 33*, 16–26.

Sidtis, J. J. & Volpe, B. T. (1988). Selective loss of complex-pitch or speech discrimination after unilateral lesion. *Brain and Language, 34*, 235–245.

Speedie, L. J., Branch Coslett, H., & Heilman, K. M. (1984). Repetition of affective prosody in mixed transcortical aphasia. *Archives of Neurology, 41*, 268–270.

Tompkins, C. A. & Flowers, C. R. (1987). Contextual mood priming following left and right hemisphere damage. *Brain and Cognition, 6*, 361–376.

Van Lancker, D. (1980). Cerebral lateralization of pitch cues in the linguistic signal. Papers in Linguistics. *International Journal of Human Communication, 13*, 201–275.

Van Lancker, D. & Fromkin, V. A. (1973). Hemispheric specialization for pitch and "tone": evidence from Thai. *Journal of Phonetics, 3*, 101–109.

Van Lancker, D. & Sidtis, J. J. (in press). The identification of affective-prosodic stimuli by left and right hemisphere damaged subjects: all errors are not equal. *Journal of Speech and Hearing Research.*

Weniger, D. (1984). Dysprosody as part of the aphasic language disorder. In F. C. Rose (Ed.), *Advances in Neurology, Vol. 42: Progress in Aphasiology. 41–50.* New York: Raven Press.

Zurif, E. & Mendelsohn, M. (1972). Hemispheric specialization for the perception of speech sounds: the influence of intonation and structure. *Perception and Psychophysics, 11*, 329–332.

Dorothea Weniger, Zürich (Switzerland)

19. Nonpropositional Speech in Aphasia

1. Introduction

'Nonpropositional speech' is a cover term for a set of heterogeneous language behaviors that lack certain linguistic attributes. These attributes have long been viewed as central and unique to human language, a perspective that was given new impetus by the publication of "Syntactic Structures" (Chomsky 1957). In this perspective, language (i. e., propositional language) is generated by the application of a finite set of grammatical rules to lexical units. Together, lexical units (or sets of lexical features) and grammatical rules (along with other constraints) generate a potentially infinite set of sentences. These processes distinguish human language from all other communication systems, and probably are, at least in some form, innate.

These essential principles of human language – stable word meanings newly arranged by specifiable grammatical rules – are precisely what nonpropositional language, in varying degrees, does not especially utilize. In nonpropositional language, conventional word meanings are weak or irrelevant to the meaning of the phrase. The phrase is the thing. And while most nonpropositional expressions may have the appearance of being grammatically well formed, this appearance is often misleading, because they do not have the flexibilitiy of a newly generated sentence, and they are familiar and 'correct' only in that form.

Assuming the validity of the distinction between propositional and nonpropositional language, at least two interesting questions follow. The first question addresses whether nonpropositional subsets in language differ importantly from one another. That is, are there characteristics that significantly differentiate idioms, proverbs, conventional sayings, speech formulas, indirect requests, and other related types of language? If so, how are these properties handled in language use? The second question relates to the first. Are there meaningful correspondences between these distinguishing properties and brain function? Thus, we can inquire whether different kinds of nonpropositional language, corresponding to their unique characteristics, are processed differently in the brain. The different types of nonpropositional language, along with their distinguishing festures, will be reviewed below.

2. Characterization of Nonpropositional Language

Nonpropositional expressions, comprising a large proportion of normal communication, are woven into the fabric of propositional language (Jespersen 1965; Bolinger 1976; Tyler 1978; Pawley/Syder 1980). A nonpropositional expression (such as a proverb, idiom, or speech formula) is defined first by default: it is not newly created from the arrangement of lexical items by grammatical rules. Instead, a nonpropositional expression is made up of a stereotyped form associated to a conventional meaning, which has been learned as a whole. Many different types occur:

(1) Idioms: *She has him eating out of her hand. Keep your nose to the grindstone. He's turning over a new leaf.*
(2) Proverbs: *Rome wasn't built in a day. People who live in glass houses shouldn't throw stones. While the cat's away, the mice will play.*
(3) Slang: *What's happenin'? Get on the stick. Grody to the max.*
(4) Cliches: *The pursuit of happiness. Have a nice day. It's a small world.*
(5) Social speech formulas: *How are you? Say when. I'll get back to you later.*
(6) Indirect requests: *Do you know what time it is? It's getting late. Would you pass the salt?*
(7) Other conventional expressions: *There's always a first time. I couldn't eat another bite. I'm stuffed.*
(8) Expletives: *God damn it. Go to hell. Son of a gun.*
(9) Sentence stems: *I'd like you to meet ... Would you be willing to ... It's quarter after ...*
(10) Memorized expressions: prayers, song lyrics, chants, poems, etc.
(11) Serial speech: lists such as numbers, alphabet, days of the week
(12) Pause-fillers: *So ... Well... Ya' know ...*

Many expressions belong in more than one subclass, but perusal of the subclasses listed above reveals differences between many of them. The idiom, the prototype of nonliteral language, is the clearest example: in most cases, idioms are not interpretable by the application of grammatical rules to usual lexical meanings (see below). Both form and meaning are learned, and idioms are not reliably interpretable when encountered without benefit of this natural learning process (for example, by the adult second language learner).

Proverbs are similar in some ways to idioms, but proverbs typically have a literal as well as a nonliteral reading. For example, *A rolling stone gathers no moss* stands as a proposition (has a literal meaning), using standard grammatical processes, but other features present in the proverb 'force' an additional more general, or nonliteral, interpretation. For unfamiliar proverbs, this second interpretation may be stimulated by the social and linguistic contextual features in which the expression is uttered, by the classic formal features of the proverb (present tense, plural or generic subjects), and by tone of voice. Acquisition of familiar proverbs remains poorly understood, and proverb interpretation has a long but uneven history in clinical testing of mental status (Gorham 1956; Delis/Kramer/Kaplan 1984) marred by imprecise test formulation (see Van Lancker 1990 a) and scoring difficulties (Andreasen 1977).

Speech formulas differ from these two types in being transparent in meaning (e. g.,

Have a nice day, How's the family? Will you respect me in the morning?), and because knowledge of sociolinguistic features is a prerequisite to their appropriate use and understanding. However, because they also have stereotyped forms and conventional meanings, many speech formulas are grammatically irregular, and they may use archaic vocabulary items: e. g., *Just in the nick of time, A chip off the old block, Easy does it.*

Indirect requests are closely related to speech formulas, as are sentence stems and other conventional utterances: they have an intended meaning not directly indicated by the words and grammatical form of the utterance. For example, *Would you pass the salt?* is not intended as a question (despite its interrogative form), but as a request to do something. Like other types of nonpropositional speech, indirect requests are closely associated with contextual features but their form is much more variable. To request that a window be closed, a number of expressions can be used (e. g., *it's getting cold in here*), and some flexibility within indirect requests is seen (e. g., *It's really getting cold in here*).

A complete typology of nonpropositional subsets of language would doubtless reveal more differences between them, as well as more similarities. The question of interest here is, are these differences reflected in structure-function correlations of brain processing? It is likely that different parts of the brain are involved. Different sites of representation in the brain for propositional versus nonpropositional language have long been assumed. There is also evidence for dissociated abilities to produce versus comprehend certain subsets of nonpropositional speech. The roles of the right hemisphere (RH) and the frontosubcortical system in nonpropositional language functions will be considered in the light of the unique properties of nonpropositional language discussed below.

Nonpropositional expressions all have an important property in common: they are familiar. To establish this fact, we need only to ask native speakers of English to select them from array that includes nonpropositional as well as propositional expressions – they do this nearly flawlessly. Similarly, when subjects fill in missing words in both kinds of expressions, agreement is seen in words in nonpropositional expressions but not in matched propositional exemplars (Table 19.1). Many propositional and nonpropositional exemplars can be reliably distinguished by acoustic cues (Van Lancker/Canter/Terbeek 1981).

While propositional language (logically) is made up of an infinite set of sentences, nonpropositional expressions comprise a finite set of relatively fixed forms associated with their conventional meanings. The number of such expressions is probably quite large. Nearly 3,000 interactional speech formulas have been catalogued (Fillmore, personal communication). More than 4,000 commonly used expressions including slang, proverbs, idioms and cliches appear in "A Dictionary of American Idioms" (Boatner/Gates/Makkai 1975). Previously receiving little attention in the linguistic, neurolinguistic and clinical literature (but see Chafe 1968; Lyons 1968; Weinreich 1969; Van Lancker 1973, 1987; Clark 1979; Gibbs 1980; Hopper 1987), more recently much has been learned about nonpropositional language.

As stated above, contrary to propositional language, nonpropositional expressions have unitary and cohesive form. They are familiar (rather than novel or newly created); they constitute a finite (although large) set; and both form and meaning are relatively fixed. Some familiar phrases are more 'frozen' than others (Van Lancker 1973; Bolinger 1976; Pawley/Syder 1980; Gibbs/Gonzales 1985; Gibbs/Nayak 1989; Gibbs/Nayak/Cutting 1989; Hopper 1987), and cohesion and conventionality in human language are best conceived as occurring in degrees, or along a continuum from newly generated to entirely fixed (Van Lancker 1987). But whatever their degree of 'frozenness,' idioms, proverbs and

Nonpropositional	Propositional
1. He has his ________ in the clouds.	1. He takes his ________ in the car.
2. Just in the ________ of time.	2. Almost to the ________ of the mountain.
3. I'll get ________ to you later.	3. He ________ up to her suddenly.

Table 19.1

social formulas differ from propositional language in being familiar and conventional in form and meaning. Applying grammatical knowledge alone to an idiom or proverb may result in mistaken comprehension, and utilizing such knowledge in the production of idioms, speech formulas, or conventional expressions may result in 'incorrect' utterances. For example, to comprehend the expression *She has him eating out of her hand*, one does not utilize lexical meanings for *eating* or *hand*, although some grammatical and lexical processing of *She has him* might be important (see Gibbs/Nayak 1989). In production, errors in familiar expressions generated by nonnative speakers of English are reflected in lexical choice and grammatical forms. Examples from nonnative speakers of English are:

That would come in helpful (for *That would come in handy*);

I wanted to get it out of my chest (for *I wanted to get it off my chest*);

I don't know how much water that holds (for *That doesn't hold water*, meaning *it's not correct*);

In summary, nonpropositional language can be conceptualized as occurring on a continuum from *reflexive* or *overlearned* at one end to *novel, newly created*, at the other (see Van Lancker 1975; 1987). In this schema, nonpropositional language is made up of subsets differing from each other in specific properties of their *fixed forms* and *conventional meanings*. The notion that propositional and nonpropositional language are mediated by disparate brain regions is supported by neurolinguistic data. Although many details remain unclear, clinical studies do suggest that types along the language continuum are differentially affected by focal brain lesions.

3. Nonpropositional Speech Production

In aphasic patients with propositional language impairments, their residual speech includes expletives, social formulas, stereotyped phrases and cliches, serial and memorized speech — the so-called 'automatic speech' often referred to by aphasiologists (Jackson 1878; 1915; Critchley 1962; 1970; Eisenson 1962; Espir/Rose 1970; Van Lancker 1973; 1975; 1987; Benson 1979; Code 1987). Aphasic patients can often fluently produce such stereotyped utterances, while being unable to produce parts of those same utterances; e. g., the patient who says *son of a bitch* cannot say the word *son* to refer to his male offspring. As the nonfluent patient recovers speech fluency, the repertory of fixed expressions may increase, progressing from a few stereotypies, through a larger number of fixed expressions, to grammatically produced (propositional) speech (Alajouanine 1956). The repertory of residual utterances varies greatly across patients (Van Lancker 1975; Code 1987). Usually short phrases are involved, but one aphasic patient reportedly produced Shakespearean and other learned quotations almost exclusively (Critchley 1970).

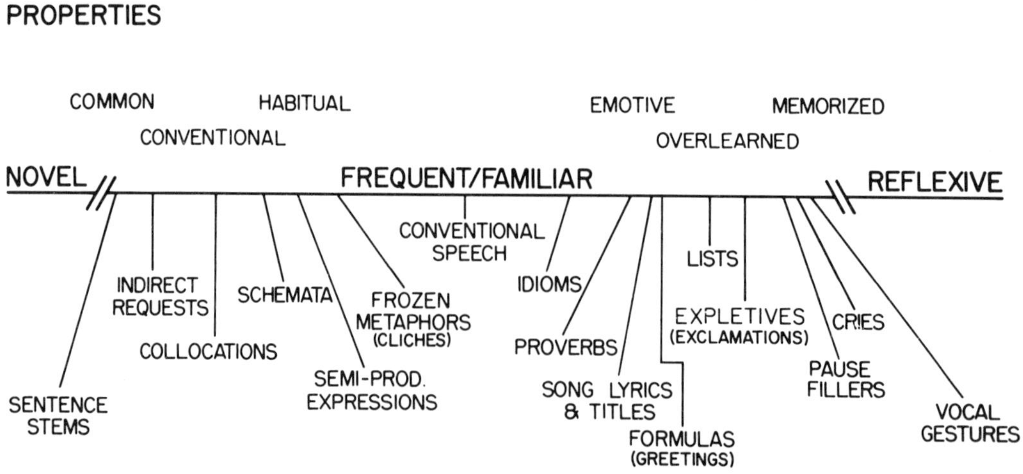

Fig. 19.1: Nonpropositional Speech in Aphasia

Specific abilities to perform better on nonpropositional than on propositional speech production tasks have been reported. Completion of idioms was reported by Geschwind/Quadfasel/Segarra (1968) and by Whitaker (1976) in patients with severe propositional language deficits. (The notion that idioms were completed because they are 'overlearned' does not account for these observations, because many idioms are heard and used only occasionally.) A patient with multiple sclerosis, who had developed severe stuttering on word-initial and syllable-initial consonants, spoke fluently and clearly when producing serial speech (1 – 30), days of the week, and memorized prayers. Thus, in this patient, development of plaques had interfered selectively with the ability to produce propositional speech but not with exemplars that have traditionally been referred to as 'automatic' speech (Van Lancker/Rorabaugh 1990).

Some nonpropositional speech is selectively preserved in Alzheimer patients, who typically have moderate to severe language deficits (Cummings 1985; Kempler 1990). Even in late stages of the disease, these patients produce interactional social formulas in casual conversation with ease and fluency, despite severely disturbed propositional language ability, and in the severely impaired Alzheimer patient, the difference between these language functions are dramatic. Consider the Alzheimer patient who cannot match single words to pictures, does not initiate speech, and is unable to answer yes-no questions or follow 1-step commands. Such patients are nonetheless able, with seeming normalcy, to use greetings such as *Nice to see you again*, leave-taking phrases such as *Thanks for all your help* and *See you all later* and other social formulas such as *Excuse me*, *Surely*, *Okay*, and so on.

Another nonpropositional subset, expletives, often seen in nonfluent aphasia, is also prominent in an illness associated with subcortical pathology: Tourette's disease. About 50% of Tourette's patients develop coprolalia at some time in the course of their disease. This symptom involves the tic-like vocalization of taboo words and phrases.

Thus, we see relatively intact production of expletives, social formulas, indirect speech acts and other conventional expressions in focal left hemisphere (LH) damage, and in the posterior cortical damage associated with Alzheimer disease. In addition, hyperactivated production of expletives occurs in subcortical pathology, as is associated with Tourette's syndrome. These observations suggest that brain structures different from those mediating propositional speech underlie these speech behaviors. The RH and frontosubcortical structures have both been implicated.

Jackson's (1878; 1915) view that propositional speech is represented in the LH and nonpropositional (or 'automatic') speech is mediated also by the RH, is still tenable. The degree of emotionality and holistic structure of much of nonpropositional speech leads one to implicate the RH. (This probably does not hold true for production of recurrent consonant-vowel 'nonsense' utterances (Kreindler/Fradis 1968; De Bleser/Poeck 1985; Code 1987).) Mouth openings differ for the two types of speech production. In their study of mouth symmetry during aphasic speech, Graves/Landis (1985) reported greater openings on the right side of the mouths of aphasic speakers for spontaneous speech, repetition, and word list generation (propositional tasks), in contrast to greater openings on the left for serial speech and singing ('automatic' speech). These reports lent physiological evidence to the notion that the RH is the source of 'automatic' speech.

The (nondominant) RH has appeared to be the site of aphasic speech in selected case reports (Cummings/Benson/Walsh/Levine 1979; Landis/Cummings/Benson 1980). Further, studies of blood flow (Knopmen/Rubens/Selnes et al. 1984) and evoked potentials (Papanicolaou/Moore/Levin/Eisenberg 1987; Papanicolaou/Moore/Deutsch et al. 1988) also point to the RH as a significant source of recovery in aphasia. Studies using the WADA procedure reported continued aphasic output during anesthetization of the left (dominant) hemisphere (Kinsbourne 1971; Czopf 1981), implying that the residual aphasic speech was produced by the right (unanesthetized) hemisphere. There have been reports of callosal-sectioned patients with linguistic expression via RH mechanisms (Butler/Norrsell 1968; Levy/Nebes/Sperry 1971; Sidtis/Volpe/Wilson et al. 1981; Gazzaniga/Sidtis/Volpe et al. 1982), but whether nonpropositional speech has been observed under such conditions is unclear. Singing without lyrics has been reported for the nonanesthetized RH during WADA testing (Bogen/Gordon 1971). More dramatically, several left (dominant) hemispherectomized adults with little or no propositional speech have been observed to produce exemplars of fluent, normally intoned expletives, counting, and singing of familiar lyrics (Crockett/Estridge 1951; Hillier 1954; Smith 1966; 1974; Bogen 1973).

Although following RH damage, alterations in nonpropositional speech have not been systematically investigated, there are anecdotal observations about deficient production of social interaction formulas and other nonliteral expressions in such patients (Jaffe 1978; Myers 1979; Foldi/Cicone/Gardner 1983). For example, a RH patient reported to this author that his wife had told him he ought to say *Goodbye* when he ends a telephone conversation. An unusual case of abnormal stimulated inner nonpropositional speech, consisting of fragments of prayers and hymns, was recently described (Ellis/Young/Critchley 1989). The onset of intrusive prayers and hymns followed bilateral, but primarily RH, injury. This case brings to mind the provocative ideas of Julian Jaynes about an evolutionarily early RH site of rehearsed and overlearned admonitions (1976; and see Van Lancker 1979).

Implication of frontosubcortical areas in production of nonpropositional forms comes from observations in Alzheimer's speech, described above. Here, the motor programs for some types of nonpropositional speech (especially speech formulas) are relatively intact. In most Alzheimer cases studied, posterior cortical areas of the brain have become involved before anterior areas; frontal cortex and basal ganglia remain relatively functional until late stages of the disease (Cummings 1982; Cummings/Benson 1983). Thus, the preserved ability to produce speech formulas may be attributable to intact frontal and/or frontosubcortical systems. In support of this view, Grafman (1989) includes the ability to engage in social communication in the set of abilities mediated by frontal lobes.

In normal subjects, RH participation in speech has been suggested by advanced radiographic methods of observing brain function during behavior, using measures of blood flow (Ingvar/Schwartz 1974; Lassen/Ingvar/Skinhoy 1978); and during automatic speech (pronouncing the days of the week), the RH, especially the anterior portion, was more active than the left (Ryding/Bradvik/Ingvar 1987).

For all the evidence suggesting RH or right frontal participation in speech production in normal and aphasic speakers, it remains a mystery that many globally aphasic patients, who have intact RHs, do not ever produce intelligible speech, nonpropositional or otherwise, beyond a few stereotyped utterances. The question of the source of nonword recurrent utterances (De Bleser/Poeck 1985; Code 1987) in residual speech also requires explanation. Although some predictable anatomical correlations of recovery from severe global aphasia have been reported (Naeser/Gaddie/Palumbo/Stiassny–Eder 1990), how active the RH or its frontal quadrant is in spontaneous production of nonpropositional speech remains to be studied, both in the recovering aphasic patient and the normal speaker.

4. Nonpropositional Language Comprehension

The role of the RH in comprehension of nonpropositional language is clearer than is the picture for production. First, it is well established that the RH recognizes linguistic stimuli, so long as phonological or grammatical analysis is not involved (Zaidel 1981; 1982). As idioms and proverbs do not require such analysis and may be processed holistically (Simon 1974; Horowitz/Manelis 1973; Osgood/Hoosain 1974), it is possible that the RH understands considerably more nonpropositional than propositional language. Indeed, it is often observed by clinicians, family members and caretakers that aphasic patients with severe language comprehension deficits seem to understand a great deal more in conversational interaction than can be demonstrated in formal testing of propositional language. Some of this comprehension is attributable to affective and gestural cues (Boller/Cole/Vrtunski et al. 1979), and the familiarity of the expressions (Van Lancker/Klein 1990; Van Lancker/Lanto/Klein et al. 1990; Van Lancker, 1991), which are natural properties of social formulas, idioms, and conventional expressions used in daily interaction. Abilities to process these properties are probably not impaired by LH damage.

Winner/Gardner (1977) were the first to report that comprehension and interpretation of idiomatic expressions such as *heavy heart* are impaired by RH damage. Since then, other clinical studies have shown that comprehension of idioms (Myers/Linebaugh 1981; Van Lancker/Kempler 1987), and proverbs (Benton 1968; Hier/Kaplan 1980) is impaired by RH damage.

Suggestive evidence for relatively intact nonpropositional language in aphasic speakers comes from Dronkers (1984). Using a paradigm adapted from Swinney/Cutler (1979), in which subjects judged whether phrases presented visually were natural English phrases or not, aphasic patients were found to make this judgment faster for nonpropositional phrases (e. g., *all of a sudden, I beg your pardon*) than propositional phrases (Dronkers 1984). (Of course, from these results on aphasic patients, whether the primary site of processing was the LH or RH cannot yet be known).

Other kinds of nonpropositional language comprehension have been associated with RH function. A deficit in comprehending indirect requests was found in RH damaged patients (Weylman/Brownell/Roman/Gardner 1989). Abilities to process verbal and situational context (Foldi/Cicone/Gardner 1983; Molloy/Brownell/Gardner 1990), important features of nonpropositional language, have also been explored. Brownell/Potter/Gardner/Bihrle (1986) found RH damaged subjects to be deficient in making the inferences required to interpret nonliteral meanings in texts, and RH damaged patients are less able than normal subjects to use context to interpret humorous meanings in jokes (Brownell/Michel/Powelson/Gardner 1983; Brownell/Gardner 1988). Deficits in familiarity perception have been associated with RH damage, such that the RH may be specialized for establishing and maintaining personal familiarity, or 'personal relevance' (Van Lancker, 1991).

A role of posterior cortical areas in idiom comprehension was suggested by a study of Alzheimer patients. Even those in mild stages of the disease were significantly more impaired in comprehension of idioms than of matched literal expressions, using a picture-pointing task (Kempler/Van Lancker 1985; Kempler/Van Lancker/Read 1988). As posterior aspects of the cortex are affected first in Alzheimer disease, and RH damage apparently uniquely affects this ability, the posterior RHs may be implicated in normal comprehension of some kinds of nonpropositional language.

5. Discussion

Aphasic speakers gave us the first clues about the uniqueness of nonpropositional speech. Now nonpropositional language is recognized as an important part of human language ability, deserving of study in normal speakers, and selectively impaired or preserved in brain damage. Expletives, serial speech, social formulas, and pause fillers are often preserved in global aphasia; deficient comprehension of idioms and indirect requests has been associated with damaged RHs; and impaired idiom comprehension was also associated with posterior cortical damage in studies of Alzheimer patients (Kempler/Van Lancker/Read 1988). Problems with proverb interpretation have been seen following RH damage (Hier/Kaplan 1980), and frontal lobe damage (Stuss/Benson 1984; Stuss/Benson 1986), especially right frontal damage (Benton 1968). From clinical observations in Alzheimer's patients, selective preservation of speech formulas has been associated with an intact frontosubcortical system.

We might speculate about what differences in left and right, and anterior and posterior brain function might account for these findings. The LH specialization for orderly sequencing of units, known for some time in studies of language, involves primarily phonology and syntax, mathematics, and phonological reading and writing. On the other hand, the RH is specialized for global processing (e. g., Bever 1975; Navon 1977), pattern recognition (Bradshaw/Nettleton 1983), apperception (Bogen 1969), and appreciation of contextual information (reviewed above). Therefore, preferential processing of nonpropositional language by the RH could be attributable to any or all of these qualities. Idioms, proverbs, speech formulas and conventional expressions may be processed primarily as patterns, although some decomposition of these phrases occurs in processing (see Gibbs/Nayak 1989). Given the LH/RH contrasts mentioned above, instances of idiom decomposition may be attributable to LH processes interacting with those of the RH.

Evidence from several different studies suggests a rich, often idiosyncratic, meaning association network in the RH (Van Lancker/Klein 1990; Van Lancker 1990 b; Sidtis/Volpe/Holtzmann et al. 1981). And RH deficits often involve problems in interpreting context: examples are topographical agnosia, topographical reduplication, and other environmental agnosias. Many of these deficits are not well studied or documented because they occur in the natural setting of the RH patient after he or she has left the hospital. For example, a patient with a right parietal lobe lesion, on recovering sufficiently to return to her apartment, insisted that the emergency number 911 be called after viewing an incident of assault in a television show in her apartment (Pappadis, 1990). This and other examples of defective appreciation of context were reported by family members. Semantic and contextual RH disabilities remain to be investigated, and better understanding will impact on information about nonpropositional language function.

In summary, because nonpropositional subsets of language are made up of familiar stereotyped forms with conventional meanings that are tied to linguistic and social context, the special abilities of the RH uniquely qualify that processing system to acquire, store, manage, and process these subsets of language. In comprehension, nonpropositional forms may be processed by pattern recognition abilities of the RH, while RH abilities for contextual and semantic inference and for familiarity judgments may be especially suited to process nonpropositional meanings. In production, the overlearned motor patterns that characterize nonpropositional speech may lead us to associate the right frontosubcortical system as a primary site of processing.

More must be learned about normal processing of nonpropositional language. At the same time, further evaluation of patients with known lesions is needed to elucidate cerebral structure-function correlations of the different types of nonpropositional language in both production and comprehension modalities.

6. References

Alajouanine, T. (1956). Verbal realization in aphasia. *Brain, 79*, 1–28.

Andreasen, N. (1977). Reliability and validity of proverb interpretation to assess mental status. *Comprehensive Psychiatry, 18*, 465–472.

Benson, D. F. (1979). Aphasia, alexia and agraphia. New York: Churchill Livingston.

Benton, A. (1968). Differential behavioral effects in frontal lobe disease. *Neuropsychologia, 6*, 53–60.

Bever, T. G. (1975). Cerebral asymmetries in humans are due to the differentiation of two compatible processes: Holistic and analytic. *Annals of the New York Academy of Science, 263*, 251–262.

Boatner, M. T., Gates, J. E., & Makkai, J. E. (1975). *A dictionary of american idioms*. New York: Barron's Educational Series, Inc.

Bogen, J. E. (1969). The other of the brain. II: An appositional mind. *Bulletin of the Los Angeles Neurological Societies, 3, 4*, 191–219.

Bogen, J. E. (1973). Movie of a hemispherectomy patient and what it all means. UCLA Conference of Cerebral Dominance, Los Angeles.

Bogen, J. E. & Gordon, H. (1971). Musical tests for functional lateralization with intracarotid amobarbitol. *Nature, 230.5295*, 524–525.

Bolinger, D. (1976). Meaning and memory. *Forum Linguisticum, 1*, 1–14.

Boller, F., Cole, M., Vrtunski, P., Patterson, M., & Kim, Y. (1979). Paralinguistic aspects of auditory comprehension in aphasia. *Brain and Language, 7*, 164–174.

Bradshaw, J. L. & Nettleton, N. C. (1983). *Human cerebral asymmetry*. Englewood Cliffs, N. J.: Prentice-Hall, Inc.

Brownell, H. H., Michel, D., Powelson, J. A., & Gardner, H. (1983). Surprise but not coherence: Sensitivity for verbal humor in right hemisphere patients. *Brain ánd Language, 18*, 20–27.

Brownell, H. H., Potter, H. H., Bihrle, A. M., & Gardner, H. (1986). Inference deficits in right brain-damaged patients. *Brain and Language, 27*, 310–312.

Brownell, H. H. & Gardner, H. (1988). Neuropsychological insights into humor. In J. Duraut & J. Miller (Eds.), *Laughing matters. 17–34*. Essex: Longman Scientific.

Bryden, M. P. (1982). Laterality: *Functional asymmetry in the human brain*. New York: Academic Press.

Butler, S. & Norrsell, N. (1968). Vocalization possibly initiated by the minor hemisphere. *Nature, 220*, 793–794.

Chafe, W. (1968). Idiomaticity as an anomaly in the Chomskyan paradigm. *Foundations of Language, 4*, 109–127.

Chomsky, N. (1957). *Syntactic structures*. The Hague: Mouton.

Clark, H. H. (1979). Responding to indirect speech acts. *Cognitive Psychology, 11*, 430–477.

Code, C. (1987). *Language, aphasia and the right hemisphere*. Chichester: John Wiley.

Critchley, M. (1962). Speech and speech loss in relation to the duality of the brain. In V. Mountcastle (Ed.), *Interhemispheric relations and cerebral dominance. 208–213*. Baltimore: Johns Hopkins University Press.

Critchley, M. (1970). *Aphasiology and other aspects of language*. London: Edward Arnold, Ltd.

Crockett, H. G. & Estridge, N. M. (1951). Cerebral hemispherectomy. *Bulletin of the Los Angeles Neurological Societies, 16*, 71–87.

Cummings, J. (1982). Cortical dementias. In D. F. Benson and D. Blumer (Eds.), *Psychiatric aspects of neurologic disease. 93–121.* New York: Grune and Stratton.

Cummings, J. (1985). *Clinical neuropsychiatry.* Orlando: Grune and Stratton.

Cummings, J. & Benson, D. F. (1983). *Dementia: A clinical approach.* Boston: Butterworths.

Cummings, J., Benson, D. F., Walsh, M. J. & Levine, H. L. (1979). Left-to-right transfer of language dominance: A case study. *Neurology, 29,* 1547–1550.

Czopf, J. (1981). Über die Rolle der nicht dominanten Hemisphäre in der Restitution der Sprache der Aphasischen. *Archiv für Psychiatrie und Nervenkrankheiten, 216,* 162–171.

De Bleser, R., Poeck, K. (1985). Analysis of prosody in the spontaneous speech of patients with CV-recurring utterances. *Cortex, 21,* 405–416.

Delis, D., Kramer, J., & Kaplan, E. (1984). *The California proverb test.* Unpublished protocol. Copyright.

Dronkers, N. F. (1984). The role of syntax in automatic speech processing. Paper presented at the 22nd Meeting of the Academy of Aphasia, Los Angeles, California.

Eisenson, J. (1962). Language and intellectual findings associated with right cerebral damage. *Language and Speech, 5,* 49–53.

Ellis, A. W., Young, A. W., & Critchley, E. M. R. (1989). Intrusive automatic or nonpropositional inner speech following bilateral cerebral injury: A case report. *Aphasiology, 3,* 581–585.

Espir, L. & Rose, F. (1970). *The basic neurology of speech.* Oxford: Blackwell Scientific Publications.

Fillmore, C. (1979). On fluency. In C. J. Fillmore, D. Kempler, & S.-Y. Wang (Eds.), *Individual differences in language ability and language behavior.* 85–103. New York: Academic Press.

Foldi, N. S., Cicone, M., & Gardner, H. (1983). Pragmatic aspects of communication in brain-damaged patients. In S. J. Segalowitz (Ed.), *Language functions and brain organization. 51–86.* New York: Academic Press.

Gazzaniga, M., Sidtis, J., Volpe, B., Smylie, C., Holtzman, J., & Wilson, D. (1982). Evidence for paracallosal verbal transfer after callosal section. *Brain, 105,* 53–63.

Geschwind, N., Quadfasel, F., & Segarra, J. (1968). Isolation of the speech area. *Neuropsychologia, 6,* 327–340.

Gibbs, R. W., Jr. (1980). Spilling the beans on understanding and memory for idioms in conversation. *Memory and Cognition, 8,* 149–156.

Gibbs, R. W. Jr. & Gonzales, G. P. (1985). Syntactic frozenness in processing and remembering idioms. *Cognition, 20,* 243–259.

Gibbs, R. W., Jr. & Nayak, N. (1989). Psycholinguistic studies on the syntactic behavior of idioms. *Cognitive Neuropsychology, 21,* 100–138.

Gibbs, R. W. Jr., Nayak, N., & Cutting, C. (1989). How to kick the bucket and not decompose: Analyzability and idiom processing. *Journal of Memory and Language, 28,* 576–593.

Gorham, D. R. (1956). A Proverbs Test for clinical and experimental use. *Psychological Reports, 1,* 1–12.

Grafman, J. (1989). Plans, actions, and mental sets: Managerial knowledge units in the frontal lobes. In E. Perecman (Ed.), *Integrating Theory and Practice in Clinical Neuropsychology. 93–138.* New Jersey: Lawrence Erlbaum.

Graves, R. & Landis, T. (1985). Hemispheric control of speech expression in aphasia: A mouth asymmetry study. *Archives of Neurology, 42,* 249–251.

Hier, D. B. & Kaplan, J. (1980). Verbal comprehension deficits after right hemisphere damage. *Applied Psycholinguistics, 1,* 279–294.

Hillier, N. E. (1954). Total left hemispherectomy for malignant glioma. *Neurology, 4,* 718–721.

Hopper, P. (1987). Emergent grammar. *Berkeley Linguistic Society, 13.* Berkeley, CA.

Horowitz, L. M. & Manelis, L. (1973). Recognition and cued recall of idioms and phrases. *Journal of Experimental Psychology, 100,* 291–296.

Ingvar, D. H. & Schwartz, M. S. (1974). Blood flow patterns induced in dominant hemisphere by speech and reading. *Brain, 79,* 273–288.

Jackson, J. H. (1878). On affections of speech from disease of the brain. *Brain, 1,* 304–330. (Reprinted in J. Taylor (Ed.), *Selected writings of John Hughlings Jackson.* New York: Basic Books, Vol. 2, 1958.)

Jackson, J. H. (1915). Affections of speech from disease of the brain. *Brain, 38,* 106–174.

Jaffe, J. (1978). Parliamentary procedure and the brain. In A. W. Siegman & S. Feldstein (Eds.), *Nonverbal behavior and communication. 55–66.* Hillsdale, N. J.: Erlbaum.

Jaynes, J. (1976). The origin of consciousness in the breakdown of the bicameral mind. Boston: Houghton-Mifflin Company.

Jespersen, O. (1965). *The philosophy of grammar.* New York: Norton.

Kempler, D. (1990). Language changes in dementia of the Alzheimer type, to appear. In R. Lubinski (Ed.), *Dementia and communication: Research and clinical implications.* Philadelphia: Decker.

Kempler, D. & Van Lancker, D. (1985). *The Familiar and Novel Language Comprehension test* (FANL-C). Unpublished; copyright.

Kempler, D., Van Lancker, D., & Read, S. (1988). Comprehension of proverbs and idioms in Alzheimer patients. *Journal of Alzheimer Disease and Associated Disorders, 2,* 38–49.

Kempler, D. & Van Lancker, D. (1992). Familiar phrases, second-language learning and the brain.

In F. R. Eckman (Ed.), *Linguistics, Second Language Aquisition and Speech-Language Pathology.* New York: John Benjamin, in press.

Kinsbourne, M. (1971). The minor cerebral hemisphere as a source of aphasic speech. *Transactions of the American Neurological Association, 96,* 141 – 145.

Knopman, D. S., Rubens, A. B., Selnes, O. A., Klassen, A. C., & Meyer, M. W. (1984). Mechanisms of recovery from aphasia: Evidence from serial xenon 133 cerebral blood flow studies. *Annals of Neurology, 15,* 530 – 535.

Kreindler, A. & Fradis, A. (1968). *Performances in aphasia.* Paris: Gautier-Villars.

Landis, T., Cummings, J. L., & Benson, D. F. (1980). Le passage de la dominance du language a l'hemishere droit: Une interpretation de la recuperation tardive lors d'aphasies globales. *Revue de la Suisse Romande, 100,* 171 – 177.

Larson, L. B., Skinhoj, E., & Lassen, N. A. (1978). Variation in regional cortical blood flow in the right and left hemisphere during automatic speech. *Brain, 101,* 198 – 209.

Lassen, N. A., Ingvar, D. H., & Skinhoj, E. (1978). Brain function and blood flow. *Scientific American, 239,* 62 – 71.

Levy, J., Nebes, R. D., & Sperry, R. W. (1971). Expressive language in the surgically separated minor hemisphere. *Cortex, 7,* 49 – 58.

Lyons, J. (1968). *Introduction to theoretical linguistics.* Cambridge, England: The University Press.

Molloy, R., Brownell, H., & Gardner, H. (1990). Discourse comprehension by right-hemisphere stroke patients: Deficits of prediction and revision. In Y. Joanette & H. Brownell (Eds.), *Discourse ability and brain damage: Theoretical and empirical perspectives.* 113 – 130. New York: Springer Verlag Publishers.

Myers, P. S. (1979). Profiles of communication deficits in patients with right cerebral hemisphere damage: Implications for diagnosis and treatment. In: R. Brookshire (Ed.), *Clinical Aphasiological Conference Proceedings. 38 – 46.* Minneapolis: BRK Publishers.

Myers, P. S. & Linebaugh, C. W. (1981). Comprehension of idiomatic expressions by right-hemisphere-damaged adults. In Brookshire (Ed.), *Clinical aphasiology proceedings.* 254 – 261.

Naeser, M. A., Gaddie, A., Palumbo, C., & Stiassny-Eder, D. (1990). Late recovery observed with subcortical temporal isthmus lesion vs Wernicke's cortical area lesion. *Archives of Neurology, 47,* 425 – 432.

Navon, D. (1977). Forest before trees: The precedence of global features in visual perception. *Cognitive Psychology, 9,* 353 – 383.

Osgood, C. & Hoosain, R. (1974). Salience of the word as a unit in the perception of language. *Perception and Psychophysics, 15,* 168 – 192.

Papanicolaou, A. C., Moore, B. D., Deutsch, G., Levin, H. S., & Eisenberg, H. M. (1988). Evidence for right-hemisphere involvement in recovery from aphasia. *Archives of Neurology, 45,* 1025 – 1029.

Papanicolaou, A. C., Moore, B. D., Levin, H. S., & Eisenberg, H. M. (1987). Evoked potential correlates of right hemisphere involvement in language recovery following stroke. *Archives of Neurology, 44,* 521 – 524.

Pappadis, T. 1990. Personal communication.

Pawley, A. & Syder, F. H. (1983). Two puzzles for linguistic theory: Nativelike selection and nativelike fluency. In J. C. Richards & R. Schmidt (Eds.), *Communicative competence.* 191 – 225. London: Longmans.

Ryding, E., Bradvik, B., & Ingvar, D. (1987). Changes of regional cerebral blood flow measured simultaneously in the right and left hemisphere during automatic speech and humming. *Brain, 110,* 1345 – 1358.

Simon, H. A. (1974). How big is a chunk? *Science, 183,* 482 – 488.

Sidtis, J. J., Volpe, B., Holtzman, J., Wilson, D., & Gazzaniga, M. (1981). Cognitive interaction after staged callosal section: Evidence for transfer of semantic activation. *Science, 212,* 344 – 346.

Sidtis, J. J., Volpe, B. T., Wilson, D. H., Rayport, M., & Gazzaniga, M. S. (1981). Variability in right hemisphere language function after callosal section: Evidence for a continuum of generative capacity. *Journal of Neuroscience, 1,* 323 – 331.

Smith, A. (1966). Speech and other functions after left (dominant) hemispherectomy. *Journal of Neurology, Neurosurgery, and Psychiatry, 29,* 467 – 471.

Smith, A. (1974). Dominant and nondominant hemispherectomy. In M. Kinsbourne & L. Smith (Eds.), *Hemisphere disconnection and cerebral function.* 37 – 68. Springfield, Illinois: Chas. E Thomas.

Stuss, D. T. & Benson, D. F. (1984). Neuropsychological studies of the frontal lobes. *Psychological Bulletin, 95,* 3 – 28.

Stuss, D. T. & Benson, D. F. (1986). *The frontal lobes.* New York: Raven Press.

Swinney, D. A. & Cutler, A. (1979). The access and processing of idiomatic expressions. *Journal of Verbal Learning and Verbal Behavior, 18,* 523 – 534.

Tyler, S. A. (1978). *The said and unsaid.* New York: Academic Press.

Van Lancker, D. (1973). Language lateralization and grammars. In J. P. Kimball (Ed.), *Studies in syntax and semantics.* 197 – 204. New York: Seminar Press.

Van Lancker, D. (1975). *Heterogeneity in language and speech: Neurolinguistic studies.* UCLA Working Papers in Phonetics 29, Los Angeles.

Van Lancker, D. (1979). Review of Julian Jaynes, "The origin of consciousness in the breakdown of the bicameral mind," *Forum Linguisticum*, IV, 72–91, August.

Van Lancker, D. (1987). Nonpropositional speech: Neurolinguistic studies. In A. E. Ellis (Ed.), *Progress in the psychology of language. 49–118.* Vol. III. Hillsdale, NJ: Lawrence Erlbaum Associates.

Van Lancker, D. (1990 a). The neurology of proverbs. *Behavioral Neurology, 3*, 169–187.

Van Lancker, D. (1990 b). A case of deep dysgraphia attributed to right hemisphere function. Academy of Aphasia, Baltimore, MD, October.

Van Lancker, D (1991). Personal relevance and the human right hemisphere. *Brain and Cognition, 17*, 64–92.

Van Lancker, D., Canter, G. J., & Terbeek, D. (1981). Disambiguation of ditropic sentences: Acoustic and phonetic cues. *Journal of Speech and Hearing Research, 24*, 330–335.

Van Lancker, D. & Kempler, D. (1987). Comprehension of familiar phrases by left- but not by right-hemisphere damaged patients. *Brain and Language, 32*, 265–277.

Van Lancker, D. & Klein, K. (1990). Preserved recognition of familiar personal names in global aphasia. *Brain and Language, 39*, 511–529.

Van Lancker, D., Lanto, A., Klein, K., Riege, W., Hanson, W., & Metter, E. J. (1991) Preferential representation of personal names in the right hemisphere. *Clinical Aphasiology, 20*, 181–189.

Van Lancker, D. & Rorabaugh, A. (1990). Preserved nonpropositional speech in a patient with multiple sclerosis. Unpublished.

Weinreich, U. (1969). Problems in the analysis of idioms. In J. Puhvel (Ed.), *Substance and structure of language*. 23–82. Los Angeles, California: University of California Press.

Weylman, S. T., Brownell, H. H., Roman, M., & Gardner, H. (1989). Appreciation of indirect requests by left- and right-brain-damaged patients: The effects of verbal context and conventionality of wording. *Brain and Language, 36*, 580–591.

Whitaker, H. (1976). A case of the isolation of the language function. In H. Whitaker and H. A. Whitaker (Eds.), *Studies in neurolinguistics: Vol. 2.* 1–58. New York: Academic Press.

Winner, E. & Gardner, H. (1977). The comprehension of metaphor in brain-damaged patients. *Brain, 100*, 719–727.

Zaidel, E. (1981). Reading by the disconnected right hemisphere: A perspective from the normal brain. In U. Kirk (Ed.), *Neuropsychology of language, reading and spelling*. Academic Press, New York, in press.

Zaidel, E. (1982). Reading by the disconnected right hemisphere: an aphasiological perspective. In Y. Zotterman (Ed.), *Dyslexia: neuronal, cognitive and linguistic aspects. 67–91.* Wenner-Gren Symposium Series, Vol. 35. Proceedings of an International Symposium held at the Wenner-Gren Center, Stockholm, June 3–4, 1980. Oxford: Pergamon Press.

Diana Van Lancker, Los Angeles, California (USA)

20. Repetitive Phenomena in Aphasia

1. Introduction

Involuntary repetition of speech segments is a fairly frequent occurrence in the verbal output of people having suffered brain damage. These patients may unintentionally repeat all or part of their own utterance or that of their speech partner. Various types of repetitive verbal behavior can therefore be distinguished on the basis of the speech segment which is repeated and the conditions under which the repetition takes place.

2. Stereotypy or Recurrent Utterance

Probably the most striking form of repetition is stereotypy or recurrent utterance. A stereotypy is a speech segment which occurs over and over again in the patient's output. Indeed, apart from interjections (such as *ha* or *er*), and a few occasional words, the patient produces nearly exclusively his particular stereotypy. This severe reduction of expressive speech has been appropriately termed 'monophasia' by Critchley (1970, 8).

The recurrent utterance in monophasia may be a syllable, a word, a neologism, a phrase, or even a complete sentence, which may or may not be anomalous. For instance, Broca's famous patient Leborgne said virtually nothing but /tã/ (Broca 1861). After repeated strokes the active vocabulary of the Russian revolutionist Lenin was reduced to the word *vot*, which means something like *look here* or *that's it* (Lebrun/Hasquin/Zouboff 1982). At the end of his life, the French poet Charles Baudelaire could only say *cré nom nom*, which was probably a debased form of the French expletive (*sacré*) *nom de Dieu* (Lebrun/Brihaye/Flament 1971). A patient of Critchley's (1970, 206) always said *on the booze*, and another *yes today*. Smith (1974) had a patient whose stereotypy was *a big house*. And for some time the French writer Valéry Larbaud could only say *Bonsoir les choses d'ici-bas* (Alajouanine 1968, 75).

A small percentage of patients have two or even three stereotypies instead of just one. For example, a monophasic patient of Hughlings Jackson's (1880) alternated between *jimmy*, *jin* and *jigger*, and a patient observed by Blanken and co-workers between /nau/ and /de:s/ (Blanken/Wallesch/Papagno 1990).

When the stereotypy is a syllable, it is generally repeated several times in a row whenever the patient attempts to express himself. More often than not, syllabic stereotypies have a simple consonant-vowel (CV) or consonant-vowel-consonant (CVC) structure. The initial consonant is frequently a plosive (Code 1982).

Stereotypies are not always uttered in the same way. They may undergo temporary phonemic variations. A Flemish patient of Lebrun's (1986) whose stereotypy was /masti:kə/ sometimes produced this neologism as /pasti:kə/. And a patient of Blanken and co-workers produced several different varieties of his stereotypy, such as /vɛdi/, /vidi/, /vɛti/ or /viri/ (Blanken/Wallesch/Papagno 1990).

2.1. Prosody

Stereotypies are not always uttered in the same tone of voice. In fact, pitch variations can often be observed in the patient's recurrent strings. Speech rate and vocal intensity may also vary. It is not at all clear, however, whether these prosodic features match the speaker's mood. It is equally uncertain whether monophasic patients utilize rising or falling intonations intentionally, among other things as a marker distinguishing questions from statements.

A number of aphasiologists, including Alajouanine/Lhermitte (1964), have expressed the view that patients with monophasia become particularly clever at using intonation to convey meaning: they skillfully modulate their stereotypy to have it express various needs, thoughts, or feelings.

Those who live with a monophasic relative hardly ever confirm this optimistic view. Rather, they find it hard to understand the patient, even though he intonates his recurrent utterance. For instance, in a letter to a friend, the mother of Charles Baudelaire reported that her son had repeatedly tried to tell her something about one of his books. But she could not grasp what his stereotypy was conveying, modulated though it was (Lebrun/Hasquin/Brihaye/Flament 1971).

As a matter of fact, a study by De Bleser/Poeck (1985) shows that monophasics tend to use a limited repertoire of intonation patterns. In aphasia with recurrent utterance, then, lexical poverty is not compensated for by enhanced use of suprasegmentals.

Monophasic patients never seem to have difficulty in uttering their stereotypy. They produce it easily, smoothly, and without apparent effort. The pronunciation is not laboured or distorted. The stereotypy is fluent. However, patients may insert a pause filler at various places in the monophasic strings they produce, as if they are having a temporary word-finding difficulty or are groping for the correct verbal formulation.

2.2. Repetition Test

As a rule, the verbal output of monophasic patients is the same in conversation as in repetition. They generally produce their stereotypy not only in attempts to communicate verbally but also when requested to reproduce the words of their speech partner. Only a few monophasic patients perform better in imitative speech than in conversation.

Interestingly, when the stereotypy is produced during a repetition task, the length of the stereotypic response often exceeds the length of the stimulus. For instance, having been requested to repeat the sentence *J'ai mangé de la viande* (= I ate (some) meat), a French-speaking patient of Lebrun's (1986) said *te te tet*, *te tet*, *te te te tet*, *te te te te tet te te te tet te te te tets* (commas indicate short pauses).

Of course, in such a case one can never be sure that the patient is simply attempting to repeat the test sentence. He may be trying to add some comment or to make a remark.

It should be pointed out, however, that when the stereotypy consists of a syllable, it is rarely produced individually, even in response to questions which would normally be answered with just *yes* or *no*. This seems to indicate that even though the stereotypy appears to be a syllable, it does not function like a syllable. Or at any rate it is not substituted for each of the successive syllables that would make up the correct answer.

On the other hand, when the stereotypy comprises several different syllables, these syllables usually cannot be produced in isolation. For instance, a patient of Bazire's quoted by Hughlings Jackson (1880) always said *sapon*. This man could not be made to say either *sap* or *pon*.

The same holds true for the real words which make up some recurrent utterances. A German patient of Liepmann's (1900, 119) could say nothing but *das kann ich nicht sagen* (= I can't say that). Liepmann never succeeded in having the patient say *das kann ich* (= I can do it). The patient proved unable to intentionally produce only the first three words of her stereotypy.

The observation that the patient is generally unable to break up his stereotypy may be one of the reasons why some authors consider stereotypes to be speech automatisms.

2.3. Written Expression

Stereotypies appear to be restricted to oral language, as no patient has ever been observed who would produce a written stereotypy when trying to express himself in writing. Monophasics' attempts at written communication usually result in illegible scribble. Some patients, however, manage to write a few words. But none have been found to produce an invariable string of letters repeated several times whenever they seek to communicate in writing (see also Blanken 1991).

2.4. 'Mitigated Monophasia'

Some patients exhibit what might be called 'mitigated monophasia'. Under a number of circumstances they are able to suppress their stereotypy and to produce a more appropriate response. For instance, a patient of Kremin's (1986) could adequately answer simple questions with *yes* or *no*. In addition, he was able to repeat isolated words and groups of two words. Further, in the confrontation naming test he would often produce approximations of the target words. However, when he attempted to speak of his own accord, he usually produced his stereotypy only.

2.5. Etiopathology

The etiopathology of the stereotypy is a matter of debate. As early as 1880 Hughlings Jackson offered an explanation for the phenomenon. He suggested that the stereotypy corresponds to the word(s) which the patient was saying or was about to say when the cerebral damage occurred. Hughlings Jackson reasoned that the lesion must have blocked the cerebral speech mechanisms to an extent which could no longer be reversed. If the stereotypy was a neologism, one had to assume that in addition to freezing the speech mechanisms, the lesion had also disturbed them.

In support of his view Hughlings Jackson adduced several clinical cases. For instance, he mentioned a woman who was taken ill while riding a donkey and whose subsequent stereotypy was *gee gee*. He assumed that she was hastening her mount when the stroke occurred.

Hughlings Jackson also mentioned "a clerk who lost speech and became paralyzed on one side, after hard work in making a catalogue: this poor fellow could only say *list complete*." A third patient could say nothing but *I want protection*. This man had incurred a cerebral trauma in a fistfight.

Hughlings Jackson's view has been adopted by many aphasiologists, although it fails to account for the fact that a number of monophasic patients change their stereotypy in the course of time. Hughlings Jackson himself (1880) described a man whose recurrent utterance was at first *dick*. After some time this stereotypy was replaced by *jimmy*, *jin* and *jigger*, used alternately. In addition, the patient would shout *bugger* when angry. Another of Hughlings Jackson's patients at first said only *wo wo* and later only *pooh pooh* (Hughlings Jackson 1874).

The theory does not provide an explanation for such changes. Neither does it explain why the stereotypy sometimes undergoes temporary phonemic variations, as in /masti:kə/ → /pasti:kə/ or /vɛdi/ → /vidi/ → /vɛti/ → /viri/.

Another observation which is difficult to reconcile with Hughlings Jackson's view is the gradual occurrence of monophasia. In children with Landau-Kleffner's syndrome, the initial aphasia may progressively evolve into monophasia as a case reported by van Dongen and co-workers shows. Their patient was a 4-year-old girl who gradually lost her active vocabulary. Eventually she became unable to say anything except /tytyt/ (Van Dongen/Van Harskamp/Loonen 1977). This progressive reduction of expressive speech to a stereotypy does not fit in well with Hughlings Jackson's etiological explanation, which implies sudden freezing of the cerebral speech mechanisms in an unalterable state.

Last but not least, in a number of cases the stereotypy appears to be not the word or phrase which the patient was using or was about to use at the moment he incurred cerebral damage, but rather the first word or phrase he uttered following a period of complete speechlessness. Critchley (1970, 208) described a woman who, "totally aphasic and in bed after her stroke, saw her daughter fiddle with her jewel-case on the dressing table. She got upset and called out *That's mine*. Thereafter the phrase *that's mine* became her recurrent utterance."

As a matter of fact, the etiopathology of stereotypy is still poorly understood. It is not clear why a number of brain-damaged patients constantly produce the same speech segment when attempting to express themselves orally. It is also uncertain to what extent these patients are conscious of their repetitive verbal behavior (Lebrun 1987).

3. Echolalia

Another repetitive behavior which can severely disrupt verbal communication is echolalia. Echolalia is the involuntary repetition of all or part of the speech partner's utterance.

The condition is referred to as 'complete echolalia' when the patient repeats the whole utterance of his speech partner. It is said to be incomplete or partial, when he repeats only part of it. In partial echolalia, it is usually the end of the partner's utterance which is repeated.

The echolalia is considered pure when the patient repeats verbatim. It is considered mitigated if he changes some of the words. The changes in mitigated echolalias usually affect personal pronouns and verb endings, as when a patient echoes *How old are you*? with *How old am I*?

In their echolalic responses some patients tend to correct minor grammatical or articulatory errors made intentionally or unintentionally by the speech partner. Such corrections may be made even by patients who usually fail to react to verbal instructions and therefore seem to have severe comprehension difficulties.

The echolalic response may immediately follow the stimulus or on the contrary take place some time later. One accordingly distinguishes between immediate and delayed echolalias.

At times the echolalic reproduces not only the partner's words but also his intonation. Also, the echolalia may begin before the patient's vis-à-vis has finished his utterance.

Some patients echo only the words which are addressed to them, others tend to also repeat verbal messages which are not directed to them.

In some cases the echolalic response is compulsive. The patient cannot help repeating the partner's words even if he totally disagrees with them. Schneider (1938) has reported the case of a 76-year-old woman who following a stroke in the left hemisphere had very little spontaneous speech and compulsively repeated the words which were adressed to her even when she utterly disapproved of them. For instance, when the examiner once said to her *You murdered your mother*, she reacted with *Oh, Oh! You murdered your mother No! No!* Similarly, she could not help repeating obscene words, but showed her deep disapproval by a facial expression of disgust.

Generally, patients whose echolalic behavior is compulsive, repeat foreign words even if they do not understand them. In some cases, their reproduction of the foreign accent is strikingly correct.

Some echolalic patients have virtually no sponteanous speech; thus they rarely express themselves verbally. When spoken to, they either remain silent or repeat (some of) the words that have been addressed to them. However, they may be able to sing whole stanzas from popular songs when prompted by the examiner or when the examiner hums the tune while they are singing. In a case observed by Geschwind and co-workers, the patient was even able to learn new songs which were played to her (Geschwind/Quadfasel/Segarra 1968).

Some patients are clearly aware of their echolalic behavior, even though they cannot repress it. Others appear not to be aware of their echolalias. Some obviously understand the words from their mother-tongue which they forcibly echo, others seem to repeat the words without comprehending them (Lebrun/Rubio/Jongen/Demol 1971).

3.1. Completion Phenomenon

When the examiner utters only the first part of an idiom or a popular expression, the echolalic patient, when familiar with the entire phrase, tends to produce the rest of it instead of repeating the beginning. For instance, when Whitaker (1976) once said to her echolalic patient "I wish you a Merry ...", the patient replied: "Christmas." This behavior is known as the completion phenomenon. The drift to complete may be as irrepressible as the drift to repeat.

Rubens (1975) has reported the case of an aphasic patient who had very little spontaneous verbal output. She was not echolalic but could not help completing well-known phrases or popular song titles when the first words were pronounced in her presence. For instance, on hospital rounds, doctors often greeted her with the question *How are things*?, and she would invariably respond with *in Glocca Morra*, thus reproducing the title of a song from a popular musical comedy. When other open-ended phrases were furnished she would shake her head in exasperation and would grimace, yet could not remain silent despite explicit instructions to the contrary. She was unable to refrain from completing unfinished phrases.

3.2. Echo-Answer

Some echolalic patients retain the ability to express themselves verbally, but in conversation frequently repeat questions before answering them. In addition, they tend to give echo-answers. An echo-answer is a verbal response in which words from the question are superfluously repeated, as when the patient answers the question *Do you live in a flat*? with *I live in a flat, yes.*

In itself, an echo-answer is not a pathological occurrence. Like mitigated echolalias, echo-answers can be observed in normal speech. Their frequency is relatively low, however, and they are always deliberate. On the contrary, in aphasic speech, they may be very frequent. Moreover, they appear unintentional, if not incoercible. Also, the patient may be unable to effect the necessary grammatical changes, as when the question *Is this your coat*? is answered with *Yes, this is your coat*, instead of *Yes, this is my coat*.

4. Contamination

At times patients inadvertently reproduce only one of the words spoken by their partners, substituting it for the appropriate word in their own utterance. Such interference is called 'contamination'. At some point in the utterance the patient's lexical choice is contaminated or defiled by the interlocutor's words.

At times the patient's choice of words is influenced not by the terms themselves which his partner uses, but by their meaning. For instance, a patient who had just been asked whether he liked movies on television and had answered negatively, was next asked what he liked to watch on television. He answered films, while he in fact meant *news bulletins*. He selected the word *films* under the influence of the word *movies* used by the examiner.

Lexical choice may even be swayed by environmental nonverbal factors. This was obviously the case in the following example. During a naming task a brain-damaged patient was presented a pair of scissors. At that very instant, water audibly flowed through a pipe in the corner of the room, and the patient called the scissors *water*.

Occasionally, contaminations may also be observed in the verbal output of healthy speakers. Certain kinds of slips of the tongue are nothing other than contaminations. As in pathological discourse, they may be literal or semantic. A German example of the former was recorded by Meringer/Mayer (1895, 45):

- Speaker A: Was soll man denn lesen? (= What should one read?)
- Speaker B: Ja, das muss man überlesen (instead of *überlegen*, i.e. One should think about it).

An example of semantic contamination was reported by Fromkin (1973, 262):

- Speaker A: When are going to have the ale?
- Speaker B: With the beer (instead of *With the dinner*)

In normal speech, contaminations are infrequent. Moreover, healthy speakers can always correct themselves when they notice a slip of the tongue or when their attention is drawn to it. On the contrary, brain-damaged patients may be unable to correct their error. In attempts to amend their utterance, they may involuntarily repeat the mistake. When patients keep repeating an erroneous word in successive attempts to correct themselves, they are in fact making a perseveration.

5. Perseveration

A perseveration consists of the inappropriate recurrence or continuance of a particular behavior. It is unintentional, and the patient may or may not be aware of his perseverative behavior.

Perseverations may occur under a variety of circumstances. For instance, the patient may react in a certain way to a stimulus and then reproduce this behavior in reaction to the next stimulus which would in fact require a different response. The classical example is that of a patient who is first asked what his name is. He says his name and is then asked where he lives. Instead of stating his address he says his name again.

A similar form of perseveration may also occur in writing. Allison/Hurwitz (1967) have published the written responses of a patient who was first asked to write his name, which he laboriously did, producing *John*. He was then requested to write his address and he wrote *John* again.

The perseveration is not always immediate. In a task involving a succession of stimuli the patient may very well repeat a response which was given several items earlier. A study by Santo Pietro/Rigrodsky (1986) shows that sometimes the stimulus which elicits a non-immediate perseveration is semantically related to the perseverate or begins with the same phoneme(s).

A perseveration may be transfered from one task to another even if the two tasks are different in nature. Buckingham (1985) described a patient who had been asked whether she had any children. She responded with a description of familial relations that was full of semantic paraphasias of kinship terminology. She was then asked whether there were lights in the room and she answered *Uh, two brother children?* To the next question *Are you in a hotel now?* her response was *No. Have any children, you said?* A repetition task ensued, in which the word *children* continued to be perseverated:

- (Chair) *Two children ... jazz children*
- (Nose) *Two children*
- (Pipe) */bra/ children*
- (Snowball) *Two children*
- (The telephone is ringing) *There's so many children ... seven children*
- (The spy fled to Greece) *Seventy-five girls or boys, did you say?*

The next test was a sentence completion task. The word *children* recurred in the patient's first answer:

- (Christmas is in the month of ...) Thirty-two children.

In this example, the perseverate *children* occurred for the first time in an answer about the patient's family. Indeed, the word had been used by the examiner himself in his question about the patient's progeny. Therefore, the first occurrence of *children* in the patient's output was probably adequate. This is not always the case, however. The first occurrence of the perseverate may be inappropriate. For instance, one day Buckingham's patient (1985) was asked to name the picture of a hand. She responded with *more drink, drink*. The word *drink* perseverated throughout the rest of the visual naming test. Its first occurrence was just as inadequate as the subsequent ones.

In serial tasks such as the picture naming test, it may happen that the patient can give no answer when a picture of, say, a bear is shown, but later on repeatedly produces the word *bear* in response to other stimuli.

At times the perseverate does not replace the correct response but blend with it. After he had been shown the picture of a fountain-pen and had named it *A kind of pen*, a patient examined by Allison/Hurwitz (1967) was shown the picture of a watch, which he called *A pen ... no ... your pen for telling the time*. In a similar test, Santo Pietro/Rigrodsky's patient (1986) correctly named a picture of a woman and a little later called a picture of a church a *churchwoman*.

Such blends are not infrequent in patients with reading and visual naming difficulties. An alexic patient of Caplan/Hedley-White (1974) gave the following answers in a picture naming test:

"(Picture of a bus) *A map, no, I know it, of course, ought to be able to say it. Not a map. (What do you do with it?) It's a road, you use it on a road. (Is it a chair, is it a car, is it a horse, is it a bus?) No. (Is it a bus?) It could be a bus, yes, yes, that's what it is, a bus.*

(Picture of a belt) *Like a map, no, I know what it is, I can't say it. (What do you do with it?) You measure something with it. (Is it a tape measure?). No. (Is it a belt?) Yes, more like a belt.)*

(Picture of a banana) *Fruit, it's a measure, no. (What do you do with it?) Eat it. (Is it an apple, a prune, a pear, a banana?) No. (Is it a banana?) No, more like a pineapple.*

(Picture of a bathtub) *It's for water, you measure water with it, a sink, no you have it near a sink like a faucet, a drain, it has another name, I know. (What do you do with it?) Take a bath in it, wash. (Is it a bathtub?) Yes, it could be, yes.*

(Picture of a cane) *It's a drain, a sink, no like a sink. (What do you do with it?) It's a ... (Is it a cane, a bed, a chair?) No. (Is it a cane?) No.*

(Picture of a cigarette) *A water, it's a water, it's a shadow, a shade. (What do you do with it?) I can't tell you. (Is it a horse, a cigarette, a chair?) No. (Is it a cigarette?) It might be a cigarette.*

(Picture of a clock) *A shade, it's a shade, I know what it is, a shade (Is it a floor, a table, a clock?) No, it's a shade."*

At times there may be some doubts as to whether the patient is making a verbal perseveration or is having a visual perseveration. Being shown a picture of a razor, the alexic patient of Lebrun/Devreux (1984) answered *A fountain-pen, a ballpoint.* Next a picture of a toothbrush was presented and she said *Fountain-pen, something to write with.* This answer allows of two interpretations. The patient may have perseverated the compound *fountain-pen* and its semantic field, *something to write with*, substituting them for the appropriate verbal response. But she may equally well have meant *fountain-pen* because she thought she was looking at a picture of a fountain-pen. In other words, she may have had a visual perseveration. She may have mistaken the razor for a fountain-pen and have had the impression that the next picture also represented something to write with.

That she did have visual perseverations at times seems beyond doubt, as she once named a picture of a pair of scissors adequately and then, being shown a picture of a knife, said *These are also scissors.* Similarly, the patient of Lhermitte/Beauvois (1973), after he had been shown a picture of a wrist watch and had named it correctly, was shown a picture of a pair of scissors, which he called *wrist watch again.*

Some patients, then, have visual perseverations in addition to making verbal perseverations. Therefore, it may at times be difficult to ascertain whether one is confronted with an instance of efferent or an instance of afferent perseveration (Lebrun/De Vreese 1991).

The tendency to make verbal perseverations may vary with the task the patient engages in. Santo Pietro/Rigrodsky (1982) found that their aphasic subjects perseverated more when they had to supply the last word of a sentence presented by the examiner or to name pictures, than when they had to read a list of isolated words aloud. Moreover, in each test the number of perseverations decreased when the time interval between successive stimuli was increased from 1 to 10 seconds. A patient of Denes and co-workers made far less perseverations when naming, or pointing to, body parts than when naming, or pointing to, pictures (Denes/Dalla Barba/Cipolotti/Semenza 1990).

Not only words but also parts of words or even single phonemes may be perseverated. For instance, in a naming-on-confrontation task, jargonaphasic patients may produce a succession of distorted or neologistic responses all beginning with the same phoneme(s), as in the following example recorded by Santo Pietro/Rigrodsky (1986):

– (Church) /sərtʃ/
– (Pumpkin) /sʌmpən/
– (Broom) /sum/
– (Harp) /sarp/
– (Owl) /saul/

Verbal perseveration may also occur in the absence of a new stimulus. Within an utterance, a speech segment may be unduly repeated and possibly substituted for the appropriate item.

Perseverations within utterances are frequent in neologistic jargonaphasia, where they often take the form of alliterations and assonances, also called *clang associations.* Many such alliterative and assonantic strings occurred in the verbal output of the patient with poly-infarct dementia and neologistic jargonaphasia described by Lebrun/Devreux/Rousseau (1987), e. g. /õe lak pãsã vẽsẽ bazãfã de bally bella babjẽ bjẽsy sãlwi/.

Strings of phonologically related neologisms are sometimes observed during partial seizures. Bell and co-workers described a patient who would utter reiterative non-words during epileptic fits. Afterwards she proved amnesic for the attack as well as for her perseveratory verbal behavior (Bell/Horner/Logue/Radtke 1990).

If the partial seizure occurs while the patient is writing, he may start producing strings of words or neologisms containing obvious repetitions. The patient is generally unaware of this deviant production. As an example, an excerpt from a letter written by a French-speaking female and published by Souques

(1928) may be quoted: "je vous remercions mercions davoir d'avoir dat vous d'avions a davoir davons vous etrions davons enrions vous irons ce que vous donniez en derrière ou vous donnez lirez en vous orniez ayez de vous de vous etiez de vez en ayez en ayez envoyez".

Perseverations may occur not only in neologistic but also in semantic jargon. In semantic jargonaphasia, the perseverate is usually an identifiable word, as in: "I don't hear you talking. I know you're talking, but I'm not talking you like I can talk you 'bout. I can see you talking that way. That's if I'm talking when I'm ... I see you talking that way then if I'm talking my head."

Buckingham (1985), who tape recorded this jargonaphasic utterance, argues that it is not mere verbigeration. On the contrary, the patient was actually trying to communicate. In fact, she had a peripheral hearing loss and was explaining that she could not hear her interlocutor well. The first two occurrences of the word *talking* therefore seem appropriate. But when it occurred for the third time it was probably substituted for *hearing* and, at the end of the utterance it appears to have replaced *turning* (the patient probably meant that when turning her better ear to the partner, she could hear him better).

Word perseverations may also occur in writing. Hughlings Jackson (1880) has published the following letter written by one of his patients: "I feel very well just know for Hurst Row I feel very well just now for thing in the first way for the thamk now. I know now I was in the first now in the first now in the Newington Road. I keep you first way in Newington Road the poor way is the best way for me is the best way for me is the best way for me is the best way the way is the best for me for ways kept for me for kept ways kept me for way kept for me."

In this case it is not at all clear what the patient was trying to impart. Indeed, it is uncertain whether at the end of the letter the perseverates stand for other words or whether the patient was unable to stop the action of writing in due time and for a while produced words involuntarily in the absence of communicative intent. If this was actually the case, then his letter is an instance of what Goldberg (1986) has called the 'interminability of verbal monologue'.

Perseverations may at times be observed in the speech of aphasic patients when they try to correct themselves. Lebrun and co-workers have mentioned a French-speaking patient with conduction aphasia who answered the question *What's your daughter's occupation?* With /kwafyz/. She in fact wanted to say /kwafyʀ/, i. e. *coiffure* (= hairdressing). Noticing her phonemic paraphasia, she attempted to correct herself but could only say /kwafyz/ again. This happend 5 times in succession. Thus, she could not help repeating her error each time she tried to correct it (Lebrun/Rétif/Kaiser 1983).

Perseverations may occasionally occur in normal speech and in normal writing. Healthy language users may inadvertently duplicate a verbal segment which they have just been using, or substitute it for the one they should use next. The perseverate may be a phoneme (or a grapheme), a part-word or a word. An example of this is a slip of the tongue recorded by Garrett (1980): *The juice is still on the table. Is that enuice?* (instead of *enough*). At times it is the semantic content which is perseverated, as in *Bel Paese with biscuits or cheese* instead of ... *or bread* (Fromkin 1973). Usually healthy speakers can easily correct their perseveration, when they notice it.

5.1. Typology

Many aphasiologists distinguish between two types of perseverations. The first type is usually called a 'repetitious' or 'recurrent perseveration'. It consists of the inappropriate repetition of all or of part of a previous behavior after some intervening event. The intervening event may be a different behavior by the patient or renewed stimulation by the partner.

When the intervening event is a new stimulus to which the patient reacts with his previous response, some aphasiologists speak of 'immediate perseveration'. When, on the contrary, the patient produces some language before he makes a perseveration, the latter is said to be 'delayed'. Shindler and her coworkers used the word *intrusion* to refer to delayed perseverations occurring after several intervening stimuli (Shindler/Caplan/Hier 1984).

Repetitious perseverations are sometimes referred to as 'intentional perseverations', because they occur during deliberate attempts to produce spoken or written language. The term may be misleading, though, as it may suggest that the perseveration itself is volitional, whereas actually an "intentional perseveration is the unintentional repetition of a previously emitted response when a new response is intended" (Sandson/Albert 1984).

Though correct, this definition sounds somewhat like a 'contradictio in terminis'.

The second type of perseveration is usually called 'continuous'. It consists of the inappropriate continuation of an action beyond the point of completion. The patient fails to terminate his activity although the purpose has been achieved. For instance, when asked to write the letter *O*, the patient draws several *O*'s on top of each other, since he is unable to end his circular writing movement in due time.

Goldberg/Tucker (1979) have called this type of perseveration 'hyperkinetic perseveration'. While there is some sense in calling 'hyperkinetic' an action which is continued beyond the point of completion, confusion may result from the fact that the adjective is also frequently used to refer to a disorder causing disruptive and often purposeless over-activity in children.

The stroke and letter duplications made by a number of right-brain damaged patients (for examples, see Lebrun 1976; 1980; 1983; 1985) are sometimes construed as continuous perseverations. The patients, it is thought, are unable to inhibit their graphomotor behavior in time and involuntarily produce several *e*'s or several *o*'s in succession, or add supernumerary down-strokes to their *n*'s or *m*'s.

This explanation does not seem to be adequate, however. For one thing, these patients make not only stroke and letter duplications but also stroke and letter deletions. Obviously, these omissions cannot be regarded as perseverations. Moreover, there is no indication that the patients have any difficulty in ending movements. In fact, it has been shown (Lebrun/Rubio 1972; Lebrun 1976; 1985) that stroke and letter reduplications and omissions in the writing of right-brain damaged patients are due to a disturbance of the visual and kinesthetic control of writing. The patients can no longer accurately ascertain how many strokes or letters they have already drawn, especially in sequences of similar strokes, as in *n* or *m*, or of similar loops, as in *ee* or *oo*. Far from resulting from a defect in motor behavior, their reduplications and omissions result from a faulty processing of incoming spatial data.

Sandson/Albert (1984) distinguish a third type of perseveration, which they call 'stuck-in-set perseveration'. It consists of the inappropriate maintenance of a framework and can sometimes be observed when two tasks are given in succession. In the first task the patient follows the instructions as given. In the second task, he continues to apply these instructions although new ones have been given. For instance, a patient of De Vreese/Motta/Toschi/Vecchi (1988) was first asked to turn active into passive sentences, which he did. He was then asked to turn positive into negative sentences. He turned them into passive sentences instead.

On the other hand, a number of aphasiologists do not distinguish between word contamination and word perseveration. Some of them use the compound *word intoxication* to refer to both types of repetitions. Actually, a perseveration is an auto-contamination. Moreover, patients who make perseverations also tend to make contaminations. From a patho-physiological point of view the two phenomena are probably closely related.

5.2. Palilalia

A particular form of continuous perseveration is called palilalia. A palilalia is the incoercible repetition of an utterance, or a large chunk of it, several times in a row. For instance, a palilalic patient of Boller/Boller/Denes et al. (1973), who had been asked why he had stopped working, said *I was tired, I was tired, I was tired, yes sir, yes sir, yes sir.* Asked what he did all day, his answer was *I stay at home all the time, all the time, all the time* (Boller/Boller/Denes et al. 1973).

The successive repetitions may take place with increasing speed and end up in *cluttering*. However, such *festination* is not always observed. The rate of delivery may very well remain constant throughout the palilalia.

Vocal volume may decrease as the palilalia takes it course. Indeed, the final repetitions may be whispered. But this is not always so. The vocal volume may remain unchanged from the beginning to the end of the palilalia. Palilalias whose end is whispered are sometimes called 'aphonic palilalias'.

At times the number of repetitions is quite impressive. A palilalic patient of Sterling's (1924) who had been asked whether he felt any pain, answered *No pain* and repeated this answer 15 times in succession.

The palilalic tendency may affect all forms of oral expression or only some of them. The patient of Boller and co-workers made palilalias in conversational speech but not when reading aloud or when singing. In serial speech he showed no palilalia within over-learned series but would often produce the required series several times in a row. Palilalia was present in imitative speech and increased in severity with the length of the utterance to be reproduced (Boller/Boller/Denes et al. 1973). A patient seen by Helm (1979), although severely palilalic in conversational speech, produced no palilalias when generating lists of words, such as names of animals. The patient of Trénel/Crinon (1912) was palilalic in conversational and in imitative speech as well as in the naming-on-confrontation test, but not when she read aloud, sang, or said her prayers.

Some patients are totally unable to suppress their palilalias. Others can do so for a while but it requires great effort. Still others can speak without palilalia only when using a instrument like the pacing board designed by Helm (1979). This board enables the patient to speak slowly, a syllable at a time, and thus to overcome his otherwise irrepressible tendency to palilalia.

Palilalia is a speech disturbance which may occur in the absence of any significant aphasia, but it may be associated with dysarthria, as in Foix/Schulmann's case (1915) or in the second case of Boller/Albert/Denes (1975). The tendency to palilalia may also be concomitant with a tendency to echo-answers as in a case reported by Souques (1928), to echopraxia, as in the patients described by Trénel/Crinon (1912) and by Dupré/Le Savoureux (1914), or to palipraxia, as in Foix/Schulmann's case (1915).

In a number of patients the palilalic behavior occurs only during seizures without loss of consciousness. The patient then repeats the sentence he was uttering when the seizure began. During the paroxysmal palilalia, speech may be produced with gradually decreasing force or may be slurred. Usually the patient is aware of his palilalic behavior but cannot control it.

At times, a paroxysmal palilalia is observed in patients who were silent when the seizure began. Falconer (1967) mentioned a patient who kept repeating *I beg your pardon* during fits. At the same time he was unresponsive to the outside world. Afterwards he had no recollection of the attack or his palilalic behavior.

A patient of Van Bogaert's (1934) had seizures during which she could answer questions but only in a palilalic way. She would give a short response and repeat it up to 20 times in a decreasing tone of voice.

Some time later, she started to have nocturnal fits. She would be found sitting up in her bed. She was staring at the ceiling and repeating a phrase or sentence. The fit could last up to two hours. The phrase or sentence varied from spell to spell but could always be related to some event in the patient's family life.

The patient remained conscious during these seizures. She was aware of her palilalias, but she could not stop them.

Involuntary repetition of a message or of a chunk of it may also take place in written language. The deviance is called 'paligraphia'. An instance of paligraphia has been reported by Lebrun/Devreux/Rousseau (1986). Their patient, who had progressive supranuclear palsy and micrographia, was once requested to write his telephone number. He scribbled the number 26 times on end. He realized what he was doing but commented afterwards that he could not stop writing.

Palilalia and paligraphia do not necessarily co-occur.

5.3. Iteration

Yet another form of continuous perseveration is iteration. Ideally, an iteration differs from a palilalia in that it involves a shorter segment which is repeated a smaller number of times. Typically in palilalia sentences or phrases are repeated several times, if not many times, on end, whereas in iterations, phonemes, part-words or words are repeated a few times in succession.

However, in quite a number of cases the distinction between palilalia and iteration is blurred, as patients tend to repeat short speech segments a great number of times. For instance, the patient of Lebrun/Devreux/Rousseau (1986) once continued to repeat the French negation *ne* for 2 min. and 24 sec. And the patient of LaPointe/Horner (1981) explained the saying *Look before you leap* as "You should look, look, look, look in, look in, look in, you should, you should look in ... ($\pm$ 52 repetitions) ... you should, you should, you should look, look, look into, into, into things, things, things before, before, before you go, you go, you go, you go into them."

When a short speech segment is repeated involuntarily a few times in succession, the iteration resembles what is commonly observed in developmental stuttering. Accordingly, continuous perseverations of phonemes, part-words or words are often called *stutter-like repetitions*.

Stutter-like repetitions are frequently observed in transcortical motor aphasia. As Luria (1970, 178) pointed out, in severe cases, the patient does not get passed the first word or first syllable which he helplessly repeats.

Iterations may sometimes be produced experimentally. Brickner (1940) has reported that electrical stimulation of the left supplementary motor cortex caused a patient of his to iterate letters during recitation of the alphabet. The iteration would last as long as the current was applied. When the stimulation was withdrawn, the patient continued reciting normally.

5.4 Neurogenic Stuttering

The speech of some brain damaged adults evidence not only iterations but also blocks and prolongations which often result from the involuntary continuance of an articulatory position such as lip closure or tongue elevation. The co-occurrence of these three perseveratory features following brain damage is generally referred to as neurogenic stuttering.

Neurogenic stuttering may mimic developmental stuttering so closely that the two conditions cannot be reliably distinguished on the basis of their symptomatology alone (Lebrun/Leleux/Rousseau/Devreux 1983; Lebrun 1991).

In a number of cases, neurogenic stuttering is concomitant with aphasia. However, the two disorders are relatively independent of one another, as one disorder may clear up while the other persists (Lebrun/Leleux/Rousseau/Devreux 1983).

5.5. Logoclonia

Fairly long repetitions of a single syllable or of a short word or short neologism are not uncommon in advanced degenerative or multi-infarct dementia. For instance, one of the 4 demented patients described by Lebrun/Devreux/Rousseau (1987) once said /ʒəʒə ʒəʒəʒəvələkələʒəʒə ʒiʒiʒiʒi fəvəvələ/.

Such iterations are often produced rapidly and without apparent effort and are usually referred to as logoclonias.

5.6. Etiopathology of Perseveration

Various explanations have been propounded for the phenomenon of perseveration. Some researchers have incriminated attention, which is known to be often defective in brain-damaged individuals.

Others have accounted for perseveration as lack of inhibition. They have reasoned that patterns of behavior which have been activated cannot be quickly switched off again and therefore tend to supersede patterns which should be called into play (repetitious perseveration) or to continue beyond the completion of the task (continuous perseveration).

In this view, perseveration is a primary disturbance. It is the lack of inhibition that causes the displacement of the adequate response by the perseverate. The opposite opinion also exists, however, especially regarding verbal perseveration. It is believed by some that verbal perseveration often results from anomia or verbal dysmnesia. The appropriate verbal item cannot be accessed and is substituted for by an item which has just been used and is therefore more rapidly accessible. In this view, perseveration is the consequence of a primary word-finding difficulty.

Liepmann (1905, 126) thought that this applied particularly to intentional perseverations. He assumed that as the current of excitation could not reach the desired pattern, it deviated to a pattern which had just been used and whose threshold of activation was therefore lowered.

In Goldstein's opinion (1948, 18) the secondary substitution was more or less deliberate, for the avoidance of a distressing failure: "We consider perseveration as a means utilized by the organism to avoid catastrophe."

Some authors hold, on the contrary, that every new activated pattern spontaneously tends to inhibit the patterns previously used. If a given pattern cannot be accessed, there is no activation and consequently no inhibition, and previously excited patterns tend to recur.

None of these views has been adequately substantiated so far. Theories of the origin of perseveration remain highly conjectural.

Partial explanations have also been offered. For instance, it has been submitted that in transcortical motor aphasia, stutter-like iterations result from a disturbance of the dynamics of speech production. The patient, it is assumed, is unable to effect a quick transition from one pattern to the next. He maintains the pattern just used instead of proceeding to the next, thus repeating the utterance instead of producing novel speech.

On the other hand, repetitious perseverations, and particularly intrusions, when they occur in word list generation, are sometimes ascribed to a defect of memory. The patient, it is thought, mentions a given item a second time because he has forgotten that this item was already mentioned a little earlier in the list.

At times, metaphors have been used in lieu of explanations. For example, as quoted by Hughlings Jackson (1880), Gairdner compared patients with severe perseverations to street musicians operating barrel organs. Once the patient has produced a given response, he monotonously reproduces it many times; it continues to recur in his speech as a leitmotiv. Buckingham/Whitaker/Whitaker (1979) have published a striking case of what Hughlings Jackson called 'barrel-organism':

- Patient: *I can see and everything, but it's funny. I can't – uh – I can't say it. It's sort of funny ... but I can't say it. It's hard to ... you now ... but I don't know, it's funny. It's a funny – uh – ... I can't – uh – know why it makes you feel ... funny.*
- Clinician: *Do they have television here?*
- Patient: *Yeah, but i's funny – uh – funny way. You can't ... uh ... it's a funny – uh – such a – uh – so funny.*
- Clinician: *But you see things all right.*
- Patient: *Yeah. I understand. Yeah, but it's funny. I just can't tell you, it's sort of funny.*

6. Conclusions

It appears that the pathogenesis of repetitive phenomena in aphasia is still poorly understood. It is not clear whether a common mechanism underlies the various clinical forms of involuntary repetitions. Perhaps some forms occur only when several factors are simultaneously present, whereas other forms have a simpler etiology. It is also possible that different patients produce repetitive speech for different reasons. Obviously, more research based on careful observation of individuals with repetitive (verbal) behaviors is needed.

7. References

Alajouanine, T. (1968). *L'aphasie et le langage pathologique*. Paris: Baillière.

Alajouanine, T. & Lhermitte, F. (1964). Non-verbal communication in aphasia. In A. De Reuck & M. O'Connor (Eds.), *Disorders of language. 168–177*. London: Churchill.

Allison, R. & Hurwitz, L. (1967). On perseveration in aphasics. *Brain, 90*, 429–448.

Bell, W., Horner, J., Logue, P., & Radtke, R. (1990). Neologistic speech automatisms during complex partial seizures. *Neurology, 40*, 49–52.

Blanken, G. (1991). The functional basis of speech automatisms (recurring utterances). *Aphasiology, 5*, 103–127.

Blanken, G., Wallesch, C., & Papagno, C. (1990). Dissociations of language functions in aphasics with speech automatisms (recurring utterances). *Cortex, 26*, 41–63.

Boller, F., Albert, M., & Denes, F. (1975). Palilalia. *British Journal of Disorders of Communication, 10*, 92–97.

Boller, F., Boller, M., Denes, G., Timberlake, W., Zieper, I., & Albert, M. (1973). Familial palilalia. *Neurology, 23*, 1117–1125.

Brickner, R. (1940). A human cortical area producing repetitive phenomena when stimulated. *Journal of Neurophysiology, 3*, 128–130.

Broca, P. (1861). Remarques sur le siège de la faculté de langage articulé, suivies d'une observation d'aphémie (perte de la parole). *Bulletin de la Société d'Anatomie, 6*, 330–357.

Buckingham, H. (1985). Perseveration in aphasia. In S. Newman & R. Epstein (Eds.), *Current perspectives in dysphasia. 113–154*. Edinburgh: Churchill Livingstone.

Buckingham, H., Whitaker, H., & Whitaker, H. (1979). On linguistic perseveration. In H. Whitaker & H. Whitaker (Eds.), *Studies in neurolinguistics 4. 329–352*. Orlando: Academic Press.

Caplan, L. & Hedley-Whyte, R. (1974). Cuing and memory dysfunction in alexia without agraphia. *Brain, 97*, 251–262.

Code, C. (1982). Neurolinguistic analysis of recurrent utterance in aphasia. *Cortex, 18*, 141–152.

Critchley, M. (1970). *Aphasiology and other aspects of language*. London: Arnold.

De Bleser, R. & Poeck, K. (1985). Analysis of prosody in the spontaneous speech of patients with CV-recurring utterances. *Cortex, 21*, 405–415.

Denes, G., Dalla Barba, G., Cipolotti, L., & Semenza, C. (1990). An unusual case of perseveration sparing body-related tasks. *Cortex, 26*, 269–273.

De Vreese, L., Neri, M., Motta, M., Toschi, A., & Vecchi, G. (1988). The right hemisphere syndrome and Alzheimer's disease: A case report. In A. Agnoli, J. Cahn, N. Lassen, & R. Mayeux (Eds.), *Senile dementias. Second International Symposium. 71–74*. Paris: John Libbey Eurotext.

Dupré, E. & Le Savoureux, X. (1914). Palilalie chez une pseudo-bulbaire. *Revue Neurologique, 25*, 453–456.

Falconer, M. (1967). Brain mechanisms suggested by neurophysiological studies. In F. Darley & C. Millikan (Eds.), *Brain mechanisms underlying speech and language. 185–203*. New York: Grune & Stratton.

Foix, C. & Schulmann, X. (1915). A propos d'un cas de palilalie. *Revue Neurologique, 26*, 779–782.

Fromkin, V. (1973). *Speech errors as linguistic evidence*. The Hague: Mouton.

Garrett, M. (1980). Levels of processing in sentence production. In B. Butterworth (Ed.), *Language production. 177–195*. London: Academic Press.

Geschwind, N., Quadfasel, F., & Segarra, J. (1968). Isolation of the speech area. *Neuropsychologia, 6*, 327–340.

Goldberg, E. (1986). Varieties of perseveration: A comparison of two taxonomies. *Journal of Clinical and Experimental Neuropsychology, 8*, 710–726.

Goldberg, E. & Tucker, D. (1979). Motor perseveration and long-term memory for visual forms. *Journal of Clinical Neuropsychology, 1*, 273–288.

Goldstein, K. (1948). *Language and language disturbances*. New York: Grune & Stratton.

Helm, N. (1979). Management of palilalia with a pacing board. *Journal of Speech and Hearing Disorders, 44*, 350–353.

Helmick, J. & Berg, C. (1976). Perseverations in brain injured adults. *Journal of Communication Disorders, 9*, 143–156.

Hughlings Jackson, J. (1874). On the nature of the duality of the brain. *Medical Press and Circular, 1*, 19–41.

Hughlings Jackson, J. (1880). On affections of speech from disease of the brain. *Brain, 2*, 203–220, 323–251.

Kremin, H. (1986). Is there more than Ah-oh-oh? Alternative strategies for writing and repeating lexically. In M. Coltheart, R. Job, & G. Sartori (Eds.), *The cognitive neuropsychology of language. 295–335*. London: Erlbaum.

LaPointe, L. & Horner, J. (1981). Palilalia: A descriptive study of pathological reiterative utterances. *Journal of Speech and Hearing Disorders, 46*, 34–38.

Lebrun, Y. (1976). Neurolinguistic models of language and speech. In H. Whitaker (Ed.), *Studies in neurolinguistics 1. 1–30*. New York: Academic Press.

Lebrun, Y. (1980). Reading, writing and drawing disorders due to right brain damage. *Acta Neurologica Latino-americana, 26*, 223–237.

Lebrun, Y. (1983). Cerebral dominance for language: A neurolinguistic approach. *Folia Phoniatrica, 35*, 13–39.

Lebrun, Y. (1985). Disturbances of written language and associated abilities following damage to the right hemisphere. *Applied Psycholinguistics, 6*, 231–260.

Lebrun, Y. (1986). Aphasia with recurrent utterance: A review. *British Journal of Disorders of Communication, 21*, 3–10.

Lebrun, Y. (1987) Anosognosia in aphasics. *Cortex, 23*, 251–263.

Lebrun, Y., Bijleveld H., & Rousseau J. (1991). A case of persistent neurogenic stuttering following a missile wound. *Journal of Fluency Disorders, 15*, 251–258.

Lebrun, Y. & De Vreese, L. (1991). Pure alexia. In M. Joshi (Ed.), *Written language disorders. 105–126*. Dordrecht: Kluwer.

Lebrun, Y. & Devreux, F. (1984). Alexia in relation to aphasia and agnosia. In R. Malatesha & H. Whitaker (Eds.), *Dyslexia: A global issue. 191–209*. The Hague: Nijhoff.

Lebrun, Y., Devreux, F., & Rousseau, J. (1986). Language and speech in a patient with clinical diagnosis of progressive supranuclear palsy. *Brain and Language, 27*, 247–256.

Lebrun, Y., Devreux, F., & Rousseau, J. (1987). Disorders of communicative behavior in degenerative dementia. *Folia Phoniatrica, 39*, 1–8.

Lebrun, Y., Hasquin, J., Brihaye, J., & Flament, J. (1971). L'aphasie de Charles Baudelaire. *Revue Neurologique, 125*, 310–316.

Lebrun, Y., Leleux, C., Rousseau, J., & Devreux, F. (1983). Acquired stuttering. *Journal of Fluency Disorders, 8*, 323–330.

Lebrun, Y., Rétif, J., & Kaiser, G. (1983). Acquired stuttering as a forerunner of motor-neuron disease. *Journal of Fluency Disorders, 8*, 161–167.

Lebrun, Y. & Rubio, S. (1972). Réduplications et omissions graphiques chez des patients atteints d'une lésion hémisphérique droite. *Neuropsychologia, 10*, 249–251.

Lebrun, Y., Rubio, S., Jongen, E., & Demol, O. (1971). On echolalia, echo-answer and contamination. *Acta Neurologica Belgica, 71*, 301–308.

Lebrun, Y. & Zouboff, A. (1982). L'aphasie chez les grands: Baudelaire et Lénine. *Médecine et Hygiène, 40*, 429–442.

Lhermitte, F. & Beauvois, M. (1973). A visual-speech disconnexion syndrome. *Brain, 96*, 695–714.

Liepmann, H. (1900). Das Krankheitsbild der Apraxie (motorische Asymbolie). *Monatsschrift für Psychiatrie und Neurologie, 8*, 15–44, 102–132, 182–197.

Liepmann, H. (1905). *Über Störungen des Handelns bei Gehirnkranken*. Berlin: Karger.

Luria, A. (1970). *Traumatic aphasia*. The Hague: Mouton.

Luria, A. (1977). *Neuropsychological studies in aphasia*. Lisse: Swets & Zeitlinger.

Meringer, R. & Mayer, K. (1895). *Versprechen und Verlesen*. Stuttgart: Göschen.

Rubens, A. (1975). Aphasia with infarction in the territory of the anterior cerebral artery. *Cortex, 11*, 239–250.

Sandson, J. & Albert, M. (1984). Varieties of perseveration. *Neuropsychologia, 22*, 715–732.

Santo Pietro, M. & Rigrodsky, S. (1982). The effects of temporal and semantic conditions on the occurrence of the error response of perseveration in adult aphasics. *Journal of Speech and Hearing Research*, *25*, 184–192.

Santo Pietro, M. & Rigrodsky, S. (1986). Patterns of oral-verbal perseverations in adult aphasics. *Brain and Language*, *29*, 1–17.

Schneider, D. (1938). The clinical syndrome of echolalia, echopraxia, grasping and sucking. *Journal of Mental and Nervous Disease*, *88*, 18–35.

Shindler, A., Caplan, L., & Hier, D. (1984). Intrusions and perseverations *Brain and Language*, *23*, 148–158.

Smith, M. (1974). Operant conditioning of syntax in aphasia. *Neuropsychologia*, *12*, 403–405.

Souques, A. (1928). Note sur les troubles de l'écriture pendant les absences épileptiques et sur l'intérêt psychologique et médico-légal de ces troubles. *Revue Neurologique*, *39*, 353–360.

Sterling, W. (1924). Palilalie et le symptome 'linguo-salivaire' dans le parkinsonisme encéphalitique. *Revue Neurologique*, *35*, 205–220.

Trenel, X. & Crinon, Y. (1912). Palilalie chez une pseudo-bulbaire. *Revue Neurologique*, *23*, 676–680.

Van Bogaert, L. (1934). Ocular paroxysms and palilalia. *The Journal of Nervous and Mental Disease*, *80*, 48–61.

Van Dongen, H., Van Harskamp, F., Loonen, M. (1977). Verworven afasie bij kinderen. *Nederlands Tijdschrift voor Geneeskunde*, *121*, 813–816.

Whitaker, H. (1976). A case of the isolation of the language function. In H. Whitaker & H. Whitaker (Eds.), *Studies in neurolinguistics 2. 1–58.* New York: Academic Press.

Yvan Lebrun, Brussels (Belgium)

21. Aphasia and Models of Language Production and Perception

1. Introduction

Models, in the sense of (comparatively) explicit accounts of some set of phenomena, often embodied in a diagram, or more recently in a computer programme, have been enormously influential in the development of science. The history of psychology is littered with the corpses of models, many of which have led brief, but useful, lives – interpreting old data, or motivating the discovery of new phenomena – before being fatally wounded in a fierce exchange of rhetoric.

In the history of aphasiological studies one model – the Wernicke-Lichtheim diagram (Lichtheim 1885) – has shown remarkable resilience, despite suffering accurate sniper fire (Freud 1891) and heavy pounding (Head 1926), since its publication. In a variety of guises, it continues to loom in the background of our thinking on aphasia and still forms an important basis for our principal diagnostic categories (e.g. Goodglass/Kaplan 1972).

In this chapter I will compare Lichtheim's model with a modern variant, and discuss some of the advantages of working with models of this type, and some of the disadvantages.

2. Lichtheim's Model

Lichtheim's model was a development of Wernicke's (1874) analysis of the anatomy and functional architecture of language processing. It was revolutionary for its time in several quite different ways. It proposed an explicit information-processing account, with distinct 'centres', or what we would call nowadays, 'components' or 'isolable subsystems' (Shallice 1984), each of which was a specialised repository for a particular type of information and carried out a different information transduction.

It was moreover formulated as a directed graph in which the direction of the flow of information was not only defined but also critical to the predictions made by the model. In addition to all this, it was an attempt to synthesise information processing with anatomy in that particular bits of cortex supported the information processing components, and particular transcortical or subcortical tracts were held to be the neutral substrate of the connexions between the components.

Even by modern standards, it is a sophisticated and detailed account of a wide range of known aphasic phenomena. But it was designed to go further than a redescription of available data: It defined syndromes in terms of damage to components of the model, exactly in the way that neuropsychologists nowadays are meant to, rather than simply as co-occurring symptoms. As Lichtheim (1885, 435) himself wrote,

> "The morbid types I intend to discuss ... have been determined, in as far as they are new, deductively: it was the task of clinical observations to test the validity of the inferences."

2.1. Dissociations

The model stressed the importance of dissociations rather than associations. This was a major methodological breakthrough, though not one appreciated by all workers in the area (e. g. Head 1926). Further, Lichtheim used single patient data to test and to modify the model when the data failed to conform to predictions derived from the model.

2.2. Inferences from the Standard Wernicke-Lichtheim Model

The usual form of the Lichtheim diagram is given in Figure 21.1. (corresponding to his Figure 1). The numbered lines represent points of potential damage — "interruptions" in Lichtheim's terminology — whose consequences are interpretable by reference to the

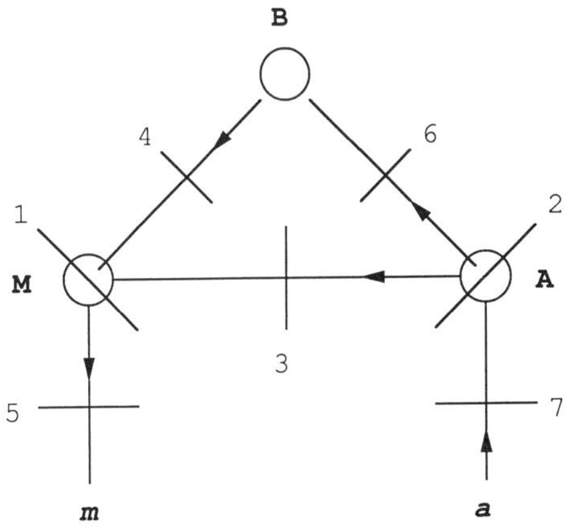

Fig. 21.1: Lichtheim's original diagram. See text for explanation (Redrawn from Lichtheim 1885, Figure 1)

model. (It is important to remember that information flow models don't do anything! They simply describe the information exchange arrangements. This is as true for modern 'box and arrow' models, as those of the past century, as will be seen below. To derive predictions about data, or to account for data in terms of this type of model, requires a rich metatheoretical interpretative apparatus, much of which will be tacit.)

Lichtheim's model distinguished in the modern manner between an input store of lexical information (auditory word images) from an output store (motor word images) (but see Allport/Funnell 1981; Butterworth 1983). A distinct expressive syndrome could thus arise from selective damage (Line 1) to the output store located in Broca's area, while a receptive syndrome could arise from selective damage (line 2) to the input store (located in what is now known as Wernicke's area). Of course, part of the predictive value of the model would be saved even if the anatomical basis of the syndromes turned out to be at fault. The differentiation between receptive and expressive difficulties was entailed by the model on the basis of information flow among component information transducers, as well as, but independently from, the anatomical locale of the components.

An important feature of the model, indeed of the whole approach, was that it was designed to predict and explain new patterns of deficit. If well-known sets of co-occurring symptoms could be explained in terms of damage to an element in the model, then the finding of new syndromes could be expected based on the selective damage of other elements in the model, in particular those held to arise from lesioning the connexions between centres. Again like the modern models that 'lesion' computer simulations (e. g. Hinton/Shallice 1991), the anatomical claims can be differentiated logically from the behavioural claims.

These 'disconnexion' syndromes required new tests to reveal quite a different set of critical symptoms, where a symptom is as importantly a spared function as a deficit. The fundamental point here is the overall pattern of deficient and spared functions.

Historically, the most important symptom was the impairment or the sparing of repetition. The model held that there existed a subcortical connexion between the auditory word images in Wernicke's area and the motor word images in Broca's area that mediated the exact repetition of heard speech, the lesioning of which (line 3) would lead to deficits on this task without other receptive or expressive difficulties. A repetition impairment, even if it had been tested previously, would have been quite obscure without this model; a selective sparing of repetition in the absence of comprehension or volitional speech in the 'transcortical' syndromes discussed below would have been even more obscure.

2.3. Levels of Deficit

The model was able to distinguish in principled way what we might now call levels of deficit. Thus speech production can be impaired because there is an impairment at the level of concepts (Centre B in the diagram), in a manner not fully explicated by Wernicke or his followers, but presumably such a deficit would affect the comprehension as well as the production of speech.

It could also be impaired on the route from concepts to Broca's area. This would produce the syndrome known as 'transcortical motor aphasia', in which concepts and comprehension are intact, repetition will be intact, as will the ability to enunciate words in, for example, a reading aloud task, but the selection of words in spontaneous speech will be affected. Actually, Lichtheim (unlike Wernicke) believed that concepts were not found in a single centre, like the motor word images, but were a set of entities spread over a considerable region of the cortex with the connexions converging on Broca's and Wernicke's area. This allowed him to predict that this type of disconnexion aphasias will be more severe the closer the lesion is to Broca's area (or to Wernicke's area) since the same sized lesion will sever more connexions. See Figure 21.2.

At a lower level, Broca's area and hence motor word images will be affected, leading, it is claimed, to effortful speech. Here repetition problems are of a kind predictable from the speech output deficit, while comprehension will be intact. Praxic and arthric difficulties will arise through damage to the peripheral route to the vocal musculature M *m* (in Fig. 21.1.).

Similarly, levels of impairment in comprehension are predictable from the model. Thus an interruption on route *a*A (in Fig. 21.1.) should result in 'pure word deafness' – a total inability to recognise a word without hearing impairment, while damage to the auditory word images in Wernicke's area should

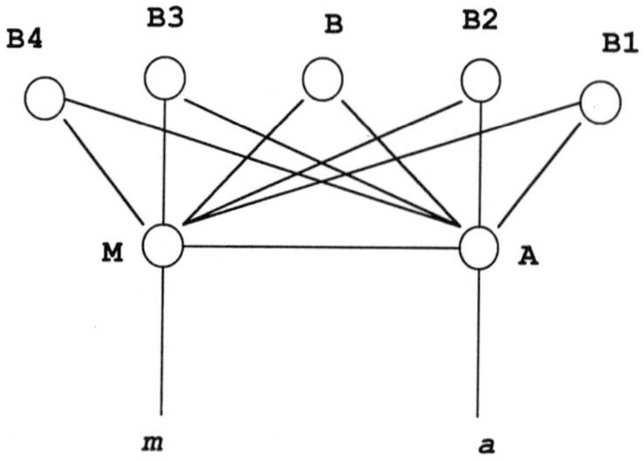

Fig. 21.2: The single concept centre, B ("Begriffe"), is replaced by concepts distributed over the cortex. (Redrawn from Lichtheim 1885, Figure 7)

result in poor word recognition, with concomitant difficulties in repetition and word understanding (with speech intact); while lesioning the pathways A B to concepts will leave repetition and word recognition intact, but with poor word comprehension ('transcortical sensory aphasia'), and as can be seen from Fig. 21.2., lesions close to Wernicke's area should yield a more severe version of this syndrome.

2.4. Lichtheim's Account of Disorders of Reading and Writing

Less familiar perhaps to most students of aphasia are Lichtheim's attempts to integrate reading and writing disorders into his scheme. It had been well-known at least since Jackson's (1879) investigations, that if writing were perfectly preserved in the absence of speech, then some kind of core language production function must be intact and that the problem must lie at a more peripheral locus. Similar arguments can be made for the sparing of reading comprehension in the absence of spoken language understanding. Figure 21.3. (Lichtheim's Figure 2) shows his first provisional version of the relation between reading ("O"), writing ("E") and the other language functions.

Lichtheim saw very clearly the necessity for specifying functional relations between the subcomponents of his system. He postulated that the meaning of a written word depended on the prior elicitation of its 'auditory image'.

> "Reading postulates the existence of visual memories of letters and groups of letters. We may learn to understand writing through the connection between such visual representations (centre O [in Figure

21.3.]) and auditory representations: by spelling aloud we bring the auditory centre into action, and thus establish a connection, through the path O A, between O and B; in reading aloud, the tract O A M *m* is thrown into activity." (Lichtheim 1885, 437)

While modern authors would like to see some experimental evidence to support this idea, Lichtheim appeared to believe that some kind of armchair task analysis ("self-observation") or armchair developmental psychology would suffice where clinical evidence was lacking. Of course, the kinds of experimental evidence available to us, but not always employed by neuropsychologists, just were not available to Lichtheim. Nevertheless the basic idea that the meaning of a read word depends on first activating its pronunciation, still has currency in attempts to model normal skilled reading (e. g. van Orden 1987).

2.5. The Theoretical Significance of Writing Disorders

A revealing test of Lichtheim's methodological approach centres on writing. The plausible account offered in Figure 21.3. was based in part on armchair task analysis, but was supported by many observations of patients with Broca-like difficulties with speech output. Certainly modern views, as we shall see, correspond with the arrangements presented in Figure 21.3.

On the other hand, if this is the route to writing, then writing difficulties should be deducible from speech difficulties. Thus Wernicke patients, with paraphasic output, should produce comparable paragraphic writing. However, the problem arises from a famous case of Wernicke's in which the patient's speech recovered while difficulties of comprehension and agraphia persisted. Lichtheim thus modified the model so that the connection M E disappears and is replaced by the path M A E in Figure 21.4.

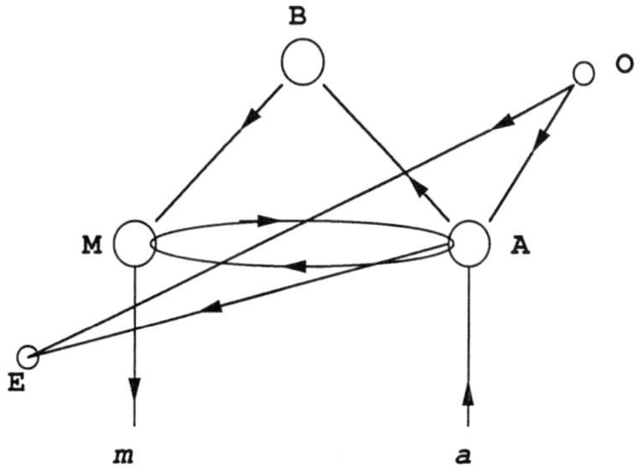

Fig. 21.4: The revised Lichtheim model incorporating reading and writing. (Redrawn from Lichtheim 1885, Figure 4)

"It is ... difficult to determine the path through which volitional or intelligent writing is executed. This tract must unite B with E, and clinical facts leave no doubt that it passes through M. There may be some doubt as to whether it leads directly to E, or passes through A on the way thither." (Lichtheim 1885, 437)

Lichtheim (1885, 444) notes that "it is not safe to draw a definite conclusion from a

Fig. 21.3: Reading and writing incorporated into Lichtheim's scheme: First attempt. (Redrawn from Lichtheim 1885, Figure 2)

single instance", and presents two further cases (his Case I and Pitres's case) to support the route M A E. The model was thus modified on the basis of the pattern of deficit found in a single case, and supported by additional observations.

2.6. A Critical Modification: The Introduction of Feedback

A potentially critical, but universally neglected, modification concerns the path A M: this now clearly operates in two directions A M and M A. There is additional motivation for this. Lichtheim, like Wernicke, was concerned that damage to A also had an impact on speech production – speech became 'paraphasic', i. e. fluent, well-formed grammatically most of the time, but full of errors. This did not seem predicted by the model. Freud (1891) made this the fulcrum of his incisive critique of the model and, incidentally, his first published consideration of speech errors. Lichtheim seems to have wanted the auditory word image to somehow monitor or support speech production. Now this idea no longer seems quite so implausible as it did to Freud, for example. Levelt (1989) has proposed that monitoring speech production, even prior to actual utterance, is carried out by the speech comprehension process – a point to which I shall return. In Interactive Activation models (e. g. Dell 1986), the activation of whole words feeds forward to activate subword elements – phonemes and or syllables –, which in turn feed back activation to the whole word nodes, and so on. This has the effect of vastly favouring the production of strings of subword elements that make up whole, real words, while preventing the production of strings that do not.

It may be possible to formulate this kind of model in such a way as to locate the word nodes on the input pathway, but connected to lower level purely production elements in the output system. (For a critical analysis of the Interactive Activation account see Butterworth 1989; Levelt/Schriefers/Vorberg et al. 1991.)

There is a more general difficulty: if a speaker has a tendency to mispronounce words, the model would seem to allow several loci for the problem – (i) there is some impairment to motor word images in M; (ii) there is an impairment in the route M *m*, or maybe (iii) there is a deficit in the feedback monitoring of output, along the M A A M pathway. In any event the problem of paraphasias, to which we will return below, is that, whatever the pathway, simple interruptions will not tell you what kind of speech error will ensue.

Whatever the failings of this model, it allowed researchers to make specific predictions about patterns of symptoms that should and should not be found. Where they were not found, the model could, indeed had to be modified – as we have seen in the case of writing. It also encouraged researchers and clinicians to look at the whole pattern of symptoms – language use in all its forms and modalities.

3. Modern Box and Arrow Models

The nearest modern equivalent that integrates across modalities is shown in Figure 21.5. This is taken from Howard/Franklin (1988, 21: Figure 1). I have chosen this version as my stalking horse not because it is in any way crass or incompetent, but rather because the authors are the most careful of the deployers of the most elaborated of a range of essentially similar models (e. g. Morton/Patterson 1980; Ellis/Young 1988, 222: Figure 8.3). It derives, historically, not from Lichtheim at all, but rather from studies of normal word recognition and production, especially those formulated in terms of Morton's logogen models (e. g. Morton 1970; 1979) and from Marshall/Newcombe's (1973) pioneering account of the acquired dyslexic syndromes, which itself initially made no reference to Lichtheim.

Broad similarities in architecture are apparent. There are separate lexicons for speech input and speech output, which correspond to Lichtheim's auditory word images and motor word images, and a direct connexion between them (corresponding presumably to the route A M in Figure 21.1.); a further loop feeding back from M to A via some more peripheral apparatus, is carefully motivated by a beautiful series of experiments on a patient who lacks this loop. This corresponds to the path M A in Lichtheim's revised diagram (see above Figure 21.4.). For both Lichtheim and Howard and Franklin, there is direct access from semantic concepts (or the cognitive system) to motor word images, and from auditory word images to semantic concepts.

Like Lichtheim's model, there are also separate stores for input visual word forms (the 'Orthographic Input Lexicon') and writing

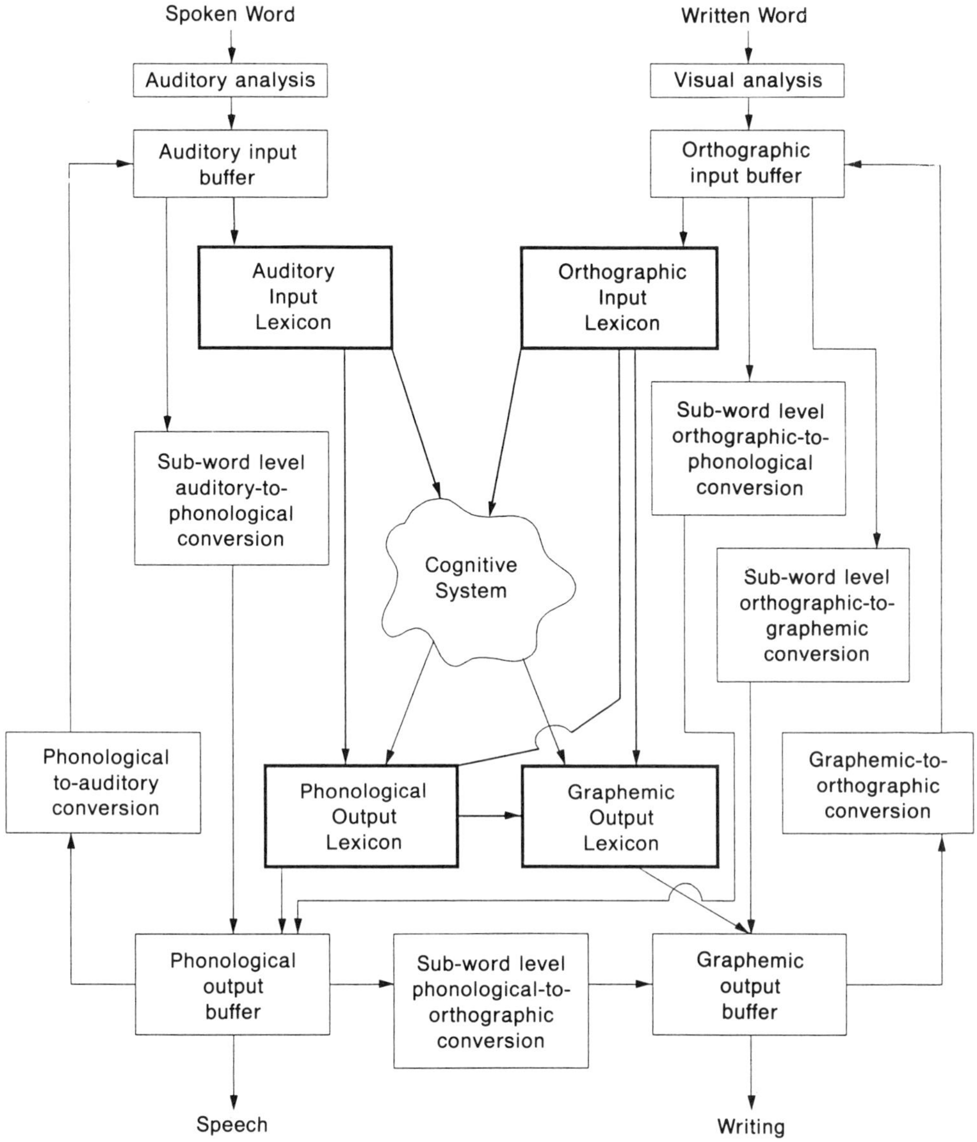

Fig. 21.5: "A simple model of single word lexical processing." (Howard/Franklin 1988, 20: Figure 1)

('Graphemic Output Lexicon'), and a direct connexion between them.

There are, however, several important differences from Lichtheim's original model, motivated in part by studies of performance by normal subjects in a wide variety of language tasks – a source of evidence unavailable to Lichtheim.

For written output, in this model but not in Lichtheim's revision (Figure 21.4.), the Phonological Output Lexicon (motor word images) maps directly onto the Graphemic Output Lexicon; and unlike Figure 21.4., there is no direct path leading from the Phonological Output Lexicon to the Auditory Input Lexicon to mediate volitional writing.

For reading, there is a direct route from the Orthographic Input Lexicon to the Phonological Output Lexicon, but no corresponding route O M in Figure 21.4.

However, the main differences are motivated by Marshall/Newcombe's (1973) idea that there could be two routes for reading a word: one which maps the whole letter string onto meaning and hence onto a pronunciation; while the second utilises the assembly of subword correspondences between letters and sounds. The former will in any case be needed for irregularly-spelled words, while the latter procedure will be needed to read aloud new words or for nonwords. In Figure 21.5., in addition to the two routes from visual input to spoken output, the idea of two routes is employed to map from visual input to written output, and from auditory input to spoken output. This basic format of both whole-word and sub-word processes is repeated where possible. As with Lichtheim, a critical test of the elements of the modern model is its ability to account for patterns of spared and impaired functioning.

The well-known dissociations in reading are a case in point. Some patients are able to read only words, but are unable – or very severely impaired in reading nonwords – the classic deep and phonological dyslexias – which is normally explained in terms of this model as an impairment to the 'subword level orthographic-to-phonological conversion route', while other reading routes are intact; while other patients are unable to read irregular words, but are good at reading aloud both regular words and nonwords. This is explained as a preservation of the 'subword level orthographic-to-phonological conversion route' with deficits to whole word reading routes. (See for example Ellis/Young 1988, Chapter 8.)

Similarly, but much less well-known, is the dual route account of repeating heard speech. According to the model, subword as well as whole word procedures can be used. The subword route enables us to repeat new words or nonwords as well as real, known words. The inability to repeat nonwords, while being able to repeat real words, was first documented by Goldstein (as P.S. in Goldstein 1906 and as Case 7 in Goldstein 1948). M.K. is a modern case described in detail by Howard/Franklin (1988), who also provide a critical summary of previously reported cases.

One further obvious difference is that while short-term memory tasks ('repetition') are mediated by the line A M in Lichtheim's diagram, they are subserved by two buffers and a loop for rehearsal in Figure 21.5. The need for more complex theoretical apparatus to deal with short-term memory is motivated largely by seemingly endless experiments on the factors determining normal memory span (Baddeley 1986).

4. A Comparison and Critique

This model however suffers from the same deficiencies as Lichtheim's. At best, it represents only static aspects of the language processing system, and then only some of these. For example, it does not specify what kind of information is stored in the lexicons, nor how it is organised. Are all the words a speaker knows separately represented, or does the speaker just store a basic form of, say, a verb (*walk*) along with rules for producing or understanding or reading aloud all the conjugations (*+s*, *+ed*, *+ing*) or both? Some Broca's aphasic patients have problems with verb endings, and deep dyslexics have problems reading aloud the endings on all types morphologically complex words (see Marshall/Newcombe 1980; Coltheart 1980); Wernicke patients, on the other hand, even those with severe jargon, can inflect spoken words correctly (Butterworth 1979; Butterworth/Howard 1987) and it has recently been found that some patients with severe word-finding problems make up words using the full range of derivational morphology to construct novel forms to fill the gaps (Semenza/Butterworth/Panzeri/Ferreri 1990). Clearly, then, prediction and diagnosis for detailed phenomena of this type will depend on hypotheses about the internal organisation of the lexical stores. Unfortunately, there is no unanimity among theorists – is there ever? – about lexical storage and retrieval. Useful reviews can be found in Butterworth (1983) and Frauenfelder/Schreuder (1991).

More strikingly, and perhaps more critically, dynamic aspects of the language processing system are not treated. Insofar as they are represented at all, they are designated by lines in the diagrams, not even by boxes. No attempt is made to say how elements in the lexical stores are accessed, how for example the pronunciation – a phonetic plan – is constructed on the basis of lexical retrieval or of some sublexical assembly procedure, and there is no awareness, apparently, that words are typically produced and received not as single units but as sentences or whole discourse. There appears to be an assumption that words in construction are a simple sum or concatenation of words in isolation, which, it has to be said, goes against everything that is known, not least by the proponents of the modern model, about language production and comprehension. For example, it is known that context profoundly affects both visual and auditory word recognition: it affects the visual exposure duration required for accurate recognition (Morton 1969), and can play a part in auditory word identification within the first 100 msecs of a heard word (Tyler 1984). In specialised models of speech recognition, like the "cohort model" (Marslen-Wilson 1987) or TRACE (McClelland/Elman 1986) contextual information is automatically invoked at the earliest stages of the recognition process. Similarly, it is known that context contributes to word-finding in spontaneous speech (Goldman-Eisler 1958; Beattie/Butterworth 1979).

These models provide no way of organising the words to form a sentence, let alone a meaningful or contextually appropriate one. There is no way for these models of the hearer to distinguish *Brutus killed Caesar* from *Caesar killed Brutus,* let alone from *Brutus was killed by Caesar*. It follows that there is no coherent way for either model to identify or explain impairments in combining words to form sentences: to distinguish agrammatic output from paragrammatic output; nor to say why a patient who can understand single words quite well is unable to understand sentences correctly. That is there is no syntax and only the sketchiest treatment of semantics.

5. A Modern Treatment of Paraphasias

Of course, modern research has made some notable advances in describing the dynamic aspects of language production since the time of Lichtheim which could be usefully incorporated into future models. One example is the process by which a stored lexical representation is realised as a string of phonemes – what is usually called, 'phonological encoding' ('PE' henceforth). The problem of paraphasias, especially phonemic paraphasias, has been critical to the assessment of the Lichtheim model. As was mentioned above, Freud made it the basis of his critique, and Lichtheim himself went through theoretical contortions to reconcile Wernicke's model with the clinical observations.

Without some idea of what actually happens inside boxes or along the arrows, it is nearly impossible to derive predictions about the fine-structure of behaviour. The idea that it has something to do with the centre for auditory word images is, at best, far too unspecific. What kind of error is likely to follow from an interruption in Auditory Word Images, even supposing these really do have something to do with mispronunciations. Similarly, interruptions in M or in the path M *m* in Figure 21.1., at most, allowed Lichtheim to distinguish speech disturbance with or without disturbance of volitional writing. In Figure 21.5., the situation is scarcely better. An interruption in the path between the Phonological Output Lexicon and the Phonological Output Buffer can be discriminated from deficits involving solely nonwords, but nothing can be said about the kinds of errors that will be made.

The model of PE that is described below will be used to attempt a diagnosis of a single paraphasic error, [semənt]. A fluent, Wernicke's aphasic patient, DJ, with largely recovered comprehension, produced mildly neologistic, but frequently paragrammatic and paraphasic speech, as in the following excerpt with the item of interest in bold:

(1) E: What do you do?
DJ: I've got a publican – publican.
E: Uh-huh. Where's that?
DJ: Old Bethnal Green Road ...
E: Are you the manager?
DJ: [dəmiəun] I'm sem- sem- What they call **[semənt]** ... Yer. Your own governor. Your own governor. I's mine.
E: Your a tenant.
DJ: I work to Truman's. But it's mine, like, you know. What I mean. Actually now I'm I'm actually the top thing you can do. You you are the – you work for the brewery as a [emnənt].
(For further case details, see Butterworth/Howard 1987)

Intuitively, the phonological encoding of a known word entails accessing a stored representation of the sound of that word, what I shall term the Phonological Lexical Representation (PLR) (a motor word image in Lichtheim's model; an entry in the phonological output lexicon in Figure 21.5.). How a PLR is itself accessed is a matter of some controversy, and will not be treated here; for, discussions see Butterworth (1989; 1992); Levelt/Schriefers/Vorberg et al. (1991).

PLR has to contain sufficient information to specify, for the word in its intended speech context, (1) the syllabic structure of the word, (2) the stress pattern of the word and (3) the segmental contents of the syllables. I leave aside entirely the question as to whether the

PLR is an 'underlying' or a 'superficial' phonological representation. (But see Caplan 1987, for arguments in favour of an underlying representation).

Following a number of authors, I will assume that these three types of information are represented separately (see Levelt 1989, chapter 9, for a review; cp. art. 1). A set of processes must then translate the information stored in the PLR into the phonetic representation appropriate to the current speech context that is ultimately passed on to the articulators. Encoding subsystems "spell out", in Levelt's (1989) useful term, information in a PLR. One can think of a PLR as containing phonological information in a condensed or abbreviated form, which requires elaborating before it can be deployed by later processes. Elaboration may involve adding information on the basis of general rules of phonology, which the (normal) speaker may be assumed to know. For example, it may involve generating allophonic variants appropriate to the current syllabic context, like lengthening a vowel before a voiced obstruent. Unfortunately, we have insufficient evidence to be precise about how this spelling out might work. Allophonic variation may already be explicitly encoded in the PLR. PLRs may also be underspecified in a more technical sense: that is, some phonetic features will systematically not be represented in the PLR, so that for example, the consonant following /s/ in *start* will be marked for place but voicing is left unspecified, and is represented instead by an archiphoneme /T/ that could be realised as either /t/ or /d/. Other types of underspecification in underlying lexical representations have been suggested in phonological theory (e. g. Kiparsky 1982; Archangeli 1985), and some of the ideas have been recruited to explain normal speech errors (Stemberger/Treiman 1986; cp. art. 5) and aphasic paraphasias (Béland 1990; cp. art. 17).

I shall follow several authors (Levelt 1989, Chapters 8 and 9; cp. art. 1; Shattuck-Hufnagel 1987) in assuming that translation processes have the form of a slot-and-filler device. The slots are defined jointly by spelling out the syllabic structure (how many syllables, and their form) and spelling out the prosodic structure — the stress (and pitch, where relevant) of each syllable. Information about the segmental content is spelled out and inserted into the appropriate slots. (This account is a considerable simplification, as well as a slight modification, of Levelt's in several ways, and the reader is urged to consult his book for a fuller description of the processes that might be at issue).

I shall assume without argument that word-forms for known words are not derived online from morphemic components (though cp. Levelt 1989). This is not to say that morphology is unrelated to the phonological form of a word (cp. Kiparsky 1982), nor that the rules for derivation and inflexion are unknown to the speaker, nor even that a PLR contains no morphological information, but only that information about morphology and lexical rules are deployed just when word search fails to retrieve a PLR meeting the retrieval specification — the phonological address.

This outline account presented diagrammatically in Figure 21.6., leaves open many details, some of which will be discussed below.

Because phonological representation and processes are implicated in, and link, lexical representations to phonetic plans for output, the presence of a speech error may be difficult to interpret with respect to candidate processes and representations.

In (1) above, our jargon aphasic patient, DJ, produced ['semənt] instead of the target, *tenant*. Single phoneme substitution paraphasias are not uncommon in aphasic speech (e. g. Fry 1959), nor indeed in normal speech (e. g. Shattuck-Hufnagel/Klatt 1979), yet a definitive locus in the production system needs to be determined. DJ may have a corrupted lexical representation for *tenant* in which the initial /t/ has been replaced by an initial /s/; or the /t/ may have lost elements of featural specification, in the PLR, so that only something like [−sonorant, +coronal] remains to specify the initial segment and additional features will need to be generated, in this case incorrectly; or the initial phoneme /t/ has just been lost in its entirety, yet syllabic structure clearly indicates that an initial consonant is required; or, like normal errors, where loss of information at the level of PLR, is not usually an option, something has gone wrong translating the PLR /t/ into the phonetic plan; or something arthric or praxic difficulty results in /t/'s, or stops more generally, being properly articulated.

To eliminate some of the candidate interpretations, one needs to see what other types of error the patient makes, in particular, one needs to see whether the patient makes the

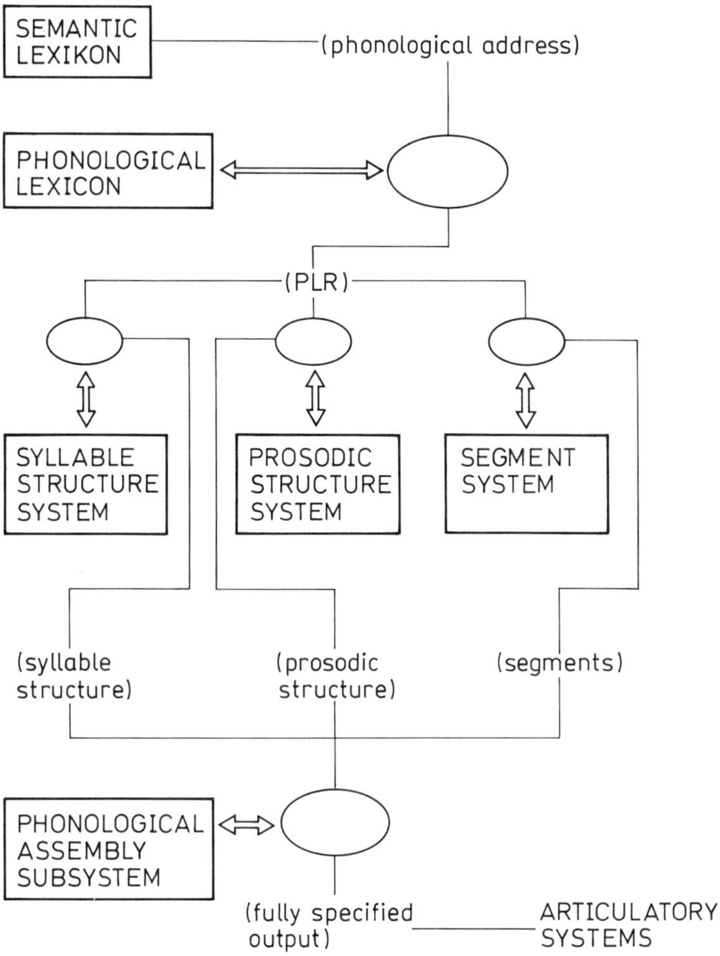

Fig. 21.6: *Outline model of phonological encoding processes.* The operation of this model can be best illustrated by stepping through the encoding of the word *tenant*, and the paraphasia ('semənt].
1. A phonological address is retrieved from the SEMANTIC LEXICON and can be thought of as an n-tuple defining a location in the PHONOLOGICAL LEXICON — e. g. ⟨2, 3, 6 ...⟩. It will have as neighbour, say, *tennis* at ⟨2, 3, 7 ...⟩. The generation of both target and paraphasia are held to start with the retrieval of the correct address.
2. The PHONOLOGICAL LEXICON associates the address with a PLR (Phonological Lexical Representation) that contains information as to how *tenant* should be pronounced — the segments it contains, and its syllable and prosodic structures. For reasons that are explained in Section 1.1, the PLR for *tenant* has not been corrupted in store.
3. This information is spelled out by dedicated, independent systems for SYLLABLE STRUCTURE, PROSODIC STRUCTURE and SEGMENTS. For the correct output, *tenant*, all the information in the PLR is correctly spelled out. For ['semənt], syllable and stress information may be fully available, though defaults could yield similar outcomes, but it is assumed that some or all of the information about the first consonant has been wholly or partly lost in transmission; the segment system generates a default segment, /s/, either from scratch, or from residual information about place of articulation, with manner information lost.
4. These are then assembled by the PHONOLOGICAL ASSEMBLY SUBSYSTEM, which fits the segments into slots in a prosodically specified syllable-structure. Thus the initial /t/, or the default /s/, is fitted into the onset position of the strong first syllable. The fully-specified output needs to include all relevant information for the ARTICULATORY SYSTEM.

The control processes, indicated by ovals, enable the generation of default information from the associated systems, or elsewhere, in the event that relevant information is missing from the PLR. For further explanation, see text. (Butterworth 1992, Figure 1)

same error every time he or she tries to produce the target.

In the case of DJ and *tenant* we do have some relevant data. As we saw in (1), DJ was a publican, working as the tenant of a brewery, a fact he was at pains to convey, since a tenant, who holds a lease on his pub, has a different, and, in DJ's view, a higher, status than a mere manager who simply operates the pub for a salary. Five examples, in two sessions, of this attempts to produce *tenant* in spontaneous conversation were recorded, and are reproduced in example (2).

(2) ['emnənt ... 'semənt ... 'tenənt ... 'tenəmən ... 'təneit]

Each attempt came from a separate sentence, so the sequence cannot be regarded as conduite d'approche. Taking the incorrect attempts as a whole, one can see that each segment, /t, e, n, ə, t/ is produced in its correct word position at least once, and no error is produced more than once; and one attempt was fully correct. It is reasonable to suppose, therefore, that the PLR of the word has not suffered permanent corruption, either through the replacement of a target segment by an intrusion, nor by the loss of a phonetic feature on one or more of the segments. Leaving aside arthric or praxis problems, from which DJ did not suffer, some problem in translating an intact PLR into a phonetic plan seems the most likely explanation, though the variability of error forms precludes proposing a specific locus in the translation process. The most likely account is that on each attempt to say the word, some of the information about the segments was lost in transmission, but in a rather unsystematic, perhaps random, way. (This is not, of course, to say that DJ had a fully preserved vocabulary that sometimes got scrambled in his attempts to talk, but only that for this target, the translation explanation appears the most consistent with the evidence so far presented.)

A similar analysis can be adduced for the syllabic structure of the PLR: in three examples it corresponds to the target – ['semənt, 'tenənt, 'təneit], while the other two show distinct error types. In ['emnənt] the structure of the syllables CVC$CVCC rather than CVC$VCC, with stress remaining on the first syllable; and in ['tenəmən], we find an additional epenthetic weak syllable, and a final syllable reduced from CVCC to CVC, though the first syllable is like the target. It is plausible to interpret this pattern also as due to variable loss in transmission from an intact PLR.

Without an examination of other attempts to say the same word the translation account of the original error, ['semənt], for this patient, would not have been adequately grounded. In the case of normal speech errors, we are entitled to assume that the target PLR is intact, unless there are good grounds for thinking otherwise, as there are for Sheridan's character, Mrs. Malaprop.

Of course, we were fortunate in finding several examples of the same identifiable target in free speech. This permitted the inference of loss of information from one intact PLR to the translation processes. However, if only one PLR resulted in this pattern of errors, then a reconsideration of this inference would be needed. To see whether other words suffered the fate of *tenant*, we tested DJ on a picture-naming task in two separate sessions one month apart. Overall, he named three pictures in Session 1 that he was unable to name in Session 2, and five pictures in Session 2 that he could not name in Session 1. The paraphasic errors indeed showed a similar pattern to the *tenant* example.

(3) Target: eskimo
  Session 1: ['esiməu]
  Session 2: ['æstiməu]
 Target: hedgehog
  Session 1: ['dɪdʒɒg]
  Session 2: [ɪg, ɒs, 'hɪdʒɒg, 'egɒg], H-E-
 Target: jacket
  Session 1: ['dʒækə, dʒæk]
  Session 2: ['dʒæk], zipper, [zɪpəweiz]

Although we found evidence that he knew all the segments of *hedgehog*, the other two examples show different errors on each occasion, as would be expected if there was variable loss in transmission, but the errors do not contain in sum the whole segmental specification of the target. Perhaps with further trials, the remaining segments would have emerged (/k/ in *eskimo*, /ɪt/ in *jacket*). With only two trials it is hard to say. However, in most studies of phonological encoding, there is only one trial for each word presented as evidence, which means that, at best, the pattern across different errors remains the only evidence to identify the locus of the deficit.

In any event, the model presented in Figure 21.6, and its interpretative apparatus, allowed us to explain the pattern of paraphasic errors in a single patient in a plausible way and it stressed the need for data on item-consistency that is usually neglected. (Cp. Butterworth 1992)

6. Conclusion

To say that a model is deficient in obvious and important ways, is not to say that it is without value to a science. Indeed, according to Lichtheim the very act of schematization in diagrammatic form (Figure 21.1.) historically turned out to be important:

> "The necessity of differentiating still further types [of disorder] struck me on attempting to schematize the forms hitherto known, for the purposes of instruction." (Lichtheim 1885, 435)

Howard/Franklin (1988, 99) note that they are using the model in Figure 21.5. "because it is the only lexical model that specifies all the word processing routines we have investigated with (the patient) MK in sufficient detail to permit a discussion" of his problem in term of a small number of information-processing impairments. They conclude that this patient has impairments to four boxes, two arrows and to the cognitive system itself (Howard/Franklin 1988, 111). Such a conclusion, if not inconceivable without this kind of diagram, would at the very least have been hard to imagine.

The neuropsychologist faces a dilemma: on the one hand, the aphasic patient arrives in the clinic with interrelated deficits in more than one modality, and to understand what is wrong, and just as importantly, what is right, a multi-modal model is needed; on the other hand, to understand the fine structure of each behavioural abnormality a detailed, dynamic model of the processes of constructing continuous speech output, or interpreting continuous speech input, will be needed.

7. References

Allport, D. A. & Funnell, E. (1981). Components of the mental lexicon. *Philosophical Transaction of the Royal Society of London, B 295*, 397–410.

Archangeli, D. B. (1985). Yokuts harmony: evidence for coplanar representation in nonlinear phonology. *Linguistic Inquiry, 16*, 335–372.

Baddeley, A. (1986). *Working Memory*. Oxford: Oxford University Press.

Beattie, G. W. & Butterworth, B. (1979). Contextual probability and word frequency as determinants of pauses and errors in spontaneous speech. *Language and Speech, 22*, 201–211.

Béland, R. (1990). Vowel epenthesis in aphasia. In J.-L. Nespoulous & P. Villard (Eds.), *Morphology, Phonology and Aphasia*. 235–252. New York: Springer-Verlag.

Brown, R. & McNeill, D. (1966). The "tip of the tongue" phenomenon. *Journal of Verbal Learning and Verbal Behavior, 5*, 325–337.

Butterworth, B. (1979). Hesitation and the production of verbal paraphasias and neologisms in jargon aphasia. *Brain and Language, 8*, 133–161.

Butterworth, B. (1983). Lexical representation. In B. Butterworth (Ed.), *Language Production, Volume 2. 257–294*. London: Academic Press.

Butterworth, B. (1985). Jargon aphasia: Processes and strategies. In S. Newman & R. Epstein (Eds.) *Current Perspectives in Dysphasia. 61–96*. Edinburgh: Churchill Livingstone.

Butterworth, B. (1989). Lexical access in speech production. In W. Marslen-Wilson (Ed.), *Lexical Representation and Process. 108–135*. Cambridge, MA: MIT Press.

Butterworth, B. (1992). Disorders of phonological encoding. *Cognition, 42*, 261–286.

Butterworth, B. & Howard, D. (1987). Paragrammatisms. *Cognition, 26*, 1–37.

Caplan, D. (1987). Phonological representations in word production. In E. Keller & M. Gopnik (Eds.), *Motor and Sensory Processes of Language. 111–124*. Hillsdale, NJ: LEA.

Coltheart, M. (1980). Deep dyslexia: A review of the syndrome. In M. Coltheart, K. Patterson (Eds.), *Deep Dyslexia*. 22–47. London: RKP.

Dell, G. (1986). A spreading-activation theory of retrieval in sentence production. *Psychological Review, 93*, 283–321.

Ellis, A. W. & Young, A. (1988). *Human Cognitive Neuropsychology*. London: LEA.

Frauenfelder, U. & Schreuder, R. (1991). Constraining psycholinguistic models of morphological processing and representation: The role of productivity. In: G. Booij & J. van Marle (Eds.), *Yearbook of Morphology 1991*. 165–183. Amsterdam: Kluwer.

Freud, S. (1891): *On Aphasia: A Critical Study*. Translated by E. Stengel. London: Imago 1953.

Fry, D. (1959). Phonemic substitutions in an aphasic patient. *Language and Speech, 2*, 52–61.

Garrett, M. (1980). Levels of processing in sentence production. In B. Butterworth (Ed.), *Language Production, Volume 1: Speech and Talk. 177–220*. London: Academic Press.

Garrett, M. (1984). The organisation of processing structure for language production: Applications to aphasic speech. In D. Caplan, A. R. Lecours & A. Smith (Eds.), *Biological Perspectives on Language. 172–193*. Cambridge, MA: MIT Press.

Goldman-Eisler, F. (1958). Speech production and the predictability of words in context. *Quarterly Journal of Experimental Psychology, 10*, 96–106.

Goldstein, K. (1906). Ein Beitrag zur Lehre von der Aphasie. *Journal für Psychologie und Neurologie, 7*, 172–188.

Goldstein, K. (1948). Language and Language Disturbances. New York: Grune & Stratton.

Goodglass, H. & Kaplan, E. (1972). *The Assessment of Aphasia and Related Disorders*. Philadelphia: Lea & Febiger.

Head, H. (1926). *Aphasia and Kindred Disorders of Speech*. Cambridge: Cambridge University Press.

Hinton, G. & Shallice, T. (1991). Lesioning an attractor network: Investigations of acquired dyslexia. *Psychological Review, 98*, 74–95.

Howard, D. & Franklin, S. (1988). *Missing the Meaning? A Cognitive Neuropsychological Study of Processing of Words by an Aphasic Patient*. Cambridge, MA: MIT Press.

Jackson, J. H. (1879). On affectations of speech from diseases of the brain. In J. Taylor (Ed.), *Selected Writings of John Hughlings Jackson*. Vol. II, 155–170. London: Hodder & Stoughton.

Kiparsky, P. (1982). From cyclic phonology to lexical phonology. In H. van der Hulst (Ed.), *The Structure of Phonological Representations: Part 1. 131–176*. Dordrecht: Foris.

Levelt, W. J. M. (1989). *Speaking. From Intention to Articulation*. Cambridge, MA: MIT Press.

Levelt, W. J. M., Schriefers, H., Vorberg, D., Meyer, A., Pechmann, T., & Havinga, J. (1991). The time course of lexical access in speech production: A study of picture naming. *Psychological Review, 98*, 122–142.

Lichtheim, L. (1885). On aphasia. *Brain, VII*, 433–484.

McClelland, J. L. (1987). The case for interactionism in language processing. In M. Coltheart (Ed.) *Attention and Performance XII: The Psychology of Reading. 3–36*. London: LEA.

McClelland, J. & Elman, J. (1986). Interactive processes in speech perception: the TRACE model. In J. L. McClelland & D. E. Rumelhart (Eds.), *Parallel Distributed Processing: Explorations in the Microstructures of Cognition. Volume 2. 58–121*. Cambridge, MA: MIT Press.

Marshall, J. C. & Newcombe, F. (1973). Patterns of paralexia. *Journal of Psycholinguistic Research, 2*, 175–199.

Marshall, J. C. & Newcombe, F. (1980). The conceptual status of deep dyslexia. In M. Coltheart, K. Patterson & J. C. Marshall (Eds.) *Deep Dyslexia*. 1–21. London: RKP.

Marslen-Wilson, W. (1987). Functional parallelism in spoken word recognition. *Cognition, 25*, 71–102.

Morton, J. (1969). The interaction of information in word recognition. *Psychological Review, 76*, 165–178.

Morton, J. (1970). A functional model for memory. In D. A. Norman (Ed.), *Models of Human Memory. 203–249*. New York: Academic Press.

Morton, J. (1979). Facilitation in word-recognition: experiments causing change in the logogen model. In P. Kolers, M. Wrolstad & H. Bouma (Eds.), *Processing of Visible Language*. 259–268. New York: Plenum.

Morton, J. & Patterson, K. E. (1980). A new attempt at an interpretation or an attempt at a new interpretation. In M. Coltheart, K. Patterson & J. C. Marshall (Eds.), *Deep Dyslexia. 91–118*. London: RKP.

Panzeri, M., Semenza, C., & Butterworth, B. (1987). Compensatory processes in the evolution of severe jargon aphasia. *Neuropsychologia, 25*, 919–933.

Patterson, K. E. (1986). Lexical but non-semantic spelling? *Cognitive Neuropsychology, 3*, 341–367.

Semenza, C., Butterworth, B., Panzeri, M. & Ferreri, T. (1990). Word-formation: New evidence from aphasia. *Neuropsychologia, 28*, 499–502.

Shallice, T. (1984). More functionally isolable subsystems but fewer 'modules'? *Cognition, 17*, 243–252.

Shattuck-Hufnagel, S. (1987). The role of word-onset consonants in speech production planning: New evidence from speech error patterns. In E. Keller & M. Gopnik (Eds.), *Motor and Sensory Processes of Language. 17–51*. Hillsdale NJ: LEA.

Shattuck-Hufnagel, S. & Klatt, D. (1979). Minimal use of features and markedness in speech production. *Journal of Verbal Learning and Verbal Behavior, 18*, 41–55.

Stemberger, J. P. & Treiman, R. (1986). The internal structure of word-initial consonant clusters. *Journal of Memory and Language, 25*, 163–180.

Tyler, L. K. (1984). The structure of the initial cohort: Evidence from gating. *Perception & Psychophysics, 36*, 417–427.

Van Orden, G. C. (1987). A ROWS is a ROSE: Spelling, sound and reading. *Memory & Cognition, 15*, 181–198.

Wernicke, C. (1874). *Der aphasische Symptomenkomplex: eine psychologische Studie auf anatomischer Basis*. Breslau: Cohn & Weigert. English translation by G. H. Eggert (1977). *Wernicke's Works on Aphasia: A Sourcebook and Review*. The Hague: Mouton.

Brian Butterworth, London (UK)

22. Acquired Disorders of Reading

1. Introduction

In 1973, Marshall and Newcombe published a paper that had a seminal influence on subsequent understanding of acquired dyslexic disorders and speeded the decline of the then dominant tradition in aphasiology that sought to relate reading impairment to lesion site and aphasia syndrome (see also Marshall/Newcombe 1966). The novelty of Marshall and Newcombe's viewpoint was in the way that they elucidated three quite different patterns of reading difficulty, carefully documented in six neurological patients, by placing them within the context of a cognitive model of normal reading. They advocated a model of single word reading in which there were two routes from print to sound, one which consisted of rule-based procedures for translating visual forms into corresponding sound forms, and another which consisted of semantically-based procedures.

Marshall and Newcombe's approach provided a way of investigating acquired reading disorders that had been obscured by the apparent lack of predictability between traditional syndrome type and nature of the reading impairment. It also opened up the possibility of a link between aphasia research and the new flowering of linguistics (e.g. Chomsky 1965). Indeed, Marshall and Newcombe's characterisation of two of the patterns of acquired reading disability, which they termed 'deep' dyslexia and 'surface' dyslexia, drew directly on the Chomskyean notion of 'deep' and 'surface' structures. In the quarter of a century since then, and particularly over the last fifteen years, there has been a proliferation of studies concerned with reading impairments in aphasia, although these have principally been undertaken from a cognitive rather than linguistic perspective. They have been driven by advances in the development of cognitive models of normal reading, an enterprise in which the study of reading impairments is regarded by many as a fruitful source of evidence with which to test such models (e. g. Coltheart 1985).

A review of acquired dyslexic disorders must therefore be set within the context of our current understanding of how normal reading – and, more precisely, written word recognition and production – is achieved. The complex network of interacting systems that is required to carry out even relatively simple skills such as recognizing what a written word is, or generating a corresponding sound form, suggests that one might expect to observe many different types and variants of disorder acquired through brain damage. This has indeed become clear with the increasing sophistication of individual case reports that document precisely the fractionation of basic distinctions between patterns of reading disorder. What follows is a brief synthesis of existing findings concerning the varieties of acquired dyslexia with reference to current models of written recognition and production.

2. Disorders of Written Word Perception and Identification

During the course of perceiving a word and recognising what it is, a written letter string must be transformed from an image on the retina into an abstract form (regardless of case, font and orientation, for example), that is compatible with a stored lexical representation. What this entails is that, with the aid of attentional processing resources (e. g. Treisman 1988), elementary visual procedures act to transform a spatial 'retino-centric' representation into a form that is independent of location in the visual field and that specifies information about letter identities and their relative positions within the string. Caramazza and his colleagues (Caramazza/Hillis 1990; Rapp/Caramazza 1991) propose three perceptual-representational levels, which draw heavily on the work of Marr (1982), and assume that the 'representational spaces' involved in visual word and object recognition are the same. At the first level, a retino-centric feature map is constructed in which a description of the edges in the projected retinal image are created from information specified by the relative discontinuities of light intensities falling across the retina.

The spatial location of the image in the visual field (that is, where it occurs on the retina) will also be reproduced in the feature map. At a second level of analysis, the shape properties of individual letters (lines, angles, curves, for example) must be recovered. At this point, at which a letter shape map is constructed, the spatial relationships of the elements of the string are stimulus-centred; that is, they specify the actual orientation of the letter shapes with respect to the stimulus (and each other), although information about absolute, retino-centric, location is lost. At a third level, letter shapes must be translated into knowledge about what the letters are. This consists of gaining access to information about abstract letter identities; that is, information that abstracts across case and font (e. g. Evett/Humphreys 1981). The form of the representation at this level is a sequence of abstractly coded letters, or graphemes. The spatial relationship between the graphemes is represented according to a 'word-centred' frame. This means that the veridical nature of the stimulus-centred letter shape map is 'normalised' to an orientation-invariant, canonical format, in which the major axis is the horizontal frame. The word-centred graphemic description can then be used by lexical processing procedures to access representations in a visual input lexicon (also sometimes referred to as a word-form system). Information about graphemes is transmitted in parallel to access lexical representations that share the same graphemes in the same relative positions (e. g. McClelland/Rumelhart 1981).

Neglect dyslexia is an acquired reading disturbance, usually associated with right parietal lesions, in which portions of the left side of text can be omitted and errors can be made in processing the beginning letters of individual words: initial letters may be omitted (e. g. *pan* → *an*), added (e. g. *pan* → *span*), or substituted (e. g. *pan* → *man*). A common assumption is that it is just one of a constellation of features associated with, and indicative of, a more general neglect of contralesional space. Neglect, itself, however, has been demonstrated to be made up of a number of discrete disturbances, each of which can occur in isolation in individual patients. That neglect dyslexia may similarly occur independently appears to be demonstrated in some cases (e. g. Baxter/Warrington 1983; Patterson/Wilson 1990; Riddoch/Humphreys/Cleton/Fery 1990; Warrington 1991). However, as Riddoch (1990) has made clear, since the task of reading may place more demands on visual processing abilities than other visuo-spatial tasks, it is possible that evidence of a more generalised neglect might have been elicited even in these 'pure' cases if more stringent testing had been undertaken (e. g. under limited exposure conditions). It is still not entirely proven, therefore, that neglect dyslexia does exist as an independent disorder; this issue bears strongly on questions concerning how far the procedures involved in general visual analysis and analysis of written input are the same.

Recent work (see individual papers in Riddoch 1990) has clearly revealed the fractionation of deficits that can occur within neglect dyslexia itself. Thus, while both word and text reading may be affected in some patients (e. g. Behrmann/Moscovitch/Black/Moser in press; Ellis/Flude/Young 1987; Kinsbourne/Warrington 1962 a; Caramazza/Hillis 1990; Young/Newcombe/Ellis 1991; Warrington 1991), reading of single words can be impaired selectively (e. g. Costello/Warrington 1987; Patterson/Wilson 1990; Riddoch/Humphreys/Cleton/Fery 1990). Evidence from a further patient who shows a selective deficit in reading text, but not individual words (Kartsounis/Warrington 1989), indicates that disturbances of word and text reading can doubly dissociate. This supports Young/Newcombe/Ellis (1991) claim that qualitatively different mechanisms underpin neglect reading errors in single words and in text. In line with this view, dissociations have also been reported which depend on the nature of the written material patients are given to read. Thus, commonly, neglect patients have greater success with words than nonwords, though this is not invariably the case (e. g. Patient VB; Ellis/Flude/Young 1987). And while it is as yet uncommon to find reports of patients who have been tested with different kinds of written material (e. g. letters, numbers, geometric shapes), a patient investigated by Patterson/Wilson (1990) was impaired in dealing with the alphanumeric stimuli, but not with strings of the geometric shapes. (It is pertinent to note, however, that this may reflect not a material-specific deficit, but simply the limited variety of geometric shapes.) Interestingly, these recent investigations also show that neglect dyslexia is not exclusively produced by right hemisphere lesions; cases reported by Caramazza/Hillis (1990), Sieroff (1990) and Warrington (1991) all had left hemisphere lesions which correspondingly affected word endings and the right side of text. Perhaps intriguingly, however, the case of Patterson/Wilson (1990) mentioned above, also displayed left hemisphere damage, but nonetheless showed a neglect that particularly affected the initial letter of words. Hemisphere of lesion does not relate in any simple way to the fractionation of deficits within neglect dyslexia, though Sieroff (1990) suggests that there are differences in the nature of attentional disturbances in left and right parietal lesions.

Neglect and neglect dyslexia have popularly been regarded as attentional disorders in which there are impairments either in engaging, moving or disengaging a general attentional resource (e. g. Humphreys/Riddoch 1990; Posner/Walker/Friedrich/Rafal 1984). Caramazza and his colleagues suggest that the patterns of performance observed in neglect dyslexia can be accounted for by positing deficits to prelexical representations that are not necessarily attentional in nature. Patient VB (Ellis/Flude/Young 1987), for example, might be considered as a candidate for either a retino-centric or stimulus-centred representational deficit. VB suffered from a general neglect of the left side of visual space. Both text and single word reading were affected. VB was also affected by the actual spatial location of the letter string and letters within the string: if a word was presented upside-down, VB continued to neglect the left-most letters, even though these were now the right-most letters in the word itself. When the word was presented vertically, however, VB did not show evidence of neglect across any letter position. In contrast, patient NG (Caramazza/Hillis 1990) continued to make errors to the left-most, initial, letters of a word whether it was presented as a mirror image, inverted, or in a vertical orientation. This suggests that the level of deficit in this patient is based not on spatial location or stimulus coordinates, but on a more abstract level of representation, namely a word-centred graphemic description. Caramazza and Hillis also attempt to explain the variety of other recent cases within their classificatory scheme. How does this account – based on the claim that these disorders are representational impairments – square with the view that the 'neglect' impairment reflects a deficit to an attentional mechanism? As Caramazza and Hillis point out, the symptomatology exhibit by their patient, NG, would appear to rule out a general attentional deficit, since processing at the retino-centric feature level and stimulus-centred shape level (gauged by her performance with differently oriented and displayed materials), seem to be intact. They conclude that, "either we assume that there are distinct attentional mechanisms operating at different levels of representation, or we reject the hypothesis that the deficit concerns an attentional mechanism" (Caramazza/Hillis 1990, 485).

Recent theory has pondered a connection between neglect dyslexia and another form of peripheral reading impairment known as **letter-by-letter reading**. Before the nature of this connection is considered, the disorder must be introduced. It is characterised by the length of time taken to read single words, which can be in the order of seconds rather than milliseconds: patient RAV (Warrington/Shallice 1980), for example, took 1.8 seconds on average simply to read words of 3 and 4 letters, while patient CH (Patterson/Kay 1982) took 16.9 seconds. The term, letter-by-letter reading, refers to the tendency of some, but by no means all, patients to spell out overtly by name each letter of the string. It is a disorder that has long been recognised and, indeed, constituted one of two major classes of acquired dyslexia distinguished by Déjerine (1892) and termed alexia without agraphia (it also appears under the guise of other names: pure word-blindness, agnosic alexia and word-form dyslexia are examples). It has been assumed that the pattern of deficits in different patients has a common locus, and debate has focussed on the nature of this disturbance. Thus, Patterson/Kay (1982) claim that the critical impairment is post-perceptual but prelexical, and concerns a failure of parallel grapheme analysis in the course of lexical access. Warrington/Shallice (1980), on the other hand, argue that the deficit is not in pre-lexical procedures but within representations in a reading lexicon, or, more precisely, a word-form system. (Note that these accounts do not run the full gamut of explanation; other views exist, some of which argue for a more general visual processing deficit (e. g. Friedman/Alexander 1984), that may involve a 'simultanagnosia' in the ability to process multiple forms (e. g. Kinsbourne/Warrington 1962 b).)

As is the case for neglect dyslexia, letter-by-letter reading also seems to fractionate into different patterns of deficit (see, for example, papers in Riddoch 1990). While there is evidence that a patient investigated by Kay/Hanley (1991) has particular difficulty in processing letters, or rather, abstract grapheme identities, in parallel (supporting the general argument of Patterson/Kay 1982), another patient reported by Reuter-Lorenz/Brunn (1990) appears to have difficulties in determining abstract grapheme identities themselves. It is claimed that a third letter-by-letter reader is impaired at an earlier, stimulus-centred, level of representation (Rapp/Caramazza 1991).

Riddoch (1990) considers the evidence for a common functional deficit in neglect dyslexia and letter-by-letter reading. At present, the data are little more than circumstantial, though perhaps instructive: Rapp and Caramazza's case showed 'neglect-like' spatial location deficits on a variety of tasks. Moreover, as Riddoch observes, the impaired perception of simultaneously presented forms, demonstrated by the patients of Kay/Hanley/Reuter-Lorenz/Brunn, is also characteristic of visual neglect (revealed by the phenomenon of extinction, for example).

Furthermore, both neglect dyslexics and letter-by-letter readers show a gradient of deficit, which in the former affects only beginning (or end) letters, but in the latter can extend across the whole string. Rapp and Caramazza suggest that these patterns may involve the same level of impairment, but result from differences in perceptual processing resources that can be marshalled during analysis. Riddoch/Humphreys/Cleton/Fery (1990) posit an attentional deficit in orienting to the 'convenient viewing position' at which we attend to words (based on computed word length and usually to the left of the centre of the string), which can be manifested in different ways. While the status of these alternatives is uncertain, and demands further examination, what one can assert with more confidence is that recent intensive investigations provide little evidence for the view that the deficit in letter-by-letter reading is at a lexical, word-form, level (Warrington/Shallice 1980).

There are reports, however, of some patients whose reading characteristics do seem to square with a lexical-level impairment. Hillis/Caramazza (1992), for example, describe a case in which the patient made almost exclusively visual errors in response to reading both words and word-like strings (and no nonword phonemic errors). The patient's reading performance is reminiscent of the pattern of disorder described by Marshall/Newcombe (1973) as **visual dyslexia**. Apart from problems with reading, the patient did not show signs of other visual and/or spatial difficulties. Unlike a neglect dyslexic, his visual errors in reading occured across all letter positions in words: on the left (e. g. *excess* → *recess*), in the centre (e. g. *moment* → *movement*), on the right (e. g. *provide* → *proverb*) and in more than one position (e. g. *vivid* → *avoid*). It is, of course, difficult to be sure that so-called 'visual' errors are not in fact phonological word errors. Phonologically-based errors might suggest that the patient had difficulties at an output rather than input level. Hillis and Caramazza report that the patient produced a number of errors, hard to explain by a phonological account, in which target and reponse shared letters but in different relative orders (the nonword *phloke* was read aloud as *polka*, for example). Furthermore, the patient had difficulty with an 'easy' lexical decision task, in which he accepted 11% of the written nonwords as words. Moreover, another task indicated that words read aloud as visually similar words were also not understood correctly. These findings suggest that the patient's difficulties led to problems in visual recognition and comprehension and were not simply problems in retrieving appropriate pronunciations.

It is also the case that visual errors in reading aloud commonly accompany other error types in other forms of acquired dyslexia. It will be argued, however, that visual errors — like other error types — can arise from a number of different levels of impairment. Patients with a disorder known as **surface dyslexia** (one of Marshall and Newcombe's original categories) sometimes make errors that appear to be visual in nature. However, Coltheart/Masterson/Byng et al. (1983) regard the key symptom of surface dyslexia as the 'regularisation' error. This means that words referred to as irregular or exceptional, because their pronunciation is difficult to predict from their spelling, are often given literal pronunciations. Words like *castle* or *two* or *mortgage*, for example, may be pronounced as *kast-ul* or *twoh* or *mortgidge*. One also sees errors in stress assignment, in which stress is shifted to an inappropriate syllable (e. g. *begin* becomes *beggin*, with stress on the first syllable). It is claimed that these errors occur because the patient is reading phonologically and not by the normal operation of lexical procedures. But what is meant by the term 'phonological reading'? Even people who are not necessarily practised readers can generally read aloud things that look as if they could be words, like *drist*, but are not. Non-words will not have full lexical specifications in the way that words have, although there must be procedures that allow plausible pronunciations for these strings to be constructed. It is claimed that surface dyslexic readers rely on such procedures, and, by this argument, their ability to read aloud nonwords should be preserved.

According to Coltheart and his co-workers, there are a number of other features, some of which are 'essential', others less essential, to the 'syndrome' of surface dyslexia. One of the symptoms is that when a word is misread, it is also miscomprehended in terms of the response – so that *gauge* might be given the regularised pronunciation, *gorge*, and defined as, *a big dip*. As Shallice (1988) points out, in defining this grouping of symptoms as a syndrome or symptom-complex, no theoretical grounds were given for *why* one characteristic was rated 'key' and others were considered 'essential' or less essential. It has since become clear that a number of different deficits may precipitate 'phonological reading' (see papers in Patterson/Marshall/Coltheart 1985). Thus, while the misreadings of some patients are also misunderstood, other patients can demonstrate appropriate understanding, even though words are misread (Kremin 1981; 1985; Goldblum 1985; Kay/Patterson 1985; Margolin/Marcel/Carlson 1985): the patient investigated by Kay and Patterson, for example, read *choir* aloud as *singing … choyer*. The first finding is consistent with a difficulty in accessing correct semantic information from a visual representation, or at a semantic level itself, while the second is consistent with a later-level impairment, perhaps in addressing output phonology from the semantic system.

Several researchers have observed that at least some surface dyslexic readers read aloud in a slow and laboured way (the patient described by Shallice/Warrington 1980, for example, took an average of 4.2 seconds to read a one-syllable word). Hand-in-hand with this finding, some surface dyslexic sound out letters in a word, trying to work out what it is, and often making errors in sounding it out (e. g. Marshall/Newcombe 1973; Newcombe/Marshall 1985). Nonword reading is also affected in similar ways. Henderson (1982) has argued that these features may indicate that what one is seeing in these patients are the products of a compensatory procedure which can tell us little about the usual operation of reading systems. Shallice (1988) goes further by claiming that this pattern of surface dyslexic reading is in fact related to letter-by-letter reading, and that both reflect the operation of compensatory mechanisms. He suggests that surface dyslexia, like letter-by-letter reading, "may well result from damage at the word-form level, at least in many patients so classified". Shallice's conjecture of a link between surface dyslexia and letter-by-letter reading may well turn out to be correct. However, there is little good evidence, as we have seen, to support the notion of impaired lexical-level representations in letter-by-letter reading and rather more in favour of the view that damage may have occurred to pre-lexical stimulus-centred or word-centred graphemic descriptions. More investigation is required to clarify the relationship between these two disorders, to elucidate the nature of the impairment, and to find why such patients differ in the extent to which they use a letter naming or sounding-out procedure in oral reading (e. g. Patterson/Kay 1982).

There are case reports of some patients who, it is claimed, read phonologically in a fast and fluent fashion (e. g. Warrington 1975; Schwartz/Saffran/Marin 1980; Shallice/Warrington/McCarthy 1983; Bub/Cancelliere/Kertesz 1985). These patients were able to read nonwords and many words aloud, even, paradoxically, if they were irregular. All the patients had extremely impoverished comprehension abilities and, arguably, were unable to use semantically mediated lexical procedures to read aloud. Patient MP, for example, described by Bub/Cancelliere/Kertesz (1985), performed at chance level on a variety of written word and picture comprehension tasks, and failed to show facilitation effects on reading latency for associatively semantically primed words. It is unlikely in MP's case that the difficulty can be attributed to a visual lexical-level impairment, since, even for those irregular words (like *leopoard*) that she could not read aloud successfully, she was able to recognise that they were words, and to reject as words, nonwords constructed from irregular words by changing one letter (e. g. *rubtle*). Shallice/Warrington/McCarthy (1983) have termed this disorder, **semantic dyslexia**, to distinguish it from surface dyslexia, while others refer to it as **direct-route**

reading, for a reason that will soon be made apparent.

Detailed investigations of these patients' performance have attempted to establish a little more about the nature of phonological reading, when it is operating in relative isolation from a lexical, semantic, route. There is continuing debate over what these phonological procedures might be and the sources of knowledge on which they act. Some theorists, for example, claim that there are separable systems of word-based and sub-word-based knowledge (e.g. Coltheart 1978; Patterson/Morton 1985). Sub-word-based knowledge is used to read phonologically, but what are the 'rules' on which the system is constructed? Coltheart (1978) proposed that the phonological reading system consists of letter-sound patterns, or, more precisely, graphemes such as <p> or <sh> that correspond with individual phonemes like /p/ and /ʃ/ (rules governing grapheme-phoneme correspondence in English have been classified by Venezky 1970). Patterson/Morton (1985) suggest that this system supplements information about sub-syllables like *-ave* in *save*, that constitute the 'body' or 'rime' of a word. Shallice and his colleagues (Shallice/Warrington/McCarthy 1983; Shallice/McCarthy 1985), on the other hand, claim that phonological reading makes use of a range of sub-word-sized units: grapheme-phoneme correspondences, sub-syllables, syllables and morphemes. Evidence from the case reports of surface dyslexia suggests that a range of spelling-sound information is indeed available in phonological reading. Thus, while a surface dyslexic patient reported by Kay/Lesser (1985) made use of grapheme-phoneme correspondences on at least some occasions in single-word reading, Shallice, Warrington/McCarthy (1983) demonstrated convincingly that another patient, given many of the same reading materials to read aloud, relied on sub-syllabic information about spelling-sound patterns. Their findings converge neatly with evidence from reaction-time studies with normal readers that show the importance of sub-syllabic knowledge in producing word and nonword pronunciations (e.g. Seidenberg/Waters/Barnes/Tanenhaus 1984; Kay/Bishop 1987).

Even more interesting for this debate is the finding that phonological readers described above, such as patient MP (Bub/Cancelliere/Kertesz 1985), were able to read aloud even irregular words that they were unable to understand. MP, for example, was able to read 77% of a set of irregular words. Bub/Cancelliere/Kertesz (1985) discovered that MP's reading performance was particularly affected by word frequency: she was faster to read aloud high frequency than low frequency words. This factor also influenced the responses that she gave to irregular words: irregular words that were also low in frequency were much more likely to be given regularised pronunciations than corresponding high frequency words. Patient WLP (Schwartz/Saffran/Marin 1980) showed even better performance than MP in reading aloud irregular words; early in her illness she read aloud 95% of a set of irregular words successfully, though her semantic comprehension skills were very poor. For example, she read the irregular word *hyena* correctly, saying, *Hyena ... hyena ... what in the heck is that?* WLP suffered from a progressive dementing disease, and later on in her illness, the percentage of irregular words that she could read decreased to 71%. At the same time, she began to produce substantial numbers of regularisation errors. Shallice and his colleagues explain findings such as these by assuming that a 'broad' phonological route, distinguishable from a semantic route, specifies information about morphemic correspondences, as well as smaller units. It is further proposed that larger units, such as morphemes, are more vulnerable to impairment, particularly if they are low in frequency. These assumptions attempt to explain why a progressive disease, such as that observed in WLP, can increasingly restrict the range of correspondences that are available.

The response of researchers who favour a phonological reading routine that operates on grapheme-phoneme correspondences and/or sub-syllable correspondences is not to concede that the routine may have a broader base, but to assume that there is more than one phonological reading system. A lexical phonological routine, which deals with lexical and morphemic representations, is added to the non-lexical one, so that, within this scheme, there are three reading routes rather than two. Shallice (1988) claims that the difference between this version of the 'standard' model and the 'multiple-levels' model is "mainly terminological", and it is certainly clear that both accounts seem equally capable of dealing with most of the findings to do with phonological reading. However, so does a third account, which is a rather more radical alternative. This approach does away with any phonological routine other than one based on word spelling and pronunciation (e.g. Marcel 1980; McClelland/Rumelhart 1981). According to this view, pronunciation can be constructed for all written letter strings – whether word or non-word – by activating spelling patterns and corresponding sound patterns in visually similar words. The difference between this general approach and a multiple-levels model is that, for the latter, a range of orthographic units are represented within a visual word-form system (with correspondences in a phonological word-form system), whereas, for the former, these units are represented only in as much as they occur in words.

3. Impairments of Phonological Reading

Some patients with surface dyslexia have difficulty with reading aloud irregular words, but are able to construct plausible pronunciations for non-words. Another variety of acquired dyslexia has been characterised as the obverse side of the same coin. In **phonological dyslexia**, the ability to read aloud nonwords is severely impaired, while word reading is affected not by regularity, but by grammatical class (Beauvois/Derouesné 1979). For example, AM, reported by Patterson (1982) was able to read only 8% of a set of nonwords, while, on the same occasion, he was able to repeat 83% of a second set. This finding indicates that the problem is not secondary to a speech production difficulty. Neither does there seem to be a problem in visually recognising nonwords to judge from the patient's normal performance on a visual lexical decision task. In contrast with his nonword reading ability, AM's performance with nouns, adjectives and verbs was substantially better (86%, 83% and 94%, respectively).

A second patient, WB, described by Funnell (1983) averaged about 85% correct in reading words aloud, while he was completely unable to read nonwords. At the same time, WB had very poor semantic understanding (he was unsure, for example, whether *mitten* or *sock* was a close associate of *glove*), suggesting that his ability to read aloud words considerably exceeded his ability to understand fully what they meant. It has been claimed that phonological dyslexic patients like WB, provide convincing evidence for a lexical route to phonology that is independent of nonlexical procedures (e.g. Coltheart 1985). (This route involves direct lexical mappings between orthography and phonology – hence the term, direct route reading.) However, the champion of the multiple-levels approach points out a potential problem for this view (Shallice 1988). As a group, phonological dyslexics tend to experience greater difficulty in reading aloud functors than other word classes: AM, for example, was able to read only 72% of functors. It is not hard to see why there might be a difficulty with functors if word reading is mediated by the semantic system ('meaningless' functors might not be represented there, for example), but if phonological dyslexic reading depends on a lexical, non-semantic, routine, then why should functors be relatively disadvantaged? This is even more surprising when one recalls that evidence from the surface dyslexic patient described by Bub/Cancelliere/Kertesz (1985), often used to support the notion of direct route reading, indicated that word frequency was an important factor in reading success by the direct route: functors are among the most frequent words in the language.

Shallice (1988) turns this question on its head and asks why it is that functors, in particular, tend to cause difficulty for phonological dyslexics. Patterson (1982) has proposed that this is because function word reading depends on intact phonological procedures (we will not go into why this may be the case here) which are not available to phonological dyslexics. This view predicts that patients who are severely impaired in reading aloud nonwords will also inevitably experience problems with functors. There is tantalising evidence that this may not be true. Both Shallice/Warrington (1980) and Funnell (1983) describe phonological dyslexic patients who did not have especial difficulty with functors, though in each of these cases a subtle speech production difficulty might actually have been responsible for the nonword reading impairment (Howard 1985; Shallice 1988).

4. Reading via Semantics

Difficulties in reading aloud nonwords have also been described in the acquired reading disturbance known as **deep dyslexia**, the third major reading impairment discussed by Marshall/Newcombe (1973). In investigating this disorder, much of the debate has centred on whether it actually constitutes a coherent syndrome or symptom-complex, and, if so, which features can be taken as 'key', 'essential' and 'less essential' (to echo the above discussion about surface dyslexia). As with the other disorders we have discussed, the answer seems to be that deep dyslexia fractionates into a variety of different underlying impairments, and that the relative importance of various features of the disorder changes with the nature of the impairment.

Word reading success in deep dyslexia is considerably lower than in phonological dyslexia and is characterised by a number of different error types. Pre-eminent among them, and taken as the defining or pathognomonic sign, is the semantic reading error (*cannibal* read aloud as *savages*, for example, or, *merry* read as *Christmas*). For a detailed discussion of the categories of semantic error that can occur, see Coltheart (1980 a). Other major error types are visual errors (e. g. *own* → *now*), which include visual and/or semantic errors (e. g. *fragment* → *segment*) and visual-then-semantic errors (e. g. *sympathy* read as *orchestra*, perhaps via the mediation of symphony), morphological errors (referred to as derivational errors) such as *free* for *freedom*, *rejected* for *rejection*, and function-word substitutions of one functor for another (e. g. *was* → *and*).

Whether a word can be read successfully critically depends on how imageable or concrete it is, rather than on how frequent it is (e. g. Richardson 1976). Much also depends on the part-of-speech to which the word belongs: nouns, for example, are read aloud correctly more often than verbs or functors. It appears, however, that this effect can also be attributable to imageability rather than to grammatical word class, since nouns tend to have higher imageability ratings than verbs or functors (e. g. Allport/Funnell 1981). (Note that this variable may not be responsible for the particular difficulty with functors experienced by phonological dyslexics, since imageability is not an important factor governing this disorder.) In addition, the ability to read nonwords is generally totally abolished, single letter naming and sounding is often severely impaired, and great difficulty is experienced in making any kind of phonological judgements from written material (e. g. Patterson/Marcel 1977).

Marshall/Newcombe's (1973) classic account argued that the absence of phonological reading in deep dyslexia precipitated the production of semantic errors; they suggested that any available phonological information would have allowed the patient to eliminate such errors. It is further suggested that the reason why semantic errors occur in the first place has to do with the inherently imprecise nature of semantic representations (Saffran/Schwartz/Marin 1976; Newcombe/Marshall 1980). Thus, deep dyslexia, it is assumed, provides a window on a semantic mechanism that is operating in a relatively normal fashion. A major difficulty with this account is that it now appears that different levels of impairment can underpin deep dyslexia and that different deficits can each result in the production of semantic reading errors.

Several authors have proposed that a 'deep dyslexic' pattern of reading in general, and the semantic error in particular, can result from different kinds of impairment (e. g. Shallice/Warrington 1980; Shallice 1988). These can be broadly summarised as a 'input' difficulty in accessing the semantic system from the visual input lexicon, a 'central' difficulty within the semantic system itself, and an 'output' difficulty in accessing lexical semantic representations within the speech output lexicon.

A large percentage of errors produced by deep dyslexics like KF (Shallice/Warrington 1975) and PS (Shallice/Coughlan 1980) were visual errors (61% and 51% respectively). The percentage of semantic errors was much lower (4% and 10% respectively). Shallice (1988) suggests that patients exhibiting a high ratio of visual-to-semantic errors may have an 'input' disorder that arises during the course of access to the semantic system. Shallice explicitly rules out an impairment to the visual input lexicon as the cause of the patients' visual errors, because here one might have expected such errors to occur on high and low imageability words alike (since the deficit would precede the semantic system). This was not the case; visual errors tended to be produced more often in response to low imageability words – the words that gave the patients most difficulty. In line with this proposed locus of impairment, both patients showed much poorer performance on written comprehension tasks than on auditory comprehension tasks.

Some deep dyslexic readers appear to have a central semantic difficulty that can affect all modalities of input and output. An example is patient GR (Newcombe/Marshall 1980) who produced semantic errors in picture-to-word matching and in spelling-to-dictation. A further example is the case of KE, recently described by Hillis/Rapp/Romani/Caramazza (1990). This patient was reported to make comparable types and rates of semantic errors across a variety of tasks: oral reading, reading and auditory comprehension, spelling-to-dictation, writing picture names and saying picture names, consistent with the proposal of a selective impairment to the semantic system.

A third type of 'output' deep dyslexic reader is characterised by patient PW (Patterson 1978). PW made considerably more semantic errors than visual errors (54% compared with 13%, respectively). His performance on comprehension tasks that did not require a verbal response was good, both for written and auditory input. His comprehension of low imageability words was also good, even though he had substantial difficulty in reading them aloud (Patterson/Besner 1984). The difficulty for this patient appears to be at the level of access to word phonology, rather than within the semantic system. A similar explanation is proposed for patient RGB, described by Hillis/Rapp/Romani/Caramazza (1990). Hillis and her colleagues suggest that intact semantic representations activate in varying degrees a set of semantically related representations in a phonological output lexicon. If the target word is inaccessible for some reason, another semantically related response may be produced instead. This proposal is similar to the 'response-blocking' explanation put forward by Morton/Patterson (1980).

These accounts of the variation that can occur in the level of impairment in deep dyslexia have recently been exploited by connectionist-based investigations of acquired dyslexic deficits (see Hinton/Shallice 1991), with some surprising yet promising findings (e. g. Plaut/Shallice 1991). This work is rooted in the view that deep dyslexia reveals certain operations of the normal reading system, with damage to some of its components. However, a radical alternative exists, which claims that deep dyslexia reflects the operation of right-hemisphere language processing systems (Coltheart 1980 b; Saffran 1980). The right-hemisphere hypothesis has attracted a good deal of controversy over the past decade (e. g. Coltheart 1983; Patterson/Besner 1984). Much of it focuses on revealing the abilities of the right hemisphere reading system in normal subjects (from laterality studies) and on comparing the reading performance of deep dyslexics with right hemisphere reading by a small group of 'split-brain' patients (patients in whom cortical connections between right and left hemisphere have been severed in an attempt to relieve intractable epilepsy). Much of it is inconclusive, as Patterson/Besner (1984) convincingly demonstrate. Indeed, the right hemisphere theory of deep dyslexia was in danger of simply trickling away: as Shallice (1988) noted, "Problems for the theory keep arising. As soon as one leak is temporarily plugged, another bursts through". However, there has been a recent upsurge of interest in the theory that stems primarily from cerebral blood-flow and PET-scan studies that show far more right than left hemisphere activation in individual deep dyslexic patients (e. g. Coltheart/Weekes/Savage et al. 1991). A challenge for the theory is to account for the fractionation of deficits that occur within the disorder.

In conclusion, a variety of different patterns of reading disturbance that can be acquired through brain damage have been described and interpreted with reference to cognitive models of single word recognition and production. Existing findings demonstrate convincingly the fractionation of the basic categories of deep, surface and visual dyslexia, though this work is firmly within the spirit of Marshall and Newcombe's original enterprise.

5. References

Allport, D. A. & Funnell, E. (1981). Components of the mental lexicon. *Philosophical Transactions of the Royal Society of London, B, 295*, 397–410.

Baxter, D. M. & Warrington, E. K. (1983). Neglect dysgraphia. *Journal of Neurology, Neurosurgery & Psychiatry, 46*, 1073–1078.

Beauvois, M.-F. & Derouesné, J. (1979). Phonological alexia: Three dissociations. *Journal of Neurology, Neurosurgery & Psychiatrie, 42*, 1115–1124.

Behrmann, M., Moscovitch, M., Black, S. E., & Moser, M. (in press). Perceptual and conceptual mechanisms in neglect dyslexia: Two contrasting case studies. *Brain.*

Bub, D., Cancelliere, A., & Kertesz, A. (1985). Whole-word and analytic translation of spelling-to-sound in a non-semantic reader. In K. E. Patterson, M. Coltheart, & J. C. Marshall (Eds.), *Surface Dyslexia. 15–34.* London: Erlbaum.

Caramazza, A. & Hillis, A. E. (1990). Levels of representation, co-ordinate frames and unilateral neglect. *Cognitive Neuropsychology, 7*, 369–389.

Chomsky, N. (1965). *Aspects of the Theory of Syntax*. Cambridge, MA.: MIT-Press.

Coltheart, M. (1978). Lexical access in simple reading tasks. In G. Underwood (Ed.), *Strategies of Information Processing*. London: Academic Press.

Coltheart, M. (1980 a). The semantic error: Types and theories. In M. Coltheart, K. E. Patterson, & J. C. Marshall (Eds.), *Deep Dyslexia. 146–159*. London: Routledge.

Coltheart, M. (1980 b). Deep dyslexia: A right-hemisphere hypothesis. In M. Coltheart, K. E. Patterson, & J. C. Marshall (Eds.), *Deep Dyslexia. 326–380*. London: Routledge.

Coltheart, M. (1983). The right hemisphere and disorders of reading. In A. W. Young (Ed.), *Functions of the Right Cerebral Hemisphere*. London: Academic Press.

Coltheart, M. (1985). Cognitive neuropsychology and the study of reading. In M. I. Posner & O. S. M. Marin (Eds.), *Attention & Performance, Vol. 11. 3–37*. Hillsdale, N. J.: Erlbaum.

Coltheart, M., Masterson, J., Byng, S., Prior, M., & Riddoch, J. (1983). Surface dyslexia. *Quarterly Journal of Experimental Psychology, 35 A*, 469–495.

Coltheart, M., Weekes, B., Savage, K., Simpson, L., Zurinsky, Y., & Gordon, E. (1991). *Deep dyslexia and right hemisphere reading: A regional cerebral bloodflow study*. Paper presented to Deep Dyslexia: 12 Years On. London, Birkbeck College.

Costello, A. de L. & Warrington, E. K. (1987). Dissociation of visuo-spatial neglect and neglect dyslexia. *Journal of Neurology, Neurosurgery & Psychiatry, 50*, 1110–1116.

Déjerine, M. J. (1892). Contribution a l'etude anatomo-pathologique et clinique des differentes varietes de cecite verbale. *Comptes Rendus des Seances et Memoires de la Societe de Biologie, 44*, 61–90.

Ellis, A. W., Flude, B. M., & Young, A. W. (1987). 'Neglect dyslexia' and the early visual processing of letters in words and nonwords. *Cognitive Neuropsychology, 4*, 439–464.

Evett, L. J. & Humphreys, G. (1981). The use of abstract graphemic information in lexical access. *Quarterly Journal of Experimental Psychology, 33 A*, 325–350.

Friedmann, R. B. & Alexander, M. P. (1984). Pictures, images and pure alexia: A case study. *Cognitive Neuropsycholoy, 1*, 9–23.

Funnell, E. (1983). Phonological processes in reading: New evidence from acquired dyslexia. *British Journal of Psychology, 74*, 159–180.

Goldblum, M. C. (1985). Word comprehension in surface dyslexia. In K. E. Patterson, M. Coltheart, & J. C. Marshall (Eds.), *Surface Dyslexia. 175–205*. London: Erlbaum.

Henderson, L. (1982). *Orthography and Word Recognition in Reading*. London: Academic Press.

Hillis, A. E. & Caramazza, A. (1992). The reading process and its disorders. In D. I. Margolin (Ed.), *Cognitive Neuropsychology in Clinical Practice*. Cary: Oxford University Press.

Hillis, A. E., Rapp, B. C., Romani, C., & Caramazza, A. (1990). Selective impairment of semantics in lexical processing. *Cognitive Neuropsychology, 7*, 191–244.

Hinton, G. & Shallice, T. (1991). Lesioning an attractor network: Investigations of acquired dyslexia. *Psychological Review, 98*, 74–95.

Howard, D. (1985). *The Semantic Organisation of the Lexicon: Evidence from Aphasia*. Unpublished doctoral dissertation. University of London.

Humphreys, G. W. & Riddoch, M. J. (1990). Interactions between object and space systems revealed through neuropsychology. In D. E. Meyer & S. Kornblum (Eds.), *Attention and Performance, Vol. 14*. Hillsdale, N. J.: Erlbaum.

Kartsounis, L. D. & Warrington, E. K. (1989). Unilateral neglect overcome by cues implicit in stimulus displays. *Journal of Neurology, Neurosurgery & Psychiatry, 52*, 1253–1259.

Kay, J. & Bishop, D. V. M. (1987). Anatomical differences between nose, palm and foot, or, the body in question. In M. Coltheart (Ed.), *Attention and Performance, Vol. 12. 449–469*. London: Erlbaum.

Kay, J. & Hanley, J. R. (1991). Simultaneous form perception and serial letter recognition in a case of letter-by-letter reading. *Cognitive Neuropsychology, 8*, 249–273.

Kay, J. & Lesser, R. (1985). The nature of phonological processing in oral reading: Evidence from surface dyslexia. *Quarterly Journal of Experimental Psychology, 37 A*, 39–81.

Kay, J. & Patterson, K. E. (1985). Routes to meaning in surface dyslexia. In K. E. Patterson, M. Coltheart, & J. C. Marshall (Eds.), *Surface Dyslexia. 79–103*. London: Erlbaum.

Kinsbourne, M. & Warrington, E. K. (1962 a). A variety of reading disability associated with right hemisphere lesions. *Journal of Neurology, Neurosurgery & Psychiatry, 25*, 339–344.

Kinsbourne,M. & Warrington, E. K. (1962 b). A disorder of simultaneous form perception. *Brain, 85*, 461–486.

Kremin, H. (1981). Deux strategies de lecture dissociable par la pathologie: Description d'un cas de dyslexie profonde et d'un cas de dyslexie de surface. In C. L. Nespoulos (Ed.), *Etudes neurolinguistiques*. Toulouse: Le Mirail.

Kremin, H. (1985). Routes and strategies in surface dyslexia and dysgraphia. In K. E. Patterson, J. C. Marshall, & M. Coltheart (Eds.), *Surface Dyslexia. Neuropsychological and Cognitive Studies of Phonological Reading. 105–137*. London: Erlbaum.

McClelland, J. L. & Rumelhart, D. E. (1981). An interactive activation model of context effects in letter perception: Part 1. An account of basic findings. *Psychological Review*, *88*, 375–407.

Marcel, A. J. (1980). Surface dyslexia and beginning reading: A revised hypothesis of the pronunciation of print and its impairments. In M. Coltheart, K. E. Patterson, & J. C. Marshall (Eds.), *Deep Dyslexia. 227–258.* London: Routledge.

Margolin, D. I., Marcel, A. J., & Carlson, N. R. (1985). Common processes in dysnomia and post-semantic dyslexia: Processing deficits and selective attention. In K. E. Patterson, M. Coltheart, & J. C. Marshall (Eds.), *Surface Dyslexia. 139–173.* London: Erlbaum.

Marr, D. (1982). *Vision.* San Francisco: Freeman.

Marshall, J. C. & Newcombe, F. (1966). Syntactic and semantic errors in paralexia. *Neuropsychologia*, *4*, 169–176.

Marshall, J. C. & Newcombe, F. (1973). Patterns of paralexia: A psycholinguistic approach. *Journal of Psycholinguistic Research*, *2*, 175–199.

Morton, J. & Patterson, K. E. (1980). A new attempt at an interpretation, or, an attempt at a new interpretation. In M. Coltheart, K. E. Patterson, & J. C. Marshall (Eds.), *Deep Dyslexia. 91–118.* London: Routledge.

Newcombe, F. & Marshall, J. C. (1980). Transcoding and lexical stabilization in deep dyslexia. In M. Coltheart, K. E. Patterson, & J. C. Marshall (Eds.), *Deep Dyslexia. 176–188.* London: Routledge.

Newcombe, F. & Marshall, J. C. (1985). Reading and writing by letter sounds. In K. E. Patterson, M. Coltheart, & J. C. Marshall (Eds.), *Surface Dyslexia. 35–51.* London: Erlbaum.

Patterson, K. E. (1978). Phonemic dyslexia: errors of meaning and meaning of errors. *Quarterly Journal of Experimental Psychology*, *30*, 587–601.

Patterson, K. E. (1982). The relation between reading and phonological coding: Further neuropsychological observations. In A. W. Ellis (Ed.), *Normality and Pathology in Cognitive Functions. 77–111.* London: Academic Press.

Patterson, K. E. & Besner, D. (1984). Is the right hemisphere literate? *Cognitive Neuropsychology*, *1*, 315–342.

Patterson, K. E. & Kay, J. (1982). Letter-by-letter reading: Psychological descriptions of a neurological syndrome. *Quarterly Journal of Experimental Psychology*, *34 A*, 411–441.

Patterson, K. E. & Marcel, A. J. (1977). Aphasia, dyslexia and the phonological coding of written words. *Quarterly Journal of Experimental Psychology*, *29*, 307–318.

Patterson, K. E. & Morton, J. (1985). From orthography to phonology: An attempt at an old interpretation. In K. E. Patterson, M. Coltheart, & J. C. Marshall (Eds.), *Surface Dyslexia. 335–359.* London: Erlbaum.

Patterson, K. E. & Wilson, B. (1990). A rose is a rose or a nose: A deficit in initial letter identification. *Cognitive Neuropsychology*, *7*, 447–479.

Patterson, K. E., Marshall, J. C., & Coltheart, M. (Eds.) (1985). *Surface Dyslexia.* London: Erlbaum.

Plaut, D. C. & Shallice, T. (1991). *Effects of abstractness in a connectionist model of deep dyslexia.* Proceedings of the 13th Annual Meeting of the Cognitive Science Society, pages 73–78. Chicago, IL.

Posner, M. I., Walker, J. A., Friedrich, F. J., & Rafal, R. D. (1984). Effects of parietal injury on covert orienting of visual attention. *Journal of Neuroscience*, *4*, 1863–1874.

Rapp, B. C. & Caramazza, A. (1991). Spatially determined deficits in letter and word processing. *Cognitive Neuropsychology*, *8*, 275–312.

Reuter-Lorenz, P. A. & Brunn, J. L. (1990). A prelexical basis for letter-by-letter reading. *Cognitive Neuropsychology*, *7*, 1–20.

Richardson, J. T. E. (1976). The effect of word imageability in acquired dyslexia. *Neuropsychologia*, *13*, 281–288.

Riddoch, M. J. (1990). Neglect and the peripheral dyslexias. *Cognitive Neuropsychology*, *7*, 369–389.

Riddoch, M. J., Humphreys, G., Cleton, P., & Fery, P. (1990). Interaction of attentional and lexical processes in neglect. *Cognitive Neuropsychology*, *7*, 479–517.

Saffran, E. M. (1980). Reading in deep dyslexia is not ideographic. *Neuropsychologia*, *18*, 219–223.

Saffran, E. M., Schwartz, M. F., & Marin, O. S. M. (1976). Semantic mechanisms in paralexia. *Brain & Language*, *3*, 255–265.

Schwartz, M. F., Saffran, E. M., & Marin, O. S. M. (1980). Fractionating the reading process in dementia: Evidence for word-specific print-to-sound associations. In M. Coltheart, K. E. Patterson, & J. C. Marshall (Eds.), *Deep Dyslexia. 259–269.* London: Routledge.

Seidenberg, M. S., Waters, G. S., Barnes, M. A., & Tanenhaus, M. K. (1984). When does irregular spelling or pronunciation influence word recognition? *Journal of Verbal Learning and Verbal Behavior*, *23*, 383–404.

Shallice, T. (1988). *From Neuropsychology to Mental Structure.* Cambridge: Cambridge University Press.

Shallice, T. & Coughlan, A. K. (1980). Modality specific word comprehension deficits in deep dyslexia. *Journal of Neurology, Neurosurgery & Psychiatry*, *43*, 866–872.

Shallice, T. & McCarthy, R. (1985). Phonological reading: From patterns of impairment to possible procedures. In K. E. Patterson, M. Coltheart, & J. C. Marshall (Eds.), *Surface Dyslexia. 361–397.* London: Erlbaum.

Shallice, T. & Warrington, E. K. (1975). Word recognition in a phonemic dyslexic patient. *Quarterly Journal of Experimental Psychology*, *27*, 187–199.

Shallice, T. & Warrington, E. K. (1980). Single and multiple component central dyslexic syndromes. In M. Coltheart, K. Patterson & J. C. Marshall (Eds.), *Deep dyslexia. 119–145*. London: Routledge.

Shallice, T., Warrington, E. K., & McCarthy, R. (1983). Reading without semantics. *Quarterly Journal of Experimental Psychology*, *35 A*, 111–138.

Sieroff, E. (1990). Focusing on/in visual-verbal stimuli in patients with parietal lesions. *Cognitive Neuropsychology*, *7*, 519–554.

Treisman, A. (1988). Features and objects: The fourteenth Bartlett Memorial Lecture. *Quarterly Journal of Psychology*, *40 A*, 201–237.

Venezky, R. L. (1970). *The Structure of English Orthography*. The Hague: Mouton.

Warrington, E. K. (1975). The selective impairment of semantic memory. *Quarterly Journal of Experimental Psychology*, *27*, 635–657.

Warrington, E. K. (1991). Right neglect dyslexia: A single case study. *Cognitive Neuropsychology*, *8*, 193–212.

Warrington, E. K. & Shallice, T. (1980). Word-form dyslexia. *Brain*, *103*, 885–896.

Young, A., Newcombe, F., & Ellis, A. W. (1991). Different impairments contribute to neglect dyslexia. *Cognitive Neuropsychology*, *8*, 177–192.

Janice Kay, Exeter (U. K.)

23. Acquired Disorders of Writing and Spelling

1. Historical Introduction

As is the case with the field of aphasiology in general, the neuropsychological study of agraphia originated with the work of nineteenth century European neurologists. Several different models and classifications of agraphia were proposed by these early investigators based on clinico-anatomical observations in patients with focal brain damage (for reviews see Leischner 1969; Marcie/Hécaen 1979). While some of these are purely anatomically based, others also focus on cognitive mechanisms and bear a striking resemblance to current linguistic information processing models of spelling (Charcot 1889; Ellis 1988). Rather than provide an exhaustive review of the various classification systems of agraphia, we will only attempt here to highlight certain historic developments relevant to our current understanding of the linguistic processes and brain mechanisms involved in writing and spelling.

Although the first discussion of writing disturbances following focal brain lesions is attributed to Marcé (1856), it was Benedikt (1865) who first used the term agraphia. Benedikt (1865) also suggested that parts of the brain that control written and spoken language may have different anatomical localization. Ogle (1867) reached a similar conclusion based on his own clinico-anatomical studies of aphasic patients: "The occasional separation of agraphia and aphasia points [...] to the existence of distinct cerebral centers for the faculties concerned in speaking and in writing; while the more frequent coincidence of the two affections leads us to infer that these centers must be closely contiguous". Ogle distinguished two types of agraphia. In "amnemonic" agraphia, letters are well-formed but are used incorrectly or one word is substituted for another. In "atactic" agraphia, letters are poorly formed and are sometimes unrecognizable. While the views about the independence of writing from speech were rejected by many (Wernicke 1874; Lichtheim 1885; Jackson 1878; Déjerine 1914), Ogle's clinical distinction between the linguistic and motor disorders of writing was universally endorsed.

The next phase of development in the study of agraphia was characterized by attempts to identify the anatomical location of the cortical centers that mediated the linguistic and motor components of writing. This was a natural direction to take, given the prevailing nineteenth century view of language function in the brain which assumed that psycholinguistic faculties were localizable to distinct cortical regions. The cortical language centers served as memory stores for specific types of linguistic or motor representations and the transmission of information between the language centers occurred via connecting neuronal pathways. These early theories of brain functioning, advocated by the so-called 'diagram makers', provided the impetus for the proliferation of connectionist models of language processing. Within this conceptual framework, Exner (1881) proposed that the cortical center of "motor graphic images" was located at the foot of the second frontal convolution, directly in front of the hand area of the primary motor cortex. The notion of a center for the motor movements of writing, analogous to the motor center for the programming of speech movements (i. e., Broca's area), was criticized on various grounds both by Wernicke (1886) and Déjerine (1914) but was accepted with only slight modifications by Charcot (1889), Pitres (1894) and Bastian (1898) among others. Despite the controversy about Exner's writing center, there was a general consensus that the motor movements of writing had to be activated by input from centers that contained linguistic information relevant to the spelling of words. These orthographic representations or "optic word images" were believed by many to be stored in the region of the dominant angular gyrus (Déjerine 1891; Pitres 1894; Henschen 1922; Pick 1931; Nielsen 1946). The putative parietal memory store of learned spellings thus plays a central role in several models of writing. Wernicke (1874; 1886), however, was of the opinion that written language always depended on spoken language and maintained that orthographic representations could only be activated indirectly via phonological representations. He also entertained the possibility that once the ability to write has been acquired, the motor movements could be activated directly from 'sound images' without the participation of visual orthographic representations.

The connectionist models of writing, in their fully developed form, were also explicit about mechanisms for the coordinated activity between the parietal center of orthographic representations and the frontal motor center for the movements of writing (Henschen 1922; Pick 1931; Nielsen 1946). The flow of information between the cortical centers of writing was generally conceptualized as a sensory-to-motor spread of excitation from posterior to anterior brain areas, similar to Wernicke's (1874) model of spoken language production. The connectionist view is perhaps best articulated by Nielsen (1946): "When one wishes to write, one starts activity in the neurons of the left angular gyrus and by this means revives memories of letters and words one wishes to write. Impulses travel for association to all posterior portions of the brain and forward in the external capsule to the writing center at the foot of the second frontal convolution [...] coordinated activity between the writing center and the angular gyrus is necessary not only for the proper execution of the movements of writing but also for the proper concept and spelling of the words".

It is interesting to note that although the connectionists generally assumed that the orthographic representations stored in the dominant angular gyrus were accessed by a whole-word retrieval process, there were also proponents of a subword level phoneme-grapheme conversion procedure in spelling. Grashey (1885), for example, postulated that the writing of words always required the serial translation of each sound unit to the corresponding grapheme. This view was later adopted by Wernicke (1886), although he originally posited that the indivisible unit of spelling was the word (Wernicke 1874). A model of spelling based on the use of sound-letter correspondence rules was also favored by Luria (1970).

Although considerable progress has been made over the years in providing more refined and comprehensive neurolinguistic accounts of the writing process, until recently there was relatively little attention devoted to the linguistic analysis of spelling errors. A notable exception in the older literature is a posthumously published paper by Arnold Pick (1925). Based on a review of previously reported cases and his own observations, Pick makes a clear distinction between phonetic and orthographic writing. Since orthographic knowledge is acquired relatively late in language development, Pick suggests that it may be especially vulnerable to brain pathology. He concludes, in agreement with the earlier views of Heilbronner (1910), that brain damage may selectively impair orthographic writing, while sparing the ability to write 'purely phonetically'. Pick also observes that many patients already have an imperfect orthographic knowledge premorbidly and that the disparity between phonetic and orthographic writing may vary considerably in different languages. Although Pick's remarkable insights received little attention at the time of publication, their relevance for current information processing models of writing is quite striking.

2. Modern Models of Writing

2.1. Neurological Models

Recent classifications of agraphia have been of two general types, neurological and linguistic. The neurological classifications have emphasized clinical-pathological correlations and the relationship between agraphia and other language disturbances, i. e., aphasia and alexia. This approach has led to the development of three general categories of acquired agraphia: aphasic agraphia, agraphia with alexia and pure agraphia.

2.1.1. Aphasic Agraphia

The emphasis on the relationship of agraphia and aphasia has been present since Lichtheim (1885) described one of the earliest neurological models of written language and even before him (Benedikt 1865; Ogle 1867) the relationship was addressed. Aphasic agraphia is usually subdivided into the agraphia of Broca's aphasia, the agraphia of conduction aphasia, the agraphia of Wernicke's aphasia and the agraphia of transcortical sensory aphasia (Benson 1979; Clark/Grossfield 1983; Kaplan/Goodglass 1981; Marcie/Hécaen 1979). The characteristics of each type of agraphia are said to be dependent upon the type of aphasia associated with it.

2.1.2. Agraphia with Alexia

This disorder is also called parietal agraphia because the two symptoms of alexia and agraphia, in the absence of significant aphasia, are said to usually occur together in patients with dominant parietal lobe lesions (Kaplan/Goodglass 1981). These patients are said to typically produce poorly formed graphemes when writing and, although in spelling aloud they pronounce letters correctly, they have difficulty spelling.

2.1.3. Pure Agraphia

In the traditional neurological models, this is a writing disorder without other significant language disturbance. Most patients with pure agraphia produce well formed graphemes or letters but make different types of spelling errors, depending upon the lesion location. Multiple lesion sites have been implicated in pure agraphia and include the second frontal convolution (Exner's area) (Aimard/Devick/Lebel et al. 1975; Vernea/Merory 1975; Hécaen/Albert 1978; Kaplan/Goodglass 1981; Marcie/Hécaen 1979) the superior parietal lobule (Auerbach/Alexander 1981; Basso/Taborielli/Vignolo 1978), the posterior perisylvian region (Rosati/DeBastiani 1981) and the region of the left caudate and internal capsule (Laine/Marttila 1981).

Pure agraphia, unlike pure alexia which is associated with a fairly consistent lesion site (the dominant occipital lobe) and a fairly consistent pattern of reading disorder (letter by letter reading or inability to read), occurs from multiple lesion sites and consists of multiple types of behavioral abnormalities. One goal of the neurological models has been an attempt to delineate anatomic loci that can be associated with pure agraphia. Although early studies emphasized various cortical regions, more recent studies have emphasized subcortical regions (Laine/Marttila 1981; Tanridag/Kirshner 1985; Kertesz/Latham/Mc Cabe 1990).

The traditional neurological approach to agraphia has helped explain some features found in agraphic patients but there are frequent inconsistencies. First, there is an overlap between syndromes in that two types of agraphia, such as one subtype of aphasic agraphia (Broca's aphasic agraphia with disturbed letter production) and the agraphia with alexia may have the same description (Kaplan/Goodglass 1981; Marcie/Hécaen 1979). Also, some patients with an agraphia defined by the neurological approach, i. e. Broca's aphasic agraphia, may have impairment of writing and spelling that more closely resembles the impaired writing and spelling of a patient with Wernicke's aphasia than the impairment found in other patients with Broca's aphasia (Roeltgen/Sevush/Heilman 1983).

In addition to the difficulties in the behavioral analysis utilizing the traditional neurologic models, there are difficulties that arise regarding attempts at clinical-pathologic correlation. One lesion locus may be associated with multiple disorders and conversely, the same disorder may be associated with multiple anatomic loci. For example, the dominant parietal lobe has been implicated in the syndrome of agraphia with alexia but has also been implicated in the syndrome of pure agraphia (Basso/Taborelli/Vignolo 1978; Hécaen/Albert 1978; Kaplan/Goodglass 1981; Leischner 1969; Marcie/Hécaen 1979), and pure agraphia has occurred in patients with lesions in various sites as noted previously.

2.2 Linguistic Models

In the past ten to fifteen years, investigators have attempted to find models that are not dependent upon other disorders and thereby develop a classification of agraphia that is more dependent upon the analysis of the agraphia rather than the co-occurrence of aphasia or alexia. This approach can best be termed linguistic because of its emphasis on patterns of linguistic performance, including both analysis of errors made by patients as well as analysis of performance on words of different linguistic type. The linguistic models also differ from the traditional models in that most put very little emphasis on clinical-pathological localization, although occasional attempts at clinical-pathological correlation have been made (Roeltgen/Sevush/Heilman 1983; Roeltgen/Heilman 1984; Roeltgen/Rothi/Heilman 1982; Iwata 1984; Kawamura/Hirayama/Hasegawa et al. 1987; Rapcsak/Rubens 1990).

Attempts at linguistic analysis of agraphia have involved two different language groups, Indo-European and Japanese. Although certain features are similar both within the disorders involved as well as the written language systems, sufficient differences exist so that they will be treated separately here.

In this chapter we discuss the various agraphias in patients with focal lesions and also senile dementia of the Alzheimer type within the framework of a linguistic processing model of spelling and review relevant anatomical data when appropriate.

2.2.1. Linguistic Studies of Agraphia in Indo-European Languages

The initial detailed linguistic studies of agraphia were performed by Shallice (1981) and Beauvois & Derouesné (1981). Since then, data from their studies and others have been used to develop linguistic models of the normal writing process. Ellis (1982) provided one of the first such models and others have followed (Margolin 1984; Roeltgen 1985; Roeltgen/Heilman 1984; Patterson 1986; Lesser 1990; Rapcsak/Rubens 1990). All of these models contain many of the same features as that first developed by Ellis, and a prototypical model is presented in Figure 23.1. Most of the differences among these models are in terminology. However, there are certain important conceptual differences that address some of the features within the model. All of the models emphasize two dissociable systems or pathways through which spellings of words could be produced, a phonological nonlexical system that requires phoneme to grapheme conversion [or phonographeme to letter (Lesser 1990) or phonological

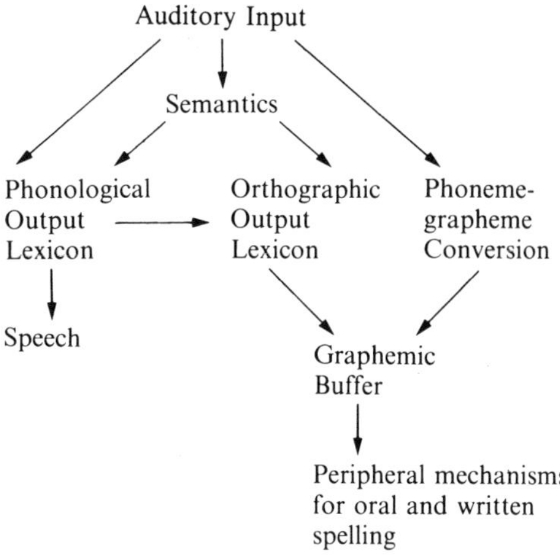

Fig. 23.1: Diagrammatic model of linguistic spelling systems. Modified after Rapcsak/Rubens (1990)

to orthographic conversion (Patterson 1986; Margolin 1984)] and a lexical (Roeltgen/Heilman 1984; Lesser 1990) [or a lexical-orthographic (Margolin 1984) or orthographic (Patterson 1986; Rapcsak/Rubens 1990)] system. In addition to these two systems, a third major component included in all of these models is a semantic system (Roeltgen/Rothi/Heilman 1986; Roeltgen 1985; Margolin 1984; Lesser 1990; Rapcsak/Rubens 1990) or what has been alternatively called the cognitive system (Patterson 1986). The phonological system is thought to be important for spelling pronounceable nonwords (e. g., *flig*) and can also serve as a back-up system for spelling regular real words, especially regular words of limited ambiguity. Ambiguity is operationally defined based on the number of alternative graphemes or letters appropriate for each of the phonemes within a word. For example, *charm* may be spelled in only one way that produces the correct pronounciation. In contrast, *cotton* may be spelled in multiple ways (e. g., *cotton, kotton, kottin*) with the same resulting phonology. Although the phonological system is usually presented as a nonlexical system of phoneme to grapheme conversion, some authors have argued that it really represents a lexically based system that allows the spelling of unknown words using analogy (Campbell 1983). The lexical system is important for production of known words and is typically necessary for spelling words that are orthographically irregular and words of high ambiguity. Irregular words are words that cannot be spelled by direct phoneme-to-grapheme conversion (e. g., *island* and *yacht*). Semantic influence, although not important for the correct spellings of words, is necessary for the incorporation of meaning into what is written by selection of words containing the correct meaning. In addition to these systems necessary for the correct letter and word selection, there is one additional cognitive component involved prior to the more peripheral or motoric components of writing or oral spelling, and that system has been labeled the graphemic or orthographic buffer (Caramazza/Micheli/Villa/Romani 1987; Hillis/Caramazza 1989; Badecker/Hillis/Caramazza 1990; Margolin 1984; Lesser 1990). This last component is defined as a temporary working memory store of abstract letters or graphemes prior to the conversion into concrete letter shapes (for written spelling) or letter names (for oral spelling) (Caramazza/Micheli/Villa/Romani 1987).

These systems or pathways that are thought to be important for the production of normal spelling have primarily been developed from the analysis of patients with acquired agraphia. Patients with these agraphias have produced patterns of performance that appear to be consistent with selective dysfunction of one of the above postulated systems. The disorders include phonological agraphia due to disruption of the nonlexical phonological or phoneme-grapheme conversion system, lexical agraphia due to disruption of the lexical or orthographic system, semantic agraphia due to disruption of the semantic system or disconnection of the semantic system from the other linguistic spelling systems and graphemic buffer agraphia, due to disruption of the graphemic buffer.

2.2.1.1. Phonological Agraphia

In 1981, Shallice described a patient who had difficulty spelling pronounceable nonwords (e. g., *flig*) but had preserved ability to write (spell) real words that were orthographically irregular. Shallice termed this syndrome phonological agraphia. Others have described patients with similar disorders (Morton 1980; Roeltgen/Sevush/Heilman 1983; Baxter/Warrington 1985; Bolla-Wilson/Speedie/Robinson 1985; Roeltgen/Heilman 1984; Goodman-Schulman/Caramazza 1987; Hatfield 1985; Nolan/Caramazza 1982; Roeltgen/Rothi/Heilman 1982). These studies include two small series described by Roeltgen and colleagues (Roeltgen/Sevush/Heilman 1983; Roeltgen/Heilman 1984) and together include more than 15 patients. Among these patients there are certain variabilities, although all patients have had decreased ability to spell or write nonwords and have had no difference in their ability to spell regular and irregular words. The variability among patients has included differing effects of word class, concreteness and imageability. Word class differences have been found in some subjects, such that they can spell or write nouns better than verbs, adverbs and adjectives, all of which are written better than function words. The question has been raised whether this word class effect can be explained merely on the basis of concreteness. However, Baxter/Warrington (1985) have shown in their subject G. O. S. that concreteness can not account for the word class effect. Many subjects also show effects of imageability in that words of high imagery (book) are written better than words of low imagery (hope) even if these words are matched for length and frequency of occurrence (Roeltgen/Rothi/Heilman 1982). A similar effect is found for concreteness, and it is possible that the effects of imageability can be explained on that basis.

In addition to the variability found in these patients based on types of words on which they make errors, there are also some differences in the quality of the errors that are produced. Many of the subjects produced real word errors that have been termed 'derivational', i. e., responses with the same free morpheme as the stimulus but different bound morphemes (e. g., hunting for hunts or closed for closes) (Roeltgen/Sevush/Heilman 1983; Baxter/Warrington 1985). A second type of error is of particular interest because it suggests the way in which the patient may be accessing the spelling of the word that they are attempting to produce. These are visual errors or errors that demonstrate partial lexical knowledge (Ellis 1982). A visual similarity between the stimuli and the responses was demonstrated by Roeltgen/Sevush/Heilman (1983) and Hatfield (1985). They concluded that at least some of their patient's preserved spelling ability was dependent upon visual representations or visual word images. Based on a different method of analysis, Morton (1980) suggested a similar mechanism. Hatfield (1985) in an in-depth analysis of a patient with phonological agraphia concluded that what was termed the lexical system or orthographic knowledge is a collection of word knowledge that has accumulated through familiarity with the understanding of sound relationships, whole word shapes, word analogies and, perhaps, certain mnemonic rules. In the discussion of lexical agraphia later in this chapter, this heterogeneous collection of abilities becomes very important.

Some patients with impaired ability to spell nonwords also make semantic paragraphias (written responses with little phonological or visual resemblance to the stimulus words, e. g., spelling *flight* when *propeller* is the stimulus. Bub/Kertesz (1982) termed this syndrome deep agraphia because of its similarity to the reading disorder, deep dyslexia. Other patients with phonological agraphia who produce semantic paragraphias have also been described by Marshall/Newcombe (1966), Assal/Buttet/Jolivet (1981), Saffran/Schwartz/Marin (1981), patient 1 of Roeltgen/Sevush/Heilman (1983), patient EB of Hatfield (1985) and Van Lancker (1990). These patients also showed effects of imagery, spelling nouns of high imagery better than nouns of low imagery and function word substitution (e. g., spelling *and* when *but* is a stimulus). Because deep agraphia includes the error patterns found in phonological agraphia, plus semantic paragraphias, it is possible that deep agraphia represents phonological agraphia plus an additional linguistic dysfunction. As in the syndrome of deep dyslexia (Coltheart 1980; Saffran/Bogyo/Schwartz/Marin 1980), the functional breakdown leading to this important additional finding is not certain. It may be related to a disturbance of the semantic area or semantic ability, an incorrect access to or from semantics or the orthographic lexicon or the utilization of alternative or compensatory right hemispheric spelling strategies (Rapcsak/Beeson/Rubens 1991).

One additional area of controversy regarding phonological agraphia is its precise definition. In a prospective study of 43 patients with acquired left hemispheric lesions, Roeltgen (1989; 1991) described patients with a wide range of impairment on nonwords and showed that this impairment in nonword ability highly correlated with overall performance on an independent test of spelling achievement. However, a few subjects had relatively selective impairment of nonword spelling without severe impairment in the spelling of real words. It is uncertain whether the most appropriate operational definition of phonological agraphia should include only the latter group of patients with relatively isolated impairment in nonwords or whether it should include those patients who perform poorly on nonwords and also have mild impairments of real word performance.

2.2.1.2. Lexical Agraphia

Similar to phonological agraphia, lexical agraphia was first defined in 1981. Beauvois/Derouesné (1981) described a patient who, in contrast to patients with phonological agraphia, spelled nonwords well but had trouble spelling words that were irregular and ambiguous. By analogy with a similar reading disorder, this selective impairment of the lexical spelling system has also been termed surface agraphia. Also, similar to phonological agraphia, more than 15 patients have been described with lexical agraphia (Beauvois/Derouesné 1981; Hatfield/Patterson 1983; Roeltgen/Heilman 1984; Goodman-Schulman/Caramazza 1987; Rapcsak/Arthur/Rubens 1988; Friedman/Alexander 1989; Rothi/Roeltgen/Kooistra 1987; Croisile/Trillet/Laurent et al. 1989; Roeltgen 1989; Alexander/Friedman/Lo Verso/Fischer 1990; Rapcsak/Rubens/Laguna 1990). In one study (Roeltgen/Heilman 1984) four patients with lexical agraphia were compared to a random selection of four patients with phonological agraphia and two groups of control patients (brain damaged and not brain damaged). The patients with lexical agraphia had more difficulty spelling irregular words than a group of matched regular words. Control patients and patients with phonological agraphia did not show this effect. The lexical agraphia patients also had more difficulty spelling words of high ambiguity than words of low ambiguity, another finding not seen in the other groups. In contrast, the lexical agraphic patient spelled nonwords as well as controls and better than the patients with phonological agraphia. Also in contrast to the patients with phonological agraphia, who made errors that were usually not phonologically correct, the patients with lexical agraphia usually made errors that were phonologically correct (e. g., spelling *gelosy* for *jealousy*). Lastly, patients with lexical agraphia have not shown word class, concreteness or imageability effects. These data are consistent with an impairment of a nonphonological, lexical or orthographic spelling system. The findings from the Roeltgen/Heilman study suggest that the lexical and phonological systems may be impaired independently. Therefore, it indicates that these systems operate in parallel. – There is a certain degree of uncertainty as to the procedure by which these patients retain some ability to spell. Two conflicting positions are the following: First, it is possible that a sublexical phonological ability that performs phoneme-grapheme translation is responsible for the preserved ability. In contrast, given the preserved ability to spell real words, the spelling could occur via a lexical level phonological system, and the nonwords could be spelled by analogy. This is an important issue as demonstrated in the discussion by Friedman/Ferguson/Robinson/Sunderland (in press) of reading in Alzheimer's patients. Their results indicated that the patients performed well on reading nonwords that were similar orthographically to real English words but performed poorly on nonwords for which there were no analogous English words. This suggests that use of an analogy system rather than a sublexical grapheme to phoneme conversion was being used by the patients in their study. Results from certain patients with lexical agraphia also supply support for the position that at least certain lexical or orthographical responses are dependent upon visual imagery or visual word images. One of the patients described by Roeltgen/Heilman (1984) stated that her impaired spelling ability was associated with an impairment in the visualization of the words she was attempting to spell. Second, subject BT of Friedman/Alexander (1989) had poor imaging ability of letters. The authors suggest that this poor imaging of letters corresponds with poor imagery of words and the impairment found in lexical agraphia.

Similar to the concern regarding the specificity of the syndrome of phonological agraphia, there is also a concern regarding the specificity of lexical agraphia. In the same prospective study of patients with left hemispheric lesions described previously, Roeltgen (1989; 1991) described a series of patients with lexical agraphia. Based on previous studies of normal control subjects, these patients did fulfill the criteria of having lexical agraphia. However, for the overall population of patients studied in this group, there was a very high correlation between premorbid education ability and post-lesion achievement ability. In addition, Roeltgen and colleagues have described patients with developmental spelling impairment who have difficulty in spelling that is qualitatively and quantitatively indistinguishable from that seen in patients with acquired lexical agraphia (Roeltgen/Tucker 1988; Blaskey/Roeltgen 1990). Based on these results, Roeltgen (1991) has questioned the degree to which premorbid ability and education contribute to the syndrome of acquired lexical agraphia. He has suggested that certain subjects, based on premorbid ability or weakness in the orthographic lexicon, may be at a much higher risk for developing lexical agraphia. Minor cerebral lesions affecting any of those cognitive abilities delineated by Hatfield (1985) (familiarity with phonological components, memorization of word shapes, word analogy and mnemonic rules) can lead to the production of lexical agraphia. If this is the case, lexical agraphia is best considered a heterogeneous syndrome, rather than a specific disorder.

2.2.1.3. Semantic Agraphia

The initial conceptualization of the linguistic components of spelling was that the two spelling systems were phonological and lexical-semantic (Hatfield/Patterson 1984; Roeltgen/Sevush/Heilman 1983). The term lexical-semantic was a consequence of the data that indicated a relationship between semantic influence and spelling in subjects with phonological agraphia. However, a series of studies have indicated that semantic influence can be dissociated from the lexical or orthographic output (Roeltgen/Rothi/Heilman 1986; Patterson 1986; Rapcsak/Rubens 1990). Patients in these studies were shown to be able to spell words but were not able to incorporate meaning into what they wrote. Also, their responses were not influenced by part of speech or regularity. The primary method used to study these patients was a homophone spelling test. For this test, a homophone was dictated and then used in a sentence. The patient was asked to spell the correct word. The patients frequently responded with correctly spelled but semantically incorrect homophones (spelling *dough* when the stimulus was *doe* or *mite* when the stimulus was *might*). In the study by Roeltgen/Rothi/Heilman (1986), the data indicated that the dissociation of the lexical system from the semantic system could be due to either a generalized disruption of semantic processing or to a disconnection of a relatively intact semantic system from the orthographic or lexical output. Also in that study, it was demonstrated that the pattern of performance on nonwords, regular words and irregular words that characterizes lexical and phonological agraphia was independent of the semantic agraphia, in that the subjects with semantic agraphia had varying types of other linguistic agraphia, including both phonological and lexical agraphia.

The patient of Rapcsak/Rubens (1990) had spared general semantic abilities. In addition, their subject had an intact phonological and lexical spelling system. Their results, together with previous results, indicate that the semantic system is dissociable from the lexical and phonological spelling systems and that semantic influence on spelling can be selectively disrupted in the absence of damage or disruption to either of the two spelling systems.

2.2.1.4. Graphemic Buffer Agraphia

Although the graphemic buffer has been proposed in multiple models of writing and spelling, only limited attempts have been made to assess patients with presumed disruption of this system. Most of the studies have been performed by Caramazza and colleagues (Caramazza/Miceli/Villa/Romani 1987; Badecker/Hillis/Caramazza 1990; Hillis/Caramazza 1989).

According to Caramazza and colleagues, subjects with disturbance of the graphemic buffer typically produce letter omissions, substitutions, insertions and transpositions in words and nonwords with written and oral spelling and in all situations including writing to dictation, spontaneous writing, written naming and delayed copying. This last task consists of showing a word to a subject for a transient period. This is followed by a delay, and the subject is asked to then write the word. Subjects with disturbances of the graphemic buffer produce errors that are not affected by linguistic factors, such as those described in the previous agraphias, including degree of concreteness or imageability, word class, frequency, or regularity. The errors are typically influenced by word length, in that more errors are made on longer words than shorter words. In addition, frequently the errors are not evenly distributed across words. Frequently, the graphs of the errors show a bow shaped curve with more errors being produced in the middle of the word than either at the end or at the beginning. Hillis/Caramazza (1989) suggest that different types of disruption of the graphemic buffer may occur and emphasize the complexity of this process. A further study (Badecker/Hillis/Caramazza 1990) found that although there was a bow shaped curve for errors, there was an influence generated by prefixes and suffixes such that there were decreased errors in these morphemes compared to the expected frequency of errors based on the error patterns in the root morpheme. Therefore, they suggested that information was passed to the buffer in morpheme-sized processing units.

A recent study by Lesser (1990) found a dissociation in spelling pattern between oral spelling and written spelling. Written spelling was influenced by whether or not the stimuli were words or nonwords, but was not influenced by the regularity of the words. In contrast, oral spelling was influenced by the regularity but not by whether the stimuli were words or nonwords. Lesser concluded that there are two buffers, one for written spelling and one for oral spelling and that each of these buffers receives input from the letter production systems, i. e., the orthographic or lexical system and the phonological system. Such a model is demonstrated in Figure 23.2 This addition to the models of writing represents the first major conceptual change in these models in the last few years.

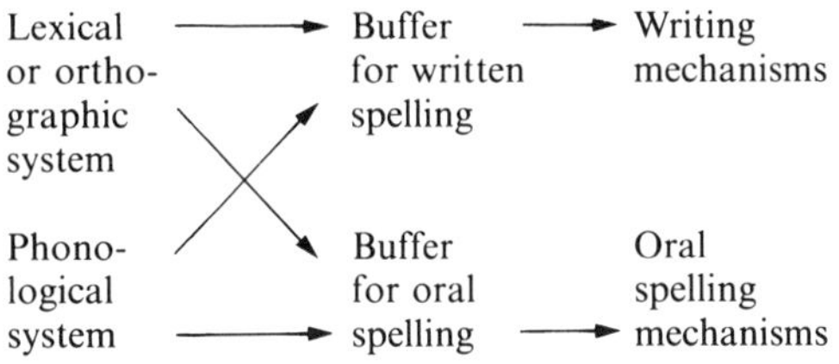

Fig. 23.2: Interaction of linguistic spelling systems and spelling buffers. Modified after Lesser (1990)

2.3. Possible Anatomic Relationships of Linguistic Agraphias

It is controversial as to whether attempts to provide clinical-pathological correlations for the linguistic agraphias is beneficial. Roeltgen/Heilman (1984) have suggested that understanding of the neuroanatomy in the context of the linguistic agraphias may allow better classifications of the agraphias and a better understanding of the nature of agraphia. In contrast, Margolin (1984) has suggested that neuroanatomical correlations, especially those based on CT scan results, should be interpreted with caution given the proximity of the areas of interest as well as variability in the topography of the human cortex. A further criticism can be raised of most previous clinical-pathological correlations of agraphias, and that is the failure to consider subcortical structures. As noted previously in this chapter, multiple recent studies have described agraphia from subcortical lesions (Laine/Marttila 1981; Tanridag/Kirshner 1985; Kertesz/Latham/Mc Cabe 1990). However, the anatomical correlations proposed principally by Roeltgen and colleagues have not considered subcortical structures (Roeltgen/Heilman 1984; Roeltgen 1985).

2.3.1. Phonological Agraphia

Roeltgen and colleagues have attempted to use CT analysis to help delineate the anatomy of phonological agraphia (Roeltgen/Rothi/Heilman 1982; Roeltgen/Heilman 1984; Roeltgen/Sevush/Heilman 1983), and these studies have been reviewed by Roeltgen/Heilman (1985). In those studies, it was suggested that patients with phonological agraphia have lesions that are typically in the area of the supramarginal gyrus or in the insula deep to that structure. Indeed, one of their subjects had an isolated phonological agraphia (with no additional language deficits) and had on CT a small focal lesion confined to the insula, or possibly extending to the surface of the supramarginal gyrus (Roeltgen/Rothi/Heilman 1982). Consistent with that hypothesis, other patients described with phonological agraphia have had lesions in the same area (Bub/Kertesz 1982; Nolan/Caramazza 1982; Shallice 1981). However, the patient described by Baxter/Warrington (1985) had a lesion that appears, based on the CT scans, in their paper to be slightly posterior to this region. In a study of a left handed patient with phonological agraphia, Bolla-Wilson/Speedie/Robinson (1985) also described a lesion of the frontal parietal area that included the supramarginal gyrus, but the lesion was in the right hemisphere. In contrast to these results, are results presented by Roeltgen (1989) in which phonological agraphia was attributed to lesions outside of this region (supramarginal gyrus and insula) and included subcortical structures. Based on those data, Roeltgen suggested that the specificity of the clinical-pathological association between phonological agraphia and the supramarginal gyrus may need to be expanded to include subcortical structures as well as individual variations in cerebral architecture and functional representation.

2.3.2. Lexical Agraphia

In data also summarized by Roeltgen/Heilman (1985), the anatomic basis for lexical agraphia was suggested to be the junction of the posterior angular gyrus and the parietal occipital lobule (the superior-lateral aspects of Brodmann's area 19). In a previous study (Roeltgen/Heilman 1984), they demonstrated that patients with phonological agraphia had lesions that did not overlap the region associated with lexical agraphia, and patients with lexical agraphia did not have lesions that overlapped the region associated with phonological agraphia. They argued that the anatomic dissociation supported the contention that phonological and lexical agraphia were dissociable, both functionally and anatomically. Since that review in 1985, additional patients have been described with lexical agraphia who have had lesions away from the left angular gyrus, including the right parietal region (in a right hander without aphasia) (Rothi/Roeltgen/Kooistra 1987), the left posterior temporal region (middle temporal gyrus) (Croisile/Trillet/Laurent et al. 1989), and the left frontal region (Rapcsak/Arthur/Rubens 1988). In the prospective study of patients with left hemispheric lesions performed by Roeltgen (1989; 1991), the localization of lesions in patients with acquired lexical agraphia was far more varied. These data plus unpublished data of Rapcsak's, have indicated that multiple sites within the left hemisphere may be associated with lexical agraphia, including the posterior angular gyrus, the dorso-lateral frontal lobe, the caudate, and the thalamus. However, these lesion sites seem to spare the immediate cortical perisylvian region, including the supramarginal gyrus. In addition, there is a suggestion that the most striking cases have angular gyrus lesions (Roeltgen/Rapcsak, unpublished data).

2.3.3. Semantic Agraphia

In their anatomically based neuropsychological model of writing, Roeltgen/Heilman (1985) indicated that their anatomic data for semantic agraphia did not appear to be as specific as were the anatomic data for the syndromes of lexical and phonological agraphia. That conclusion was based on the study of semantic agraphia by Roeltgen/Rothi/Heilman (1986). Their patients had lesions involving the cortical watershed area, the caudate, the internal capsule and frontal subcortical region, and bilateral medial-frontal and medial-parietal areas and the thalamus. Roeltgen/Rothi/Heilman (1986) suggested that the lesions did not overlap anatomically but were in areas frequently associated with transcortical aphasias with impaired comprehension. Consistent with the nonspecificity associated with semantic agraphia is a recent study by Rapcsak/Rubens (1990) in which a left prefrontal lesion was associated with a disruption of semantic influence on writing. Given the variability in the presentation of the clinical syndrome of semantic agraphia and previous studies of semantic ability in aphasia that have indicated multiple ways that semantics can be disrupted, such results are not surprising.

2.3.4. Graphemic Buffer Agraphia

Given that the linguistic studies of patients with agraphia due to the disruption of the graphemic buffer have indicated varying types of impairment, a consistent clinical-pathological correlation with this syndrome would be unexpected. There are, in fact, a wide variety of lesions described in patients with proposed dysfunction of the graphemic buffer, including the left frontal-parietal region (Hillis/Caramazza 1989; Lesser 1990), the left frontal region (Miceli//Silveri/Caramazza 1985) and the right frontal-parietal-temporal region (Hillis/Caramazza 1989). Therefore, conclusions regarding clinical-pathological correlation for this syndrome are similar to those for semantic agraphia.

2.4. Linguistic Agraphia in Japanese

2.4.1. Background

There are two written language systems that are used in Japanese, Kanji and Kana. Kanji has been traditionally described as ideogram writing, but a more precise description would be morphogram writing because the symbols have both semantic and phonetic value, although there is no systematic relationship between the Kanji and speech sound. The symbols, which are primarily used for nouns and stems of verbs, adjectives and adverbs, number up to 10,000 in the Japanese language. However, it is expected that only approximately 1,900 of these are learned by the end of the ninth grade and some errors in Kanji writing are common even in educated Japanese individuals (Tanaka/Yamadori/Murata 1987; Iwata 1984; Kawamura/Hirayama/Hasegawa et al. 1987; Soma/Sugishta/Kitamura et al. 1989; Iwata/Sugishta/Toyokura 1981).

Kana, in contrast, consists of a limited number of syllabic characters (102) (Paradis/Hagiwara/Hildebrandt 1985) that are usually learned by the first grade and can be used for writing any of the words in the Japanese language. Kana symbols are typically termed phonograms but are probably better described as syllabograms. Each Kana character has a one-to-one correspondence to a syllable. Kana characters are typically used for writing conjugated endings of verbs, adjectives and adverbs and function words. These grammatical morphemes can only be written using Kana, whereas major lexical items can be written in Kanji and Kana.

2.4.2. Kanji Agraphia

Agraphias for both Kanji and Kana have been reported, but the most frequently reported dissociation is impaired Kanji with normal or relatively normal Kana. Most patients with Kanji agraphia have an associated alexia and a brain lesion that is typically associated, in Indo-European languages, with pure alexia (left occipital lobe). However, pure Kanji agraphia has been described from lesions of the posterior left temporal regions and the junction of the posterior temporal region with the lateral occipital or the angular gyrus (Kawahata/Nagata 1988) and the left inferior temporal gyrus (Kawamura/Hirayma/Hasegawa et al. 1987).

There are limited descriptions of the errors produced by patients with Kanji agraphia. However, the most commonly reported errors include distortion of the grapheme, production of a partial grapheme, simplification of the grapheme and "graphical confusion" (Mochizuki/Ohtomo 1988; Yokoto/Ishiai/Furukawa/Tsukagoshi 1990; Iwata/Sugishita/Toyokura 1981). The last error type, graphical confusion, are incorrect graphemes with portions replaced by correctly formed but incorrect grapheme components. Despite the striking 'visual' or 'visual-spatial' character of these errors, they are not typically associated with impairment on constructive tasks (Iwata/Sugishita/Toyokura 1981).

2.4.3. Kana Agraphia

The occurrence of selective Kana agraphia is very rare and it has been suggested by some authors (Soma/Sugishita/Kitamura et al. 1989) that there have been no cases of pure Kana agraphia reported. The description that is closest to a case of pure Kana agraphia is the patient reported by Tanaka/Yamadori/Murata (1987) who described a patient with relatively normal Kanji writing ability but impaired Kana writing ability. In writing

Kana characters, the patient showed frequent substitutions of other graphemes, as well as perseverations. In addition, when writing words using Kana, there was a very striking length effect such that Kana symbols at the ends of the words were written correctly much less frequently than those at the beginnings of the words. Their patient had a lesion of the left inferior parietal lobe, as well as a small lesion in the left corona radiata. These authors interpreted the performance as indicating a difficulty in translating acoustic word images into graphemic forms.

2.4.4. Models of Agraphia in Japanese

Based on studies of Japanese agraphia, Iwata/Sugishita/Toyokura (1981) have offered both an information processing model, as well as an anatomical model, in an attempt to explain Japanese writing. They suggest that in writing Kana, the auditory representation of a word is activated and it in turn activates a 'somesthetic' representation and subsequently produces the Kana output. In contrast, they suggest that for Kanji writing, the auditory representation may or may not be activated prior to the activation of a visual-semantic representation of the word.

The anatomical model proposed by Iwata (1984) suggests two separate anatomic pathways for Kanji and Kana. For Kanji, he suggests that the pathway is from Wernicke's area to or through the posterior inferior temporal region, into the occipital lobe and from there to the angular gyrus before the information flow accesses the peripheral writing mechanisms. In contrast, he suggests that for Kana writing, the information flow is directly from Wernicke's area to the angular gyrus.

2.4.5. Relationship of Agraphia in Japanese and Agraphia in Indo-European Languages

Soma/Sugishita/Kitamura et al. (1989) have suggested that there is an important behavioral similarity between the agraphias in these two language systems and that Kanji agraphia represents lexical agraphia in Japanese. In contrast, Tanaka/Yamadori/Murata (1987) argue that it is difficult to establish differences or similarities between the two writing systems. In order to address this controversy, it is important to review those similarities and differences that are present.

In comparing and contrasting Kanji writing and writing of irregular words, there are certain similarities. Both Kanji and irregular words have semantic, orthographic and phonological information. Both may be misspelled by normal highly educated people and agraphias associated with these words have been reported following nonperisylvan lesions. However, they differ in important ways as well. They perform different functions in each of the languages. The irregular words in Indo-European languages may be of any word class or any word type, including both highly concrete and richly semantic words (e. g., *yacht*) or words that are primarily grammatical in nature (e. g., *though*). Kanji characters, highly concrete words with rich semantic content, on the other hand, are only used to represent major lexical morphemes. In addition, irregular words in Indo-European languages frequently incorporate the conjugated portion of the word within the morpheme itself, rather than utilizing the addition of separate components. For example, *caught* an irregular English word carries both the information of the route morpheme (*catch*) as well as the past tense. A Japanese conjugated form contains both the Kanji and Kana components. From the neuropsychological standpoint, Kanji and lexical agraphia also differ in that Kanji agraphia almost always occurs in the context of alexia. In contrast, in our prospective study of agraphia containing 43 subjects, there were four patients with pure agraphia and three of these four had lexical agraphia (Roeltgen 1989; 1991). Furthermore, of the six patients in the study with lexical agraphia, four had no alexia of any type.

Comparison of Kana and phonological spelling is difficult because of the levels of function represented by these systems. Kana spelling incorporates phonograms, whereas nonword spelling incorporates phonemes. However, there are certain similarities. First, the ability to produce Kana spelling and nonword spelling utilizes sound to grapheme conversion. Also, both Kana graphemes and letters lack semantic representation. The major difference is that the agraphia associated with each of these is defined very differently. Kana agraphia is defined by dysfunction at the grapheme level, in that Kana graphemes are not produced. In contrast, phonological agraphia is defined at the word level in that nonwords are not produced correctly.

Given some of the difficulties in comparing Kanji and irregular words and Kana and nonwords, and consequently lexical agraphia with Kanji agraphia and phonological agraphia with Kana agraphia, we are inclined to agree with Tanaka/Yamadori/Murata (1987) that comparison or discussion of similarities in agraphias of the two different language systems is difficult.

3. Agraphia in Alzheimer's Disease

In his original report, Alzheimer (1907) described a patient with a progressive dementing illness who, in addition to aphasia and alexia, also demonstrated agraphia. Pick (1925) observed that disorders of orthography were indeed often associated with dementia and that orthographic errors increased with the progression of the disease. Several investigators have since confirmed that agraphia is a common feature in Alzheimer's disease (AD) (Appell/Kertesz/Fisman 1982; Cummings/Benson/Hill/Read 1985; Murdoch/Chenery/Wilks/Boyle 1987; Bayles/Kaszniak 1987; Faber-Langendoen/Morris/Knesevich et al. 1988; Horner/Heyman/Dawson/Rogers 1988). It is apparent from these studies that both the linguistic and motor components of writing may become compromised in the course of the illness. Although most agraphic AD patients are also aphasic, the writing impairment is often more severe than the spoken language deficit and at times may precede it (Appell/Kertesz/Fisman 1982; Cummings/Benson/Hill/Read 1985; Faber-Langendoen/Morris/Knesevich et al. 1988; Homen/Heyman/Dawson/Rogers 1989).

More recent studies of agraphia in AD have attempted to determine the nature of the cognitive-linguistic breakdown in the writing process. Impairments have now been documented at several different levels. At the pragmatic/semantic level, the written narrative of AD patients is often poorly organized, repetitive, irrelevant, uninformative or 'empty' and there is a paucity of written output (Neils/Boller/Gerdeman/Cole 1989; Glosser/Kaplan 1989; Horner/Heyman/Dawson/Rogers 1988; Neils/Kavrie 1990). However, the basic syntactic frame of the sentences is relatively well preserved (Glosser/Kaplan 1989). At the single word level, Rapcsak/Arthur/Bliklen/Rubens (1989) found that AD patients spelled regular words and nonwords significantly better than irregular words. In addition, the spelling errors of AD patients on irregular words were frequently phonologically plausible. Rapcsak/Arthur/Bliklen/Rubens (1989) proposed that these findings were consistent with an impairment of the lexical spelling system in AD, and reflected either a loss of word representations from the orthographic lexicon or an inability to access these representations. On the other hand, spelling by the phonological spelling system (i. e., phoneme-grapheme conversion) was relatively spared. Others have also documented that irregular words are especially difficult for AD patients and that their spelling errors are often phonologically accurate (Smith/Snyder/Meeks 1991; Glosser/Kaplan 1989). However, Smith/Snyder/Meeks (1991) also provided evidence that in some AD patients phonological spelling by phoneme-grapheme conversion may not be entirely intact either.

Although the studies reviewed above are not directly comparable since they have used different methodologies and have included subjects at various stages of dementia, it is our impression that agraphia in AD does have certain characteristic cognitive-linguistic features that seem to follow a typical pattern of progression. In the earliest stages, the writing disturbance is characterized by a general disruption of semantic processing but relative preservation of basic syntactic form. The semantic impairment will adversely affect performance on all writing tasks that require semantic mediation. These include spontaneous or descriptive writing, written naming and homophone spelling. With the exception of homophones, however, writing to dictation in early AD may be relatively intact, since this task can be performed without semantic processing (Roeltgen/Rothi/Heilman 1986; Glosser/Kaplan 1989). The next stage of the writing disturbance is characterized by additional impairment at the level of single word orthography. Initially, the orthographic impairment is most severe for irregular words, since these can only be spelled lexically. At this stage, the phonological spelling system (i. e., phoneme-grapheme conversion) is still operational and thus regular word and nonword spelling can still be performed with relative success. Consistent with the relative sparing of the phonological spelling system, spelling errors on irregular words are likely to be phonologically plausible. In more advanced stages of the illness, however, the phonological spelling system may also become compromised. It is apparent from this general outline that, depending on the stage of the illness, a given patient or group of patients might exhibit dysfunction at the level of overall pragmatic/semantic organization and at the level of single word orthography simultaneously. In addition to the linguistic impairment, the peripheral motor mechanisms of writing may also fail even in patients with only mild to moderate dementia (Rapcsak/Arthur/Bliklen/Rubens 1989; Horner/Heyman/Dawson/Rogers 1988).

Whether the progression of the cognitive-linguistic impairment in the writing process conforms to the pattern we have outlined above is yet to be determined by longitudinal studies of agraphia in AD. However, this model is consistent with general observations that language deterioration in AD predominantly affects lexical-semantic and pragmatic abilities, while phonological and syntactic operations are relatively spared until the later stages of the illness (Irigaray 1973; Schwartz/Marin/Saffran 1979; Appell/Kertesz/Fisman 1982; Bayles 1982; Obler 1983). We emphasize that our model does not address explicitly the relationship of memory impairment and agraphia in AD (e. g., storage or access disorders of semantic memory and possible impairment of putative working memory systems for the temporary storage of linguistic items such as the phonological and graphemic output buffers). The impairment of different memory systems and attentional deficits are likely to contribute significantly to agraphia in all stages of AD and require further study.

Pick (1892) was the first to suggest that specific aphasic syndromes, similar to those seen following focal brain lesions, may occur in senile atrophy of the brain. He believed that these syndromes were caused by the "local accentuation of a diffuse process". The pattern of language impairment in AD indeed correlates well with the distribution of neuropathological changes in the cerebral cortex. Several anatomical and histological studies have demonstrated that the degenerative process affects the multimodal association cortex of the temporo-parieto-occipital junction most severely and most consistently (Brun/Gustafson 1976; Brun/Englund 1981; Kemper 1984). The neuropathological findings are paralleled by cerebral blood flow and positron emission tomographic studies in AD that show a marked reduction in metabolic activity in the temporo-parieto-occipital areas, as well as an inability to activate these regions during cognitive effort (Hagberg/Ingvar 1976; Ingvar/Risberg/Schwartz 1975; Friedland/Bundinger/Ganz et al. 1983; Chase/Foster/Fedio et al. 1984; Friedland/Budinger/Koss/Ober 1985; Friedland/Brun/Budinger 1985). Furthermore, in AD patients with aphasia, alexia and agraphia, the most significant reduction of metabolic activity is in the temporo-parieto-occipital region on the left side (Gustafson/Hagberg/Ingvar 1978; Foster/Chase/Fedio et al. 1983; Haxby/Duara/Grady et al. 1985). Given the above considerations, it is not surprising that language dysfunction is a consistent feature in AD (Appell/Kertesz 1982; Cummings/Benson/Hill/Read 1985; Bayles/Kaszniak 1987) and that the pattern of language impairment closely resembles the aphasic syndromes that are seen following focal lesions of the left temporo-parietal association cortex (Obler/Albert 1981; Benson/Cummings/Tsai 1982). As pointed out by Luria (1974), damage to these cortical regions severely disturbs lexical-semantic linguistic operations. By the same token, it is likely that the frequently observed preservation of phonological and syntactic abilities in AD reflects the relative sparing of immediate perisylvian language areas by the disease process (Whitaker 1976).

In terms of the writing disturbance in AD, the involvement of the left temporo-parietal region by the degenerative process is likely to be responsible for the disruption of lexical-semantic processing that is evident in tasks of spontaneous or descriptive writing, written naming and homophone spelling. As we have seen earlier, the left angular gyrus is also an important neural substrate of lexical spelling, and the frequent involvement of this region in AD probably accounts for the word-level orthographic impairment (i. e., lexical agraphia). Phonological spelling, on the other hand, depends on the integrity of the immediate perisylvian language zone (the supramarginal gyrus and insula, in particular) (Roeltgen/Sevush/Heilman 1983), and the sparing of these regions until later in the disease process may account for the relative preservation of spelling by phoneme-grapheme conversion.

4. References

Aimard, G., Devick, M., Lebel, M., Trouillas, M., & Boisson, D. (1975). Agraphie pure (dynamique?) origine frontale. *Revue Neurologique, 7*, 505–512.

Alexander, M. P., Friedman, R., Lo Verso, F., & Fischer, R. (1990). Anatomic correlates of lexical agraphia. Presented at *The Academy of Aphasia*. Baltimore, MD.

Alzheimer, A. (1907). A unique illness involving the cerebral cortex. In D. A. Rottenberg & F. H. Hochberg, (Eds.), *Neurological classics in modern translation*. 41–43. New York: Hafner Press.

Appell, J., Kertesz, A., & Fisman, M. (1982). A study of language functioning in Alzheimer's patients. *Brain and Language, 17*, 73–91.

Assal, G., Buttet, J., & Jolivet, R. (1981). Dissociations in aphasia: A case report. *Brain and Language, 13*, 223–240.

Auerbach, S. H. & Alexander, M. P. (1981). Pure agraphia and unilateral optic ataxia associated with a left superior parietal lobule lesion. *Journal of Neurology, Neurosurgery and Psychiatry, 5*, 430–432.

Badecker, W., Hillis, A., & Caramazza, A. (1990). Lexical morphology and its role in the writing process: Evidence from a case of acquired dysgraphia. *Cognition, 35*, 205–243.

Basso, A., Taborielli, A., & Vignolo, L. A. (1978). Dissociated disorders of speaking and writing in aphasia. *Journal of Neurology, Neurosurgery and Psychiatry, 6* 556–563.

Bastian, H. C. (1898). *Treatise on aphasia and other speech defects*. London: H. K. Lewis.

Baxter, D. M. & Warrington, E. K. (1985). Category specific phonological dysgraphia. *Neuropsychologia, 23*, 653–666.

Bayles, K. A. (1982). Language function in senile dementia. *Brain and Language, 16*, 265–280.

Bayles, K. A. & Kaszniak, A. W. (1987). *Communication and cognition in normal aging and dementia.* Boston: Little Brown & Co.

Beauvois, M. F. & Derouesné, J. (1981). Lexical or orthographic agraphia. *Brain, 104*, 21–49.

Benedikt, M. (1865). *Über Aphasie, Agraphie und verwandte pathologische Zustände. Wiener medizinische Presse, 6*, 897–899; 923–926.

Benson, D. F. (1979). *Aphasia, alexia and agraphia.* New York: Churchill Livingston.

Benson, D. F., Cummings, J. L., & Tsai, S. Y. (1982). Angular gyrus syndrome simulating Alzheimer's disease. *Archives of Neurology, 39*, 616–620.

Blaskey & Roeltgen (1990). Mild phonological (alphabetic) impairment in children who are good readers and poor spellers. *Journal of Clinical and Experimental Neuropsychology, 12*, 100.

Bolla-Wilson, K., Speedie, L. J., & Robinson, R. G. (1985). Phonologic agraphia in a left-handed patient after a right-hemisphere lesion. *Neurology, 35*, 1778–1781.

Brun, A. & Englund, E. (1981). Regional pattern of degeneration in Alzheimer's disease: neuronal loss and histopathological grading. *Histopathology, 5*, 549–564.

Brun, A. & Gustafson, L. (1976). Distribution of cerebral degeneration in Alzheimer's disease: a clinico-pathological study. *Arch. Psychiatr. Nervenkrank, 223*, 15–33.

Bub, D. & Kertesz, A. (1982). Deep agraphia. *Brain and Language, 17*, 146–165.

Campbell, R. (1983). Writing nonwords to dictation. *Brain and Language, 19*, 153–178.

Caramazza, A., Miceli, G., Villa, G., & Romani, C. (1987). The role of the graphemic buffer in spelling: Evidence from a case of acquired dysgraphia. *Cognition, 26*, 59–85.

Charcot, J. M. (1889). *Clinical lectures on diseases of the nervous system. Vol. 3.* London: New Syndenham Society.

Chase, T. N., Foster, N. L. Fedio, P., Brooks, R., Mansi, L., & Di Chiro, G. (1984). Regional cortical dysfunction in Alzheimer's disease as determined by positron emission tomography. *Annals of Neurology, 15* (Suppl.), 170–174.

Clark, L. W. & Grossfield, M. L. (1983). Nature of spelling errors in transcortical sensory aphasia: A case study. *Brain and Language, 18*, 47–56.

Coltheart, M. (1980). Deep dyslexia: A right hemisphere hypothesis. In M. Coltheart, K. E. Patterson, & J. C. Marshall (Eds.), *Deep dyslexia. Ch. 16, 326–380.* London: Routledge and Kegan Paul.

Croisile, B., Trillet, M., Laurent, B., Latombe, D., & Schott, B. (1989). Agraphie lexicale par hematome temporo-parietal gauche. *Revue Neurologique (Paris), 145* (4), 287–292.

Cummings, J. L., Benson, D. F., Hill, M. A., & Read, S. (1985). Aphasia in dementia of the Alzheimer type. *Neurology, 35*, 394–397.

Déjerine, J. (1891). Sur un cas de cécité verbale avec agraphie, suivi d'autopsie. *Mem. Soc. Biol., 3.*, 197–201.

Déjerine, J. (1914). *Sémiologie des affections du système nerveux.* Masson: Paris.

Ellis, A. W. (1982). Spelling and writing (and reading and speaking). In A. W. Ellis (Ed.), *Normality and pathology in cognitive functions. 113–146.* London: Erlbaum.

Ellis, A. W. (1988). Modelling the writing process. In G. Denes, C. Semenza, & P. Bisiacchi (Eds.), *Perspectives in cognitive neuropsychology. 189–214.* Hove and London: Erlbaum.

Exner, S. (1881). *Untersuchungen über die Lokalisation der Funktionen in der Grosshirnrinde des Menschen.* Wien: Wilhelm Braumüller.

Faber-Langendoen, K., Morris, J. C., Knesevich, J. W., La Barge, E., Miller, J. P., & Berg, R. (1988). Aphasia in senile dementia of the Alzheimer type. *Annals of Neurology, 23.* 365–370.

Foster, N. L., Chase, T. N., Fedio, P., Patronas, J. N., Brooks, R. A., & Di Chiro, G. (1983). Alzheimer's disease: focal cortical changes shown by positron emission tomography. *Neurology, 33*, 961–965.

Friedland, R. P., Brun, A., & Budinger, T. F. (1985). Pathological and positron emission tomographic correlations in Alzheimer's disease. *Lancet, 1*, 228.

Friedland, R. P., Budinger, T. F., Koss, E., & Ober, B. A. (1985). Alzheimer's disease: anterior-posterior and lateral hemispheric alterations in cortical glucose utilization. *Neuroscience Letters, 53*, 235–240.

Friedland, R. P., Budinger, T. F., Ganz, E., Yano, Y., Mathis, C. A., Koss, B., Ober, B. A., Huesman, R. H., & Derenzo, S. E. (1983). Regional cerebral metabolic alterations in dementia of the Alzheimer type: positron emission tomography with [18 F] fluorodeoxyglucose. *Journal of Computer Assisted Tomography, 7*, 590–598.

Friedman, R. B. & Alexander, M. P. (1989). Written spelling agraphia. *Brain and Language, 36*, 503–517.

Friedman, R. B., Ferguson, S., Robinson, S., & Sunderland, T. (in press). Mechanisms of reading in Alzheimer's disease. *Neurology*.

Glosser, G. & Kaplan, E. (1989). Linguistic and nonlinguistic impairments in writing: a comparison of patients with focal and multifocal CNS disorders. *Brain and Language, 37*, 357–380.

Goodman-Schulman, R. & Caramazza, A. (1987). Patterns of dysgraphia and the nonlexical spelling process. *Cortex, 23*, 143–148.

Grashey, H. (1885). Über Aphasie und ihre Beziehungen zur Wahrnehmung. *Archiv für Psychiatrie und Nervenkrankheiten, 16*, 654–688. (Translated by R. De Bleser (1989), Cognitive Neuropsychology, 6, 515–546).

Gustafson, L., Hagberg, B., & Ingvar D. H. (1978). Speech disturbances in presenile dementia related to local cerebral blood flow abnormalities in the dominant hemisphere. *Brain and Language, 5*, 103–118.

Hagberg, B. & Ingvar, D. H. (1976). Cognitive reduction in presenile dementia related to regional abnormalities of the cerebral blood flow. *British Journal of Psychiatry, 128*, 209–222.

Hatfield, F. M. (1985). Visual and phonological factors in acquired dysgraphia. *Neuropsychologia, 23*, 13–29.

Hatfield, F. M. & Patterson, K. E. (1984). Interpretations of spelling disorders in aphasia: impact of recent developments in cognitive psychology. In C. E. Rose (Ed.), *Advances in neurology. Vol. 42 Progress in aphasiology* New York: Raven Press.

Hatfield, F. & Patterson, K. E. (1983). Phonological spelling. *Quarterly Journal of Experimental Psychology, 35 A*, 451–468.

Haxby, J. V., Duara, R., Grady, C. L., Cutler, N. R., & Rapoport, S. I. (1985). Relations between neuropsychological and cerebral metabolic abnormalities in early Alzheimer's disease. *Journal of Cerebral Blood Flow and Metabolism, 5*, 193–200.

Hécaen, H. & Albert, M. L. (1978). *Human neuropsychology*. New York: John Wiley and Sons.

Heilbronner, K. (1910). Die aphasischen, apraktischen und agnostischen Störungen. Im M. Lewandowsky (Ed.), *Handbuch der Neurologie* Berlin: Springer Verlag.

Henschen, S. E. (1922). *Klinische und anatomische Beiträge zur Pathologie des Gehirns. VII. Über motorische Aphasie und Agraphie*. Stockholm: Nordiska Bokhandel.

Hillis, A. E. & Caramazza, A. (1989). The graphemic buffer and attentional mechanisms. *Brain and Language, 36*, 208–235.

Horner, J., Heyman, A., Dawson, D., & Rogers, H. (1988). The relationship of agraphia to the severity of dementia in Alzheimer's disease. *Archives of Neurology, 45*, 760–763.

Ingvar, D. H., Risberg, J., & Schwartz, M. S. (1975). Evidence of subnormal function of association cortex in presenile dementia. *Neurology, 25*, 964–974.

Irigaray, L. (1973). *Le langage des dements*. The Hague: Mouton.

Iwata, M. (1984). Neuropsychological correlates of the Japanese writing system. *Trends in Neurosciences, 7*, 290–293.

Iwata, M., Sugishita, M., & Toyokura, Y. (1981). The Japanese writing system and functional hemispheric specialization. In *Neurology, Proceedings of the 12 th World Congress of Neurology*. Amsterdam-Oxford-Princeton: Excerpta Medica.

Jackson, J. H. (1878). On affections of speech from disease of the brain. *Brain, 1*, 305–330.

Kaplan, E. & Goodglass, H. (1981). Aphasia-related disorders. In M. T. Sarno (Ed.), *Acquired aphasia*. New York: Academic Press.

Kawahata, N. & Nagata, K. (1988). Alexia with agraphia due to the left posterior inferior temporal lobe lesion – Neuropsychological analysis and its pathogenetic mechanisms. *Brain and Language, 33*, 296–310.

Kawamura, M., Hirayama, K., Hasegawa, K., Takahashi, N., & Yamaura, A. (1987). Alexia with agraphia of Kanji (Japanese morphograms). *Journal of Neurology, Neurosurgery, and Psychiatry, 50*, 1125–1129.

Kemper, T. (1984). Neuroanatomical and neuropathological changes in normal aging and dementia. In M. L. Albert (Ed.), *Clinical neurology of aging*. 9–52. New York: Oxford University Press.

Kertesz, A., Latham, N., & McCabe, P. (1990). Subcortical agraphia. *Neurology, 40* (1), 172.

Laine, T. N. & Marttila, R. J. (1981). Pure agraphia: a case study. *Neuropsychologia, 19*, 311–316.

Leischner, A. (1969). The agraphias. In P. J. Vinken & G. W. Bruyn (Eds.), *Disorders of speech, perception and symbolic behaviour. 141–180*. Amsterdam: North-Holland.

Lesser, R. (1990). Superior oral to written spelling: Evidence for separate buffers? *Cognitive Neuropsychology, 7* (4), 347–366.

Lichtheim, L. (1885). On aphasia. *Brain, 7*, 433–485.

Luria, A. R. (1970). *Traumatic aphasia.* The Hague: Mouton.

Luria, A. R. (1974). Language and brain: Towards the basic problems of neurolinguistics. *Brain and Language, 1,* 1–14.

Marcé, M. (1856). Mémoire sur quelques observations de physiologie pathologique tendant à démontrer l'existence d'un principe coordinateur de l'écriture. *Compte-rendu de la Société Biologie (Paris), 3,* 93–115.

Marcie, P. & Hécaen, H. (1979). Agraphia. In K. M. Heilman & E. Valenstein (Eds.), *Clinical neuropsychology* (1st Edit.). *Ch. 4. 92–127.* New York: Oxford University Press.

Margolin, D. I. (1984). The neuropsychology of writing and spelling: Semantic, phonological, motor, and perceptual processes. *The Quarterly Journal of Experimental Psychology, 36 A,* 459–489.

Marshall, J. & Newcombe, F. (1966). Syntactic and semantic errors in paralexia. *Neuropsychologica, 4,* 169–176.

Miceli, G., Silveri M. C., & Caramazza, A. (1985). Cognitive analysis of a case of pure dysgraphia. *Brain and Language, 25,* 187–212.

Mochizuki, H. & Ohtomo, R. (1988). Pure alexia in Japanese and agraphia without alexia in Kanji. *Archives of Neurology, 45,* 1157–1159.

Morton, J. (1980). The logogen model and orthographic structure. In U. Frith (Ed.), *Cognitive processes in spelling. 117–133.* London: Academic Press.

Murdoch, B. E., Chenery, H. J., Wilks, V., & Boyle, R. S. (1987). Language disorder in dementia of the Alzheimer type. *Brain and Language, 31,* 122–137.

Neils, J., Boller, F., Gerdeman, B., & Cole, M. (1989). Descriptive writing abilities in Alzheimer's disease. *Journal of Clinical and Experimental Neuropsychology, 11,* 692–698.

Neils, J. & Kavrie, S. (1990). Dysgraphia in early Alzheimer's disease. *Journal of Clinical and Experimental Neuropsychology, 12,* 398.

Nielsen, J. M. (1946). *Agnosia, apraxia, aphasia: Their value in cerebral localization.* New York: Paul B. Hoeber.

Nolan, K. A., & Caramazza, A. (1982). Modality-independent impairments in word processing in a deep dyslexic patient. *Brain and Language, 16,* 236–264.

Obler, L. K. (1983). Language and brain dysfunction in dementia. In S. J. Segalowitz (Ed.), *Language functions and brain organization, 267–282.* Orlando: Academic Press.

Obler, L. K. & Albert, M. L. (1981). Language in the elderly aphasic and the dementing patient. In M. T. Sarno (Ed.), *Acquired aphasia. 385–398.* Orlando: Academic Press.

Ogle, J. W. (1867). Aphasia and agraphia. *Report of the Medical Research Counsel of St. George's Hospital (London), 2,* 83–122.

Paradis, M., Hagiwara, H., & Hildebrandt, N. (1985). *Neurolinguistic aspects of the Japanese writing system.* Orlando: Academic Press.

Patterson, K. (1986). Lexical but nonsemantic spelling? *Cognitive Neuropsychology, 3* (3), 341–367.

Pick, A. (1931). Aphasie. In O. Bumke & O. Foerster (Eds.), *Handbuch der normalen und pathologischen Physiologie.* (Vol. XV). Berlin: Springer.

Pick, A. (1892). On the relation of aphasia and senile atrophy of the brain. In D. A. Rottenberg & F. H. Hochberg (Eds.), *Neurological classics in modern translation.* 34–40. New York: Hafner Press.

Pick, A. (1925). Zur Pathologie der Rechtschreibung. *Zeitschrift für die gesamte Neurologie und Psychiatrie, 95,* 234–247. (Translated by R. De Bleser (1989), Cognitive Neuropsychology, 6, 571–586).

Pitres, A. (1894). *Rapport sur la question des agraphies.* Bordeaux.: Congres Francais de Médecine Interne.

Rapcsak, S. Z., Arthur, S. A., & Rubens, A. B. (1988). Lexical agraphia from focal lesion of the left precentral gyrus. *Neurology, 38,* 1119–1123.

Rapcsak, S. Z., Arthur, S. A., Bliklen, D. A., & Rubens, A. B. (1989). Lexical agraphia in Alzheimer's disease. *Archives of Neurology, 46,* 65–68.

Rapcsak, S. Z., Beeson, P. M., & Rubens, A. B. (1991). Writing with the right hemisphere. *Brain and Language, 41,* 510–530.

Rapcsak, S. Z. & Rubens, A. B. (1990). Disruption of semantic influence on writing following a left prefrontal lesion. *Brain and Language, 38,* 334–344.

Rapcsak, S. Z., Rubens, A. B., & Laguna, J. F. (1990). From letters to words: Procedures for word recognition in letter-by-letter reading. *Brain and Language, 38,* 504–514.

Roeltgen, D. P. (1985). Agraphia. In K. M. Heilman & E. Valenstein (Eds.), *Clinical neuropsychology* (2 nd). 75–96. New York: Oxford University Press.

Roeltgen, D. P. (1989). Prospective analysis of a model of writing, anatomic aspects. Presented at *The Academy of Aphasia,* Santa Fe, New Mexico.

Roeltgen, D. P. (1991). Prospective analysis of writing and spelling. Part II: Results not related to localization. *Journal of Clinical and Experimental Neuropsychology, 13,* 48.

Roeltgen, D. P. & Heilman, K. M. (1984). Lexical agraphia, further support for the two system hypothesis of linguistic agraphia. *Brain, 107,* 811–827.

Roeltgen, D. P. & Heilman, K. M. (1985). Review of agraphia and a proposal for an anatomically based neuropsychological model of writing. *Applied Psycholinguistics, 6*, 205–230.

Roeltgen, D. P., Rothi, L. J. G., & Heilman, K. M. (1982). Isolated phonological agraphia from a focal lesion. Presented at *The Academy of Aphasia*, New Paltz.

Roeltgen, D. P., Rothi, L. G., & Heilman, K. M. (1986). Linguistic semantic agraphia. *Brain and Language, 27*, 257–280.

Roeltgen, D. P., Sevush, S., & Heilman, K. M. (1983). Phonological agraphia: writing by the lexical-semantic route. *Neurology, 33*, 733–757.

Roeltgen, D. P. & Tucker, D. M. (1988). Developmental phonological and lexical agraphia in adults. *Brain and Language, 35*, 287–300.

Rosati, G. & De Bastiani, P. (1981). Pure agraphia: a discreet form of aphasia. *Journal of Neurology, Neurosurgery and Psychiatry, 3*, 266–269.

Rothi, L. J. G., Roeltgen, D. P., & Kooistra, C. A. (1987). Isolated lexical agraphia in a right-handed patient with a posterior lesion of the right cerebral hemisphere. *Brain and Language, 30*, 181–190.

Saffran, E. M., Bogyo, L. C., Schwartz, M. F., & Marin, O. S. M. (1980). Does deep dyslexia reflect right-hemisphere reading? In M. Coltheart, K. E. Patterson, & J. C. Marshall (Eds.), *Deep dyslexia*. 381–406. London: Routledge and Kegan Paul.

Saffran, E. M., Schwartz, M. F., & Marin, O. S. M. (1981). Semantic mechanisms in paralexia. *Brain and Language, 13*, 255–265.

Schwartz, M. F., Marin, O. S. M., & Saffran, E. M. (1979). Dissociations of language function in dementia: A case study. *Brain and Language, 7*, 277–306.

Shallice, T. (1981). Phonological agraphia and the lexical route in writing. *Brain, 104*, 412–429.

Smith, S. T., Snyder, W. B., & Meeks, L. M. (1991). Agraphia in Alzheimer's disease. *Journal of Clinical and Experimental Neuropsychology, 13*, 71.

Soma, Y., Sugishita, M., Kitamura, K., Maruyama, S., & Imanaga, H. (1989). Lexical agraphia in the Japanese language. *Brain, 112*, 1549–1561.

Tanaka, Y., Yamadori, A., & Murata, S. (1987). Selective Kana agraphia: A case report. *Cortex, 23*, 679–684.

Tanridag, O. & Kirshner, H. S. (1985). Aphasia and agraphia in lesions of the posterior internal capsule and putamen. *Neurology, 35*, 1797–1801.

Van Lancker, D. (1990). A case of deep dysgraphia attributed to right hemispheric function. Presented at *The Academy of Aphasia*. Baltimore, MD.

Vernea, J. J. & Merory, J. (1975). Frontal agraphia, (including a case report). *Proceedings of the Australian Association of Neurologists, 12*, 93–99.

Wernicke, C. (1874). *Der aphasische Symptomencomplex*. Breslau: Max Cohn & Weigert.

Wernicke, C. (1886). Nervenheilkunde. Die neueren Arbeiten über Aphasie. *Fortschritte der Medizin, 4*, 463–482. (Translated by R. De Bleser (1989), Cognitive Neuropsychology, 6, 547–569).

Whitaker, H. (1976). A case of isolation of the language function. In H. Whitaker & H. A. Whitaker (Eds.), *Studies in neurolinguistics, vol. 2*. 1–58. Orlando: Academic Press.

Yokota, T., Ishiai, S., Furukawa, T., & Tsukagoshi, H. (1990). Pure agraphia of kanji due to thrombosis of the Labbe vein. *Journal of Neurology, Neurosurgery, and Psychiatry, 53*, 335–338.

David P. Roeltgen/Steven Z. Rapcsak, Philadelphia, Pennsylvania (USA)/ Tucson, Arizona (USA)

24. Multilingualism and Aphasia

1. Introduction

The basic question in the neuropsychology of bilingualism has been whether the cerebral representation of language in bilinguals differs from that in unilinguals, and if so, in what specific ways. Some researchers have turned to aphasia in bilinguals for evidence in support of their hypotheses. Others have developed models in an attempt to explain the observed phenomena, in particular the patterns of recovery of the various languages of bilingual and multilingual aphasic patients.

2. Patterns of Recovery

Six basic patterns of recovery have been observed over the past century: Parallel, when all languages are recovered at the same time and to the same extent; differential, when one is recovered better than the other(s); successive, when one is not recovered at all until the other(s) has/have been maximally recovered; selective, when one language is never recovered; antagonistic, when only one language is initially recovered, then is eventually replaced by another language; and mixed, when two languages are systematically mixed intrasententially (and even sometimes intramorphemically) at the level of phonology, morphology, syntax and/or the lexicon (Paradis 1977).

Some patients exhibiting a selective recovery have been reported to have retained comprehension in the language that was selectively unavailable for production tasks. The available language in some cases of antagonistic recovery has been reported to alternate over periods ranging from 24 hours to 3 weeks (Paradis/Goldblum/Abidi 1982; Nilipour/Ashayeri 1989) or even 8 months (Paradis/Goldblum 1989). Moreover, these six patterns are not mutually exclusive: A recovery may change from one pattern into another over time, e. g., from successive to antagonistic (Minkowski 1928), or different patterns may coexist relative to different languages, e. g., alternating antagonism between two languages with successive recovery of a third (Nilipour/Ashayeri 1989). Selective aphasia (aphasia in one language with no measurable deficits in the other(s)), and selective recovery (when one language remains permanently inaccessible) have been interpreted as representing opposite poles on a continuum of differential aphasia (Paradis/Goldblum 1989).

In addition, three cases have been interpreted as exhibiting differential aphasia, i. e., a different aphasic syndrome in each language (Albert/Obler 1978; Silverberg/Gordon 1979). However, one of them (Silverberg/Gordon, case 1) can really be considered a standard case of selective recovery. The patient is reported to have exhibited conduction aphasia in his native Russian and global aphasia in the little Hebrew he had attempted to acquire with very little success over the previous few years. The other two patients were believed to present with Broca's aphasia in one language and Wernicke's aphasia in the other. In both cases Hebrew was the language in which the patients were said to have exhibited Wernicke's aphasia, as reflected by their paraphasias in Hebrew. Their respective native languages were English and Spanish, in which they exhibited typical agrammatism. However, closer study of these cases suggests that the patients actually exhibited agrammatism in both of their languages, and that the symptoms of substitution in Hebrew were erroneously interpreted as evidence of paragrammatism (Paradis 1988). It is also possible that the apparent dissociation of aphasic symptoms might have reflected the patient's differential mastery of the various components of each language before the aphasia. Indeed, some non-brain-damaged speakers of foreign languages can easily pass for Broca or Wernicke patients. It is not unlikely that, given what we now know about the form that agrammatism takes in Hebrew (Grodzinsky 1984), the authors who initially reported cases of differential aphasia would no longer interpret them as such, but as cases of agrammatism in both languages, with possibly different degree of severity in each.

Finally, a number of cases have been reported to exhibit paradoxical translation (Paradis/Goldblum/Abidi 1982; De Vreese/Mota/Toshi 1988) and compulsive translation behavior (Veyrac 1931; Weisenburg/McBride 1935; Jakobson 1964; Schulze 1968; Perecman 1984; De Vreese/Mota/Toshi 1988). Patients are said to exhibit paradoxical behavior when they are able to translate into a language that is not available for spontaneous speech or any other production task, but are unable to do the reverse, i. e., to translate from a language which they do understand (though which they cannot speak spontaneously) into a language which is available for spontaneous speech. Compulsive translation refers to the patient's unsolicited spontaneous translation of what they say or of what is said to them. Inability to translate in either direction has also been reported (Goldstein 1948).

3. Three Questions about Language Representation in the Brain

These various recovery patterns raise three questions that have not always been kept distinct: (1) How is it that these patterns are possible in the first place? (2) Why does one particular pattern obtain rather than another in a given patient? (3) Why is one specific language (say, English) preferentially recovered rather than another (say, Japanese)? More specifically, one may ask what neurophysiological mechanisms are responsible for the fact that one language can be temporarily or permanently unavailable while the other(s) remain(s) relatively accessible; how it is possible that only one language is accessible for a period of time, and subsequently only the other language is; and what provokes systematic mixing. Assuming that we have a satisfactory explanation for the very possibility of the occurrence of all recovery patterns, the next step is to ascertain under what circumstances which of the possible recovery patterns will obtain. Then, assuming that we can explain the mechanism(s) underlying the various patterns of recovery and that we know the circumstances that determine the particular type of recovery, we may further ask, given any nonparallel pattern, why one specific language is preferentially recovered rather than the other. Most early studies have attempted to answer the third question. A few have attempted to answer the first. None have addressed the second, except, possibly, those that have tried to localize a switch mechanism (see below).

3.1. How are the Various Patterns Possible?

The first substantive monograph on aphasia in polyglots is that of Pitres (1895). Pitres addressed two questions. How are the various patterns possible? And what determines which language will be recovered first or best? Most of the literature of the subsequent 80 years has concentrated on his contribution to the latter question. On the basis of his review of the literature and of eight cases of his own, Pitres concluded that, contrary to what his precursor Ribot (1881) had proposed in a two-line incidental remark in a book otherwise devoted to diseases of memory, the language preferentially recovered is not the native language (by virtue of the fact that its acquisition is less recent), but is the language most familiar to the patient at the time of insult. This language in many cases indeed happens to be the mother tongue, but then it is recovered not because it was the first acquired, but because it happens also to be the most familiar. This came to be known as "Pitres' rule", and was then contrasted with "Ribot's rule" in a lively debate for years to come (Sträussler 1912; Schwalbe 1920; Pick 1921; Hegler 1931; Smirnov/Faktorovich 1949; Lambert/Fillenbaum 1959; Obler/Albert 1977). Papers that claimed to refute either Ribot's or Pitres' rule, or both, appeared in quick succession, and other tentative explanations for patterns of loss and recovery were then proposed.

Minkowski (1927; 1928), for instance, suggested that the language to be preferentially recovered was the one for which the patient had the strongest positive affective ties. However, exceptions to this proposal abound (Halpern 1950). Moreover, it is very difficult to interpret affective impact. If one wishes to take into account negative as well as positive affect, then just about every case could be interpreted in this light. Yet, in some cases, it is difficult to determine what kind of differential affect there might exist between two languages (e. g., the case described by Zangwill 1979). Pötzl (1925) suggested that the preferentially recovered language was the language most needed by the patient, while Goldstein (1948) proposed that it was the language of the environment, most often that of the hospital. However, while some patients recovered the language of the environment rather than their mother tongue or their most fluent language, just as many did not recover the language of the environment even if it was both their native and most familiar language.

3.1.1. Differential Localization

The first question, namely how the various patterns are possible, was formulated most clearly by Scoresby Jackson (1867) who, when referring to the case of "a gentleman who, after a blow on the head, lost his knowledge of Greek and did not appear to have lost anything else," asked: "Where was that gentleman's Greek deposited that it could be blotted out by a single stroke, whilst his native language and all else remained?" (p. 705). In an effort to explain this phenomenon, while quickly adding that it was "of course, mere speculation" on his part, Scoresby Jackson surmised that an individual might acquire his native language "by the aid of the posterior third of his left frontal convolution" and that, with the addition of other languages, "more and more of the convolution is utilized." (p. 704). This amounted to suggesting that different languages were subserved by different areas of cortex. Pitres (1895) argued at length against the mere hint of such hypothetical new centres specifically assigned to each of the languages learned by polyglot subjects and, although no one actually proposed that different languages were represented in different locations in the brain, authors continued to argue against this view for a long time

(Pötzl 1925; Minkowski 1927; Veyrac 1931; Ombredane 1951; Penfield 1953; Penfield/Roberts 1959; Gloning/Gloning 1965), until the notion was revived in a slightly different form by Albert/Obler (1978) who suggested that there was greater participation of the right hemisphere in the acquisition and use of a second language (Albert/Obler 1978), and by Ojemann/Whitaker (1978) in their interpretation of their electro-cortical stimulation findings.

However, there is only contradictory experimental evidence and no clinical evidence in support of differential lateralization of language in bilinguals (Mendelsohn 1988; Solin 1989; Paradis 1990 a). In addition, according to Ojemann/Whitaker, the more automatized language is subserved by a less extensive area of cortex than the less fluent language. That is, both languages share the core areas of the classical language zone, but the less automatic language is also represented in additional areas at the periphery of the language area. Rapport/Tan/Whitaker (1983) reported additional evidence in support of this hypothesis. So did Berthier/Starkstein/Lylyk/Leiguarda (1990), except that upon closer examination, it can be seen that the latter findings actually provide counter-evidence to such a proposal (Paradis 1990 b). In any case, it may be premature, for methodological reasons, to interpret these results as indicative of differential localization. The electrodes used by Ojemann/Whitaker (1978) for cortical stimulation were bipolar, with electrodes 5 millimetres apart, which, with some spreading at each end, must have interfered with an area of about 20 square millimetres. It is therefore difficult to be sure that exactly the same area of cortex was stimulated on separate occassions. (The various loci were marked by numbered tags that were manually removed for subsequent stimulation at a later time.) A more likely explanation seems to be that, within the core of the language area, language was interfered with every time, but at the periphery, sometimes it was, sometimes it was not, depending on whether the electrodes actually touched the language area, or were displaced from it by a millimetre or so.

3.1.2. The Switch Mechanism

Rejecting the notion of a different location for each particular language, Pötzl (1925) proposed that there was a cerebral switch mechanism allowing transition from one language to another. Based on his observation that there was a correlation between selective recovery and damage to the left supramarginal gyrus and adjacent temporo-parietal area, Pötzl (1930) concluded that this area subserved that distributing device. Kauders (1929) and Leischner (1948) reached similar conclusions: damage to the switch mechanism causes a patient either to be able to speak only one language or to switch uncontrollably between languages. Yet patients with switching difficulties or mixing in the context of a lesion in the anterior language area – and an intact temporo-parietal region (Minkowski 1927; Stengel/Zelmanovitch 1933; Gloning/Gloning 1965, L'Hermitte/Hécaen 1966) as well as patients without switching disturbances in the context of a damaged temporo-parietal area (Gloning/Gloning 1965; L'Hermitte/Hécaen/Dubois 1966; Schulze 1968) have been reported. Thus, if there is a specific bilingual switch mechanism, it is not likely to be localized in the supramarginal gyrus or adjacent temporo-parietal area. In fact, there is no need to postulate anatomical localization or even a type of functional language organization specific to bilinguals other than that which allows every unilingual speaker to switch between register or to select a passive over a cleft construction.

3.1.3. Inhibition/Disinhibition

Pitres (1895) proposed a different explanation, namely, that the unrecovered language is not lost, but temporarily or permanently inhibited. This hypothesis allows for two or more languages to be subserved by the same cortical areas, while remaining neurofunctionally distinct and even possibly subserved by different neural circuits, but inextricably intertwined within the same gross anatomical area. The inaccessibility of one of the languages would thus not be caused by the physical destruction of its substrate, but by the neurophysiological inhibition of its neural network. This account has the merit of being compatible with a wide range of data. In fact, it is compatible with all bilingual aphasia recovery patterns. It may also be used to explain normal bilingual verbal behaviour, such as the ability to speak one language at a time, to switch between them, and to mix them at will. In addition, it may be assumed that inhibition is not an all-or-nothing phenomenon. The underlying cerebral substrate of a given item is unable to "fire" (i.e., be activated) when inhibition exceeds a certain level. When a language item is selected for production, it receives excitatory impulses while its competitors are inhibited, or, more accurately, the activation threshold of its competitors is raised (i.e., more excitatory impulses are necessary to cause these items to fire). It may be further assumed that the activation threshold of an item is lower for comprehension than for production (i.e., for a response to an external stimulus in contrast to self-activation).

4. Neurofunctional Organization of More Than One Language

Therefore, in an effort to account for all reported clinical as well as normal (i.e., non-pathological) phenomena, we will attempt to integrate the subsystems hypothesis (Paradis 1981) and the activation threshold hypothesis (Paradis 1984; 1985) within Green's (1986) activation, control and resource framework. This should help shed some light on how a speaker-hearer has control over two language systems and avoids interference while retaining the ability to mix at will and to translate from one language to another.

4.1. The Organization of Cerebral Substratum

At least four hypotheses have been formulated with respect to the way in which two languages are organized in their neuroanatomical and neurophysiological representation (Paradis 1981). The extended system hypothesis holds that the languages are undifferentiated in their representations. The bilingual system is in all respects similar to a single language system except that it simply contains more phonemes, morphemes, lexical entries and syntactic rules. These are subserved as additional elements of the same kind within the system and are integrated into it. The syntactic rules of both languages are stored in the same way as the various syntactic rules within a single language. For example, the same mechanism that allows a speaker to select an active rather than a passive or a cleft construction allows the bilingual speaker to select the English over the Japanese structure, the selection of *broccoli* over *cauliflower* is of the same nature as the selection of *chou-fleur* over *cauliflower* or *Blumenkohl*. The dual system hypothesis holds that each language is subserved by an altogether different neural system. That is, an independent network of neural connections underlies each language. Phonemes, morphemes and syntactic rules of one language are thus subserved by a separate system of connections, independent of the one which subserves the other language. The tripartite system hypothesis holds that those items which are identical in both languages are represented in a common underlying neural substrate, while those that are different are represented in their respective language-specific neural substrates. The Subsystems hypothesis holds that each language is subserved as a subsystem of the larger system known as linguistic competence. Language functions form a cognitive system separate from other cognitive systems, and each language forms a distinct subset of that system. Language as a system is susceptible to inhibition as a whole, but each subsystem is also susceptible to selective inhibition (as well as parts of each subsystem). It is important to note that the subsystems hypothesis is the only one compatible with all the observed phenomena. While it is compatible with all patterns of recovery as well as with the ability to mix languages at will, it nevertheless needs additional experimental and/or clinical support.

4.2. The Activation Threshold Hypothesis

The activation threshold hypothesis holds that comprehension and production are subserved by the same neural substrate, but that it takes more 'energy' (or more numerous neural impulses) to voluntarily self-activate a trace (or 'engram' or 'address', depending on one's metaphor) than to activate it as a result of impulses triggered by external stimuli. In the normal course of events, the threshold of activation (i.e., the propensity to be activated) of any given trace is a function, among other factors, of frequency and recency of activation. The more frequently a given trace is used, the lower its threshold of activation, hence the easier it is to activate it again and the lesser the amount of energy needed to activate it. The longer it has been since a trace was last activated, the higher its threshold of activation, that is the more difficult it is to activate, and the greater the amount of energy needed to activate it. However, pathology may disrupt the normal pattern of activation threshold.

All things being equal, when an item is not activated, its threshold slowly rises until it is activated again, at which time the threshold is lowered and starts rising slowly again from that point on. If the item is not activated for a very long time, its threshold becomes too high for self-activation, but it can still be activated by external stimulation, thus allowing for comprehension though not for voluntary recall. When a whole language system has not been used for many years, as can occur when one emigrates for instance, the speaker is generally said to have retained a "passive knowledge" of that language, namely the ability to understand it without necessarily being able to speak it anymore (because of massive word-finding difficulty as well as morphosyntactic interference from the currently used language). If the period of disuse has not been too lengthy, and if that system is sufficiently reactivated through extensive interaction with speakers of that language, it will become active, namely its activation threshold will be sufficiently lowered for it to be self-activated. If the period of disuse has extended beyond a certain length (which may vary with the age at which the speaker ceased using the language – in subjects who ceased using the language at a younger age, the language has been reported to have become permanently unavailable after shorter periods of time than in subjects who used it until an older age) the activation threshold will have been raised so high that the subject will have lost even the ability to understand that language.

It is assumed that the selection of a particular item requires that its activation exceed that of any possible alternatives (Luria 1973; Green 1986). In order to ensure this, its competitors must be inhibited, i. e., their activation threshold must be raised. Thus, as an item is targeted for activation, its competitors are simultaneously inhibited, that is, their activation threshold is raised and consequently more energy is required to activate them (though it is not usually raised so high as to prevent comprehension of incoming signals). In other words, the appropriate item is activated by the raising of the activation threshold of competing items (i. e., all other possible candidates) as much as by actually activating it. Since the availability of an item is a function of the frequency and recency of its activation (Luria 1974), expressions may be more available (because they have been activated more often and/or more recently) in one language than in another. A word (or any other linguistic item) must reach a certain level of activation in order to become available for use. The activation threshold for the internal representation of specific words (or independently for their semantic and morphosyntactic properties on the one hand, and for their phonological form on the other), or of any other item (e. g., a syntactic or morphological rule) may differ from that of other items within the system.

It is further assumed that when a bilingual speaker elects to speak one language rather than another, the nonselected language is partly deactivated. That is, the activation threshold of the nonselected language is raised. In cases of aphasia, it sometimes becomes impossible to disinhibit (i. e., to sufficiently lower the activation threshold of) one of the languages, either permanently (as in selective recovery), temporarily (as in successive recovery), or alternatingly (as in antagonistic recovery). The activation threshold may be higher for one language than for the other (differential recovery). Deactivation of one language (raising its activation threshold) may be difficult, resulting in abundant inadvertant mixing or hybridization.

4.3. Different Grammars for Comprehension and Production?

Polyglot speakers have been reported to understand, after insult, a language they are no longer able to speak. Contrary to Albert/Obler's (1978, 220) and Green's (1986, 211) suggestion, such a situation does not necessarily indicate that different functional systems underly the comprehension and production of language (beyond the obvious peripheral auditory and motor involvement). A different threshold of activation is sufficient to account for the occassionally observed clinical dissociation, as well as for the fact that comprehension skills precede production skills during the early stages of language development (Bloom 1974); that perceptual knowledge of a second language is more advanced than productive knowledge (Tarone 1974; Tremaine 1974); that when language is not practiced, production deteriorates more quickly than comprehension (Leopold 1949; Kinzel 1964; Cohen 1989); that in amnestic aphasia, comprehension is recovered before expression (Pitres 1895; Lecours 1975); and that although it is possible for a bilingual to choose to speak either language, it is not possible to choose *not* to understand either one under any circumstance, as evidenced in all bilingual Stroop tests (Obler/Albert 1978).

In addition to the difference in activation threshold, a good deal of comprehension need not involve linguistic (e. g., morphosyntactic) decoding, but educated guessing based on the situational, linguistic, and paralinguistic contexts of the speech event, as well as general knowledge (Bloom 1974). The activation threshold hypothesis would also explain why recognition is easier than reconstruction, which is easier than evocation or recall (Florès 1970; Piaget 1970). In terms of language use, recognition corresponds to comprehension; reconstruction to comprehension from a degraded stimulus, or part of a stimulus; and recall to the self-activation of the cerebral representation of an item for production (or for inner speech) in the absence of an external stimulus.

There is therefore no need to postulate the destruction of an 'output system' independent of an 'input system' (Green 1986) in addition to the modality-specific peripheral systems in order to account for the dissociation between comprehension and production. The cerebral systems subserving the comprehension and production of language may be assumed to be separable only in that they are dependent on different activation thresholds. On the other hand, different functional systems must be assumed to underlie different languages, since double dissociations between them have been amply documented.

4.4. Resources in the Control of the Use of Language Systems

Non-parallel recovery in bilingual aphasia has been postulated since Pitres (1895) not to be the result of selective destruction of the cerebral representation of one language system, but of its temporary or permanent inhibition. Green (1986) argues in favor of this position and underscores the energy dimension of the cerebral control over the use of language systems. He maintains that regulation of inhibition/disinhibition (or, in our terms, the respective activation threshold) involves the use (and hence possible depletion) of energy resources.

The model assumes the following. When an utterance is produced, the appropriate item comes to dominate other possible candidates by reducing their level of activation, i. e., by inhibiting them (Luria 1973; Luria/Hutton 1977; Green 1986). When a bilingual speaker elects to speak one language rather than another, the nonselected language is not completely deactivated (Green 1986; Grosjean/Soares 1986); in other words, the threshold of activation is raised sufficiently to prevent interference during production, but not sufficiently to preclude borrowing and mixing, or comprehension in the other language. Practice could probably make a difference. Individuals used to mixing must have developed a lower activation threshold for the nonselected language than individuals who speak each language to different unilingual groups of people and thus never have occasion to mix, in which case the two languages are rigorously kept separate at all times and hence the threshold of the nonselected language is likely to be high.

Green (1986) then goes on to assume that words possess particular 'tags' that label each item as belonging to one or the other language. Alternatively, we may consider that items in a given language are part of a specific subsystem, and items of another language part of a different subsystem, each subsystem being subserved by a different neural network. These different networks need not be represented in different anatomical locations; they are indeed more likely to be intricately interwoven within the same cortical areas. In any case, Green rightly points out that selection of items in a particular language is partly a matter of increasing the activation of that language but also a matter of suppressing the activation of items in the other language.

To further clarify, during the voluntary use of L_A, L_B is inhibited by L_A. Dysfluencies will occur in L_A whenever there is an L_B expression which is more available than its equivalent in L_A, e. g., when a concept is more "verbalizable" (Clark/Clark 1977) or "codable" (Brown/Lenneberg 1954) in L_B than in L_A, or when it has been recently used more frequently. In a bilingual speech mode (Grosjean 1985) the speaker will not attempt to suppress the more readily available expression in the other language, and will switch to that language. In a unilingual mode, however, the expression in the other language cannot be produced, and the speaker will continue the search for an expression in the appropriate language, i. e., the speaker will try to inhibit the response in L_B in order to activate that in L_A, thus possibly causing some dysfluency (the same type of dysfluency would be expected by a unilingual having word-finding difficulty). This model also accounts for the fact that the time required to name simple objects is greater for trilinguals than for bilingual speakers (Mägiste 1986), as L_A must externally suppress the activity of the L_C system as well as that of L_B. In any case there are more competitors to be inhibited (synonyms/translation equivalents) in a trilingual than in a bilingual, and in a bilingual than in a unilingual – though a unilingual person with a very extensive lexicon also has more competing items than one with a more limited lexicon. It is interesting to note that Mägiste's data show some overlap between some unilinguals and bilinguals, possibly reflecting the fact that some unilinguals in the sample may have had very large lexicons, potentially as large as the sum of the two (relatively restricted) lexicons of some bilinguals. (A more complex form of regulation is proposed by Green (1986) in the case of translation. Two kinds of inhibition are postulated: internal inhibition of the system by itself, and external inhibition of the antagonistic system. When one is translating from L_B to L_A, L_B needs to be inhibited internally. This issue will not be considered in the limited space available here.)

Within Green's (1986) framework, which we tentatively adopt here, it is assumed that brain damage may limit the availability of the means both to excite and to inhibit a system. The kinds of output produced depend on the relative balance of the means to excite or inhibit a system. Resources are not available for language in general but independently for each specific language, so that the use of one language does not deplete the resources available to the other language(s). The inhibitory system of each language is thus susceptible to selective impairment.

The question that remains unanswered is why the (partially depleted) available resources are sometimes equally distributed among the two languages (as in parallel recovery), sometimes more in one than in the other (as in differential recovery), sometimes all in one and none in the other (as in selective recovery), or sometimes alternating between one and the other (as in successive and antagonistic recovery). That is, what determines the type of pattern? In addition, in non-parallel cases, why does L_A lack resources rather than L_B (or vice versa)? On what basis are resources assigned to one language rather than to the other, or on what basis are resources shared equally between them? In addition to the question of means (resource, energy), there is the question of automatic control: How, and on what basis, does the mechanism that controls the distribution of inhibitory resources function? These two fundamental questions remain unanswered. But they can now be rephrased as follows: What factors induce the control mechanism to assign all resources to one language and not the other (instead of distributing them equally), and why to L_A rather than to L_B? Inhibitory resources allow the regulation of active systems. But what is it that regulates and assigns inhibitory resources? And what assigns them in one way rather than in another (reflecting a specific pattern of recovery), and once the pattern is determined, what determines that one language rather than another will be allocated more inhibitory resources?

The non-recovered language remains active in some bilingual aphasic patients but not in others. That is, either comprehension is retained in the absence of production, or both are unavailable. In cases when not even comprehension is possible in one of the languages (i. e., when that language is not active, in Green's terms), it may be assumed that the threshold of activation for that language has been raised so high that it even prevents activation from outside stimuli. Indeed, some patients have been reported to have lost access to one of their premorbidly fluent languages to such an extent that it appeared as though they had never been acquainted with it before, not only having lost comprehension, but not even being able to repeat sentences in that language any better than someone who was hearing the language for the first time.

While some patterns of recovery are indeed explained by inhibition/disinhibition phenomena (i. e., the raising and lowering of the activation threshold), it must be conceded that, in some cases, when the neural substrate subserving the grammar has been physically destroyed or surgically removed, the grammar (i. e., linguistic competence, the implicit knowledge of the language) is simply no longer there. It is extremely unlikely, however, that this could result in the loss of only one of the patient's languages, as there is no evidence that two languages are not subserved by circuits within the same (macro-)anatomical area (i. e., in terms of cubic millimeters), even if we allow for possible micro-anatomical differences (in terms of cubic microns), and a fortiori if the very same neurons are involved, albeit in a different neural network. Green's model, in conjunction with the activation threshold hypothesis, offers a reasonable account of how the various observed phenomena *can* occur. Why one rather any other phenomenon *does* occur remains to be explained, however. We may hope that the assessment of large numbers of bilingual aphasic patients, permitting correlational analyses of recovery patterns and the numerous linguistic, physiological and pathological variables, will eventually provide us with sufficient data to arrive at an answer.

5. The Measure of Deficits

Such a project is underway with the systematic collection of data from every nonunilingual aphasic patient seen in various hospitals around the world, using the *Bilingual Aphasia Test* (BAT). The BAT is currently available in over 60 languages and 100 language pair combinations. The various language versions are not mere translations of each other but transpositions that are as linguistically and culturally equivalent as possible. The criterion of equivalence between the different versions varies with each task. The BAT comprises a questionnaire (Part A) to ascertain the context of acquisition and use and the degree of mastery of each language. It measures performance (Part B) at the level of the word, the sentence and the paragraph. Results are grouped according to skill (comprehension, repetition, judgment, lexical access, propositionizing, reading and writing), as well as to level of linguistic structure (phonology, morphology, syntax, lexicon, and semantics). For specific language-pairs (Part C), there are word recognition, translation, and grammaticality judgment tasks. (For a thorough description of the BAT, see Paradis/Libben 1987.)

6. Conclusion

The data thus collected over the next few years should allow us to determine whether the organization of two languages in one brain is a function of the structural distance between the languages concerned, and/or of their context of acquisition and/or use, the relative degree to which they have been mastered, the type of aphasia, the severity of the insult, or of any other variable that has been suspected of playing a potential role. In addition to answering questions about patterns of recovery, the systematic collection of data with the BAT should also eventually give us some indications as to whether two languages are represented in the brain as an extended system, two separate systems, a tripartite system, or as two subsystems of the language system.

7. References

Albert M. L. & Obler, L. K. (1978). *The bilingual brain.* New York: Academic Press.

Berthier, M. L, Starkstein, S. E, Lylyk, P., & Leiguarda, R. 1990. Differential recovery of languages in a bilingual patient: A case study using selective amytal test. *Brain and Language, 38*, 449–453.

Bloom, L. (1974). Talking, understanding and thinking. In L. Schiefelbusch & L. Lloyd (Eds.), *Language perspectives.* Baltimore: University Park Press.

Brown, R. & Lenneberg, E. H. (1954). A study in language and cognition. *Journal of Abnormal and Social Psychology, 49*, 454–62.

Clark, H. H. & Clark, E. V. (1977). *Psychology and language.* New York: Harcourt Brace Jovanovich.

Cohen, A. (1989). Attrition in the productive lexicon of two Portuguese third language speakers. *Applied Psycholinguistics, 20*, 135–147.

De Vreese, L., Mota, M., & Toshi, A. (1988). Compulsive and paradoxical translation behaviour in a case of presenile dementia of the Alzheimer type. *Journal of Neurolinguistics, 3*, 233–259.

Florès, C. (1970). Mémoire à court terme et mémoire à long terme. In B. Bovet et collaborateurs, *La mémoire.* Paris: Presses Universitaires de France.

Gloning, I. & Gloning, K. (1965). Aphasien bei Polyglotten. Beitrag zur Dynamik des Sprachabbaus sowie zur Lokalisationsfrage dieser Störungen. *Wiener Zeitschrift für Nervenheilkunde, 22*, 362–97. (Translated in Paradis 1983, 681–716.)

Goldstein, K. (1948). Disturbances of language in polyglot individuals with aphasia. In *Language and language disturbances.* New York: Grune and Stratton. 138–146.

Green, D. (1986). Control, activation, and resource: A framework and a model for the control of speech in bilinguals. *Brain and Language, 27*, 210–223.

Grodzinsky, Y. (1984). The syntactic characterization of agrammatism. *Cognition, 16*, 99–120.

Grosjean, F. (1985). The bilingual as a competent but specific speaker-hearer. *Journal of Multilingual and Multicultural Development, 6*, 467–477.

Grosjean, F. & Soares, C. (1986). Processing mixed language: some preliminary findings. In J. Vaid (Ed.), *Language processing in bilinguals. 145–179.* Hillsdale, N. J.: Lawrence Erlbaum Associates.

Halpern, L. (1950). Observations on sensory aphasia and its restitution in a Hebrew polyglot. *Monatsschrift für Psychiatrie und Neurologie, 119*, 156–173.

Hegler, C. (1931). Zur Aphasie bei Polyglotten. *Deutsche Zeitschrift für Nervenheilkunde, 117*, 236–239. (Translated in Paradis 1983, 317–319.)

Jakobson, R. (1964). General discussion. In A. De Reuck & M. O'Connor (Eds.), *Disorders of language.* Boston: Little, Brown.

Kauders, O. (1929). Über polyglotte Reaktionen bei einer sensorischen Aphasie. *Zeitschrift für die gesamte Neurologie und Psychiatrie, 122,* 651–666. (Translated in Paradis 1983, 286–300.)

Kinzel, P. (1964). *Lexical and grammatical interference in the speech of a bilingual child.* Seattle: University of Washington Press.

Lambert, W. E. & Fillenbaum, S. (1959). A pilot study of aphasia among bilinguals. *Canadian Journal of Psychology, 13,* 28–34.

Lecours, A. R. (1975). Aphasie. In *Encyclopédie médico-chirurgicale (système nerveux).* Paris: EMC, 17019, ALO 7–1975, 7–26.

Leischner, A. (1948). Über die Aphasie der Mehrsprachigen. *Archiv für Psychiatrie und Nervenkrankheiten, 180,* 731–775. (Translated in Paradis 1983, 456–502.)

Leopold, W. (1949). *Speech development of a bilingual child.* Evanston, III.: Northwestern University Press.

L'Hermitte, R., Hécaen, H., Dubois, J., Cuoli, A., & Tabouret-Keller, A. (1966). Le problème de l'aphasie des polyglottes: Remarques sur quelques observations. *Neuropsychologia, 4,* 315–329. (Translated in Paradis 1983, 727–743.)

Luria, A. R. (1973). Two basic kinds of aphasic disorders. *Linguistics, 115,* 57–66.

Luria, A. R. (1974). Basic problems of neurolinguistics. In T. A. Sebeok (Ed.), *Current trends in linguistics, vol. 12., 2561–2593.* The Hague: Mouton.

Luria, A. R. & Hutton, J. T. (1977). A modern assessment of the basic forms of aphasia. *Brain and Language, 4,* 129–151.

Mägiste, E. (1986). Selected issues in second and third language learning., In J. Vaid (Ed.), *Language processing in bilinguals. 97–122.* Hillsdale, N.J.: Lawrence Erlbaum Associates.

Mendelsohn, S. (1988). Language lateralization in bilinguals: Facts and fantasy. *Journal of Neurolinguistics, 3,* 261–292.

Minkowski, M. (1927). Klinischer Beitrag zur Aphasie bei Polyglotten, speziell im Hinblick aufs Schweizerdeutsche. *Schweizer Archiv für Neurologie und Psychiatrie, 21,* 43–72. (Translated in Paradis, 1983, 205–232.)

Minkowski, M. (1928). Sur un cas d'aphasie chez un polyglotte. *Revue Neurologique, 49,* 361–366. (Translated in Paradis 1983, 274–279.)

Nilipour, R. & Ashayeri, H. (1989). Alternating antagonism between two languages with successive recovery in a third in a trilingual aphasic patient. *Brain and Language, 36,* 23–48.

Obler, L. K. & Albert, M. L. (1977). Influence of aging on recovery from aphasia in polyglots. *Brain and Language, 4,* 460–463.

Obler, L. K. & Albert, M. L. (1978). A monitor system for bilingual language processing. In M. Paradis (Ed.), *Aspects of bilingualism.* Columbia, NC.: Hornbeam Press.

Ojemann, G. A. & Whitaker, H. A. 1978. The bilingual brain. *Archives of Neurology, 35,* 409–412.

Ombredane, A. (1951). *L'aphasie et l'élaboration de la pensée explicite.* Paris: Presses Universitaires de France.

Paradis, M. (1977). Bilingualism and aphasia. In H. Whitaker & H. A. Whitaker (Eds.), *Studies in neurolinguistics, vol. 3. 65–121.* New York: Academic Press.

Paradis, M. (1981). Neurolinguistic organization of a bilingual's two languages. *The LACUS Forum, 7,* 486–494.

Paradis, M. (Ed.) (1983). *Readings on aphasia in bilinguals and polyglots.* Montréal: Marcel Didier.

Paradis, M. (1984). Aphasie et traduction. *Μετα: Translators' Journal, 29,* 57–67.

Paradis, M. (1985). On the representation of two languages in one brain. *Language Sciences, 7,* 1–39.

Paradis, M. (1988). Recent developments in the study of agrammatism: their import for the assessment of bilingual aphasia. *Journal of Neurolinguistics, 3,* 127–160.

Paradis, M. (1989). Bilingual and polyglot aphasia. In F. Boller & J. Grafman (Eds.) *Handbook of neuropsychology, vol. 2. 117–140.* Amsterdam: Elsevier.

Paradis. M. (1990 a). Language lateralization in bilinguals: Enough already! *Brain and Language, 39,* 576–586.

Paradis, M. (1990 b). Differential recovery of languages in a bilingual patient following selective amytal injection: A comment on Berthier et al. (1990). *Brain and Language, 39,* 469–470.

Paradis, M., Goldblum, M.-C., & Abidi, R. (1982). Alternate antagonism with paradoxical translation behavior in two bilingual aphasic patients. *Brain and Language, 15,* 55–69.

Paradis, M. & Goldblum, M.-C. (1989). Selected crossed aphasia in a trilingual aphasic patient followed by reciprocal antagonism. *Brain and Language, 36,* 62–75.

Paradis, M. & Libben, G. (1987). *The assessment of bilingual aphasia.* Hillsdale, N.J.: LEA.

Penfield, W. (1953). A consideration of the neurophysiological mechanism of speech and some educational consequences. *Proceedings of the American Academy of Arts and Sciences, 82,* 199–214.

Penfield W. & Roberts, L. (1959). *Speech and brain-mechanisms.* Princeton, N.J.: Princeton University Press.

Perecman, E. (1984). Spontaneous translation and language mixing in a polyglot aphasic. *Brain and Language, 23*, 43–63.

Piaget, J. (1970). Mémoire et intelligence. In B. Bovet et collaborateurs, *La mémoire*. Paris: Presses Universitaires de France.

Pick, A. (1921). Zur Erklärung gewisser Ausnahmen von der sogenannten Ribotschen Regel. (Translated in Paradis 1983, 156–168.)

Pitres, A. (1895). Etude de l'aphasie chez les polyglottes. *Revue de Médecine, 15*, 873–899. (Translated in Paradis 1983, 26–49.)

Pötzl, O. (1925). Über die parietal bedingte Aphasie und ihren Einfluss auf das Sprechen mehrerer Sprachen. *Zeitschrift für die gesamte Neurologie und Psychiatrie, 96*, 100–124. (Translated in Paradis 1983, 176–198.)

Pötzl, O. (1930). Aphasie und Mehrsprachigkeit. *Zeitschrift für die gesamte Neurologie und Psychiatrie, 124*, 145–162. (Translated in Paradis 1983, 301–316)

Rapport, R. L., Tan, C. T., & Whitaker, H. A. (1983). Language function and dysfunction among Chinese- and English-speaking polyglots: cortical stimulation, Wada testing, and clinical studies. *Brain and Language, 18*, 342–366.

Ribot, Th. (1881). *Les maladies de la mémoire*, Paris: G. Baillère.

Schulze, H. (1968). Unterschiedliche Rückbildung einer sensorischen und einer ideokinetischen motorischen Aphasie bei einem Polyglotten. *Psychiatrie, Neurologie und medizinische Psychologie, 20*, 441–445. (Translated in Paradis 1983, 753–760.)

Schwalbe, J. (1920). Über die Aphasie bei Polyglotten. *Neurologisches Zentralblatt, 39*, 265. (Translated in Paradis 1983, 155.)

Scoresby Jackson, R. (1867). Case of aphasia with right hemiplegia. *Edinburgh Medical Journal, 12*, 696–706.

Silverberg, R. & Gordon, H. W. (1979). Differential aphasia in two bilingual individuals. *Neurology, 29*, 51–55.

Smirnov, B. & Faktorovitch, N. (1949). K voprosu ob afazii u poliglotov. *Nevropatologiia Psikhiatria, 18*, 26–28. (Translated in Paradis 1983, 535–538.)

Stengel, E. & Zelmanowicz, J. (1933). Über polyglotte motorische Aphasie. *Zeitschrift für die gesamte Neurologie und Psychiatrie, 149*, 292–311. (Translated in Paradis 1983, 356–375.)

Sträussler, E. (1912). Ein Fall von passagerer systematischer Sprachstörung bei einem Polyglotten, verbunden mit rechtsseitigen transitorischen Gehörshalluzinationen. *Zeitschrift für die gesamte Neurologie und Psychiatrie, 9*, 503–511. (Translated in Paradis 1983, 94–101.)

Tarone, E. (1974). Speech perception in second language acquisition: A suggested model. *Language Learning, 24*, 223–233.

Tremaine, R. V. (1975). *Syntax and Piagetian operational thought*. Washington, D. C.: Georgetown University Press.

Veyrac, G.-J. (1931). Etude de l'aphasie chez les sujets polyglottes. *Thèse pour le doctorat en médecine*, Université de Paris. (Translated in Paradis 1983, 320–338.)

Weisenburg, Th. & McBride, K. 1935. Aphasia: A clinical and psychological study. New York: Hofner (case 4, 160–182) (Translated in Paradis 1983, 376.)

Zangwill, O. L. (1979). Two cases of crossed aphasia in dextrals. *Neuropsychologia, 17*, 167–172.

Michel Paradis, Montréal, Québec (Canada)

25. Communicative Behavior in Aphasia

1. Introduction

Language use has considerably improved the communicative ability of human beings and in a first approximation, one may presume that under its diverse forms, aphasia necessarily entails an impairment in the capacity to interact with other people. This intuition does not follow sound reasoning rules, however, and it deserves several qualifications.

Communication is not limited to language. Animals, infants, as well as normal adult subjects are endowed with a wealth of devices enabling social exchanges by nonverbal means. Inversely, some uses of language are not directed toward a social partner. Internal speech, for instance, may serve self-regulatory or mnemonic functions. Speech impairments as assessed in aphasia examinations are typically observed in tasks like confrontation naming whose aim is to elicit expected standard responses, not to test the capability to perform the speech act of reference appropriately. Thus, one may wonder whether aphasic subjects retain communicative skills and more particularly, whether they compensate for language disorders by nonverbal behavior. The alternative hypothesis assumes a supramodal impairment which may concern various aspects of communication (see discussions in Feyereisen 1988; 1991).

Communication and language processing involve several components which may be selectively impaired in cases of brain damage. Current models of information processing attempt to describe these components by breaking down complex behavior into elementary operations. Discussing the details of these models is beyond the scope of this chapter but some critical features of the information processing approach to language may nevertheless be stressed. First, in keeping with the distinction between several components of verbal behavior, multiple forms of aphasia can be described in addition to cases of global aphasia in which all the aspects of language processing are impaired. Accordingly, the term 'aphasia' should not be used in the singular form; instead the heterogeneity of the pathologies should be considered (Caramazza 1986; Shallice 1988). Second, language impairments of diverse kinds have different consequences for communication. For the sake of clarity, it is convenient to distinguish between the processes of comprehension and production though they are narrowly linked in natural use of language. Thus, communication may be analyzed into modality-specific components, dealing with input and output processing and with verbal and nonverbal information. Furthermore, during comprehension, different pieces of knowledge are identified and progressively integrated within the conceptual system. For instance, speech understanding involves sublexical processes, word recognition, and semantic activation. Expression relies on operations of a different nature. The intention of the message is activated within the conceptual system, the modality is selected and the form is gradually specified in relation to contextual constraints. There are thus 'central' operations dealing with the meaning of the message and more domain-specific processes involved in categorical perception of various classes of stimuli and motor control of various responses. At least in some aphasic subjects, the central cognitive system is spared, thus leaving communication to rely on intact conceptual processing. For instance, ability to repeat and to understand verbal material is retained in certain patients with anomia, who consequently are less impaired in communication than patients suffering from impairments of the semantic memory. In other cases, written and oral language processing may dissociate. Similarly, unless they suffer from ideomotor apraxia or pantomime agnosia, aphasics may use gestures in order to communicate. Accordingly, ability to process different kinds of verbal and nonverbal information must be assessed empirically on an individual basis and cannot be inferred from, for example, lesion localization or associated deficits.

The impaired components of the communication system may nevertheless function with a reduced efficiency. Not every component of an information-processing system works in an all-or-nothing way, but it may operate at varying levels of efficiency. Thus, some residual abilities may be retained even in the domain of the impairment. For example, anomic speakers may still have access to the most frequent lexical items and agrammatic subjects may be able to process simple syntactic structures. Likewise, in comprehension tasks, aphasic subjects can often respond correctly to some stimuli and incorrectly to others. Furthermore, some automatic processing may be spared even when more controlled access to information is disturbed (see a recent demonstration by Chenery/Ingram/Murdoch 1990). Thus, language use is not completely abolished by left-hemisphere lesions. Different tasks, as defined by the input to and the output from the system, may be impaired at various degrees because they are more or less demanding. To use an insightful analogy, the term 'resource' has been borrowed from microeconomics to name these task demands. In cognitive psychology, this term refers to attention, to controlled processing, or to load in working memory, all notions that refer to the means the subject can devote to the task. An alternative account assumes data limitations and thus, variations of performance in relation to characteristics of input that may be degraded or, to the contrary, enriched. Then, task difficulty may depend on resource-limited and data-limited processes. Parallelly, severity of aphasia may be characterized either by variation in the amount of resource or data available for a given task (for a related discussion, see Shallice 1988, Chapter 10).

In order to communicate, aphasic subjects have to adapt to resource limitations and input degradation, and in this respect, communication involves problem solving. Besides compensations which use the spared components of the system, other communicative strategies exploit the residual capacity of the impaired mechanisms and result in performance that demands fewer resources. Multiple routes exist from an idea to its expression and, for instance, a periphrase may convey the same meaning as a precise term. Sentence production results from the selection of a particular frame among alternative ways to express a propositional content. This selection is influenced by contextual constraints since some circumstances require more or less elaborate formulations. The activation of a surface form is also sensitive to contextual influences of a different nature, and on another level, the motor execution of the utterance necessitates local accomodations, too. Thus, if a formulation is momentarily unavailable, it is possible to adapt using other methods. Strategic use of linguistic devices like ellipsis, anaphora, or paraphrase allows the aphasic speaker to bypass lexical and syntactic impairments. Especially agrammatism has been interpreted from such a perspective (Kolk/Heeschen 1990). Similarly, there are several contributions to the activation of the meaning of a spoken utterance. Language comprehension is achieved by the interaction of several sources, input processing (phonological analysis, word recognition, syntactic parsing) and inferential, integrative procedures. Thus, residual speech comprehension can not only be explained by intact conceptual processing, but also by reduced processing demands and by contextual influences when multiple sources of information, verbal and nonverbal, combine.

Communication is a collaborative process between at least two subjects. Current models of conversation stress the need for cooperation between different partners to achieve mutual understanding (see e. g. Clark/Schaefer 1989). The normal partner may assist the aphasic subject by supplying missing words, by requesting confirmation, or by asking yes-no questions. Rate of speech, intonation, lexical selection and mean length of utterance can be adapted to the assumed residual capabilities of the disabled speech partner. Furthermore, ill-formed utterances like telegraphic speech or phonetic and phonemic paraphasias may nevertheless be interpreted. Thus, communicative effectiveness of aphasic subjects sometimes depends on support by an attentive healthy listener. Communication also results from a matter of convention. Familiarity with the partner allows the use of simpler or shorter forms because previous experience supplies further, implicit information to the message. The spouse and after some time, the speech therapist of the aphasic subject probably gain some expertise in dealing with distorted utterances. Reciprocally, one may wonder whether aphasic subjects benefit from repeated exposures to situations of communication.

Overview. These diverse elements of discussion make the treatment of the issue of 'communication and aphasia' more complex. Several accounts of the impairments in communication and of the spared communicative ability of aphasic subjects are made possible. From a structural point of view, selective impairments which spare the nonverbal modalities or some components of the verbal information processing system can be described. More particularly, if the central cognitive processes are intact, the subject will remain able to use encyclopaedic and social knowledge for the purpose of communication. From a dynamic perspective, the development of compensatory, heuristic stategies can be described as adaptations to a reduction of processing resources and impoverishment of input, or resulting from reliance on a healthy partner. In the next section, experimental literature on the communicative behavior of aphasic subjects, first in its receptive, then in its expressive aspects, will be reviewed in relation to the theoretical issues raised in this introduction. Due to space limitations, this review will focus on those recent studies, not treated in the chapter by Foldi/Cicone/Gardner (1983). In a final section, the clinical implications of these findings will be discussed, as far as assessment and rehabilitation of aphasia are concerned.

2. Review of the Experimental Evidence

2.1. Comprehension

Do comprehension disorders in aphasia result from selective impairments of verbal information processing or from a more general deficit which also affects other modalities? Does the nonverbal context facilitate understanding of speech? Does grasping the intention of a message dissociate from presemantic processing like phonological analysis? Unfortunately, these questions have not yet elicited studies on comprehension in interactive situations and on on-line processing of speech. The main evidence available results from experiments dealing with metacommunicative abilities and, in that domain, with the processing of prosody and gestures, among the multiple cues that may facilitate speech comprehension.

2.1.1. Nonverbal Comprehension in Aphasia

2.1.1.1. Auditory Processing

Most studies on the reception of vocal cues by brain-damaged subjects were conducted upon the assumption of a right-hemisphere dominance in the processing of emotion and of the nonpropositional aspects of speech. Right-hemisphere damaged subjects may be impaired in several tasks that require prosody to be processed such as voice recognition, perception of linguistic stress and interrogation marks, and comprehension of emotional expressions. However, some left-hemisphere damaged subjects are also impaired in the processing of affective and nonaffective prosody, often in relation to disorders in spoken-language comprehension. These data converge with the results of dichotic listening studies in normal subjects to show that both hemispheres contribute to prosody processing. It does not mean that the left and the right parts of brain are equally sensitive to the same components of the auditory input. However, the characteristics of the signal for the processing of which one cerebral region is specialized remain to be identified (see, e. g., Hartje/Willmes/Weniger 1985; Heilman/Bowers/Speedie/Coslett 1984; Tompkins/Flowers 1985; for a review, see Van Lancker 1987).

2.1.1.2. Visual Processing

Several studies reported impairments in the perception of facial expressions of emotions in aphasic as compared to normal subjects though in this domain, right hemisphere-damaged subjects are often even more severely impaired (for reviews, see Feyereisen 1986; 1989). Likewise, in gesture-to-picture matching tasks, aphasics perform worse than control subjects, and the extent of the deficit correlates with the severity of naming and auditory comprehension deficits (see e. g., Duffy/Duffy 1981; Rothi/Heilman/Watson 1985; Feyereisen 1988 for a review). The most frequent error involves the choice of a picture that has something in common with the correct response. Thus, impaired aphasics understand a part of the meaning of the gesture but not enough to discriminate related concepts (Duffy/Watkins 1984; Varney/Benton 1982). Similarly, impaired subjects can understand some gestures, while failing to understand others (e. g., Daniloff/Noll/Fristoe/Lloyd 1982; Netsu/Marquardt 1984). Thus, aphasic subjects show similar impairments in the processing of vocal and gestural signals and in the processing of words and pictures in semantic decision or categorization tasks. But, although the existence of nonverbal disorders after left-hemisphere damage is not controverted, the problem remains to identify the impaired mechanism in relation to a model of the operations involved in the task. More particularly, the deficit could involve central semantic processes or result from the association of several modality-specific impairments affecting the presemantic encoding operations. Progress in the neuropsychological analysis of nonverbal comprehension is likely to be made from detailed single case studies. Modality-specificity of some disorders is suggested by the observation of impaired discrimination and comprehension of gestures in left-hemisphere damaged subjects without speech comprehension deficits (Rothi/Mack/Heilman 1986). Cases showing the inverse dissociation were also mentioned in some group studies (Varney 1982; Varney/Damasio/Adler 1989). Retained comprehension of gestures when speech comprehension is impaired might relate to similar dissociations between written and spoken language processing.

2.1.2. Integration of Verbal and Nonverbal Information

2.1.2.1. Auditory Information

Several vocal cues may facilitate speech comprehension in aphasia. In a word monitoring task, stressed words were responded to faster than unstressed ones (Swinney/Zurif/Cutler 1980). Aphasic subjects suffering from mild or moderate comprehension disorders also performed better in answering yes-no questions when the critical information was emphasized by intonation (Kimelman/Mc Neil 1987). Another kind of interaction between verbal and nonverbal comprehension was demonstrated in experiments bearing on the comprehension of emotional cues. When the verbal content itself conveyed affective meaning, left-hemisphere damaged like control subjects performed better if intonation and meaning were congruent and worse when the message was incongruent (Bowers/Coslett/Bauer et al. 1987; Seron/Van der Kaa/Van der Linden/Remits/Feyereisen 1982; Tompkins/Flowers 1987).

2.1.2.2. Auditory and Visual Information: Pictures and Gestures

In the recent years, the interaction of visual and auditory information during lip reading has been analyzed mainly in cases of word meaning deafness who, typically, have no problem in understanding written language (Campbell/Garwood/Franklin et al. 1990; Shindo/Kaga/Tanaka 1991). Likewise, little or nothing is known about the visual processing of pictorial or actual scenes during sentence comprehension. However, illustrations have been shown to facilitate speech processing in some experimental tasks. In the verification of sentences like *a fish is smaller than a whale*, the presentation of pictures showing the two arguments reduced the number of errors, even when the verification bore on a less picturable property such as weight (Nicholas/Brookshire 1981). Pictures as well as verbal contexts also facilitated answering questions about sentences but the contextual influences were qualified by interactions with subject and sentence characteristics (Pierce/Beekman 1985). Reciprocally, semantic decisions about pictures were more accurate when a written word cued the relevant semantic feature (Koemeda-Lutz/Cohen/Meier 1987). Thus, aphasic subjects may benefit from the redundancy of verbal and pictorial information or from focussing of attention on critical aspects of the task.

There are few comparable studies on the influence of the gestural context. Better performances in object manipulation tasks after gestural than after oral instructions might simply reflect advantages of imitation over verbal request in the control of motor activity (see, e. g., Beukelman/Yorkston/Waugh 1980). Only two studies have experimentally examined the facilitation of auditory comprehension by gestural cues in word-to-picture matching tasks. Venus/Canter (1987) did not find aphasic subjects performing better in processing words with a concurring gestural cue than in control conditions. This result, however, stems from an analysis of a group performance and the gestural context may facilitate speech comprehension in specific cases. In the other study, greater attention was paid to the description of comprehension disorders in the individual aphasic subjects (Feyereisen/Hazan 1991; see also a summary report in Feyereisen 1991). However, no case of dissociation between visual and auditory comprehension was present in the group and no specific effect of gestural facilitation was observed.

2.1.3. Heuristic Procedures in Speech Comprehension: the Use of "Context"

In a word recognition task, phonemic errors are more frequent when the target word is part of a sentence with an incongruous meaning (Beck 1984). Interactive models of speech comprehension may account for such a result by assuming retroactive influence of semantic activation on speech perception. Similarly, in spoken sentence-to-picture matching tasks, partial processing of content words and of visual, nonverbal information probably activates general knowledge of the world on which the subjects rely on for their responses. Sentences that describe highly improbable events are typically more difficult to understand than those which respect semantic rules of selection or common sense. A bias toward the correct understanding of metaphors instead of their literal interpretation may probably be explained in the same way: presented with several possible responses corresponding to different events, aphasic subjects would adopt the general strategy of selecting the most plausible alternative (see, e. g., Caramazza/Zurif 1976; Deloche/Seron 1981; Huber 1990; see also discussions in Caramazza 1988; Grodzinsky/Marek 1988; Sherman/Schweickert 1989).

A different account of residual comprehension is proposed by Van Lancker (1987) who suggested that different processes may underlie sentence comprehension. Some aphasic subjects would recognize overlearned, familiar sentences as a whole in the same way single words are processed whereas right brain-damaged subjects would parse the sentence into its constituents. As a result, a double dissociation is demonstrated in the processing of idioms like *while the cat's away, the mice will play* and of quite novel sentences that require analysis (Van Lancker/Kempler 1987). Performances in the comprehension of frozen metaphors that are presented out of context may be explained in the same way. From a slightly different perspective, one may also assume that aphasic subjects would have access to the connotative meaning of the lexical items. They would therefore be able to identify the appropriate meaning of potentially ambiguous metaphors (Brownell 1988; Brownell/Simpson/Bihrle et al. 1990).

Still other mechanisms are demonstrated with different experimental procedures. In a task of answering questions about directly stated or indirectly suggested items, no difference was observed in relation to the nature of the response and thus, aphasic subjects were shown able to infer information from the sentential context (Brookshire/Nicholas 1984). Their comprehension of sentences was also facilitated by a narrative context by which some constituents were cued, even if this context did not allow a prediction of the event described in the sentence (Hough/Pierce/Cannito 1989). These compensatory strategies present shortcomings, however, because there are circumstances in which guessing leads to error. For example, 'prestimulation', i. e. giving some elements of a sentence before the complete sentence itself, did not affect the number of correct choices among related pictures when all the proposed pictures showed primed items along with distractors (Waller/Darley 1979). Predictibility of a word from context also increased the probability of making semantic errors in answering questions about this word (Pierce/De Stefano 1987).

Heuristic procedures, which aphasic subjects employ to fill in some gaps in comprehension, have mainly been studied for indirect speech acts and linguistic indicators of implicit attitudes (for a more extensive review, see Weylman/Brownell/Gardner 1988).

2.1.3.1. The Comprehension of Indirect Requests

The first experimental demonstration of access to contextually conveyed meaning by aphasic subjects was provided in the study of Wilcox/Davis/Leonard (1978). Subjects were presented short videotaped segments in which two characters interacted. One uttered a sentence of the form *Will you open the door?* or *Must you bite the pen?*. The other behaved either in an appropriate way, by doing or stopping to do something, or in an inappropriate way. The task was to answer yes or no in accordance to the appropriateness of this behavior. As a group, aphasic subjects with high scores in standard tests of auditory comprehension performed better than subjects with low scores and, on the whole, the correlation between the experimental result and the clinical assessment was significant. However, the subjects' performance was found much better in the experimental task than in comprehension testing. The worse score was 74 % of correct responses, much higher than the chance level of 50 %. Furthermore, performances were influenced by the presented material. Two variables interacted, sentence formulation and behavior appropriateness. The subjects were globally more often correct when judging a request to do something than to stop something, and in this case, when judging the continuation of action inappropriate rather than its requested cessation appropriate. Thus, the major difficulty was in approving the stopping of an undesirable activity. A plausible interpretation of this result is that subjects were mainly influenced by congruity of action in context and the nonverbal reactions of the speaker but not by the adequacy of the behavior to the verbally expressed request. In that sense, aphasic subjects might have direct access to the intended meaning as infered from context without processing the literal meaning of the verbal message. That hypothesis was supported in another study using a similar procedure. Sentences of the kind *Can you ...* were presented either as requests or as questions, i. e. in contexts from which either the performance of the appropriate action or the answer *yes* was expected. In a sample of five 'anterior' aphasics, subjects were found unable to process the literal meaning of the questions, and they were more often correct in inferring the intended meaning of requests, probably from the nonverbal context (Hirst/Ledoux/Stein 1984).

Further studies did not use videotapes in their procedures, so the influence of the nonverbal context was reduced. Hence, a different conclusion was drawn and the comprehension was found to be more influenced by linguistic processing than in the previous experiments. Foldi (1987) had subjects rate the likelihood of different dialogs; the verbal responses were illustrated by pictures. Left brain-damaged subjects gave more appropriate responses than right brain-damaged subjects but in the two groups, understanding an indirect request was more difficult than processing direct commands or wh-questions. In another study, only a verbal material was presented and subjects had to identify the most appropriate answer to a verbal request. Aphasic subjects were more often correct, when the context suggested that the literal meaning of the sentence was intended. They were also influenced by the surface form of the questions, and more often correct when the conventional formulations *Can you* or *Could you* were used than with sentences like *Is it possible for you* ... or *Are you able* ... (Weylman/Brownell/Roman/Gardner 1989).

2.1.3.2. Processing the Indicators of Implicit Attitudes

The use of many lexical items relies on pragmatic, context-dependent decisions. For instance, the definite article *the* is appropriate when the referent is unique in nature, is specified in the remainder of the sentence, or has been mentioned previously. By choosing such a form, the speaker assumes the partner may know something about the referent. Otherwise, the undefinite form *a* is prefered. Sentences that obey appropriateness rules are typically easier to understand than other ones. For example, in front of a sample array of one square and two circles, normal subjects are expected to take longer time to respond to a request like *Take the round one* than to that in which the undefinite article is used. Furthermore, in that situation, subjects are expected to reduce the ambiguity of the sentence by relying on another, nonnamed dimension like the colour of the figure and to select the round figure that is unique to this respect. This pattern of performance was observed in anomic subjects without comprehension disorders but not in other aphasic subjects (Goodenough/Zurif/Weintraub 1977). In these controlled conditions, linguistic impairments prevented access to the implicit meaning of the message because the data for the inference process were limited. A similar conclusion was reached in another experiment. In several respects, sentence comprehension requires reliance on some knowledge shared by the partners. This is also the case with the processing of adverbs like *even*, *also*, and *mainly* used in explicit statements by which some other part of the information is implicitly conveyed. For instance, the sentence *Even Alice came* refers both to the Alices's presence and to its somewhat unexpected character, i. e. a propositional attitude assumed by both the speaker and the listener toward the stated fact. In an experimental situation, nonverbal communication may be prevented and the implicit attitude may be expressed by the surface form of the sentence only. One may thus predict that aphasic subjects who are impaired in the processing of these parts of speech will also be unable to decide about the contextual appropriateness of sentences using words of that class. That hypothesis was tested in a sentence-to-picture matching task (Hupet/Seron/Frederix 1986). The sentences refered to the color of a figure and the pictures, actually simple rectangles, varied by the number and the size of parts of different colors. Several patterns of performance were observed. Some aphasics behaved like normal subjects whereas other aphasics did not process the adverb and generally selected the figure with the largest surface of the asserted color. Finally, a third subset of aphasic subjects selected a rectangle with a high amount of the asserted color but not necessarily the highest. They were thus appropriate with the sentences using *mainly*, but not with *even* sentences. These performances did not systematically relate to aphasia type but it is now clear than even within a selected sample of so-called agrammatic patients, a great heterogeneity exists in the processing of the function words. Some agrammatic subjects have no comprehension problems and others may be impaired in the comprehension of some function words only.

2.1.4. Conclusions

The several possible accounts of residual comprehension in aphasia do not receive equal support from the literature. Experimental studies do not offer compelling evidence in favour of the nonverbal compensation hypothesis. However, nonverbal deficites do only concern a subgroup of the aphasic population and their assessment remains an empirical matter, preferably in detailed analyses of single cases. Another hypothesis has been the dissociation of pragmatic and linguistic domains, perhaps in relation to different competencies of the right and left cerebral hemispheres in each of these functions. However, if we can admit the possibility that communicative skills may be impaired in cases of brain damage without aphasia, it is much more difficult to understand how aphasic subjects could obtain direct access the speaker's intention without processing of the message linguistically. Actually, some residual verbal ability is needed and this favors explanations in terms of processing resource. Such an account is also consistent with the frequent superiority of receptive abilities over expressive ones if we consider that responses in comprehension tasks are less demanding with regard to number of alternatives or complexity of execution.

2.2. Expression

2.2.1. Channel Use in Communication: Speech, Vocalizations and Gestures

From current models of information processing, it may be predicted that a breakdown of the central, conceptual system should impair communication in different modalities whereas more specific disorders like an inability to access a word form from its semantic activation may spare nonverbal expression. Accordingly, expressive skills must be assessed empirically in brain-damaged subjects whose drawing, gesturing, writing, and speaking abilities may be impaired to different extent (see, e. g., Gainotti/Silveri/Villa/Caltagirone 1984; Grossman 1988). A great interindividual variability and the specificity of the different nonverbal modalities (that is their independence from language processing) can explain why, for instance, contradictory findings have been reported about the expression of emotion by aphasic subjects in the vocal and facial channels (Borod/Koff/Perlman-Lorch/Nicholas 1985 and 1986; Mammucari/Caltagirone/Ekman et al. 1988; Ryalls/Behrens 1988).

From such a perspective, how should one approach the question as to whether aphasic subjects show similar impairments in performing conversational gestures, as in naming, and in apraxia examination? From some pilot studies, it was concluded that linguistic and gestural abilities dissolve simultaneously in aphasia and that left-hemisphere lesions disrupt communication both in the verbal and the gestural modality (e. g. Glosser/Wiener/Kaplan 1986; see discussions in Feyereisen 1987; 1991; Mc Neill 1985; 1987; 1989). However, other studies contradicted these observations and aphasic subjects were found to display higher manual activity than normal control subjects. Highest gesture rates have been observed either in nonfluent or in fluent aphasics. Proportion of representational gestures was usually higher in nonfluent aphasics but these subjects sometimes performed more batonic (i. e., nonrepresentational) gestures than fluent aphasics (Feyereisen 1983; Le May/David/Thomas 1988; Smith 1987 a, b). In a heterogeneous group of 11 aphasics, appropriate usage of gestures did not relate to measures of verbal skills but fluent aphasics tended to perform gestures which supported oral expression while nonfluent aphasics more often substituted gestures for verbal communication (Behrmann/Penn 1984). In another study, higher reliance on gestural mode of communication was observed in severe nonfluent aphasics (Broca's and global aphasics) as compared to their normal partners and during referential communication task, more gestures were performed by the more severely impaired aphasics whose residual language was less efficient (Feyereisen/Barter/Goossens/Clerebaut 1988; Herrmann/Reichle/Lucius-Hoene et al. 1988). Furthermore, there is some evidence that aphasic subjects control their gestural behavior in relation to communication functions since fewer gestures were performed when visual access to the partner was prevented (Glosser/Wiener/Kaplan 1988).

In summary, only one study has shown reduced gestural activity in aphasics as compared to control (Glosser/Wiener/Kaplan 1986) while several others have shown increased gestural activity in cases of language impairment. Actually, very different patterns of association between gestures and speech may be found in a heterogeneous sample of aphasic subjects and this variability does not relate to speech characteristics like fluency or use of content words. Furthermore, variability also exists among normal subjects who sometimes perform no hand gesture while speaking. Due to the lack of constraints on gestural performance, 'errors' cannot be easily identified in brain-damaged subjects. For these different reasons, greatest insight is expected from single cases studies undertaken in more controlled situation than natural conversations (Feyereisen/Bouchat/Déry/Ruiz 1990).

2.2.2. The Role of Context

2.2.2.1. Cueing

In normal subjects, the selection of syntactic forms and of the lexical items can be influenced by the sentences previously heard or spoken and by associations to this material (see e. g. Bock 1987). This clarifies the common clinical experience that oral performances of aphasic subjects may be improved by contextual cues. For instance, providing open ended sentences increases the proportion of correct naming of pictures (Pease/

Goodglass 1978). Nevertheless, there is little experimental evidence that speech production is less impaired in natural settings than during out-of-context formal examinations. Semantic priming has been demonstrated in lexical decision task but not in naming tasks. Semantic cues such as priming the word *camel* with complete sentences like *it lives in the desert* or *it carries heavy loads* are generally less effective than a phonemic cue (e.g. Li/Williams 1990). Similarly, presenting pictures of objects in their functional context or among items of the same semantic category did not significantly facilitate naming whereas objects integrated in composite pictures but without strong semantic links are more often correctly named than isolated objects, at least in some subjects (Hatfield/Howard/Barber et al. 1977; Seron/Monsel/Van der Kaa et al. 1980; Williams/Canter 1982; 1987). It must be emphasized, however, that priming effects were often qualified by interactions with aphasia subtype and that, anyway, large individual differences are observed in the ability to take advantage of the primes. Accordingly, contextual facilitation might better be demonstrated in single-cases than in heterogeneous samples (see e.g. Zingeser/Berndt 1988).

2.2.2.2. Topicalization

During sentence production, the speakers select lexical items and syntactic frames in function of assumption about the knowledge shared by their partners. Mental dispositions are infered from the situation, from previous interactions, or from the content of the preceding utterances. These presuppositions shape the surface structure of the sentence: use of the definite/indefinite article, pronominalization, word order in active, passive, and cleft sentence, etc. One study dealt with these aspects of sentence production in aphasia (Bates/Hanby/Zurif 1983). Ten subjects (five Broca's and five Wernicke's aphasics) were given nine series of three pictures to be verbally described. In each array, only one element, for instance, the agent of the action, varied and the other remained constant. Similar to normal subjects, aphasics increased lexicalization for the variable information and ellipsis for the constant elements. The aphasics also used the definite article more often with the constant term. In contrast, pronominalization was little affected by pragmatic constraints. These results were replicated in a crosslinguistic study (e.g. Wulfeck/Bates/Juarez et al. 1989).

2.2.3. Communicative Effectiveness and Compensatory Strategies

The referential communication task provides an experimental model by which the structure, the development, and the breakdown of conversation skills may be analyzed (Clark/Wilkes-Gibbs 1986; Krauss/Glucksberg 1977). Two subjects are given similar arrays of pictures and are instructed to communicate in the most convenient way in order to arrange the pictures in the same way or to identify the same target picture. Performance is assessed based on speed and accuracy rather than by formal criteria like sentence structure or lexical diversity. This procedure was used in several studies with aphasic subjects. The main result was that these subjects generally succeeded in the task despite their verbal impairments and thus, communicative effectiveness was demonstrated in that population (Busch/Brookshire/Nicholas 1988; Feyereisen/Barter/Goossens/Clerebaut 1988; Meuse/Marquardt 1985).

Several aspects of the task have to be taken into account in order to qualify that conclusion. First, peculiarities of task requirements must be underlined. In order to communicate, the subject has to give some cues in order to pinpoint the referent among the distractors. Gestures, onomatopoeias, phonemic approximations, or periphrases may be used, all responses that would be considered incorrect in a naming task. Likewise, gestures that are rated as poor performances in apraxia examination may nevertheless be efficient in the referential task (Feyereisen/Barter/Goossens/Clerebaut 1988). Second, the pictures presented in the task define a common ground of knowledge and limit the range of possible meanings of the message. It should be easier to find the best match between the provided cues and the different pictures than to identify a referent without any context. However, experimental support for such a hypothesis is still lacking. Third, communication requires a cooperative partner who may facilitate the transmission of information by asking yes-no questions, by commenting on possible confusions, and by suggesting appropriate formulations. This dimension of the performance remains to be systematically controlled by comparing expert and nonexpert partner or by providing different kinds of model and feedback to the aphasic subject.

2.2.4. Conclusions

If "aphasics communicate better than they speak", which theoretical proposal can account for spared communicative ability despite impaired verbal expression? One suggestion is that to some extent, nonverbal devices may supply alternative means of expression. Another explanation is the reliance on contextual influences which facilitate speech production in interactive situations, as compared to the formal setting of aphasia examination. However, there is no clear demonstration of independence between verbal and nonverbal modalities of communication nor is there firm experimental evidence supporting the contextual facilitation hypothesis on the aphasic population level. Actually, in many cases of aphasia, verbal and nonverbal behavior is impaired by motor and cognitive deficits, but gestural expression is less severely disturbed than oral expression. Thus, the best explanation for the residual capacities of severe aphasic subjects seems to be the reduced task demand to produce understandable messages. First, to express oneself is less difficult than to produce the specific form required in aphasia or apraxia examination; second, manual signs are probably relatively easier to perform than the verbal ones and third, the partner is contributing to dialogue.

3. Clinical Implications

Experimental studies on communication in aphasia have renewed the clinical approach to aphasic subjects by suggesting higher consideration than in the past of the pragmatic aspects in language assessment and therapy.

3.1. Assessment

Unlike thought disorders manifested in schizophrenia and senile dementia, aphasia is usually assumed to spare the highest-level mechanisms concerning the message elaboration and reception and to impair only the instruments of communication. It remains useful, however, to evaluate the incidence of these instrumental deficits on social interactions because communication problems may be the greatest cause of suffering in aphasic subjects and their main motivation to undergo a rehabilitation process. Questionnaires about the complains of brain-damaged patients and about their functionning in home environment signal needs for help in several domains and thus, reliance on communicating with healthy partners (Shewan/Cameron 1984; Smith 1985).

Three kinds of procedure have been proposed to assess communicative ability of aphasic subjects.

3.1.1. Naturalistic Observations

Holland (1982) trained observers to note in a reliable way instances of behavior like "asking questions" and "using spatial indicators" by aphasic subjects in their home environment. Most of these communicative acts were found successful. However, aphasic subjects differed in the amount of communication attempted and in the proportion of failures. Auditory comprehension disorders especially resulted in inappropriate behavior.

3.1.2. Role Playing

Aphasic subjects might avoid situations in which they encounter difficulties and thus, it is useful to elicit communicative acts in a greater variety of situations than those observed at home. Communicative competence may be assessed in simulations of daily-life interactions (Blomert/Koster/Van Mier/Kean 1987). The performance of control subjects indicates what is expected from the situation. For instance, in front of a ticket counter at the station, a 'request' with the mention of the destination is a necessary component of the appropriate behavior. The precision "second class" may be optional. In the sample studied by Blomert et al., aphasic subjects were found to produce the necessary information normally but less than control subjects the non-essential components. These performances were largely independent from assessment of speech in standard aphasia testing.

3.1.3. Rating Scales and Checklists

From the literature on pragmatics, Prutting/Kirchner (1987) compiled a list of 30 items, which therapists rated for appropriateness based on their observation of spontaneous communication. The list bears on verbal and nonverbal aspects of communication like "maintaining the coherence of topic across the discourse" and "using gestures to support, complement, or replace verbal behavior". In a sample of 11 left brain-damaged subjects, some parameters like physical distance and mutual gaze between the partners were never found inappropriate whereas all subjects were inappropriate in specificity and accuracy of their vocabulary. Another list of 16 items was proposed by Lomas/Pichard/Bester et al. (1989) from direct observations of performances in daily life. The patients' spouses or other familiar people were asked to rate the subject's ability at different activities like "getting somebody's attention" and "communicating his/her emotion". In another approach to communicative skills in aphasia, subjects were rated on their responses to 20 questions of a standardized interview. One scale dealt with the adequacy of each response and another with the strategy used by the subject (using compensatory paraverbal or nonverbal behavior, asking support, etc.). These performances correlated only moderately with the results of the aphasia examination and non-significantly with the results of the Token test (Herrmann/Koch/Johannsen-Horbach/Wallesch 1989). Copeland's (1989) Conversation Assessment focussed on 20 speech functions like requesting, agreeing, warning, etc. Prompts were prepared to elicit these speech acts during a 15 minute conversation with the subject. Each function was rated on a five-point rating scale. More specific scales were also proposed, for example, about the spontaneous gestural behavior as estimated by people involved with the aphasic subject. However, the validity of the instrument remains to be assessed by relating these clinical ratings to the actual performances of the subject (Borod/Fitzpatrick/Helm-Estabrooks/Goodglass 1989).

3.2. Therapy

3.2.1. Nonvocal Rehabilitation Techniques

Attempts to teach nonvocal communication systems in aphasia therapy have a long history. In one direction, artificial 'languages' using icons or geometric forms were devised to meet the main communication needs of the subject. These methods are now becoming more sophisticated through the increased availability of microcomputers and the development of programs by which use visual systems. They may be helpful for global aphasics who have not retained any expressive means (see, e. g. Steele/Weinrich/Wertz et al. 1989). In another direction, aphasic subjects are trained to use manual systems like the American Sign Language or the Amerind. An apparent paradox in these techniques is that they rely on nonverbal abilities which are often impaired in cases of aphasia. Sign acquisition in speechless subjects may be explained, however, if one considers that performing a gesture is less difficult than uttering the corresponding message vocally. A support for such a suggestion can be found in the analysis of individual differences. To some degree of severity of the language impairment, manual signs may still be learned whereas spoken words do not (see e. g. Coelho/Duffy 1987; 1990). Another evidence stems from the analysis of sign characteristics like transparency, iconicity, and motor complexity. Even in the gestural modality, some signs are more easily acquired than others (Coelho/Duffy 1986; Daniloff/Fritelli/Buckingham et al. 1986; for reviews, see Christopoulou/Bonvillian 1985; Helm-Estabrook/Emery 1988; Peterson/Kirshner 1981; Rowley 1983).

A crucial issue in devising a nonverbal communication system is to evaluate the benefit of the training against its cost for the patient and the healthy partners. From such a point of view, learning a more efficient use of residual verbal abilities may be less expensive if the same objectives can be achieved. This problem was systematically addressed by Funnell/Allport (1989) in a study on the use of Blissymbolics, a visual logographic system, by two aphasic subjects. The subjects were clearly able to learn associations between the geometric symbols of the system and pictures of objects. However, acquisition of symbols for function words was much less successful. Actually, these performances mirrored the results of language examinations showing spared ability in auditory-visual matching of concrete nouns and severe impairments in processing function words and meaningless syllables. The authors concluded that symbols were simply equivalent to their written counterparts and that there was no benefit in the learning of an artificial system. Treatment was re-oriented towards a better exploitation by the subjects of their residual abilities in processing written language, abilities which have been demonstrated in careful pretherapeutic examinations.

3.2.2. Promoting Aphasic Communicative Effectiveness (PACE)

PACE therapy focusses on the incorporation of natural conversation parameters in order to improve communicative ability of aphasic subjects. Four aspects are emphasized and contrasted with traditional rehabilitation techniques: (a) Both the clinician and the patient take active parts as senders and receivers. (b) The exchanged messages bring new information. (c) Any communication modality may be used to convey messages. (d) Performances are rated for communicative effectiveness rather than according to formal criteria (Davis 1989; Davis/Wilcox 1978; 1985). Actually, the PACE therapy relies on an extensive training to referential communication tasks (see section 2.2.3.). The clinician plays an important role in modelling effective messages, for instance, by showing the utility of nonverbal signals, and in inhibiting ineffective ways to transmit information like the inappropriate expansion in some cases of fluent aphasias (see also Penn 1987). Along the same lines, the healthy partner may be given advice in order to improve collaboration to discourse: slowing down speech tempo, using short sentences, reformulating the message, etc. (Green 1984).

4. General Conclusions

Considerable advances in the pragmatic approach to aphasia have been realized in the recent years. Systematic studies have attempted to analyse the processes involved in communication and therapeutic implications have been brought out. Increased attention is being paid to individual differences in language impairments and communicative skills. No general claim about 'communication and aphasia' is risked here. Instead, heterogeneity of performances is exploited to demonstrate the separability of components forming the cognitive system. Some operations deal with modality-specific input and output processes. Accordingly, the first empirical question addressing the aphasic is about his or her ability to recognize and produce manual and vocal gestures, pictures of objects, spoken and written words, etc. Other processes are implied in the integration of information from different modalities, in using knowledge acquired from past experience, and in selecting the appropriate means to achieve communication goals. A more precise description of this adaptative behavior should be the aim of further research, and finding the best way to improve it, the endeavour of speech therapists.

Acknowledgments

Pierre Feyereisen is presently supported as a Research Associate by the National Fund for Scientific Research (Belgium). Gratitude is expressed to Michel Hupet for helpful comments on a previous version of the manuscript. Parts of the chapter were presented in a keynote paper at the Fourth International Aphasia Rehabilitation Congress at Edinburgh on September 4, 1990.

5. References

Bates, E., Hamby, S., & Zurif, E. (1983). The effects of focal brain damage on pragmatic expression. *Canadian Journal of Psychology, 37*, 59–84.

Beck, A. R. (1984). The processing of the sounds and meanings of ongoing speech by aphasic subjects. *Brain and Language, 22*, 320–338.

Behrmann, M. & Penn, C. (1984). Non-verbal communication of aphasic patients. *British Journal of Disorders of Communication, 19*, 155–168.

Beukelman, D. R., Yorkston, K. M. & Waugh, P. F. (1980). Communication in severe aphasia: Effectiveness of three instruction modalities. *Archives of Physical Medicine and Rehabilitation, 61*, 248–252.

Blomert, L., Koster, C., Van Mier, H., & Kean, M.-L. (1987). Verbal communication abilities of aphasic patients: The everyday language test. *Aphasiology, 1*, 463–474.

Bock, J. K. (1987). Co-ordinating words and syntax in speech plans. In A. W. Ellis (Ed.), *Progress in the psychology of language, vol. 3. 337–390*. London/Hillsdale, N. J.: Lawrence Erlbaum.

Borod, J. C., Fitzpatrick, P. M., Helm-Estabrooks, N., & Goodglass, H. (1989). The relationship between limb apraxia and the spontaneous use of communicative gesture in aphasia. *Brain and Cognition, 10*, 121–131.

Borod, J. C., Koff, E., Perlman-Lorch, M., & Nicholas, M. (1985). Channels of emotional expressions in patients with unilateral brain damage. *Archives of Neurology, 42*, 345–348.

Borod, J. C., Koff, E., Perlman-Lorch, M., & Nicholas, M. (1986). The expression and perception of facial emotion in brain-damaged patients. *Neuropsychologia, 24*, 169–180.

Bowers, D., Coslett, H. B., Bauer, R. M., Speedie, L. J., & Heilman, K. M. (1987). Comprehension of emotional prosody following unilateral hemispheric lesions: Processing defect versus distraction defect. *Neuropsychologia, 25*, 317–328.

Brookshire, R. H. & Nicholas, L. E. (1984). Comprehension of directly and indirectly stated main ideas and details in discourse by brain-damaged and non-brain-damaged listeners. *Brain and Language, 21*, 21–36.

Brownell, H. H. (1988). Appreciation of metaphoric and connotative word meaning by brain-damaged patients. In C. Chiarello (Ed.), *Right hemisphere contributions to lexical semantics. 19–31*. Berlin/Heidelberg/New York: Springer.

Brownell, H. H., Simpson, T. L., Bihrle, A. M., Potter, H. H., & Gardner, H. (1990). Appreciations of metaphoric alternative word meaning by left and right brain-damaged patients. *Neuropsychologia, 28*, 375–383.

Busch, C. R., Brookshire, R. H., & Nicholas, L. E. (1988). Referential communication by aphasic and nonaphasic adults. *Journal of Speech and Hearing Disorders, 53*, 475–482.

Campbell, R., Garwood, J., Franklin, S., Howard, D., Landis, T., & Regard, M. (1990). Neuropsychological studies of auditory-visual fusion illusions. Four case studies and their implications. *Neuropsychologia, 28*, 787–802.

Caramazza, A. (1986). On drawing inferences about the structure of normal cognitive systems from the analysis of patterns of impaired performances: The case for single patients studies. *Brain and Cognition, 5*, 41–66.

Caramazza, A. (1988). When is enough, enough? A comment of Grodzinsky and Marek's "Algorithmic and heuristic processes revisited". *Brain and Language, 33*, 390–399.

Caramazza, A. & Zurif, E. (1976). Dissociation of algorithmic and heuristic processes in language comprehension: Evidence from aphasia. *Brain and Language, 3*, 572–582.

Chenery, H. J., Ingram J. C. L., & Murdoch B. E. (1990). Automatic and volitional semantic processing in aphasia. *Brain and Language, 38*, 215–232.

Christopoulou, C. & Bonvillian, J. D. (1985). Sign language, pantomime, and gestural processing in aphasic persons: A review. *Journal of Communication Disorders, 18*, 1–20.

Clark, H. H. & Wilkes-Gibbs, D. (1986). Referring as a collaborative process. *Cognition, 22*, 1–40.

Clark, H. H. & Schaefer, E. F. (1989). Contributing to discourse. *Cognitive Science, 13*, 259–294.

Coelho, C. A. & Duffy, R. J. (1986). Effects of iconicity, motoric complexity, and linguistic function on sign acquisition in severe aphasia. *Perceptual and Motor Skills, 63*, 519–530.

Coelho, C. A. & Duffy, R. J. (1987). The relationship of the acquisition of manual signs to severity of aphasia: A training study. *Brain and Language, 31*, 328–345.

Coelho, C. A. & Duffy, R. J. (1990). Sign acquisition in two aphasic subjects with limb apraxia. *Aphasiology, 4*, 1–8.

Copeland, M. (1989). An assessment of natural conversation with Broca's aphasics. *Aphasiology, 3*, 301–306.

Daniloff, J. K., Fritelli, G., Buckingham, H. W., Hoffman, P. R., & Daniloff, R. G. (1986). Amer-Ind versus ASL: Recognition and imitation in aphasic subjects. *Brain and Language, 28*, 95–113.

Daniloff, J. K., Noll, J. D., Fristoe, M., & Lloyd, L. L. (1982). Gesture recognition in patients with aphasia. *Journal of Speech and Hearing Disorders, 47*, 43–49.

Davis, G. A. (1989). Pragmatics and cognition in treatment of language disorders. In X. Seron & G. Deloche (Eds.), *Cognitive approaches in neuropsychological rehabilitation, 317–353*. Hillsdale, N. J.: Lawrence Erlbaum.

Davis, G. A. & Wilcox, M. J. (1978). Incorporating parameters of natural conversation in aphasia treatment. In R. Chapey (Ed.), *Language intervention strategies in adult aphasia. 169–193*. Baltimore: Williams & Wilkins.

Davis, G. A. & Wilcox, M. J. (1985). *Adult aphasia rehabilitation: Applied pragmatics*. London: Nfer/Nelson.

Deloche, G. & Seron, X. (1981). Sentence understanding and knowledge of the world: Evidences from a sentence-picture matching task performed by aphasic patients. *Brain and Language, 14*, 57–69.

Duffy, J. R. & Watkins, L. B. (1984). The effect of response choice relatedness on pantomime and verbal recognition ability in aphasic patients. *Brain and Language, 21*, 291–306.

Duffy, R. J. & Duffy, J. R. (1981). Three studies of deficits in pantomimic expression and pantomimic recognition in aphasia. *Journal of Speech and Hearing Research, 24*, 70–84.

Feyereisen, P. (1983). Manual activity during speaking in aphasic subjects. *International Journal of Psychology, 18*, 545–556.

Feyereisen, P. (1986). Production and comprehension of emotional facial expressions in brain-damaged subjects. In R. Bruyer (Ed.), *The neuropsychology of face perception and facial expression. 221–245*. Hillsdale, N. J.: Lawrence Erlbaum Associates.

Feyereisen P. (1987). Gestures and speech, interactions and separations: A reply to Mc Neill (1985). *Psychological Review, 94*, 493–498.

Feyereisen P. (1988). Nonverbal communication. In F. C. Rose, R. Whurr, & M. A. Wyke (Eds.), *Aphasia. 46–81*. London: Whurr.

Feyereisen, P. (1989). What can be learned from lateral differences in emotional processing? In G. Gainotti & C. Caltagirone (Eds.), *Emotions and the dual brain. 121–146*. Experimental Brain Research Series, Vol. 18. Berlin/Heidelberg/New York: Springer.

Feyereisen, P. (1991). Brain pathology, lateralization, and nonverbal behavior. In R. S. Feldman & B. Rimé (Eds.), *Fundamentals of nonverbal behavior. 31–70*. Cambridge/New York: Cambridge University Press.

Feyereisen, P., Barter, D., Goossens, M., & Clerebaut, N. (1988). Gestures and speech in referential communication by aphasic subjects: Channel use and efficiency. *Aphasiology, 2*, 21–32.

Feyereisen. P., Bouchat, M. P., Déry, D., & Ruiz, M. (1990). The concomitance of speech and manual gesture in aphasic subjects. In G. R. Hammond

(Ed.), *The cerebral control of speech and limb movements. 279–301.* Amsterdam/New York/Oxford: North-Holland.

Feyereisen. P. & Hazan, K. (1991). Les gestes facilitent-ils chez les sujets aphasiques la compréhension de mots présentés oralement? *Revue de Neuropsychologie, 1*, 367–391.

Foldi, N. S. (1987). Appreciation of pragmatic interpretations of indirect commands: Comparison of right and left hemisphere brain-damaged patients. *Brain and Language, 31*, 88–108.

Foldi, N. S., Cicone, M., & Gardner, H. (1983). Pragmatic aspects of communication in brain-damaged patients. In S. J. Segalowitz (Ed.), *Language functions and brain organization. 51–85.* New York: Academic Press.

Funnell, E. & Allport, A. (1989). Symbolically speaking: Communicating with Blissymbols in aphasia. *Aphasiology, 3*, 279–300.

Gainotti, G., Silveri, M. C., Villa, G., & Caltagirone, C. (1984). Drawing objects from memory in aphasia. *Brain, 106*, 613–622.

Glosser, G., Wiener, M., & Kaplan, E. (1986). Communicative gestures in aphasia. *Brain and Language, 27*, 345–359.

Glosser, G., Wiener, M., & Kaplan, E. (1988). Variations in aphasic language behaviors. *Journal of Speech and Hearing Disorders, 53*, 115–124.

Goodenough, C., Zurif, E. B., & Weintraub, S. (1977). Aphasics' attention to grammatical morphemes. *Language and Speech, 20*, 11–19.

Green, G. (1984). Communication in aphasia therapy: Some of the procedures and issues involved. *British Journal of Disorders of Communication, 19*, 35–46.

Grodzinsky, Y. & Marek, A. (1988). Algorithmic and heuristic processes revisited. *Brain and Language, 33*, 216–225.

Grossman, M. (1988). Drawing deficits in brain-damaged patient's freehand pictures. *Brain and Cognition, 8*, 189–205.

Hartje, W., Willmes, K., & Weniger, D. (1985). Is there parallel and independent hemispheric processing of intonational and phonetic components of dichotic speech stimuli? *Brain and Language, 24*, 83–99.

Hatfield, F. M., Howard, D., Barber, J., Jones, C. & Morton, J. (1977). Object naming in aphasics: The lack of effect of context or realism. *Neuropsychologia, 15*, 717–728.

Heilman, K. M., Bowers, D., Speedie, L., & Coslett, H. B. (1984). Comprehension of affective and nonaffective prosody. *Neurology, 34*, 917–921.

Helm-Estabrooks, N. & Emery, P. A. (1988). Nonvocal approaches to aphasia rehabilitation. In F. C. Rose, R. Whurr, & M. A. Wyke (Eds.), *Aphasia. 473–488.* London: Whurr.

Herrmann, M., Koch, U., Johannsen-Horbach, H., & Wallesch, C. W. (1989). Communicative skills in chronic and severe nonfluent aphasia. *Brain and Language, 37*, 339–352.

Herrmann, M., Reichle, T., Lucius-Hoene, G., Wallesch, C. W., & Johannsen-Horbach, H. (1988). Nonverbal communication as a compensative strategy for severely nonfluent aphasics? A quantitative approach. *Brain and Language, 33*, 41–54.

Hirst, W., Ledoux, J., & Stein, S. (1984). Constraints on the processing of indirect speech acts: Evidence from aphasiology. *Brain and Language, 23*, 26–33.

Holland, A. L. (1982). Observing functional communication of aphasic adults. *Journal of Speech and Hearing Disorders, 47*, 50–56.

Hough, M. S., Pierce, R. S., & Cannito, M. P. (1989). Contextual influences in aphasia: Effects of predictive versus nonpredictive narratives. *Brain and Language, 36*, 325–334.

Huber, W. (1990). Text comprehension and production in aphasia: Analysis in terms of micro- and macroprocessing. In Y. Joanette & H. H. Brownell (Eds.), *Discourse ability and brain damage. 154–179.* New York/Berlin/Heidelberg: Springer.

Hupet, M., Seron, X., & Frederix, M. (1986). Aphasics' sensitivity to contextual appropriateness conditions for pragmatic indicators. *Brain and Language, 28*, 126–140.

Kimelman, M. D. Z., & Mc Neil, M. R. (1987). An investigation of emphatic stress comprehension in adult aphasia: A replication. *Journal of Speech and Hearing Research, 30*, 295–300.

Koemeda-Lutz, M., Cohen, R., & Meier, E. (1987). Organization of and access to semantic memory in aphasia. *Brain and Language, 30*, 321–337.

Kolk, H. & Heeschen, C. (1990). Adaptation symptoms and impairment symptoms in Broca's aphasia. *Aphasiology, 4*, 221–231.

Krauss, R. M. & Glucksberg, S. (1977). Social and nonsocial speech. *Scientific American, 236.2*, 100–105.

Le May, A., David, R., & Thomas, A. P. (1988). The use of spontaneous gesture by aphasic patients. *Aphasiology, 2*, 137–145.

Li, E. C. & Williams, S. E. (1990). The effects of grammatical class and cue type on cuing responsiveness in aphasia. *Brain and Language, 38*, 48–60.

Lomas, J., Pichard, L., Bester, S., Elbard, H., Finlayson, A., & Zoghaib, C. (1989). The communicative effectiveness index: Development and psychometric evaluation of a functional communication measure for adult aphasia. *Journal of Speech and Hearing Disorders, 54*, 113–124.

Mammucari, A., Caltagirone, C., Ekman, P., Friesen, W., Gainotti, G., Pizzamiglio, L., & Zoccolotti, P. (1988). Spontaneous facial expression of emotions in brain damaged patients. *Cortex, 24*, 521–533.

McNeill, D. (1985). So you think gestures are nonverbal? *Psychological Review, 92*, 350–371.

McNeill, D. (1987). So you do think gestures are nonverbal! Reply to Feyereisen (1987). *Psychological Review, 94*, 499–504.

McNeill, D. (1989). A straight path – to where? Reply to Butterworth and Hadar. *Psychological Review, 96*, 175–179.

Meuse, S. & Marquardt, T. P. (1985). Communicative effectiveness in Broca's aphasia. *Journal of Communication Disorders, 18*, 11–24.

Netsu, R. & Marquardt, T. P. (1984). Pantomime in aphasia: Effects of stimulus characteristics. *Journal of Communication Disorders, 17*, 37–46.

Nicholas, L. E. & Brookshire, R. H. (1981). Effects of pictures and picturability on sentence verification by aphasic and nonaphasic subjects. *Journal of Speech and Hearing Research, 24*, 292–298.

Pease, D. M. & Goodglass, H. (1978). The effects of cuing on picture naming in aphasia. *Cortex, 14* 178–189.

Penn, C. (1987). Compensation and language recovery in the chronic aphasic patient. *Aphasiology, 1*, 235–245.

Peterson, L. N. & Kirshner, H. S. (1981). Gestural impairment and gestural ability in aphasia: A review. *Brain and Language, 14*, 333–348.

Pierce, R. S. & Beekman, L. A. (1985). Effects of linguistic and extralinguistic context on semantic and syntactic processing in aphasia. *Journal of Speech and Hearing Research, 28*, 250–254.

Pierce, R. S. & DeStefano, C. C. (1987). The interactive nature of auditory comprehension in aphasia. *Journal of Communication Disorders, 20*, 15–24.

Prutting, C. A. & Kirchner, D. M. (1987). A clinical appraisal of the pragmatic aspects of language. *Journal of Speech and Hearing Disorders, 52*, 105–119.

Rothi, L. J. G., Heilman, K. M., & Watson, R. T. (1985). Pantomime comprehension and ideomotor apraxia. *Journal of Neurology, Neurosurgery, and Psychiatry, 48*, 207–210.

Rothi, L. J. G., Mack, L., & Heilman, K. M. (1986). Pantomime agnosia. *Journal of Neurology, Neurosurgery, and Psychiatry, 49*, 451–454.

Rowley, D. T. (1983). Artificial languages and communication aids in aphasia therapy. In C. Code & D. J. Müller (Eds.), *Aphasia therapy. 171–177.* London: Arnold.

Ryalls, J. H. & Behrens, S. J. (1988). An overview of changes in fundamental frequency associated with cortical insult. *Aphasiology, 2*, 107–115.

Seron, X., Monsel, Y., Van der Kaa, M. A., Remits, A., & Vanderlinden, M. (1980). La dénomination d'images chez des patients aphasiques: mesure de l'influence de trois contextes non-verbaux différents. *Psychologica Belgica, 20*, 205–213.

Seron, X., Van der Kaa, M. A., Vanderlinden, M., Remits, A., & Feyereisen, P. (1982). Decoding paralinguistic signals: Effect of semantic and prosodic cues on aphasic comprehension. *Journal of Communication Disorders, 15*, 223–231.

Shallice, T. (1988). *From neuropsychology to mental structure.* Cambridge: Cambridge University Press.

Sherman, J. C. & Schweickert, J. (1989). Syntactic and semantic contributions to sentence comprehension in agrammatism. *Brain and Language, 37*, 419–439.

Shewan, C. M. & Cameron, C. (1984). Communication and related problems as perceived by aphasic individuals and their spouses. *Journal of Communication Disorders, 17*, 175–187.

Shindo, M., Kaga, K., & Tanaka, Y. (1991). Speech discrimination and lip reading in patients with word deafness or auditory agnosia. *Brain and Language, 40*, 153–161.

Smith, L. (1985). Communicative activities of dysphasic adults: A survey. *British Journal of Disorders of Communication, 20*, 31–44.

Smith, L. (1987 a). Nonverbal competency in aphasic stroke patients' conversation. *Aphasiology, 1*, 127–139.

Smith, L. (1987 b). Fluency and severity of aphasia and non-verbal competency. *Aphasiology, 1*, 291–295.

Steele, R. D., Weinrich, M., Wertz, R. T., Kleczewska, M., & Carlson, G. (1989). Computer-based visual communication in aphasia. *Neuropsychologia, 27*, 409–426.

Swinney, D. A., Zurif, E. B., & Cutler, A. (1989). Effects of sentential stress and word class upon comprehension in Broca's aphasics. *Brain and Language, 10*, 132–144.

Tompkins, C. A. & Flowers, C. R. (1985). Perception of emotional intonation by brain-damaged adults: The influence of task processing levels. *Journal of Speech and Hearing Research, 28*, 527–538.

Tompkins, C. A. & Flowers, C. R. (1987). Contextual mood priming following left and right hemisphere damage. *Brain and Cognition, 6*, 361–376.

Tompkins, C. A. & Mateer, C. A. (1985). Right hemisphere appreciation of prosodic and linguistic indications of implicit attitude. *Brain and Language, 24*, 185–203.

Van Lancker, D. (1987). Nonpropositional speech: Neurolinguistic studies. In A. W. Ellis (Ed.), *Progress in the psychology of language, vol. 3. 49–118.* London/Hillsdale, N. J.: Lawrence Erlbaum.

Van Lancker, D. & Kempler, D. (1987). Comprehension of familiar phrases by left- but not by right-hemisphere-damaged patients. *Brain and Language, 32*, 265–277.

Varney, N. R. (1982). Pantomime recognition defect in aphasia: Implications for the concept of asymbolia. *Brain and Language, 15*, 32–39.

Varney, N. R. & Benton, A. L. (1982). Qualitative aspects of pantomime recognition defect in aphasia. *Brain and Cognition, 1*, 132–139.

Varney, N. R., Damasio, H., & Adler, S. (1989). The role of individual difference in determining the nature of comprehension defects in aphasia. *Cortex, 25*, 47–55.

Venus, C. A. & Canter, G. J. (1987). The effect of redundant cues on comprehension of spoken messages by aphasic adults. *Journal of Communication Disorders, 20*, 477–491.

Waller, M. R. & Darley, F. L. (1979). Effect of prestimulation on sentence comprehension by aphasic subjects. *Journal of Communication Disorders, 12*, 461–469.

Weylman, S. T., Brownell, H. H., & Gardner, H. (1988). "It's what you mean, not what you say": Pragmatic language use in brain-damaged patients. In F. Plum (Ed.), *Language, communication, and the brain. 229–243.* New York: Raven.

Weylman, S. T., Brownell, H. H., Roman, M., & Gardner, H. (1989). Appreciation of indirect requests by left- and right-brain-damaged patients: The effects of verbal context and conventionality of wording. *Brain and Language, 36*, 580–591.

Wilcox, M. J., Davis, G. A., & Leonard, L. B. (1978). Aphasics' comprehension of contextually conveyed meaning. *Brain and Language, 6*, 362–377.

Williams, S. E. & Canter, G. J. (1982). The influence of situational context on naming performance in aphasic syndromes. *Brain and Language, 17*, 92–106.

Williams, S. E. & Canter, G. J. (1987). Action naming performance in four syndromes of aphasia. *Brain and Language, 32*, 124–136.

Wulfeck, B., Bates, E., Juarez, L., Opie, M., Friederici, A., MacWhinney, B., & Zurif, E. (1989). Pragmatics in aphasia: Crosslinguistic evidence. *Language and Speech, 32*, 315–336.

Zingeser, L. B. & Berndt, R. S. (1988). Grammatical class and context effects in a case of pure anomia: Implications for models of language production. *Cognitive Neuropsychology, 5*, 473–516.

Pierre Feyereisen, Louvain-la-Neuve (Belgium)

26. Text Processing in Aphasia

1. Introduction

Information relevant to text processing in aphasia has emerged primarily from two perspectives, one related to text representation and the other related to how cognitive and linguistic processes operate on the representation of text. The representation of text and processing of text are closely related; however, for theoretical purposes the two can be discussed separately. For this paper, the terms 'text' and 'discourse' are used interchangeably to refer to both oral and written forms of connected language.

Researchers of text representation attempt to characterize (1) the features that distinguish text from non-text, as well as (2) the features that differentiate the various types of text. At a general level, text is defined as connected language. Connected language is frequently characterized as a series of ideas which form an integrated, complete message. That is, text represents a corpus of interrelated chunks of information. In contrast, a unrelated string of sentences or ideas would not typically be labelled as text.

A word of caution, however, against too stringent definitional criteria for text is necessary. This bias toward a loose definition for text is particularly relevant when dealing with aphasic populations with marked linguistic disturbances. Impairment of certain linguistic devices interferes with surface level marking of semantic relations across sentences comprising text. Thus, aphasic patients may produce 'texts' in which ideas are adjoined but seem only vaguely related since these patients do not have the linguistic devices to signal relations. With this concern in mind, it is important to interpret 'text' produced by aphasics using pragmatic criteria of communicative intent rather than surface level criteria. Justification for a pragmatic basis for defining text is supported by Halliday/Hasan (1976), who suggest that any passage should be interpreted as text if there is the remotest possibility of doing so.

At a more specific level, texts are classified according to the particular genre/s represented, e. g. narrative, procedural, conversational and expository text. Research efforts have been directed toward identifying the unique properties of different text-types in terms of characteristic components, unique organizational structure, and elements of meaning.

In contrast to text representation, researchers of text processing focus on the processes involved in manipulating language for purposes of communication. Processing of text covers both production and comprehension, in spoken and written modalities. These two modalities are of interest since they entail different processing demands. Spoken language, for example, typically unfolds as it is being formulated. Written text, on the other hand, can be produced over a long period of time with some planning. Processing requirements for text depend on the type of discourse genre and the nature of the task. Processing demands will vary, depending on whether the text is spontaneously-generated, recalled, paraphrased, summarized or reinterpreted in some way.

Characterization of text representation is not a simple, straightforward matter, since text processing entails the interactive contribution of multiple components, some realized at a sentential level and others at a discourse level. At a sentential level, both lexical and syntactic variables contribute to text organization. For example, manipulation of clauses within sentences is important to the foregrounding and backgrounding of certain information. At a discourse level, unique properties of text operate above and beyond the sentence level. The dilemma in characterizing text lies in sorting out the aspects of text that depend on sentence-level grammars from those aspects of text that operate independently of sentence-level features.

The primary purpose of this chapter is to review the literature relevant to text representation and processing in aphasia. As will be evident from the review, text processing relies on multiple components, some realized by linguistic structures, some by information structures, and others by the interaction of both types. The specific components addressed in this chapter include: (1) sentential level aspects, (2) text level aspects, and (3) constructs which involve the interaction between these two levels of language. The aspects of text representation which combine both sentential and text level structures are conceptualized by the abstract constructs of cohesion, coherence and macrostructure.

Our main objective is to demonstrate that explanations for selective disturbances of text processing in aphasia will be derived from approaches that seek to characterize both the interactions and the dissociations across the components of text comprehension and production. At present, the nature of the interaction across components is not well understood. However, recent studies on cohesion and coherence suggest that breakthroughs are being made in this area. Approaches that seek to identify the interdependencies across language levels will complement and clarify previous documentation of dissociations between levels of language processing.

2. Sentence Level within Text

Early studies of text processing in aphasia adopted sentential level measures to characterize discourse performance. Specifically, the individual sentences comprising text were analyzed. The justification for such an approach was the belief that higher levels of language were dependent on intactness of lower levels of language. That is, sentential abilities were felt to be dependent on lexicosyntactic abilities, and discourse abilities were based on sentential ability. This perspective of language processing predicted that discourse difficulties could be explained by problems at a sentential level.

The findings of studies of sentential level abilities within texts confirmed deficits in aphasia which were previously identified on isolated sentential measures (Ulatowska/North/Macaluso-Haynes 1981; Ulatowska/Freedman-Stern/Doyel et al. 1983). However, these sentential measures failed to account for discourse level performance. Observations were made that aphasic patients were able to communicate at a text level better than could be predicted from their performance on sentential measures, suggesting an inverse dissociation between language levels. Unexpectedly, higher levels of language appeared to be better preserved than lower levels. This inverse dissociation between lower and higher levels of language performance observed in aphasic patients suggested that a 'bottom-up' theory of language processing was inadequate to explain the observed behavioral phenomena in aphasia. Consequently, researches began to focus on how to objectively document text performance beyond sentence level measures.

One of the earliest studies to document a dissociation between text structure and sentential level performance was a single case study of the written discourse of a Wernicke's aphasic patient (Ulatowska/Freedman-Stern 1978; Freedman-Stern/Ulatowska/Baker/DeLacoste 1984). Linguistic analyses revealed sentential level errors in morphology and syntax. Analyses at a discourse level revealed relative preservation of narrative structure in that the necessary components were present. Interestingly, the impairment of linguistic structures within sentences did not preclude effective manipulation of linguistic devices at a discourse level to signal aspects of information structure. For example, the patient was able to linguistically signal digressions from the main story line.

This early study demonstrated a way in which textual structure could be evaluated above and beyond the individual sentences that comprised the text. Subsequently, a number of studies were undertaken to characterize text processing in aphasia. The following section summarizes the general findings from these studies.

3. Text Level Processing

The majority of investigations of text processing in aphasia have examined narrative discourse. These investigations of narrative discourse have been instigated for various reasons. For one, narratives represent the most basic discourse genre from which other discourse genres, e. g. procedural, are derived. Additionally, the organizational structure of narratives has been the most extensively characterized of all the discourse types. Knowledge of the specific structure provides a theoretical framework for evaluating the disruption of structure above a sentential level.

3.1. Text Production

The findings from studies of text processing suggested that aphasic subjects processed the most important information contained in a discourse sample, on both production and comprehension measures. Production studies of simple narrative discourse revealed that discourse structure was relatively preserved for mildly and moderately impaired aphasic subjects. The subject populations included both Broca's and Wernicke's aphasic patients. Evidence for preservation of discourse structure on production measures was reported both in single case studies (Freedman-Stern/Ulatowska/Baker/DeLacoste 1984; Ulatowska/Freedman-Stern 1978) and in small group studies (Dressler/Pleh 1988; Ulatowska/North/Macaluso-Haynes 1981; Ulatowska/Weiss Boyel/Freedman-Stern et al. 1983; Ulatowska/Freedman-Stern/Doyel 1983). Narrative structure was analyzed using discourse superstructure and sequence of events. Narrative superstructure delineates the components of a narrative, e. g. setting, complicating action and resolution. The sequence of events refers to the temporal unfolding of events in a chronological sequence.

In contrast to the relative preservation of narrative superstructure for mildly and moderately impaired aphasic subjects, discourse structure for severely impaired aphasic subjects was not preserved. At this increased severity level, narrative structure was found to be impaired both in terms of omission of the essential superstructure components and disrupted temporal sequence of events (Bond/Ulatowska/Macaluso-Haynes/May 1983). These results suggest that a certain amount of language is necessary to support discourse structure. The mechanisms underlying the disruption, however, are not well understood.

The disruptions in superstructure and event sequence for severely impaired aphasic subjects were attributed to the severe reduction of language rather than a primary underlying conceptual deficit. The evidence given to support this claim was an apparent intactness of an internal representation of the story in the subject's mind, manifested in two ways. First, the severely impaired aphasic subjects used formulaic initiators (e. g. *once upon a time*) and terminators (e. g. *the end*) to mark the story boundaries. Second, the severely impaired aphasic subjects were able to sequence picture stories on a nonverbal picture arrangement task. These performances supported a preserved conceptual organization for story structure and sequence, at least for the small population of severely impaired aphasic subjects studied.

The disruption in narrative text processing for severely impaired aphasic subjects was less marked in conversational discourse. In conversational discourse, discourse structure as manifested by range and sequence of speech acts was preserved. Severely-impaired aphasic subjects were able to maintain the discourse structure in a conversation task with only rudimentary sentential language. A possible explanation for preservation of conversation at a discourse level is that many speech acts can be conveyed with only a single word or phrase, and/or because in conversation the structure is a cooperative process (Ulatowska/Allard/Reyes/Chapman 1988). These findings must be interpreted cautiously as the sample size was small. Also, alternative analyses may prove to be more sensitive to elucidating disruptions of conversational discourse.

3.2. Text Comprehension

On measures of text comprehension, aphasic subjects were found to comprehend main ideas embedded in narrative discourse better than less important details. A similar pattern of enhanced comprehension for the main ideas was found for non-brain-damaged control subjects (Brookshire/Nicholas 1984). Comprehension of the most critical information could not be predicted by performance on isolated sentential measures nor by degree of coherency of the text (Wegner/Brookshire/Nicholas 1984). The findings from other studies on text comprehension in aphasia suggested that aphasic subjects comprehended text level material better than sentential level material. Aphasic subjects apparently benefit from linguistic context in the comprehension of spoken narratives as contrasted with the more limited linguistic context a variable in isolated sentences (Stachowiak/Huber/Poeck/Kerschensteiner 1977). The predominant explanation for the enhancement of textual processing (as compared to the processing of isolated sentences) is that aphasic subjects benefit from the redundancy of information provided by text which is not available in isolated sentences (Cannito/Jarecki/Pierce 1986; Hough/Pierce/Cannito 1989; Huber/Gleber 1982).

4. Dissociation between Language Levels

Documentation of relatively preserved discourse structure in aphasic patients for both comprehension and production measures (for simple narratives) stood in sharp contrast to well documented impairment of sentential structures. This evidence provided insight into how aphasic patients could be communicatively viable despite severe disruption of sentential level abilities. From a theoretical perspective, the findings documented a dissociation between discourse and sentential level abilities on objective measures. From a methodological perspective, this research demonstrated the value of applying certain theoretical constructs for evaluating discourse structure above the sentential level.

As with many new findings, however, the documentation of relative preservation of discourse structure raised more questions than it answered. While processing of text in aphasia may be preserved relative to sentential processing, there is no question that a relationship between sentential and text processing exists. Although a dissociation between these two levels was established for mildly and moderately impaired aphasic subjects, certain findings support that a relationship exists between sentential and discourse level performance in aphasia. Subjective ratings of narrative discourse were lower for aphasic subjects as compared to normals (Ulatowska/Hayashi/Cannito/Fleming 1986). Specifically, aphasic subjects' discourses were consistently rated as aberrant on clarity and coherence of spoken narratives despite preservation of narrative superstructure. Furthermore, quantitative differences were found between aphasic and normal subjects' discourses. Compared to normals, aphasic subjects' discourses showed reduction of information, reduced sentential and discourse complexity, and increased discourse and sentential errors (Berko-Gleason/Goodglass/Obler et al. 1980; Dressler/Pleh 1988; Ulatowska/Hayashi/Cannito/Fleming 1986; Ulatowska/North/Macaluso-Haynes 1981).

One specific pattern which supported a relation between sentential and text level factors was the disruption of reference. Reference in this case refers to the identification of the actors throughout a story by nouns and pronouns. Reference operates across sentences at a textual level, and it is realized through nouns/pronouns at a sentential level. Errors of reference occur when the identification of a particular actor is ambiguous or unclear. Instances of referential ambiguity were traced to increased use of pronouns in mildly and moderately impaired aphasic subjects (Ulatowska/North/Macaluso-Haynes 1981; Ulatowska/Weiss Boyel/Freedman-Stern et al.

1983; Ulatowska/Freedman-Stern/Doyel et al. 1983).

For severely impaired aphasic subjects, the relation between sentential reduction and quality of discourse was more obvious. The reduction of sentential language was deemed responsible for discourse collapse (Bond/Ulatowska/Macalusco-Haynes/May 1983). A certain level of sentential intactness and complexity appears to be necessary for supporting discourse structure.

In sum, the above examples demonstrate that the relationship between discourse and sentence level structures is important to understanding selective disturbances in text processing in aphasia. As is evident, the relationship is extremely complex. Currently, the most promising approaches to elucidate the impairment and preservation of text processing in aphasia are those that seek to identify the constructs that are critical to text. These approaches utilize the constructs of cohesion and coherence of text and macrostructures. Information relevant to these constructs are summarized below.

5. Relationship between Language Levels

5.1. Cohesion and Coherence of Text

The prime mediator between sentential and discourse level structures is cohesion. Cohesion refers to surface level linkages across sentences or even across larger units of text. Cohesion is achieved by manipulation of various linguistic devices that serve to bind parts of a text into a coherent whole. These devices are called cohesive ties. Cohesive ties form what is called 'cohesive chains' as continuity of meaning is found throughout text.

Coherence operates at a more conceptual level than the surface markings of cohesion. Nonetheless, cohesive devices contribute directly to coherence, since the ability to produce coherent text requires facility with cohesive devices. The relationship between coherence and cohesion varies depending on the complexity and type of text. For discourse genres with more conventional structures (e.g. narratives), coherence is easier to achieve even when linguistic disturbances of cohesive devices exist. However, as the discourse complexity increases or when discourse genres with less conventional structures (e.g. expository discourse) are utilized, it is more difficult to produce coherent text when cohesive devices are disturbed.

Studies of cohesion in aphasic texts have been performed using two different types of analyses, one objective and the other subjective. Objective studies utilized quantitative analyses of cohesive ties. Berko-Gleason/Goodglass/Obler et al. (1980), for example, counted cohesive ties of reference and found that reference was differentially impaired for Wernicke's and Broca's aphasic patients. Wernicke's aphasic subjects showed increased frequency of deictic pronouns, whereas Broca's aphasic subjects exhibited reduced frequency of both deictic and personal pronouns. This same pattern of impairment was confirmed in later discourse studies (Ulatowska/North/Macaluso-Haynes 1981; Ulatowska/Weiss Boyel/Freedman-Stern et al. 1983; Ulatowska/Freedman-Stern/Doyel et al. 1983).

More recent work on text cohesion of aphasic language has applied a schema developed by Halliday/Hasan (1976) for evaluating cohesion (Armstrong 1987; 1989; Mathews 1987; Piehler/Holland 1984). Using the Halliday and Hasan framework, researchers identified: 1) reduced use of cohesive ties, 2) poor use of local connectors, 3) greater use of deictics, and 4) increased use of pronouns without antecedents or referents in aphasics' texts as compared to normals'. Additionally, amount and type of cohesive ties were utilized to document different profiles of recovery for a Broca's and Wernicke's aphasic patient (Piehler/Holland 1984).

One important implication of studies of cohesion was that cohesive ties are not equal in terms of their contribution to cohesion of text. In fact, cohesive ties operate differently in text, although by definition, all cohesive devices provide continuity in meaning across sentences. For example, both reference and connectives are markers of continuity of ideas. However, linguistic devices of reference do not in themselves reveal anything about the relationship among ideas, whereas connectives explicitly mark relations between ideas. This distinction was evident in an in-depth descriptive study of written text for one Wernicke's patient. The texts produced by this patient exhibited skillfull manipulation of reference but marked disruption in use of connectives (Freedman-Stern/Ulatowska/Baker/DeLacoste 1984).

At present, it is apparent that quantitative measures of cohesive devices alone are inadequate for measuring cohesion in text production. Evidence from a study by Huber/Gleber (1982) supports the view that surface level cohesive ties do not necessarily improve quality of text. In this study, degree of textual cohesion had no impact on comprehension for aphasic subjects, contrary to expectations. It was argued that the surface level markings of cohesion may not account for overall coherence of the texts. The difficulty in interpreting quantitative measures of cohesive devices is amplified by the lack of data concerning normal cohesion patterns for comparison with cohesion in aphasia.

A second type of cohesion analysis, subjective evaluation, can complement quantitative measures in order to clarify the quality of discourse in relation to cohesion. Subjective analyses incorporated ratings of overall cohesion and clarity of discourse for aphasic subjects (Ulatowska/North/Mocaluso-Haynes 1981; Ulatowska/Weiss Boyel/Freedman-Stern et al. 1983; Ulatowska/Freedman-Stern/Doyel et al. 1983). However, to date, limited evidence exists concerning correlations between language ratings and counts of cohesive devices. As is evident from the above discussion, quantitative counts of cohesive ties and subjective ratings provide only a partial picture of the relationship between sentence and text level processing. Some recent evidence suggests that this relationship may be clarified by examining clusters of cohesive devices that contribute to key aspects of coherence. For example, two specific features essential to the production of coherent text of the narrative type include temporality and reference. A number of cohesive devices contribute to effective marking of temporality and reference. Temporality and reference operate at a global level, and yet both are realized through linguistic markers of cohesion that operate at a sentential level. Because of this codependence of sentential and text levels, these two aspects may provide additional insight into the interdependency between the two levels of language.

6. Macrostructure in Text Processing

The construct of macrostructure denotes the global semantic meaning of a discourse (van Dijk 1972). Textual macrostructures are represented by the main ideas of a text and are associated with notions such as theme, gist and topic (Mross 1990). The constructs of macrostructure and superstructure are often confused primarily because there is some degree of overlap. Both macrostructure and superstructures operate much like an 'outline,' providing a global schema for organizing information, both in comprehension and production. On the other hand, superstructures provide the organizational structure, whereas macrostructures provide the semantic content in terms of amount, type and distribution of information (van Dijk 1977). Macrostructure can be tapped at two levels. First, the content of the text itself can be used to evaluate intactness of macrostructure by examining (1) relevant and irrelevant content, (2) distribution of information within superstructure components, and (3) distribution of important information and details. Additionally, macrostructure can be tapped with tasks soliciting titles, summaries, and outlines for texts. These latter tasks require preservation of meaning with reduction of information. It is of interest to note that these tasks can be produced with relatively simple language. For example, titles consist of few words relative to the entire text and represent the global meaning of the story. Outlines are easily expressed in telegraphic language and represent the most important ideas.

Research on macrostructure processing in aphasia indicated that macrostructure was impaired as measured by alterations in title and summary productions in comparison to normals (Ulatowska/Freedman-Stern/Weiss Doyel/Macaluso-Haynes 1983). Aphasic patients produced concrete titles that failed to grasp the global meaning of the story at an abstract level. However, these findings should not be generalized to aphasic patients, at large, since some patients produced acceptable titles.

A disruption in macrostructure was not as readily apparent in aphasic patients for simple narrative productions. Amount of language and information was reduced for aphasic patients. This reduction was selective in that the most important information was retained, and less important details were omitted. Perhaps a disruption in narrative macrostructure was obscured because there were not enough details to depart from the macrostructure. The probability of observing impairment of macrostructure for narrative discourse is more likely in posteriorly aphasic patients as compared to anterior patients, since more detail exists in their discourse.

While previous evidence suggested that narrative structure was preserved in aphasia

(Ulatowska/North/Macaluso-Haynes 1981; Ulatowska/Freedman-Stern/Doyel et al. 1983), this pattern referred to superstructure and not macrostructure. Narrative structure may appear intact for aphasic patients because superstructure drives the ongoing processing of narratives. This is to say that superstructure replaces macrostructure in guiding aphasic patients' narrative structure. Superstructure is more global, less demanding and conceptually simpler than macrostructure. Further evidence to suggest that superstructure replaces macrostructure in narrative processing for aphasic patients is the finding that these patients cannot produce discourse genres with less conventionalized superstructures, e. g. expository. There appears to be a restriction in discourse genres available in aphasia in that expository discourse becomes either narrative or descriptive discourse, and narrative discourse becomes conversational genre. Additionally, aphasic subjects have considerable difficulty combining discourse types. For example, they exhibit problems shifting from conversational to narrative discourse. (Ulatowska/Sadowska 1992).

7. Conclusion

Most of the earlier text studies in aphasia were done from the perspective of documenting dissociations. Historically, dissociation phenomena of various language components in aphasia have been of great interest both theoretically and clinically, since these phenomena showed selectivity of impairment of particular language functions as a result of an insult to a specific part of the brain. Studies have documented dissociations within morphology, between morphology and syntax, and between syntax and semantics (MacWhinney/Bates 1989; Zurif/Caramazza 1976). In text studies, the dissociation between sentence level language and discourse has been described (Freedman-Stern/Ulatowska/Baker/DeLacoste 1984).

This chapter has emphasized the interrelationships that exist between levels of language. This new direction may prove to be more revealing in accounting for both impairments and preservations in aphasic discourse and in characterizing the nature of cohesion and coherence in aphasic texts. This approach may one day substantiate the intuition of one of our aphasic patients who remarked: "It took me four hours tp produce this page and a half but it is not a composition but just a collection of individual sentences."

8. References

Armstrong, E. (1987). Cohesive harmony in aphasic discourse and its significance to listener perception of coherence. In R. H. Brookshire (Ed.), *Clinical aphasiology*, Vol. 17. 210–215. Minneapolis, MN: BRK Publishers.

Armstrong, E. (1989). The potential of cohesion analysis in the assessment of aphasic discourse. Paper presented at the American Speech-Language Hearing Association Annual Convention.

Berko-Gleason, J., Goodglass, H., Obler, L., Green, E., Hyde, M. R., & Weintraub, S. (1980). Narrative strategies of aphasic and normal speaking subjects. *Journal of Speech and Hearing Research, 23*, 370–382.

Bond, S. L., Ulatowska, H. K., Macaluso-Haynes, S., & May, E. B. (1983). Discourse production in aphasia: Relationship to severity of impairment. In R. H. Brookshire (Ed.), *Proceedings of the clinical aphasiology conference*. 202–210. Minneapolis: BRK Publishers.

Brookshire, R. H. & Nicholas, L. E. (1984). Comprehension of directly and indirectly stated main ideas and details in discourse by brain-damaged and non-brain-damaged listeners. *Brain and Language, 21*, 21–36.

Cannito, M., Jarecki, J., & Pierce, R. S. (1986). Effects of thematic structure on syntactic comprehension in aphasia. *Brain and Language, 27*, 38–49.

Dressler, W. U. & Pleh, C. (1988). On text disturbances in aphasia. In W. U. Dressler & J. A. Stark (Eds.), *Linguistic analyses of aphasic language. 151–177.* New York: Springer-Verlag.

Freedman-Stern, R., Ulatowska, H. K., Baker, T., & DeLacoste, C. (1984). Disruption of written language in aphasia: A case study. *Brain and Language, 21*, 181–205.

Halliday, M. A. K. & Hasan, R. (1976). *Cohesion in English*. London: Longman.

Hough, M. S., Pierce, R. S., & Cannito, M. P. (1989). Contextual influences in aphasia: Effects of predictive versus nonpredictive narratives. *Brain and Language, 36*, 325–334.

Huber, W. & Gleber, J. (1982). Linguistic and non-linguistic processing of narratives in aphasia. *Brain and Language, 16*, 1–18.

MacWhinney, B. & Bates, E. (1989). *Crosslinguistic studies of sentence processing*. Cambridge University Press.

Mathews, C. (1987). Discourse before and after the onset of aphasia. Paper presented at Clinical Aphasiology Conference.

Mross, E. F. (1990). Text Analysis: Macro- and microstructural aspects of discourse processing. In Y. Joanette & H. H. Brownell (Eds.), *Discourse ability and brain damage. 50–68.* New York: Springer-Verlag.

Piehler, M. & Holland, A. (1984). Cohesion in aphasic language. Paper presented at the Clinical Aphasiology Conference.

Stachowiak, F. J., Huber, W., Poeck, K., & Kerschensteiner, M. (1977). Text comprehension in aphasia. *Brain and Language, 4*, 177–195.

Ulatowska, H. K., Allard, L., Donnell, A., Bristow, J., Haynes, S. M., Flower, A., & North, A. J. (1988). Discourse performance in subjects with dementia of the Alzheimer type. In H. A. Whitaker (Ed.), *Neuropsychological studies of non-focal brain damage: Trauma and dementia. 108–131.* New York: Springer-Verlag.

Ulatowska, H. K. & Freedman-Stern, R. (1978). Analysis of aphasic writing. Paper delivered at the Aphasia Research Group, World Federation of Neurologists, University of Iowa, Iowa City.

Ulatowska, H. K., Freedman-Stern, R., Doyel, A., Macaluso-Haynes, S., & North, A. T. (1983). Production of narrative discourse in aphasia. *Brain and Language, 19*, 317–334.

Ulatowska, H. K., Hayashi, M. M., Cannito, M. P., & Fleming, S. G. (1986). Disruption of reference in aging. *Brain and Language, 28*, 24–41.

Ulatowska, H. K., North, A. J., & Macaluso-Haynes, S. (1981). Production of narrative and procedural discourse in aphasia. *Brain and Language, 13*, 345–371.

Ulatowska, H. K. & Sadowska, M. (1992). Some observations on aphasic texts. In: Hwang, S. J. & Merrifield, W. R. (eds.). Language in context: Essays for Robert E. Longacre. Arlington: The Summer Institute of Linguistics and The University of Texas at Arlington, 51–66.

Ulatowska, H. K., Weiss Boyel, A., Freedman-Stern, R., Macaluso-Haynes, S., & North, A. T. (1983). Production of procedural discourse in aphasia. *Brain and Language, 18*, 315–341.

van Dijk, T. A. (1972). *Some aspects of text grammar.* The Hague: Mouton Press.

van Dijk, T. A. (1977). *Text and context. Explorations in the semantics and pragmatics of discourse.* London: Longman.

Wegner, M. L., Brookshire, R. H., & Nicholas, L. E. (1984). Comprehension of main ideas and details in coherent and noncoherent discourse by aphasic and non-aphasic listeners. *Brain and Language, 21*, 37–51.

Zurif, E. B. & Caramazza, A. (1976). Psycholinguistic structures in aphasia: Studies in syntax and semantics. In H. Whitaker & H. A. Whitaker (Eds.), *Studies in neurolinguistics*. Vol. 1. New York: Academic Press.

Hanna K. Ulatowska/Sandra Chapman, Dallas, Texas (USA)

27. Aphasia and Intelligence

> When Wertheimer (1945) told Einstein that "many report that their thinking is always in words, he only laughed."

1. Introduction

Even the most cursory literature search for references to cognitive or intellectual status in the aphasias will reveal a curious dichotomy of theoretical presuppositions. On the one hand, there is a long tradition of testing patients who have sustained unilateral left or right hemisphere damage with materials originally devised to measure individual differences in 'general intelligence' within the 'normal' population. The first substantial work of this nature was Weisenburg/McBride (1935), and there have subsequently been a number of excellent surveys of conceptual impairment in aphasic patients (Zangwill 1969; Hamsher 1981; Kertesz 1988; Vignolo 1989) that update the research consensus (or lack thereof). All these chapters include fairly full reviews of how well or badly different samples of indisputably aphasic patients perform on standard tests of psychometric intelligence.

On the other hand, most of the major textbooks of cognitive neuropsychology that include extensive discussion of aphasic phenomena make no mention of intelligence. The very term cannot be found in the subject indexes of Ellis/Young (1988), Caplan (1987), Shallice

(1988), or McCarthy/Warrington (1990), for example. Research papers within the tradition of which these books are representative do sometimes (but far from invariably) give psychometric scores on the patients who are then the subjects of detailed cognitive investigation. The Wechsler Adult Intelligence Scale (WAIS; Wechsler 1958), Progressive Matrices (Raven 1965), and the New Adult Reading Test (Nelson/O'Connell 1978) seem to be the most frequently reported measures; the latter test is widely used as an indicant of premorbid general intelligence (for those patients without significant dyslexic impairment). In (almost) all cases, however, this psychometric information is given in the 'clinical background' section of the paper and subsequently ignored in the design and interpretation of the experiments that document the nature of the patient's cognitive deficit.

What, then, is the likely cause of this striking discrepancy between two research traditions? Are there substantive empirical and theoretical issues at stake? If so, how do they relate to the methodology of competent investigations of the patient and to practical management?

2. Intelligence or Intelligences?

Two extreme positions with respect to the *nature* of intelligence could be taken up: One is that intelligence is unitary, the other that it is multiple. Although the absolute extremes are not occupied by any reputable psychometrician, very different relative positions have been advanced (and continue to be debated). Spearman (1927) held that the important component of human intelligence was general intelligence or g. Ex hypothesi, g plays a significant role in all activities deemed (pre-theoretically) to involve the exercise of intellectual capacity. Thurstone (1938), by contrast, laid far greater stress upon the notion of a set of primary abilities that are *relatively* independent of each other. In Thurstone's hierarchical model, general intelligence is just one component that contributes to otherwise distinct primary abilities, which in turn contribute to more restricted task-specific factors. Psychometric testing was never primarily intended to shed light upon the patterns of impaired or preserved ability in cases of demonstrable brain pathology (either acquired or developmental). The intent was rather to measure the spread of ability (or abilities) within normal populations of different ages. 'Subnormal' (or 'supernormal') within this framework has no meaning other than scoring significantly below (or above) the average ('norm') for a particular reference group (the general population at given ages). Tests were constructed (i. e. items selected) in order to yield a 'normal distribution' of scores that permitted statistical analysis of the correlations between tests. To a first approximation, Spearman's g can be regarded as a construct that captures the extent of positive correlation between all tests. Different individual tests are then found to correlate differentially with g. Those that correlate most highly with g include Vocabulary and General Information (from the verbal section of the WAIS), Block Design (from the performance section of the WAIS) and Raven's Progressive Matrices. These tests are accordingly regarded as the 'purest' measures of g. We stress again that psychometric tests are standardized on the general population.

Neuropsychological inquiry originated in a context that could not be more different. Gall's theory of 'multiple intelligences' was explicitly founded upon the study of *extreme* differences between individuals who could in no way be regarded as representative of the 'general population' (Marshall 1984). The samples of concern to Gall were saints and mass murderers, idiots and geniuses, psychotics and supermen. It was the investigation of people with extreme talents (for good or ill) that led Gall to postulate that all basic human competencies had a discrete, responsible organ in the brain. The relatively sizes of these organs in the individual then determined the pattern of domain-specific psychological strengths and weaknesses in that individual.

That Gall initially based his theory upon the somewhat shaky base of craniology is irrelevant. Since it rapidly became clear that injury to different regions of the brain produced qualitatively different patterns of cognitive impairment, the term 'localization of function' could replace 'cerebral organology' without necessitating any conceptual shift. From the moment that Hughlings Jackson (1876) formulated the central dogma of human neuropsychology – the left hemisphere is 'leading' for verbal ideation, the right hemisphere for visuo-spatial ideation – the hypothesis that there could be a 'brain-centre' for 'general intelligence' began to lose any plausibility. From there it was but a short step to argue that the notion of 'general intelligence' was in itself ill-conceived. Under attack from many quarters, general intelligence (and other IQ measures) came to be seen by some psychologists and many neuropsychologists as the mere reification of test scores subjected to factor-analysis.

After brain injury, patients with focal (or diffuse) damage are no more representative of the general population than are Gall's extreme cases (irrespective of how 'normal' they may have been before sustaining that damage.) Neuropsychological inquiry has accordingly placed great stress upon demonstrating the existence of 'double dissociations' as an indicant of the existence of discrete cognitive modules devoted to specialized domains. If on two tasks A and B, patient X scores well on A but poorly on B, while patient Y scores poorly on A and well on B, this is prima facie evidence for the involvement of two distinct 'intelligences' responsible for the two tasks (Shallice 1988). For purposes of discovering the structure of mentation, it is simply irrelevant that within the normal population, performance on the two tasks may correlate highly (and that both tasks load highly on g).

Lezak (1988) therefore argues that in neuropsychological practice, the use of IQ measures "and that of any scores representing sums or averages of disparate data obtained from tests of brain functions and mental abilities can obscure specific facets of a subject's neuropsychological status and can misrepresent it generally."

It might be thought that the above arguments apply only to Spearman's conception of intelligence and not to Thurstone's. And this is how Margolin (1992) seems to interpret the issue. The notion of human intelligence as a "unidimensional monolithic attribute or capacity" has been "officially pronounced dead" and replaced by "the concept of intelligence as a multifaceted multidimensional array of capacities" (Margolin 1992). Descriptively, this is indeed the case (Gardner 1983), although even with respect to Thurstone's position, the concerns of the psychometrician and of the cognitive neuropsychologist are actually diametrically opposed. In the following section we outline the nature of that opposition, with reference to both Spearman and Thurstone.

3. Intelligence and Information-Processing

One obvious problem in any discussion of intellectual status in the aphasias (or other language disorders) is how to avoid trivializing the relationship between language and intelligence. If, for example, intelligence is defined as that which conventional IQ tests measure, then it will almost invariably be the case that aphasic patients will have a low verbal intelligence quotient (VIQ).

Consider, for example, some sample items from the WAIS. It would hardly be surprising if most (or indeed all) patients with a moderately severe aphasia had difficulty in answering the question *How does yeast cause dough to rise?* (an item from the Information subtest). Likewise, such patients would be expected to have problems in explaining what *encumber* means (an item from Vocabulary), or explicating how *poem* and *statue* are alike (Similarities). Similarly, digit span is usually (but not inevitably) impaired after aphasia-provoking lesions, and arithmetic likewise. It is accordingly difficult to imagine an aphasic patient who would score well on the question *If eight machines are needed to finish a job in six days, how many machines would be needed to finish the job in one-half day?* (Arithmetic subtest).

Now, it is of course possible to report lowered scores on such tests in aphasic patients as poor VIQs – the tests were after all taken from a standard IQ test. But does the 'IQ' in such descriptions mean anything over and above the 'V' for verbal? To say that aphasic patients have language (verbal) disorders is to give a (rough) definition of 'aphasia'; it is not to make a discovery about aphasia.

From the viewpoint of genuine intelligence testing (in the normal population), however, the 'IQ' component of VIQ is meaningful. Recall that, within Spearman's framework, Vocabulary and Information have very high loadings on g. It would then follow that the aphasic patient who scores poorly on these tests could have suffered a precipitous fall in g or an impairment to whatever specific abilities are involved in good performance on Vocabulary and Information: no test could measure g and nothing but g; all tests demand information-processing pertinent to the specific task that is given. To show that an interpretation based upon impairment to g is false, it suffices to demonstrate that there is some other task that also loads highly on g (e. g. Block Design) on which the patient performs well.

And if, contrariwise, the patient scored badly on Block Design, there would still be no support for the hypothesis that g had been diminished by brain damage: the patient could simply have conjoint impairment of both sets of disjoint abilities required for Vocabulary and Block Design, respectively. Studies of 'dementia' have often been bedevilled by illegitimate reification of g. Thus Hamsher (1981), for example, argues that "The concept of dementia may be viewed as a pathological counterpart to g." It is, of course, true that 'dementia' has often been defined clinically as an impairment to three (or more) cognitive domains. But if a patient manifests aphasia, agnosia and amnesia, it is not clear what is gained by postulating that he or she has suffered "a significant decline in g" (Hamsher 1981) rather than (conjointly) exhibiting a disorder of language, perception, and memory. Further discussion of this issue can be found in Schwartz (1990) and Gurd/Marshall (1991).

Exactly the same argument goes through with respect to Thurstone's primary abilities (or group factors). Good performance on one task that loads highly on a particular group factor in conjunction with poor performance on another task that also loads highly on this same factor indicates that a (reified) primary ability has not been impaired. Conjointly impaired performance can likewise indicate that the neuronal instanciation of mechanisms involved in two specific factors have both suffered damage.

If it is the case empirically that association of impairment for tasks belonging to a common primary ability is more frequent than dissociation, the finding would most likely reflect an anatomical constraint rather than neuropsychological support for Thurstone's factorial theory. That is, competences that are psychologically similar seem often to be represented in neighbouring regions of the brain (Lashley 1937).

It remains, however, a logical point (not a matter of empirical observation) that behavioural studies of the patterns of impaired and preserved performance after brain damage can never support claims for the existence of g or any other more specific psychometric construct. From the standpoint of neuropsychology, it is purely accidental that the vocabulary items to be defined on the WAIS are part of an intelligence test and not part of an aphasia battery. It is also the case that the nature of the questions asked by neuropsychologists has little overlap with the nature of those asked in psychometric IQ testing.

From the latter standpoint, it suffices to know whether or not the subject can correctly answer the question (e.g. *How does yeast cause dough to rise?*). For the aphasiologist, however, failure to provide the correct answer is only the starting point of the inquiry. The relevant issues here include: Does the patient have a disorder of phonemic hearing sufficient to block or distort adequate perceptual input? Can the patient access function word vocabulary (*how, to*)? Can abstract verbs (*cause*) be understood? The examiner must be able to answer all such questions before it even makes sense to inquire whether the patient has a disorder of semantic memory such that he or she no longer knows how yeast causes dough to rise.

In short, the question *How does yeast cause dough to rise*? is not (from the examiner's standpoint) the same question when given to a 50 year-old who has sustained a left middle cerebral artery stroke and a healthy 50 year-old member of the general population. Even if the answer is an indicant of 'intelligence' in the latter case, it cannot be so in the former. The distinction is fairly obvious for this particular constrast, but there are other cases where we believe that the same or similar points hold but have gone unrecognized.

For example: in a series of publications, Dennis and her colleagues have argued that syntactic comprehension is more impaired after left than right surgical hemidecortication for infantile cerebral injury (see Dennis 1980). Dennis interprets these results as showing that the 'equipotentiality' hypothesis – that the right hemisphere can mediate language as adequately as the left if one hemisphere is removed early enough – is false. Bishop (1983) points out (correctly) that there are a number of statistical inadequacies in the analysis of the data (and some overgenerous generalizations therefrom). However, Bishop also argues that Dennis's results – the failure of some children to comprehend reversible passives – can be explained by the relatively low 'mental age' (or 'intellectual level') of the children in question. In support of this hypothesis, Bishop (1983) reports that (in normal children) there is a significant positive association between mental age and performance on reversible passives. Mental age was assessed using the Peabody Picture Vocabulary Test (Dunn 1965). What we find odd about this strategem is the notion that performance on one language task, the PPVT – a measure of receptive vocabulary – can be used to explain performance on another language task – syntactic comprehension. The superficial semblance of explanation is consequent upon nothing more than calling the PPVT scores a measure of 'mental age' and then assuming that mental age has explanatory power. This just cannot be right: the undoubted fact that the receptive vocabulary of the normal child increases with chronological age is a datum to be explained. No definition of 'mental age' based upon the similarly undisputed fact that the vocabulary of some children increases faster than that of others can turn mental age into an explanation of anything.

A related example of pseudo-explanation can be found in the literature on language deficits in Parkinson's disease (PD). A number of authors (including Gurd/Ward 1989) have reported that many patients with PD show deficits on verbal fluency – producing sequences of words within a particular semantic category (e.g. animals) or beginning with a specified letter. Patients produce fewer items than controls and do so at a slower rate. Hanley/Dewick/Davies et al. (1990) replicated this finding. They then showed that the difference between the patient and control samples disappeared if "present verbal ability" was entered into an analysis of covariance. Hanley/Dewick/Davies et al. argue that it is possible that the poor performance of the PD patients on verbal fluency tests "is due to lower general verbal ability." Their measure of general verbal ability is the Mill Hill Synonyms Test (Raven 1943), a test of knowledge of word meanings.

Again, however, it is unclear how a deficit on one verbal test (Mill Hill Synonyms) can be regarded as an explanation of a deficit on another verbal test (fluency). Any association between test scores in either normal or brain-damaged populations is a datum in search of explanation. In the latter population, a theoretically-significant association will be explained by proposing an information-processing account of how the two tasks (that yield the test scores) depend upon common mechanisms. That account will always be subject to revision if some patients show a strong double-dissociation between task performances that cannot be 'explained away' by convincing differential strategic adaptations to a common underlying impairment. The interpretation of correlated impairments after brain damage as due to a decrement in 'general intelligence' or 'general verbal ability' will always be pseudo-explanatory.

4. Aphasia and Non-Verbal Deficits

There are a number of seemingly non-verbal tests on which some (but not all) aphasic patients have been reported to perform very poorly. The most notable are Gottschaldt's Hidden Figures Test (Teuber/Weinstein 1956), Progressive Matrices (Basso/De Renzi/Faglioni et al. 1973; Basso/Capitani/Luzzatti/Spinnler 1981), and varied tests for the comprehension of gesture and pantomime (Duffy/Duffy 1981). The existence of these associations has sometimes been interpreted as indicating that the aphasias are not solely disorders of language.

The basic idea that underlies all the different versions of this claim is that some forms of aphasia reflect a breakdown of conceptual thought and reasoning that is not intrinsically tied to a linguistic code (lexical semantics, syntax, and phonology). The notion has been variously expressed as a failure to adopt an 'abstract attitude' (Goldstein 1948), loss of general intelligence (Marie 1906), and impairment of 'categorical thinking' (Vignolo 1989). Both Hughlings Jackson (1878) and Finkelnburg (1870) regarded the symptomatology of aphasia itself as a deficit of "symbolic formulation and expression" (Hughlings Jackson, 1878), or "asymbolia" as Finkelnburg (1870) phrases it.

Finkelnburg (1870) explicitly relates aphasia to an impairment of the facultas signatrix (Kant 1798), a faculty that occupies "a kind of middle ground between sensory perception and conceptual thought" (Duffy/Liles 1979).

While these ideas are of some interest (and perhaps heuristic value), it is not easy to see how they could be expressed sufficiently clearly to allow empirical data to be brought to bear upon them. In some instances the relevant data-base is itself far from consistent.

For example, both Teuber/Weinstein (1956) and Orgass/Poeck/Kerschensteiner/Hartje (1972) found an impairment on the Gottschaldt Hidden Figures Test that was specific to patients with aphasia after left hemisphere damage. But, by contrast, Meyers (1948) and Bauer/Beck (1954) could find no such impairment in aphasics as compared to control subjects. The only conclusion that can be drawn at present is that we do not understand the information-processing demands of the test.

With respect to Progressive Matrices, the primary data are similarly conflicting, and

Zangwill (1964) has emphasized the poor correlation between severity of aphasia and performance on Matrices. Kertesz/McCabe (1975) have reported that many global aphasics are impaired on Matrices and that poor comprehension is the best predictor of that impairment. This conclusion is supported by the results of Gainotti/d'Erme/Villa/Caltagirone (1986). On the other hand, Kinsbourne/Warrington (1963) and Kertesz (1988) have documented the fact that some aphasics with very poor comprehension can nonetheless obtain well above average scores on Matrices.

The most plausible account of the numerous discrepancies between different studies of Matrices is that many of the individual items can be solved by either verbal strategies, visuo-spatial strategies (or some combination thereof). This conclusion is strongly supported by the work of Zaidel/Sperry (1973) who administered Matrices to a series of patients with cerebral commissurotomy. Each independent hemisphere scored well above chance, but each used "different strategies of approach and different modes of central processing." Costa, (1976) has likewise shown, in patients with left or right unilateral damage, that some items are more easily solved by perceptual matching (Part A) while others place more verbal demands on the deduction of analogies. While these results make good sense, it remains unclear why some authors (e. g. Zaidel/Zaidel/Sperry 1981) wish to impose a psychometric interpretation upon them. The claim that "'g' may contain at least two independent factors, gl and gr", or that "the data better support the primary abilities model of intelligence" (Zaidel/Zaidel/Sperry 1981) adds little to the results by way of either description or explanation.

From a purely psychometric standpoint, Matrices loads highly on g and on a specific spatial factor. The moral, however, is that many supposedly visuo-spatial problems can be solved by verbal means and will be so attempted by some people (not including Einstein). The same point can be made in reverse by the three-term series problem. If one is told that *Tom is taller than Dick and Harry is shorter than Dick* and then asked *Who is tallest*?, the problem is explicitly verbal and can be solved by logico-linguistic reasoning. It is nonetheless more easily solved by constructing a mental image of the three heights and reading off the answer directly from the 'visual' code (Wason/Johnson-Laird 1972).

With respect to the facultas signatrix, Duffy/Duffy (1981) interpret results on pantomime expression and recognition in aphasia as support for the "hypothesis of a generic symbolic ability or process which is prerequisite to, and underlies the use of, specific verbal and nonverbal communicative behaviors." But this conclusion is surely both too strong and too weak. It is too strong because there are double-dissociations between the two domains. Thus Alajouanine/Lhermitte (1964) have described some severely aphasic patients with essentially intact nonverbal communicative skills; and Hécaen (1978) has shown that conventional gesture codes can be impaired in the absence of equivalent disorders of the linguistic system. As Alajouanine/Lhermitte (1964) conclude: "Aphasia appears not to bear any necessary relationship to the presence or absence of extralinguistic disorder."

The hypothesis of impaired 'generic symbolic activity' is too weak in that it provides no account of the specific linguistic patterns of aphasic language (Caplan 1987). While the explication of the functional architecture of communicative gesture and pantomime is an interesting problem in its own right (Seron/van der Kaa/Remitz/van der Linden 1979), it seems fundamentally misguided to conflate communication by gesture and by language.

5. Conclusions

The main thrust of this chapter has been to argue that psychometric definitions of intelligence are irrelevant to any understanding of the functional architecture of language skills and their breakdown in aphasia. Language, we have argued, must be regarded as a specific cognitive module (Chomsky 1980; Fodor 1983) and investigated as such. The Gallist philosophy is correct, however much has yet to be discovered in order to give substance to the modular approach.

We should nevertheless reiterate that our arguments against the reification of intelligence concern only the extremely odd view that psychometric intelligence (= score on a behavioural test or tests) can be regarded as an explanatory construct. We have provided no grounds for disbelief in the existence of 'biological intelligence' as currently conceived by Eysenck (1986). It could well be true that IQ scores show remarkably high correlations with synaptic transmission fidelity as assessed by 'string' measures of averaged evoked responses to flashes of light or pure tones (Blinkhorn/Hendrickson 1982). The validity of such results would, however, shed no light on the structure of language, the character of the processing mechanisms deployed in the use thereof, or the nature of the neuronal instanciation of linguistic capacity.

6. References

Alajouanine, T. & Lhermitte, F. (1964). Non-verbal communication in aphasia. In A. de Reuck & M. O'Connor (Eds.), *Disorders of Language. 168–182.* London: Churchill.

Basso, A., Capitani, E., Luzzatti, C., & Spinnler, H. (1981). Intelligence and left hemisphere disease. *Brain, 104*, 721–734.

Basso, A., De Renzi, E., Faglioni, P., Scotti, G., & Spinnler, H. (1973). Neuropsychological evidence for the existence of cerebral areas critical to the performance of intelligence tasks. *Brain, 96*, 715–728.

Bauer, K. & Beck, D. (1954). Intellect after cerebrovascular accident. *Journal of Nervous and Mental Disorders, 120*, 379–395.

Bishop, D. V. M. (1983). Linguistic impairment after left hemidecortication for infantile hemiplegia? A reappraisal. *Quarterly Journal of Experimental Psychology, 35A*, 199–207.

Blinkhorn, S. F. & Hendrickson, D. E. (1982). Averaged evoked responses and psychometric intelligence. *Nature, 295*, 596–597.

Caplan, D. (1987). *Neurolinguistics and Linguistic Aphasiology: An Introduction.* Cambridge: Cambridge University Press.

Chomsky, N. (1980). Rules and representations. *The Behavioral and Brain Sciences, 3*, 1–61.

Costa, L. D. (1976). Intertest variability on the Raven Coloured Progressive Matrices as an indicator of specific ability deficit in brain lesioned patients. *Cortex, 12*, 31–40.

Dennis, M. (1980). Capacity and strategy for syntactic comprehension after left and right hemidecortication. *Brain and Language, 10*, 287–317.

Duffy, R. J. & Duffy, J. R. (1981). Three studies of deficits in pantomimic expression and pantomimic recognition in aphasia. *Journal of Speech and Hearing Research, 46*, 70–84.

Duffy, R. J. & Liles, B. Z. (1979). A translation of Finkelnburg's (1870) lecture on aphasia as 'asymbolia' with commentary. *Journal of Speech and Hearing Disorders, 44*, 156–168.

Dunn, L. N. (1965). *Expanded Manual for the Peabody Picture Vocabulary Test.* Minnesota: American Guidance Service Inc.

Ellis, A. W. & Young, A. W. (1988). *Human Cognitive Neuropsychology.* London: Lawrence Erlbaum.

Eysenck, H. J. (1986). Toward a new model of intelligence. *Personality and Individual Differences, 7*, 731–736.

Finkelnburg, F. (1870). Niederrheinische Gesellschaft. Sitzung vom 21. März in Bonn. *Berliner Klinische Wochenschrift, 8*, 449–450, 460–462.

Fodor, J. A. (1983). *The Modularity of Mind.* Cambridge, Mass.: MIT Press.

Gainotti, G., D'Erme, P., Villa, G., & Caltagirone, C. (1986). Focal brain lesions and intelligence: a study with a new version of Raven's colored matrices. *Journal of Clinical and Experimental Neuropsychology, 8*, 37–50.

Gardner, H. (1983). *Frames of Mind: The Theory of Multiple Intelligences.* New York: Basic Books.

Goldstein, K. (1948). *Language and Language Disturbances.* New York: Grune and Stratton.

Gurd, J. M. & Marshall, J. C. (1991). Neuropsychology: Cognitive status in progressive neurological illness. *Current Opinion in Psychiatry, 4*, 612–615.

Gurd, J. M. & Ward, C. D. (1989). Retrieval from semantic and letter-initial categories in patients with Parkinson's disease. *Neuropsychologia, 27*, 743–746.

Hamsher, K. (1981). Intelligence and aphasia. In M. T. Sarno (Ed.), *Acquired Aphasia.* 327–359. New York: Academic Press.

Hanley, J. R., Dewick, H. C., Davies, A. D. M., Playfer, J. & Turnbull, C. (1990). Verbal fluency in Parkinson's disease. *Neuropsychologia, 28*, 737–741.

Hécaen, H. (1978). Les apraxies idéomotrices: Essai de dissociation. In H. Hécaen & M. Jeannerod (Eds.), *Du Controle Moteur à l'Organisation du Geste. 343–358.* Paris: Masson.

Jackson, J. H. (1876). Case of large cerebral tumor without optic neuritis and with left hemiplegia and imperception. *Royal London Ophthalmic Hospital Reports, 8*, 434–440.

Jackson, J. H. (1878). On affections of speech from disease of the brain. *Brain, 1*, 304–330.

Kant, I. (1798). *Anthropologie in pragmatischer Hinsicht.* Königsberg: Nicolvius.

Kertesz, A. (1988). Cognitive function in severe aphasia. In L. Weiskrantz (Ed.), *Thought without Language. 451–463.* Oxford: Clarendon Press.

Kertesz, A. & McCabe, P. (1975). Intelligence and aphasia: Performance of aphasics on Raven's Coloured Progressive Matrices (RCPM). *Brain and Language, 2*, 387–395.

Kinsbourne, M. & Warrington, E. K. (1963). Jargon aphasia. *Neuropsychologia, 1*, 27–37.

Lashley, K. S. (1937). Functional determinants of cerebral localization. *Archives of Neurology and Psychiatry, 38*, 371–387.

Lezak, D. (1988). IQ: R. I. P. *Journal of Clinical and Experimental Neuropsychology, 10*, 40.

Margolin, D. I. (1992). Clinical cognitive neuropsychology: An emerging speciality. In D. I. Margolin (Ed.), *Cognitive Neuropsychology in Clinical Practice. 9–17.* Oxford: Oxford University Press.

Marie, P. (1906). Revision de la question de l'aphasie: La troisième convolution frontale gauche ne joue acun role spéciale dans la fonction du language. *Semaine Médicale, 21,* 241–247.

Marshall, J. C. (1984). Multiple perspectives on modularity. *Cognition, 17,* 209–242.

Meyers, R. (1948). Relation of 'thinking' and language: an experimental approach using dysphasic patients. *Archives of Neurology and Psychiatry, 60,* 119–139.

McCarthy, R. A. & Warrington, E. K. (1990). *Cognitive Neuropsychology: A Clinical Introduction.* New York: Academic Press.

Nelson, H. E. & O'Connell, A. (1978). Dementia: The estimation of premorbid intelligence levels using the new adult reading test. *Cortex, 14,* 234–244.

Orgass, B., Poeck, K., Kerschensteiner, M., & Hartje, W. (1972). Visuocognitive performances in patients with unilateral hemispheric lesions. An investigation with three factorial reference tests. *Zeitschrift für Neurologie, 202,* 177–195.

Raven, J. C. (1943). *The Mill Hill Vocabulary Scale.* London: H. K. Lewis.

Raven, J. C. (1965). *Guide to Using the Coloured Progressive Matrices.* London: H. K. Lewis.

Schwartz, M. F. (Ed.) (1990). *Modular Deficits in Alzheimer-Type Dementia.* Cambridge, Mass.: MIT Press.

Seron, X., van der Kaa, M., Remits, A., & van der Linden, M. (1979). Pantomimic interpretation and aphasia. *Neuropsychologia, 17,* 661–668.

Shallice, T. (1988). *From Neuropsychology to Mental Structure.* Cambridge: Cambridge University Press.

Spearman, C. (1927). *The Abilities of Man.* New York: Macmillan.

Teuber, H.-L. & Weinstein, S. (1956). Ability to discover hidden figures after cerebral lesions. *Archives of Neurology and Psychiatry, 76,* 369–379.

Thurstone, L. L. (1938). *Primary Mental Abilities.* Chicago: Chicago University Press.

Vignolo, L. A. (1989). Non-verbal conceptual impairment in aphasia. In F. Boller & J. Grafman (Eds.), *Handbook of Neuropsychology, Vol. 2. 185–206.* Amsterdam: Elsevier.

Wason, P. C. & Johnson-Laird, P. N. (1972). *Psychology of Reasoning: Structure and Content.* London: Batsford.

Wechsler, D. (1958). *The Measurement and Appraisal of Adult Intelligence,* Baltimore: Williams and Wilkins.

Weisenburg, T. & McBride, K. E. (1935). *Aphasia: A Clinical and Psychological Study.* New York: The Commonwealth Fund.

Wertheimer, M. (1945).*Productive Thinking.* New York: Harper.

Zaidel, D. & Sperry, R. W. (1973). Performance on the Raven's colored progressive matrices test by subjects with cerebral commissurotomy. *Cortex, 9,* 34–39.

Zaidel, E., Zaidel, D. W., & Sperry, R. W. (1981). Left and right intelligence: Case studies of Raven's progressive matrices following brain bisection and hemidecortication. *Cortex, 17,* 167–186.

Zangwill, O. L. (1964). Intelligence in aphasia. In A. V. S. de Reuck & M. O'Connor (Eds.), *Disorders of Language. 261–284.* London: Churchill.

Zangwill, O. L. (1969). Intellectual status in aphasia. In P. J. Vinken & G. W. Bruyn (Eds.), *Handbook of Clinical Neurology, Vol 4. 105–111.* Amsterdam: North-Holland.

Jennifer M. Gurd/John C. Marshall, Oxford (UK)

28. Aphasia and Apraxia

1. Introduction

Like the aphasias, the variants of motor apraxia are among the classic syndromes in human neuropsychology. In the vast majority of cases, apraxia arises after lesions in the language-dominant hemisphere. In those rather rare cases in which language is organized in the right hemisphere, apraxia can also develop after a right-sided brain lesion (Poeck/Kerschensteiner 1971; Poeck/Lehmkuhl 1980). A dissociation of hemispheric dominance for praxis and language has been discussed only in exceptional single cases (Heilman/Coyle/Gonyea/Geschwind 1973; Heilman/Gonyea/Geschwind 1974). Also, aphasia and apraxia occur very frequently together following a single (either large or small) left hemispheric brain lesion.

1.1. These observations might indicate that the apraxias are language dependent syndromes. The term language dependent in this context is ambiguous: on the one hand, it can imply that a symptom or syndrome is the direct consequence of the aphasic language deficit. Characteristic examples are the inability of aphasic patients to discriminate verbally between left and right (Poeck/Orgass 1967; 1971) or to identify individual fingers verbally (Poeck/Orgass 1969). However the fact that aphasia and apraxia can vary independently of each other argues against this kind of language dependency. That is, after a lesion of the language-dominant hemisphere, apraxia may improve or disappear, whereas aphasia persists. The reverse is also possible. Handedness is not particularly helpful to explain left brain dominance for praxis, since apraxia, with only a few anatomically defined exceptions, affects both hands and feet.

On the other hand 'Language dependency' may also mean that a symptom or a syndrome is brought about by an interruption of fiber tracts between a specific cortical area and the language region (Geschwind 1965). This view would imply that the language region of the brain has conceptual functions beyond those involved in linguistic expression and comprehension. This assumption is, to a certain extent, supported by the observation that users of American Sign Language are reported to develop different types of sign language aphasia, corresponding to Broca's and Wernicke's aphasia, respectively, following lesions in anterior or posterior parts of the language region (Poizner/Klima/Bellugi 1990). However, such a disconnection model is difficult to prove in detail. Furthermore, there are no autopsy studies available for large patient groups. And finally the spatial resolution of available imaging methods as yet is certainly not fine enough to document complete interruption of specific fiber tracts.

1.2. If apraxia is not language dependent in the restricted sense considered above, then the striking association between disorders of language and of praxis might be explained in a different way. Other possibilities are:

- The two disorders are independent and their frequent association is due to the proximity of the cortical areas within which lesions produce the disturbances.
- The two disorders are the expression of a common underlying deficit of communication affecting linguistic and gestural behavior in a general sense. This hypothesis recalls Finkelnburg's (1870) concept of asymbolia. In contrast one might assume a disturbance of motor control mechanisms governing both limb and speech musculature.

The last hypothesis, however, does not account for the linguistic aspects of language disturbances associated with lesions of the left hemisphere. In addition, apraxia also affects movements that have neither symbolic value, nor communicative function, such as cutting an apple or drinking a cup of tea.

1.3. The relationship between aphasia and apraxia was aptly discussed as early as the beginning of this century. Liepmann (1913), for one, had already observed that aphasia and apraxia are frequently associated. He linked this association to either impairment in neighboring neural structures or, and this was his preferred position, to disturbances of the same kind ("wesensgleich"). Liepmann stressed that he had conceived of the aphasia in one of his patients as "apraxia of the musculature of speech". He compared the planning of purposeful movements with the planning of words and sentences, both termed 'ideation'. Whereas in purposeful movements the ideation had temporal, spatial, as well as visual aspects, in language the ideation had temporal-acoustic ones. Thus, according to Liepmann, only the temporal aspect is common to both activities. Liepmann equated limb-kinetic apraxia with Broca's aphasia, and he stressed the similarity between various kinds of parapraxic distortions of movements with paraphasic alterations of the motor aspects of language. In particular, he mentioned perseveration, elision, repetition, anticipation, and confusion of semantically similar words or movements. For example, semantically different finite movements reminded him of semantic paraphasias, and the motoric counterpart to word finding disturbances were problems producing the correct movement. Liepmann also stressed that it is difficult to distinguish mnestic and executional disturbances, a consideration which is reminiscent of Geschwind's seminal paper on the variety of naming disorders (Geschwind 1967).

2. Brain Localization

Under the aspect of cerebral localization, there is strong overlap between areas involved in the control of speech and of movement. The most interesting of these areas is the Supplementary Motor Area, situated in the medial part of area 6. Indeed, recordings of SMA neuronal activity in conscious, behaving monkeys have demonstrated that SMA's role in movement control is different from that of the primary motor area in area 4 of the precentral gyrus (Brinkman 1981). The results seem to point to the SMA's possible role in programming movement. The SMA might actually modulate primary motor area activity, since it is, in fact, located 'upstream' from the primary motor area. Correspondingly, in monkeys Brinkman found a deficiency in bimanual coordination after unilateral SMA lesions. That is to say that both hands tended to be used in a symmetrical manner instead of sharing the work load between them. Furthermore, the apraxics showed a disability in adjusting their hands for catching purposes which Brinkman interpreted as an inability to sequence flexion and extension components of the movement.

Freund (1985) has reported, that in humans, lesion of the mediofrontal cortex including SMA leads to a notable decrease in spontaneous motor activity in the contralateral limbs. These lesions also result in a decrease in language activity, corresponding to Luria's "dynamic aphasia" (1980) or to 'transcortical motor aphasia'.

3. Apraxia and Type of Aphasia

Studies associating motor apraxia with the various subtypes of aphasia will not be discussed in detail here, since in my view, these studies are not very productive, and their results have little, if any, explanatory value. In keeping with this objection, in a large scale study, Lehmkuhl/Poeck/Willmes (1983) were unable to associate presence or absence of apraxia with subtypes of aphasia in any way.

An obvious misconception arising from studies such as those mentioned above is the claim that oral apraxia is directly related to Broca's aphasia. In fact, there actually is a very strong positive correlation between the occurrence of phonemic paraphrasias (omission, substitution, anticipation, perseveration and reversal of phonemes) in the setting of any aphasic syndrome and apraxic distortions of nonspeech oral movements (DeRenzi/Pieczuro/Vignolo 1966). Oral apraxia is a regular feature of syndromes like conduction aphasia or Wernicke's aphasia. The underlying brain lesions are localized, according to Vignolo (1977) in the perisylvian region as opposed to, in Vignolo's terminology, marginal, i.e. more peripheral, parts of the language area. This close correlation between oral apraxia and phonemic paraphasias suggests that indeed similar brain mechanisms subserve intricate sequential movements in the oral sphere during speech as well as nonspeech motor activity.

4. Modality Specific Apraxia

In addition to the standard aphasias (Broca's, Wernicke's, Global, Amnesic), several nonstandard types of aphasia have been described. From the perspective of brain mechanisms, the modality specific naming disorders are the most interesting. For instance, there are optic aphasia, or naming deficits on visual stimulation, as well as tactile aphasia in conjunction with Braille aphasia. Localization of lesion strongly suggests a disconnection mechanism in these cases.

De Renzi/Faglioni/Sorgato (1982) have described modality specific mechanisms in apraxia, in other words, apraxia depending on the kind of stimulus that was given to elicit the gesture. They found a dissociation between the ability to correctly use objects when the stimulus was verbal, visual or tactile, respectively. They concluded that these cases of apraxia resulted from disconnection between cerebral areas where the sensory information is processed and those areas, where movements are programmed.

5. Testing for Apraxia

At the present stage, studies in apraxia suffer from a regrettable lack of standardized and generally accepted testing procedures. In contrast to existing reliable aphasia test batteries, as of yet there is neither an apraxia test on record based on item analysis, nor on test-retest reliability, nor on interrater stability.

Furthermore, many researchers base the diagnosis of apraxia on a rather arbitrary cut-off score instead of establishing a cut-off range.

6. 'Linguistic' Description and Analysis of Parapractic Errors

Until a few years ago, most investigators limited themselves to rating the performance of their patients on apraxia test simply as pass or fail. A more detailed insight into the nature of motor apraxia became possible only when the parapractic movement sequences were subjected to a qualitative analysis.

6.1. Early work on a normal population became available from Efron (1941), who made use of highly differentiated methods of describing movements in a study on gestures. Efron had already noted certain analogies between verbal and gestural behavior, and he used the term 'linguistic' to describe the referential aspects of symbolic movements. Unfortunately, he limited his analysis to finite movement sequences and chose not to describe their individual components. This is also true of Ekman/Friesen's studies (1969; 1972) on the repertoire of nonverbal behavior, in particular of their transcultural investigation of gestural movements.

6.2. The methods of structural linguistics were first applied to normal movements by Birdwhistle (1970), who recognized that body posture, movements, and gestural expression can have fixed patterns, which he catalogued in a hierarchy of elements, similar to the description of language units. Just as phonemes and morphemes are distinguished in linguistics, Birdwhistle differentiated between motor elements he termed 'kinemes' and 'kinemorphes', and he used a notation system that permitted the exact description of individual elements in a motor sequence. In a field that he called 'kinesics', he suggested studying the group of movements that is significant for communicative processes.

6.3. Ulatowska/Kumin/Kaplan (1974) also attempted to categorize errors in an investigation of symbolic gestural behavior (so-called emblems) in aphasic patients and in normal subjects.

6.4. On the basis of these earlier studies, we (Kerschensteiner/Poeck 1974; Poeck/Kerschensteiner 1975) developed a method that permitted the coding of those individual components that constitute apractic movements. That is, we were able to transcribe these components into graphic symbols that could then be analyzed qualitatively and quantitatively. The goal was to describe the 'vocabulary' of apraxia in a manner similar to that of aphasia research, while seeking regularities characteristic either for individual patients or for subtypes of apraxia in certain subtypes of aphasia. The following groups of errors have been distinguished: a) Substitutions: The requested movement is replaced by a finite motor response or by a verbal or sound response. b) Augmentations: The patient makes additional movements or sounds. c) Omissions: These consist either of complete failure to respond or of fragmentary execution of the response. d) Other errors: This is not a uniform category. It includes behaviors that are similar to the 'conduite d'approche' of aphasic patients when they try to correct phonological or semantic paraphasias by means of different degrees of approximation. Similarly, apractic patients, when asked to make a hissing noise, may first whistle, then alternate between whistling and a movement by which they inhale air through half-closed lips, before they finally perform the correct movement. Amorphous movements do not fit into any of the categories just named. In our experience, the significance of such movements for the apraxias is less important than what has been reported in the literature.

A final very important element of ideomotor apraxia is perseveration. This consists not only of repetition of entire movements, but also of inappropriate introduction of elements of a movement that the patient had performed earlier. The patient perseverates not only from one movement to the immediately following one; rather the tendency to perseverate can be so strong that an element that had been performed correctly (or incorrectly) earlier, recurs eight or ten tasks later.

This overview would be too lengthy, if details of the coding and the interpretation of our qualitative analysis of ideomotor-apractic movement sequences were presented here, particularly in relation to aphasic syndromes; the reader is therefore referred to the original publications. One finding, however, deserves special attention. The individual subtypes of aphasia are not accompanied by distinct subtypes of apraxia. Not a single type of ideomotor apraxia characterized by certain kinds of apractic errors can be distinguished (see also Lehmkuhl/Poeck/Willmes 1983).

7. Receptive Aspects of Apraxia

7.1. The receptive aspects of apraxia have rarely been investigated thoroughly. Gonzales Rothi/Heilman/Watson (1985) were able to demonstrate that apractic patients with retrorolandic lesions including the parietal areas were impaired in the differential recognition of gestures. They presented videos of pantomimes, and the subjects had to indicate their meaning by chosing the corresponding illustration from a multiple choice set. The drawings were of the kind that if the pantomime was of hammering, one drawing was of a nail, and three were foils. Similarly, in an earlier paper Heilman/Rothi/Valenstein (1982) found that ideomotor apraxic patients with posterior lesions had a gestural discrimination deficit, whereas anterior apraxics did not.

Several studies have demonstrated that some aphasics do not recognize gestures. Ferro/Martins/Mariano/Castro-Caldas (1983) studied this performance in 65 left hemispheric stroke patients whose lesions were located by CT scan. In the acute stage frontal lobe and basal ganglia were frequently involved in patients showing inability to recognize gestures. In the later and chronic stages parietal lobe involvement was important. Lesions producing gesture recognition impairment were larger, had more extensive and more frequent parietal involvement and produced less temporal lobe damage than those causing verbal comprehension defects. The latter finding underscores the importance of the multimodal parietal lobe for gesture recognition.

7.2. As indicated above, one of the major issues in gestural behavioral studies is whether the frequent occurrence of gestural impairment after posterior left hemisphere lesions is due to the anatomical coincidence of areas serving both functions or due to an impairment of an underlying general communicative or cognitive ability. Correlation between gesture and language comprehension varies with type of aphasia. For instance, whereas it is highly significant in global aphasia, it is nonsignificant in Wernicke's aphasia (Ferro/Santos/Castro-Caldas/Mariano 1980). Moreover, among those aphasics with similar language impairments some are impaired in gesture recognition, while others are not. Involvement of centroparietal white matter can cause gesture comprehension disturbance while sparing auditory comprehension at least at the word level. In contrast, severe comprehension defect without gesture recognition disturbance has been associated with temporal lesions and the relative sparing of the parietal lobe. Also, the size of the lesions was shown to play an important role. The loci specifically associated with gesture recognition impairment correspond to parietal supramodal cortical areas that can integrate visual and somesthetic information and the exploration of extrapersonal space.

Certain brain areas are mainly associated either with gesture or with language comprehension defects. For other areas (for example part of Wernicke's area and supramarginal gyrus), both disturbances can be found with comparable frequency. This partial overlap of the areas crucial to those two functions explains some of the striking discrepancies in the literature.

All in all, lesions producing auditory comprehension defects are smaller than those causing gesture recognition impairment, suggesting a multicomponent cortical representation of gestures.

8. Sequential Aspects of Aphasia and Apraxia

On several occasions Poeck/Huber (1977) found evidence that the left hemisphere of humans is particularly involved in the sequential organization of certain types of motor behavior. Based on the results of interestingly devised experiments, Kimura and colleagues (1970; 1973; 1974) had reached the same conclusion. She has elaborated this concept into the assumption that sequential behavior is a supramodal left hemisphere function. In view of this conviction, Kimura/Archibald (1974) have noted "that speaking is another activity characterized by a high degree of precision of movement". The authors speculate that "it is quite possible that speech disturbances and apraxia are simply (spacing mine) different manifestations of an impairment of motor sequencing" and that it is "not specifically a symbolic, or language system which is affected in aphasia, but the speech system". Also on another occasion,

Kimura maintained that "language is a sequential activity".

Contrary to this view, Poeck/Huber (1977) have pointed out that a very important characteristic of the speech code is that the same part of the acoustic signal relays diverse items of information about successive phonemic segments of the message simultaneously. In support of this assumption MacNeilage (1970) demonstrated that this information processing cannot be achieved simply by serial ordering of fixed articulatory instructions. Language is described in most linguistic models on different levels. Certainly, the information is not processed on each level in isolation, rather it is available from different levels simultaneously. However, sequential activity is certainly characteristic for operations at the phonemic level. Alterations in the sequential order, like anticipation, perseveration, omission, substitution or reversal of phonemes change the meaning of a morpheme profoundly or lead to a meaningless utterance. This holds true for speech errors of normal individuals (Fromkin 1973) as well as for those of aphasics. Up to this point, there are obvious parallels between operations in the realm of speech and gestures, even though reversal of the elements of a movement has rarely, if ever, been demonstrated. However, even at the phonemic level, sequential ordering is only part of the operations performed. The use of phonemes also obeys principles of selection. To my knowledge it has not been possible to demonstrate comparable principles of selection in gestures, even though their elements do have a sequential order. Also, out of the roughly 200 phonetically different phonemes identified in all known languages, the inventory of English includes only some 40 of these (Heike 1972). There are neither dialects, nor different languages in movements, rather individual variations that, by themselves, can vary from one instance to the other and still produce a purposeful or expressive movement. Of course, there are no selection restrictions in gestures; yet even selection restrictions cannot be explained by sequential activity. Severe phonemic jargon in aphasia exhibits both, distortion of the inventory and/or violation of the permitted combinations of phonemes. Parapraxic movements exhibit obvious distortions of the inventory and incorrect combinations of these, but there is no binding or obligatory combinations of kinemes that can be violated.

Speech errors certainly are not arbitrary, but rather obey certain linguistic regulations. For instance, two reversed phonemes always belong to the same category (vowels or consonants), and they usually differ in only one or two phonemic features.

Similar basic differences between language and movement have been established by Poeck/Huber (1977) for the lexical and the semantic/syntactical level as well as for pragmatic factors that play a great role in language. Thus the claim that aphasic language can be explained solely, in analogy to apraxic errors in movement, as a failure in sequencing cannot be supported. This is not to negate the fact that the left hemisphere plays an important role in the processing of temporal qualities of motor activities as well as of sensory stimuli (Efron 1963).

9. Linguistic Models of Aphasia in Relation to Apraxia

9.1. Garrett's model of speech production (1980) distinguishes a general conceptual level, a language specific sentence level and a motor level of articulatory control (see Roy/Square (1985, 9.2.). The conceptual or message level contains processes that are based on the speaker's perceptual and affective state and his or her general knowledge of the world. Language production takes place under message level control. The message level is the intended locus of the inferential processes that determine structured discourse. At the articulatory level there is the translation from sentence level structures to articulatory structures including those responsible for respiration.

9.2. Roy/Square (1985) describe control mechanisms in limb praxis on the basis of two control systems, the conceptual and the production system. For the conceptual system they stress the notion of action fields which surround objects and comprise functional information such as descriptions of purposes and usage. Further, other information, important for categorical knowledge, e. g. perceptual attributes then develops from this functional core. The perceptual attributes of tools and objects provide one source of information. The performer learns through experience with objects that certain perceptual features enable certain actions. The perceptual attributes enable assessment of which actions are possible. The other source of information concerns the environmental/situational context in which tools are normally used. Thus, one possible type of error is a failure to discriminate, as when the performer confuses contextual or perceptual aspects of objects.

The production system is concerned with effecting action on the environment. Errors arise principally when the performer is not attending to the unfolding action. These errors occur at 'key choice points'.

The perceptual attributes of tools at surfaces bring about certain restrictions, e. g. the way a pen has to be held in the hand for the act of writing. The performance of actions involves a delicate balance between processes subserved by higher level systems which demand attention and the more autonomous operations subserved at lower levels.

Thus, Roy's theories are based on limb praxis as motor activity involving use of objects.

9.3. Dell (1988) has reviewed a model of retrieval processes in speech production that makes predictions about the factors influencing speech errors possible. For example, the regularities that govern the exchange of phonemes in speech errors are the dimensions of similarity. Also, the major rule systems associated with a linguistic level are usually not violated by an error occurring at such a low level. In other words, the resulting non-words are always phonologically 'legal' sequences and adhere to the phonological rules of the language. Likewise, errors involving lexical items tend to produce sequences that are syntactically coherent. Thus, there is strong control over errors emanating from the systematic organization of language.

Exchange, anticipation, perseveration are phenomena common to aphasia, to speech errors of non-brain lesioned patients and to apraxia. To me it seems to be impossible to draw parallels between the research into speech errors (which betray certain regularities observed by Fromkin (1973) as well as Garrett (1989)) and sequencing errors in apraxic movements which do not follow any recognizable regularity. The problem appears to be that there are rules for the production of language, but there is an almost infinite variety of movements other than emblems. In language production it is possible either to deviate from or adhere to a given grammatical category. The same is not true for movements, however.

Regularities such as increase in the number of perseverations when people are rushed are not observed in apraxia. Also there is no recognized correspondence to intended syllables or words. Furthermore, deviations from the intended movement also do not have common features like rhyming, and rarely do parapraxias belong to the same class as the intended movement. Slips of the tongue frequently create meaningful expressions, which is not often the case in parapraxias. Finally, the similarity of target items plays an important role in determining the frequency of slips, but not of parapraxias. It must be added, however, that the influence of speed on movement has not been studied to the extent of its influence on speaking rate.

10. Conclusions

The common interhemispheric and the similar intrahemispheric localization of the underlying brain lesions calls for consideration of a possible structural relationship between the two syndromes. It is true that both activities, language and speech as well as praxis share certain communicative functions. However, praxis also embraces many non-communicative activities.

The rules that govern language and speech are not valid for praxis. Consequently, apraxia cannot be described in terms of violation of inherent rules. Movements may well draw from an inventory of motor elements that one might metaphorically term lexicon, and there are elements of movements that might be equated to phonemes, but here the analogy ends. There is no syntax of movements, and the present author doubts that one will ever be discovered.

11. References

Birdwhistle, R. L. (1970). *Kinemics and Context*. Philadelphia: University of Pennsylvania Press.

Brinkman, C. (1981). Lesions in supplementary motor area interfere with monkey's performance of a bimanual coordination task. *Neurosciences Letters, 27*, 267–270.

Dell, G. S. (1988). The retrieval of phonological forms in production: Tests of Prediction from a Connectionist Model. *Journal of Memory and Language, 27*, 124–142.

De Renzi, E., Faglioni, P., & Sorgato, P. (1982). Modality-specific and supramodal mechanisms of apraxia. *Brain, 105*, 301–312.

De Renzi, E., Pieczuro, A., & Vignolo, L. A. (1966). Oral apraxia and aphasia. *Cortex, 2*, 60–73.

Efron, D. (1941). *Gesture and Environment*. New York: King's Crown.

Efron, R. (1963). Temporal perception, aphasia and déja vu. *Brain, 86*, 403–424.

Ekman, P. & Friesen, W. (1969). The repertoire of nonverbal behaviour: Categories, origins, usage and coding. *Semiotica, 1*, 49–98.

Ekman, P. & Friesen, W. (1982). Hand movements. *Journal of Communication, 22*, 353–374.

Ferro, J. M., Martins, I. P., Mariano, G., & Castro-Caldas, A. (1983). CT scan correlates of gesture recognition. *Journal of Neurology, Neurosurgery, and Psychiatry, 46*, 943–952.

Ferro, J. M., Santos, M. E., Castro-Caldas, A., & Mariano, G. (1980). Gesture recognition in aphasia. *Journal of Clinical Neuropsychology, 2*, 277–292.

Finkelnburg, R. (1870). Vortrag in der Niederrhein. Gesellschaft der Ärzte. Bonn, Berlin, *Klinische Wochenschrift, 7*, 449.

Freund, H.-J. (1985). Clinical aspects of premotor function. *Behavioural Brain Research, 18*, 187–191.

Fromkin, V. A. (1973). Introduction. In V. A. Fromkin (Ed.), *Speech errors as linguistic evidence. 11–45*. The Hague: Mouton.

Garrett, M. F. (1980). Levels of processing in sentence production. In B. Butterworth (Ed.), *Language Production, vol. 1. 177–220*. London: Academic Press.

Geschwind, N. (1965). Disconnexion syndromes in animals and man, 2. *Brain, 88*, 585–644.

Geschwind, N. (1967). The varieties of naming errors. *Cortex, 3*, 97–112.

Gonzalez Rothi, L. J., Heilman, K. M., & Watson, R. T. (1985). Pantomime comprehension and ideomotor apraxia. *Journal of Neurology, Neurosurgery, and Psychiatry, 48*, 207–210.

Heike, G. (1972). *Phonologie*. Stuttgart: Metzler.

Heilman, K. M., Coyle, J. M., Gonyea, E. F., & Geschwind, N. (1973). Apraxia and agraphia in a left-hander. *Brain, 96*, 21–28.

Heilman, K. M., Gonyea, E. F., & Geschwind, N. (1974). Apraxia and agraphia in a right-hander. *Cortex, 10*, 284–288.

Heilman, K. M., Rothi, L. J., & Valenstein, E. (1982). Two forms of ideomotor apraxia. *Neurology, 32*, 342–346.

Kerschensteiner, M. & Poeck, K. (1974). Bewegungsanalyse bei buccofacialer Apraxie. *Nervenarzt, 45*, 9–15.

Kimura, D. (1973). Manual activity during speaking. I. Right handers. *Neuropsychologia, 11*, 45–50.

Kimura, D. & Archibald, Y. (1974). Motor functions of the left hemisphere. *Brain, 97*, 337–350.

Kimura, D. & Vanderwolf, C. H. (1970). The relation between hand preference and the performance of individual finger movements by left and right hands. *Brain, 93*, 769–774.

Lehmkuhl, G., Poeck, K., & Willmes, K. (1983). Ideomotor apraxia and aphasia: An examination of types and manifestations of apraxic symptoms. *Neuropsychologia, 21*, 199–212.

Liepmann, H. (1913). Motorische Aphasie und Apraxie. *Monatsschrift für Psychiatrie und Neurologie, 34*, 485–494.

Luria, A. R. (1980). *Higher cortical functions in man*. 2nd edition. New York: Basic Books, Inc.

MacNeilage, P. F. (1970). Motor control of serial ordering of speech. *Psychology Review, 77*, 182–196.

Poeck, K. & Huber, W. (1977). To what extent is language a sequential activity? *Neuropsychologia, 15*, 359–363.

Poeck, K. & Kerschensteiner, M. (1971). Ideomotor apraxia following right-sided cerebral lesions in a left-handed subject. *Neuropsychologia, 9*, 359–361.

Poeck, K. & Kerschensteiner, M. (1975). Analysis of the sequential motor events in oral apraxia. In K. J. Zülch, O. Creutzfeldt, & G. C. Galbraith (Eds.), *Cerebral Localization. 98–111*. Berlin/Heidelberg/New York: Springer.

Poeck, K. & Lehmkul, G. (1980). Ideatory apraxia in a left-handed patient with right-sided brain lesion. *Cortex, 16*, 273–284.

Poeck, K. & Orgass, B. (1967). Über Störungen der Rechts-Links-Orientierung. *Nervenarzt, 38*, 285–291.

Poeck, K., & Orgass, B. (1969). An experimental investigation of finger agnosia. *Neurology, 19*, 801–807.

Poeck, K. & Orgass, B. (1971). The concept of the body schema: A critical review and some experimental results. *Cortex, 7*, 254–277.

Poizner, H., Klima, E., & Bellugi, H. (1987). *What the hands reveal about the brain*. Boston: MIT.

Roy, E. A. & Square, P. A. (1985). Common considerations in the study of limb, verbal and oral apraxia. In E. A. Roy (Ed.), *Advances in Psychology*, vol. 23. Neuropsychological Studies of Apraxia and Related Disorders. *111–161*. Amsterdam/New York/Oxford: North-Holland.

Ulatowska, H. K., Kumin, L., & Kaplan, E. (1974). Symbolic gestural behavior of aphasics and normals under three task conditions. Unpublished manuscript.

Vignolo, L. A. (1977). Le Sindromi Afasiche. In *Neuropsicologia Clinica*, 11–42. Milano: Franco Angeli Editore.

Klaus Poeck, Aachen (Germany)

29. Aphasia and Acalculia

1. Overview

The observation that aphasia often coincides with acalculia has spurned attempts to relate two higher cortical functions, language and calculation. In this article, I shall not present new experiments and data linking aphasia and acalculia. Instead, for each theoretical issue, I will try to integrate the relevant pieces of information available from past research as well as from developmental and neuropsychological literature. In the course of this article, it will become progressively clear that it currently makes little if any sense to look for general, necessary conditions relating the two domains. Rather, it will be proposed that number processing and calculation be viewed as operations performed on symbolic systems. Under certain circumstances, such operations can contribute to understanding aspects of other high-level cognitive activities. Indeed, compared to language, arithmetical notations and skills are quite easy to model. This simplicity may highlight some issues under discussion in other more complex domains to be formalized. In such a way, some limited functional relations may be expected from in-depth analysis of single subjects' language and mathematical processing. I will conclude with some current theoretical issues in the domains of language, memory, etc. which might benefit from this cautious approach.

2. Introduction

Since oral language is usually required to process and calculate numbers, and orthographic numbers are indispensible when writing cheques, it is easy to see how disturbances to language can also have an impact on mathematical operations. Moreover, this question goes far beyond the simple instrumental aspect of language, since arithmetical abilities have been acquired, developed, automated in close relation to language. For instance, one must master counting words before one can learn to add (Secada/Fuson/Hall 1983) and subtract (Fuson 1984), and one learns the multiplication tables by rote. The issue thus also involves the potential effects of acquired language disorders due to brain damage on the more or less autonomous calculation process in adults.

First, it is important to note that from a methodological point of view, the question of the relation between aphasia and acalculia may receive quite different answers depending on its level of generality and maybe also on individual factors. The first point refers to the varieties of the taxonomies used for classifying language disturbances on the one hand and calculation deficits on the other hand. The second point simply draws attention to the fact that inter-individual variations in cognitive styles and skills may result in different architectural relations between language and calculation.

I shall now review and comment on different ways of formulating the question of the relationship between aphasia and acalculia. At each step, it must of course be kept in mind that whereas there are two modalities in language (oral, written), there are at least three symbolic systems for the notation of numbers (the same two as in language, plus the Arabic digit ideographic system, not to mention Roman numerals). For an historical review, see Boller/Grafman (1983).

3. Is there a Functional Relation between Aphasia and Acalculia?

The answer to this question depends on how narrowly one defines functional relation and on whether one seeks such a relation among brain-damaged patients as a group or as different single cases, and on whether one regards aphasia and acalculia as entities or presenting different syndromes.

Up to Henschen (1919), number processing and calculation disorders were simply interpreted within the symptom complex of aphasia. His careful review of patients' performance in language and calculation established that there was no mandatory relationship between the occurrence of aphasia and the concomitant presence of calculation impairments. From Henschen's point of view, such findings indicated the possible independence of calculation and language, thus justifying coining the term 'acalculia' for referring to the effects of brain damage on this 'new' higher cortical function. Within the modern theoretical and methodological information processing approach, this conclusion is still valid since double dissociations of preserved/impaired abilities in one domain, with the reverse pattern of results in the other domain experimentally demonstrates their functional independence. More recently, Ardila/Rosselli (1990) have proposed a classification of acalculias into 6 different types, one of which being "aphasic acalculia". The existence of the 5 other types thus constitutes an a contrario argument in support of the non-deterministic relation between the occurrence of aphasia and acalculia and the effects of the former disorder on the latter deficit.

Despite the fact that the answer to this first question, viewed at the general level, is clearly no, the issue may still be considered in more detail when the neuropsychological examination of patients establishes both aphasia and acalculia. The question then becomes: are there relationships between types of aphasia and varieties of acalculia? Is it worth mentioning that Grewel's studies (1952; 1969) on this topic seem to have also progressed from the general question to the more specific question regarding different syndromes since the title of the first study was "Acalculia", whereas 17 years later it changed to "The Acalculias". Before such detailed analyses can be made, serious methodological problems must be considered. First, neither language nor calculation disorders have been classified in an unambiguous, theoretically motivated, and universally accepted manner. For instance, the taxonomies of mathematical disabilities vary according to the scientific domain (education, psychology ...), the area of mathematics concerned (simple calculations, problem solving ...), the level of descriptions of impairments and framework of reference (lesional, functional ...), the etiology of disorders (developmental, acquired ...), the syndromes they may constitute (Gerstmann, Alzheimer ...) and other factors (Kosc 1980). The second difficulty is due to the great diversity of the aspects of number processing and calculation abilities. The assessment batteries for calculation try to tap these different facets by presenting a large variety of subtests: production of more or less automated sequences of counting words; transcoding quantities from one notation system into another (Arabic digits, oral or written numbers); counting, enumeration, estimation of quantities or dot patterns perceptually structured in different ways; access to, and manipulation of the semantic representations of numbers in magnitude comparison or in placing numbers on some analogic number line ...; numerical knowledge, number facts; performing operations with carrying and borrowing; knowledge of mathematical algorithms, problem solving, numerical reasoning ... (See for instance the batteries devised by Hécaen/Angelergues/Houillier 1961; Hitch 1978; Claros-Salinas/von Cramon 1987; Rosselli/Ardila 1989; Deloche/Seron 1989; Deloche/Seron/Bergego 1989). As a consequence of the diversity of tasks, mathematical abilities can be impaired in a variety of different ways. Furthermore, computing correlations between calculation error types of so many tasks and the types of aphasia, tends to become venturous, all the more so as there is not as yet any general unified model of number processing and calculation which could account for all tasks. Such a model could enable error types to be defined and identified on theoretically motivated grounds. Such difficulties are clearly indicated by the analysis of the results reported in studies by Dahmen/Hartje/Büssing/Sturm (1982) and Rosselli/Ardila (1989). In the former case, sophisticated statistical analysis first seemed to indicate a linguistic factor and a visuo-perceptual factor contributing to calculation errors observed in Broca's and Wernicke's aphasics, respectively. However, there was in fact significant interaction between types of aphasia and task-groups factors. In the second study, groups of patients were very small (from 3 to 13). Correlations were also task-dependent and their interpretations were not based on theory.

Finally, if some functional relationship between aphasia and acalculia were to hold in any patient, then the patients' abilities in the two domains should evolve in the same direction. This was clearly not the case of patient *8 in the study by Cohn (1971) since "the patient had recovered more effective language function, but his calculating ability had become more disturbed".

If there is any conclusion to be drawn from this body of arguments and findings, it seems to be that neither at a general level, nor at the level of particular aphasic syndromes, should there necessarily exist a simple relation between language deficits and calculation impairments.

4. Can Individual Factors Affect Relations between Aphasia and Acalculia?

In addition to the variety of mathematical tasks, to the diffuseness of the classifications of language and calculation disturbances and to the single or group study approach discussed above, it may well be that differences in the cognitive styles of patients affect the tentatively proposed relation between aphasia and acalculia.

In fact, identical lesions can result in different forms of acalculia because of the premorbid differences in the ways of performing mental calculations (Grewel 1969). Leonhard (1979) identified three quite different calculation styles followed by normals. Some people operate automatically on overt or covert verbal number forms. In such cases, a language disorder affecting the verbal sphere should secondarily induce a calculation disorder. This type of relation between aphasia and acalculia was actually reported in two patients with Gerstmann syndrome, their calculation errors being caused by verbal paraphasias (Benson/Denckla 1969). However, the functional relationship between paraphasic speech and paraphasias in the domain of number names was in fact clearly observed only in case 1 which presented paraphasic English jargon, but not in case 2 where no overt aphasia was noticed in a minimal lexical disorder marked by a slight wordfinding difficulty. Other normal people report "writing in their mind" the figures involved in calculation. They seem to manipulate numbers in the very same way they would perform operations on Arabic number forms on a sheet of paper. In such cases, alexia or agraphia for letters or words should extend to isolated digits or multidigit numbers. It must, however, be pointed out that the parallel between digits and letters is not yet clear. First, except when producing Arabic numbers in response to numbers presented in the same notation system, all other number processing or calculation tasks oblige these subjects to transcode either stimuli or responses (or both) into or from the figure system they operate upon. Following brain damage, such transcoding may of course be impaired, thus introducing an extra source of calculation error. Second, there is a difference between the nature of language and Arabic numbers since the latter system is an ideographic one, a characteristic which is highly relevant for brain machinery (see for instance Besner/Coltheart 1979 for separate orthographic and ideographic processing in normals). In fact, alexia and agraphia do not always co-occur in the two systems (Grewel 1952). But when dissociations were observed, descriptions of the premorbid calculation style of patients were unfortunately lacking, thus rendering the dissociation argument inconclusive. However, the potential role of what people write in their mind is clearly illustrated by Japanese studies showing that in mental calculation verification tasks expert abacus operators may be confused by numbers corresponding to the intermediate configuration steps of the abacus algorithm, whereas non experts were not disturbed (Hatano/Miyake/Binks 1977). Finally, there is a minority of normal people who refer to some kind of visual stereotyped diagrams as internal representations of integer number (Galton 1880 a, b; Seron/Pesenti/Deloche et al. 1992). Such subjects may also have visual diagrams for positioning other sorts of structured serial-ordered verbal material like the months of the year. Lesions of the brain affecting visuo-spatial abilities should induce acalculia as a consequence of the general visuo-spatial deficits, since their normal number-representation system and/or the procedures operating on it become impaired. Such a case was reported in which a left-sided occipito-parietal gunshot wound had impaired the patient's topographical sense, and calculation abilities, resulting in only slight speech difficulties that could not be invoked to explain the calculation disorder (Spalding/Zangwill 1950).

In the discussion of the role of premorbid idiosyncratic calculation strategies on the type of functional relation between impaired higher cortical functions (mainly language, occasionally spatial processes) and calculation thus far, it was assumed that each individual had developed just one path to master calculation. However, the possible influence of other functions like memory on both language and calculation has not yet been mentioned. Indeed, the first point has no empirical support from developmental psychology (Lawler 1981) nor from the psychology of normal (Gonzalez/Kolers 1982) or brain-damaged adults (Campbell/Clark 1988). On the contrary, these domains seem to indicate that cognitive structures depend, on the one hand, on the specific experiences encountered bearing in mind that there are many ways of dealing with numbers. On the other hand cognitive structures also interact with each other. Such interactions might involve attention (Grewel 1952), serial order processing (Benson/Weir 1972), perseverations (Grewel 1969), body schema, finger agnosia, visuo-constructive abilities (Collignon/Leclercq/Mahy 1977), and processing capacities (Benson/Weir 1972). The latter authors reported a case where the patient's deficit appeared only when a number of steps had to be carried out simultaneously; the patient had no difficulties performing single steps or other mental operations.

Ideally, the question of relating aphasia and acalculia should also consider the two deficits in relation to some theory of spontaneous recovery and of neuropsychological rehabilitation, since what is observed following brain damage is not produced by an intact brain, and consequently does not necessarily reflect the premorbid architecture of functions of that brain. In other words, depending on the post-onset neurophysiological processes (structural redundancy, closing of the diaschisis, vicariance) that subserve behavioral modifications (restoration of functions, reteaching previous knowledge, building new strategies) the relation between aphasia and acalculia in a patient might equally well fail to mirror the prior hypothetical functional relation between language and calculation in a normal subject.

5. Are there Functional Relations between Disturbed Language and Calculation Components at the Higher Level of Semiotic Systems?

As mentioned above, there are a lot of arguments which imply that there are hardly any mandatory functional relationships between aphasia and acalculia. But these conclusions might be misleading for the simple reason that the analyses of data did not consider the relevant formalization levels in the two domains.

Grewel (1952) pointed out that the different notation systems used for representing quantities by different number forms should be considered as semiotic systems with their own distinctive features. Accordingly, each numerical system is broken down into several components: (i) the set of symbols used; (ii) the semantic interpretation of numbers; and (iii) the syntactic rules for combining and manipulating numbers (Grewel 1969). He concluded that the three semiotic systems (Arabic digits, verbal and orthographic numbers) might be independently affected by brain damage since "they represent different symbolic systems with a different syntax". Having thus situated acalculia within the paradigm of semiotic disorders, the initial question of its relation to aphasia may be reformulated. The relationships should be considered between the three different components (lexicon, semantics, syntax and computational rules) of each number notation system (arabic, orthographic, verbal numbers) on the one hand, and the corresponding components of language and speech on the other. From a general as well as a formal point of view, divergencies in the linguistic structures of verbal numbers should constitute different sources of difficulty and therefore induce different disturbances in calculation. Grewel (1952) illustrated this point on the different systems for teens in English and French. We have reported data in the same direction, for instance in the transcoding of 75 into the Wallonian regular decade-unit structure (*septante* (70) *cinq* (5)), as compared to the more complicated phonographic form in French (*soixante* (60) *quinze* (15)); see Deloche/Seron (1984 a).

In some ways, the semiotic level approach is linked to Finkelnburg's (1870) (see Duffy/Liles 1979 for translation) theory of asymbolia. Within such unitary views, different semiotic systems should be subserved by common mechanisms, and consequently brain damage should not cause system-specific deficits, but should affect many symbolic usages. Ferro/Bothelo (1980) have reported the case of two patients with asymbolic acalculia whose only deficit in numerical abilities was the misidentification of arithmetic signs. But contrary to expectations in the theoretical framework of asymbolia, patient *1 clearly showed no extension of impaired processing for other symbolic systems like letters, numbers, traffic signs, playing cards, emblems of political parties, horoscope signs, and so on.

The authors interpreted their patients' disorders as cases of alexia for a special lexicon, arithmetical signs.

Therefore the semiotic level analysis, originally formulated by Grewel (1952) for numerical systems, does not seem to provide a theoretical framework which reveals simple relations between the consequences of brain damage on the different components described in language and speech on the one hand and their formal corresponding relations in calculation on the other.

6. Are there Functional Relations between Language and Calculation Components at the Level of Formal Languages?

Stated in contemporary terms of formal language theory, the three components of the different numerical semiotic systems described by Grewel (1952; 1969) would refer to the following classification:

The set of symbols used in a notation system is its lexicon, the interpretation of numbers is its semantics, and the rules governing the well-formedness of lexical primitives into legal number forms is its syntax. It seems that Grewel (1952; 1969) considered syntax to involve not only the integration of the elements of lexicons into well-formed numbers, but also to extend to the computational rules for performing operations like borrowing from and carrying over. At the level of formal languages, such computational knowledge should not be included in the syntactical systems of the different number notations (Arabic digits, phonographic number forms).

Such a formal approach to numerical systems is intriguing because it identifies components strictly parallel to those described in language and speech, and because the numerical components are far more simple to analyse and formalize than those manipulated in natural languages. Lexicons contain only few primitives (the ten digits from 0 to 9 for Arabic numbers, less than thirty words for verbal and orthographic integers). The semantics of numbers are also straightforward; namely, the meaning of a number is the quantity it refers to. And syntaxes are limited to a few grammatical rules (see for instance Deloche/Seron 1986). Moreover, there is a one-to-one correspondence between the different notation forms of any number, which is by no means the case between two different natural languages with the problems due to lexical ambiguities, idiomatic expressions and so on. Several authors have thus proposed explicit descriptions of numerical lexicons, syntaxes and semantics, and applied them to transcoding processes between Arabic numbers and verbal or orthographic number forms (Power/Longuet-Higgins 1978; Deloche/Seron 1982 a; Mc Closkey/Caramazza 1987; Cohen/Dehaene 1991).

From this standpoint, we have looked for some formal parallels between the level of deficits (lexical, syntactic) in language on the one hand, and numerical transcoding errors in aphasic patients on the other hand in both group studies (Deloche/Seron 1982 b; 1986; Seron/Deloche 1984), and in single cases (Deloche/Seron 1984 b; 1985). The group studies seem to indicate some very gross relations between lexical/syntactical language processing preserved/impaired abilities of Broca's or Wernicke's aphasics and their types of numerical transcoding impairments. However, the numbers of patients with Broca's or Wernicke's aphasia were small, and thus firm conclusions could not be established. The double dissociation paradigm seems more appropriate for indicating parallels, in preserved/impaired lexical/syntactical performances of brain damaged patients, between language and calculation performances.

This line of research of functional relations between language and calculation, aphasia and acalculia may seem promising. However, this relation is not mandatory for lexical processing, since as already indicated alexia and agraphia for letters may occur without corresponding impairments for digits. At the semantic level, the assumption of a unique semantic representation for each number seems quite unrealistic when one considers the constellation of usages and meanings for numbers, which ranges from such items as cardinality, prices, or private bank account numbers, room numbers in an hotel, bus line numbers in the city to nursery rhymes and numbers in idiomatic expressions. However, the results seem more encouraging for syntax. In this domain, we have reported the case of an agrammatic patient where data from linguistic tasks and from (Roman and Arabic) number processing supported Grossman's (1980) hypothesis of a central processor for hierarchically structured material in different notation systems (Deloche/Seron 1985).

7. Some Tentatively Concluding Remarks

On the one hand, I have presented some methodological and theoretical arguments that seem to indicate that at present a general functional relation between aphasia and acalculia cannot be clearly established. The factors to be considered include the type of idiosyncratic calculation style premorbidly developed by subjects, the potentially differential effects of brain damage on the architectures of language processing and of calculation, the formal levels of analyses (and diffuseness of classification deficits) where relations between the two domains may be studied, the diversity of meanings attached to numbers depending on context of usage, the ideographic or phonographic natures of notation systems, the degrees of generalities expected from single cases or group studies and so forth.

On the other hand, since calculation and number processing are well learned and extensively used in everyday life, and because of the relative simplicity of the different notation systems, one of which is ideographic and almost universal (Arabic numbers), the other being phonographic and thus related to each language, the domain of calculation presents many interesting aspects in developmental psychology, psychology, neuropsychology, artificial intelligence and more generally in the field of cognitive sciences. It seems to me that looking for correlations in order to investigate the lawfulness of mental processes in different domains should first be restricted to the study of many single cases. It is in this way that preserved/impaired calculation abilities may highlight some theoretical issues of concern generally studied in other high level cognitive activities. Among others such issues may encompass the distinctions between operative and figurative cognition (Gardner/Strub/Albert 1975), between conscious and automatic processing (Leleux/Kaiser/Lebrun 1979), between autonomous and non autonomous mechanisms (Zbrodoff/Logan 1986), between procedural and declarative knowledge in the field of memory (Squire 1987), between single abstract format-independent representations in modular systems (Sokol/Goodman-Schulman/McCloskey 1989) and integrated networks with format-specific representations and procedures (Campbell/Clark 1988). Multiple single case analyses conducted in such directions should not consider calculation to be representative of the other higher cortical functions, but they should nonetheless provide some insights into the different areas of cognition and thus contribute to significant advances in disentangling the intricacy of human cognitive machinery.

8. References

Ardila, A. & Rosseli, M. (1990). Acalculias. *Behavioural Neurology, 3*, 39–48.

Benson, D. F. & Denckla, M. B. (1969). Verbal paraphasia as a cause of calculation disturbances. *Archives of Neurology, 21*, 96–102.

Benson, D. F. & Weir, W. F. (1972). Acalculia: Acquired anarithmetia. *Cortex, 8 (4)*, 465–472.

Besner, D. & Coltheart, M. (1979). Ideographic and alphabetic processing in skilled readers of English. *Neuropsychologia, 14*, 467–472.

Boller, F. & Grafman, J. (1983). Acalculia: Historical development and current significance. *Brain and Language, 2*, 205–223.

Campbell, J. I. D. & Clark J. M. (1988). An encoding-complex view of cognitive number processing: Comments on Mc Closkey, Sokol, and Goodman (1986). *Journal of Experimental Psychology: General, 117 (2)*, 204–214.

Claros-Salinas, D. & von Cramon, D. (1987). Diagnostik von Störungen im Umgang mit Zahlen (Akalkulie). *Fortschr. Neurologie Psychiatrie, 55*, 239–248.

Cohen, L. & Dehaene, S. (1991). Neglect dyslexia for numbers? A case report. *Cognitive Neuropsychology, 8 (1)*, 39–58.

Cohn, R. (1971). Arithmetic and learning disabilities. In H. R. Myklebust (Ed.), *Progress in Learning Disabilities. 322–389.* New York: Grune & Sratton.

Collignon, R., Leclercq, C., & Mahy, J. (1977). Etude de la sémiologie des troubles du calcul observés au cours des lésions corticales. *Acta Neurologica Belgica, 77*, 257–275.

Dahmen, W., Hartje, W., Büssing, A., & Sturm, W. (1982). Disorders of calculation in aphasic patients – spatial and verbal components. *Neuropsychologia, 20*, 145–153.

Deloche, G. & Seron, X. (1982 a). From one to 1: An analysis of a transcoding process by means of neuropsychological data. *Cognition, 12*, 119–149.

Deloche, G. & Seron, X. (1982 b). From three to 3: A differential analysis of skills in transcoding quantities between patients with Broca's and Wernicke's aphasia. *Brain, 105*, 719–733.

Deloche, G. & Seron, X. (1984 a). Some linguistic components of acalculia. In F. C. Rose (Ed.), *Advances in Neurology, Vol. 42: Progress in Aphasiology. 215–222.* New York: Raven Press.

Deloche, G. & Seron, X. (1984 b). Semantic errors reconsidered in the procedural light of stack concepts. *Brain and Language, 21*, 59–71.

Deloche, G. & Seron, X. (1985). Syntactical knowledge in a case of agrammatism: Evidence from transcoding Roman to Arabic numerals. *Brain and Language, 25*, 234–245.

Deloche, G. & Seron, X. (1986). Grammaticality judgments by aphasics of alphabetically written numeral forms. *Psychologica Belgica, 36 (1)*, 17–42.

Deloche, G. & Seron, X. (1989). *Protocole de dépistage des troubles du calcul et du traitement des nombres, EC 301*. Paris: La Salpêtrière Hospital.

Deloche, G., Seron, X., & Bergego, C. (1989). Traitement des nombres et calcul: Données théoriques et perspectives thérapeutiques. *Annales de Réadaptation et de Médecine Physique, 32*, 627–637.

Duffy, R. J. & Liles, B. Z. (1979). A translation of Finkelnburg's (1870) lecture on aphasia as "asymbolia" with commentary. *Journal of Speech and Hearing Disorders, 44*, 156–168.

Ferro, J. M. & Bothelo, M.A.S. (1980). Alexia for arithmetical signs: A cause of disturbed calculation. *Cortex, 16*, 175–180.

Fuson, K. (1984). More complexities in substraction. *Journal of Research in Mathematics Education, 15 (3)*, 214–225.

Galton, F. (1880 a). Visualised numerals. *Nature, 21*, 252–256.

Galton, F. (1880 b). Visualised numerals. *Nature, 21*, 494–495.

Gardner, H., Strub, R., & Albert, M. L. (1975). A unimodal deficit in operational thinking. *Brain and Language, 2*, 333–344.

Gonzalez, E. G. & Kolers, P. A. (1982). Mental manipulation of arithmetic symbols. *Journal of Experimental Psychology: Learning, Memory and Cognition, 8 (4)*, 308–319.

Grewel, F. (1952). Acalculia. *Brain, 75*, 397–407.

Grewel, F. (1969). The Acalculias. In P. J. Vinken & G. Bruyn (Eds.), *Handbook of Clinical Neurology, 3. 181–196*. Amsterdam: North Holland.

Grossman, M. (1980). A central processor for hierarchically structured material: Evidence from Broca's aphasia. *Neuropsychologia, 18*, 299–308.

Hatano, G., Miyake, Y., & Binks, M. G. (1977). Performance of expert abacus operators. *Cognition, 5*, 57–71.

Hécaen, H., Angelergues, R., & Houillier, S. (1961). Les variétés cliniques des acalculies au cours des lésions rétrorolandiques: Approche statistique du problème. *Revue Neurologique, 105*, 85–103.

Henschen, S. E. (1919). Über Sprache, Musik und Rechenmechanismen und ihre Lokalisationen im Großhirn. *Zeitschrift für die gesamte Neurologie und Psychiatrie, 52*, 273–298.

Hitch, G. J. (1978). The numerical abilities of industrial trainee apprentices. *Journal of Occupational Psychology, 51*, 163–176.

Kosc, L. (1980). To the problem of diffuseness in terminology in the field of disturbances and disorders of mathematical abilities. *Focus on Learning Problems in Mathematics, 2 (4)*, 79–83.

Lawler, R. W. (1981). The progressive construction of mind. *Cognitive Science, 5*, 1–30.

Leleux, C., Kaiser, G., & Lebrun, Y. (1979). Dyscalculia in a right-handed teacher of mathematics with right cerebral damage. In Y. Lebrun & R. Hoops (Eds.), *Problems in Aphasia: Neurolinguistics, 9. 141–158*. Lisse: Swets & Zeitlinger B. V.

Leonhard, K. (1979). Ideokinetic aphasia and related disorders. In Y. Lebrun & R. Hoops (Eds.), *Problems in Aphasia: Neurolinguistics, 9. 11–77*. Lisse: Swets and Zeitlinger.

McCloskey, M. & Caramazza, A. (1987). Cognitive mechanisms in normal and impaired number processing. In G. Deloche & X. Seron (Eds.), *Mathematical Disabilities: A Cognitive Neuropsychological Perspective. 201–219*. Hillsdale: Lawrence Erlbaum Associates.

Power, R. J. D. & Longuet-Higgins, F. R. S. (1978). Learning to count: A computational model of language acquisition, *Proceedings of the Royal Society London, 200*, 391–417.

Rosseli, M. & Ardila, A. (1989). Calculation deficits in patients with right and left hemisphere damage. *Neuropsychologia, 27*, 607–618.

Secada, W. G., Fuson, K. C., & Halls, J. W. (1983). The transition from counting-all to counting-on in addition. *Journal for Research in Mathematics Education, 14 (1)*, 47–57.

Seron, X. & Deloche, G. (1984). From 2 to two: An analysis of a transcoding process by means of neuropsychological evidence. *Journal of Psycholinguistic Research, 13* , 215–236.

Seron, X., Pesenti, M., Noel, M. P., Deloche, G., & Cornet, J. (1992). Images of numbers, or when 98 is upper left and 6 sky blue. *Cognition, 44*. 159–196.

Sokol, S. M., Goodman-Schulman, A. R., & McCloskey, M. (1989). In defense of a modular architecture for the number processing system: Reply to Campbell and Clark. *Journal of Experimental Psychology: General, 111 (1)*, 105–110.

Spalding, J. M. K. & Zangwill, O. L. (1950). Disturbance of numberform in a case of brain injury. *Journal of Neurology, Neurosurgery and Psychiatry, 13*, 24–29.

Squire, L. R. (1987). *Memory and Brain*. New York: Oxford University Press.

Zbrodoff, N. J. & Logan, G. D. (1986). On the autonomy of mental processes: A case study of arithmetic. *Journal of Experimental Psychology: General, 115 (2)*, 118–130.

Gérard Deloche, Paris (France)

30. Short-Term Memory in Aphasia

1. Introduction

There is no doubt that language processing is highly complex. It involves at least the coordinated execution of multiple linguistic processes that subserve each of several segmental types of information represented in language. It is possible, however, that even a fully elaborated account of these linguistic processes may not be adequate to explain our efficient use of language material. Thus, our ability to understand, repeat or express a sentence may turn as well on some facility with processes not typically thought to be 'linguistic' such as learning and memory. Several studies have begun to probe whether memory plays a role in sentence processing, and more recently, to incorporate memory in some specific fashion in a model of sentence processing. The ultimate goal is that a more realistic processing account of language use can be achieved, that is, a description of the cognitive and linguistic elements that interact in order for us to understand, repeat, or express a sentence.

This review will specifically examine whether short-term memory plays a role in sentence processing. In order to focus the scope of such a review, I will concentrate on data obtained from observations of adults with brain damage attempting to process sentence material. Space limitations prevent a discussion of the cerebral topographic representation or neurotransmitter basis for memory functioning in language. The data discussed below can be interpreted to support the claim that short-term memory plays a role in sentence processing, and in some cases may even be said to play a specific role in a particular language task, but it may be premature to state that memory deficits can account entirely for impaired sentence comprehension, repetition, or expression.

2. Memory Disorders in Aphasic Patients

There is ample evidence that aphasics have a memory impairment. Some of this evidence will be reviewed below. It is unclear, however, whether this memory deficit necessarily contributes to aphasics' language difficulties, or whether the memory impairment is a bystander that happens to co-occur but without any direct impact on language processing. Indeed, it is possible that an aphasic disorder may prevent patients from learning or recalling verbal material.

2.1. Do Aphasics Have a Memory Impairment?

The technique of Peterson/Peterson (1959) has frequently been used to document a short-term memory (STM) impairment. This involves the presentation of the stimulus material, following which the subject performs a task such as mental arithmetic for a specified period of time, and then stimulus recall is probed. The mental arithmetic prevents explicit rehearsal of the stimulus material prior to recall, and the length of time between presentation and recall establishes the decay characteristics of the memory trace.

Consider some representative early studies of memory in aphasia. Butters/Samuels/Goodglass/Brody (1970) found that aphasics are significantly impaired in their recognition of visual and auditory single phonemes and consonant trigrams using the Peterson/Peterson (1959) technique. Goodglass/Gleason/Hyde (1970) asked aphasics to point to a series of pictures corresponding to a list of nouns read to them. Anomic, conduction, and Wernicke's types of aphasics exhibited significantly better pointing span scores than so-called Broca's aphasics. Although not without fault, findings such as these have been taken as evidence that a verbal memory impairment can be seen in aphasic patients.

Consider in more detail the significance of these memory deficits in aphasics. It is possible that the memory impairment reflects some general properties of the language material which may be difficult for aphasics. For example, some have focused on the observation that words are sequentially ordered in a sentence, and it may be difficulty remembering this sequential order that accounts in part for aphasics' sentence processing difficulty. De Renzi/Nichelli (1975) asked brain-damaged patients to repeat a series of digits orally, point to a written sequence of orally presented digits, and point to a series of pictures corresponding to an orally presented series of words. Broca's, Wernicke's and global types of aphasics were significantly more impaired than non-aphasic patients with left hemisphere insult on all of these span tasks. However, aphasic and non-aphasic groups did not differ in their ability to repeat a spatially-presented pointing sequence. These authors argued that aphasic patients' deficits are due to difficulty holding verbal information in a specific sequence or order. However, such an account would have to explain how non-aphasic patients with frontal lobe insult also exhibit deficits in the temporal organization of information in memory (Milner/Petrides/Smith 1985). Within the domain of language, moreover, there are language processing devices represented in the grammatical or semantic features of a language processor which help circumvent dependence on the linear character of the input string.

Another approach has been adopted by Cermak and his associates. Cermak has cast aphasics' memory impairment within a general model of memory. Cermak/Moreines (1976) presented a list of words to aphasics, and asked the patients to indicate when a word had been repeated in the list. Aphasics encountered increasing difficulty recognizing a repeated word as the number of words between the initial presentation and the subsequent repetition increased. Cermak/Tarlow (1978; also Riege/Metter/Hanson 1980) attempted to prove the specificity of this finding for language processing by demonstrating the effect only for the presentation of verbal material but not non-verbal material. Cermak/Moreines (1976; Cermak/Stiassny/Uhly 1984) also found that aphasics were even more compromised when asked to detect repeated rhymes or repeated words from the same semantic category. When patients were allowed more processing time or given instructions prior to list presentation, improvement was seen in the detection of semantically similar items but not rhymes. Riege/Metter/Hanson (1980) performed an analysis of patients' errors on their detection task, and found that many false positives were phonemically-based.

Results such as these have been interpreted within the framework of a 'depth of processing' approach (e.g. Craik/Lockhart 1972) that suggests a differential impairment in the encoding of phonemic information in comparison to semantic information. It may be possible, however, to explain patterns of results such as these without relying on an independent theory of memory. Thus, these data do not rule out the possibility of a compromised language processing device where access to a phonologically-based code for a word is relatively compromised when compared to access via a semantically-based code (Blumstein/Baker/Goodglass 1977).

Others have taken this type of criticism quite seriously. These investigators have suggested that the aphasic patients' memory system is relatively intact, but that their language impairment may lead to the appearance of a deficit on certain memory tasks. Rothi/Hutchinson (1981), for example, found that aphasics encounter difficulty encoding the verbal information represented in the stimulus material used for their assessment of word list memory. Locke/Deck (1978) found that superspan list learning varied depending on whether or not the lists were composed of words that the patients could use for naming. Ostergaard/Meudell (1984; also Heilman/Scholes/Watson 1976) found that Broca's aphasics and Wernicke's aphasics are severely compromised on a word span task. An assessment of the locus of patients' errors indicated that Broca's aphasics do not exhibit a primacy effect. The rehearsal of encoded material may be troublesome for Broca's aphasics because of their 'expression' difficulty (Martin 1990).

It is important to point out that aphasic patients' memory impairments are not necessarily restricted to the verbal domain. Boller/De Renzi (1967; Gainotti/Caltagirone/Miceli 1978) found that left hemisphere-damaged patients are significantly more impaired than right hemisphere-damaged patients in their recall of visually presented information such as meaningful and meaningless pictures. Kelter/Cohen/Engel (1977) found that fluent aphasics are impaired in their recall of meaningful pictures as well as snowflake patterns, while non-fluent aphasics encounter difficulty only in their recall of the snowflake patterns. Ostergaard/Meudell (1984) found that Broca's aphasics encountered difficulty remembering faces. Goodglass/Denes/Calderon (1974) have suggested that aphasics are unable to use any form of covert verbal mediation to support their participation in non-linguistic processes such as their memory of non-verbal material. These observations call to question the material specificity of aphasics' memory disorder and the role which this type of memory impairment may play in aphasics' language processing difficulties.

Episodic memory thus may be impaired in aphasics. Does this mean that this memory disorder plays a causal role in their language deficit? It is possible that it is actually the aphasia that interferes with the ability to acquire, encode, and/or retrieve the verbal material. Indeed, even if aphasics do have an episodic memory impairment, this is not restricted to the verbal domain and thus may not be related to their language difficulty.

3. Do Memory Impairments Play a Specific Role in Sentence Repetition, Comprehension, and Expression?

One of the general problems potentially limiting our ability to specify the relationship between memory and language is that the verbal material used in the above assessments of memory may not be truly 'linguistic' in nature. Though elegant experimentally, it may be difficult to leap from the random lists of letters or words to the highly organized phonologic or grammatical information which is so critical to our daily language. This problem may be circumvented by manipulating sentence material instead of consonants and trigrams. A second general problem is the type of memory evaluated in these studies. The conscious attempt to learn and recall specific facts is generally referred to as 'episodic memory'. When trying to understand or express a sentence, however, we do not ordinarily try to remember the sentence as we might learn a fact. Instead, there may be a transient mental representation of a sentence while it is being processed or otherwise manipulated mentally. It is this fleeting trace of a sentence which is addressed below.

3.1. Working Memory in Sentence Processing

The theory often implicated in sentence processing is the model of 'working memory' described by Baddeley (1986). A 'central executive' is said to manage the selective input of a stimulus into an information processing system. One component of the central executive regulates the distribution of finite attentional resources. There is also a limited storage component. When this is overwhelmed, either because of excessive processing demands or a large volume of input data, excess information can be stored temporarily in an associated slave system. The specific salve system which is recruited varies depending on the modality or material of the input data, and in the case of language is thought to be an 'articulatory loop'. The articulatory loop in turn is composed of two elements – a phonological store and an articulatory rehearsal mechanism. The rehearsal mechanism can refresh the content of the phonological store. Working memory thus may serve as a interface between a perceptual device and a computational mechanism such as a sentence parser.

While remarkably powerful and clearly capable of accounting for a wide variety of phenomena, it is just this universal applicability that may prove to be a shortcoming of the working memory model. The roles of short-term memory (STM) postulated in sentence comprehension, repetition, and sentence expression often appear to be quite similar, but this is not necessarily the case. Sentence processing may be supported by a general purpose STM such as the working memory model, or there may be a series of special-purpose STM processors with slightly different characteristics that are particularly suited to the needs of, say, a grammatical processing device (e.g. Berwick/Weinberg 1984; Marcus 1980). Below I explore the possibilities that language-impaired patients have deficits in working memory that interfere with language functioning, and that amnesic patients with deficits in working memory have language disorders.

3.2. The Role of Short-Term Memory in Sentence Repetition

One type of task where language and memory are thought to interact is sentence repetition. In repeating a sentence, the subject must remember the initial parts of the sentence while the remainder of the sentence continues to be presented. In a sense, then, one part of a sentence may be playing the role of filler material that interferes with active rehearsal during the process of remembering the entire sentence. From this perspective, sentence repetition may resemble the Peterson/Peterson technique. Nevertheless, sentence repetition is sensitive to the processing of linguistic material that has phonologic, grammatical, and semantic attributes. It is for this reason that sentence repetition differs from the repetition of an equally long list of unrelated words.

Analyses of performance profiles in conduction aphasia have served as the natural arena for studying the relative role of these mnestic and linguistic processes in sentence repetition. Green/Howes (1977) reviewed the clinical features of the 52 cases of conduction aphasia in the literature at the time of their report. According to these authors, the major characteristics of conduction aphasia include a severe impairment in repetition despite normal or mildly impaired auditory comprehension and mild to moderate deficits of spontaneous speech. Secondary deficits include mild to moderate difficulty with reading comprehension and serial speech, but moderate to severe deficits in oral reading, writing, and naming. An error analysis indicates that literal and verbal paraphasias, jargon, and grammatical errors occur in equal proportions in conduction aphasics' repetition, spontaneous speech, naming, and oral reading.

While there may be some agreement on the broad clinical picture of conduction aphasia, there is little consensus on the nature of the disrupted mechanism that underlies the repetition deficit. The classic explanation roughly states that there is limited information transfer from an input device to an output device (Geschwind 1965; Kinsbourne 1972). Goldstein (1948) specifically suggested that there may be a disruption of 'inner speech' which results in difficulty relating non-verbal mental phenomena to external speech. Relatedly, Alajouanine/Lhermitte (1964) have characterized the repetition impairment in terms of an unstable phonological trace. Hecaen/Dell/Roger (1955; Dubois/Hecaen/Angelergues et al. 1964) elaborated these claims by specifying that thoughts may have structural attributes that can be ordered, selected, and otherwise regulated. It is argued by these investigators that conduction aphasics cannot appreciate the sequence of mental forms constituting the information which must be repeated. Moreover, certain types of words appear to be particularly difficult for conduction aphasics to repeat in an utterance or to use in spontaneous speech. For example, low frequency words are said to be more difficult to repeat than high frequency words, sentences with conjunctions and complex structures may be more difficult than simple utterances, and verbs may be more difficult than nouns which are more difficult than initial articles.

Shallice/Warrington (1977), Warrington/Logue/Pratt (1971), and Warrington/Shallice (1969) have published an elegant series of case descriptions which point to an entirely different type of explanation for the repetition deficit in conduction aphasia. These investigators have suggested that the repetition deficit is due to an auditory-verbal STM impairment. This type of explanation is a direct extension of Baddeley's (1986) working memory model, applied in this case to the auditory-verbal domain. Specifically, these authors found that their patients are profoundly limited in their auditory digit span, a standardized task that has been taken to measure STM. Moreover, this impairment was much more evident in the auditory modality than when equivalent strings were presented in the visual modality. Using the Peterson/Peterson technique, a decrement in performance was observed at longer delay conditions. The authors were careful to rule out several other possible explanations for their patients' impairments, demonstrating that the deficit can not be attributed to a perceptual, comprehension, or expression deficit. Tests of long-term memory such as paired associate learning and logical memory subtests of the Wechsler Memory Scale failed to reveal significant abnormalities, suggesting a relatively specific STM problem. On the basis of these findings, it was claimed that the repetition deficit in conduction aphasia can be attributed to a selective defect of auditory-verbal STM.

Tzortzis/Albert (1974) and Strub/Gardner (1974) have seized on several inconsistencies in these observations in an attempt to demonstrate that the deficit in conduction aphasia is linguistic in nature rather than mnestic. Conduction aphasics' performance on digit span tasks replicated the results described above. However, Tzortzis/Albert (1974) and Strub/Gardner (1974) emphasized that there is more difficultly repeating items in the correct sequence than simply reproducing the items regardless of the sequence. A decrement in performance was also seen with more rapid rates of presentation. Strub/Gardner's analysis of incorrect responses indicated many paraphasic errors rather than the omission of items that might be expected in a memory impairment. Patients demonstrated an advantage for the repetition of meaningful and more familiar material, and they were able to recognize whether paired sequences of digits are similar. Characteristics such as these do not support strong claims that the deficit in conduction aphasia is due to a STM impairment. Conduction aphasics also encountered difficulty on tasks assessing structural aspects of linguistic material such as later portions of the Token Test. Impairments in the repetition of non-verbal material such as musical notes, meaningful sounds, and rhythms called to question the specificity of the memory disorder for language material. There were also impairments on perceptual identification tasks, suggesting reduced appreciation of the input stream.

Focusing on the relative difficulty repeating sequences correctly compared to the relative success repeating items in an order-free fashion, Tzortzis/Albert (1974) supported Hecaen/Dell/Roger's (1955) claim that conduction aphasics are compromised because of difficulty reproducing the organizational attributes of the target material. However, this type of explanation fails to account for the patients' consistent ability to repeat visually-presented material more accurately than auditory material. Strub/Gardner (1974) felt that conduction aphasics exhibit difficulty decoding the auditory input signal for transformation into phonological shapes. This was based in part on the finding of a significant decrement in performance with more rapid rates of presentation and the difficulty with perceptual identification tasks.

Caramazza/Berndt/Basili/Koller (1981) attempted to compare the mnestic and linguistic hypotheses in their examination of a conduction aphasic MC. Unfortunately, there was not a clear outcome supporting one hypothesis or the other. MC exhibited a reduced digit span, as did the other patients described above. The pattern of MC's errors revealed more sensitivity to list length than to the length of the delay between presentation and response, interpreted as support for a STM impairment. An analysis of repetition errors revealed a primacy effect but not a recency effect, consistent with the STM hypothesis, but a recognition task probing each of the serial positions in a digit sequence revealed equivalent treatment of initial and terminal items. An advantage for visually-presented sequences over auditorily-presented sequences of material was seen in MC's memory performance, consistent with the Warrington/Shallice data and Strub/Gardner's observations, but there was also better repetition performance when scored in an order-free fashion as compared to scoring that penalized for incorrect sequencing of material. A material-specific repetition effect was seen for the presentation of some auditory materials but not others. Thus, lists of functors were repeated very poorly compared to lists of nouns, but high frequency noun sequences were repeated as accurately as low frequency noun sequences. While MC exhibited impairments on assessments of structural aspects of language material such as grammar, he exhibited little difficulty on tasks requiring lexical processing. Caramazza tentatively concluded that the STM hypothesis is the best available account of conduction aphasia.

Allport (1984) also compared the mnestic and linguistic hypotheses in several conduction aphasics. As with Strub/Gardner (1974), but unlike Caramazza/Berndt/Basili/Koller (1981), Allport found an effect for word frequency. There was also an effect for word imagability, but no disadvantage for the repetition of functors. An auditory discrimination task revealed significant difficulty, and an analysis of repetition errors revealed many literal paraphasias. In contrast to Caramazza/Berndt/Basili/Koller (1981), Allport (1984) concluded that the repetition deficit in conduction aphasia is due to an impairment decoding the auditory input signal, and that this impairment in fact underlies the STM deficit.

It is difficult to resolve competing claims such as these. Several tasks such as digit span have been administered to all of the cases discussed above. However, a common set of baseline tasks and a common method of analysis have not been identified. Without this common body of information, it remains difficult to determine whether there are two populations of conduction aphasics, as suggested by Shallice/Warrington (1977). These authors indicate that one group of conduction aphasics may have a prominent 'reproduction' deficit, that is, difficulty specifically repeating single words composed of many syllables (see below), but the second group may have a 'true repetition' deficit. Moreover, while the above studies correlated performance on STM tasks with repetition performance, there has been very little manipulation or qualitative analysis of the sentential material which conduction aphasics are attempting to repeat.

Ostrin/Schwartz (1986) responded to this challenge in their study of sentence repetition in six agrammatic aphasics. Their patients had difficulty repeating a target sentence, but their detailed analysis in fact indicated an important interaction between linguistic elements and the retained memory trace of the target. The NP_1-V-NP_2 sentences that were presented as targets varied in terms of a grammatical variable (they were in the active voice or passive voice) and the sentences varied in terms of a semantic variable (they were reversible sentences (NP_1 and NP_2 could be interchanged) or non-reversible sentences (NP_1 and NP_2 could be interchanged) or non-reversible sentences (NP_1 could not be exchanged with NP_2) which were either plausible or implausible). It should be noted that a change in the voice of an implausible item would make the item plausible. The results revealed that subjects made more errors in their attempts to repeat passive than active sentences, and most errors were in the repetition of closed class items. These findings alone are ambiguous with respect to the mnestic and linguistic hypotheses: Passive voice items are longer, and difficulty here may be due in part to a limited STM, but the material – specific difficulty with closed class items appears more consistent with a linguistically-based impairment. An error analysis revealed different types of responses to the semantic variable depending on the voice of the target, and this analysis suggests one possible resolution of the mnestic-linguistic conflict. In the active voice, omissions of free grammatical morphemes accounted for the errors in reversible and plausible items, but mixed morphology errors (combining together elements of active and passive voice) were seen in implausible items. The order of major sentential constituents was maintained.

Ostrin/Schwartz argued that, for the mixed morphology type of error to occur in the implausible items, patients must have a memory trace of the target after which they can pattern their responses. This must consist of some mental representation of surface word order or its argument structure. The authors go on to state that patients must also have a bias toward producing semantically coherent sentences. In order to maintain word order while respecting semantic coherency, patients apparently add an element of the passive voice to their responses on implausible items presented in the active voice. That is, patients attempt to modify the voice of an active implausible item toward the passive in order to make the item seem plausible. The same type of explanation is used to account for the mixed morphology errors in the passive voice. The authors did not state whether the patients are told beforehand that they will hear some implausible items, nor did they monitor whether the patients are aware of the anomalous nature of the implausible items. Thus, the role of a decoding deficit in these patients is not clear. Nevertheless, in terms of defining the role of mnestic and linguistic processes in sentence repetition, the important point of this study is that an analysis of patients' repetitions suggests an interaction of partially compromised grammatical and STM processors.

3.3. The Role of Short-Term Memory in Sentence Comprehension

While a potential role for memory in sentence repetition seems fairly obvious, it has become apparent only more recently that STM may also contribute significantly to sentence comprehension. It is somewhat trivial to state that memory may be a factor in the comprehension of very long sentences, but recent observations suggest the possibility that STM may also play a role in supporting the comprehension of certain grammatical features of a sentence regardless of sentence length.

3.3.1. Sentence Comprehension in Stroke Patients

Linguistic analyses of the aphasias have often led to characterizations of so-called Broca's aphasics as agrammatic. Thus, these patients were said to omit grammatical morphemes from their spontaneous speech and to express themselves with utterances consisting of one or two nouns and possibly a verb – so-called telegraphic speech. This was thought to be a characteristic of their writing, repetition, and oral reading as well. In comprehension, moreover, it was claimed that Broca's aphasics encounter considerable difficulty interpreting sentences which turn on grammatically-specified relationships between the words constituting the utterance. While there have been some observations of modality-specific grammatical impairments (Miceli/Mazzucchi/Menn/Goodglass 1983; Nespoulous/Dordain/Perron et al. 1988), the hypothesis has nevertheless been forwarded that Broca's aphasics may not be competent with respect to syntactic appreciation (Berndt/Caramazza 1980).

This 'syntactic loss' hypothesis has recently been called to question. One type of objection has focussed on the difficulty which this theory has for the different levels of performance that are seen across different sentence types: If a syntactic capacity is lost, it is argued, then it ought to be lost across-the-board. Kolk/van Grunsven (1985) examined eleven Dutch-speaking aphasics who were generally representative of patients with a so-called Broca's aphasia. On a sentence-picture matching task where active, locative, and passive sentences were used, they observed differing levels of accuracy for each sentence type across patients. A second type of objection has focused on the observation that each patient exhibits a varying degree of impairment depending on the sentence type. Relatedly, variability has been observed across identical sets of items administered to the same subject repeatedly, such as on successive days. Kolk/van Grunsven argued that inter-subject and intra-subject variability such as this are incompatible with the 'syntactic loss' hypothesis.

Several attempts to explain these types of variability have been proposed. Since these are not 'on-line' tasks, it is possible that patients can rely on a variety of non-specific 'strategies' to understand sentences. Caramazza/Zurif (1976) pointed out that Broca's aphasics can reliably match a sentence to a picture if non-reversible nouns are used in the sentence's arguments. This allows only one possible semantic interpretation of the sentence, even if the sentence is relatively complex grammatically. Bootstrapping strategies such as reliance on SVO word-ordering (which is typical in English) and dependence on sentential relations derived from thematic roles have also been proposed (e. g. Caplan 1983). It can be countered that these heuristic strategies may be very tedious, and their intricacy can potentially occupy a large amount of processing space, so they may not be very efficient or even useable in the real world. There is also evidence arguing against the likelihood that patients use even simple word order or semantic bootstrapping strategies (Kolk/van Grunsven 1985; Schwartz/Saffran/Marin 1980).

Another approach to the problem of variability has been to attribute sentence comprehension impairments to a deficit at some performance level of processing such as short-term memory. It is not difficult to conceive of a working memory mechanism which takes as its input the speech signal and retains a mental representation on which further processing may be performed (Clark/Clark 1977). A STM disorder could easily account for the variability in intra-subject and inter-subject performance, for example, since sentence comprehension performance would vary depending on the limited number of features of the sentence that happened to be remembered. This type of STM mechanism was first investigated in conduction aphasics' sentence comprehension (Saffran/Marin 1975; Heilman/Scholes/Watson 1976; Caramazza/Basili/Koller/Berndt 1981). The comprehension deficit in conduction aphasia was attributed to the auditory-verbal STM impairment thought to underlie their repetition.

More recently, studies of agrammatic aphasics have been performed to determine whether agrammatic comprehension can be attributed to an auditory-verbal STM impairment. Linebarger/Schwartz/Saffran (1983) asked four agrammatic aphasics to make grammaticality judgments of sentences containing a wide variety of grammatical structures. While their patients were generally quite successful, two types of sentences proved inordinately difficult. These grammatical constructions seemed to require that the entire sentence be held in memory since information presented at the beginning of the sentence and at the end of the sentence had to be compared (e. g. *The little boy fell down, didn't it?*). Linebarger/Schwartz/Saffran questioned the 'syntactic loss' hypothesis, and emphasized the role of a STM mechanism in the appreciation of some aspects of the grammar of a sentence. Similarly, in the Kolk/van Grunsven (1985) study mentioned above, the authors did not find that the grammatical features of the sentences discriminated between successful and poor sentence comprehension. Instead, their agrammatic patients encountered more difficulty on longer sentences than shorter sentences, regardless of grammatical complexity. Kolk/van Gunsven attributed poor performance to the greater processing demands made by longer sentences on a defective STM device.

Others have cast some doubt on sweeping claims such as these, and have underlined the importance of determining the precise role which a STM mechanism may play in sentence comprehension. Martin (1987), for example, evaluated three nonfluent patients whose speech was consistently and severely agrammatic and three nonfluent aphasics who were judged not to be agrammatic since their speech included some simple sentences that were grammatically correct (two patients) or consisted only of stereotyped utterances (the third patient). On a sentence-picture matching task using active, passive and relative-clause types of sentences, the agrammatic patients performed at worse levels than the nonfluent patients who were not agrammatic. All nonfluent patients had equally reduced digit spans. Martin argued that the disrupted STM mechanism reflected in reduced digit span is not necessarily the same mechanism proposed to support sentence comprehension (also Caplan/Vanier/Baker 1986).

Martin / Wetzel / Blossom-Stach / Feher (1989) attempted to test the relative success of the syntactic loss hypothesis and the STM hypothesis at explaning agrammatic aphasics' sentence comprehension impairment. Three sentence-picture matching paradigms were used where active and passive sentences of varying lengths were presented. Foils included reversals (subject and object depicted in the incorrect role) or lexical substitutions (an unmentioned bit of information depicted in a picture choice). Martin argued that the 'syntactic loss' hypothesis would predict better performance on active sentences than passives, but that the STM hypothesis would predict better performance on shorter sentences than longer sentences. The results revealed that the vast majority of errors were due to the incorrect selection of reversal foils. In this context, three of the four aphasics encountered significantly more difficulty on passive items than active items. However, only one of the four patients actually performed at chance levels in sentence-picture matching. None of the patients demonstrated significantly better performance on the shorter items than the longer items, but the small number of errors involving lexical substitution foils occurred exclusively on longer sentences, suggesting a partial memory deficit. The patterns of performance seen in this study thus failed to provide support for strong versions of either the syntactic loss hypothesis or the STM hypothesis.

The role of memory in grammatical comprehension has also been evaluated by examining the ability of agrammatic patients to learn a new word. Grossman/Carey (1987) taught a low frequency word *bice* – an adjective referring to the dark green portion of the color spectrum – to seven patients who were classified as Broca's aphasics by the Boston Diagnostic Aphasia Examination (Goodglass/Kaplan 1983). This was accomplished by first exposing each patient to the new word, paired with a dark green pen and a brown pen, in the sentence *Take the bice pen – not the brown pen but the bice pen – and draw a picture of some clothes*. This statement in this context provided all of the information necessary for patients to learn the new word's phonological shape (*bice*), the new word's meaning (that it refers not to brown but to dark green), and the new word's grammatical form class (in the phrase *the bice pen, bice* modifies the noun *pen* so it is an adjective). About ten minutes after the exposure period, patients were probed for their knowledge of the new word's grammatical form class and its meaning. To assess the ability to learn the new word's grammatical form class, patients were asked to judge sentences where bice was used in an adjectival slot or a verb slot. This was compared with their judgments of sentences containing a known adjective or a nonsense syllable in adjectival or verb slots. It was found that each of the Broca's aphasics encountered significant difficulty demonstrating that they had learned the new word's form class.

This failure to learn that bice was a kind of adjective also had ramifications for their mental representation of the meaning of bice. In order to assess what they learned about the meaning of the new word, patients were asked to classify as *bice* or *not bice* objects that were bice-colored, bice-related in color (e. g. focal green, dark blue), or unequivocally not bice-colored (e. g. orange, red). In addition, the objects were different shapes: long and-thin (as in the initial pen used to illustrate bice), round or oblong (an object that was not pen-shaped), and shapeless swatches of colored paper. All but one of the Broca's aphasics exhibited a graded judgment criteria for classifying the objects. They classified bice-colored objects as *bice* more often than bice-related objects, which in turn were more often considered *bice* than objects which were unrelated in color to bice. This differed from their classification of green-colored objects, where there was a sharp discontinuity between objects considered green and non-green objects. All but one of the Broca's aphasics also classified long-and-thin-shaped objects as *bice* more often than roundish objects, which in turn were classified as *bice* more often than color swatches. The authors reasoned that these patients hadn't learned that the word was an adjective, so they also hadn't learned that the word referred to a single property of the objects they were sorting. Findings such as these can be interpreted as indicating that a selective decoding impairment may have a significant impact on what can be learned or remembered. However, there is an alternate explanation – that a compromised attention component of the central executive may be limited in its ability to focus on the important features that should be captured for lexical acquisition. Both of the accounts stand in contrast to the role often attributed to STM in sentence processing – a mechanism that supports time-consuming process such as mapping across representational formats, or a post-interpretive process that supports the clarification of ambiguous material (Caplan/Waters 1990; McCarthy/Warrington 1987; Saffran/Martin 1990). Regardless of the correct interpretation, these observations could not be made without a word learning technique that eliminates bootstrapping strategies.

Taken together, there is some evidence that sentence comprehension deficits may be due in part to a STM impairment. This evidence is far from definitive. Indeed, the alternate argument remains to be excluded. Caplan/Waters (1990) have argued that STM has a marginal role in normal sentence comprehension, and a selective linguistic impairment in decoding the input string or performing the necessary grammatical computations may determine in part what can be remembered. One additional way to evaluate the role of STM in language processing is to assess amnesic patients who have a sentence comprehension deficit. To the extent that selective aspects of STM may be compromised in different groups of amnesics, these evaluations may also help us understand the precise role of each STM component in sentence comprehension.

3.3.2. Sentence Comprehension in Amnesic Patients

Assessments of aphasics have not provided a definitive picture of the role of STM in sentence comprehension. Other investigators have focussed instead on the evaluation of sentence comprehension in patients with STM impairments. Vallar/Baddeley (1984; 1987) described PV, a patient with a very limited phonological STM, no articulatory rehearsal capacity, and apparently little ability to recode visually presented information. PV has considerable difficulty understanding relatively long sentences where the subject and object are reversible, and she has difficulty detecting errors of anaphoric reference where one or two sentences are placed between the item and its subsequent reference. A second patient, TB, also has very limited phonological STM, despite normal phonological processing. He has profound difficulty verifying complex or lengthy sentences presented auditorily, but improves somewhat with visual presentation. Both patients are without obvious syntactic deficits in their spoken language, and both can understand a range of syntactic structures in short sentences. It is argued that a syntactic deficit per se can not explain the difficulties experienced by these patients, and that their sentence comprehension impairment is attributable to a compromised STM mechanism.

Findings such as these have been called to question. Butterworth/Campbell/Howard (1986) and Howard/Butterworth (1989) have reported a patient RE with an auditory-verbal STM impairment who has little difficulty understanding sentences. In reviewing the literature, these authors argue that many of these STM-impaired patients may have sentence comprehension impairments for other reasons, such as an independent grammatical processing deficit, and indeed that there is great heterogeneity across patients with so-called STM deficits. It is also possible that several of the STM-impaired patients may not have a STM impairment which is exclusively phonologic and/or auditory: TB, for example, also has a reduced visual digit span. In sum, there is debate about the need for a STM processor in sentence comprehension based on assessments of patients with discrete STM deficits.

3.3.3. Sentence Comprehension in Alzheimer's Disease

STM has also been shown to be compromised in patients with probable dementia of the Alzheimer type (pDAT). Thus, several experiments have demonstrated a reduction in immediate serial recall of digits (Kaszniak/Garron/Fox 1979), letters (Morris 1984), and words (Corkin 1982). This is due in part to a moderate decrease in the recency effect (Martin/Brouwers/Cox/Fedio 1985). In order to define the locus of this impairment within the STM mechanism, each of the components of working memory have been examined in more detail. Morris (1984) demonstrated that pDAT patients are as sensitive to the effects of phonological similarity on a letter list recall task as control subjects, suggesting that the phonological store is relatively preserved in pDAT. Morris (1987) has shown that short words are recalled better than long words on a memory span task, and that concurrent articulation suppresses this effect, both paralleling the effects seen in neurologically-intact adults. This suggests that the articulatory loop rehearsal mechanism is relatively intact. By comparison, Baddeley/Logie/Bressi et al.

(1986) have shown that pDAT patients' performance on immediate recall tasks suffers when they are asked to perform concurrent tasks. Using the Peterson/Peterson (1959) technique with different types of intervening material, Morris (1986) claimed that dividing their attention with increasingly difficult task results in progressively inferior performance. These findings have been taken as support for the argument that the central executive is compromised in pDAT. It should be noted, however, that alternate explanations have been offered for results such as these (Broadbent 1983; Monsell 1984). Moreover, memory span deficits are also seen on a pointing span task (Corkin 1982), suggesting that these phenomena are not specific to a language processing system. Careful analyses of errors on span tasks have also revealed a reduction in the primacy effect (Martin/Brouwers/Cox/Fedio 1985), and there is a strong correlation between performance on span tasks and the overall degree of dementia (Corkin 1982; Kopelman 1985). The central executive component of working memory may be compromised in pDAT, but these data must be interpreted cautiously.

In this context, there have been several assessments of sentence comprehension in pDAT. Clinically, it is claimed that grammatical structure in language expression is impaired late in the disease process in some patients, including inappropriate tense agreement and the breakdown of phrase markers in spontaneous speech (Constantinidis/Richard/de Ajuriaguerra 1978; Irigaray 1967). Observations of mildly and moderately impaired patients seem to support the claim that the bulk of patients' difficulty is in the processing of semantic aspects of sentences. Appell/Kertesz/Fisman (1982) and Cummings/Benson/Hill/Read (1985) administered aphasia screening batteries to pDAT patients, for example, and found relatively profound impairments in the domains of naming/word-finding and lexical semantic comprehension/expression. Kertesz/Appell/Fisman (1986) directly compared the language performance patterns of pDAT patients with stroke patients, and found that pDAT patients resembled aphasics with Wernicke's, transcortical sensory, and anomic syndromic profiles, but that none of the demented patients resemble so-called Broca's aphasics or transcortical motor aphasics. Bayles (1982) has also suggested relatively preserved appreciation of a sentence's grammatical features in pDAT, since pDAT patients were able to correct 'syntactic' errors in sentences but not 'semantic' errors. It should be noted that the sentences with semantic errors used by Bayles apparently violated syntactic rules as well, including strict subcategorization and argument structure constraints. Nebes (1989) asked pDAT patients to recall short sentences that were normal, that exhibited disrupted semantic structure, and/or had disrupted syntactic structure. They found that recall of the syntactically disrupted sentences is similar in pDAT and normal subjects. However, they also found that semantic disruption did not differentially affect pDAT and control subjects.

While these findings suggested relatively preserved grammatical processing, Appel/Kertesz/Fisman (1982) found significant impairments on the 'sequential commands' subtest of the Western Aphasia Battery (Kertesz 1982), and Cummings/Benson/Hill/Read (1985) found significant impairments on the 'complex commands' subtest of the Boston Diagnostic Aphasia Examination (Goodglass/Kaplan 1983). Hier/Hagenlocker/Shindler (1985), analyzing pDAT patients' descriptions of "The Cookie Theft Scene" (Goodglass/Kaplan 1983), found that the mean length of utterances, the use of subordinate clauses, and the use of prepositional phrases are all reduced. Findings such as these may be consistent with a grammatical processing impairment, but the extent to which these deficits may also be attributed to an impaired working memory system or to some other cognitive impairment in pDAT remains unclear.

One recent study, however, has found specific impairments on a sentence comprehension task that implicate difficulty with grammatical aspects of sentence comprehension (Chawluk/Grossman/Calcano-Perez et al. 1991). These investigators administered an extensive set of sentences to six pDAT patients who were mildly impaired according to the MMSE, had digit spans of about 5, and were relatively intact in their sentence repetition. The sentences, composed of high frequency nouns and verbs, were cast in three syntactic frames: Simple, terminal subordinate where a relative clause was placed at the end of a simple sentence, and center-embedded subordinate where a relative clause was placed in the center of a simple sentence. Half of each type of sentence was in the active voice and the remainder in the passive voice.

The information in each sentence was probed with a simple question that was in the active or passive voice (e. g. *The eagle chased the hawk. Which bird was chased?*). The results revealed an error rate of 26%, significantly inferior to the performance of control subjects. A detailed analysis of the error pattern revealed that pDAT patients responded randomly on items where the voice of the sentence did not correspond to the voice of the question. Given their ability to repeat sentences such as these, one possible interpretation of this finding is that a compromised central executive was overwhelmed by the mental manipulation required to compare thematic roles in the sentence and its question when these did not correspond in voice. Alternate explanations include attributing the deficit to a non-specific effect of limited information processing or a defect in performing the necessary grammatical comutations. Regardless of the specific explanation, the finding of a sentence processing impairment in Alzheimer's disease opens the way to characterizing the nature of sentence processing that may occur in the setting of a compromised central executive.

3.3.4. Sentence Comprehension in Parkinson's Disease

Parkinson's disease (PD) is a common neurodegenerative condition that results in a movement disorder consisting of tremor, rigidity, and bradykinesia. It has been stated that the cognitive impairment in PD can be characterized as a so-called subcortical dementia, where deficits can be seen in the domains of memory, visuo-spatial processing, executive functioning such as attention and organizational capacity, and bradyphrenia (Cummings 1990). An aphasia is said to be among the exclusionary criteria of subcortical dementia (Cummings/Darkins/Mendez et al. 1988). Thus, the presence of a language processing deficit in PD ought to be attributable to some non-linguistic cognitive impairment, such as limited STM.

Lieberman/Friedman/Feldman (1990) administered the Rhode Island Test of Language Structure to PD patients who had a moderate motor disorder. Several of their patients had high rates of comprehension errors on sentences that were moderately complex syntactically. The impaired patients also were demented, but the authors did not characterize the dementia or report the results of memory measures. Grossman/Carvell/Gollomp et al. (1991, 1992) assessed the ability of mildly impaired, non-demented PD patients to answer simple questions about target sentences such as *The eagle chased the hawk that was fast. Which bird was chased?*. The sentences varied in terms of phrase structure, voice, and semantic constraint. Probes were also designed to assess the ability to compare information from adjacent and non-adjacent segments of the target sentence. Patients were also asked to detect errors in some similarly constructed sentences.

Significant impairments in PD patients' overall performance were found when compared with control subjects. Indeed, discriminant analyses revealed that 65% of PD patients differ from control subjects. Performance on sentences deteriorated as they became more demanding grammatically, an order of difficulty seen in 83% of the patients. There was little effect for sentence length, and errors occurred regardless of whether the information being probed could be found in adjacent or non-adjacent portions of the sentence. These negative findings argued against the possibility that a limitation in the size of a STM buffer can explain their impairment. However, the PD patients encountered difficulty detecting the presence and nature of errors in grammatical morphemes in the sentences. This suggested that a compromised attentional mechanism within a grammatical processor may be contributing to PD patients' sentence comprehension difficulties.

Geyer/Grossman (submitted) confirmed this type of sentence processing impairment in another group of mildly impaired, non-demented PD patients. In this experiment, patients were asked to make truth verification judgments of probes that followed sentences (e. g. *The pirate sank the ship. The ship sank – True or False*). The items contained one of two types of verbs: a simple transitive verb, where its subject in a transitive sentence is also its subject in an intransitive sentence; or a lexical causative verb, where its object in a transitive sentence is its subject in an intransitive sentence, as in the above example. These verbs were embedded in active voice, passive voice, or periphrasic (as in *The pirate made the ship sink*) sentential frames. All PD patients performed at normal levels on a short version of the Token Test. Sixty percent of PD patients encountered significant difficulty determining the accuracy of probes about sentences containing lexical causative verbs, and compromised individuals exhibited similar performance profiles with equivalent levels of absolute impairment in all but one case. While lexical causatives were more difficult than simple transitives in both active and passive voice sentences, the 2 verb types were treated equivalently when embedded in the periphrastic type of sentence. Moreover, lexical causatives in the periphrastic voice were easier to understand than lexical causatives in the passive voice. These findings suggest that a defect in performing grammatical computations cannot fully account for PD patients' sentence comprehension difficulties. The periphrasic voice may have helped PD patients disambiguate the atypical mapping from syntactic roles to thematic roles in lexical causative verbs, a kind of process that is said to be subserved by working memory (Berndt/Salasoo/Mitchum/Blumstein 1988; Saffran/Martin 1990; Schwartz/Saffran/Marin 1980).

Grossman/Carvell/Peltzer (submitted) assessed the role of working memory and a mapping function in grammatical comprehension in PD as well. In the first experiment, non-demented patients with mild PD were asked to judge sentences containing a mass noun (e. g. *water*) or a count noun (e. g. *pencil*) modified by a quantifier such as *much* or *few*. In half of the items, the noun was modified appropriately by a mass adjective or a count adjective, but in the remainder the noun and the adjective did not agree. In half of each type of count item, moreover, the 's' modifying the noun was used appropriately and in the remainder inappropriately. In the second experiment, patients were asked to match a sentence containing a count term or a mass term (e. g. *Point to the container with many*) with one of four pictures (a large amount of a mass substance, a large amount of a count substance, a small amount of a mass substance, or a small amount of a count substance).

The results revealed on the first experiment that 45% of PD patients encounter significant difficulty detecting sentences where a noun and its adjective do not agree. In these patients, the impairment was due to difficulty detecting an adjective-noun mismatch or difficulty identifying an inappropriate use of a modifying 's'. Importantly, sentences exhibiting both types of errors simultaneously were judged accurately by PD patients. This effect is not consistent with a grammatical computation impairment, but instead suggests a threshold effect as might be seen in a limited working memory. On the second experiment 70% of PD patients were impaired, indicating significant difficulty mapping sentences onto pictures. An error analysis indicated that patients frequently err by choosing the wrong type of substance, but they rarely err by choosing the wrong amount of substance. These findings emphasize the difficulty experienced by these patients in mapping syntactic roles onto thematic roles, lending support to the claim that working memory may play a role in the sentence comprehension deficits of PD patients.

In sum, there is some evidence that STM may play a role in sentence comprehension. This conclusion, however, is far from unequivocal. In aphasics, for example, the nature of the interaction between mnestic and linguistic factors remains to be established. It is also unclear whether the role is as simple as a limitation in the size of a STM buffer or involves a more dynamic process such as actively attending to appropriate grammatical information. Such a role may be linked to a so-called central executive, as suggested by the data from Alzheimer's disease patients.

3.4. The Role of Memory in Sentence Expression

The traditional treatment of sentence expression difficulty has emphasized the identification of the modality through which expression cannot be accomplished. For example, alexia is used to refer to an impairment in reading written material, and agraphia refers to an impairment in written expression. The initial descriptions of these phenomena were concerned with determining whether an alexia or agraphia occurred in isolation (so-called 'alexia without agraphia' or 'pure agraphia') or the two deficits co-occurred.

More recent clinical descriptions of neurologically-impaired adults have described alexic and agraphic impairments in more detail. Thus, surface alexia or agraphia (Hatfield/Patterson 1983; Patterson/Marshall/Coltheart 1985) is said to describe that group of patients where known words with unusual spelling patterns cannot be read or written accurately (e. g. *who, said*). By comparison, words and novel lexemes with transparent grapheme-phoneme correspondence rules are read and written accurately (e. g. *stad, lif*). Their reading and writing errors are often regularizations of irregular words (e. g. *guest* → *'just'*). Moreover, they are more likely to read mildly irregular words correctly in comparison to very irregular words (e.g. *yacht*) and are influenced by word frequency, letter frequency, and part-of-speech (Bub/Cancelliere/Kertesz 1985; Goodman/Caramazza 1986; Shallice/Warrington/McCarthy 1983). Graded irregularity and frequency effects such as these have suggested the possibility of reading and writing models which turn on the use of units that are larger than the grapheme or phoneme, and may even entail reading/writing by analogy to known words that are similar in appearance to the target word (Marcel 1980; Friedman 1988; Patterson/Morton 1985).

The reverse pattern of performance is called phonological alexia or agraphia (Beauvois/Desrouesne 1979; Funnell 1983; Roeltgen/Heilman 1984). These individuals find it difficult to read and write novel words with transparent grapheme-phoneme correspondence rules, but are accurate at reading or writing known words even if their spelling pattern is quite irregular. Some of these patients nevertheless find functors difficult to read and write (Bub/Kertesz 1982; Patterson 1982). Among the alternate explanations is the proposal that the word includes form class or other category-specific information that can be used to mediate some aspects of reading and writing (Bub/Chertkow 1988; Friedman 1988).

On the basis of observations such as these, a minimal computational apparatus for reading and writing can be hypothesized. This may include a phonological output lexicon to mediate oral reading of known words, a graphemic output lexicon for writing known words, and a set of grapheme-phoneme correspondence rules to mediate the oral reading of novel written words and the writing of novel dictated words. The overall architecture of this expression mechanism, although widely held, may not be computationally adequate to support oral or written expression or account for the entire spectrum of impairments said to occur in neurologically-impaired patients with reading and writing disorders. The most common strategy has been to postulate additional processing elements, such as a memory component (Ellis 1982; Miceli/Silveri/Villa 1985; Morton 1980; Newcombe/Marshall 1980). A STM buffer such as this may be needed to retain the code of an output lexicon while the identity of each letter or sound is chosen prior to expression.

Consider some of the case studies of acquired dysgraphia that underline the necessity for hypothesizing a STM buffer mechanism. A graphemic buffer, for example, is said to hold the information from a graphemic output lexicon while a letter name conversion mechanism translates the abstract graphemic representation into an orally spelled word or an allographic conversion mechanism translates the graphemic representation into a written word. Caramazza/Miceli/Villa/Romani (1987) described a patient LB who was thought to have a functional lesion to the graphemic buffer. LB made the same types of errors in writing, typing, and oral spelling, suggesting that the deficit was due to an impairment prior to the planning and execution of a motor program. LB also erred when asked to write spontaneously, write dictated words, and produce the written name of an object, suggesting that the deficit occurred after the orthographic information had been retrieved. Spelling errors were not responsive to any lexical properties such as imagability, word frequency, or grammatical form class. Similarly, error types did not reflect any consistent semantic, morphologic, or phonologic characteristics, consistent with the possibility that the graphemic buffer is a post-lexical mechanism. Errors consisted of letter deletions that became increasingly frequent as the word was longer, and they were more likely to occur in the middle of a word.

Related patterns of spelling errors have been described in other patients (Hillis/Caramazza 1989; Posteraro/Zinelli/Mazzucchi 1988). These recent observations, as well as additional analyses of LB, have suggested that the original characterization of the graphemic buffer must be recast. Caramazza/Miceli (1990) provided additional descriptions of LB that indicated the sensitivity of his spelling errors to the syllabic context in which they occurred. For example, LB made more errors on words with complex consonant-vowel patterns (e.g. CCVCVV) than words with a, regular consonant-vowel pattern (e.g. CVCVCV). Errors in the regular-CV words were overwhelmingly transpositions and substitutions, but deletions and insertions were equally frequent for complex-CV words. LB also tended to apply doubled letters to the incorrect consonant within a word (e.g. *sorella* → *sorrela*), although a letter-doubling error rarely occurred in words that did not already have a doubled letter. Findings such as these suggested that the graphemic buffer does not simply hold an ordered sequence of graphemes, but must also be sensitive to certain rule-determined properties of words. Thus, the graphemic buffer apparently represents the consonant-vowel status of graphemes and the graphosyllabic structure of words. Similarly, based on detailed analyses of spelling errors in morphologically complex words, Badecker/Hillis/Caramazza (1990) have also demonstrated that information is stored in the graphemic buffer in morpheme-sized packages.

There is additional evidence that the graphemic buffer may not simply be a passive storage vehicle. The distribution of types of errors in words and non-words was quite similar in these patients, for example, but some had more difficulty spelling non-words than words. Some patients were also affected by lexical factors such as word frequency. Observations such as these suggest that other factors may contribute to the functioning of the graphemic buffer, and again raise the specific possibility of a role for writing by analogy to the corpus of words in the patient's written vocabulary. Errors were also differentially distributed in words as a function of the location of the causative brain lesion in some patients (Hillis/Caramazza 1989). This effect for spatial location suggests a role for an attentional mechanism in the graphemic buffer. Several of the individuals exhibited impairments in other cognitive domains which bear an important family resemblance to their language expression deficit. Consider, for example, the errors in drawing abstract figures from memory made by DH (Hillis/Caramazza 1989) and the dyscalculia, drawing apraxia, and poor verbal memory of SE (Posteraro/Zinelli/Mazzucchi 1988). These additional neuropsychological deficits call to question the specificity of something like a graphemic buffer for language expression. Thus, there is considerable evidence for the existence of a buffer mechanism that holds a transient mental representation of a word during its spelling, but many questions remain about the specific nature of this buffer.

A phonologic buffer has been postulated to hold phonologic material while a conversion mechanism prepares the material for expression. A phonologic buffer plays a role in 3 expressive modalities: writing words to dictation, mediated by the phonologic output lexicon; reading non-words orally, mediated by a grapheme-phoneme conversion mechanism; and repeating non-words orally. In the case of written output, material is held in the phonologic buffer while a phoneme-grapheme conversion system transcodes phonemes for the graphemic buffer. For oral output, the phonologic buffer retains the set of phonemes while an articulatory process prepares the information for expression.

Evidence for a functional lesion of the phonologic buffer would come from the converging inability to perform all 3 of these expression tasks in the face of an ability to write known words to copy or dictation, that is, expression tasks that depend only on the graphemic buffer. Caramazza/Miceli/Villa (1986) present such converging evidence from patient IGR. Errors were more evident in longer words and overwhelmingly consisted of single letter substitutions. Similarly, many errors were made in the repetition of non-words (data are not provided for the repetition of familiar words), and errors were typically single phoneme substitutions. These findings are largely consistent with the proposed location of the phonologic buffer in the language expression system. Findings inconsistent with the proposed characteristics of this STM mechanism included that this patient made many more errors writing non-words than words. Moreover, the length of delay on a delayed writing task did not have an effect. Errors in oral reading resembled the target response phonologically and consisted of deviations by 1 or 2 letters, also consistent with some expected properties of the phonologic buffer. However, oral reading errors were more common for non-words than words, a finding inconsistent with the proposed location and role of the phonologic buffer. An examination of the ordinal location of errors indicated a relative predominance of reading errors at a word's initial position when compared to writing and repetition, but errors otherwise occurred in the middle positions of words. Since IGR had a right hemisphere lesion, it is possible that this patient was displaying some left-sided inattention. As with the graphemic buffer, there may be some influence of an attentional mechanism on the phonologic buffer. Moreover, the persistent finding of inferior performance with non-words emphasizes the need to incorporate additional attributes in these buffers or develop an alternate functional architecture that can incorporate this finding.

Additional evidence for a phonological buffer may come from an analysis of patients with a so-called reproduction conduction aphasia (Caplan/Vanier/Baker 1986; Kohn 1984; McCarthy/Warrington 1984). These individuals are affected by word length and produce many phonemic paraphasias that often consist of single phoneme errors, characteristics thought to be associated with a phonologic buffer. The 'output' nature of their disorder is emphasized by the fact that they often repeat words multiple times in an attempt to reproduce the target, and their performance on span tasks is generally quite good. As with IGR, the patients of Caplan and McCarthy/Warrington had much more difficulty with non-words than words, suggesting that other factors involving alternate procedural and/or computational mechanisms must be taken into consideration in the characterization of the phonologic buffer. Moreover, a study by Pate/Saffran/Martin (1987) found that errors occurred differentially depending on the context and nature of the phonologic material being repeated (e. g. *murderous* vs *murder us*). This suggested that the phonologic buffer is not a passive reservoir but may be sensitive to the nature of the information being represented. As in the case of the graphemic buffer, then, additional word has begun to suggest some of the internal characteristics of outout buffer mechanisms that retain information in preparation for oral expression.

In sum, there is some evidence from a handful of case studies that suggests the existence of graphemic and phonologic output buffer mechanisms for language expression. The nature of these buffers, however, is far from clear. While some observations have begun to clarify the internal nature of these devices, others have suggested that we are far from the point of feeling confident about the precise role of these devices in the functional architecture underlying expression. There has not been an adequate interpretation of the persistent advantage of words over nonwords, for example.

4. Summary

Do memory impairments play a role in the language processing deficits seen in aphasia? Investigators interested in memory and language initially treated sentential material as but one example of a broader set of stimuli. Thus, the sequence of words in a sentence was taken to be representative of any type of sequence, and difficulties were thought to occur because of the compromised appreciation of the ordered material (De Renzi/Nichelli 1975). Aphasiologists often felt that reasonably detailed linguistic analyses would probably be adequate for an appropriate schema characterizing sentence processing. Indeed, there was even some reason in ignore claims about the potential impact of aphasics' memory impairments on their language performance since several studies had indicated that memory deficits were not restricted to the verbal domain (Boller/De Renzi 1967; Gainotti/Caltagirone/Miceli 1978).

More recently, investigations of sentence repetition in conduction aphasia have served as a forum for debating whether a linguistic deficit or mnestic deficit can explain the repetition difficulty (Caramazza/Berndt/Basili/Koller 1981; Shallice/Warrington 1977; Strub/Gardner 1974). Linguists have pointed to several shortcomings in the arguments of the 'memory loss' advocates; mnemonists have also pointed out inconsistencies in the thinking of the 'linguistic loss' advocates. Fortunately, more recent work (Ostrin/Schwartz 1986) has adopted the rational view that both linguistic and STM processors probably contribute to sentence repetition. This work has thus initiated the next step in our attempts to characterize a reasonable model of sentence processing, that is, determining how memory and language processes may work together in supporting sentence repetition. One hypothesis is that there may be a partial memory trace of the sentence which the patient is attempting to repeat. The semantic and grammatical capabilities of the listener may bias the content of the memory trace.

Other studies have considered the role of memory in sentence comprehension. Again, there has been a contrast between, on the one hand, 'syntactic loss' advocates who have observed sentence comprehension impairments to increase in correlation with increasing grammatical complexity in a sentence (Benson/Geschwind 1986; Berndt/Caramazza 1980), and on the other hand, 'memory loss' advocates who see increasingly frequent sentence comprehension impairments as the sentences become longer and therefore more difficult to remember (Kolk/van Grunsven 1985; Linebarger/Schwartz/Saffran 1983). One possible resolution may be that a working memory device within the grammatical processor is compromised (Grossman/Carvell submitted; Kolk/van Grunsven 1985). This may prevent appropriate identification of grammatical morphemes, the storage of appropriate information in a STM buffer, and thus degrade the quality of grammatical computations.

It also appears that STM processors may be necessary for language expression. Earlier characterizations of these STM devices suggested only slave buffers that interface 2 processing components. However, even these mechanisms appear to have internal characteristics indicating that they actively participate in the exchange of information from processor to processor. It is noteworthy, as implied throughout the discussion, that the STM devices involved in comprehension, repetition, and expression are quite different in many respects. The variability depends in large part on the nature of the task being performed. Such non-uniformity is inconsistent with 'working memory' as conceived by Baddeley (1986) in that a single working memory mechanism does not appear to subserve these diverse manifestations of STM in language processing.

I should briefly mention that this componential approach to the role of memory in sentence processing assumes a great deal about the overall architecture of the cognitive elements contributing to these language tasks. A very different approach has recently been developed – parallel distributed processing (McClelland/Rumelhart 1986). According to this model, a layered device using large numbers of densely interconnected units 'learns' about the probabilities inherent in a corpus based on several exposures to the material. During each learning session, feedback is given to the device in response to its answers to questions. The task-specific device then modifies the weights on the set of internal connections between layers. The learning-feedback cycle is repeated many times until the device's answers approach 100% accuracy.

This radically different approach has proven extraordinarily powerful. In one experiment intended to model dyslexia, for example, the number of units in the middle layer of a three-layered device was decreased. This modified processor appeared 'dyslexic' in that it was less capable of making appropriate decisions about the acceptability of letter strings as words despite an equal number of learning sessions (Patterson/Seidenberg/McClelland 1988). More remarkable yet was the finding that the "lesioned" device produced the same pattern of errors that is seen clinically in phonologic alexia. Despite the power of this approach, there are many potential problems (Pinker/Prince 1988). The middle layers of these devices are 'hidden', for example, so that the precise cognitive role played by these layers is far from clear. Detailed examinations of various linguistic constructs claimed to be learned by parallel distributed processing devices – such as the regular versus irregular past – in fact may not be reliably represented. With respect to dyslexia, it is unclear why only one form of dyslexia has emerged from lesioned devices. Despite these shortcomings, the 'parallel distributed processing' approach represents an important alternative to the componential model.

In sum, the data suggest that memory probably plays a role in sentence processing – probably an important role. The strong forms of arguments characterizing memory as explanatory for all aspects of sentence processing impairment may not be supported over the long run. Instead, the data are beginning to outline some of the specific ways in which mnestic and linguistic processes may interact in our attempts to appreciate a sentence. It is the precise description of this interaction which holds the hope of providing a computationally adequate characterization of the processes subserving sentence appreciation.

Author's note: This work was supported in part by the United States Public Health Service (DC00039 and AG09399) and by the McCabe Foundation. I would like to express my appreciation to Patricia Giampapa for her help with preparing this manuscript.

5. References

Alajouanine, T. & Lhermitte, F. (1964). Les composantes phonemiques et semantiques de la jargonaphasie. *International Journal of Neurology, 4*, 277–286.

Allport, D. A. (1984). Auditory-verbal short-term memory and conduction aphasia. In H. Bouma & D. G. Bowhuis (Eds.), *Attention and performance X*. New York: Academic Press.

Appell, J., Kertesz, A., & Fisman, M. (1982). A study of language functioning in Alzheimer patients. *Brain and Language, 17*, 73–91.

Baddeley, A. D. (1986). *Working memory*. Oxford: Oxford University Press.

Baddeley, A. D., Logie, R., Bressi, S., Della Sala, S., & Spinnler, H. (1986). Dementia and working memory. *Quarterly Journal of Experimental Psychology, 38A*, 603–618.

Badecker, W., Hillis, A., & Caramazza, A. (1990). Lexical morphology and its role in the writing process: Evidence from a case of acquired dysgraphia. *Cognition, 35,* 205–243.

Bayles, K. A. (1982). Language function in senile dementia. *Brain and Language, 16,* 265–280.

Beauvois, M. F. & Desrouesne, J. (1979). Phonological alexia: Three dissociations. *Journal of Neurology, Neurosurgery, & Psychiatry, 42,* 1115–1124.

Benson, D. F. & Geschwind, N. (1986). Aphasia and related disorders: A clinical approach. In M. M. Mesulam (Ed.), *Principles of behavioral neurology.* 193–238. Philadelphia: F. A. Davis, Inc.

Berndt, R. S. & Caramazza, A. (1980). A redefinition of the syndrome of Broca's aphasia: Implications for a neuropsychological model of language. *Applied Psycholinguistics, 1,* 225–278.

Berndt, R. S., Salasoo, A., Mitchum, C. C., & Blumstein, S. E. (1988). The role of intonation cues in aphasic patients' performance of the grammatical judgment task. *Brain and Language, 34,* 65–97.

Berwick, R. C. & Weinberg, A. (1984). *The grammatical basis of linguistic performance: Language use and acquisition.* Cambridge: MIT Press.

Blumstein, S. E., Baker, E., & Goodglass, H. (1977). Phonological factors in auditory comprehension in aphasia. *Neuropsychologia, 15,* 19–30.

Boller, F. & De Renzi, E. (1967). Relationship between visual memory defects and hemispheric locus of insult. *Neurology, 17,* 1052–1058.

Broadbent, D. E. (1983). The functional approach to memory. *Philosophical Transactions of the Royal Society of London, B302,* 239–249.

Bub, D. N., Cancelliere, A., & Kertesz, A. (1985). Whole-word and analytic translation of spelling to sound in a non-semantic reader. In K. E. Patterson, J. C. Marshall, & M. Coltheart (Eds.), *Surface dyslexia.* 15–34. London: Lawrence Erlbaum.

Bub, D. N. & Chertkow, H. (1988). Agraphia. In F. Boller, J. Grafman (Eds.), *Handbook of neuropsychology, volume 1.* 393–414. Amsterdam: Elsevier.

Bub, D. N. & Kertesz, A. (1982). Deep agraphia. *Brain and Language, 17,* 146–165.

Butters, N., Samuels, I., Goodglass, H., & Brody, B. A. (1970). Short term visual and auditory memory disorders after parietal and frontal lobe damage. *Cortex, 6,* 440–459.

Butterworth, B., Campbell, R., & Howard, D. (1986). The uses of short-term memory: A case study. *Quarterly Journal of Experimental Psychology, 38A,* 705–737.

Caplan, D. (1983). A note on the "Word Order Problem" in agrammatism. *Brain and Language, 20,* 155–165.

Caplan, D., Vanier, M., & Baker, C. (1986). A case of reproduction aphasia. II. Sentence comprehension. *Cognitive Neuropsychology, 3,* 129–146.

Caplan, D., Vanier, M., & Baker, C. (1986). A case study of reproduction conduction aphasia, I. Word production. *Cognitive Neuropsychology, 3,* 99–128.

Caplan, D. & Waters, G. S. (1990). Short-term memory and language comprehension: A critical review of the neuropsychological literature. In G. Vallar & T. Shallice (Eds.), *Neuropsychological impairments of short-term memory.* 337–389. New York: Cambridge University Press.

Caramazza, A., Basili, A. G., Koller, J. J., & Berndt, R. S. (1981). An investigation of repetition and language processing in a case of conduction aphasia. *Brain and Language, 14,* 235–271.

Caramazza, A., Berndt, R. S. Basili, A. G., & Koller, J. J. (1981). Syntactic processing deficits in aphasia. *Cortex, 17,* 333–348.

Caramazza, A. & Miceli, G. (1990). The structure of graphemic representations. *Cognition, 37,* 243–297.

Caramazza, A., Miceli, G. & Villa, G. (1986). The role of the (output) phonological butter in reading, writing, and repetition. *Cognitive Neuropsychology, 3,* 37–76.

Caramazza, A., Miceli, G., Villa, G., & Romani, C. (1987). The role of the graphemic buffer in spelling: Evidence from a case of acquired dysgraphia. *Cognition, 26,* 59–85.

Caramazza, A. & Zurif, E. B. (1976). Dissociations of algorithmic and heuristic processes in language comprehension: Evidence from Broca's aphasia. *Brain and Language, 3,* 572–582.

Cermak, L. S. & Moreines, J. (1976). Verbal retention deficits in aphasic and amnesic patients. *Brain and Language, 3,* 16–27.

Cermak, L. S., Stiassny, D., & Uhly, B. (1984). Reconstructive retrieval deficits in Broca's aphasia. *Brain and Language, 21,* 95–104.

Cermak, L. S. & Tarlow, S. (1978). Aphasic and amnesic patients' verbal vs. nonverbal retentive abilities. *Cortex, 14,* 32–40.

Chawluk, J. B., Grossman, M., Calcano-Perez, J. A., Alavi, A., Hurtig, H. I., & Reivich, M. (1991). Positron emission tomography studies of cerebral metabolism in Alzheimer's disease: A critical review stressing current and future neuropsychological methodology. In M. F. Schwartz (Ed.). *Modular deficits in Alzheimer-type dementia.* 101–142. Cambridge: MIT Press.

Clark, H. H. & Clark, E. V. (1977). *Psychology and language.* New York: Harcourt Brace Jovanovich.

Constantinidis, J., Richard, J., & de Ajuriaguerra, J. (1978). Dementias with senile plaques and neurofibrillary tangles. In A. Isaacs & F. Post (Eds.). *Studies in geriatric psychiatry.* Toronto: Wiley.

Corkin, S. (1982). Some relationships between global amnesias and the memory impairments in Alzheimer's disease. In S. Corkin, K. L. Davis, J. H. Growdon, E. Usdin, & R. J. Wurtman (Eds.), *Alzheimer's disease: A report of research in progress.* 149–164. New York: Raven Press.

Craik, F. I. M. & Lockhart, R. S. (1972). Levels of processing: A framework for memory research. *Journal of Verbal Learning and Verbal Behavior, 11,* 671–684.

Cummings, J. L. (1990). *Subcortical dementia.* New York: Oxford University Press.

Cummings, J. L., Benson, D. F., Hill, M. A., & Read, S. (1985). Aphasia in dementia of the Alzheimer type. *Neurology, 35,* 394–397.

Cummings, J. L., Darkins, A., Mendez, M., Hill, M. A., & Benson, D. F. (1988). Alzheimer's disease and Parkinson's disease: Comparison of speech and language alteration. *Neurology, 38,* 680–684.

De Renzi, E. & Nichelli, P. (1975). Verbal and nonverbal short-term memory impairment following hemispheric damage. *Cortex, 11,* 341–354.

Dubois, J., Hecaen, J., Angelergues, R., de Chatelier, A., & Marcie, P. (1964). Etude neurolinguistique de l'aphasie de conduction. *Neuropsychologia, 2,* 9–24.

Ellis, A. W. (1982). Spelling and writing (and reading and speaking). In A. W. Ellis (Ed.), *Normality and pathology in cognitive functions.* New York: Academic Press.

Friedman, R. B. (1988). Acquired alexia. In F. Boller, & J. Grafman (Eds.), *Handbook of neuropsychology, volume 1.* 377–391. Amsterdam: Elsevier.

Funnell, E. (1983). Phonological processes in reading: New evidence from acquired alexia. *British Journal of Psychology, 74,* 159–180.

Gainotti, G., Caltagirone, C., & Miceli, G. (1978). Immediate visual-spatial memory in hemisphere-damaged patients: Impairments of verbal coding and of perceptual processing. *Neuropsychologia, 16,* 501–507.

Geschwind, N. (1965). Dysconnexion syndromes in animals and man. *Brain, 88,* 237–294, 585–644.

Geyer, H. & Grossman, M. (submitted). A grammatical impairment for lexical causative verbs in Parkinson's disease.

Goldstein, K. (1948). *Language and language disturbances.* New York: Grune and Stratton.

Goodglass, H., Denes, G., & Calderon, M. (1974). The absence of covert verbal mediation in aphasia. *Cortex, 10,* 264–269.

Goodglass, H., Gleason, J. B., & Hyde, M. R. (1970). Some dimensions of auditory language comprehension in aphasia. *Journal of Speech and Hearing Research, 13,* 595–606.

Goodglass, H. & Kaplan, E. (1983). *The assessment of aphasia and related disorders.* Philadelphia: Lea & Febiger.

Goodman, R. A. & Caramazza, A. (1986). Aspects of the spelling process: Evidence from a case of acquired dysgraphia. *Language and Cognitive Processes, 1,* 263–296.

Green, E. & Howes, D. H. (1977). The nature of conduction aphasia: A study of anatomic and clinical features and of underlying mechanisms. In H. Whitaker & H. Whitaker (Eds.), *Studies in neurolinguistics, vol. 3.* New York: Academic Press.

Grossman, M. & Carey, S. (1987). Selective word-learning deficits in aphasia. *Brain and Language, 32,* 306–324.

Grossman, M. & Carvell, S. (submitted). Verb learning in Parkinson's disease.

Grossman, M., Carvell, S., Gollomp, S., Stern, M. B., Vernon, G., & Hurtig, H. I. (1991). Sentence comprehension and praxic deficits in mild Parkinson's disease: Exclusionary criteria for subcortical dementia? *Neurology, 41,* 1620–1626.

Grossman, M., Carvell, S., Stern, M. B., Gollomp, S., & Hurtig, H. I. (1992). Sentence comprehension in Parkinson's disease: The role of attention and memory. *Brain and Language, 42,* 347–384.

Grossman, M., Carvell, S., Stern, M. B., Gollomp, S., Vernon, G., & Hurtig, H. I. (1990). The frequency of dementia in mild Parkinson's disease. *Movement Disorders, 5,* 71.

Grossman, M., Carvell, S., & Peltzer, L. (submitted). The sum and substance of it: Lexical subcategorization and the appreciation mass/count adjective/noun agreement in Parkinson's disease.

Hatfield, F. M. & Patterson, K. (1983). Phonological spelling. *Quarterly Journal of Experimental Psychology, 35A,* 451–468.

Hécean, H., Dell, M., & Roger, A. (1955). L'aphasie de conduction. *Encephale, 2,* 170–195.

Heilman, K. M., Scholes, R., & Watson, R. T. (1976). Defects of immediate memory in Broca's and conduction aphasia. *Brain and Language, 25,* 117–133.

Hier, D. B., Hagenlocker, K., & Shindler, A. G. (1985). Language disintegration in dementia. Effects of etiology and severity. *Brain and Language, 25,* 117–133.

Hillis, A. E. & Caramazza, A. (1989). The graphemic buffer and attentional mechanisms. *Brain and Language, 36,* 208–235.

Howard, D. & Butterworth, B. (1989). Short-term memory and sentence comprehension: A reply to Vallar and Baddeley, 1987. *Cognitive Neuropsychology, 6,* 455–463.

Irigaray, L. (1967). Approche psycholinguistique du language des dements. *Neuropsychologia, 5,* 25–52.

Kaszniak, A. W., Garron, D. C., & Fox, J. (1979). Differential aspects of age and cerebral atrophy upon span of immediate recall and paired associate learning in older subjects with suspected dementia. *Cortex, 15,* 285–295.

Kelter, S., Cohen, R., Engel, D., List, G., & Strohner, H. (1977). Verbal coding and visual memory in aphasics. *Neuropsychologia, 15,* 51–60.

Kertesz, A. (1982). *The western aphasia battery.* New York: Grune and Stratton..

Kertesz, A., Appell, J., & Fisman, M. (1986). The dissolution of language in Alzheimer's disease. *Canadian Journal of Neurological Sciences, 13,* 415–418.

Kinsbourne, M. (1972). Behavioral analysis of the repetition deficit in conduction aphasia. *Neurology, 22,* 1126–1132.

Kohn, S. (1984). The nature of the phonologic disorder in conduction aphasia. *Brain and Language, 23,* 97–115.

Kolk, H. H. J. & van Grunsven, M. M. F. (1985). Agrammatism as a variable phenomenon. *Cognitive Neuropsychology, 2,* 347–384.

Kopelman, M. D. (1985). Rates of forgetting in Alzheimer-type dementia and Korsakoff's syndrome. *Neuropsychologia, 23,* 623–638.

Lieberman, P., Friedman, J., & Feldman, L. S., (1990). Syntax comprehension deficits in Parkinson's disease. *Journal of Nervous and Mental Disease, 178,* 360–365.

Linebarger, M. C., Schwartz, M. F., & Saffran, E. M. (1983). Sensitivity to grammatical structure in so-called agrammatic aphasics. *Cognition, 13,* 361–392.

Locke, J. L. & Deck, J. W. (1978). Retrieval failure, rehearsal deficiency, and short-term memory loss in the aphasic adult. *Brain and Language, 5,* 227–235.

Marcel, A. J. (1980). Surface dyslexia and beginning reading: A revised hypothesis of the pronunciation of print and its impairments. In M. Coltheart, K. Patterson, & J. C. Marshall (Eds.), *Deep dyslexia.* 227–258. London: Routledge and Kegan Paul.

Marcus, M. P. (1980). *A theory of syntactic recognition for natural language.* Cambridge: MIT Press.

Martin, R. C. (1987). Articulatory and phonological deficits in short-term memory and their relation to syntactic processing. *Brain and Language, 32,* 159–192.

Martin, R. C. (1990). Neuropsychological evidence on the role of short-term memory in sentence processing. In G. Vallar & T. Shallice (Eds.), *Neuropsychological impairments of short-term memory.* 390–427. Cambridge: Cambridge U. Press.

Martin, A., Brouwers, P., Cox, C., & Fedio, P. (1985). On the nature of the verbal memory deficit in Alzheimer's disease. *Brain and Language, 25,* 323–341.

Martin, R. C., Wetzel, W. F., Blossom-Stach, C., & Feher, E. (1989). Syntactic comprehension deficits. *Cognition, 32,* 157–191.

McCarthy, R. & Warrington, E. (1984). A two-route model of speech production: Evidence from aphasia. *Brain, 107,* 463–485.

McCarthy, R. A. & Warrington, E. K. (1987). Understanding: A function of short-term memory? *Brain, 110,* 1565–1578.

McClelland, J. L. & Rumelhart, D. E. (1986). *Parallel distributed processing: Explorations in the microstructure of cognition.* Vol. 2. Cambridge: MIT Press.

Miceli, G., Mazzucchi, A., Menn, L., & Goodglass, H. (1983). Contrasting cases of Italian agrammatic aphasia without comprehension disorder. *Brain and Language, 18,* 65–97.

Miceli, G., Silveri, M. C., & Villa, G. (1985). Cognitive analysis of a case of pure dysgraphia. *Brain and Language, 25,* 187–196.

Milner, B., Petrides, M., & Smith, M. L. (1985). Frontal lobe and the temporal organization of memory. *Human Neurobiology, 4,* 137–142.

Monsell, S. (1984). Components of working memory underlying verbal skills: A "distributed capacities" view. In H. Bouman & D. G. Bouwhuis (Eds.), *Attention and performance X.* Hillsdale NJ: Lawrence Erlbaum Associates.

Morris, R. G. (1984). Dementia and the functioning of the articulatory loop system. *Cognitive Neuropsychology, 1,* 143–157.

Morris, R. G. (1986). Short-term forgetting in senile dementia of the Alzheimer type. *Cognitive Neuropsychology, 3,* 77–97.

Morris, R. G. (1987). Articulatory rehearsal in Alzheimer-type dementia. *Brain and Language, 30,* 351–362.

Morris, R. G. & Kopelman, M. D. (1986). The memory deficits in Alzheimer-type dementia: A review. *Quarterly Journal of Experimental Psychology, 38A,* 575–602.

Morton, J. (1980). The logogen model and orthographic structure. In U. Frith (Ed.), *Cognitive processes in spelling.* 117–134. New York: Academic Press.

Nebes, R. D. (1989). Semantic memory in Alzheimer's disease. *Psychological Bulletin, 106,* 377–394.

Nebes, R. D. & Brady, C. B. (1989). Focused and divided attention in Alzheimer's disease. *Cortex, 25,* 3–5–315.

Nespoulos, J. L., Dordain, M., Perron, C., Ska, B., Bub, D., Caplan, D., Mehler, J., & Lecours, A. R. (1988). Agrammatism in sentence production without comprehension deficits: Reduction availability of syntactic structures and/or of grammatical morphemes? A case study. *Brain and Language, 33,* 273–295.

Newcombe, F. & Marshall, J. C. (1980). Transcoding and lexical stabilization. In M. Coltheart, K. E. Patterson, & J. C. Marshall (Eds.), *Deep dyslexia.* London: Routledge and Kegan Paul.

Ostergaard, A. L. & Meudell, P. R. (1984). Immediate memory span, recognition memory for subspan series of words, and serial positoin effects in recognition memory for supraspan series of verbal and nonverbal items in Broca's and Wernicke's aphasia. *Brain and Language, 22,* 1–13.

Ostrin, R. K. & Schwartz, M. F. (1986). Reconstructing from a degraded trace: A study of sentence repetition in agrammatism. *Brain and Language, 28,* 328–345.

Pate, D. S., Saffran, E. M., & Martin, N. (1987). Specifying the locus of the production impairment in conduction aphasia. *Language and Cognitive Processes, 2,* 43–84.

Patterson, K. E. (1982). The relation between reading and phonological coding: Further neuropsychological observations. In A. W. Ellis (Ed.), *Normality and pathology in cognitive functioning.* 77–111. London: Academic Press.

Patterson, K. E., Marshall, J. C., & Coltheart, M. (Eds.), (1985). *Surface dyslexia.* London: Lawrence Erlbaum.

Patterson, K. E. & Morton, J. (1985). From orthography to phonology: An attempt at an old interpretation. In K. E. Patterson, J. C. Marshall, & M. Coltheart (Eds.), *Surface dyslexia.* 335–360. London: Lawrence Erlbaum.

Patterson, K. E., Seidenberg, M. S., & McClelland, J. L. (1988). Reading acquisition and dyslexia: A connectionist perspective. In P. Morris (Ed.), *Connectionism: The Oxford perspective.* Oxford: Oxford University Press.

Peterson, L. R. & Peterson, J. J. (1959). Short term retention of individual verbal items. *Journal of Experimental Psychology, 58,* 193–198.

Pinker, S. & Prince, A. (1988). Rules and connections in human language. *Cognition, 28,* 73–193.

Posteraro, L., Zinelli, P., & Mazzucchi, A. (1988). Selective impairment of the graphemic buffer in acquired dysgraphia: A case study. *Brain and Language, 35,* 274–286.

Riege, W. H., Metter, E. J., & Hanson, W. R. (1980). Verbal and nonverbal recognition memory in aphasic and nonaphasic stroke patients. *Brain and Language, 10,* 60–70.

Roeltgen, D. P. & Heilman, K. (1984). Lexical agraphia. *Brain, 107,* 811–827.

Rothi, L. J. & Hutchinson, E. C. (1981). Retention of verbal information by rehearsal in relation to the fluency of verbal output in aphasia. *Brain and Language, 12,* 347–359.

Saffran, E. M. & Marin, O. S. M. (1975). Immediate memory for word lists and sentences in a patient with deficient auditory short-term memory. *Brain and Language, 2,* 420–433.

Saffran, E. M. & Martin, N. (1990). Short-term memory impairment and sentence processing: A case study. In G. Vallar & T. Shallice (Eds.). *Neuropsychological impairment of short-term memory.* Cambridge: Cambridge University Press.

Schwartz, M. F., Saffran, E. M., & Marin, O. S. M. (1980). The word order problem in agrammatism. I. Comprehension. *Brain and Language, 10,* 263–280.

Shallice, T. & Warrington, E. K. (1977). Auditory-verbal short-term memory impairment and conduction aphasia. *Brain and Language, 34,* 235–245.

Shallice, T., Warrington, E. K., & McCarthy, R. (1983). Reading without semantics. *Quarterly Journal of Experimental Psychology, 35A,* 111–138.

Strub, R. L. & Gardner, H. (1974). The repetition defect in conduction aphasia: Mnestic or linguistic? *Brain and Language, 1,* 241–255.

Tzortzis, C. & Albert, M. L. (1974). Impairment of memory for sequences in conduction aphasia. *Neuropsychologia, 12,* 355–366.

Vallar, G. & Baddeley, A. D. (1984). Phonological short-term store, phonological processing and sentence comprehension: A neuropsychological case study. *Cognitive Neuropsychology, 1,* 121–141.

Vallar, G. & Baddeley, A. D. (1987). Phonological short-term store and sentence processing. *Cognitive Neuropsychology, 4,* 417–438.

Warrington, E. K., Logue, V., & Pratt, R. T. (1971). The anatomical localization of selective impairment of auditory-verbal short-term memory. *Neuropsychologia, 9,* 377–387.

Warrington, E. K. & Shallice, T. (1969). The selective impairment of auditory-verbal short-term memory. *Brain, 92,* 885–896.

Murray Grossman, Philadelphia, Pennsylvania (USA)

31. Aphasia Therapy

1. Introduction

A spate of research papers and editorials published in medical journals in the UK in the late 1970s and early 1980s prompted a new examination of the practice and evaluation of aphasia therapy, the ripples from which spread around the world. Three papers in particular (David/Enderby/Bainton 1982; Lincoln/McGuirk/Mulley et al. 1984; Meikle/Wechsler/Tupper et al. 1979) came to the conclusion that the therapy for aphasic patients provided as part of the speech therapy service in Britain was not effective, or at least was no more effective than the help which volunteers could provide if given some advice.

Coming at a time of economic cutbacks, and pressures on health services to work within cost-effective budgets, these papers evoked strong reactions. One, taken by some physicians, health managers and their advisers, was to question the need for referring aphasic patients for specialist help, and to promote interest in catering for the needs of this section of the population by encouraging volunteer helpers. There was also discussion of increasing the numbers of paid 'speech therapy assistants', and of creating generic therapists who could cope at a basic level with a range of 'paramedical' needs, such as social work, physical therapy, speech therapy and occupational therapy. A second, more reasoned, reaction was to examine the methodological validity of the studies. It was argued that they were applying, inexactly and inappropriately, a design of randomised controlled trials developed for other purposes, which presumed, in particular, that the subjects used were homogeneous in respect of the critical variable (aphasia), and that the treatment engaged was similarly homogeneous and exactly specified. Neither of these conditions had in fact applied (Howard 1986; Pring 1986). Randomised allocation of aphasic subjects to the different treatment conditions rests on the questionable assumption that aphasia is essentially a unitary condition. Treatment regimes in all these studies were described vaguely as classical, traditional, conventional, or as flexibly adapted to the patient's needs, but with no further information. Replication of the studies, on these grounds alone, would therefore be impossible.

1.1. A Paradigm Shift?

The result of such heart-searching has been to accelerate a paradigm shift in the study of therapy for aphasia (therapy here being used in its broadest sense of any kind of intervention aimed at alleviating the patient's communicative dysfunction). It consolidated the moves which were already being made on three fronts towards a more scholarly approach to the examination of aphasia therapy. These were: first, the matching of defined categories of patients with therapy programmes which were published in detail and were replicable; second, the application of psycholinguistic models of language processing to the examination of aphasic individuals, with a model-based specification of the disorder and of the aims of therapy; and third, the systemization of therapy which focusses on communication rather than language, and which therefore also gives primacy to the aphasic individuals' partners in everyday life. What all these approaches have in common, and what justifies the claim of a paradigm shift, is the emphasis on systematic analysis, though the methods used depend on the discipline with which each approach is allied. For these three 'schools' of therapy they are, respectively, the disciplines of neurology, cognitive psychology and sociolinguistics. In all these schools, aphasia therapy is not seen as intuitive and ad hoc, but as based on motivated and recursive assessment of the individual, systematically testing hypotheses about the nature of the disorder. This assessment is not necessarily psychometric in its nature (cf. also art. 11.), and the discussion of each of these three schools of therapy will attempt to show how the approach to assessment, as well as to therapy, differs.

2. Intuitive Therapies

Before we look at these three particular schools, however, a word of explanation is needed as to how the circumstances should have arisen which lead to the articles mentioned at the beginning of this chapter, in which aphasia therapists lent themselves to what they believed was an honest exposure of the inadequacies of the service they were offering. Their conclusions seemed to support the recommendation that, since it appeared that face-to-face therapy with aphasic patients could be conducted as effectively by guided volunteers as by skilled therapists, therapists' roles should become those of assessors and supervisors of less-qualified helpers rather than direct practitioners of therapy. The reason was that, for some time, the dominant practice of aphasia therapy had been intuitive, with therapists responding reactively to patients' patterns of language behavior. Therapy required, not so much expert knowledge, as a sympathetic rapport, good judgement as to when to encourage and when to hold back, and a stock of language exercises, classed as to whether they were aimed at helping speech, auditory comprehension, reading or writing. Specialised postgraduate training in aphasia therapy was short on the ground (and still is). The only attempts at theories of aphasia were unitary theory (which proposed that aphasia could not be divided into types) or neurologically-based theories. The only one of these that had direct relevance to therapy was that of Luria (1970) which was little known outside Eastern Europe until the 1980s. Very little experimental work had been published on the effectiveness of different types of therapy for different types of aphasic patients. With a predominantly intuitive and empirical approach to therapy, therefore, the difference between many speech therapists (for whom aphasia was just one of their areas of practice) and dedicated, experienced volunteers was less great at this time than the professional/amateur boundary might suggest.

2.1. Stimulation Therapy

This is not to imply that there had not been any attempts to introduce a systematic rationale to aphasia therapy before the 1970s (in addition to the delayed world-wide impact of the Lurian approach, to which we shall refer later) (see Howard/Hatfield 1987, for an excellent review of the history of aphasia therapy). One of these was developed by the 'stimulation' school of aphasia therapy, initiated by Wepman (1951) and developed by Schuell/Jenkins/Jiménez-Pabón (1964). This was based on a quasi-physiological concept of brain damage, in which it was held that the language system in the brain operated with reduced efficiency, and that stimulation was the only means by which the therapist could make complex events occur in this damaged brain system. This unitary conception of brain function was mirrored in a unitary conception of aphasia, the defining characteristics of which were a reduction in available vocabulary and in comprehension. Vocabulary items were not lost, but were inaccessible at will. This conceptualisation of aphasia, and its consequent implications for remediation, differed from the earlier emphasis, which had focussed on speech production difficulties, and assumed that abilities were lost and had to be re-taught. In the stimulation school of therapy the key to remediation for all aphasic patients was intensive auditory stimulation, predominantly at word rather than sentence level, from which the patient's own responses would be produced as an overflow rather than being forced. The therapist was encouraged to repeat words to the patient over and over again – to the order of 20 times. The obvious surface differences between individual aphasic patients was explained by saying that they had (or had not) additional peripheral disorders overlaid on the 'simple' aphasia which was the true, unitary aphasia – peripheral disorders which could be visual affecting reading, visuospatial affecting writing, sensorimotor affecting the praxis of articulation, for example. The full therapeutic repertoire, therefore, incorporated exercises using all modalities. The aim was to build on automatic production in order to develop voluntary control. Despite the current unpopularity of unitary theory, the stimulation approach remains influential in clinical practice, although now much modified from the stress on intensive repetition of words by the therapist. At the time of its introduction the popularity of this therapy can be attributed to several features. It was linked with the first comprehensive assessment to be designed specifically for aphasia (the Minnesota Test for the Differential Diagnosis of Aphasia), and to a formal proposition about the nature of aphasia based on results from this test. It provided advice on a number of therapeutic exercises and on interactions with the patient. The book in which it was popularised, with authors from the disciplines of psychology and neurology as well as speech pathology (Schuell/Jenkins/Jiménez-Pabón 1964), reveals a warmth and insightfulness into the care of aphasic people, and a respect for their courage, which makes it attractive to members of a caring profession.

We can see the changes that have occurred in therapy derived from this school in the recommendations for therapy published by Shewan/Bandur (1986). Although in reporting the group results of 28 patients who received Language Oriented Therapy (LOT), these therapists used the Boston classification (Broca's, Wernicke's aphasia etc.), the types of treatment used were not married to these syndromes. The schemes of treatment (specified in commendable detail, and with materials and procedures provided in the book) were modality based in a similar way to Schuell's recommendations i. e. they are classed as treatments for auditory processing, visual processing, gestural/gestural-verbal communication, oral expression and graphic expression. The patient is to be assessed on a standard test or otherwise, so that deficits in these language behaviors can be recorded, and individual therapy programmes then be targeted at the deficits in the modalities. The general philosophy of aphasia is similar to that of Schuell i. e. that the language system is impaired or disturbed and that access to it is also faulty. Although in its lack of a specific match of treatment to theory, we feel justified in classing this approach still under the heading of 'intuitive', it represents a serious attempt to provide a clinically practicable methodology for therapy and to evaluate the effectiveness of the approach used.

2.2. Behavioral Therapy

Where earlier approaches to therapy had assumed that language had to be retaught or to be reactivated through stimulation, behavior therapy as applied to aphasia rests on the intuition that language is essentially intact, and can be revealed if the behavioral blockages are removed. Much of the influence of behaviorism in the 1960s and early 1970s was on applying the principles of behavior modification such as shaping and reinforcement as a teaching method using programmed learning, often with teaching machines (Holland 1970; Sarno/Silverman/Sands 1970). This aspect of behaviorism has its most modern form in the more flexible use of microcomputers and interactive discs as teaching machines. Robertson has reviewed the development of computers as a medium of therapy, commenting that their use for teaching precise aspects of language to aphasic patients has so far been restricted "Because of the lingering adherence to more generalized notions of wide-ranging and non-specific language reabilitation" (Robertson 1990, 388). He does, however, cite an unpublished study by Stachowiak and his colleagues in Bonn in which results from a large randomized controlled trial suggested that adding extra hours of general computerized speech therapy improved effectiveness. As well as providing a medium through which therapy can be delivered in clinic or home (Petherham 1991), microcomputers can also, of course, provide an alternative means of communication (see Kraat 1990) for a review) or a supplement to communication, as in providing word-finding prompts (Bruce/Howard 1987; Colby/Christinaz/Parkison et al. 1981). Behaviorism provided more than ideas for improving the teaching media used in rehabilitation. It influenced the content of therapy through its tenet that language behavior, like other behaviors, could be shaped by modelling and reinforcement by tokens, praise, or simply accurate feedback as to success (Goodkin 1969; Goldstein/Ruthven 1983). In some cases also, aphasia could be accompanied by learned fears of communicating, and could therefore be reduced by the same desensitization techniques that were used with stutterers or people with phobias (Ince 1968; Damon/Lesser/Woods 1979). Similarly relaxation (Marshall/Watts 1976), laughter (Potter/Goodman 1983) or hypnosis (Thompson/Hall/Sison 1986) might be effective as facilitators. Behaviorism's most significant influence on aphasiology in the 1970s was probably in its stress on quantification and 'objectivity', an overtly anti-theoretical perspective, as expressed by Sidman (1971, 413): "The phenomena of aphasia can be classified empirically, without biassing the observations by preconceptions of what language 'really' is. The data will then be available to any theory". One result of this attempt at empirical objectivity was the categorisation of patients by their quantifiable production of speech rather than by their more-difficult-to-measure comprehension, as fluent or non-fluent. Another was the formulation of tests which aimed to meet the standards laid down for psychological tests (Porch 1967) and to compare stimulus and response systematically (Sidman 1971). But its influence on therapy also remains. Porch (1986), maintaining like Schuell that aphasia represents a reduction in the processing efficiency of the brain, describes how the results of his test can be used in therapy. But his recommendations relate to general management and are atheoretical. Patterns of performance within subtests ('slowrise' compared with rapid fatiguability) and across subtests can be used to predict the potential which the patient could achieve; therapy should be directed at parallel items to those in the subtests in which the patient was able to perform accurately but only after delay or further prompts.

An effective recent application of behavioral principles in aphasia therapy was reported by Doyle/Goldstein/Bourgeois/Nakles (1989). It is particularly interesting because it overtly marries behaviorism with some of the tenets of functional communication therapy, which we shall describe later. It remains, however, within what we have called intuitive approaches to therapy, in that the therapy was not based on a rationale which distinguished individual patients' patterns of aphasia, or on a coherent theory of the nature of aphasia. Doyle/Goldstein/Bourgeois/Nakles's paper describes how four stroke patients with Broca's aphasia were trained to ask questions. The technique was primarily to "give the subject an opportunity to talk" on one of three topics (health, leisure and personal information). The patients were told explicitly to ask as many questions of their conversational partner as they could. They were praised if they asked an intelligible (however ungrammatical) question, and were also 'rewarded' with an answer. If the patient had not formulated a request for information within 20 seconds despite the partner's nonverbal encouragement through eye contact, the partner modelled a request for the patient to imitate; cue cards could be used if necessary. To maintain the naturalness of the requests for information on the topics, a large number of volunteers were used as partners, as well as three therapists who functioned as the trainers. The researchers report that "following the initiation of treatment, all subjects demonstrated a rapid and marked increase in the use of requests during trainer probes" (Doyle/Goldstein/Bourgeois/Nakles 1989, 165) i.e. during 5-minute conversation samples in a nontreatment setting. The patients were also rated as being significantly more talkative, after the initiation of treatment, by a group of 12 students who were asked to assess videotaped samples presented in random order. The criterion for success was functional communication, not language structure, and the authors note that "improved efficiency of requesting occurred within the context of negative effects with regard to grammatical completeness and question morpheme usage" (Doyle/Goldstein/Bourgeois/Nakles 1989, 169). The behavioral philosophy behind this approach to therapy is that aphasic patients can communicate if instructed to do so and given appropriate modelling and reinforcement. This successful study indicates that this may apply at the level of the social and pragmatic use of language, but does not necessarily circumvent the aphasic person's difficulties with language structure as such. It suggests, in fact, a trade-off between the two, with the implication that an emphasis on grammatical structure in therapy could even make functional communication less effective.

The various alternative visual communication systems which have been used with aphasic patients, such as Blissymbols, VIC and its computerised adaptation C-VIC have concentrated on communication of the message, with minimal loading on grammatical effort other than word or symbol order (Gardner/Zurif/Berry/Baker 1976; Funnell/Allport 1989; Weinrich 1991).

Two of the formalised programmes of therapy which have recently emerged from the influential Boston group also apply the behaviorist philosophy that language can be brought under control by instruction and feedback, i.e Voluntary Control of Involuntary Utterances (VCIU) and Treatment of Aphasic Perseveration (TAP). In VCIU (Helm-Estabrooks 1983b) patients whose speech is largely restricted to stereotypies are asked to read voluntarily any words they have been heard to read involuntarily, as in semantic paralexias. The list is supplemented by emotional words, which are usually considered to be better preserved; the patients are then asked to use these words in other ways, thus moving to voluntary production of them. TAP (Helm-Estabrooks/Emery/Albert 1987) employs strategies to avoid perseveration in naming such as drawing patients' attention to the phenomenon and explaining it, slowing the pace of presentation of items and tearing up a piece of paper which has the perseverated word written on it. A more radical approach to preventing perseveration is to avoid circumstances which promote it in some patients, such as the rather unnatural task of naming pictures.

3. Model-Based Approaches

In contrast to the approaches we have reviewed so far, three model-based approaches have been developed, which attempt to relate individual patients' symptoms to coherent models of aphasia. Two of these are neurological in motivation, one psychological.

3.1. Syndrome-Linked (Lurian)

Luria's physiologically based concept of the operation of mind proposed a system of distributed neural networks which served the 'higher cortical functions' such as language. Such a network has a degree of plasticity; if one component is damaged, a similar output from it can sometimes be achieved through reconstitution of the network using the other components. Whereas the approaches to therapy we reviewed above can be categorised as re-teaching, reactivating or revealing, the Lurian approach is essentially one of reconstitution through re-organization. With such a theory of potential plasticity, and working often with young head-injured soldiers, Luria had a much more active interest and participation in aphasia therapy than currently do most Western neurologists. Luria's techniques, however, though developed in the 1930s and described in Russian in the 1940s, were not made available in English until the 1960s (Luria 1963; 1966), and were therefore influential on clinical practice predominantly only in Eastern Europe until recently. Luria developed a classification of aphasias into (originally) six syndromes, associated with neuroanatomical sites according to the location in which damage interrupted the network. His proposals for therapy were therefore the first to be syndrome-linked and matched to the underlying concept of the nature of that particular disorder. With afferent motor aphasia, for example, the underlying disorder was considered to be in the kinaesthetic basis of the articulation of speech; therapy included substituting visual input for the kinaesthetic feedback through diagrams of articulatory gestures. This externally assisted reorganisation could then become internalised and automatised as part of the reconstituted network. Similarly visual input could be helpful in the impairment of phonological discrimination which underlay sensory aphasia. A well-known application of therapy for efferent motor aphasia by a student of Luria's is the "preventive method" (Beyn/Shokhor-Trotskaya 1966), which stresses the need to use predicative words and phrases early in therapy, so as to avoid the development of telegrammatic speech. A more recent adaptation of the Lurian approach in Finland has taken the notion of reorganisation as applying more generally to the whole language system, and has resulted in the development of an integrated multi-modal Language Enrichment Therapy programme (Salonen 1980), which shares some similarities with the general stimulation approach.

3.2. Syndrome-Linked (Bostonian)

The most structured syndrome-linked therapies for aphasia have been developed in the last two decades at the Boston V. A. Hospital in Massachusetts. From this base the neurologist Geschwind (1965) repopularised the classical localizationist doctrines of the late 19th century, and the division into aphasia of the syndromes of Broca's, Wernicke's, conduction, anomic, transcortical and global aphasias. The syndromes were linked with linguistic levels by the clinical psychologists Goodglass/Kaplan (1972), with Broca's aphasia identified (as well as with articulatory disorder) with a disorder of syntax, Wernicke's with a lexical-semantic disorder, conduction with an output phonological deficit particularly affecting repetition, and anomic with difficulty in lexical retrieval. Transcortical aphasia (in its isolation, motor and sensory forms) was a complete or partial separation of the whole language system from thought. The speech pathologists at Boston have published a number of formal programmes aimed at ameliorating some of these syndromes. Melodic Intonation Therapy (MIT) is used for patients with a Broca's aphasia in which the 'articulation' difficulties of apraxia of speech are prominent (Helm-Estabrooks 1983a). This draws on the theory that the right cerebral hemisphere, considered to be the neural substrate for some aspects of music, may take over some language functions after severe left hemisphere damage, or may be able to assist recovery in the left hemisphere. (An extreme form of therapy based on this notion is Brain Function Therapy (Buffery/Burton 1982) in which multimodal stimulation is directed at the right hemisphere with masking stimuli to the left hemisphere; other, more pragmatic "right-brain stimulation" therapies for aphasia use drawing (Pillon/Signoret/Van Eeckhout/Lhermitte 1980) and visual imagery (Fitch-

West 1983)). For the syntactic aspects of Broca's aphasia, Helm-Estabrooks (1981) has devised the Helm Elicited Language Syntax Stimulation (HELPSS) programme, which provides graded exercises aimed at eliciting sentences of different complexities, first with modelling, then with a lead-in prompt. Like other forms of stimulation therapy this is based on the premise that patients have not lost a particular ability (in this case the use of syntax) but need practice in accessing it. The comprehension problems of Wernicke's aphasia can be tackled by another Boston programme, Sentence Level Auditory Comprehension (SLAC) (Naeser/Haas/Mazurski/Laughlin 1986), in which the focus is on making phonemic discriminations between pairs of words, first-presented without, then with, a sentence context. This uses a tape playback system, the Language Master, and is suitable for self-teaching for some patients, as feedback as to correctness is provided. For globally aphasic patients, Visual Action Therapy (VAT) (Helm-Estabrooks/Fitzpatrick/Barresi 1981) may be suitable, as a preliminary to other therapies. This has the aim of reintegrating the patient's mental functioning, in order to cope with the processing of stimulus, symbol and response. It therefore has a rather different purpose from the direct teaching of the use of a sign system such as AmerInd (Skelly 1979) or a visual system of communication, such as we have described earlier, as an alternative means of communication – whatever secondary effect these may have on the language system itself. With VAT patients learn to associate representational drawings (first of their own hand and then of a series of objects) with the objects themselves and with gestures indicating the use of these objects. The programme culminates in the patient making a gesture to indicate an object which is out of sight. Since this is a re-integrating therapy, globally aphasic patients are expected to improve not only in the use of gesture but in auditory comprehension and other aspects of language as well. Helm-Estabrooks (1983b) indicates that VAT may be particularly suitable for a sub-type of 'global' aphasia which can be identified as secondary to subcortical damage. In the same edited book as Helm-Estabrooks' paper, several other authors offer their general guidelines for syndrome-linked therapy, applying the Boston classification. As sub-types of syndromes have emerged, programmes have become more directly targeted. Kohn/Smith/Arsenault (1990), for example, give an account of the successful use of sentence repetition as a means of treatment for a patient with the type of conduction aphasia which is characterised by "a general speech production deficit in phonemic planning" (Kohn/Smith/Arsenault 1990, 58) rather than reduced auditory verbal short-term memory.

Also emerging from Boston, though at present less closely identified with its syndromes, is pharmacological therapy for aphasia (Bachman/Albert 1990). This is not a novel approach (it was, for example, one advocated by Luria, and Bachman/Albert cite more recent studies in Russia, Romania and Germany), but it has recently been reactivated in Boston. So far only uncontrolled studies of the use of bromocriptine have been reported, using patients classed as having a chronic non-fluent aphasia. Some improvement in naming and vocabulary, with a reduction in pauses in spontaneous speech, has been reported in most cases, with a dramatic improvement in one individual. Bachman and Albert's anatomo-physiological explanation for such a recovery is that dopaminergic centres in the midbrain project to the supplementary motor area in the dorsal-medial part of the left frontal lobe. If the dysfluency or initiation difficulties result from damage to this area or the projections to it, replacement therapy with a dopamine agonist such as bromocriptine may be of benefit. The syndrome that this particular pharmacological therapy would be linked with in this case would be transcortical motor aphasia.

The Boston classification is currently in use world-wide, and other programmes have emerged elsewhere which have been linked loosely to these syndromes, as they have become more closely aligned with linguistic levels of language. Howard/Hatfield (1987) review a number of studies from Germany which describe specific therapies for impaired phonemic organisation, agrammatism and global aphasia, and are suggested as appropriate for groups of patients who share these distinctive linguistic deficits. Many of these programmes have been influenced by linguists, and Howard/Hatfield distinguish these European aphasiologists as forming a 'neurolinguistic' school of therapy. The syndrome-linked therapy of MIT has also been developed for use with French aphasic patients (Van Eeckhout/Pillon/Signoret et al. 1982).

3.3. Cognitive Neuropsychological

The model which underlies the therapies described in the last two sections is primarily a neurological one, with some sophistication introduced by linguists in elaborating it by incorporating linguistic levels. The psycholinguistic approach to therapy (or cognitive neuropsychological, as it is often called in order to distinguish it from the non-specific use of 'psycholinguistic' by therapists such as Shewan and Bandur) is based on models which have a different root i. e. in cognitive psychology. Since these models are reviewed in another chapter of this volume (cf. art. 21) they will be only briefly referred to here. They are best developed as models of cross-modality single-word processing, originally as models of the processes which intervene between seeing a printed word and reading it aloud but with later incorporation of auditory and graphic processes. Nevertheless they are still agreed to be seriously underspecified (Ellis/Young 1988), and have faced more radical criticisms (e. g. Seidenberg 1988). This applies both to models of single word processing and sentence processing. Nevertheless they act as working hypotheses as to how the mind processes these restricted aspects of language and offer a framework through which to test a rationale for direct therapy.

What these models provide is not a prescription for aphasia therapy, but a method of examining an individual patient's disturbances in language processing in such a way as to be able to select from existing therapeutic tasks those ones which, at a first pass, would seem to have some prospect of ameliorating or circumventing the condition. These tasks may be drawn from any of the methods previously described, and from the trial and error techniques which have been built up through the intuitive approach to aphasia therapy. What is different in the psycholinguistically based approach is the individual selection of specific techniques based on a hypothesis about the nature of the cognitive changes the patient has undergone. The approach used may be reteaching, reactivatory, reorganisational or substitutory, depending on what aspects of the language processing system are considered to be malfunctioning. Since one of the tenets of cognitive neuropsychology is the modularity of mental processing, the dominant approaches are reorganisational and substitutory, in which the aim is to bypass a malfunctioning module by drawing on alternative routes. With reorganisation, as in the Lurian philosophy, the substitution becomes internalized, and is absorbed into the new functioning system. Some substitutions require the continuing use of an external prosthesis, for example, the use of computers as a word-finding prompt (Colby/Christinaz/Parkison et al. 1981; Bruce/Howard 1987). Nevertheless, other approaches besides the reorganisational and substitutory may be justified, and remain consistent with the theory of mental modularity. For example, if the patient appears to have a specific impairment of some semantic categories (as has been reported by a number of investigators, notably Warrington/McCarthy 1987), an appropriate approach for the therapist to consider may be reteaching of items in these categories. If, as may be more comon, the semantic disorder seems to be a more general blurring of fine semantic distinctions, a reactivatory approach, using exercises which stimulate the patient's residual awareness of word meanings, may be attempted. This method was used by Howard/Patterson/Franklin et al. (1985) and shown to be effective in improving patients' naming abilities, and to have an influence which lasted at least 24 hours, in contrast to facilitating naming by phonemic cuing. The improvement was achieved, moreover, without the patients themselves having any practice in producing spoken names, a result consistent with the proposed psycholinguistic model, in which the semantic system is conceived of as a module essentially independent of word form. The model also implies that different types of therapeutic exercises should be appropriate for different types of anomic difficulties: semantic exercises may be effective with patients with semantic degradation, while exercises which emphasise word-form may be effective for patients whose impairment is not essentially semantic, but is in retrieving lexical form (Lesser 1989). This hypothesis has been tested in a therapy study by Nettleton/Lesser (1991), and received some support.

Since the application of psycholinguistic modelling in neuropsychology was first made in reading, it is not suprising that the first detailed applications of cognitive neuropsychologically based rehabilitation in aphasia were directed at the same behavior, with writing not far behind. In what was probably the first paper to review specifically the relationship between (cognitive) neuropsychology and therapy, Beauvois/Derouesné (1982) describe the model-based therapy they used with four aphasic patients. With one (with an aphasia categorised as dynamic in Luria's classification) therapy was directed at elaboration of ideas rather than at language. With another (with tactile aphasia), help was given in the form of encouragement to visualise held objects which he could not name. But the most detailed programmes described were devised for two patients with reading disorders, one with a pure alexia and optic aphasia for colours, one with phonological alexia. Assessment indicated in the first patient, M. P., that the traditional therapy for such an alexia – retraining in reading through using the intact writing system by tracing letters during reading – would not be successful. M. P. appeared to have a visuo-verbal dissociation such that any direct association of what she saw with language was not possible. Accordingly she was trained to use a roundabout strategy to link seen letters with their names; the seen letter was associated with an arbitrary gesture, the seen gesture was then identified with a verbal code, and this verbal code was then translated into the name of the letter. After five months of this therapy (begun two years after her stroke) there were highly significant improvements in her ability to read letters and words. Four years later she was reading novels, slowly, but as her main relaxation. The other patient, R. G., with phonological alexia, was unable to read nonwords aloud, and made errors on reading aloud sentences which suggested he was snatching at their gist rather than reading them exactly. His errors were particularly noticeable on function words. The therapists interpreted this pattern of reading as an inability to override contextual expectations, and encouraged him to read sentences as a series of isolated words. After a month of practice in this programme R. G. 's reading of words in sentence contexts, and particularly of function words, had improved highly significantly.

At about the same time, Hatfield (1983) was also applying to therapy for agraphia the insights from the then current two-route models which Beauvois and Derouesné had applied to alexia (the two routes being the lexical-semantic and the phonological-graphemic). Hatfield reports her application of the two-route model of writing to four aphasic patients. Three of them were diagnosed as having deep agraphia (i. e. they could write to dictation only by means of the lexical-semantic route, and made more errors on function words than on content words). Therapy drew on their superior ability to write the content word rather than the function word member of a pair of homophonic words. The patients learned to associate such homophonic pairs as *bean/been* and *hymn/him,* with the function word always being associated with a content word which they could already spell. By use of this strategy all three patients showed some improvement in the ability to spell the targeted function words. The fourth patient was diagnosed as having a surface agraphia and as spelling to dictation by using a simple phoneme-to grapheme translation, with loss of the lexical memory of the written form of many words. The therapy programme devised for her was to teach her some of the rules of spelling in English, so as to compensate for her lack of knowledge of lexical form by the ability to reconstitute words by rule. This was an overtly didactic approach. A similar approach has been used in Italian by Carlomagno/Parlato (1989) with a patient in whom both the lexical and the nonlexical routes to writing were considered to be seriously damaged. Reading disorders have similarly been treated by the use of an overtly didactic approach. De Partz (1986; Bachy-Languedock/de Partz 1989) found that the teaching of the grapheme-to-phoneme correspondence rules of French to a patient with deep dyslexia was so effective that his much improved reading, after nine months, showed the features of surface dyslexia in its reliance on pronunciation rules. A therapy for surface dyslexia, using memonic by-pass strategies like those effective with Hatfield's deep dysgraphic patients, is reported by Coltheart/Byng (1989). A head-injured postal-worker, E. E., showed the subtype of surface dyslexia that indicates that meaning is accessed only through the sound of misread words, and not directly from visual input through a lexical-semantic route. In therapy he learned to read correctly 24 words, all ending in *-ough*, by practising associating them with pictures of the words. A similar strategy of pairing other written words with symbols helped him to learn further sets of high frequency words.

In all these studies it is notable that conventional clinic techniques are used. The extent to which the actual techniques selected are dependent on interpretation of the patient's disorder through a psycholinguistic model has also been questioned (Caramazza 1989; Basso 1989). For example the use of analogy with homophonic content words for the spelling of function words is a technique which originated in clinics long before psycholinguistic models were fashioned in their present form. The value of the cognitive neuropsychological approach to aphasia therapy, therefore, does not lie (at least at present) in its proposing innovative techniques of intervention. The question is whether it can be demonstrated that it has contributed guidance of the selection of a particular technique beyond that of an experienced clinician's observation. This could be as much in indicating which techniques would not be expected to address the deficit, as in indicating which would. For example the type of remediation used with a nurse with a surface dyslexia by Scott/Byng (1989), i.e. judging the correctness of homophones presented in sentences on a computer, would not be appropriate for a patient in whom the surface dyslexic symtoms are due to an impairment in the lexical route which occurs after semantic access rather than before it. Psycholinguistic models have the advantage of providing a coherent framework, which is so far supported by experimental studies, through which aphasia therapists can understand some aspects of their patients' disorders (not least by keeping track of them through a visual diagram). They also provide justifications for not using certain enshrined clinical practices unselectively, for example in not endorsing spoken naming drills for those anomic patients whose disorder is predominantly semantic.

They are also of potential help with other levels of language than single words, in particular, with sentence grammar, although psycholinguistic models at the sentence level (and at the higher level of discourse) are at present even less well specified than lexical models. The sentence level model which has so far been applied in aphasia therapy is based on an adaptation of Garrett's model by Schwartz (1987), with a particular emphasis on mapping between syntactic and semantic representations through the establishment of thematic roles in sentences. Linebarger (1990) has proposed that the difficulties some agrammatic speakers have is in this mapping between syntax and semantics. Two studies of therapy have reported the application of this notion to treatment (Jones 1986; Byng/Coltheart 1986; Byng 1988). Both employed not only a teaching method but one that was overtly metalinguistic, in that the two patients concerned were taught about thematic roles and their relationship to word order in English. Byng/Coltheart used sentences incorporating locative prepositional phrases (e.g. *the pan is in the jug*), which had to be distinguished from those where the lexical items were in reversed roles, as illustrated in pictures. Jones used a more varied approach, getting her patient first to identify the verb in sentences, and then to distinguish various thematic roles, such as who or what was the doer, whom or what the theme, where the setting was and so on. This therapy, conducted with a patient with Broca's aphasia who had failed to improve after some years of therapy on spoken language, specifically discouraged attempts at sentence production, to the patient's relief. The theoretical account offered for his disorder is that his mapping disorder was bidirectional, and that work on comprehension should therefore result in improvement in speech. The outcome supported this account. Both with Jones' and with Byng/Coltheart's patients, after the therapy aimed at improving comprehension of thematic roles, agrammatic speech was ameliorated. This is not, of course, a prescription for all types of agrammatism, and Garrett's model would indeed imply that disturbances could apply at other levels of sentence production, for which direct work on speech (such as generating syntactic trees and lexical insertion) might be appropriate. It is germane to the cognitive neuropsychological approach to aphasia therapy that a prerequiste is the detailed analysis of the patient's discorder, and the specification of in what module or process the deficits appear to lie.

The emphasis in cognitive neuropsychology on individual assessment and individual variability is so strong that many of its practitioners advocate the abandonment of syndromes, and even subdivisions of the classical syndromes as in agrammatism (Badecker/Caramazza 1985; Ellis 1987; Howard/Patterson 1987). They are bolstered in this by the independence of psycholinguistic models from theories of localization, such as dominate the approaches we described in the last two sections. So far only limited attempts have been made to map the abstract level of psycholinguistic modelling onto areas of the brain (for an example of this, see Petersen/Fox//Posner et al. 1988), though as neuroscience comes closer to neuropsychology we may expect the development of an interdisciplinary field. Not only this, but clinical convenience, implies the use of grouped patients identified by some convenient label. Therapies are therefore becoming identified with what have been described as symptom-complexes rather than syndromes. This characterizes the therapy as directed at specific symptoms related to a model, without the implication that the patient shows all the other features that can be associated with a syndrome. Replication of therapy studies may thus be undertaken on other individuals who share the same critical symptoms for that procedure to be proposed as appropriate.

4. Communication Therapy

Emphasis on the needs of the individual is also paramount in the final approach to aphasia therapy that we shall discuss, though here the individuals are assessed as members of their social network. If the cognitive neuropsychological approach to therapy has independence from a medical model, so even more emphatically does this one, drawing primarily on sociolinguistic ethnomethodology, the study of language and communication in their everyday settings. Functional communication therapy has sometimes been contrasted with the cognitive neuropsychological approach in that it focusses on the patients' use of their assets, whereas the latter tends to be directed towards remedying deficits. This contrast is somewhat artificial in that, as we have seen, the logic of the reorganisation and substitution methods in applying a psycholinguistic model is to capitalise on retained routes. In a more global way, however, functional communication therapy aims to develop the patients' communicative assets. This type of approach to therapy is two-pronged. One prong relates to direct intervention with patients, generally in clinical settings (as with the other approaches to therapy we have described). The other is indirect, following the logic that, if communication is necessarily an activity involving at least two people, aphasic patients' communication can be improved by directing intervention at their partners.

4.1. Direct Intervention

In 1972, Wepman, a respected American speech pathologist who had played a major role in the development of stimulation therapy, published a paper advocating the cessation of formalised work on language exercises, with switching of both the therapist's and the patient's attention to the meaning of the message rather than the medium. He cited the case of a lawyer who had failed to respond to formal clinical exercises, but whose communication was transformed when the therapist discussed with him the legal briefs that he had been engaged on at work. To some extent this may seem to be simply an extension of the classical clinical principle of using materials which are pertinent and motivating to the patient. Wepman, however, went beyond such an interpretation. He proposed that aphasic patients' language difficulties may be due to an impairment in thought (a notion which also has a long history e. g. Marie 1906), and that "thought-centred therapy" is therefore a logical way to approach their problem. As Howard/Hatfield (1987, 71) comment "This proposal at first sight is so vague that it seems to be a recipe for almost total non-therapy; you could do almost anything and maintain that this was thought stimulation". We come back again to the question raised at the beginning of this chapter, whether there are any reasons to expect the therapist's intervention to be more beneficial than that of volunteers or family members. As Howard/Hatfield point out, however, there is a cognitive neuropsychological justification for Wepman's claim that this form of therapy could be successful for some patients: this conception of the aphasic disorder comes close to the interpretation of agrammatic comprehension as a failure to map the syntactic operation of word order onto meaning, the 'mapping hypothesis' of agrammatism. In such a case, at the very least the therapist's assessment of whether this would be an appropriate regime for an individual patient at a particular time is critical.

A more general reaction to statements such as Wepman's was one encouraged by the development of interest in pragmatics by linguistics in the 1970s (see Levinson 1983, for a review). The formalizing of notions about pragmatics offered a way of structuring clinical programmes so as to maximize communicative effectiveness (including nonverbal communication, and verbal communication by other means than speech). Two of the first ideas to be adopted were the notion from conversational analysis of turn-taking, and, from a then currently popular notion in linguistics, of 'speech acts'. The latter drew attention to the way in which spoken or written language in itself can perform behavioral acts (e. g. *I promise*) rather than reporting on them. Most importantly it emphazied the variety of speech acts – not only performatives, but requests, questions, commands and so on

– and the frequent discrepancy between the literal form of words and the speaker's intent. We have already described Doyle/Goldstein/Bourgeois et al.'s (1989) therapy programme for aphasic patients, aimed at eliciting requests for information. Another well-established clinical procedure is aimed at facilitating patients' conveying of information, in a situation which mimics the turn-taking of natural conversation. In Promoting Aphasics' Communicative Efficiency (PACE) (Davis/Wilcox 1985), therapist and patient take turns at conveying (through any means, verbal or non-verbal) what is represented on a stack of cards. The therapist models what is expected to be productive for the patient, but there is no direct instruction, so as not to spoil what is implied to be the 'naturalness' of the reciprocal communication. This procedure may be useful as practice for the patient in applying strategies which have already been drilled, such as the use of symbolic gesture, but this is different from what the authors claim to be one of the principles of PACE – that there should be a free choice of channels of communication. The extent to which 'new' information is being conveyed in such a situation is questionable, since therapists may feel the need to prime themselves with some knowledge of the set of cards to be used. The emphasis on turn-taking may also be unnecessary, since the only type of aphasia in which this seems to be in question is fluent aphasia with press-of-speech, and there is no reason to expect a disruption of awareness of turn-taking in aphasia in general. The theory base of such an approach is therefore slender, and the extent to which it reproduces a natural situation is questionable.

An overtly instructional method is used in Holland's system of Conversational Coaching (Holland 1991). This aims to maximize communicative effectiveness by analysing, in co-operation with the patients, their most productive strategies, and rehearsing the use of these through individually prepared scripts appropriate to their interests and abilities. The scripts could convey some item of news or gossip. After rehearsal with the therapist, a relative or helper is brought into the room, so that the patient can relay the information in the script. This meeting is usually videotaped, for later analysis by the therapist, relative and patient of the means by which effective communication was or could be achieved (this brings in the further dimension of communication therapy – indirect intervention – which we shall discuss in the next section). The Conversational Coaching programme is then extended by calling in a stranger to the patient, to whom the script's message can also be conveyed. This is a promising approach in communication therapy, but its value rests upon the skilled analysis of strategies. At present this is in the very early stages of systematic investigation, and so far predominantly only in respect of the analysis of the spoken elements of conversation. In present clinical practice, therefore, the analysis of communication strategies remains largely unformalized, although advice on it is plentiful (see, for example, Aten 1986) as we describe shortly.

What we have described so far is predominantly one-to-one direct therapy between patient and therapist. There is an inherent contradiction in applying this to functional communication, in that the patient's communicative needs with this one partner in a clinical setting are limited. The situation is one in which therapist and patient have inherently different roles, however much the therapist may be motivated to engage the patient as a principal in sharing ideas. Advocates of functional communication therapy, therefore, frequently utilise groups. There are two main types of this therapy, game-playing and role-playing. Stroke groups run by volunteers or social workers generally involve the patients in language-related games, as well as social outings, and the use of games has also been proposed as a part of therapist-directed treatment (Davis/Wilcox 1985). The effectiveness of such an approach in improving communication is difficult to evaluate, although patients and their relatives may derive other benefits (Lesser/Watt 1978). Aten/Caligiuri/Holland (1982), however, have demonstrated positive benefits on communication through role play in group activities, in which patients discussed and applied strategies they could use in a variety of situations such as shopping. This approach has also been claimed to improve self-confidence and motivation as well as the specific use of language itself (Tsvetkova 1980).

4.2. Indirect (Communication)

A more radical divergence in communication therapy is the focussing of therapy on the aphasic person's communicative partners, rather than on the patient. This is an application of the principle that communication is a social activity and that the enhancement of communication can be achieved by improving the partner's own use of co-operative strategies with the patient. This is different from the psychotherapeutic counselling of the patients' relatives, to which we shall refer in the next section. It was first explicitly advocated in aphasia in respect of a form usually neglected by the more classical treatments, jargonaphasia (Martin 1981). Amongst Martin's recommendations are to provide the partner with as much information about the patient's disorder as possible, perhaps by inclusion in therapy sessions, to demonstrate that it is possible to understand the patient as well as to be understood, and to train in specific techniques of modelling and encouraging monitoring. Like most other advocates of communication therapy, Martin saw this kind of approach as complementary to direct help from the therapist on communication and language. Holland (1991) makes the same point in discussing communication therapy, that it does not need to exclude direct work on language where this is indicated. By analogy with practice in the education of the deaf, this combined approach has sometimes been referred to as Total Communication. Other therapists have focussed more on naturalistic communication in everyday settings. Green (1984, 41) states that "management programmes should place a greater emphasis upon the u s a g e of language within naturalistic contexts". She describes an interactional approach to aphasia therapy based on detailed observation of family conversations. Ideally, given that utterances are always dependent on the contexts in which they are uttered, this should be within the patient's own environment, although she admits that home-like conditions may need to be simulated in clinic settings, for practical reasons. She cites examples of productive strategies which have been observed and which can be utilized by aphasic people's partners: slowing of rate, pausing, use of less ambiguous sentences, construction of sentences so that key words are at the end, changes of topic, use of alerters, stress and gesture and rephrasing. Green's and Marshall's (1987) recommendations concern strategies to improve the patient's comprehension. But this kind of approach has also led to a burgeoning interest in the application to aphasia of techniques of conversational analysis derived from sociolinguistics, such as study of the collaborative use of repair in word-finding difficulties (Lesser/Milroy 1993). This development holds the promise of tailoring recommendations for management to the individual's communicative needs, in the same way that the cognitive neuropsychological approach provides specification of the individual's psycholinguistic characteristics as a basis for selection of appropriate direct therapies for improving lexical and sentence skills.

4.3. Indirect (Psychotherapeutic)

The approaches described in the last two sections come clearly within the province of the aphasia therapist's work, in that they draw upon the specialized applications of linguistics which form part of this profession's training. Aphasia therapists normally also include a limited element of counselling in their responsibilities, aware of the needs of both the patient and the family members for support for the psychological and psychosocial consequences of brain damage (Brumfitt/Clarke 1983). Indeed one study (Hartman/Landau 1987) suggests that counselling therapy provided by speech therapists may be as effective as 'conventional' aphasia therapy, at least during the period of recovery between one and seven months post onset of aphasia. 'Family therapy' for aphasia, however, as formulated by Wahrborg (1989) is seen as an outgrowth of psychotherapy which requires a specialized training. Although it shares with the therapy we have just been describing the aim of improving the families' communication skills, it also has the aim of avoiding emotional disorders and psychological deterioration. This deals, therefore, with communication skills in a different sense from that with which linguistics is concerned, but includes family dynamics and the emotional contexts of communication. Wahrborg/Borenstein (1990, 374) conclude that there is evidence to support the "assumption that families and family life have an impact on the rehabilitation outcome", and that what happens psychologically and communicatively within aphasia families needs to be analysed. One such system for undertaking this has been proposed by Mulhall (1988). This is a computerized, questionnaire-based analysis of the dynamics of spouse-aphasic relationships. It can be used in rehabilitation, in providing the partners with insight into these dynamics, with a later re-assessment of the effects of achieving this insight.

5. Evaluation

Although the use of many of these approaches to therapy has not been evaluated in ways which stand up to close inspection, the paradigm shift we referred to earlier as having taken place since the 1980s has led to much closer attention being paid to methodologically-sound experimental designs for evaluating the effects of intervention. Group designs have continued to have their practitioners (e.g. Wertz/Weiss/Aten et al. 1986; Shewan/Bandur 1986), but the majority of efforts have been directed at single-case studies. Group designs may be necessary at some stage for confirming hypotheses about the nature of aphasia itself (Zurif/Gardner/Brownell 1989; Fitz-Gibbon 1986), but since therapy should be based on a detailed analysis of an individual's disorder, and the predominant form of intervention used is one-to-one, it is single-case studies that now dominate the approach to research into aphasia therapy.

There are several descriptions of appropriate designs in single-case studies of aphasia therapy (see for example Coltheart 1983; Pring 1986; Howard/Hatfield 1987; Willmes 1990). An important question is the extent to which these can be applied in routine clinical practice, or are suitable only for researchers into aphasia therapy. Designs which require more time than the working practitioner can spare, and can therefore only be used by researchers, still have their value; they can indicate what the results of therapy can be expected to be for specific types of patients, provided that the study identifies their characteristics in sufficient detail for them to be applied to other cases. As we have seen, also, one previous obstacle to applying the results of earlier (group) studies, that of underspecification of the actual treatments used, need no longer apply. But, given the present weakness of knowledge of brain-behavior relationship, there is still a pressing need for the practising therapist to be able to evaluate the actual (as opposed to the predicted) consequences of interventions undertaken with individual patients. Without this the therapist remains uncertain as to whether any good is actually being done and whether the patient has reached, even temporarily, a plateau in recovery.

Lapointe (1977) proposed a method, Base-10, specifically for use in routine clinical work. This is a framework which can be used with a variety of contents, and therefore matched to what are thought to be the patients' specific needs. It proposes that 10 items should be identified in respect of a particular therapeutic task, measured over about three occasions to establish a baseline, and then worked upon in therapy for 10 sessions, so that progress, if any, can be graphed. Progress on 10 items drilled in such a format is commonly shown to occur, and the graph can often be used in motivating the patient. Such a formula, however, provides no real evidence that the therapy is effective in itself. The patient may be improving spontaneously, and a three-point baseline is not sufficient to test this. Nor is there any evidence to show that the change is not due to friendly support and the feeling that someone is now interested in alleviating the aphasia (the 'placebo effect'). Two precautions have been suggested to overcome the first criticism, i.e. the taking of a longer base-line measurement (Pring 1986), and the use of this design only with patients past the period of spontaneous recovery. Sarno (1981) comments on the lack of consensus as to what this period is; the greatest recovery is likely to take place during the first three months, but studies of evaluation generally take at least six months as the period over which spontaneous recovery could significantly influence the results. Neither of these precautions is helpful to the practizing aphasia therapist. The criticism that the effect of the intervention may be a nonspecific one due to the feeling that someone is taking an interest has been tackled in a different way. Designs have been suggested which are aimed at controlling for this. One is to use a cross-over design (Coltheart 1983). For this two tasks need to be identified, to which the patient is expected to respond differently. Performance on both tasks is re-measured after a period of therapy on one. Attention in therapy is then switched to the second task, with performance on both tasks measured again at the end of this period. Getting clear results from such a design does indeed depend on the theoretical distinctiveness of the two tasks; despite the postulated modularity of language processes, it is not infrequent to find improvement on both tasks when only one has been treated (consistent with the unitary nature of aphasia proposed by Schuell). A second design, which can be used where effects are expected to be specific to items, is to split the list of items into two matched or random sets, and to work only on one (Howard/Patterson/Franklin et al. 1985). If, as predicted, the improvement occurs only on the treated set, it can be claimed that the intervention was not due to a placebo effect or to spontaneous recovery. Again it is more common to find some effects on the untreated list; in addition to the other two possible reasons for this (placebo or spontaneous recovery), it may be due to generalization – a desirable consequence for the patient, but ambiguous for proving that the result was due to the therapy itself. Nevertheless it is essential to have some comparison of the effect of treatment with non-treatment (even when initially non-treated items or tasks are to be the subject of later therapy). If the effect is shown only to occur with treatment, this is real evidence of its effectiveness, and the absence of generalization can be supportive of the model of psycholinguistic processing applied (Byng/Coltheart 1986). Assessing the value of the intervention to the patient also requires the measurement of how long the effects of treatment last, and many designs incorporate remeasurement after a period without treatment to test their stability. Howard/Patterson/Franklin et al. (1985) indeed refer to effects on naming which last less than 24 hours as being due only to facilitation, which they distinguish from therapy. It is also often desirable to include a measure of functional communication to examine whether or not the hoped-for extension of clinical work into something useful in everyday life has occurred. Such measures range from formal assessment of communication using a standardized test (such as Holland's Communicative Activities in Daily Living 1980), through a detailed conversational analysis (Lesser/Milroy 1993) to a rapid questionnaire for use by carers (such as the Communicative Effectiveness Index of Lomas/Pickard/Bester et al. 1989).

In routine clinical work it may be possible to incorporate some of these designs. Given that it is generally good practice to work on more than one aspect of language at a time, and to use more than one method of intervention in order to maintain the patient's interest and reduce fatigue, it should be possible to use cross-over designs, both in comparing tasks and in comparing methods. As Howard/Hatfield (1987, 121) comment, use of these designs is "a potential and largely unexploited source of sound empirical data on the effectiveness of therapeutic techniques".

6. Delivery of Services

No review of aphasia therapy could claim adequate coverage without some comment on the actual delivery of the interventions described in earlier sections of this chapter. Aphasia therapy takes place in many settings: hospital for in-patients and out-patients, specialized units for different types of aetiologies such as head-injury and stroke, rehabilitation units specialized for young or old age-groups, patients' own homes, health clinics, adult literacy centres (Parr 1985), and residential colleges (Borenstein/Wahrborg/Linell et al. 1987). In some countries volunteer-run clubs also provide substantial help for aphasic and other stroke patients (Griffith/Miller 1980; Lesser/Watt 1978), though this is not always integrated with the speech therapy service, and may not provide 'aphasia therapy' in the sense that we have been using this term in this chapter. The provision of professional therapy for aphasic people varies widely around the world, and, even in countries where it is well established although the supply of therapists is limited, therapy for aphasic adults tends to take second place to the more pressing demands of children with developmental speech and language disorders (Rossiter/McInally 1989). With increasing interest in cost-effectiveness in public health services, there has therefore been considerable discussion of three issues. The first is whether or not certain types of aphasic patients should be given priority of treatment over others. Another is whether the pattern of delivery of therapy as intensive or distributed, or as group or one-to-one, influences its effectiveness. The third is the one we referred to at the beginning of this chapter i. e. the extent to which unpaid volunteers or modestly-paid assistants can be used as supplements (or alternatives) to qualified therapists.

6.1. Priorities in Treatment

Enderby/Davies (1989) have suggested that aphasic patients can be divided into three groups according to the severity of the disorder. They propose that maximum therapeutic effort should be directed at the middle group, which, they argue, is the most likely to benefit. Severely impaired chronic aphasic people have been reported as having an "irreversible syndrome" (Schuell/Jenkins/Jiménez-Pabón 1964; Sarno/Silverman/Sands 1970), and, in times of stringency, it has been argued that therapists' time with them may not be well spent. This, however, is based on a notion of aphasia therapy as being concerned only with the restoration of spoken language. If functional communication is the target of therapy, achieving some improvement in global aphasia may make the difference between adequate coping in everyday life or not, reducing the stress on the family and perhaps avoiding more serious breakdowns (Edelman 1987). Similarly there have been arguments for concentrating more therapeutic effort on the mildly impaired, on the grounds that these are the people who may be able to return to work, if given a relatively modest amount of therapy (Marshall 1987). Since there is no consensus of opinion on this matter, and little research, in practice aphasia therapists tend to make their own decisions based on such parameters as estimated motivation of the patient, availability of supportive family members to assist with home assignments, ability to travel to the clinic and so on.

6.2. Pattern of Delivery

It has been proposed that aphasia therapy has to be intensive for it to be effective. David (1983, 22), for example, concludes from a review of several studies that "Very intensive therapy (18 – 25 hours per week) seems to be more effective than a more intermittent exposure". It has also been noted that, in the British studies which reported that therapy from speech therapists was no more effective than either no therapy or the help given by volunteers, the amount of contact the patients had with their speech therapists was only about two hours a week. The typical pattern of therapy in some countries is more intensive than this, perhaps due to limits on time for insurance cover, or the greater use of residential centres. Hagen's (1973) and Wertz/Weiss/Aten et al.'s (1986) reports on successful therapy in the USA, for example, refer to between 8 and 18 hours of therapy per week. The claim that intensive therapy is superior to non-intensive therapy was examined in a study by Brindley/Copeland/Demain/Martyn (1989). Five men and five women with a Broca's aphasia of between 18 and 130 months duration were given three months of intensive residential therapy (25 hours a week, given by a team of therapists, helped by a volunteer) sandwiched between three-month periods of non-intensive therapy. The measures of change were a Functional Communication Profile (FCP), grammatical analysis and a questionnaire to relatives. Although the patients' group results showed a significant inprovement in speech rating on the FCP and on the grammatical analysis after the period of intensive therapy, compared to ratings made after the first period of non-intensive therapy, the conclusion that intensive therapy is superior may not be justified. The number of hours of treatment in the two conditions differed by a factor of more than 10. Moreover the non-intensive treatment consisted of 'conventional therapy' by various therapists, while the intensive therapy followed specific programmes and was conducted by a team. The appropriateness of intensive therapy may also depend on the duration and severity of aphasia. Except when the disability is mild, the therapist's intervention immediately post onset may need to be primarily in counselling and assessing rather than in direct treatment.

One study has compared group treatment with individual treatment. Wertz/Collins/Weiss et al. (1981) compared two sets of patients who received eight hours of treatment a week between four and 48 weeks post onset. Taking the results of patients who were at least six months post onset (and arguably past the period of significant spontaneous recovery) Wertz and his colleagues indicate that both group and individual therapy were effective. Fawcus (1983, 118) concluded that "at present there are no data to support the claim that group work is potentially a more successful learning situation than the individual treatment session", and warns that, when provision of speech therapy services is inadequate, groups may be used as a substitute for individual treatment rather than a complement to it. Kearns' (1986) review of group therapy for aphasia also complains of the lack of research into the efficacy of such an approach; he comments that it evolved as a practical response to the large influx of head-injured soldiers after the second World War, and that about three quarters of therapists who use group therapy have no specialist training in this method.

6.3. Stretching the Service

Other ways of stretching the service are to extend the amount of the patient's therapy time which does not require the direct supervision of a therapist. We have already referred to the use of microcomputers in therapy. An example of the use of microcomputers supplied for home use to work through standard programmes is in the work of Petherham

(1991). The use of computers to provide an expert system to aid therapists in assessment and selection of therapeutic exercises has also been proposed (Guyard/Masson/Quinious 1990), although this has been suggested as premature in the light of our current understanding of aphasia (Hirson/Chiat 1990). Videodiscs have also begun to be used in therapy (Bruckert/Gonon/Michel/Bez 1989). Other technical innovations have been pioneered by Vaughn in Birmingham, Alabama. She first developed a system of therapy delivery by telephone, including remote control of writing, later adding telecomputer treatment (Fitch/Cross 1983). This is offered as a way of geographically stretching the service to rural areas.

At first glance the use of assistants (and even more economically volunteers) may seem to be another way of making speech therapists' work more effective in an understaffed service. Wade (1983) has pointed out, however, that engaging, training and supervising volunteers may be very demanding on therapists. Marshall/Wertz/Weiss et al.'s (1989) analysis of the Wertz/Weiss/Aten et al. (1986) study in which "home therapists" (predominantly relatives) were used emphasizes the considerable amount of time and effort which the professional speech therapists spent in training them and in monitoring their efforts. A study by Quinteros/Williams/White/Pickering (1984) examined the costs of using volunteers as part of an aphasia therapy service. Twenty four patients were allocated to either hospital or community speech therapy, and as part of the latter each was paired with a volunteer. The community group received monthly speech therapy at home, together with monthly practice sessions at home with the volunteer and fortnightly attendance at a speech therapy group. This proved one and a half times more costly than the hospital treatment, which comprised only monthly sessions. There were signs, however, that the community programme resulted in more improvement in the patients than did the hospital programme. Moreover the difference in costs would be reversed if the number of patients were to be somewhat larger, and the amount of hospital-based therapy increased to match the contact experienced by the community programme. Some of the cost was in training the volunteers – a recurrent cost, given the high turn-over to be expected of volunteer helpers. This suggests that the use of already trained and paid assistants might be beneficial. This notion has been taken up by the Health Service in England and Wales, with a proposal to develop training for therapy assistants, ranging from generic helpers to assistants with specific training relevant to different paramedical therapies. Such assistants would not be substitutes for volunteers, in that their relationships with patients would differ from that of 'equal friends' by virtue of their semi-professional role; nor is it likely that they would be employed as home-sitters to give relatives relief, a useful role for volunteers. They could, however, relieve therapists of some ancillary duties, such as taking care of the patients' welfare outside the therapy session and assisting in therapy exercises under supervision. The distinction between a high-grade assistant and a qualified therapist will give cause for some close scrutiny. One essential difference will lie in the therapist's capacity to initiate and undertake research – not only in studies for publication, but in the day-to-day interaction with the patient. If aphasia therapy is seen as a continuing process of forming hypotheses about a patient's disorder, testing these through therapy and making adjustments to provide more effective therapy (Jones/Byng 1989), research is an inherent component of the day-to-day treatment and management of aphasia. With the extension of numbers of speech therapy assistants, it will be important for therapists not to see themselves as predominantly directing their expertise to assessment, preparation of programmes, supervision of therapy-implementing assistants and counselling. In order to understand aphasia and the aphasic individuals to whom they are committed, and in order to learn more about the therapeutic process itself, they will need to maintain direct and continuing contact with the patients themselves. As the other chapters on aphasia in this volume testify, the study of acquired language disorders is ever-increasing in its range, depth and complexity. The application of this knowledge to therapy needs the expertise of specialist therapists, who can not only understand and contribute to theories but extrapolate from them to practice. But no theory of aphasia is yet fully justified, and it is also important that therapists maintain their close contact with patients as a source of data and further insights through which to moderate both theory and practice.

7. Conclusion

Very often the tasks which aphasia therapists undertake with patients seem simple. As this review has tried to indicate, the simplicity is illusory. The essence of the therapist's skill is in the selection of the right task for the right patient at the right time, the sensitive interaction with the patient during its execution, and the delicate interpretation of its outcome. Despite the theoretical weakness of many approaches to therapy, the still yawning gap between psycholinguistic models and neuroscience, and the infancy of the systematic application of sociolinguistic principles to our understanding of aphasic language, the practice of aphasia therapy has been transformed over the last decade in those areas where an enlightened service has made this possible. As the theory base of aphasiology extends, it is important that services for patients follow suit in applying these insights to their welfare.

8. References

Aten, J. L. (1986). Functional communication treatment. In R. Chapey (Ed.), *Language intervention strategies in adult aphasia. 266–276.* Baltimore: Williams & Wilkins.

Aten, J. L., Caligiuri, M. P., & Holland, A. L. (1982). The efficacy of functional communication therapy for chronic aphasic patients. *Journal of Speech and Hearing Disorders, 47,* 93–96.

Bachman, D. L. & Albert, M. L. (1990). The pharmacotherapy of aphasia: historical perspective and directions for future research. *Aphasiology, 4,* 407–413.

Bachy-Languedock, N. & de Partz, M.-P. (1989). Coordination of two reorganization therapies in a deep dyslexic patient with oral naming disorder. In X. Seron & G. Deloche (Eds.), *Cognitive approaches in neuropsychological rehabilitation. 211–247.* Hove: Lawrence Erlbaum Associates.

Badecker, W. & Caramazza, A. (1985). On considerations of method and theory governing the use of clinical categories in neurolinguistics and cognitive neuropsychology: the case against agrammatism. *Cognition, 20,* 97–125.

Basso, A. (1989). Spontaneous recovery and language rehabilitation. In X. Seron & G. Deloche (Eds.), *Cognitive approaches in neuropsychological rehabilitation. 17–37.* Hove: Lawrence Erlbaum Associates.

Beauvois, M. F. & Derouesné, J. (1982). Recherche en neuropsychologie et rééducation: quels rapports? In X. Seron & C. Laterre (Eds.), *Rééduquer le cerveau. 163–189.* Brussels: Mardaga.

Beyn, E. S. & Shokhor-Trotskaya, M. K. (1966). The preventive method of speech rehabilitation in aphasia. *Cortex, 2,* 96–108.

Borenstein, P., Wahrborg, P., Linell, S, Hedberg, E., Asking, M., & Ahlsen, E. (1987). Education in 'Folk High School' for younger aphasic people. *Aphasiology, 1,* 263–266.

Brindley, P., Copeland, M., Demain, C., & Martyn, P. (1989). A comparison of the speech of ten chronic Broca's aphasics following intensive and non-intensive periods of therapy. *Aphasiology, 3,* 695–707.

Bruce, C. & Howard, D. (1987). Computer-generated phonemic cues: an effective aid for naming in aphasia. *British Journal of Disorders of Communication, 22,* 191–201.

Bruckert, R., Gonon, M.-A. H., Michel, F., & Bez, M. (1989). The use of a computer driven videodisc for the assessment and rehabilitation of aphasia. *Aphasiology, 3,* 473–478.

Brumfitt, S. & Clarke, P. (1983). An application of psychotherapeutic techniques to the management of aphasia. In C. Code & D. J. Muller (Eds.), *Aphasia therapy. 89–100.* London: Edward Arnold.

Buffery, A. W. H. & Burton, A. (1982). Information processing and redevelopment: towards a science of neuropsychological rehabilitation. In A. Burton (Ed.), *The pathology and psychology of cognition. 253–292.* London: Methuen.

Byng, S. (1988). Sentence processing deficits: theory and therapy. *Cognitive Neuropsychology, 5,* 629–676.

Byng, S. & Coltheart, M. (1986). Aphasia therapy research: methodological requirements and illustrative results. In E. Hjelmquist & L. B. Nilsson (Eds.), *Communication and handicap. 191–213.* Amsterdam: North Holland.

Caramazza, A. (1989). Cognitive neuropsychology and rehabilitation: an unfulfilled promise? In X. Seron & G. Deloche (Eds.), *Cognitive approaches in neuropsychological rehabilitation. 383–398.* Hove: Lawrence Erlbaum Associates.

Carlomagno, S. & Parlato, V. (1989). Writing rehabilitation in brain damaged adult patients: a cognitive approach. In X. Seron & G. Deloche (Eds.), *Cognitive approaches in neuropsychological rehabilitation. 175–209.* Hove: Lawrence Erlbaum Associates.

Colby, K. M., Christinaz, D., Parkison, R. C., Graham, S., & Karpf, C. (1981). A word-finding computer program with a dynamic lexical-semantic memory for patients with anomia using an intelligent speech prosthesis. *Brain and Language, 14,* 272–281.

Coltheart, M. (1983). Aphasia therapy research: a single-case study approach. In C. Code & D. J. Muller (Eds.), *Aphasia therapy. 193–202.* London: Edward Arnold.

Coltheart, M. & Byng, S. (1989). A treatment for surface dyslexia. In X. Seron & G. Deloche (Eds.), *Cognitive approaches in neuropsychological rehabilitation. 159–174.* Hove: Lawrence Erlbaum Associates.

Damon, S. G., Lesser, R., & Woods, R.T. (1979). Behavioural treatment of social difficulties in an aphasic woman and a dysarthric man. *British Journal of Disorders of Communication, 14,* 31–38.

David, R. M. (1983). Researching into the efficacy of aphasia therapy. In C. Code & D. Muller (Eds.), *Aphasia therapy. 15–24.* London: Edward Arnold.

David, R. M., Enderby, P., & Bainton, D. (1982). Treatment of acquired aphasia: speech therapists and volunteers compared. *Journal of Neurology, Neurosurgery and Psychiatry, 45,* 957–961.

Davis, G. A. & Wilcox, M. J. (1985). *Adult aphasia rehabilitation: applied pragmatics.* Windsor: NFER-Nelson.

de Partz, M. P. (1986). Reeducation of a deep dyslexic patient: rationale of the method and results. *Cognitive Neuropsychology, 3,* 149–177.

Doyle, P. J., Goldstein, H., Bourgeois, M. S., & Nakles, K. O. (1989). Facilitating generalized requesting behavior in Broca's aphasia: an experimental analysis of a generalization training program. *Journal of Applied Behavior Analysis, 22,* 159–170.

Edelman, G. (1987). Global aphasia: the case for treatment. *Aphasiology, 1,* 75–79.

Ellis, A.W. (1987). Intimations of modularity, or, the modelarity of mind: doing cognitive neuropsychology without syndromes. In M. Coltheart, G. Sartori, & R. Job (Eds.), *The cognitive neuropsychology of language. 397–408.* Hove: Lawrence Erlbaum Associates.

Ellis, A.W. & Young, A.W. (1988). *Human cognitive neuropsychology.* Hove: Lawrence Erlbaum Associates.

Enderby, P. & Davies, P. (1989). Communication disorders: planning a service to meed the needs. *British Journal of Disorders of Communication, 24,* 301–331.

Fawcus, M. (1983). Group therapy: a learning situation. In C. Code & D. J. Muller (Eds.), *Aphasia therapy. 113–119.* London: Edward Arnold.

Fitch, J. L. & Cross, S. (1983). Telecomputer treatment for aphasia. *Journal of Speech and Hearing Disorder, 48,* 335–336.

Fitch-West, J. (1983). Heightening visual imagery: a new approach to aphasia therapy. In E. Perecman (Ed.), *Cognitive processing in the right hemisphere. 215–228.* New York: Academic Press.

Fitz-Gibbon, C.T. (1986). In defence of randomised controlled trials, with suggestions about the possible use of meta-analysis. *British Journal of Disorders of Communication, 21,* 117–124.

Funnell, E. & Allport, A. (1989). Symbolically speaking: communicating with Blissymbols in aphasia. *Aphasiology, 3,* 279–300.

Gardner, H., Zurif, E. B., Berry, T., & Baker, E. (1976). Visual communication in aphasia. *Neuropsychologia, 14,* 275–292.

Geschwind, N. (1965). Disconnexion syndromes in animals and man. *Brain, 88,* 237–294, 585–644.

Goldstein, G. & Ruthven, L. (1983). Rehabilitation of the brain-damaged adult and behaviour therapy. In G. Goldstein & L. Ruthven (Eds.), *Rehabilitation of the brain-damaged adult. 118–158.* New York: Plenum.

Goodglass, H. & Kaplan, E. (1972). *Assessment of aphasia and related disorders.* Philadelphia: Lea and Febiger.

Goodkin, R. (1969). Changes in word production, sentence production and relevance in an aphasic through verbal conditioning. *Behavior Research and Therapy, 7,* 93–99.

Green, G. (1984). Communication in aphasia therapy: some of the procedures and issues involved. *British Journal of Disorders of Communication, 19,* 35–46.

Griffith, V. E. & Miller, C. L. (1980). Volunteer stroke scheme for dysphasic patients with stroke. *British Medical Journal, 281,* 1605–1607.

Guyard, H., Masson, V., & Quinious, R. (1990). Computer-based aphasia treatment meets artificial intelligence. *Aphasiology, 4,* 599–613.

Hagen, C. (1973). Communication abilities in hemiplegia: effect of speech therapy. *Archives of Physical Medicine and Rehabilitation, 54,* 154–158.

Hartman, J. & Landau, W. M. (1987). Comparison of formal language therapy with supportive counseling for aphasia due to acute vascular accident. *Archives of Neurology, 44,* 646–649.

Hatfield, F. M. (1983). Aspects of acquired dysgraphia and implications for re-education. In C. Code & D. J. Muller (Eds.), *Aphasia therapy. 157–169.* London: Edward Arnold.

Helm-Estabrooks, N. (1981). *Helm Elicited Language Program for Syntax Stimulation.* Austin, Texas: Pro-ed.

Helm-Estabrooks, N. A. (1983a). Exploiting the right hemisphere for language rehabilitation: melodic intonation therapy. In E. Perecman (Ed.), *Cognitive processing in the right hemisphere. 229–240.* New York: Academic Press.

Helm-Estabrooks, N. (1983b). Treatment of subcortical aphasias. In W. H. Perkins (Ed.), *Language handicaps in adults. 97–103.* New York: Thieme-Stratton.

Helm-Estabrooks, N., Emery, P., & Albert, M. L. (1987). Treatment of aphasic perseveration (TAP) program. *Archives of Neurology, 44,* 1253–1255.

Helm-Estabrooks, N., Fitzpatrick, P. M., & Barresi, B. (1981). Visual action therapy for global aphasia. *Journal of Speech and Hearing Disorders, 47,* 385–389.

Hirson, A. & Chiat, S. (1990). Where the intelligent therapist fears to tread: a commentary on Guyard et al. *Aphasiology, 4,* 615–619.

Holland, A. L. (1970). Case studies in aphasia rehabilitation using programmed instruction. *Journal of Speech and Hearning Disorders, 35,* 11–16.

Holland, A. L. (1980). *Communicative abilities in daily living.* Baltimore: University Park Press.

Holland, A. L. (1991). Pragmatic aspects of intervention in aphasia. *Journal of Neurolinguistics, 6,* 197–211.

Howard, D. (1986). Beyond randomised controlled trials: the case for effective case studies of the effects of treatment in aphasia. *British Journal of Disorders of Communication, 21,* 89–102.

Howard, D. & Hatfield, F. M. (1987). *Aphasia therapy: historical and contemporary issues.* Hove: Lawrence Erlbaum Associates.

Howard, D. & Patterson, K. (1987). Models for therapy. In X. Seron & G. Deloche (Eds.), *Cognitive approaches in neuropsychological rehabilitation. 39–64.* Hove: Lawrence Erlbaum Associates.

Howard, D., Patterson, K., Franklin, S., Orchard-Lisle, V. M., & Morton, J. (1985). The treatment of word-retrieval deficits in aphasia: a comparison of two therapy methods. *Brain, 108,* 817–829.

Ince, L. P. (1968). Desensitization with an aphasic patient. *Behavior Research and Therapy, 6,* 235–237.

Jones, E. V. (1986). Building the foundations for sentence production in a non-fluent aphasia. *British Journal of Disorders of Communication, 21,* 63–82.

Jones, E. V. & Byng, S. (1989). The practice of aphasia therapy: an opinion. *Bulletin of the College of Speech Therapists,* September 1989, 2–4.

Kearns, K. P. (1986). Group therapy for aphasia: theoretical and practical considerations. In R. Chapey (Ed.), *Language intervention strategies in adult aphasia. 304–318.* Baltimore: Williams and Wilkins.

Kohn, S. E., Smith, K. L., & Arsenault, J. K. (1990). The remediation of conduction aphasia via sentence repetition: a case study. *British Journal of Disorders of Communication, 25,* 45–60.

Kraat, A. W. (1990). Augmentative and alternative communication: does it have a future in aphasia rehabilitation? *Aphasiology, 4,* 321–338.

Lapointe, L. L. (1977). Base-10 programmed stimulation: task specification, scoring and plotting performance in aphasia therapy. *Journal of Speech and Hearing Disorders, 42,* 90–105.

Lesser, R. (1987). Cognitive neuropsychological influences on aphasia therapy. *Aphasiology, 1,* 189–200.

Lesser, R. (1989). Some issues in the neuropsychological rehabilitation of anomia. In X. Seron & G. Deloche (Eds.), *Cognitive approaches in neuropsychological rehabilitation. 65–104.* Hove: Lawrence Erlbaum Associates.

Lesser, R. & Milroy, A. L. (1993). *Linguistics and aphasia: psycholinguistic and pragmatic aspects of intervention.* London: Longman.

Lesser, R. & Watt, M. (1978). Untrained community help in the rehabilitation of stroke sufferers with language disorders. *British Medical Journal, 2,* 1045–1048.

Levinson, S. C. (1983). *Pragmatics.* Cambridge: Cambridge University Press.

Lincoln, N. B., McGuirk, E., Mulley, G. P., Lendrem, W., Jones, A. G., & Mitchell, J. R. A. (1984). Effectiveness of speech therapy for aphasic stroke patients: a randomised controlled trial. *Lancet, 1,* 1197–1200.

Linebarger, M. C. (1990). Neuropsychology of sentence parsing. In A. Caramazza (Ed.), *Cognitive neuropsychology and neurolinguistics: advances in models of cognitive function and impairment. 55–122.* Hillsdale: Lawrence Erlbaum Associates.

Lomas, J., Pickard, L., Bester, S., Elbard, H., Finlayson, A., & Zoghaib, C. (1989). The communicative effectiveness index: development and psychometric evaluation of a functional communication measure for adult aphasia. *Journal of Speech and Hearing Disorders, 54,* 113–124.

Luria, A. R. (1963). *Restoration of function after brain injury.* Oxford: Pergamon.

Luria, A. R. (1966). *Higher cortical functions in man.* London: Tavistock.

Luria, A. R. (1970). *Traumatic aphasia.* Le Hague: Mouton.

Marie, P. (1906). The third left frontal convolution plays no special role in the function of language. In M. F. Cole & M. Cole (Eds.), (1971), *Piere Marie's papers on speech disorders.* New York: Hafner.

Marshall, R. C. (1987). Reapportioning time for aphasia rehabilitation: a point of view. *Aphasiology, 1,* 59–73.

Marshall, R. C. & Watts, M. (1976). Relaxation training: effects on the communicative ability of aphasic adults. *Archives of Physical Medicine and Rehabilitation, 57,* 464–467.

Marshall, R. C., Wertz, R. T., Weiss, D. et al. (1989). Home treatment for aphasic patients by trained nonprofessionals. *Journal of Speech and Hearing Disorders, 54,* 462–470.

Martin, A. D. (1981). Therapy with the jargon-aphasic. In J. W. Brown (Ed.), *Jargonaphasia. 305–326.* New York: Academic Press.

Meikle, M., Wechsler, E., Tupper, A., Benenson, M., Butler, J., Mulhall, D., & Stern, G. (1979). Comparative trial of volunteer and professional treatments of dysphasia after stroke. *British Medical Journal, 2,* 87–89.

Mulhall, D. J. (1988). The management of the aphasic patient. In F. C. Rose, R. Whurr & M. A. Wyke (Eds.), *Aphasia. 489–517.* London: Whurr.

Naeser, M. A., Haas, G., Mazurski, P., & Laughlin, S. (1986). Sentence level auditory comprehension treatment program for aphasic adults. *Archives of Physical Medicine and Rehabilitation, 67,* 393–399.

Nettleton, J. & Lesser, R. (1991). Application of a cognitive neuropsychological model to therapy for naming difficulties. *Journal of Neurolinguistics, 6,* 139–157.

Parr, S. (1985). Are you using your adult literacy resources? *Bulletin of the College of Speech Therapists, 398,* 11–12.

Petersen, S. E., Fox, P. T., Posner, M. I., Mintun, M., & Raichle, M. E. (1988). Positron emission tomographic studies of the cortical anatomy of single-word processing. *Nature, 331,* 585–589.

Petherham, B. (1991). Microcomputers as a supplement to aphasia therapy. *Journal of Neurolinguistics, 6,* 177–195.

Pillon, B., Signoret, J. L., Van Eeckhout, P., & Lhermitte, F. (1980). Le dessin chez un aphasique: incidence possible sur le langage et sa rééducation. *Revue Neurologique, 136,* 699–710.

Porch, B. E. (1967). *Porch Index of Communicative Ability.* Palo Alto: Consulting Psychologists Press.

Porch, B. E. (1986). Therapy subsequent to the Porch Index of Communicative Ability (PICA). In R. Chapey (Ed.), *Language intervention strategies in adult aphasia. 295–303.* Baltimore: Williams & Wilkins.

Potter, R. E. & Goodman, N. J. (1983). The implementation of laughter as a therapy facilitator with adult aphasics. *Journal of Communication Disorders, 16,* 41–48.

Pring, T. R. (1986). Evaluating the effects of speech therapy for aphasics and volunteers: developing the single case methodology. *British Journal of Disorders of Communication, 21,* 103–115.

Quinteros, B., Williams, D. R. R., White, C. A. M., & Pickering, M. (1984). The costs of using trained and supervised volunteers as part of a speech therapy service for dysphasic patients. *British Journal of Disorders of Communication, 19,* 205–212.

Robertson, I. (1990). Does computerized cognitive rehabilitation work? A review. *Aphasiology, 4,* 381–405.

Rossiter, D. & McInally, K. (1989). Aphasia services: provision or privation? *Bulletin of the College of Speech Therapists, 449,* 4–6.

Salonen, L. (1980). The language enriched individual therapy program for aphasic patients. In M. T. Sarno & O. Hook (Eds.), *Aphasia: assessment and treatment. 105–115.* Stockholm: Almqvist & Wiksell.

Sarno, M. T. (1981). Recovery and rehabilitation in aphasia. In M. T. Sarno (Ed.), *Acquired aphasia. 485–529.* New York: Academic.

Sarno, M. T., Silverman, M., & Sands, E. (1970). Speech therapy and language recovery in severe aphasia. *Journal of Speech and Hearing Research, 13,* 607–623.

Schuell, H. M., Jenkins, J. J., & Jiménez-Pabón, E. (1964). *Aphasia in adults: diagnosis, prognosis and treatment.* New York, Harper & Row.

Schwartz, M. (1987). Patterns of speech production deficit within and across aphasia syndromes: application of a psycholinguistic model. In M. Coltheart, G. Sartori & R. Job (Eds.), *The cognitive neuropsychology of language. 163–199.* Hove: Lawrence Erlbaum Associates.

Scott, C. & Byng, S. (1989). Computer assisted remediation of a homophone comprehension disorder in surface dyslexia. *Aphasiology, 3,* 301–320.

Seidenberg, M. (1988). Cognitive neuropsychology and language: the state of the art. *Cognitive Neuropsychology, 5,* 403–426.

Shewan, C. M. & Bandur, D. L. (1986). *Treatment of aphasia: a language-oriented approach.* London: Taylor & Francis.

Sidman, M. (1971). The behavioral analysis of aphasia. *Journal of Psychiatric Research, 8,* 413–422.

Skelly, M. (1979). *Amerind gestural code based on universal American Indian handtalk.* New York: Elsevier.

Thompson, C. K., Hall, H. R., & Sison, C. E. (1986). Effects of hypnosis and imagery training on naming behavior in aphasia. *Brain and Language, 28,* 141–153.

Tsvetkova, L. S. (1980) Some ways of optimisation of aphasics' rehabilitation. *International Journal of Rehabilitation Research, 3,* 183–190.

Van Eeckhout, P., Pillon, B., Signoret, J.-L., Deloche, G., & Seron, X. (1982). Rééducation des réductions sévères de l'expression orale: la "therapie melodique et rythmée". In X. Seron & C. Laterre (Eds.), *Rééduquer le cerveau: logopedie, psychologie, neurologie. 109–121.* Brussels: Mardaga.

Wade, D. T. (1983). Can aphasic patients with stroke do without speech therapy? *British Medical Journal, 286,* 50.

Wahrborg, P. (1989). Aphasia and family therapy. *Aphasiology, 3,* 479–482.

Wahrborg, P. & Borenstein, P. (1990). The aphasic person and his/her family: what about the future? *Aphasiology, 4,* 371–379.

Warrington, E. K. & McCarthy, R. A. (1987). Categories of knowledge: further fractionations and an attempted integration. *Brain, 110,* 1273–1296.

Weinrich, M. (1991). Computerized visual communication as an alternative communication system and therapeutic tool. *Journal of Neurolinguistics, 6,* 159–176.

Wepman, J. M. (1951). *Recovery from aphasia.* New York: Ronald.

Wepman, J. M. (1972). Aphasia therapy: a new look. *Journal of Speech and Hearing Disorders, 37,* 203–214.

Wertz, R. T., Collins, M. J., Weiss, D., Kurtze, J. F., Friden, T., Brookshire, R. H., Pierce, J., Hotzapple, P., Hubbard, D. J., Porch, B. E., West, J. A., Davis, L., Matovitch, V., Morley, G. K., & Resurreccion, E. (1981). Veterans Administration cooperative study on aphasia: a comparison of individual and group treatment. *Journal of Speech and Hearing Research, 24,* 580–594.

Wertz, R. T., Weiss, D. G., Aten, J. L., Brookshire, R. H., Garcia-Bunuel, L., Holland, A. L., Kurtze, J. F., Lapointe, L. L., Milianti, F. J., Brannegan, R., Greenbaum, H., Marshall, R. C., Vogel, D., Carter, J., Barnes, N. S., & Goodman, R. (1986). Comparison of clinic, home and deferred language treatment for aphasia. *Archives of Neurology, 43,* 653–658.

Willmes, K. (1990). Statistical methods for a single-case study approach to aphasia research. *Aphasiology, 4,* 415–436.

Zurif, E. B., Gardner, H., & Brownell, H. H. (1989). The case against the case against group studies. *Brain and Cognition, 10,* 237–255.

Ruth Lesser, Newcastle upon Tyne (UK)

32. Psychosocial Aspects of Aphasia

1. A Framework for Psychosocial Studies

1.1. The Background

The origins of research into the psychological and psychiatric rehabilitation of aphasic individuals stems from the pioneering work of Goldstein (1942). His work with individuals with brain injuries resulting from combat, highlighted both the cognitive and personality changes resulting from such damage. The therapeutic implications of this work were emphasized by Wepman (1951). The focus of much of the earlier research in this field was on the social and emotional changes resulting from aphasia (e. g. Biorn-Hansen 1957). This led to a series of studies on the psychiatric aspects of aphasia. The results of much of this research have been drawn together in a major review by Starkstein/Robinson (1988) which concludes that depressed aphasic individuals show a lower rate of recovery and significantly higher levels of cognitive impairment than non-depressed patients. It is however, only relatively recently that consideration has been given to the relationship between individual changes in the emotional behavior of aphasic individuals and their subsequent adjustment to their families and the wider social context (Buck 1968). It is now critical that the study of psychosocial adjustment to aphasia is seen as a distinctive research area in it own right in which the focus is on rehabilitation rather than the emotional responses of aphasic individuals. The aim of this review is to help define this distinctive area, to review significant research in this field and to highlight areas requiring further investigation.

1.2. Psychosocial Aspects

The study of psychosocial aspects is concerned with rehabilitation and adjustment to the disability rather than investigation into the nature of the impairment itself. As Code/Müller (1983) have noted, the psychosocial perspective in aphasia therapy remains the most underdeveloped and yet is fundamental in the rehabilitation process. Psychosocial adjustment concerns not only coming to terms with a totally new set of circumstances for the individual experiencing aphasia, but has wider implications within the social network in which the individual lives, and in particular on the family. The prime focus of research into psychosocial adjustment is to understand better how to facilitate psychological well being in aphasic individuals; the effects an aphasic individual has on significant others and implications for the family and the broader social network; and the extent to which society in its broadest sense is able to respond and accommodate these changes in a positive manner. From the perspective of the individual aphasic person, it is the study of the extent to which the loss of communication, and hence personhood, can be compensated through coping strategies which lead to a regaining of control over the environment and adjustment to the disability. This directs study to the rehabilitation process and hence incorporates those factors which affect psychosocial adjustment.

2. Adjusting to the Social Context

2.1. The Effects on the Family Network

It is now well established that aphasia is a family problem. Spouses of aphasic people have been shown to suffer marked changes in their well being both physical and psychological. Early studies by Malone/Ptacek/Malone (1970) and Artes/Hoops (1976) have all shown the difficulties faced by spouses. As well as more predictable disturbances such as lack of sleep and tiredness through having to provide constant care, there is also some indication that children within the family situation receive less time and therefore find it difficult to adjust to the new situation. A study by Biorn-Hansen (1957) has suggested that spouses may at times reject their aphasic partners and indeed show some distaste towards them. There is also evidence to suggest that spouses may be overprotective (Malone/Ptacek/Malone 1970). The cyclic nature of the familial relationship has been demonstrated by Mulhall (1978) who has shown how frustration in the aphasic person can lead to anger in the spouse which in turn leads to rejection and a subsequent break-down in communication. The work of Kinsella/Duffy (1979) has highlighted a range of difficulties in adjustment. They found that from a sample of 79 couples, 42% of the spouses were suffering from clinical depression and that 78% of them were either taking tranquilisers or sleeping pills. Furthermore, 83% of the couples had ceased to have sexual intercourse although it was judged there was no physical disability preventing it. Taken together these studies demonstrate that marital relationships between aphasic individuals and their partners are characterised by problems of interpersonal communication, diminished sexual satisfaction and loss of partnership, as well as individual responses including isolation, anxiety and susceptibility to minor psychiatric disorders. More recent studies have confirmed these findings (e.g. Christensen/Anderson 1989) and highlighted the difficulties posed by role changes that often involve making medical and financial descisions as well as offering personal care. As Woodhouse/Müller have shown (1987), the majority of those providing care are female and are normally spouses or daughters of the aphasic person. A study by Oranen/Sihvonen/Äystö/Hagfors (1987) identified five patterns of coping and showed that the best adjusted families were characterised by an optimistic coping approach and the least well adjusted through depressive or nervous coping patterns. Similar results have been found in studies of brain injured individuals suffering from aphasia which is indicative that aphasia is a causal factor in adjustment by spouses and partners (Rosenbaum/Majenson 1976). In a recent review Wahrborg (1991) has concluded that family members of aphasic individuals are prone to developing minor psychiatric disorders; that this alters the nature and quality of the interaction between the spouse and the aphasic partner; and that in general a lack of knowledge about the disability further accentuates the problem. These important conclusions reflect significant research efforts during the last two decades which have provided clear evidence of the detrimental effects on the aphasic individual and the family network.

2.2. Interpersonal and Professional Perceptions

There have been relatively few studies of differences in the perception of disability and prognosis by the individual aphasic persons themselves, their family members and the professional concerned. Skelly (1975) has shown that aphasic people are often approached by nursing and medical personnel in a way that they perceive as insulting or degrading which can lead to a loss of interest in the rehabilitation process. A series of studies has investigated how relatives and aphasia therapists perceive the individual aphasic person's communication skills. Helmick/Watamori/Palmer (1976) in comparing test results with the judgments made by spouses as regards the language disability, concluded that spouses of aphasic persons view communication to be less impaired than it actually is. It was suggested that spouses may have unrealistic expectations of future improvements. However, Holland (1970), in discussing the study by Helmick and colleagues, argued that the spouse is better able to make use of contextual cues and might in fact be in a better position to assess the communicative abilities of the aphasic person. As Helmick/Watamori/Palmer (1977) re-affirm there is often a discrepancy between the spouses and the clinician perception. A study by Müller/Code/Mugford (1983) using the Code-Müller psychosocial scale of adjustment (Müller/Code 1983; Code/Müller 1992) showed that relatives and indeed aphasic persons themselves, view psychosocial adjustment more optimistically than the clinicians involved. Herrmann/Wallesch (1989) using a more sophisticated version of the Code/Müller scale of psychosocial adjustment, demonstrated that patients and relatives suffer considerable psychosocial strain and that they rated the probability of an improvement in psychosocial adjustment as being significantly higher than did clinicians. Shewan/Cameron (1984) have shown that there is limited agreement between aphasic individuals and their spouses as regards communication and related problems. Herrmann/Wallesch found considerable psychosocial changes in aphasic individuals including differences in job opportunities, household work and the administration of income and property, as well as social changes affecting in particular recreational activities and holidays. Using this same scale Herrmann/Wallesch (1990) investigated the perception of different professional groups using a Multiattribute Utility Technique in the investigation of physiosocial factors. Little agreement was found between a wide range of professional groups including occupational therapists, psychotherapists, neuropsychologists, neurologists and speech therapists. This highlights the importance of undertaking individual assessment and therapy within a specific rehabilitative context in order to provide effective intervention for aphasic individuals.

3. Intervention and Rehabilitation

3.1. Counselling and Social Perspectives

There have been few evaluative studies on the effectiveness of intervention directed specifically at psychosocial adjustment. This research has been hampered to some extent by there being only a limited range of appropriate assessment procedures available. This remains an important research field. There have however, been a number of approaches to the use of groups as a means of improving psychosocial behaviour. Fawcus (1983) and Pachalska (1991) have strongly advocated the use of groups and have developed a wide range of clinical techniques to provide a supportive environment for aphasic individuals. The difficulties of providing empirical data on the effectiveness of group therapy have been noted by Kearns (1986). As yet there is no definitive answer to this question. Brumfitt/Clarke (1983) initiated the application of psychotherapeutic techniques derived broadly from psychotherapy to the management of aphasia. Wiig (1973) has offered guidelines on sexual counselling and in terms of integrating aphasic individuals more widely into society, Borenstein/Linell/Wahrborg (1987) have evaluated the effectiveness of a structured one week course involving social contact outside of the hospital environment. This was shown to be beneficial and was followed up by a study integrating younger aphasic people into a 'Folk High School' which resulted in evidence to show an improvement in psychosocial and linguistic functioning (Borenstein/Wahrborg/Linell et al. 1987). There remains however difficulties in evaluating studies of naturalistic approaches to therapy.

3.2. Family Support and Involvement

There is tentative evidence to suggest that the spouse exerts influence on the recovery and rehabilitation pattern of aphasic people (Buxbaum 1967). Rollin (1987) has brought together a diverse literature in promoting the involvement of families in aphasia rehabilitation and in particular the introduction of family therapy. He advocates that trained family therapists with a knowledge of aphasia or speech-language pathologists trained in family therapy can positively influence the rehabilitation process by undertaking systematic family therapy involving all significant others as well as the individual aphasic person. A great deal of this work is derived from his own experience as a family therapist. A short empirical report by Wahrborg/Borenstein (1989) tentatively suggests that family therapy relieves depression and provides social and emotional support. In a more wide ranging debate concerning the benefits of family therapy, Wahrborg (1991) argues that training programmes in family therapy should be provided for those professionals involved in aphasia rehabilitation. There are however reservations as regards the efficacy of family therapy and the extent to which speech and language therapists should be trained as counsellors. There is increasing recognition of the importance of family members in the rehabilitation process but a need to ascertain more precisely how best to utilise their skills.

3.3. Spouse and Carer Adjustment

The need to provide support for the spouses and partners of aphasic individuals is clearly supported by the studies set out above. In particular the deterioration in general health and psychological wellbeing can be seen as likely to further disrupt the family relationship. It has been argued that it is appropriate for speech and language pathologists to initiate intervention on the grounds that they have a specialist knowledge not only of the language impairment and methods of rehabilitation but of those problems faced by aphasic individuals. Bowling (1977) offered unstructured social support to individuals to attend a group as and when they felt fit. Although attendance was spasmodic, a third of the subjects did indicate that the group had been beneficial to them, although the evidence presented is incomplete. A study by Bevington (1985) offered a structured programme of a specific educational nature. Again there is some evidence to suggest an improvement in knowledge for those regularly attending the group. A non-directive, open-ended group programme offered by Bernstein (1979), was in the end rather poorly attended and no systematic measures of the psychosocial benefits gained were taken. Nevertheless, there was sufficient evidence from the studies to encourage Rice/Paull/Müller (1987) to carry out an evaluation study of a social support group for spouses of aphasic partners. The group offered both emotional support and structured educational activities. Comparison between good and poor attenders on measures of psychosocial adjustment showed significant improvement on tests of social dysfunction, somatic symptoms, anxiety and psychological well being for those attending. There is a need for work of this kind to be followed up and for a wider variety of intervention techniques to be evaluated.

4. Future Perspectives

4.1. Research Issues

4.1.1. The Perceptions of Children

Although there has been some mention of children in the research literature (Kinsella/Duffy 1979) there has been little systematic research of the effects on children of there being an aphasic individual in the family. Starch (1990) has evaluated an educational programme targeted at young children aged between four and seven. There remain however significant gaps in our knowledge of how children experience and adjust to adult aphasia. This is an important area for future research to inform the rehabilitation process.

4.1.2. Measurements of Psychosocial Change

There is a recognised need to develop more sophisticated and sensitive measures of psychosocial adjustment which can determine change over time. It may prove beneficial to extend single case study methodology to include psychosocial factors.

4.1.3. Psychosocial Adjustment and Linguistic Performance

There is a need to determine the extent to which a high level of psychosocial adjustment is a causal factor in linguistic improvement in aphasic individuals. There is as yet no clear evidence from those research studies which have begun to address this issue (e. g. Buxbaum 1967).

4.1.4. Efficacy of Intervention with Aphasic Individuals

There is a need to undertake a series of efficacy studies to determine the extent to which psychosocial adjustment can be facilitated. There is some evidence to suggest that clinically orientated approaches are not effective (Lincoln/Jones/Mulley 1985), and future researchers need to evaluate the extent to which family members and other social networks can have psychologically beneficial effects.

4.1.5. Effective Provision of Spouse and Family Support

In recognising the psychosocial consequences for spouses, partners, and other family members, it is necessary to undertake research reviewing how best to support them. Currently, there are very few studies addressing this issue and insufficient resource prioritisation for this group.

4.1.6. Integration into Society

There is little information available concerning the extent to which aphasic individuals and their families are fully integrated into society. It is difficult to obtain information of how many aphasic individuals could be helped to return to work and how best to support them (Ramsing/Blomstrand/Sullivan 1991).

4.1.7. Policy Implications

The extent to which aphasic individuals and their families adjust to society has wider implications for government policy and the long term provision of health care (Frattali 1992). Although rehabilitation is managed differently on an international basis there is a need to develop and evaluate good practice in the provision of health care. This might best be facilitated by developing measures of the quality of life derived from aphasic individuals themselves (Lomas/Pickard/Mohide 1987).

4.2. Longitudinal Studies

In order to fully resolve a number of the research issues highlighted above it would prove to be of enormous benefit to undertake longitudinal studies. The field of aphasia research has rarely attracted sufficient funding to enable work of this kind to be carried out and there are very few studies which have assessed changes for a period of longer than one year. Those studies which have been published have focused on the assessment of language function rather than psychosocial factors (Hanson/Metter/Riege 1989). There is good evidence to show that aphasia results in long term family problems and therefore the extended rehabilitation process extends over a considerable period. Longitudinal interdisciplinary and multi-international research into the most effective models of rehabilitation for aphasic individuals and their families, is the next important stage in furthering our understanding of psychosocial adjustment in aphasia.

5. References

Artes, R. & Hoops, R. (1976). Problems of aphasic and non-aphasic stroke patients as identified and evaluated by patients' wives. In Y. Lebrun & R. Hoops (Eds.), *Recovery in Aphasics*. 31–45. Amsterdam: Swets and Zeitlinger.

Bernstein, J. C. (1979). A supportive group for spouses of stroke patients. *Aphasia, Apraxia, Agnosia, 1*, 30–35.

Bevington, L. J. (1985). The effect of a structured education programme on relatives' knowledge of communication with stroke patients. *Australian Journal of Communication Disorders, 5*, 29–41.

Biorn-Hansen, V. (1957). Social and emotional aspects of aphasia. *Journal of Speech and Hearing Research, 22*, 53–59.

Borenstein, P., Linell, S., & Wahrborg, P. (1987). An innovative therapeutic program for aphasic patients and their relatives. *Scandinavian Journal of Rehabilitation Medicine, 19*, 51–56.

Borenstein, P., Wahrborg, P., Linell S., Hedberg, E., Asking, M., & Ahlsen, E. (1987). Education in Folk High School for younger aphasic people. *Aphasiology, 1*, 263–266.

Bowling, J. H. (1977). Emotional problems of relatives of dysphasic patients. *Australian Journal of Communication Disorders, 5*, 29–41.

Brumfitt, S. & Clarke, P. (1983). In C. Code & D. J. Müller (Eds.), *Aphasia Therapy*. An application of psychotherapeutic techniques to the management of aphasia. 89–100. London: Edward Arnold.

Buck, M. (1968). *Dysphasia: Professional Guidance for Family and Patient*. Englewood Cliffs, New Jersey: Prentice-Hall.

Buxbaum, J. (1967). Effect of nurturance on wives' appraisals of their marital satisfaction and the degree of their husbands' aphasia. *Journal of Consulting Psychology, 31*, 240–243.

Christensen, J. M. & Anderson, J. D. (1989). Spouse adjustment to stroke: aphasic versus non aphasic partners. *Journal of Communication Disorders, 22*, 225–231.

Code, C. & Müller, D. J. (1983). Perspectives in aphasia therapy: an overview. In C. Code & D. J. Müller (Eds.), *Aphasia Therapy*. 3–13. London: Edward Arnold.

Code, C. & Müller, D. J. (1992). The Code-Müller Protocols: Assessing Perceptions of Psychological Adjustment to Aphasia. Kibworth: Far Communications.

Fawcus, M. (1983). Group therapy: a learning situation. In C. Code & D. J. Müller (Eds.), *Aphasia Therapy*. 113–119. London: Edward Arnold.

Frattali, C. M. (in press). Functional assessment of communication: merging public policy with clinical views. *Aphasiology*, 6, 63–83.

Goldstein, K. (1942). *Aftereffects of Brain Injuries in War*. New York: Grune and Stratton.

Hanson, W. R., Metter, E. J. & Riege, W. H. (1989). The course of chronic aphasia. *Aphasiology, 1*, 19–29.

Helmick, J. W., Watamori, T. S., & Palmer, J. M., (1976). Spouses' understanding of the communication disabilities of aphasic patients. *Journal of Speech and Hearing Disorders, 41*, 238–243.

Helmick, J. W., Watamori, T. S., & Palmer, J. M. (1977). Reply to Holland's comment on 'Spouses' understanding of the communication disabilities of aphasic patients'. *Journal of Speech and Hearing Disorders, 42*, 308–310.

Herrmann, M. & Wallesch, C. W. (1989). Psychosocial changes and psychosocial adjustment with chronic severe aphasia. *Aphasiology, 3*, 513–526.

Herrmann, M. & Wallesch, C. W. (1990). Expectations of psychosocial adjustment in aphasia: a

MAUT study with the Code-Müller Scale of Psychosocial Adjustment. *Aphasiology, 4*, 527–538.

Holland, A. (1970). Comment on 'Spouses' understanding of the communication disabilities of aphasic patients'. *Journal of Speech and Hearing Disorders, 42*, 307–308.

Kearns, K. P. (1986). Group therapy for aphasia: theoretical and practical considerations. In R. Chapey (Ed.), *Language Intervention Strategies in Adult Aphasia*. 304–318. Baltimore: Williams and Wilkins (2nd Edition).

Kinsella, G. & Duffy, F. D. (1979). Psychosocial readjustment in the spouses of aphasic patients. *Scandinavian Journal of Rehabilitation Medicine, 11*, 129–132.

Lincoln, N. B., Jones, A. C., & Mulley, G. P. (1985). Psychological effects of speech therapy. *Journal of Psychosomatic Research, 29*, 467–474.

Lomas, J., Pickard, L., & Mohide, A. (1987). Patient versus clinician item generation for quality-of-life measures. *Medical Care, 25*, 764–769.

Malone, R., Ptacek, P., & Malone, M. (1970). Attitudes expressed by families of aphasics. *British Journal of Disorders of Communication, 5*, 174–179.

Mulhall, D. J. (1978). Dysphasic stroke patients and the influence of their relatives. *British Journal of Disorders of Communication, 13*, 127–134.

Müller, D. J. & Code, C. (1983). Interpersonal perceptions of psychosocial adjustment to aphasia. In C. Code & D. J. Müller (Eds.), *Aphasia Therapy*. 101–112. London: Edward Arnold.

Müller, D. J., Code, C., & Mugford, J. (1983). Predicting psychosocial adjustment to aphasia. *British Journal of Disorders of Communication, 18*, 23–29.

Oranen, M., Sihvonen, R., Aysto, S. & Hagfors, C. (1987). Different coping patterns in the families of aphasic people. *Aphasiology, 1*, 277–281.

Pachalska, M. (1991). Group therapy for aphasic patients. *Aphasiology*, 5, 541–554.

Ramsing, S., Blomstrand, C., & Sullivan, M. (1991). Prognostic factors for return to work in stroke patients with aphasia. *Aphasiology, 5*, 583–588.

Rice, B., Paull, A., & Müller, D. J. (1987). An evaluation of a social support group for spouses and aphasic adults. *Aphasiology, 3*, 247–256.

Rollin, W. J. (1987). *The Psychology of Communication Disorders in Individuals and their Families.* Englewood Cliffs, New Jersey: Prentice-Hall.

Rosenbaum, M. & Majenson, T. (1976). Changes in life patterns and symptoms of low mood as reported by wives of severely brain-injured soldiers. *Journal of Consulting and Clinical Psychology, 44*, 881–888.

Shewan, C. M. & Cameron, H. (1984). Communication and related problems as perceived by aphasic individuals and their spouses. *Journal of Communication Disorders, 17*, 175–187.

Skelly, M. (1975). Aphasic patients talk back. *American Journal of Hearing, 7*, 1140–1142.

Starch, S. A. (1990). Increasing young children's understanding of aphasia: a unique educational approach. In T. E. Prescott (Ed.), *Clinical Aphasiology, Volume 20*. Austin, T. X.: Pro Ed.

Starkstein, S. E. & Robinson, R. G. (1988). Aphasia and depression. *Aphasiology, 2*, 1–20.

Wahrborg, P. (1991). *Assessment and Management of Emotional and Psychosocial Reactions to Brain Damage and Aphasia*. London: Whurr.

Wahrborg, P. & Borenstein, P. (1989). Family therapy in families with an aphasic member. *Aphasiology, 1*, 93–98.

Wepman, J. M. (1951). *Recovery From Aphasia.* New York: Ronald Press.

Wiig, E. H. (1973). Counselling the adult aphasic for sexual readjustment. *Rehabilitation Counselling Bulletin, 17*, 110–119.

Williams, S. E. & Freer, C. A. (1986). Aphasia: its effect on marital relationships. *Archives Physical Medicine and Rehabilitation, 67*, 250–252.

Woodhouse, L. & Müller, D. J. (1987). Caring for the carers: support levels for families of dysphasic adults. *Journal of the Royal Society of Health, 107*, 49–50.

Dave Müller, Ipswich, Suffolk (United Kingdom)

33. Pathology of Nonaphasic Language Behavior after Focal Left Hemispheric Damage

In the present chapter I will discuss some language disorders due to focal pathology of the left hemisphere which can be considered nonaphasic for either or both of the following reasons. First, a disorder may be classified as nonaphasic *on theoretical grounds*, when it does not (at least overtly) involve the main levels of language organization according to current linguistic descriptions (phonology, morphology, syntax, lexical semantics). This definition includes several different varieties of impairment of language use, which are (supposedly) associated with a 'normal' linguistic competence, and which usually appear following damage to frontal regions of the left hemisphere. Second, a language impairment may be grouped as nonaphasic *on clinical grounds*, if it is not apparent on standard language examination, but some definite impairments are perceived subjectively by the patient, and can be demonstrated with appropriate, in-depth testing. Such disorders usually affect lexical-semantic abilities, nonliteral and creative language use and have been labelled 'minimal dysphasia' in a seminal paper by Macdonald Critchley (1972). A disorder of this type can be observed both in the acute stage after non-perisylvian lesions and in patients who have recovered from a 'standard' aphasia.

1. Frontal Lobe Language Disorders

A discussion of 'nonaphasic' frontal language disorders must include several different conditions, each of which affects the ability of the patient to express him or herself. One such condition, the total suppression of vocalization and speech, known as 'mutism', is frequently observed immediately after frontal damage. Mutism has innumerable causes and several different pathophysiological mechanisms (see Table 33.1). Leaving aside peripheral conditions, even in the case of disease to the central nervous system the patient may be unable to speak for various reasons. For instance, bilateral damage to the opercular regions is sufficient to give rise to permanent mutism. Detailed testing proves some of these patients to be totally proficient in auditory comprehension and written communication and therefore nonaphasic (Villa/Caltagirone 1984; Cappa/Guidotti/Papagno/Vignolo 1987). Mutism in these cases is probably as-

A. Peripheral
  - Laryngeal disease
  - Neuromuscular disorders

B. Central
  - Bulbar disorders
    - Motor neuron disease
    - Brainstem infarction, neoplasm, trauma or infection
  - Pseudobulbar disorders
    - Opercular syndrome (Foix-Chavany-Marie)
    - Motor neuron disease
    - Multiple sclerosis
  - Other causes
    - Advanced extrapyramidal disorders
      - Progressive supranuclear palsy
      - Parkinson's disease
      - Huntington's disease
      - Dystonia
      - Wilson's disease
    - Advanced dementing disorders
      - Alzheimer's disease
      - Pick's disease
      - Multi-infarct dementia
    - Transient mutism after closed head injury
    - Transient mutism with aphasia
      - Broca's aphasia
      - Transcortical motor aphasia
      - Dynamic aphasia
      - Global aphasia
      - Subcortical aphasia
    - Aphemia
    - Akinetic mutism
    - Post-callosotomy mutism

C. Psychiatric disorders
  - Depression
  - Schizophrenia
  - Hysteria

Table 33.1: Differential Diagnosis of Mutism (modified from Cummings/Benson/Houlihan/Gosenfeld 1983)

sociated with a pseudobulbar impairment of phonation and articulation (Foix/Chavany/Marie 1926), the responsible lesions being less extensive in the left hemisphere, with partial sparing of the inferior frontal gyrus. In contrast, transient mutism is associated with lesions limited to the left frontal lobe. The outcome of this complete but temporary suppression of speech can take two different directions. First, it may lead to a lasting impairment of speech production, due to articulatory disruption, without any disturbance of language, referred to as 'aphemia'. Second, it can cause a reduction of spontaneous speech, usually connected to subtle impairment in complex language tasks termed 'transcortical motor aphasia'. Both 'aphemia' and 'transcortical motor aphasia' are distinct clinical syndromes, which can be observed in relatively pure form and are associated with different lesion locations. Aphemia generally coincides with damage to the inferior precentral gyrus with variable extension to the posterior operculum (Schiff/Alexander/Naeser/Galaburda 1983) and is best considered as a neurophonetic disorder. Therefore, I will now devote my attention to the syndrome of transcortical motor aphasia (TMA), which (at least as it is used to indicate a subgroup of patients) probably corresponds to the theoretical criteria for a nonaphasic language disorder indicated in the introduction.

This time-honored taxonomical label, originally introduced by Lichtheim (1885), is generally used to indicate a clinical picture characterized by two distinguishing features, namely, a severe quantitative reduction of spontaneous speech in combination with a preserved ability to repeat. Other names have also been used to designate this syndrome (dynamic aphasia, verbal akinesia, verbal adynamia, and so on). As is usually the case, however, all of these terms are used to refer to an extremely diverse clinical picture. This diversity is reflected by the proposal, starting from Kleist (1934) through Goldstein (1948) to de Lacy Costello/Warrington (1989), to distinguish 'subtypes' of TMA. A basic distinction, which respects differences in lesion location and (possibly) in pathophysiological mechanisms, is between the relatively seldom 'pure' form, and other more common cases involving more widespread linguistic impairment. In the 'pure' form of TMA, only monologic speech is impaired, while confrontation naming, repetition and auditory comprehension are preserved. One major problem in the assessment of these patients is that spontaneous speech or naming are sometimes only as unimpaired as one is able to judge from their very limited production. The 'pure' form of TMA has been connected to lesions of the medial frontal lobe, which, after a transient period of mutism, leave the patient with severely reduced spontaneous speech but normal naming and reading aloud (Masdeu/Schoene/Funkenstein 1978). An extension to the cingulate regions is usually associated with a severe reduction of all motor activity, including spontaneous speech, which is called akinetic mutism (Buge/Escourolle/Rancurel/Poisson 1975). In contrast, in the more common cases of TMA, disorders in naming as well as at the phonologic and/or the morphosyntactic level of production are evident. Such clinical pictures usually coincide with other lesion sites, which share the characteristic of sparing the perisylvian language area. For example, in the left frontal lobe, the lesion usually involves the dorsolateral cortex in front of Broca's area or the dorsomedial cortex, including the supplementary motor area (see Freedman/Alexander/Naeser 1984 for a review); articulatory disturbances or mild disorders of auditory comprehension are present if the damage encroaches on the perisylvian language areas. Another cause of TMA-type impairments can be subcortical lesions, involving deep grey structures and white matter: they will be discusses later on. – Several interpretations have been proposed for the pathophysiology of TMA. Kleist (1934) propagated that the syndrome is the result of an 'Antriebsmangel der Sprache' (loss of the impulse to communicate) which fits well with the later proposal of a 'fronto-limbic' disconnection (Rubens/Kertesz 1983). Recently, a variant of this interpretation has been offered in neurochemical terms, suggesting that an interruption of the mesofrontal dopaminergic projections could be responsible for this syndrome (Albert/Bachman/Morgan/Helm-Estabrooks 1988). Another closely related interpretation was originally proposed by Botez/Barbeau (1971). They ascribed the suppression or quantitative reduction of spontaneous speech to a lesion in a complex network of subcortical and frontal structures which constituted the "starting mechanism of speech". Several psycholinguistic theories have been proposed to account for the syndrome. Their origin too can be traced back to Lichtheim's original postulation of such a clinical picture

(1885). Rephrased in present day terminology (McCarthy/Warrington 1984), the syndrome may be interpreted as the result of the interruption of the direct connection between semantic analysis and speech production, with preservation of the phonological route. In a very influential account Luria/Tsvetkova (1967) provided experimental evidence for an impairment in propositionalizing. They attributed the impairment to defective formation of the linear scheme of the sentence, which the patient could correct when external cues were available. For example, the patient was given a linear array of pieces of paper corresponding in number to the units he or she had to arrange in the sentence in order to produce a coherent narrative. Unable to duplicate Luria and Tsvetkova's results, de Lacy Costello/Warrington (1989) have suggested a more 'central' defect in the process of sentence production, at the level of verbal planning. These two interpretations can be mapped to two different levels of Garrett's model of sentence production (1984). Luria and Tsvetkova's findings suggest a defect in the stage of verbal planning where the syntactic form of the sentence is produced (positional level representation). On the other hand according to De Lacy Costello and Warrington the impairment in TMA is at the stage where lexical-semantic representations of words are accessed and the argument structure of verbs is specified (functional level representation).

The relatively well defined picture of TMA should be kept distinct from other disorders of verbal communication, which can be observed in patients with extensive damage to the frontal lobes (Stuss/Benson 1986). In the latter cases, the disorder is not specific for language, but it may include not only features of TMA (quantitative reduction, perseverations) but also disorders of contextual language utilization (which may be more fruitfully described at the pragmatic level, such as appropriateness of response to the interlocutor, narrative coherence, sensitivity to the social context). A general impairment of goal-directed behavior is a crucial feature of the so called frontal syndrome, and, as originally proposed by Luria (1966), language plays a basic role in the regulation of human activity.

Even if a full-fledged frontal syndrome is not present, patients with left frontal damage, in comparison to those with right frontal damage and normals, show a definite impairment on complex verbal reasoning and verbal memory tasks (Novoa/Ardila 1987). This impairment is qualitatively similar to the latent dysphasia of nonaphasic left hemisphere patients, which will be discussed below.

2. 'Latent Dysphasia' after Non-perisylvian Cortical Damage

Originally, 'minimal aphasia' was defined by Critchley (1972) on strictly semeiological grounds, as a syndrome characterized by poverty of spontaneous speech, difficulty in the comprehension of complex sentences or nonliteral language (metaphors, idioms) and impairment of creative language usage. At this time, no one attempted to specify underlying physiopathological mechanisms. The disorder thus referred to several different conditions: patients who had recovered from severe aphasia, individuals with highly developed language skills and mild language disturbances, subtle language disorders due to increased intracranial pressure or slowly progressive degenerative pathology. In the present context, I will focus on a more restricted aspect, i. e. on the subtle language disorders which can be observed, on appropriate testing, in individuals with a recent acute vascular lesion of the left hemisphere. In a recent study (Vallar/Cappa/Papagno 1988) we selected a group of patients with a recent left hemispheric stroke who had no signs of aphasia on a 'standard' language assessment test (Basso/Capitani/Vignolo 1979) and scored within normal limits on two sensitive language tasks (Token test by De Renzi/Vignolo 1962, in the reduced version by De Renzi/Faglioni 1978, and Reporter test by De Renzi/Ferrari 1978). They were submitted to a further extensive assessment of language, including measures of phonological, lexical-semantic and syntactic abilities, and of verbal memory, and their performance was compared with right hemisphere-damaged subjects and normal controls. The 'nonaphasic' patients showed a mild, but clear-cut impairment in word comprehension and word retrieval, associated with a defect in verbal long-term memory. It is noteworthy that in a subsequent study of a larger sample of right hemisphere-damaged subjects (Cappa/Papagno/Vallar 1990), a similar pattern of mild lexical-semantic impairment was found only in a minority of subjects. An analysis of lesion site, as shown by CT scan, in left hemisphere-damaged subjects showed two possible anatomical patterns: either a) cortical lesions, confined to the medial temporal lobe and occipital regions, or b) small subcortical lesions involving the thalamus, the basal ganglia or the white matter (see below). None of the lesions involved the perisylvian language areas, associated with 'standard' aphasic syndromes, or the anterior frontal lobe, the involvement of which produces the patterns of language impairment described in the previous section. Patients with lesions of the posterior cerebral artery territory were particularly represented in the cortical group. This lesion site is often associated not only with the well-known syndrome of alexia without agraphia (Dejerine 1892) and with verbal long-term memory impairment (Benson/Marsden/Meadows 1974) but, as shown recently in a systematic study by De Renzi/Zambolin/Crisi (1987), with failure on naming tasks, independent of modality of presentation and of presence of alexia.

3. Subcortical Language Disorders

While there is a lively debate about the physiopathological mechanisms underlying subcortical aphasia (see Perani/Vallar/Cappa et al. 1987 for a discussion), it is generally accepted nowadays that clear-cut aphasic syndromes can be observed after lesions confined to the thalamus, the basal ganglia and/or the neighboring white matter tracts (see Wallesch/Papagno 1988, for a review). On the other hand, it has been observed that in subcortical lesions it is quite difficult to predict the presence and characteristics of aphasia after damage to a given location (Cappa/Cavallotti/Guidotti et al. 1982). A key factor for the appearance of aphasia is lesion size. In a recent study (Perani/Vallar/Cappa et al. 1987) the lesions associated with both severe hypoperfusion in the ipsilateral cortex and clinical evidence of aphasia were of a significantly larger size than those associated with negative cases. However, small lesions in some critical locations are concomitant with aphasia. A typical example is the TMA observed after infarction in the anterior choroidal artery territory (Wallesch 1985; Cappa/Sterzi 1990), though it is probably a transient disorder with rapid recovery. Moreover, there is some evidence that, within the thalamus, anterior lesions are more commonly associated with aphasia, while posterior lesions are not (Graff Radford/Damasio/Yamada et al. 1985; Cappa/Papagno/Vallar/Vignolo 1986). However, evidence also exists that in patients with subcortical lesions, who are not clinically aphasic, there are some subtle language impairments apparent on detailed testing. In the previously described series of recent left hemisphere lesions without aphasia, (Vallar/Papagno/Cappa 1988) five out of eleven patients had a subcortical lesion. In the chronic stage Wallesch and his coworkers (Wallesch/Kornhuber/Brunner et al. 1983; Wallesch/Kornhuber/Kunz/Brunner 1983) have shown mild language defects in patients with basal ganglia, but not with thalamic lesions.

4. Conclusion

In this article, several aspects of language impairment after focal left hemisphere pathology which could not fit in a standard definition of aphasia have been reviewed. The only conclusion which can be drawn is that incursions in this 'no man's land' between language modules and the 'cognitive cloud' have been fragmentary and have often lacked any sound theoretical framework. Concepts from neurological aphasiology and descriptive linguistics appear to be of limited usefulness in this area. A better understanding of the disorders of language described in this chapter is extremely important not only for theoretical considerations, but also from the practical standpoint of rehabilitation. Indeed, it is a common experience that traditional methods of aphasia therapy are ineffective in the treatment of the so-called 'inertia' of TMA (Huntley/Gonzalez Rothi 1988) and in dealing with the subjective complaints of those patients classified as nonaphasic after conventional testing.

Acknowledgement: I wish to thank Prof. Luigi A. Vignolo for his helpful reading of this chapter and Dr. Giuseppe Vallar for many fruitful discussions.

5. References

Albert, M. L., Bachman, D. L., Morgan, A., & Helm-Estabrooks, N. (1988). Pharmacotherapy of aphasia. *Neurology*, *38*, 877–879.

Basso, A., Capitani, E., & Vignolo, L. A. (1979). Influence of rehabilitation on language skills in aphasic patients. *Archives of Neurology*, *36*, 190–196.

Benson, D. F., Marsden, C. D., & Meadows, J. C. (1974). The amnesic syndrome of posterior cerebral artery occlusion. *Acta Neurologica Scandinavica*, *50*, 133–145.

Botez, M. I. & Barbeau, A. (1971). Role of subcortical structures and particularly of the thalamus in the mechanisms of speech and language. *International Journal of Neurology*, *8*, 300–320.

Buge, A., Escourolle, R., Rancurel, G., & Poisson, M. (1975). "Mutisme akinétique" et ramollissement bicingulaire. Trois observations anatomo-cliniques. *Revue Neurologique*, *131*, 121–137.

Cappa, S. F., Cavallotti, G., Guidotti, M., Papagno, C., & Vignolo, L. A. (1982). Subcortical aphasia: two clinical-CT scan correlation studies. *Cortex*, *19*, 227–242.

Cappa, S. F., Guidotti, M., Papagno, C., & Vignolo, L. A. (1987). Speechlessness with occasional vocalizations after bilateral opercular damage. *Aphasiology*, *1*, 35–39.

Cappa, S. F., Papagno, C., & Vallar, G. (1990). Language and verbal memory after right hemispheric stroke. A clinical-CT study. *Neuropsychologia*, *28*, 503–509.

Cappa, S. F., Papagno, C., Vallar, G., & Vignolo, L. A. (1986). Aphasia does not always follow left thalamic hemorrhage: a study of five negative cases. *Cortex*, *22*, 639–647.

Cappa, S. F. & Sterzi, R. (1990). Infarction in the territory of the anterior choroidal artery: a cause of transcortical motor aphasia. *Aphasiology*, *4*, 213–217.

Critchley, M. (1972). Communication: recognition of its minimal impairment. In M. Critchley, J. L. O'Leary, & B. Jennet (Eds.), *Scientific foundations of neurology. 221–227.* London: Heinemann.

Cummings, J. L., Benson, F. D., Houlihan, J. P., & Gosenfeld, L. F. (1983). Mutism: loss of neocortical and limbic vocalization. *Journal of Nervous and Mental Diseases*, *171*, 255–259.

Dejerine, J. (1892). Contributions à l'étude anatomopathologique et clinique des différentes variétés de cécité verbale. *Mémoires de la Société de Biologie*, *4*, 61–90.

de Lacy Costello, A. & Warrington, E. K. (1989). Dynamic aphasia: the selective impairment of verbal planning. *Cortex*, *25*, 103–114.

De Renzi, E. & Faglioni, P. (1978). Normative data and screening power of a shortened version of the token test. *Cortex*, *14*, 41–49.

De Renzi, E. & Ferrari, C. (1978). The reporter's test – a sensitive test to detect expressive disturbances in aphasics. *Cortex*, *14*, 279–293.

De Renzi, E. & Vignolo, L. A. (1962). The token test: a sensitive test to detect receptive disturbances in aphasics. *Brain*, *85*, 665–678.

De Renzi, E., Zambolin, A., & Crisi, G. (1987). The pattern of neuropsychological impairment associated with left posterior cerebral artery infarcts. *Brain*, *110*, 1099–1116.

Foix, C., Chavany, J. A., & Marie, P. (1926). Diplegie facio-linguo-masticatrice d'origin corticosouscortical sans paralyse des membres. *Revue Neurologique*, *33*, 214–219.

Freedman, M., Alexander, M. P., & Naeser, M. A. (1984). Anatomical basis of transcortical motor aphasia. *Neurology*, *34*, 409–417.

Garret, M. F. (1984). The organization of processing structure for language production. Applications to aphasic speech. In D. Caplan, A. R. Lecours, & A. Smith (Eds.), *Biological perspectives on language. 172–193.* Cambridge MA: MIT Press.

Goldstein, K. (1948). *Language and language disturbances.* New York: Grune and Stratton.

Graff Radford, N. R., Damasio, H., Yamada, T., Eslinger, P. J., & Damasio, A. R. (1985). Nonhemorrhagic thalamic infarction: clinical, neuropsychological and electrophysiological findings in four anatomical groups defined by computerized tomography. *Brain*, *108*, 485–516.

Huntley, R. A. & Gonzalez Rothi, L. J. (1988). Treatment of verbal akinesia in a case of transcortical motor aphasia. *Aphasiology*, *2*, 55–66.

Kleist, K. (1934). Gehirnpathologie. Berlin: Springer.

Lichtheim, L. (1885). On aphasia. *Brain*, *7*, 433–484.

Luria, A. R. (1966). *Higher cortical functions in man.* New York: Basic Books.

Luria, A. R. & Tsvetkova, L. (1967). The mechanism of "dynamic aphasia". *Foundations of Language 4*, 296–307.

Masdeu, J. C., Schoene, W. C., & Funkenstein, H. (1978). Aphasia following infarction of the supplementary motor area. A clinicopathologic study. *Neurology*, *28*, 1220–1223.

McCarthy, R. & Warrington, E. K. (1984). A two-route model of speech production. Evidence from aphasia. *Brain*, *107*, 463–485.

Novoa, O. P. & Ardila, A. (1987). Linguistic abilities in patients with prefrontal damage. *Brain and Language*, *30*, 206–225.

Perani, D., Vallar, G., Cappa, S. F., Messa, C., & Fazio, F. (1987). Aphasia and neglect after subcortical stroke. *Brain*, *110*, 1211–1229.

Rubens, A. B. & Kertesz, A. (1983). The localization of lesions in transcortical aphasias. In A. Kertesz (Ed.), *Localization in neuropsychology. 245–268.* New York: Academic Press.

Schiff, H. B., Alexander, M. P., Naeser, M. A., & Galaburda, A. M. (1983). Aphemia. Clinical-anatomic correlations. *Archives of Neurology*, *40*, 720–727.

Stuss, D. T. & Benson, D. F. (1986). *The frontal lobes.* New York: Raven Press.

Vallar, G., Papagno, C., & Cappa, S. F. (1988). Latent dysphasia after left hemisphere lesions: a lexical-semantic and verbal memory defect. *Aphasiology*, *2*, 463–478.

Villa, G. P. & Caltagirone, C. (1984). Speech suppression without aphasia after bilateral perisylvian softenings (bilateral rolandic operculum damage). *Italian Journal of Neurological Science*, *5*, 77–83.

Wallesch, C. W. (1985). Two syndromes of aphasia occurring with ischemic lesions involving the left basal ganglia. *Brain and Language*, *25*, 357–361.

Wallesch, C. W., Kornhuber, H. H., Brunner, R. J., Kunz, T., Hollerbach, B., & Suger, G. (1983). Lesions of the basal ganglia, thalamus and deep white matter: differential effects on language functions. *Brain and Language*, *20*, 286–304.

Wallesch, C. W., Kornhuber, H. H., Kunz, T., & Brunner, R. J. (1983). Neuropsychological deficits associated with small unilateral thalamic lesions. *Brain*, *106*, 141–152.

Wallesch, C. W. & Papagno. C. (1988). Subcortical aphasia. In F. C. Rose, R. Whurr, & M. A. Wyke (Eds.), *Aphasia. 256–287*. London: Whurr Publishers.

Stefano F. Cappa, Brescia (Italy)

34. Verbal Communication Deficits after Right-Hemisphere Damage

Apart from exceptional cases of crossed aphasia, right-hemisphere lesions can result in verbal communication problems that do not compose an aphasia proper, but that can nevertheless affect the individual's relations with others. Since these disorders only rarely affect phonological, morphological or syntactical components of language, the present chapter will focus instead on impairments of prosody, lexical-semantics, text-level performance and pragmatic ability. Finally, the specificity and the incidence of these impairments will be considered.

1. Prosody

Linguistic prosody refers to the use of intonation to realize lexical and emphatic stress and to express different modalities such as exclamation. In contrast, emotional *prosody* denotes emotional states, such as happiness. Both types of prosody can be disturbed in right-brain damaged patients (RBDs). Left-hemisphere lesions can also affect prosody. However, RBDs exhibit more difficulties with the processing of emotional prosody than left-brain-damaged patients (LBDs) do. As far as the more basic acoustic parameters of prosody are concerned, either for linguistic or for emotional prosody, a left-hemisphere lesion interferes more with the local and rapid processing of acoustic information, whereas a right-hemisphere lesion impairs processing of acoustic events distributed over longer periods of time (Perecman/Kellar 1981).

One of the strongest assumptions with regard to RBDs is that the taxonomy of prosodic deficits parallels that of aphasic deficiencies. Looking at the ability to produce, understand, and repeat emotionally-loaded prosodic patterns, Elliot Ross (1981) attempted to identify syndromes such as m o t o r aprosodia, s e n s o r y aprosodia, t r a n s - c o r t i c a l - s e n s o r y aprosodia, g l o b a l aprosodia and other aphasia-like clinical manifestations. However, Ross' proposal bears some problems: (a) the subjectivity of the examination protocol used, (b) the postulate that aphasia taxonomy in itself is well-ascertained and unanimously accepted, (c) the fact that the disorders reported were mostly present in the first three days following the insult, thus possibly confused with the patients initial reaction to the disease, and (d) the overly optimistic attitude of Ross who even states that he had never seen a perisylvian RBD patient without a prosodic deficit. Despite the fact that emotional prosody appears to be quite regularly affected in RBD patients as a group, there is still no clear global taxonomical conceptualization of those deficits. Among the problems encountered, are the methodological difficulties of evaluating the emotional component of prosody.

RBDs show deficits in comprehension of emotional prosody even when the basic linguistic components of the message have been removed through filtering (Heilman/Bowers/

Speedie/Coslett 1984). A left-hemisphere damage also results in such deficits. However, right-hemisphere lesions affect the processing of the prosodic cues themselves whereas deficits caused by left-hemisphere-lesions essentially reflect the complexity of the task (Tompkins/Flowers 1985). These facts suggest that the deficits RBDs have in understanding emotional prosody originate more from disturbances in the processing of prosody itself than from disturbances in the processing of its emotional component.

Concerning the production of emotional prosody, no satisfactory study of the ability of RBDs to spontaneously produce emotion through prosody have been conducted so far. There exists only a strong clinical impression that some RBDs exhibit flattened monotonous speech. To what extent this characteristic reflects a prosodic impairment *per se* or a more global indifference remains to be seen.

Deficits for the comprehension of lexical stress can occur in RBDs, but also in left-brain-damaged aphasics. RBDs also show deficits in understanding emphatic stress as well as in processing intonation-based modalities. However, in the latter case, RBDs are significantly more impaired than aphasics, who are in turn more impaired compared to controls (Grant/Dingwall 1985).

Most studies examining the expression of linguistic prosody have aimed at identifying the most relevant acoustic parameter involved in such a production. An important finding is the striking discrepancy between the subjective and the instrumental analysis of expressed linguistic prosody (Dordain/Degos/Dordain 1971). These results emphasize both the limits of a subjective approach *and* the difficulties of obtaining relevant acoustical parameters.

2. Lexical Semantics

RBDs can have difficulties completing sentences, providing word definitions (Eisenson 1973), and naming objects which are related to their hospitalization or incapacities (Weinstein 1964). They also have difficulties selecting the object corresponding to an orally-presented word from an array of associated responses. However, according to Gainotti/Caltagirone/Miceli (1983) and Bishop/Byng (1984) these impairments might be attributed to a nonspecific mental deterioration or to visuoperceptual disorders. According to Gainotti/Caltagirone/Miceli (1983), RBDs make many more visuosemantic errors than normal controls on picture-naming tasks. However, Coughlan/Warrington (1978) reported that RBDs performed normally on a visual object-naming task and on a naming task involving orally-described objects.

RBDs have problems in judging antonymic relationships (Gardner/Silverman/Wapner/Zurif 1978) but not in processing synonymy (Goulet/Joanette 1988). They score poorly, when they have to process the connotative or the metaphorical meanings of words presented in a triad including a target word associated literally with one word of the triad and metaphorically with the other word (Brownell 1988). However, it is not clear if the poorer performance is due to the incapacity to process the nonliteral meaning of words, or to a greater attraction of the literal meanings of words. RBDs have been said to be sensitive to cohyponymic relationships and to be able (Goulet/Joanette/Gagnon/Sabourin 1989; Wilkins/Moscovitch 1978) to judge whether drawings or words represent natural or man-made objects. But below average sensitivity to cohyponymic relationships has also been reported (Chiarello/Church 1986; Gagnon/Goulet/Joanette 1989).

When they occur, lexical-semantic errors made by RBDs reflect disruptions in effortful activation or processing of the lexical-semantic information rather than in impairments of this lexical-semantic knowledge. Indeed, RBDs have been shown to be impaired for the controlled processing of the connotative meaning of words and cohyponymic relationships but not in an automatic priming experiment involving these two types of material (Gagnon/Goulet/Joanette 1989; Tompkins 1990).

The contradictory results mentioned above demonstrate that the presence as well as the nature of the lexical-semantic impairments in RBDs is debatable. This contradiction is also evident in RBDs performance on verbal fluency tasks. The use of formal criteria (words beginning with a predetermined letter) revealed that RBDs performed normally in some studies but not in others (Joanette/Goulet/Hannequin 1990). Generally, reduced verbal fluency scores are either attributed to a frontal sydrome or to a nonspecific lesion effect. They have also been related to a reduced I.Q. Testing for semantic criteria (e. g., animal names), also brought about opposing results. For example, Newcombe (1974, 314) reported that RBDs produce as many words as normals, whereas Boller (1968) attributed the reduction of verbal fluency performance of the RBDs to a nonspecific lesion effect. Grossman (1981) failed to find that RBDs produce a smaller number of words but reported that RBDs employed word-finding strategies that differed from those used by LBDs and normals. Interestingly, Lifrak/Novelly (1984) showed that RBDs were impaired when they had to supply words respecting semantic criteria but not when no criteria were used (free production). In the same vein, it has been reported that RBDs performed less well than normals when semantic criteria were used but not when formal criteria were used (Joanette/Goulet 1986; Laine/Niemi 1988). This finding has been interpreted as an indication that word-finding problems observed in RBDs are of a semantic nature. In contrast, Cappa/Papagno/Vallar (1987) found that a right-hemisphere lesion did not alter verbal-fluency performance based on either formal or semantic criteria. Controlling for the degree of productivity associated with each type of criteria, Sabourin/Goulet/Joanette (1988) showed that RBDs were impaired when highly productive criteria were used, be it semantic or formal.

3. Text and Pragmatics

RBDs may also exhibit deficits in understanding or producing a text. Furthermore, disturbances in the processing of the pragmatic aspects of verbal communication are among the most typical symptoms after a right-hemisphere lesion.

Processing of the emotional and spatial information integrated in stories is impaired in RBDs (Wapner/Hamby/Gardner 1981). In addition, they have difficulty rejecting minimally plausible incongruous events by reference to a given story, a finding which borders on pragmatics. These patients also have difficulties in the re-organization of sentences into a coherent story despite the presence of temporal or spatial clues (Delis/Wapner/Gardner/Moses 1983; Huber/Gleber 1982). When RBDs have to match sentences or pictures on the basis of their emotional meaning, their errors seem to result more from difficulties to establish unexpected links between the pictures or the sentences, than from an erroneous processing of emotional content itself (Cicone/Wapner/Gardner 1980). Moreover, RBDs have also been shown to have problems in synthesizing and interpreting the information explicitly or implicitly contained in a text in order to find the moral of a fable (Gardner/Brownell/Wapner/Michelow 1983).

According to Joanette/Goulet (1990), RBDs, as a group, produce narratives which are comparable to those of non-brain-damaged individuals in the number of words as well as lexical and syntactic cues, but they do show some difficulties with cohesion and coherence of narratives. 50% of the RBDs in this study produced narratives containing a smaller amount of information as compared to those of controls.

RBDs are impaired by comparison to normals when they have to process some very specific texts whose understanding is context-dependant such as humorous, sarcastic and ironic texts (Joanette/Goulet/Hannequin 1990). However, whether this impairment is primarily directed towards the processing of humor, sarcasm or irony *per se* or whether it reflects RBDs' difficulties in accessing non-literal information, or being able to reject minimally plausible choices in a multiple-choice task is a matter for further research.

In addition, RBDs exhibit problems in their ability to understand indirect speech acts (Weylman/Brownell/Roman/Gardner 1989). Some RBDs have difficulties in accessing the non-literal meaning of an indirect request, even though there might be differences according to the nature of indirect requests. However, it is not clear if this impairment is to be attributed to a lowered sensitivity to context-induced constraints or to a difficulty in accessing second-level meaning of the message given these constraints.

RBDs also perform poorly when asked to interpret metaphoric texts or phrases. They tend to choose the literal meaning of metaphors more often than normal controls. However, these results cannot yet be isolated from a possible impairment of RBDs in rejecting minimally plausible events. Moreover, the distinctive nature of the metaphors such as their degree of *frozeness*, has yet to be taken into consideration. Only then will it be possible to know if the problem lies with the nature of the tasks used in the past or if there is a real deficit in metaphorisation abilities.

Many of the above-mentioned deficits among RBDs have indicated the possibility that these patients might have inferencing difficulties (Brownell/Potter/Bihrle/Gardner 1986). However, such difficulties have not been clearly demonstrated. Some studies have shown that RBDs have problems with logical inferencing or syllogistic reasoning (e. g. Read 1981) while another failed to demonstrate such problems (Joanette/Goulet 1987). Problems found have been attributed to impairments of spatial abilities, but the tasks used never allowed a clear distinction between linguistic and spatial problems. The literature is also incongruent concerning RBDs' capacities to make inferences based upon short narrations. For instance, inferencing deficits have been reported in three studies (Brownell/Potter/Bihrle/Gardner 1986; Goodenough-Trépanier/Powelson/Zurif 1982; Tompkins/Mateer 1985) while no such deficits have been reported in three other studies (Brookshire/Nicholas 1984; Joanette/Goulet 1987; McDonald/Wales 1986). Interestingly in one study reporting inferencing deficits (Brownell/Potter/Bihrle/Gardner 1986) and in one study failing to find such deficits (McDonald/Wales 1986), the main problem of RBDs was rejecting false statements.

4. Specificity of the Verbal Communication Disorders

None of the impairments mentioned here have been clearly established as being specific to a right-hemisphere lesion. Another aspect of the specificity of these impairments lies in their linguistic nature. Impairments of many cognitive processes, other than linguistic ones, could contribute to these deficits.

5. Incidence of Verbal Communication Deficits

Only half of the studies examining similar aspects of verbal communication with similar tasks reported an impairment of RBDs (Joanette/Goulet/Daoust 1991). The sole exceptions are those studies evaluating emotional prosody; all of them reported such an impairment. Moreover, many studies reported a breakdown of their patients into those with and those without an impairment. In those studies, approximately half of the RBDs exhibit a deficit. Among impaired RBDs, there can be different contrastive patterns leading to double dissociations: for example, some are impaired in a verbal-fluency task but not in a narrative task, and vice-versa. The frequency of such impairments might be linked to how much a given individual's right hemisphere contributed to verbal communication before the insult. For example, a focal right hemisphere lesion has been shown to result in more verbal communication deficits when the individual right hander has a familial history of left-handedness and when he or she is less educated (Joanette/Lecours/Lepage/Lamoureux 1983). Such factors are in line with the notion of a less-marked lateralization to the left in right-handers in the presence of a familial sinistrality or a lower level of education. Another explanation would be the localization of the lesion as suggested by Joanette/Lecours/Lepage/Lamoureux (1983).

6. References

Bishop, D. & Byng, S. (1984). Assessing semantic comprehension: Methodological considerations, and a new clinical test. *Cognitive Neuropsychology, 1*, 233–243.

Boller, F. (1968). Latent aphasia: right and left "non aphasic" brain-damaged-patients compared. *Cortex, 4*, 245–256.

Brookshire, R. H. & Nicholas, L. E. (1984). Comprehension of directly and indirectly stated main ideas and details in discourse by brain-damaged and non-brain-damaged listeners. *Brain and Language, 21*, 21–36.

Brownell, H. H. (1988). Appreciation of metaphoric and connotative word meaning by brain-damaged patients. In C. Chiarello (Ed.), *Right hemisphere contributions to lexical semantics. 19–32*. New York: Springer-Verlag.

Brownell, H. H., Potter, H. H., Bihrle, A. M., & Gardner, H. (1986). Inference deficits in right brain-damaged patients. *Brain and Language, 27*, 310–321.

Cappa, S. F., Papagno, C., & Vallar, G. (1987). Language and verbal memory in right-brain-damaged patients (RBD): a comparison with left-brain-damaged (LBD) with aphasia. *Journal of Clinical and Experimental Neuropsychology, 9*, 263.

Chiarello, C. & Church, K. L. (1986). Lexical judgements after right- or left-hemisphere injury. *Neuropsychologia, 24*, 623–630.

Cicone, M., Wapner, W., & Gardner, H. (1980). Sensitivity to emotional expressions and situations in organic patients. *Cortex, 16*, 145–158.

Coughlan, A. K. & Warrington, E. K. (1978). Word-comprehension and word-retrieval in patients with localized cerebral lesions. *Brain, 10*, 163–185.

Delis, D. C., Wapner, W., Gardner, H., & Moses, J. A. (1983). The contribution of the right hemisphere to the organization of paragraphs. *Cortex, 19*, 43–50.

Dordain, M., Degos, J. D., & Dordain, G. (1971). Troubles de la voix dans les hémiplégies gauches. *Revue de Laryngologie, 3–4*, 178–187.

Eisenson, J. (1973). Right-brain damage and higher intellectual functions. In J. Eisenson (Ed.), *Adult aphasia. 38–41*. Prentice-Hall: Appleton-Century-Crofts.

Gagnon, J., Goulet, P., & Joanette, Y. (1969). Activation automatique et contrôlée du savoir lexico-sémantique chez les cérébrolésés droits. *Langages, 96*, 95–111.

Gainotti, G., Caltagirone, C., & Miceli, G. (1983). Selective impairment of semantic-lexical discrimination in right-brain-damaged patients. In E. Perecman (Ed.), *Cognitive Processing in the right hemisphere. 149–167*. New York: Academic Press.

Gardner, H., Brownell, H. H., Wapner, W., & Michelow, D. (1983). Missing the point: The role of the right hemisphere in the processing of complex linguistic materials. In E. Perecman (Ed.), *Cognitive Processing in the right hemisphere. 169–191*. New York: Academic Press.

Gardner, H., Silvermann, J., Wapner, W., & Zurif, E. (1978). The appreciation of antonomic contrasts in aphasia. *Brain and Language, 6*, 301–317.

Goodenough-Trépanier, C., Powelson, J., & Zurif, E. (1982). *Bridging in right hemisphere patients*. Presented at the Academy of Aphasia Annual Meeting, Lake Mohonk, New York.

Goulet, P. & Joanette, Y. (1988). Semantic processing of abstract words in right brain-damaged patient. *Journal of Clinical and Experimental Neuropsychology*, 10, 312.

Goulet, P., Joanette, Y., Gagnon, J., & Sabourin, L. (1989). Semantics in right-brain-damaged right-handers. *Journal of Clinical and Experimental Neuropsychology, 11*, 353.

Grant, S. R. & Dingwall, W. O. (1985). *The role of the right hemisphere in processing linguistic prosody*. Presented at the 13th Annual Meeting of the International Neuropsychological Society, San Diego.

Grossman, M. (1981). A bird is a bird: Making reference within and without superordinate categories. *Brain and Language, 12*, 313–331.

Heilman, K. M., Bowers, D., Speedie, L., & Coslett, H. B. (1984). Comprehension of affective and nonaffective prosody. *Neurology, 34*, 917–921.

Huber, W. & Gleber, J. (1982). Linguistic and non-linguistic processing of narratives in aphasia. *Brain and Language, 16*, 1–18.

Joanette, Y. & Goulet, P. (1986). Criterion-specific reduction of verbal fluency in right brain-damaged right-handers. *Neuropsychologia, 24*, 875–879.

Joanette, Y. & Goulet, P. (1987). *Inferencing deficit in right brain-damaged: absence of evidence*. Presented at the 10th European Conference of the International neuropsychological Society, Barcelona.

Joanette, Y. & Goulet, P. (1990). Narrative discourse in right-brain-damaged right-handers. In Y. Joanette & H. H. Brownell (Eds.), *Discourse ability and brain damage. 131–153*. New York: Springer-Verlag.

Joanette, Y., Goulet, P., & Daoust, H. (1991). Incidence et profils des troubles de la communication verbale chez les cérébrolésés droits. *Revue de Neuropsychologie, 1*, 3–27.

Joanette, Y., Goulet, P., & Hannequin, D. (1990). *Right hemisphere and verbal communication*. New York: Springer-Verlag.

Joanette, Y., Lecours, A. R., Lepage, Y., & Lamoureux, M. (1983). Language in right-handers with right-hemisphere lesions: a preliminary study including anatomical, genetic, and social factors. *Brain and Language, 20*, 217–248.

Laine, M. & Niemi, J. (1988). Word fluency production strategies of neurological patterns: semantic and phonological clustering. *Journal of Clinical and Experimental Neuropsychology, 10*, 28.

Lifrak, M. D. & Novelly, R. A. (1984). *Language deficits in patients with temporal lobectomy for complex-partial epilepsy*. Presented at the 12th annual meeting of the International Neuropsychological Society, Houston.

McDonald, S. & Wales, R. (1986). An investigation of the ability to process inferences in language following right hemisphere brain damage. *Brain and Language, 29*, 68–80.

Newcombe, F. (1974). Selective deficits after focal cerebral injury. In S. J. Dimond & J. G. Beaumont (Eds.), *Hemisphere function in the human brain. 311–334*. New York: J. Wiley.

Perecman, E. & Kellar, P. (1981). The effect of voice and place among aphasics, non aphasic right-damaged, and normal subjects on a metalinguistic task. *Brain and Language, 12*, 213–223.

Read, D. E. (1981). Solving deductive reasoning problems after unilateral temporal lobectomy. *Brain and Language, 12*, 92–100.

Ross, E. (1981). The aprosodias: Functional-anatomical organization of the affective components of language in the right hemisphere. *Archives of Neurology, 38*, 561–569.

Sabourin, L., Goulet, P., & Joanette, Y. (1988). La disponibilité lexicale chez les cérébrolésés droits. *Canadian Psychology, 29*, 2 a.

Tompkins, C. & Mateer, C. A. (1985). Right hemisphere appreciation of prosodic and linguistic indications of implicit attitude. *Brain and Language, 24*, 185–203.

Tompkins, C. A. & Flowers, C. R. (1985). Perception of emotional intonation by brain-damaged adults: the influence of task processing levels. *Journal of Speech and Hearing Research, 28*, 527–538.

Tompkins, C. A. (1990).- Knowledge and strategies for processing lexical metaphor after right or left hemisphere brain damage. *Journal of speech and hearing research, 33*, 307–316.

Wapner, W., Hamby, S., & Gardner, H. (1981). The role of the right hemisphere in the apprehension of complex linguistic materials. *Brain and Language, 14*, 15–33.

Weinstein, E. A. (1964). Affections of speech with lesions of the non-dominant hemisphere. *Research Publications of the Association for Research in Nervous and Mental Disease, 42*, 220–228.

Weylman, S. T., Brownell, H. H., Roman, M., & Gardner, H. (1986). Appreciation of indirect request by left and right-brain-damaged patients: The effects of verbal context and conventionality of wording. *Brain and Language, 36*, 580–591.

Wilkins, A. & Moscovitch, M. (1978). Selective impairment of semantic memory after temporal lobectomy. *Neuropsychologia, 16*, 73–79.

Yves Joanette/Pierre Goulet, Lab. Th.-Alajouanine, Montréal, Québec (Canada)
Didier Hannequin, C. H. U. de Rouen (France)

35. Pathology of Language Behavior in Dementia

1. Introduction

The syndrome of dementia produces deterioration of intellect, memory, communicative function, and personality, sufficient to interfere with social and occupational responsibilities (American Psychiatric Association 1987). It is associated with myriad diseases and conditions, some of which are reversible.

The most common cause of dementia is Alzheimer's disease (AD), an irreversible neurodegenerative disease which accounts for approximately 50 % of dementia cases. The incidence of AD is greatest in senescence, with a steep increase from 60 to 89 years (Rorsman/Hagnell/Lanke 1986), and because of the 'graying' of the earth's population, the number of AD patients is rising dramatically.

Throughout the world, health professionals are challenged by the needs of dementia patients and their families. Vital to their care is understanding disease effects on language and the ability to communicate, a need which has motivated much research in the last decade. Before reviewing this research, it is appropriate to define the term language, however defining language is not necessarily a straight forward enterprise. Consider that individuals, who have trouble naming, are diagnosed as having a 'language problem'. If the words for the to-be-named objects have been lost from the mind of the anomic individual, then it is a language problem. However, if the individual has knowledge of the object and its name, but cannot access the name, some would describe this as a memory problem. What has sometimes been called a language problem can be explained as a deficit in attention or other nonlinguistic cognitive system. Certainly the expression of linguistic knowledge is affected by other nonlinguistic functions such as perception, attention, and memory, but these deficits differ from those caused by a loss of linguistic knowledge.

Linguists distinguish between loss of language knowledge and errors in the application of language knowledge, referring to the former as a competency problem and the latter a performance problem (Slobin 1971). They emphasize that impaired linguistic performance does not necessarily mean that the individual lacks linguistic competence because linguistic performance is an amalgam of many functions, some of which are nonlinguistic.

For the purpose of this chapter, language refers to (a) linguistic knowledge comprising phonologic, syntactic, semantic, and pragmatic rules, and (b) the use of these rules in the production and comprehension of meaningful expressions. The different types of linguistic knowledge appear to be represented brain areas and the processes by which they are manipulated appear to be subserved by different neuronal systems. Whereas the production and comprehension of phonologic and syntactic information are likely carried out within a modular system (see Fodor 1983 for criteria for modularity), semantic and pragmatic analyses likely are not. The distribution of neuropathology of the etiologically different dementing diseases may affect the neuroanatomical substrates important for certain types of linguistic knowledge and processes and spare others. Knowledge of the brain areas affected in the various dementing diseases and disease effects on neuropsychological function are requisite to understanding the communication abilities of dementia patients. Thus, in the ensuing text, specification will be made of the neuropathology and neuropsychology of Alzheimer's, Pick's, Parkinson's, and Huntington's diseases, AD, PKD, PD, and HD respectively to provide a foundation for appreciating the communication disorders.

2. Alzheimer's Disease

2.1. Neuropathology

The diagnosis of AD requires the presence of characteristic morphological changes in the brain, notably, neurofibrillary tangles (NFTs), neuritic plaques, granulovacuolar degeneration (GVD), Hirano Bodies, and amyloid deposits in leptomeningeal and cortical blood vessels (Henderson/Finch 1989). These cellular changes, together with cell loss, occur within the neocortex, hippocampi, basal forebrain, amygdalae, nucleus locus ceruleus, and the brainstem raphe nuclei.

Of these morphological changes, the NFT is the most characteristic. NFTs are intraneural fibrillary structures that appear as clusters of unbranched fibrillary structures twisted into a helix (Kidd/Allsop/Landon 1985). Within the medial temporal lobe NFTs tend to proliferate in entorhinal neurons (Hooper/Vogel 1976). Within the neocortex, NFTs have a predilection for pyramidal cells within layers II and V of multimodal associations areas that are reciprocally related to the limbic cortex and hippocampus. Primary motor and sensory areas are typically spared (Lewis/Campbell/Terry/Morrison 1987). PET studies show decreased glucose metabolism within association cortex, more so in temporoparietal than frontal regions (Duara/Grady/Haxby et al. 1986). In some individuals the degree of hypometabolism is more severe in one of the hemispheres, a fact that has neuropsychological consequences (Grady/Haxby/Schlageter et al. 1986).

Occurring in the same neural structures as NFTs are neuritic plaques, sometimes called senile plaques. They are clumps of degenerating neurons which surround a core containing deposits of amyloid (Kidd 1964) and aluminosilicates (Candy/Oakley/Klinowski et al. 1986). The clumps occur within neuropil and contain abnormal, distended, unmyelinated neurites.

GVD is a descriptive term referring to the existence of one or more clear spherical vacuoles that contains granular debris. GVD is most commonly observed in hippocampal pyramidal neurons.

Hirano bodies are rod-shaped structures occurring within neurites and perikarya of hippocampal neurons. They were originally reported in patients with the parkinsonian dementia/amyotrophic lateral sclerosis complex of Guam (Hirano/Dembitzer/Kurland/Zimmerman 1968).

Concerning biochemical alterations, decrements in brain concentrations of many neurotransmitters and related enzymes occur in individuals with AD. Best known of the neurotransmitter decrements is the cholinergic deficit in cells within the basal nucleus that project to the cortex. Also affected are the noradrenergic neurons of the brain-stem locus ceruleus, and the serotonergic cells of the raphe nucleus. Of the neuropeptides, somatostatin has been reported to dramatically decline (Davies/Wolozin 1987). As pointed out by Henderson/Finch (1989), deficits in such widely projecting subcortical nuclear areas can be expected to have far-reaching effects on a variety of cognitive functions. For example, the noradrenergic system has been linked to vigilance and selective attention, and the cholinergic system to memory.

2.2. Neuropsychology

Neuropsychologically, AD patients exhibit progressive deterioration in memory, intellect, and personality. Most studied are disease effects on memory. Using terminology popularized by Baddeley (1987), Squire (1987), Mishkin/Appenzeller (1987) and others, Alzheimer's disease can be said to particularly impair working and declarative memory systems (the latter comprising episodic and semantic memory) while sparing procedural memory (memory for learned skills).

The most common early symptom is episodic memory deficit in the form of an inability to remember a recent episode such as where the car was parked, or what was eaten for dinner the previous night (Bayles/Kaszniak 1987). Less obvious to casual observers are concomitant changes in working memory, notably the attenuation of span and the diminished efficiency of the central executive systems. Deficits in span and attention result in poor encoding of new information and therefore difficulty in developing new long-term memory for episodes and facts.

As the disease progresses, individuals appear to lose their knowledge of the world (declarative memory) and the ability to manipulate it. In sharp contrast, they retain the ability to perform procedures such as hitting a golf ball or driving a car. An explanation for this apparent dissociation is the distribution of neuropathology in the disease. Declarative memory is impaired because of its reliance upon the preservation of cortical association areas in which neuropathological changes are prominent; procedural memory is spared because of its putative reliance upon the preservation of basal ganglia and its connections.

The progressively poor performance of AD patients on mental status tests reflects their growing memory deficits. Early in the disease, the affected individual is disoriented for time, later for place, finally, for person. In the late stages, patients may no longer recognize their faces in the mirror.

Although deficits in visuoperceptual and visuospatial abilities have been reported (Pirozzolo/Hansch/Mortimer et al. 1982), these abilities are less studied than memory. Abnormalities have been noted with visuoconstructional tasks, maze tests, map reading, and the performance subtests of the Wechsler Adult Intelligence Scale (Becker/Huff/Nebes et al. 1988; Storandt/Botwinick/Danziger et al. 1984). Visuoperceptual discrimination for meaningful and nonmeaningful stimuli has been demonstrated to decline in AD patients (Brouwers/Cox/Martin et al. 1984; Eslinger/Benton 1983), as has the ability to identify the spatial orientation of lines in relation to a model. Finally, AD patients have difficulty drawing and copying.

AD profoundly affects personality. Thal (1988) observed that the symptoms often include easy distractibility, difficulties with work, problems with directions or taking trips. According to primary caregivers, the most common early symptoms were difficulty handling finances, forgetting the location of objects, and becoming less aware of recent events (Bayles 1991b). Rubin/Morris/Storandt/Berg (1987) reported the common occurrence of agitation, apathy, and self-centeredness. Petry/Cummings/Hill/Shapira (1988) reported that AD patients are less reasonable, energetic, happy, affectionate, and easygoing. Drevets/Rubin (1989) observed the frequent occurrence of delusions, misidentifications, and hallucinations throughout the disease course. In this study, rates of psychosis ranged from 42 % to 84 % among moderate and severely demented subjects. These authors state that at least half the individuals with AD will display psychosis at some point during the disease.

2.3. Effects on Language

By definition, the aforementioned neuropsychological and personality changes affect communicative function and language performance. At issue in this section is whether AD affects language knowledge.

When summarizing the effects of AD on language, it is important to consider whether distinct clinical subgroups of AD patients exist in whom language is differently affected. Subgroups for whom disease effects on language may differ are defined by: age at onset; family history of disease; presence of extrapyramidal symptomatology; and distribution of neuropathology.

Age-at-onset: The presenile form of AD has been associated with more severe cognitive deficits (Capitani/Della Sala/Spinnler 1990), among them language deficit. Many investigators report such a relation (Seltzer/Sherwin 1983; Faber-Langendoen/Morris et al. 1988; Filley/Kelley/Heaton 1986; Chui/Teng/Henderson/Moy 1985). However, these reports have been debated by other investigators. Selnes/Carson/Rovner/Gordon (1988) did not find a significant relation between age-at-onset and language deficit. Nor did Cummings/Benson/Hill/Read (1985), who observed language impairment in AD patients to be proportional to dementia severity.

Bayles (1991a) observed that investigators of the relation of age-at-onset to degree of language deficit failed to use methodology whereby the AD subjects' language score(s) were controlled for the effects of dementia severity. This is a necessary control because of the well established relation between dementia severity and language performance scores (Selnes/Carson/Rovner/Gordon 1988; Cummings/Benson/Hill/Read 1985). Bayles controlled for disease severity effects in a study of 86 Alzheimer's patients and found age-at-onset to be related to degree of language deficit, but in such a way that the older the age-at-onset the greater the language deficit.

Bayles constructed a general linear model to assess the extent to which performance on the Global Deterioration Scale (Reisberg/Ferris/De Leon/Crook 1982), Mini-Mental State Examination (Folstein/Folstein/McHugh 1975) place and time questions and figure copying task predicted language performance. By first considering the severity variables, the effects of disease duration and age-at-onset on language were evaluated after effects of disease severity were removed. To assess the possibility that the observed relation between age-at-onset and language performance was caused by the effects of normal aging, the language tests were administered to normal subjects of similar ages who scored perfectly on dementia severity measures. Bayles failed to find convincing evidence that performance on the four linguistically oriented tasks declines with normal aging.

Family history. Family history has also been linked with special clinical characteristics. Folstein/Breitner (1981) determined that the presence of aphasia or agraphia in AD patients was highly predictive of dementia in first-degree relatives. In 1984 Breitner/Folstein reported language disturbance and apraxia in 78 % of their familial cases and a sevenfold increase in lifetime dementia risk for relative of language disordered AD probands versus control subjects. In a study published in the same year, Heyman/Wilkinson/Stafford et al. (1984) reported a failure to document a relation between family history and language performance. Further, they reported that the frequency and severity of linguistic deficits in AD patients was associated to duration of illness. Chui/Teng/Henderson/Moy (1985) found no association between family history of AD and aphasia, and Knesevich/Toro/Morris/La Barge (1985) observed that a lack of aphasia was associated with a higher prevalence of familial cases.

Presence of extrapyramidal symptomatology: The clinical heterogeneity of AD with regard to the presence of extrapyramidal features, primarily rigidity and hypokinesia has been noted (Pearce 1974; Sulkava 1982; Molsa/Martilla/Rinne 1984; Chui/Teng/Henderson/Moy 1985; Mayeux/Stern/Spanton 1985). However, as yet, it is unclear whether the coexistence of extrapyramidal symptomatology has consequences for either linguistic competence or performance.

Distribution of neuropathology: As previously noted, the neuropathology of AD may be greater in one cerebral hemisphere. In fact, the possibility has been raised that the left hemisphere is particularly vulnerable to disease effects (Sourander/Sjogren 1970; Seltzer/Sherwin 1983; Seltzer/Burres/Sherwin 1984). Using PET, several investigators have found that individuals with AD vary in the degree of hypometabolism in homologous regions of the cerebral hemispheres (Chase/Fedio/Foster et al. 1984; Friedland/Budinger/Ganz et al. 1983; Haxby/Duara/Grady et al. 1985). Individuals with greater left than right hypometabolism had greater language deficits (Haxby/Duara/Grady et al. 1985). Chase/Fedio/Foster et al. (1984) noted a close association between WAIS verbal IQ scores and cortical metabolism in the left cerebral hemisphere, especially in the left temporal lobe.

Martin/Cox/Brouwers/Fedio (1985) observed that whereas the majority of their 43 AD subjects were proportionately impaired in retrieval and use of semantic knowledge and visuoconstructional skill, a subset of patients presented with deficits limited to one of these domains of functioning. Nine AD subjects had severely impaired naming and verbal fluency skills relative to visuo-constructional skills.

Subsequently, Martin/Brouwers/Lalonde et al. (1986) reported results of principal component and cluster analyses of the performance data of 42 of the 43 AD patients described in the 1985 study. Five subject clusters were identified, one of which contained the nine patients in whom dysnomia was disproportionate to severity of dementia. These subjects were described as having poor word-finding skills concurrent with intact visual perceptual and construction skills. A second cluster of eight individuals exhibited the opposite pattern, disproportionately poor visual perceptual and constructional skills compared to word-finding. Individuals in the three other clusters exhibited relatively equal deficits on all measures.

Becker/Huff/Nebes et al. (1988) attempted replication of the findings of Martin and associates. The performance data of their 86 probable AD patients were analyzed and similar results obtained. Eleven patients in the sample were described as having focal 'lexical/semantic impairments' and four had focal 'visuoconstructional impairments.'

The results of these investigators call into question the appropriateness of the stage model as a basis for predicting language performance. Therefore, Bayles/Trosset (1991) attempted to evaluate its efficacy for predicting naming disorder. Their data were interpreted as demonstrating the inadequacy of dementia severity for predicting naming performance in many AD patients, but, nonetheless, failed to offer support for defining these patients as comprising statistically distinct subgroups.

Bayles/Trosset (1992) analyzed the confrontation naming performance data of 102 probable AD patients. Severity of dementia was defined by rating on the Global Deterioration Scale (GDS) (Reisberg/Ferris/de Leon/Crook 1982) and performance on the Mini-Mental State Examination (Folstein/Folstein/Mc Hugh 1975) questions related to time and place orientation and ability to copy a figure. The GDS was chosen because language ability does not prominently influence judgments of dementia severity. Using a hierarchical general linear model to predict naming performance on the basis of perceived dementia severity, dementia severity was found to account for approximately one-third of performance variability. Additional contributions due to age-at-onset, duration, and family history were negligible. Less than one-quarter of the unexplained variation could be attributed to measurement error. Therefore, naming ability can be argued to have a subcomponent not subsumed by overall cognitive ability. Nonetheless, no statistical evidence was found to suggest that this subcomponent decomposes the AD population into clinically distinct subgroups. The picture that emerged was of a single population characterized by considerable variability. With the caveat in mind that within the population of AD patients clinical subgroups may exist, the literature about the effects of AD on language will be reviewed.

2.3.1. Form

Until the late stages, the form of language is relatively intact in individuals with AD. Their verbal and written constructions are grammatical though sometimes simplified (Hier/Hagenlocker/Shindler 1985). This is in vivid constrast to the progressive loss of content. Preservation of grammar has been frequently observed (Kempler/Curtiss/Jackson 1987; Schwartz/Marin/Saffran 1979; Appell/Kertesz/Fisman 1982) and was memorably described by Whitaker (1976) whose severely demented patient spontaneously corrected syntactic and phonologic errors in sentences she repeated. In no case did she correct a semantic error. Bayles/Boone (1982) documented that the ability of spontaneously correct grammar and phonology was not idiosyncratic to Whitaker's patient but a common phenomenon in moderately and severely demented AD patients.

2.3.2. Content Production

Glaringly affected in AD is the ability to produce meaningful content. Consider the following discourse samples of patients in different stages of the disease who were asked to describe a common object.

Subject # 1. *Moderately severe AD patient describing an orange pencil.* "We have a pencil here to use. One that I have selected to use is one that is involved with the color of orange, and we have used this so much that it's been cut again by the cutter. Have to get another pen that will match the color so that everybody that has used one of our pencils."

Subject # 2. *Severe AD patient describing an orange pencil.* "Yeah, up. Safe together and trot around so we could get same short thing that we have for the small short thing but still by making the various corrections as we're going along. We can always make corrections that vary in there, too. And they can be a correction you all have plenty of time for that."

The deficits observed by many investigators in the connected speech of AD patients can be seen in these samples. For example, numerous investigators have described the discourse of AD patients to be impoverished in content (Hart 1985; Hier/Hagenlocker/Shindler 1985; Nicholas/Obler/Albert/Helm-Estabrooks 1985; Bayles/Tomoeda/Kaszniak et al. 1985; Appell et al. 1982). Miller/Hague (1975) observed, however, that the free speech of AD patients did not indicate selective loss of rare words.

The aforementioned preservation of the grammatical form of language is apparent in these discourse samples, a phenomenon observed by Ulatowska/Allard/Donnell et al. (1988) who studied the discourse performance of AD patients. Ulatowska/Allard/Donnell et al.'s (1988, 122) ten AD patients revealed "preservation of sentential level and discourse level linguistic structures, as evidenced by the absence of significant differences between DAT [AD] and normal subjects either in the amount of complexity of language, or in the manipulation of narrative superstructure."

However, they were impaired in ability to provide a summary and moral for a story, exhibited deficits in content and reference, and provided more irrelevant information.

In the next series of examples, the same patient is describing the Normal Rockwell Easter Morning Picture two years apart.

First Testing: "This appears to be a family picture with uh three women that are involved in the picture and the young boy plus what looks to be the father of the rest of the family. The father, the mother, the daughter, the son and all are dressed up neatly for a Sunday program at church. And um the father is taking the time to read the Sunday morning paper and the first thing he looks at in it is the section of comics which are now spread around the floor and uh there daddy is there with his cup of coffee for Sunday. The father is taking life very easy with a uh robe and keeping his eyes closely on what might happen next here before he gets ready for church. Daddy sits in a very comfortable chair waiting for everybody maybe to go on to church without him."

Second Testing: "That's what I was trying to figure, and I was thinking because they were telling me how much these were worth and what they can do for you. And they had a little bitty, what looks like a very small clearance area, and, that's how much he picked up on this way last night home and the rest of it's back there at the back end, pretty much so that it came back home."

These samples were obtained in a study by Tomoeda/Bayles (1992) in which descriptive discourse was elicited once a year for five years from 3 AD patients and 3 age- and education-matched control subjects by having them describe a Norman Rockwell picture. The discourse samples were analyzed in terms of total number of words, information units, conciseness, circumlocutions, frustrations, revisions, aborted phrases, and ideational repetitions. Of these, total number of words, conciseness, and information units significantly decreased over the five year period. Thus, whether the discourse data are examined cross-sectionally or longitudinally, the production of meaningful content can be seen to diminish.

2.3.3. Content Comprehension

Hart (1985) reported decrements in the ability of AD patients to respond to the auditory commands of the Token Test (De Renzi/Faglioni 1978) which gradually increase in complexity. Hart's data indicated that the performance of AD patients on a 36-item version of the Token Test correlated significantly with that on the Wechsler Memory Scale and the Wechsler Adult Intelligence Scale (WAIS). Hart acknowledges that because correlation does not necessarily imply causation, the relation between memory and language impairment remains to be determined. It was noted that subjects in this study sometimes failed items in the final segment of the test which, although linguistically more complex, are of shorter verbal span and require less complex motor programming than commands in the penultimate section. Reading comprehension is affected relatively early but the mechanics of reading are retained until the advanced stages of the disease (Hart/Smith/Swash 1986; Vance/Bayles 1990). Vance/Bayles observed that the mechanics of reading were among the last skills to be retained in severely demented individuals and persisted long after loss of the ability to comprehend the written material. According to Hart (1988), the preservation of reading, particularly the ability to read irregularly spelled words suggests that the lexicon remains relatively intact.

Benson/Cummings/Tsai (1982) suggest that the dissociation between the ability to read aloud and read for meaning in AD patients distinguishes them from individuals with angular gyrus syndrome in whom reading aloud and reading for meaning are affected.

Many investigators have explored the question of whether lexical-semantic information is lost or inaccessible in AD patients by studying the effects of manipulating semantic context on the ability of patients to make decisions about words. The assumption in such studies is that semantic memory is an associative network and the activation of an item results in the spreading of activation to related items. For example, it can be shown that prior exposure to a related item, for example the word *lemon*, causes subjects to respond faster to the word *lime* in a paradigm in which subjects are asked to decide whether two stimuli are both real words. This effect is called semantic priming and occurs if the first word is presented simultaneously or precedes the second word (Fischler 1977a) and can occur if the two stimulus words are semantically related or associated (Fischler 1977b). Activation of semantically related items within the network occurs automatically and without an individual's conscious awareness. If, in AD, semantic memory has deteriorated and lexical-semantic knowledge is lost, one would expect to see a loss of the semantic priming effect. The results of semantic priming studies are mixed. Some investigators report that AD patients are as sensitive to semantic context as normals (Nebes/Martin/Horn 1984; Nebes/Boller/Holland 1986; Hartman 1987; Margolin 1987; Albert/Milberg 1989; Nebes/Brady/Huff 1989). Other investigators report the lack of semantic priming in a lexical decision task (Ober/Shenaut 1988), and the lack of associative priming (Huff/Mack/Mahlmann/Greenberg 1988; Salmon/Shimamura/Butters/Smith 1988). Yet others report hyperpriming, or greater response from the prior exposure to a semantically related item (Chertkow/Bub/Seidenberg 1989; Chertkow/Bub 1990).

The variability in the results of these priming studies has yet to be fully appreciated but may occur because of differences in the strength of association or semantic relation between stimuli, the length of interval between the prime and target, the task the subject was asked to perform (lexical decision, stem completion, word reading, etc.), and the subject's stage of dementia. Early stage AD patients, in whom semantic memory is mildly affected, may be primeable. Late-stage patients, in whom semantic memory is likely to be severely affected, may not be benefitted by primes.

2.3.4. Use of Language

The effects of AD on the use of language in conversation are well-recognized though few investigators have undertaken the difficult task of quantifying these effects. Critchley (1964) observed that AD patients seem to form appropriate semantic intentions, but as their episodic memory worsens, these intentions are forgotten, hence they stop midway in their utterances. Slauson/Bayles/Tomoeda (1987) noted that AD patients have difficulty sustaining conversation and severely demented individuals fail to greet, respond to compliments, correct statements made by their conversational partners, and appropriately close conversations. Golder (1988) studied the ability of two AD patients to engage in conversation and observed turn-taking violations, interruptions, inappropriate silences, and topic shifts.

Results of a longitudinal study of the effects of AD on linguistic communication by Bayles/Tomoeda/Kazniak/Trosset (1991) suggest that how language is used plays a crucial part in lexical/semantic access and retrieval. The central question in this longitudinal study was whether conceptual knowledge is lost or the ability to use conceptual knowledge. The investigators reasoned that if AD patients lost conceptual knowledge, they should miss the same concepts across tasks. And, indeed other investigators have reported error consistency across tasks (Henderson/Mack/Freed et al. in press; Warrington 1975; Huff/Corkin/Growdon 1986; Flicker/Ferris/Crook/Bartus 1987; Gainotti/Daniele/Nocentini/Silveri in press; Chertkow/Bub 1990). To test their hypothesis, Bayles/Tomoeda/Kaszniak/Trosset (1991) devised a paradigm in which 69 AD subjects were administered the following 11 tasks, each using the same 13 concepts: confrontation naming, auditory comprehension, dictation, oral reading, definition, reading comprehension, coordinate naming, superordinate naming, superordinate identification, pantomime expression, and pantomime recognition. Thus, the paradigm generated data about the ability to use language in these myriad ways.

Data analysis revealed only a few instances in which a concept was missed across all 11 tasks. When performance on the oral reading and dictation tasks were removed from analysis, because of their questionable reliance on semantic memory, the number of missed concepts rose only modestly. A substantial rise in the number of missed concepts occurred, however, when performances on the four multiple choice tasks were removed. Bayles and associates argue that interpreting the larger number of missed concepts on the five remaining semantic tasks as evidence of item-specific loss in semantic memory is problematic, nonetheless, because these generative semantic tasks were among the hardest in the battery and the frequency with which an individual subject missed a concept across all tasks accorded with the subject's dementia severity level. Results demonstrate that task difficulty, more than concept specificity, predict whether a concept is missed. Overall, results suggest that a concept will "disappear" when all of the tasks in which it is a stimulus become too hard for the patient to perform. These data indict the practice of addressing the question of loss of knowledge or loss of access by using batteries of effortful, attention-demanding tasks.

Working on the assumption that for each concept, the abilities to perform a fixed set of tasks deteriorate in the same fixed order, and that this order defines relative task difficulty, Bayles and colleagues analyzed the data. Because the sample was of insufficient size to consider the order of deterioration of all tasks simultaneously, subsets were considered and the following observation made:

(a) Auditory comprehension and reading comprehension are almost identically difficult;

(b) dictation is almost invariably more difficult than oral reading;

(c) confrontation naming is decisively easier than either coordinate or subordinate naming;

(d) definitions, pantomime expression, and pantomime recognition are of roughly comparable difficulty.

Summary: Communication and language performance problems are omnipresent in individuals with AD. Deficits in linguistic knowledge occur primarily in semantics and pragmatics with sparing of syntax and phonology.

2.4. Gaps in the Literature

The primary gap in the literature is the dearth of longitudinal data on the effects of AD on linguistic communication. However, the Arizona study and others are nearing conclusion and data will soon be forthcoming. The issue of whether AD comprises subgroups of patients who are linguistically unique continues to be debated. Then too, the debate continues as to whether the disease affects linguistic competence as well as performance. Among those who believe that AD eventuates in a loss of lexical-semantic knowledge, disagreement exists as to whether the loss is from the bottom up or top down. Bottom-up theorists argue that AD patients lose knowledge of attributes of objects before categorical knowledge of objects. Finally, virtually no one has been able to relate changes in linguistic communication seen in life to distribution of pathology at post-mortem. For example, do late-stage patients who are mute differ in distribution of pathology from those who are echolalic?

3. Parkinson's Disease

3.1. Neuropathology

Parkinson's disease is a cluster of signs associated with a variety of causes. Four variants of the parkinsonian syndrome account for the majority of cases: idiopathic, drug-induced, post-encephalitic, and arteriosclerotic. By far the most common variant is idiopathic meaning that the etiology is unknown.

Degenerative changes in the basal ganglia, basal nucleus, neocortex, and nucleus locus ceruleus cause the classic symptomatology of tremor at rest, muscular rigidity, and bradykinesia. The most conspicuous neuropathologic alteration is depigmentation of the substantia nigra in the basal ganglia and loss of the neurotransmitter dopamine. Lewy bodies, which are dense spherical intracytoplasmic inclusion bodies, are diagnostic of the disease. Associated with these degenerative changes is diffuse cortical atrophy occurring in approximately 60 % of PD patients (Alvord/Forno/Kusske et al. 1974; Becker/Grau/Schneider et al. 1976; Selby 1968). A result of these degenerative changes is a significant reduction in cerebral blood flow (Lavy/Melamed/Cooper et al. 1979).

3.2. Neuropsychology

Considerable variation exists in the neuropsychological status of PD patients. Whereas some individuals experience little, if any, cognitive deficits, others develop dementia. Estimates of the incidence of dementia in PD in the literature vary dramatically from 2 % to 77 % (Celesia/Wanamaker 1972). More recently, Lees/Smith (1983) reviewed the early literature to determine the incidence of dementia if DSM-III criteria were used to define its existence. They reported approximately 15 % of PD patients to have dementia. Although the majority of PD patients do not appear to develop dementia, they experience some intellectual deficit (Pirozzolo 1982).

The cause of dementia in PD patients is unknown. Some theoreticians argue that it is caused by the coexistence of AD, and indeed, AD-like neuropathology has been reported in many demented PD patients (Hakim/Mathieson 1979; Boller/Mizutani/Roessmann/Gambetti 1980). Other theoreticians assert that basal ganglia and other subcortical structures are sufficiently important to normal cognitive function that damage to them results in dementia even when the cortex is spared (de la Monte/Wells/Hedley-Whyte/Growdon 1989; Cools/van den Bercken/Horstink et al. 1984; Lees/Smith 1983; Stern 1983; Mortimer/Pirozzolo/Maletta 1982).

For dementia to be diagnosed, the PD patient must exhibit memory and intellectual deterioration sufficient to interfere with occupational and social functioning, thus meeting the DSM-III criteria for dementia. Some clinicians report that the dementia in PD patients is qualitatively similar to that observed in AD patients (Boller 1980; Pirozzolo/Hansch/Mortimer et al. 1982). Others, like Alexander/Geschwind (1984), Cummings/Darkins/Mendez et al. (1988), and Albert (1978) argue that they differ qualitatively.

Cognitive deficits of PD patients: According to Brown/Marsden (1990) consensus is developing that PD patients have difficulty with: shifting mental sets, recall memory (Alexander/Geschwind 1984; Boller 1980; El-Awar/Becker/Hammond et al. 1987; Albert 1978; Wilson/Kaszniak/Klawans/Garron 1980; Pirozzolo/Hansch/Mortimer et al. 1982; Huber/Shuttleworth/Paulson 1986), internal control of attention (Brown/Marsden 1988), sequencing, temporal ordering and recency discrimination (Sagar/Sullivan/Gabrieli et al. 1988; Sullivan/Sagar/Gabrieli et al. 1985), and effort-demanding tasks (Weingartner/Burns/Diebel/Le Witt 1984).

An intriguing potential difference between the memory impairment in PD and AD may be in the degree to which procedural memory is affected. Recall that the neuropathology of AD typically spares procedural memory which is reliant upon the integrity of the basal ganglia. Because the neuropathology of PD primarily affects the basal ganglia, procedural memory is thought to be particularly vulnerable (Saint-Cyr/Taylor/Lang 1988).

Another differentiating characteristic of PD may be slowness in thinking (bradyphrenia) (Naville 1922) and motor function (bradykinesia). Both may contribute to a diminished performance in the PD patients.

Depression is a common part of the disease, the incidence of which has been estimated to range from 30 % (Lieberman/Dziatolowski/Kupersmith et al. 1979) to 76 % (Alexander/Geschwind 1984). As yet it is unclear to what degree the depression is exogenous, endogenous, or both.

3.3. Effects on Language

As is clear from the literature reviewed in the previous section, PD patients are not a homogenous group. Some develop dementia, the majority appear to have some type of intellectual deficit, and a subset remains intellectually normal. Those individuals who develop dementia always have communication deficits. The intellectual deterioration that defines the dementia substantially diminishes the ability to meaningfully communicate. However, whether these individuals also lose linguistic knowledge is unclear because deficits in perception, attention, executive function and memory counfound the evaluation of linguistic competency.

In the nondemented but intellectually diminished PD patient, evaluating linguistic competence may be somewhat easier. However, linguistic incompetence and nonlinguistic intellectual deficit also can be confounded. To date, few investigators have studied language competence and performance in either group of PD patients. The studies that have been done are subclassified according to whether they provide information about disease effects on language form, content (semantics), and use.

3.3.1. Form

No deficits in phonologic knowledge have been reported in either demented or nondemented patients. Neither are there reports of loss of syntactic knowledge. However, two reports exist of simplification of grammar in PD patients. Cummings/Darkins/Mendez et al. (1988) used the Boston Diagnostic Aphasia Examination (Goodglass/Kaplan 1976) to evaluate the grammatical form of phrases in a discourse sample from demented and nondemented PD patients. Nondemented and demented PD patients were observed to produce simpler constructions compared to normal control subjects and Alzheimer's patients respectively. Illes/Metter/Hanson/Iritani (1988) also noted a decrease in the syntactic complexity in the spontaneous utterances of patients with mild compared to moderate PD.

3.3.2. Content

Conceptual or semantic knowledge has been evaluated with naming, vocabulary, and auditory comprehension tests. Freedman/Rivoria/Butters et al. (1984) and Levin/Llabre/Weiner (1989) reported normal naming in nondemented PD patients on the Boston Naming Test (Kaplan/Goodglass/Weintraub 1983). However, Matison/Mayeux/Rosen/Fahn (1982) did not. In the Matison study, nondemented PD subjects scored one standard deviation below normal subjects. Globus/Mildworf/Melamed (1985) noted only mild deterioration in naming.

More consistency exists in the reports of PD patients on generative naming or verbal fluency tasks. In these tasks, individuals are instructed to generate exemplars of items in a category, such as modes of transportation, names of animals, or words beginning with a particular letter. Most, but not all, researchers report significant impairments in nondemented PD patients (Matison/Mayeux/Rosen/Fahn 1982). Lees/Smith (1983) observed a significant decrement in only one of three stimulus categories, specifically, words beginning with the letter M but not with D or B. Miller (1985) discerned no difference in naming words beginning with the letters F, A, and S between PD patients and age-matched controls. Levin/Llabre/Weiner (1989) administered three generative naming tasks to 41 PD patients who were impaired only in the ability to generate names of food.

Another approach to the study of semantic knowledge is having subjects decide, as quickly as possible, whether a string of letters shown on a television screen is a real word. The reactions can be biased by the prior presentation of semantically related words. Hines/Volpe (1985) administered such a task to 15 PD patients. Although PD patients were slower than normal subjects, their reaction times were faster when the target was preceded by a semantically associated word, leading Hines and Volpe to conclude that "Parkinson's disease seems to have no effect on the final level of activation in semantic memory" (Hines/Volpe 1985, 106).

Some evidence has been published that suggests semantic deficits. Tweedy/Langer/Mc Dowell (1982) observed impairment in the recall and recognition of verbal information in 35 nondemented PD patients. Further, the PD patients benefitted less from semantic recall cues than normals and right-brain damaged individuals. The PD patients also were noted to have difficulty identifying synonyms of previously seen words. Scholtz/Sastry (1985) described disturbance in the ability of PD patients to cluster verbal material to facilitate recall. Levin/Llabre/Weiner (1989) evaluated immediate and delayed recall of discourse material using the Logical Memory Passages of the Wechsler Memory Scale. PD subjects performed significantly below normals in both recall conditions.

Several investigators have tested semantic knowledge using vocabulary tests, but none report decrements in nondemented PD patients (Matison/Mayeux/Rosen/Fahn 1982; Huber/Shuttleworth/Paulson 1986; Pirozzolo/Hansch/Mortimer et al. 1982). To the contrary, Matison and colleagues using the Vocabulary Subtest of the Wechsler Adult Intelligence Scale (WAIS) (Wechsler 1955) reported a mean performance that was above the average of the national and old-aged samples.

A report of the auditory comprehension ability of PD patients was published by Cummings/Darkins/Mendez et al. (1988). Using subtests from the BDAE, deficits were observed in the comprehension of complex commands in nondemented PD patients which were more severe in demented PD patients. When comparison was made of the performance of demented PD and AD patients, the groups were "... not distinguished by auditory comprehension ... reading comprehension, [or] repetition ..." (Cummings/Darkins/Mendez, C 682).

Bayles (1990) studied the performance of 12 nondemented PD patients on four linguistically oriented tasks: the Peabody Picture Vocabulary Test (Dunn 1959); an oral object description task (Bayles 1982); the Similarities subtest of the WAIS (Wechsler 1955); and a story-retelling task (Bayles 1982). A composite score was formed to reflect performance on the four tasks. After controlling for the effects of disease severity, a significant effect was observed for the presence of PD suggesting that PD does affect linguistic competence and/or performance. However, when the additional effects of performance on the Block Design subtest of the WAIS were controlled, the PD effect was of borderline significance. These results are reminiscent of those in the literature. Whereas nondemented PD patients can be demonstrated to perform significantly more poorly on linguistically oriented tasks, the performance deficit cannot be conclusively demonstrated to result from a language deficit per se.

Discourse sample: The following is a sample of discourse from a mildly demented PD patient who was asked first to describe a safety pin and then a match.

Sample # 1: Stimulus: Safety Pin "This is a metallic object. It's compressible. It is one of the two lengths of the object which are, which are parallel to each other. It is compressible into these lengths, and it's compressible. And, uh, it is available to be compressed and kept in a catch ..."

Sample # 2: Stimulus: Matches "This is a light cardboard folder which encl-, encloses a dozen or more longitudinal bodies tipped each one tipped with a red, chalky material substance. The rest of the each of the bodies is made apparently of cardboard and is colored dark, faded blue ... On the opposite side the folded bodies uh folded match case is a black band of uh safety matches phosphorus for illumination purposes."

As was the case with AD patients, the discourse of the demented PD patients is disordered primarily in content and not form. The discourse of nondemented PD patients appears to be normal. Bayles (1991) analyzed the oral discourse of 36 nondemented PD patients and 27 normal control subjects and found no significant differences in total number of words, information units, revisions, aborted phrases, ideational repetitions, and conciseness.

3.3.3. Use

As yet, there are no published reports of possible disease effects on standardized tests of pragmatic knowledge. However, the ability to use language for various purposes can be studied by observing patients in everyday situations. Although a subtle deficit cannot be ruled out by this less rigorous approach, observation of 60 PD patients in the Arizona longitudinal study has not revealed impairment in their ability to use language purposefully in everyday life.

Summary: The evidence for a language deficit per se comes from reports of diminished performance on generative naming tasks and the recall of verbal information. In the former, what appears to be a language deficit may be a decrement in the cognitive processes that influence language production, such as executive function or mental flexibility. In the latter, what appears to be a linguistic deficit may be a problem in the memory processes of retrieval and encoding and unrelated to the fact that the information being remembered is linguistic. Before it can be concluded that an individual has a linguistic competency problem, it must be established that the apparent deficit is not a linguistic performance problem. To conclude that PD patients have a deficit in linguistic performance, it must be established that the apparent deficit is not being caused by a deficit in a more elemental nonlinguistic function that influences linguistic performance.

3.4. Gaps in the Literature

Yet to be determined are the consequences, if any, of the circumscribed intellectual deficits experienced by nondemented PD patients on linguistic communication. Hand-in-hand with this issue is whether the disease affects language as well as nonlinguistic functions. As was the cause with AD, no data are published on the longitudinal effects of PD on language in either demented or nondemented PD. Finally, as yet it is unclear whether the dementia of PD affects linguistic communication differently from the dementia of AD.

4. Huntington's Disease

4.1. Neuropathology

The neostriatum and frontal lobes are the site of pathology in early HD, an autosomal dominant genetic disorder that always causes dementia. The brain atrophy and neurochemical deficiencies that characterize the disease cause chorea and dementia. Atrophy is prominent in the caudate nucleus and putamen of the basal ganglia, the cortex, and the substantia nigra. Early in the disease degeneration occurs in the small Golgi type II neurons within the caudate and putamen. These cells function to inhibit movement. Later in the disease, larger neurons in these areas are affected (Vonsattel/Meyers/Stevens et al. 1985; Lange 1981; Lange/Thorner/Hopf/Schroder 1976). In the cortex, most notably in frontal and occipital areas, diffuse neuronal loss occurs. In conjunction with these abnormalities are neurochemical depletions, specifically of gamma-aminobutyric acid and acetylcholine and their respective synthesizing enzymes within the caudate nucleus.

Neuronal degeneration is detected by radiographic changes in striatal glucose metabolism on PET (Kuhl/Metter/Riege/Markham 1984; Hayden/Martin/Stoessl et al. 1986; Young/Penney/Starosta-Rubinstein et al. 1986). Later disease effects are apparent by computed tomography (Terrance/DeLaney/Alberts 1977; Barr/Heinze/Dobben et al. 1978; Neophytides/Di Chiro/Barron/Chase 1979).

4.2. Neuropsychology

Chorea precedes dementia in HD, though there are exceptions. The motor dysfunction begins as unsteadiness, and fidgeting in the extremities, face, and neck. Ultimately the irregular, jerky, and stretching movements of the full blown chorea affect the whole body. Patients are described as having a shuffling, jerky gait in which the upper body seems to move ahead of the hips and legs.

A variety of affective changes have been observed including depression, mania, irritability, impulsivity, apathy, and in many patients psychosis develops (Caine/Hunt/Weingartner/Ebert 1978). Suicide is high, approximately 7 %, among those recently diagnosed (Reed/Chandler 1958).

HD patients always become demented. The dementia is characterized by deficits in attention, memory, visuospatial processing, and planning. HD patients have difficulty sustaining performance on motor and cognitive tasks (Fedio/Cox/Neophytides et al. 1979; Fisher/Kennedy/Caine/Shoulson 1983). Subtle declines in intellectual functioning begin years before the occurrence of motor symptoms (Lyle/Gottesman 1977). When motor symptoms are evident, so also are deficits in memory, attention, and the ability to organize and sequence information (Josiassen/Curry/Roemer et al. 1982). Later, when the dementia is florid, HD patients perform inferiorly to normals on all subtests of intellectual tests (Butters/Sax/Montgomery/Tarlow 1978; Josiassen/Curry/Roemer et al. 1982).

Butters/Sax/Montgomery/Tarlow (1978) describe early anterograde memory impairment and report that poor performance on short-term memory tasks is more the result of impaired retrieval than faulty encoding. Evidence for this view is that HD patients perform disproportionately better on recognition than free-recall tasks (Butters 1984; Butters/Wolfe/Granholm/Martone 1986). Further, HD patients have been reported to successfully employ verbal mediators to improve memory for pictorial materials (Butters/Albert/Sax 1983). Nonetheless, HD patients are recognized to ultimately suffer deficits in their ability to encode and elaborate information (Caine/Ebert/Weingartner 1977; Weingartner/Caine/Ebert 1979).

Unlike AD patients, HD patients are reported to be impaired in the acquisition of new procedures, a phenomenon explained by disease effects of the basal ganglia.

Performance deficits of HD patients on WAIS subtests measuring visuoconstructional and visuomotor abilities have been reported early (Josiassen/Curry/Mancall 1983; Moses/Golden/Berger/Wisniewski 1981; Fedio/Cox/Neophytides et al. 1979). According to Potegal (1971), HD patients also have difficulty defining their position in space related to a fixed point. Fedio/Cox/Neophytides et al. (1979) observed difficulty on tasks requiring right-left discrimination.

Because connections between prefrontal cortex and the caudate nucleus form a circuit, disease in the caudate could be expected to affect frontal lobe function, specifically executive function and indeed several reports exist of executive dysfunction. These deficits take the form of difficulty planning (Caine/Hunt/Weingartner/Ebert 1978; Fedio/Cox/Neophytides et al. 1979), loss of mental flexibility, and increased perseveration (Josiassen/Curry/Roemer et al. 1982), and impairment in set shifting (Fedio/Cox/Neophytides et al. 1979). Tests that assess planning and sequencing and visuospatial functions were those with greatest discriminative power in distinguishing between patients with stage I and II HD, according to Shoulson (1986). Further, the Stroop and Trails B tests were the most powerful correlates of the indexes of caudate atrophy.

4.3. Effects on Language

HD patients have generally been characterized as having intact language. Folstein/Brandt/Folstein (1990, 97) note, "Patients with HD do not have clinically significant language disorders such as would be seen in patients with cortical lesions of the dominant hemisphere or those with cortical dementias (e. g., DAT)." Certainly HD patients have speech problems secondary to striatal degeneration (Ludlow/Connor/Bassich 1987).

4.3.1. Form

The form of language is appropriate throughout most of the course of the disease, though it may be simplified (Podoll/Caspary/Lange/Noth 1988; Wallesch/Fehrenbach 1988; Gordon/Illes 1987). Only in severely demented individuals is form arguably affected, but in their case, the decimation of the ability to think and the lack of content may make discourse appear to be disordered in form. Wallesch/Fehrenbach (1988) analyzed spontaneous discourse of 18 HD patients and observed "few if any linguistic errors," no semantic paraphasias and few agrammatical and paragrammatical errors. Podoll/Caspary/Lange/Noth (1988) noted that syntactic structures of spontaneous speech were typically reduced to short, simple sentence constructions. Verbal stereotypes were rare and occurred late.

4.3.2. Content and Use

When reviewed, the performance of HD patients on linguistically oriented tasks seem more appropriately interpreted as indicative of a deficit in linguistic performance than competence, at least in the early and middle stages of the disease. For example, the impairment seen on generative naming, or verbal fluency tasks, has been attributed to lexical access problems (Folstein/Brandt/Folstein 1990; Wexler 1979; Smith/Butters/White et al. 1988).

Results of a study by Bayles (1985) document performance deficits but resist interpretation as evidence of loss of linguistic knowledge. Twenty-one HD patients were administered a variety of linguistically oriented tests (naming, PPVT, Similarities subtest of WAIS, FAS verbal fluency test, a sentence judgment and correction task, verbal description, storyretelling, sentence disambiguation, and a pragmatics task.) Performance of HD subjects was compared to those of AD and PD patients with dementia (Bayles/Kaszniak 1987). Comparably demented mild HD and AD patients differed on only a sentence disambiguation task with the HD patients performing more poorly. When moderately demented groups were compared, no significant differences were obtained between moderate AD and PD patients and moderate PD and HD patients. As was the case with the comparison of mildly demented individuals, the only significant differences were between AD and HD patients, in this case, on the verbal description and confrontation naming. On both tasks, AD patients performed more poorly.

Smith/Butters/Granholm (1988) administered naming, verbal fluency, and vocabulary tests to HD subjects and a significantly poorer performance was observed in mild HD patients compared with normal control subjects on all measures, results similar to those in the Bayles study. Smith/Butters/Granholm (1988) caution that although these data suggest that HD may involve a breakdown in the organization of the lexical-semantic representation system, it is impossible to rule out possible influences of general performance factors, such as active retrieval ability. Thus, it seems clear that HD affects the ability to communicate but may not cause a loss of linguistic knowledge per se.

According to Butters/Wolfe/Granholm/Martone (1986), HD patients have a preserved capacity to store new verbal information but are extremely deficient in initiating systematic retrieval strategies when asked to recall information from either episodic or semantic memory.

Certain of the data have been interpreted as evidence of a loss in the system of activation of semantic knowledge but not loss of semantic knowledge. Smith/Butters/White et al. (1988) studied the integrity of semantic or conceptual knowledge in HD patients and attempted to minimize the influence of performance factors. They used a free association paradigm in which target responses to particular stimulus items were primed. Both free association and priming activities are considered largely automatic and do not require active manipulation of knowledge (Posner/Snyder 1975; Hasher/Zacks 1979). A positive priming effect was found for mild HD, moderate HD, and normal subjects regardless of the strength of association or type of relation. However, whereas HD subjects showed no impairment in the ability to prime, there was a progressive decline in the degree to which association strengths of word pairs affected priming of semantic relations. This change represents a qualitative difference between subjects in the way activation of semantic relations is established and maintained over time. Smith/Butters/White et al. (1988, 274) write, "Although these results do not support the view that HD involves an actual loss of representation of concepts in semantic networks, they are consistent with the notion that the dementia of HD involves a deterioration in the system of activation of concepts and relations in a network."

Discourse samples: The following samples are from a moderately demented HD patient who was asked to describe common objects.

Sample # 1: Stimulus: Nail "Nail, that's a nail. Boxing, five penny boxer. It's a quart less than a five penny. That's a quarter long."

Sample # 2: stimulus: Button "That's a button. Has holes in it. Has a ..."

Sample # 3: stimulus: Envelope "Envelope. It's bent. It's a sending for a letter. It's for letter."

The lack of "productivity" and "generativity" that Rosselli/Rosselli/Penagos/Ardila (1987) describe in later stage HD is apparent. The individuals have difficulty generating a set of meaningful descriptors. As noted by Gordon/Illes (1987), there is diminished phrase length and a reduction in the number of words that would be expected in a normal description.

Linguistic communication pattern by stage of disease: Several investigators report less deterioration in language abilities than other aspects of cognitive function (Taylor/Hansotia 1983; Josiassen/Curry/Mancall

1983). Josiassen/Curry/Mancall (1983) administered 36 measures to seven recently diagnosed HD patients, nine moderately advanced HD patients, and 48 individuals at risk but asymtomatic. Verbal performance scores on the WAIS did not discriminate between the groups. Taylor/Hansotia (1983) did observe markedly lower verbal IQ scores in a sample of 16 HD patients, but they were not as low as performance IQ.

4.4. Gaps in the Literature

As was the case with AD and PD, it is unclear whether HD affects linguistic competence as well as performance. If linguistic competence is compromised, is it a bottom-up deterioration phenomenon as AD has been theorized to be? Then too, as with AD and PD, longitudinal data of disease effects on language are nonexistant.

5. Pick's Disease

5.1. Neuropathology

Pick's disease is a relatively rare neurodegenerative disease that affects women twice as often as men (Sjogren/Sjogren/Lindgren 1952). Onset is typically between the ages of 50 and 60 (Mahendra 1987). It is characterized by severe cell loss and subsequent atrophy primarily in the frontal lobes and anterior portions of the temporal lobes but also in the amygdala, basal ganglia, and thalamus. Relatively spared are the pre- and post-central gyri and the posterior superior temporal gyrus (Cummings/Duchen 1981; Uhl/Hilt/Whitehouse/Price 1983). Occasional reports exist of severe degeneration in the basal nucleus (Uhl/Hilt/Whitehouse/Price 1983).

Gustafson/Brun/Risberg (1990) published results of a longitudinal study of four Pick's patients whose brains came to postmortem examination. Three of the four had frontotemporal atrophy with slight predominance in the temporal lobes in two. One case had atrophy only in the frontal lobes. Degeneration was somewhat asymmetric in three cases. The central lobes were slightly affected in all cases and the parietal lobes in three. All cases had inflated cells and inclusions. A few neuritic plaques and neurofibrillary tangles were found in one elder individual, but none in the others.

5.2. Neuropsychology

The early involvement of the frontal lobes is associated with early changes in personality and aberrant social behavior. Affected individuals may be disinhibited, tactless, and insensitive. Typically there is a loss of insight. Kluver-Bucy syndrome tends to occur early. Severe dyspraxia develops later in the disease (Gustafson/Brun/Risberg 1990).

Although Pick's disease is often confused with AD, memory dysfunction typically is observed at a later stage as are visuospatial and constructional deficits (Cummings/Duchen 1981; Wechsler/Verity/Rosenschein et al. 1982). Then too, Kluver-Bucy syndrome is more prominant in Pick's patients.

5.3. Effects on Language

Feher/Inbody/Nolan/Pirozzolo (1988) write that language deficits are likely to be greater in Pick's disease patients than in AD. Cummings (1988) notes that transcortical sensory aphasia occurs in both AD and Pick's disease. However, Cummings (1988, 99) notes, the anomia of Pick's is often of the semantic type with "inability to recall the correct name and concomitant inability to recognize the target word when supplied by the examiner." Cummings goes on to say that Pick's patients are more repetitive, have a greater tendency to use verbal stereotypes, and become echolalic or mute in late stage.

Gustafson/Brun/Risberg (1990) compared Pick's and AD patients in a longitudinal study and observed logoclonia to be uncommon. Then too, the combination of mutism and preserved receptive language was more common in Pick's and severe comprehension deficits with paraphasias and jargon were more common in AD patients.

Holland / Mc Burney / Moossy / Reinmuth (1985) provide the most in-depth description of the deterioration of language in Pick's patient, a man known as Mr. E. They conducted a retrospective study of his language ability from the time of his first speaking difficulty in 1967 until his death 12 years later. Early in the disease his speech slowed, becoming more deliberate. He substituted lower for higher frequency words, a tendency that continued through the language deterioration period. In 1971 he was known to have language formulation and word finding problems though his responses were clear and concise. He exhibited an auditory agnosia and after 1971 became progressively more reluctant to talk. He preferred to write notes to communicate. His notes reveal that he retained memory for names of many friends and places he had been. In the final two years of life, Mr. E. had marked personality changes. He was passive, impulsive, and exhibited poor judgment.

5.3.1. Form

Whereas the AD patient had preserved form, Mr. E's form deteriorated. He lost the formal syntactic elements of language but retained access to the semantic store throughout the disease course.

5.3.2. Content and Use

Although no investigators have studied the effects of Pick's disease on the content and use of language per se, it is possible to infer effects from the anecdotal literature and our knowledge of the distribution of neuropathology. The performance of Mr. E suggests that content is less affected than in AD, and indeed, Pick's disease tends to spare the posterior portions of the temporal lobes and temporoparietal areas. Use of language likely is affected, however, because of frontal lobe pathology and personality changes.

Discourse sample: The following is the last typewritten letter from Mr. E. (Holland/McBurney/Moosy et al. 1985, p. 48).

"Dear Ruth and Bob,
I cannot compose The letter, not speak, language is good, hearing is good, not sense, noise. Stroke 1970.
Note not Mary Jane, and XX Tammy.
Envelope none Roger.
Sincerely"

5.4. Gaps in Literature

Limited data are available about the neurolinguistic effects of Pick's disease. Most of what is known comes from the anecdotal literature. Diagnosis of this relatively rare disease is problematic making large sample longitudinal investigations difficult.

6. Progressive Aphasia and Dementia

Progressive aphasia may be the presenting symptom of Pick's disease (Wechsler/Verity/Rosenschein et al. 1982), Alzheimer's disease (Pogacar/Williams 1984; Green/Morris/Sandson et al. 1990), and Creutzfeldt-Jakob disease (Shuttleworth/Yates/Paltan-Ortiz 1985). It has been reported in individuals ranging in age from the late forties to the mid-seventies. In a study of eight individuals by Green/Morris/Sandson et al. (1990), the mean age was 62.8 (S.D. = 9.4).

Not all of the progressive aphasia patients reported in the literature have developed dementia; however, not all of these patients have been followed longitudinally. Green et al. did study their eight patients longitudinally and seven developed mild dementia after five years. The eight subjects showed deterioration in performance on nonverbal psychometric measures although it was insufficient to be characterized as dementia. Poeck/Luzzatti (1988) followed three patients longitudinally and demonstrated cognitive decline in all three after five years.

In the patients described in the literature (and reviewed by Poeck/Luzzatti 1988), a broad spectrum of language disorders were present from Broca's aphasia to fluent semantic jargon. Nonetheless, the majority had amnesic aphasia which evolved to severe semantic breakdown. Dysnomia, agrammatism, dysprosody, hesitancy of speech, and other nonfluent characteristics were observed in the eight patients in the study by Green and colleagues.

Kirshner/Webb/Kelly/Wells (1984) suggested that there may be a spectrum of disorders associated with progressive aphasia with AD on one end and non-AD-like changes confined to language cortex at the other end. Graff-Radford/Damasio/Hyman et al. (1990) described a progressive aphasia patient whose post-mortem examination confirmed Pick's disease with neuronal loss and glioses in left anterior temporal cortices. The 59-year-old man was anomic and had difficulty recalling the names of people that he knew well and difficulty learning the names of new acquaintances. Scheltens/Hazenberg/Lindeboom et al. (1990) also described a 59-year-old progressive aphasia patient whose aphasia started with misunderstandings of spoken words and spontaneous paraphasias. Striking atrophy of both temporal lobes was seen on MRI and CT nine years after the onset of aphasia. This case was thought to represent a temporal lobe variant of Pick's disease. Results of Green/Morris/Sandson et al.'s (1990) study of eight patients suggest that progressive aphasia cases more commonly evolve to AD than other disorders. Poeck/Luzzatti (1988) concur that progressive aphasia patients are most likely a variant of AD.

7. References

Albert, M. L. (1978). Subcortical dementia. In R. Katzman, R. D. Terry, & K. L. Bick (Eds.), *Aging: Volume 7. Alzheimer's disease: Senile dementia and related disorders, 173–180.* New York: Raven Press.

Albert, M. L. & Milberg, W. (1989). Semantic processing in patients with Alzheimer's disease. *Brain and Language, 37*, 163–171.

Alexander, M. P. & Geschwind, N. (1984). Dementia in the elderly. In M. L. Albert (Ed.), *Clinical neurology of aging, 254–276.* New York: Oxford University Press.

Alvord, E. C., Forno, L. S., Kusske, J. A., Kauffman, R. J., Rhodes, J. S., & Goetowski, C. R. (1974). The pathology of Parkinsonism: A comparison of degenerations in cerebral cortex and brainstem. In F. H. McDowell & A. Barbeau (Eds.), *Advances in Neurology: Volume 5. Second Canadian-American Conference on Parkinson's disease. 175–193.* New York: Raven Press.

American Psychiatric Association (1987). *Diagnostic and statistical manual – III – R.* Washington D. C.: authors.

Appell, J., Kertesz, A., & Fisman, M. (1982). A study of language functioning in Alzheimer patients. *Brain and Language, 17*, 73–91.

Baddeley, A. (1987). *Working memory.* New York: Oxford University Press.

Barr, A. N., Heinze, W. J., Dobben, G. D., Valvassori, G. E., & Sugar, O. (1978). Bicaudate index in computed tomography of Huntington disease and cerebral atrophy. *Neurology, 28*, 1196–1200.

Bayles, K. A. (1982). Language function in senile dementia. *Brain and Language, 16*, 265–280.

Bayles, K. A. (1985). *Effects of dementing illnesses on communicative function.* Paper presented as part of a symposium at the International Neuropsychological Society meeting, San Diego, CA.

Bayles, K. A. (1990). Language and Parkinson disease. *Alzheimer Disease and Associated Disorders, 4*, 171–180.

Bayles, K. A. (1991a). Age at onset of Alzheimer's disease: Relation to language dysfunction. *Archives of Neurology, 48*, 155–159.

Bayles, K. A. (1991b). Alzheimer's disease symptoms: Prevalence and order of appearance. *Journal of Applied Gerontology*, 10, 919–930.

Bayles, K. A. & Boone, D. R. (1982). The potential of language tasks for identifying senile dementia. *Journal of Speech and Hearing Disorders, 47*, 210–217.

Bayles, K. A. & Kaszniak, A. W. (1987). *Communication and cognition in normal aging and dementia.* Boston, MA: College-Hill Press/Little, Brown.

Bayles, K. A., Tomoeda, C. K., Kaszniak, A. W., Stern, L. Z., & Eagans, K. K. (1985). Verbal perseveration of dementia patients. *Brain and Language, 25*, 102–116.

Bayles, K. A., Tomoeda, C. K., Kaszniak, A. W., & Trosset, M. W. (1991). Alzheimer's disease effects on semantic memory: Loss of structure or impaired processing? *Journal of Cognitive Neuroscience, 3*, 166–182.

Bayles, K. A. & Trosset, M. W. (1992). Confrontation naming in Alzheimer's patients: Relation to disease severity. *Psychology and Aging, 7*, 197–203.

Becker, J. T., Grau, H., Schneider, E., Fischer, P. A., & Hacker, H. (1976). CT examination series of Parkinson patients. In W. Lauksch & E. Kazner (Eds.), *Cranial computerized tomography.* 249–251. New York: Springer-Verlag.

Becker, J. T., Huff, F. J., Nebes, R. D., Holland, A., & Boller, F. (1988). Neuropsychological function in Alzheimer's disease: Pattern of impairment and rates of progression. *Archives of Neurology, 45*, 263–268.

Benson, D. F., Cummings, J. L., & Tsai, S. Y. (1982). Angular gyrus syndrome simulating Alzheimer disease. *Archives of Neurology, 39*, 616–620.

Boles, L. & Bayles, K. A. (1991). *Discourse in nondemented Parkinson's disease patients.* Manuscript submitted for publication.

Boller, F. (1980). Mental status of patients with Parkinson disease. *Journal of Clinical Neuropsychology, 2*, 157–172.

Boller, F., Mizutani, T., Roessmann, U., & Gambetti, P. (1980). Parkinson's disease, dementia, and Alzheimer's disease: Clinicopathological correlations. *Annals of Neurology, 7*, 329–335.

Breitner, J. C. S. & Folstein, M. F. (1984). Familial Alzheimer dementia: A prevalent disorder with specific clinical features. *Psychological Medicine, 14*, 63–80.

Brouwers, P., Cox, C., Martin, A., Chase, T., & Fedio, P. (1984). Differential perceptual-spatial impairment in Huntington's and Alzheimer's dementia. *Archives of Neurology, 41*, 1073–1076.

Brown, R. G. & Marsden, C. D. (1988). Internal versus external cues and the control of attention in Parkinson's disease. *Brain, 111*, 323–345.

Brown, R. G. & Marsden, C. D. (1990). Cognitive function in Parkinson's disease: From description to theory. *TINS, 13*, 21–29.

Butters, N. (1984). The clinical aspects of memory disorders: Contributions from experimental studies of amnesia and dementia. *Journal of Clinical Neuropsychology, 6*, 17–36.

Butters, N., Albert, M. S., Sax, D. S., Miliotis, P., Nagode, J., & Sterste, A. (1983). The effects of verbal mediators on the pictorial memory of brain-damaged patients. *Neuropsychologia, 21*, 307–323.

Butters, N., Sax, D., Montgomery, K., & Tarlow, S. (1978). Comparison of the neuropsychological deficits associated with early and advanced Huntington's disease. *Archives of Neurology, 35*, 585–589.

Butters, N., Wolfe, J., Granholm, E., & Martone, M. (1986). An assessment of verbal recall, recognition and fluencey abilities in patients with Huntington's disease. *Cortex, 22*, 11–32.

Caine, E. D., Hunt, R. D., Weingartner, H., & Ebert, M. H. (1978). Huntington's dementia: Clinical and neuropsychological features. *Archives of General Psychiatry, 35*, 378–384.

Caine, E. D., Ebert, M., & Weingartner, H. (1977). An outline for the analysis of dementia: The memory disorder of Huntington's disease. *Neurology, 27*, 1087–1092.

Candy, J. M., Oakley, A. E., Klinowski, J., Carpenter, T. A., Perry, R. H., Atack, J. R., Perry, E. K., Blessed, G., Fairbairn, A., & Edwardson, J. A. (1986). Aluminosilicates and senile plaque formation in Alzheimer's disease. *Lancet, 1*, 354–356.

Capitani, E., Della Sala, S., & Spinnler, H. (1990). Controversial neuropsychological issues in Alzheimer's disease: Influence of onset-age and hemispheric asymmetry of impairment. *Cortex, 26*, 133–145.

Celesia, G. G., & Wanamaker, W. M. (1972). Psychiatric disturbances in Parkinson's disease. *Diseases of the Nervous System, 33*, 577–583.

Chase, T. N., Fedio, P., Foster, N. L., Brooks, R., Di Chiro, G., & Mansi, L. (1984). Wechsler Adult Intelligence Scale performance. Cortical localization by flourodeoxyglucoseF 18-positron emission tomography. *Archives of Neurology, 41*, 1244–1247.

Chertkow, H. & Bub, D. (1990). Semantic memory loss in dementia of the Alzheimer's type. *Brain, 113*, 397–417.

Chertkow, H., Bub, D., & Seidenberg, M. (1989). Priming and semantic memory loss in Alzheimer's disease. *Brain and Language, 36*, 420–446.

Chui, H. C., Teng, E. L., Henderson, V. W., & Moy, A. C. (1985). Clinical subtypes of dementia of the Alzheimer's type. *Neurology, 35*, 1544–1550.

Cools, A. R., van den Bercken, J. H. L., Horstink, M. W. I., van Spaendonck, K. P. M., & Berger, H. J. C. (1984). Cognitive and motor shifting aptitude disorder in Parkinson's disease. *Journal of Neurology, Neurosurgery, and Psychiatry, 47*, 443–453.

Critchley, M. (1964). The neurology of psychotic speech. *British Journal of Psychiatry, 110*, 353–364.

Cummings, J. L. (1988). Dementia of the Alzheimer type: Challenges of definition and clinical diagnosis. In H. A. Whitaker (Ed.). *Neuropsychological studies of nonfocal brain damage*, 86–107. New York: Springer-Verlag.

Cummings, J. L., Benson, F., Hill, M. A., & Read, S. (1985). Aphasia in dementia of the Alzheimer's type. *Neurology, 35*, 394–397.

Cummings, J. L., Darkins, A., Mendez, M., Hill, M. A., & Benson, D. F. (1988). Alzheimer's disease and Parkinson's disease: Comparison of speech and language alterations. *Neurology, 38*, 1415–1422.

Cummings, J. L. & Duchen, L. W. (1981). Kluver-Bucy syndrome in Picks disease: Clinical and pathological correlations. *Neurology, 31*, 1415–1422.

Davies, P. & Wolozin, B. L. (1987). Recent advances in the neurochemistry of Alzheimer's disease. *Journal of Clinical Psychiatry, 48 (5, suppl.)*, 23–30.

De la Monte, S., Wells, S. E., Hedley-Whyte, E. T., & Growdon, J. H. (1989). Neuropathological distinction between Parkinson's dementia and Parkinson's plus Alzheimer's disease. *Annals of Neurology, 26*, 309–320.

De Renzi, E. & Faglioni, P. (1978). Normative data and screening power of a shortened version of the Token Test. *Cortex, 14*, 41–49.

Drevets, W. C. & Rubin, E. H. (1989). Psychotic symptoms and the longitudinal course of senile dementia of the Alzheimer type. *Biological Psychiatry, 25*, 39–48.

Duara R., Grady, C., Haxby, J., Sundaram, M., Cutler, N. R., Heston, L., Moore, A., Schlageter, N. L., Larson, S., & Rapoport, S. I. (1986). Positron emission tomography in Alzheimer's disease. *Neurology, 36*. 879–887.

Dunn, L. M. (1959). *Peabody Picture Vocabulary Test*. Circle Pines: American Guidance Service.

El-Awar, M., Becker, J. T., Hammond, K. M., Nebes, R. D., & Boller, F. (1987). Learning deficit in Parkinson's disease: Comparison with Alzheimer's disease and normal aging. *Archives of Neurology, 44*, 180–184.

Eslinger, P. J. & Benton, A. L. (1983). Visuoperceptual performances in aging and dementia: Clinical and theoretical implications. *Journal of Clinical Neuropsychology, 5*, 213–220.

Faber-Langendoen, K., Morris, J. C., Knesevich, J. W., La Barge, E., Miller, J. P., & Berg, L. (1988). Aphasia in senile dementia of the Alzheimer type. *Annals of Neurology, 23*, 365–370.

Fedio, P., Cox, C., Neophytides, A., Canal-Fredrick, G. & Chase, T. N. (1979). Neuropsychological profile in Huntington's disease: Patients and those at risk. In T. N. Chase, N. S. Wexler, & A. Barbeau (Eds.), *Advances in neurology: Volume 23. Huntington's disease*. 239–255. New York: Raven Press.

Feher, E. P., Inbody, S. B., Nolan, B., & Pirozzolo, F. J. (1988). Other neurologic diseases with dementia as a sequela. *Clinics in Geriatric Medicine, 4*, 799–814.

Filley, C. M., Kelley, J., Heaton, R. K. (1986). Neuropsychological features of early- and late-onset Alzheimer's disease. *Archives of Neurology, 43*, 574–576.

Fischler, I. (1977 a). Associative facilitation without expectancy in a lexical decision task. *Journal of Experimental Psychology: Human Perception and Performance, 3*, 18–26.

Fischler, I. (1977 b). Semantic facilitation without association in a lexical decision task. *Memory and Cognition, 5*, 335–339.

Fisher, J. M., Kennedy, J. L., Caine, E. D., & Shoulson, I. (1983). Dementia in Huntington's disease: A cross-sectional analysis of intellectual decline. In R. Mayeux & W. G. Rosen (Eds.), *The dementias. 229–238*. New York: Raven Press.

Flicker, C., Ferris, S., Crook, T., & Bartus, S. (1987). Implication of memory and language dysfunction in the naming deficit of senile dementia. *Brain and Language, 31*, 187–200.

Fodor, J. A. (1983). *Modularity of mind*. Cambridge, MA: The MIT Press.

Folstein, S. E., Brandt, J., & Folstein, M. F. (1990). Huntington's disease. In J. L. Cummings (Ed.), *Subcortical dementia. 87–107*. New York: Oxford University Press.

Folstein, M. F. & Breitner, J. C. S. (1981). Language disorder predicts familial Alzheimer's disease. *Johns Hopkins Medical Journal, 149*, 145–147.

Folstein, M. F., Folstein, S. E., & Mc Hugh, P. R. (1975). "Mini-mental state": A practical method for grading the mental state of patients for the clinician. *Journal of Psychiatric Research, 12*, 189–198.

Freedman, M., Rivoria, P., Butters, N., Sax, D. S., & Feldman, R. G. (1984). Retrograde amnesia in Parkinson's disease. *Canadian Journal of Neurology, 11*, 297–301.

Friedland, R. P., Budinger, T. F., Ganz, E., Yano, Y., Mathis, C. A., Koss, B., Ober, B. A., Huesman, R. H., & Derenzo, S. E. (1983). Regional cerebral metabolic alterations in dementia of the Alzheimer type: Positron emission tomography with (18 F) fluorodeoxyglucose. *Journal of Computer Assisted Tomography, 7*, 590–598.

Gainotti, G., Daniele, A., Nocentini, U., & Silveri, M. C. (in press). The nature of lexical-semantic impairment in Alzheimer's disease. *Journal of Neurolinguistics*.

Globus, M., Mildworf, B., & Melamed, E. (1985). Cerebral blood flow and cognitive impairment in Parkinson's disease. *Neurology, 35*, 1135–1139.

Golder, H. K. (1988). Structured conversational interaction tasks, turn-taking and topic shift in Alzheimer's disease subjects. Unpublished B. Sc. (Hons.) dissertation. University of Newcastle upon Tyne.

Goodglass, H. & Kaplan, E. (1976). *The assessment of aphasia and related disorders*. Philadelphia: Lea & Gebiger.

Gordon, W. P. & Illes, J. (1987). Neurolinguistic characteristics of language production in Huntington's disease: A preliminary report. *Brain and Language, 31*, 1–10.

Grady, C. L., Haxby, J. V., Schlageter, N. L., Berg, G., & Rapoport, S. I. (1986). Stability of metabolic and neuropsychological asymmetries in dementia of the Alzheimer's type. *Neurology, 36*, 1390–1392.

Green, J., Morris, J. C., Sandson, J., Mc Keel, D. W., & Miller, J. W. (1990). Progressive aphasia: A precursor of global dementia? *Neurology, 40*, 423–429.

Graff-Radford, N. R., Damasio, A. R., Hyman, B. T., Hart, M. N., Tranel, D., Damasio, H., Van Hoesen, G. W., & Rezai, K. (1990). Progressive aphasia in a patient with Pick's disease: A neuropsychological, radiologic, and anatomic study. *Neurology, 40*, 620–626.

Gustafson, L., Brun, A., & Risberg, J. (1990). Frontal lobe dementia of non-Alzheimer type. In R. J. Wurtman, S. Corkin, J. H. Growdon & E. Ritter-Walker (Eds.), *Advances in neurology: Vol. 51. Alzheimer's disease*. New York: Raven Press, Ltd.

Hakim, A. M. & Mathieson, G. (1979). Dementia in Parkinson's disease: A neuropathologic study. *Neurology, 29*, 1209–1214.

Hart, S. (1985). *Explorations of cognitive dysfunction in dementia of the Alzheimer type*. Unpublished Ph. D. thesis. University of London.

Hart, S. (1988). Language and dementia: A review. *Psychological Medicine, 18*, 99–112.

Hart, S., Smith, C. M., & Swash, M. (1986). Assessing intellectual deterioration. *British Journal of Clinical Psychology, 25*, 119–124.

Hartman, M. D. (1987). A cognitive-neuropsychological study of semantic representation in dementia of the Alzheimer type (Doctoral dissertation, University of Minnesota, 1987). *Dissertation Abstracts International, 48*, 2781 B.

Hasher, L. & Zacks, R. T. (1979). Automatic and effortful processes in memory. *Journal of Experimental Psychology: General, 108*, 356–388.

Haxby, J. V., Duara, R., Grady, C. L., Cutler, N. R., & Rapoport, S. I. (1985). Relations between neuropsychological and cerebral metabolic asymmetries in early Alzheimer's disease. *Journal of Cerebral Blood Flow and Metabolism, 5*, 193–200.

Hayden, M. R., Martin, W. R. W, Stoessl, A. J., Clark, C., Hollenberg, S., Adam, M. J., Anmann, W., Harrap, R., Rogers, J., Ruth, T., Sayre, C., & Pate, B. D. (1986). Positron emission tomography in the early diagnosis of Huntington's disease. *Neurology, 36*, 888–894.

Henderson, V. W. & Finch, C. E. (1989). The neurobiology of Alzheimer's disease. *Journal of Neurosurgery, 70*, 335–353.

Henderson, V. W., Mack, W., Freed, D. M., Kempler, D., & Anderson, E. S. (1990). Naming consistency in Alzheimer's disease. *Brain and Language, 39*, 530–538.

Heyman, A., Wilkinson, W. E., Stafford, J. A., Helms, M. J., Sigmon, A. H., & Weinberg, T. (1984). Alzheimer's disease: A study of epidemiological aspects. *Annals of Neurology, 15*, 335–341.

Hier, D. B., Hagenlocker, K., & Shindler, A. G. (1985). Language disintegration in dementia: Effects of etiology and severity. *Brain and Language, 25,* 117–133.

Hines, T. M. & Volpe, B. T. (1985). Semantic activation in patients with Parkinson's disease. *Experimental Aging Research, 11,* 105–107.

Hirano, A., Dembitzer, H. M., Kurland, L. T., & Zimmerman, H. M. (1968). The fine structure of some intraganglionic alterations: Neurofibrillary tangles, granulovacuolar bodies and "rod like" structures as seen in Guam amyotrophic lateral sclerosis and Parkinsonism-dementia complex. *Journal of Neuropathology and Experimental Neurology, 27,* 167–182.

Holland, A., Mc Burney, P. H., Moossy, H., & Reinmuth, O. M. (1985). The dissolution of language in Pick's disease with neurofibrillary tangles: A case study. *Brain and Language, 24,* 36–58.

Hooper, M. W. & Vogel, F. S. (1976). The limbic system in Alzheimer's disease. A neuropathologic investigation. *American Journal of Pathology, 85,* 1–19.

Huber, S. J., Shuttleworth, E. C., & Paulson, G. W. (1986). Dementia in Parkinson's disease. *Archives of Neurology, 43,* 987–990.

Huff, F. J., Corkin, S., & Growdon, J. (1986). Semantic impairment and anomia in Alzheimer's disease. *Brain and Language, 28,* 235–249.

Huff, F. J., Mack, L., Mahlmann, J., & Greenberg, S. (1988). A comparison of lexical-semantic impairments in left-hemisphere stroke and Alzheimer's disease. *Brain and Language, 34,* 262–278.

Illes, J., Metter, E. J., Hanson, W. R., & Iritani, S. (1988). Language production in Parkinson's disease: Acoustic and linguistic considerations. *Brain and Language, 33,* 146–160.

Josiassen, R. C., Curry, L. M., & Mancall, E. L. (1983). Development of neuropsychological deficits in Huntington's disease. *Archives of Neurology, 40,* 791–796.

Josiassen, R. C., Curry, L., Roemer, R. A., DeBease, C., & Mancall, E. L. (1982). Patterns of intellectual deficit in Huntington's disease. *Journal of Clinical Neuropsychology, 4,* 173–183.

Kaplan, E., Goodglass, H., & Weintraub, S. (1983). *Boston Naming Test.* Philadelphia: Lea & Febinger.

Kempler, D., Curtiss, S., & Jackson, C. (1987). Syntactic preservation in Alzheimer's disease. *Journal of Speech and Hearing Research, 30,* 343–350.

Kidd, M. (1964). Alzheimer's disease-an electron microscopical study. *Brain, 87,* 307–320.

Kidd, M., Allsop, D., & Landon, M. (1985). Senile plaque amyloid, paired helical filaments, and cerebrovascular amyloid in Alzheimer's disease are all deposits of the same protein. *Lancet, 1,* 278.

Kirshner, H. S., Webb, W. G., Kelly, M. P., & Wells, C. E. (1984). Language disturbance: An initial symptom of cortical degeneration and dementia. *Archives of Neurology, 41,* 491–496.

Knesevich, J. W., Toro, F. R., Morris, J. C., & La Barge, E. (1985). Aphasia, family history, and the longitudinal course of senile dementia of the Alzheimer type. *Psychiatry Research, 14,* 255–263.

Kuhl, D. E., Metter, E. J., Riege, W. H., & Markham, C. H. (1984). Patterns of cerebral glucose utilization in Parkinson's disease and Huntington's disease. *Annals of Neurology, 15,* 119–125.

Lange, H. W. (1981). Quantitative changes of telencephalon, diencephalon, and mesencephalon in Huntington's chorea, post-encephalitic, and idiopathic parkinsonism. *Verhandlungen der anatomischen Gesellschaft, 75,* 923–925.

Lange, H. W., Thorner, G., Hopf, A., & Schroder, K. F. (1976). Morphometric studies of the neuropathological changes in choreatic disease. *Journal of Neurological Sciences, 28,* 401–425.

Lavy, S., Melamed, E., Cooper, G., Bentin, S., & Rinot, Y. (1979). Regional cerebral blood flow in patients with Parkinson's disease. *Archives of Neurology, 36,* 344–348.

Lees, A. J. & Smith, E. (1983). Cognitive deficits in the early stages of Parkinson's disease. *Brain, 106,* 257–270.

Levin, B. E., Llabre, M. M., & Weiner, W. J. (1989). Cognitive impairments associated with early Parkinson's disease. *Neurology, 39,* 557–561.

Lewis, D. A., Campbell, M. J., Terry, R. D., & Morrison, J. H. (1987). Laminar and regional distributions of neurofibrillary tangles and neuritic plaques in Alzheimer's disease: A quantitative study of visual and auditory cortices. *Journal of Neurosciences, 7,* 1799–1808.

Lieberman, A., Dziatolowski, M., Kupersmith, M., Serby, M., Goodgold, A., Korein, J., & Goldstein, M. (1979). Dementia in Parkinson's disease. *Annals of Neurology, 6,* 355–359.

Ludlow, C. L., Connor, N. P., & Bassich, C. J. (1987). Speech timing in Parkinson's and Huntington's disease. *Brain and Language, 32,* 195–214.

Lyle, O. & Gottesman, I. (1977). Premorbid psychometric indicators of the gene for Huntington's desease. *Journal of Consulting Clinical Psychology, 45,* 1011–1022.

Mahendra, B. (1987). *Dementia: A survey of the syndrome of dementia.* Norwell, MA: MTP Press.

Margolin, D. I. (1987). *Lexical priming by pictures and words in aging, stroke and dementia.* Unpublished doctoral dissertation. University of Oregon.

Martin, A., Cox, C., Brouwers, P., & Fedio, P. (1985). A note on different patterns of impaired and preserved cognitive abilities and their relation to episodic memory deficits in Alzheimer's patients. *Brain and Language, 26,* 118–185.

Martin, A., Brouwers, P., La Londe, F., Cox, C., Teleska, P., & Fedio, P. (1986). Towards a behavioral topology of Alzheimer's patients. *Journal of Clinical and Experimental Neuropsychology, 8*, 594–610.

Matison, R., Mayeux, R., Rosen, J., & Fahn, S. (1982). "Tip-of-the-tongue" phenomenon in Parkinson disease. *Neurology, 32*, 567–570.

Mayeux, R., Stern, Y., & Spanton, S. (1985). Heterogeneity in dementia of the Alzheimer type: Evidence of subgroups. *Neurology, 34*, 453–461.

Miller, E. (1985). Possible frontal impairments in Parkinson's disease: A test using a measure of verbal fluency. *British Journal of Clinical Psychology, 24*, 211–212.

Miller, E. & Hague, F. (1975). Some characteristics of verbal behavior in presenile dementia. *Psychological Medicine, 5*, 255–259.

Mishkin, M. & Appenzeller, T. (1987). The anatomy of memory. *Scientific American, 256*, 80–89.

Molsa, P. K., Martilla, R. J., & Rinne, U. K. (1984). Extrapyramidal signs in Alzheimer's disease. *Neurology, 34*, 1114–1116.

Mortimer, J. A., Pirozzolo, F. J., & Maletta, G. J. (1982). Overview of the aging motor system. In J. A. Mortimer, F. J. Pirozzolo, & G. J. Maletta (Eds.), *The aging motor system* (1–6). New York: Preger.

Moses, J. A., Golden, C. J., Berger, P. A., & Wisniewski, A. M. (1981). Neuropsychological deficits in early, middle, and late stage Huntington's disease as measured by the Luria-Nebraska Neuropsychological battery. *International Journal of Neuroscience, 14*, 95–100.

Naville, F. (1922). Etudes sur les complications et les sequelles mentales de l'encephalite epidemique. La Bradyphrenie, Encephale, Par. 1922, XVII, 369; 423.

Nebes, R. D., Boller, F., & Holland, A. (1986). Use of semantic context by patients with Alzheimer's disease. *Psychology and Aging, 1*, 261–269.

Nebes, R. D., Brady, C. B., & Huff, F. J. (1989). Automatic and attentional mechanisms of semantic priming in Alzheimer's disease. *Journal of Clinical and Experimental Neuropsychology, 11*, 219–230.

Nebes, R. D., Martin, D. C., & Horn, L. C. (1984). Sparing of semantic memory in Alzheimer's disease. *Journal of Abnormal Psychology, 93*, 321–330.

Neophytides, A. N., Di Chiro, B., Barron, S. A., & Chase, T. (1979). Computed axial tomography in Huntington's disease and persons at risk for Huntington's disease. *Advances in Neurology, 23*, 185–191.

Nicholas, M., Obler, L K., Albert, M. L., & Helm-Estabrooks, N. (1985). Empty speech in Alzheimer's disease and fluent aphasia. *Journal of Speech and Hearing Research, 28*, 405–410.

Ober, B. A. & Shenaut, G. K. (1988). Lexical decision and priming in Alzheimer's disease. *Neuropsychologia, 26*, 273–286.

Pearce, J. (1974). The extrapyramidal disorder of Alzheimer's disease. *European Neurology, 12*, 94–103.

Petry, S., Cummings, J. L., Hill, M. A., & Shapira, J. (1988). Personality alterations in dementia of the Alzheimer's type. *Archives of Neurology, 45*, 1187–1190.

Pirozzolo, F. J. (1982). Neuropsychological assessment of dementia. *Neurology Clinics, 4*, 12–18.

Pirozzolo, F. J., Hansch, E. C., Mortimer, J. A., Webster, D. D., & Kuskowski, M. A. (1982). Dementia in Parkinson's disease: A neuropsychological analysis. *Brain and Cognition, 1*, 72–83.

Podoll, K., Caspary, P., Lange, H. W., & Noth, J. (1988). Language functions in Huntington's disease. *Brain, 111*, 1475–1503.

Poeck, K. & Luzzatti, C. (1988). Slowly progressive aphasia in three patients. *Brain, 111*, 151–168.

Pogacar, S. & Williams, R. S. (1984). Alzheimer's disease presenting as slowly progressive aphasia. *Rhode Island Medical Journal, 67*, 181–185.

Posner, M. I. & Snyder, C. R. (1975). Attention and cognitive control. In R. L. Solso (Ed.), *Information and cognition. 55–85.* Hillsdale, NJ: Erlbaum.

Potegal, M. (1971). A note on spatial-motor deficits in patients with Huntington's disease: Test of a hypothesis. *Neuropsychologia, 9*, 233–235.

Reed, T. & Chandler, J. (1958). Huntington's chorea in Michigan. I. Demography and genetics. *American Journal of Human Genetics, 10*, 201–225.

Reisberg, B., Ferris, S. H., de Leon, M. J., & Crook, T. (1982). The global deterioration scale (GDS): An instrument for the assessment of primary degenerative dementia (PDD). *American Journal of Psychiatry, 139*, 1136–1139.

Rorsman, B., Hagnell, O. & Lanke, J. (1986). Prevalence and incidence of senile and multi-infarct dementia in the Lundby study: A comparison between the time periods 1947–1957 and 1957–1972. *Neuropsychobiology, 15*, 122–129.

Rosselli, D., Rosselli, M., Penagos, B., & Ardila, A. (1987). Huntington's disease in Colombia: A neuropsychological analysis. *International Journal of Neuroscience, 32*, 933–942.

Rubin, E. H., Morris, J. C., Storandt, M., & Berg, L. (1987). Behavioral changes in patients with mild senile dementia of the Alzheimer's type. *Psychiatric Research, 21*, 55–62.

Sagar, H. J., Sullivan, E. V., Gabrieli, J. D. E., Corkin, S., & Growdon, J. H. (1988). Temporal ordering and short-term memory deficits in Parkinson's disease. *Brain, 111*, 525–539.

Saint-Cyr, J. A., Taylor, A. E., & Lang, A. E. (1988). Procedural learning and neostriatal dysfunction in man. *Brain, 111*, 941–959.

Salmon, D. P., Shimamura, A. P., Butters, N., & Smith, S. (1988). Lexical and semantic priming deficits in patients with Alzheimer's disease. *Journal of Clinical and Experimental Neuropsychology, 10* 477–494.

Scheltens, Ph., Hazenberg, G. J., Lindeboom, J., Valk, J., & Wolters, E. Ch. (1990). A case of progressive aphasia without dementia: "temporal" Pick's disease? *Journal of Neurology, Neurosurgery and Psychiatry, 53*, 79–80.

Scholtz, O. B. & Sastry, M. (1985). Memory characteristics in Parkinson's disease. *International Journal of Neuroscience, 27*, 229–234.

Schwartz, M. F., Marin, O. S. M., & Saffran, E. M. (1979). Dissociations of language function in dementia: A case study. *Brain and Language, 7*, 277–306.

Selby, G. (1968). Cerebral atrophy in Parkinsonism. *Journal of the Neurological Sciences, 6*, 517–559.

Selnes, O. A., Carson, K., Rovner B., & Gordon B. (1988). Language dysfunction in early- and late-onset possible Alzheimer's disease. *Neurology, 38*, 1053–1056.

Seltzer, B. Burres, M. J. K., & Sherwin, I. (1984). Left-handedness in early and late-onset dementia. *Neurology, 34*, 267–369.

Seltzer, B. & Sherwin, I. (1983). A comparison of clinical features in early- and late-onset primary degenerative dementia: One entity or two? *Archives of Neurology, 40*, 143–146.

Shoulson, I. (1986). Huntington's disease. In A. K. Asbury, G. M. McKhann & W. McDonald (Eds.), *Diseases of the nervous system. 1258–1267.* Philadelphia: Ardmore Medical Books (WB Saunders).

Shuttleworth, E. C., Yates, A. J., & Paltan-Ortiz, J. D. (1985). Creutzfeld-Jakob disease presenting as progressive aphasia. *Journal of the National Medical Association, 77*, 649–655.

Sjogren, T., Sjogren, H. & Lindgren, A. G. H. (1952). Morbus Alzheimer and morbus Pick: Genetic, clinical and patho-anatomical study. *Acta Psychiatrica et Neurologica Scandinavica Supplimentum*, (Suppl. 82), 1–152.

Slauson, T. J., Bayles, K. A., & Tomoeda, C. K. (1987). *Communication disorders in late-stage Alzheimer's disease.* Paper presented at the annual meeting of the American Speech-Language-Hearing Association, New Orleans, LA.

Slobin, D. I. (1971), *Psycholinguistics.* Glenview, Illinois: Scott, Foresman, and Company.

Smith, S., Butters, N., & Granholm, E. (1988). Activation of semantic relations in Alzheimer's and Huntington's disease. In H. A. Whitaker (Ed.), *Neuropsychological studies of nonfocal brain damage. 265–285.* New York: Springer-Verlag.

Smith, S., Butters, N., White, R., Lyon, L., & Granholm, E. (1988). Priming semantic relations in patients with Huntington's disease. *Brain and Language, 33*, 27–40.

Sourander, P. & Sjogren, H. (1970). The concept of Alzheimer's disease and its clinical implications. In G. E. W. Wolstenholme M. O'Connor (Eds.), *Alzheimer's disease and related conditions. 11–36.* London: Churchill Livingstone.

Squire, L. R. (1987). *Memory and brain.* New York: Oxford University Press.

Stern, Y. (1983). Behavior and the basal ganglia. In R. Mayeux & W. G. Rosen (Eds.), *The dementias. 195–209.* New York: Raven Press.

Storandt, M., Botwinick, J., Danziger, W. L., Berg, L., & Hughes, C. P. (1984). Psychometric differentiation of mild senile dementia of the Alzheimer type. *Archives of Neurology, 41*, 497–499.

Sulkava, R. (1982). Alzheimer's disease and senile dementia of Alzheimer type: A comparative study. *Acta Neurologica Scandinavica, 65*, 636–650.

Sullivan, E. V., Sagar, H. J., Gabrieli, J. D. E., Corkin, S., & Growdon, J. H. (1985). Different cognitive profiles on standard behavioral tests in Parkinson's disease and Alzheimer's disease. *Journal of Clinical and Experimental Neuropsychology, 7*, 160.

Taylor, H. G. & Hansotia, P. (1983). Neuropsychological testing of Huntington's patients: Clues to progression. *The Journal of Nervous and Mental Disease, 171*, 492–496.

Terrence, C. F., DeLaney, J. F., & Alberts, M. C. (1977). Computerized tomography for Huntington's disease. *Neuroradiology, 13*, 173–175.

Thal, L. J. (1988). Dementia update: Diagnostic and neuropsychiatric aspects. *Journal of Clinical Psychiatry, 49* (suppl.), 5–7.

Tomoeda, C. K. & Bayles, K. A. (1992). *Longitudinal effects of Alzheimer's disease on discourse production.* Manuscript submitted for publication.

Tweedy, J. R., Langer, K. G., & McDowell, F. H. (1982). The effect of semantic relations on the memory deficit associated with Parkinson's disease. *Journal of Clinical Neuropsychology, 4*, 235–237.

Uhl, G. R., Hilt, D. C., Whitehouse, P. J., & Price, D. L. (1983). Pick's disease (lobar sclerosis): Depletion of neurons in the nucleus basalis of Meynert. *Neurology, 33*, 1470–1473.

Ulatowska, H. K., Allard, L., Donnell, A., Bristow, J., Haynes, S. M., Flower, A., & North, A. J. (1988). Discourse performance in subjects with dementia of the Alzheimer type. In H. A. Whitaker (Ed.), *Neuropsychological studies of nonfocal brain damage. 108–131.* New York: Springer-Verlag.

Vance, K. T. & Bayles, K. A. (1990). *Dissociation of oral reading and semantic information in advanced Alzheimer's disease patients.* Paper presented at the meeting of the Rocky Mountain Psychological Association, Tucson, AZ.

Vonsattel, J. P., Meyers, R. H., Stevens, T. J., Ferrante, R. J., Bird, E. D., & Richardson, P. (1985). Neuropathological classification of Huntington's disease. *Journal of Neuropathology and Experimental Neurology, 44*, 559–577.

Wallesch, C. W. & Fehrenbach, R. A. (1988). On the neurolinguistic nature of language abnormalities in Huntington's disease. *Journal of Neurology, Neurosurgery, and Psychiatry, 51*, 367–373.

Warrington, E. K. (1975). The selective impairment of semantic memory. *Quarterly Journal of Experimental Psychology, 27*, 635–657.

Wechsler, A. F., Verity, M. A., Rosenschein, S., Fried, I., & Scheibel, A. B. (1982). Pick's disease: A clinical, computed tomographic, and histological study with Golgi impregnation observations. *Archives of Neurology, 39*, 287–290.

Wechsler, D. (1955). *Manual for the Wechsler Adult Intelligence Scale.* New York: The Psychological Corporation.

Weingartner, H., Burns, S., Diebel, R., & Le Witt, P. A. (1984). Cognitive impairments in Parkinson's disease: Distinguishing between effort-demanding and automatic cognitive processes. *Psychiatry Research, 11*, 223–235.

Weingartner, H., Caine, E. D., & Ebert, M. H. (1979). Encoding processes, learning, and recall in Huntington's disease. In T. N. Chase, N. S. Wexler, & A. Barbeau (Eds.), *Advances in Neurology, Volume 23: Huntington's Disease, 215–226.* New York: Raven Press.

Wexler, N. S. (1979). Perceptual-motor, cognitive, and emotional characteristics of persons at-risk for Huntington's disease. In T. N. Chase, N. S. Wexler, & A. Barbeau (Eds.), *Advances in neurology, Volume 23: Huntington's disease. 257–271.* New York: Raven Press.

Whitaker, H. A. (1976). A case of isolation of the language function. In H. Whitaker & H. A. Whitaker (Eds.), *Studies in neurolinguistics: Volume 2. 1–58.* New York: Academic Press.

Wilson, R. S., Kaszniak, A. W., Klawans, H. L., & Garron, D. C. (1980). High speed memory scanning in Parkinsonism. *Cortex, 16*, 67–72.

Young, A. B., Penney, J. P., Starosta-Rubinstein, S., Markel, D. S., Barent, S., Giordan, B., Ehrenkaufer, R., Jewett, D., & Hichwa, R. (1986). PET scan investigations of Huntington's disease: Metabolic correlates of neurologic features and functional decline. *Annals of Neurology, 20*, 296–303.

Kathryn A. Bayles, Tucson, Arizona (USA)

36. Language Disorders with Diffuse Brain Disease of Acute Onset

1. Introduction

The study of neurologically-based language impairment in adults has evolved from examination of disorders with focal lesions to research and clinical concerns with disorders of more diffuse neurological substrates. Where aphasia received primary attention in the past, literature now highlights linguistic and communicative deficits in patients suffering closed head trauma, right hemisphere impairment, and dementia. Narrow considerations of purely linguistic phenomena have given way to broader models of behavioral deficit that encompass the full array of neuropsychological domains and acknowledge the cognitive underpinnings of some communicative deficits.

It is surprising, therefore, to find that almost no language-based research or clinical attention has been paid to one subset of the neurologically-impaired population – individuals who have suffered some form of anoxic encephalopathy with relatively acute onset. Parkin/Miller/Vincent (1987, 655) define anoxic encephalopathy as a diffuse "... deterioration in brain function following disruption or cessation of the brain's vascular supply".

The causes of anoxic encephalopathy may vary. Relatively unusual incidents such as near-drownings, failed hangings, anesthesia complications or induced hypotension, and carbon monoxide poisoning account for a small percentage of known cases, along with encephalopathy of unknown origin. However, the vast majority of individuals with acute onset anoxic encephalopathy are those who have suffered cardiac arrest followed by cardiopulmonary resuscitation. It is projected that between 100,000 and 200,000 out-of-hospital resuscitations are attempted yearly in this country (Safar 1986; Krause/White/Aust et al. 1988), with an additional unknown number of resuscitations attempted within the confines of the hospital setting. Although survival-to-discharge rates remain low (between 6% and 35%) for out-of-hospital resuscitations, thousands of individuals survive to be at-risk for disorders of linguistic and cognitive function.

Neurological outcome, however continues to be defined in rather broad terms that may obscure deficit. Volpe/Holtzmann/Hirst (1986, 408) state that, "Cognitive abnormalities are often not defined, or defined only as inability to return to former occupation". Thus, linguistic and communicative quality of life issues for persons with anoxic encephalopathy of acute onset are rarely addressed, and a systematic framework for clinical assessment and service delivery is lacking.

This chapter briefly reviews general neurological outcomes in patients with anoxic encephalopathies of acute onset, neurophysiological mechanisms presumed to be responsible for deficit, and recent literature concerning language consequences of such encephalopathies. Findings from a six month neuropsychological follow-up of 39 cardiac arrest patients are summarized.

2. General Neurological Outcomes

Safar (1988) notes that initial concerns with simple survival and restoration of healthy cardiac function following resuscitation have given way in the last two decades to a preoccupation with quality of survival. Research emphases have shifted to epidemiological analyses of neurological outcomes, clinical trials of specific treatment regimes designed to improve cerebral status, and exploration of subject or treatment factors influencing neurological outcomes.

Neurological outcome data tend to substantiate Krause/White/Aust et al.'s (1988, 714) claim that, "Neurologic injury is the major limitation of cardiac resuscitation". However, there are marked discrepancies with respect to the proportion of resuscitated individuals who experience return to normal cerebral function, with estimates ranging from 93% (Bedell/Delbanco/Cook/Epstein 1983) to percentages as low as 13% (Bass 1985; BRCT I Study Group 1986).

Differences in sample characteristics may account for some of these discrepancies. However the more fundamental problem concerns a definition of good cerebral recovery. In recent work, measures such as the Glasgow Outcome Performance Scales (BRCT II Study Group 1989) assign "good cerebral performance" to individuals who may still be experiencing minor psychologic or neurologic deficits, including mild aphasia or cranial nerve abnormalities. Thus, the scale would classify individuals who have suffered mild cerebral dysfunction as having made good neurological recovery. It is not surprising that Kotila/Kajaste (1984) plead for greater attention to the identification of neuropsychological deficits in patients who appear outwardly normal or recovered. To address such deficits, the underlying neurophysiological mechanisms that might be expected to contribute to impaired functioning must be examined.

3. Underlying Neurophysiological Mechanisms

Cerebral damage may result from two aspects of the arrest/resuscitation cycle. The more obvious aspect of the cycle is that there are finite limits to the amount of time neuronal tissue can withstand sustained lack of oxygenation before irreversible damage or neuronal death occurs (Safar 1988). In addition, the reperfusion and reoxygenation measures necessary to restore metabolism and cell viability initiate a postresuscitation syndrome after a period of five minutes without blood flow.

Initial anoxia coupled with ensuing resuscitation efforts lead to cell death in predictable regions, including the phylogenetically older regions of the brain in general and particularly the basal ganglia, hippocampus, cerebellum, occipital lobe, and "border zone" or watershed regions of the parietotemporal cortex (c. f., Safar 1988; Parkin/Miller/Vincent 1987; Bigler/Alfano 1988). Reperfusion efforts and failures may also lead to a variety of organ and cell derangements.

Neuropsychological deficits in survivors of anoxic encephalopathy might be predicted to reflect pervasive alterations in basic cognitive processes (e. g., attention and orientation) coupled with more specific deficits in motor functioning (cerebellum, basal ganglia), memory (hippocampus), visual skills (occipital lobe), and perceptual processes and language (temperoparietal regions). These predictions are supported in the linguistic and neuropsychological literature.

4. Language Characteristics of Patients with Diffuse Brain Disease of Acute Onset

The neuropsychological literature concerning dysfunction in patients with anoxic encephalopathies is scattered through a variety of sources and relies heavily upon case studies (for review, see Shadden/Holland 1990). The earliest case study reports tended to focus upon the range of memory impairments in survivors, with particular attention to Korsakoff-like dementia traits. Concern with memory deficits continues to the present day (c.f., Cermak 1976; Cummings/Tomiyasu/Read/Benson 1984). There appears to be reliable evidence that at least one subgroup of cardiac arrest or anoxic encephalopathic patients is characterized by pronounced impairment of memory skills in the absence of notable deficit in other aspects of cognitive functioning. When neuroradiological or postmortem data are available, amnesic deficits are usually traced to hippocampal lesions (Cermak 1976; Cummings/Tomiyasu/Read/Benson 1984; Bigler/Alfano 1988).

A variety of deficits in visual perception (including cortical blindness) are documented in virtually every study of neuropsychological consequences of anoxic encephalopathy. Reports of orientation and attentional deficits are common.

It is interesting to note that memory and visual perceptual skills underpin many language behaviors, yet the presence of linguistic deficits in a number of these studies is either ignored, controlled for, or denied. For example, Parkin/Miller/Vincent (1987) concluded that language functions were well preserved in the context of pronounced perceptual and memory deficits despite their reports of word-finding deficits and acquired dyslexia in the patient they studied. Anomalous treatment of language performance is also evident when one considers that memory measures in a number of studies traditionally include forward and backward digit span. Similar measures of auditory memory span can be found in aphasia tests.

In general, reference to speech and language dysfunction in many studies is incidental or anecdotal. For example, Caronna/Finklestein (1978) noted one subject out of four with motor speech and language comprehension deficits, and Yarnell (1976) indicated that two out of four survivors remaining in a vegetative state retained some ability to comprehend and follow simple commands. Rose/Symonds (1960) described their subject's problems in repeating sentences and in auditory memory span; one of Willanger/Klee/Lindeneg/Jorgensen's (1970) young patients desplayed total alexia and severe acalculia. In fact, even early reports examining Korsakoff-like symptoms of cases with anoxic encephalopathy stressed the presence of confabulation and verbosity.

More recent investigations of neuropsychological sequelae of cardiac arrest and resuscitation have begun to examine a broader range of cognitive functions. In addition to the Parkin/Miller/Vincent (1987), Volpe/Hirst (1983), and Volpe/Holtzmann/Hirst (1986) works, Armengol/Moes (1986) describe neuropsychological profiles of nine patients with anoxic encephalopathy of varying origins. They reported that linguistic and visuospatial skills were impaired in all subjects, with deficits in attention, memory, orientation, and task behavior noted in seven of the nine. Similarly, Kotila/Kajaste (1984) identified dysphasia in four out of ten patients who had suffered out-of-hospital cardiac arrest.

The work of Bigler/Alfano (1988) is probably one of the most comprehensive neuropsychological evaluations to date. They explored profiles of 12 patients who were at least nine months post anoxic brain injury with an initial deep coma and abnormal EEG's. An extensive neuropsychological test battery was administered, including language-based measures such as the Rey Auditory Verbal Learning Task. Only results of WAIS-R, Wechsler Memory Scale, and Halstead-Reitan administrations were discussed in the paper. Experimental subjects were compared with a matched control group of closed head injured patients. Premorbid IQ was estimated.

Although the anoxic brain damage group scored within the normal range on the Verbal portion of the Aphasia Screening Exam subtest of the Halstead-Reitan, postmorbid Verbal IQs on the WAIS-R were significantly lower than those of the control group. The anoxic group also performed more poorly on all verbal subtests of the WAIS-R, suggesting that skills such as auditory memory span, vocabulary, and comprehension were im-

vocabulary, and comprehension were impaired considerably. As in earlier studies, greatest deficits continued to be noted in the memory domain. The authors concluded that, "the clinician assessing the anoxic encephalopathy patient needs to utilize a wide spectrum of neuropsychological measures along with specific tests of memory function" (Bigler/Alfano 1988, 396).

The preceding overview of the neuropsychological literature concerning linguistic impairment with anoxic encephalopathy is remarkable for its very few comprehensive studies of neuropsychologic functions and its relative inattention to language. The largest number of subjects considered in any one study was 22 (Bengtsson/Holmberg/Jansson 1969), of whom a much smaller number received the designated psychologic/psychiatric battery. Subject selectivity is also apparent. Few studies measure behaviors in an entire sample of survivors. There are a limited number of experimental studies of either the nature of or underlying processes involved in observed deficits.

In general, detailed descriptions of spontaneous naming and verbal expression characteristics of this population are lacking. The word finding deficits mentioned specifically by Bengtsson/Holmberg/Jansson (1969) and Parkin/Miller/Vincent (1987), among others, appear to resemble the tip-of-the-tongue phenomena noted in both aphasia and some forms of dementia. However, impaired word-retrieval processes are not described in any depth. Expressive language disturbances are either labeled aphasia or described relatively consistently as reflecting verbosity, impulsivity, perseveration, and irrelevance. There are no controlled comparisons of naming or broader communicative functions in patients with anoxic encephalopathy, aphasia, and dementia.

In response to some of these concerns, a neuropsychological protocol was developed to provide a mechanism for longitudinal screening of a broad range of deficits and to supplement more traditional outcome measures such as the Glasgow Outcome Performance Scales. Analysis has recently been completed on neuropsychological screening examination data gathered from 39 subjects at two weeks and six months post cardiac arrest. These data represent outcomes for the largest body of resuscitated individuals to date that have received a consistent battery of neuropsychological measures in any one study.

The Neuropsychological Screening Instrument (NPSI) developed for this investigation is a 48 point examination designed for brevity, ease of administration, and capability of translation into different languages. Although brief, it contains tasks well within the normal performance range and samples a range of neuropsychologic performance areas. The 16 different tasks comprising the instrument sample aspects of orientation, long-term memory, procedural memory, delayed recall, verbal language comprehension (following commands, answering simple factual questions), verbal expression (picture naming, sentence repetition, word fluency), reading comprehension, writing, drawing and copying, and visuospatial and visuomotor attention and sequencing. For analysis, items were grouped into three categories: Orientation and Memory, Visuospatial Perception and Attention, and Language.

Subjects were drawn from the 516 participants in the Pittsburgh School of Medicine's multi-site Brain Resuscitation Clinical Trial II (BRCT II) data base (BRCT II Study Group 1989). BRCT II is a randomized, double-masked clinical trial study comparing the effects of lidoflazine with placebo on recovery of cerebral function post cardiac arrest. The Neuropsychological Screening Instrument (NPSI) was administered to all subjects judged able to cooperate at two weeks and six months, with only the 39 subjects tested at both intervals forming the primary data base. A group of 20 control subjects matched for age decade, sex, and gender distribution also completed the NPSI. Data were available with respect to demographics, arrest causes and times, and regular monitoring of coma severity, functional level, and Glasgow Outcome Performance Categories which reflect levels of cerebral and overall performance functioning.

In this discussion, only key language-related findings will be highlighted, although visuospatial perception and attentional processes were clearly impaired in the cardiac arrest group as compared with a group of controls. It should be noted, however, that NPSI-tested subjects received consistently higher ratings than non-tested subjects on the Glasgow Outcome Performance Categories at both two weeks and six months, reflecting their status as the highest functioning component of the survivor group.

With respect to language functioning, the following findings are of interest. First, cardiac arrest survivors scored significantly lower than control subjects on the combined Language Cluster at both two and six weeks. In fact, at both intervals, more subjects fell below the one standard deviation cut-off score in the Language Cluster than in any other cluster of subtests. Of the five most consistently discriminating individual subtests, three were in the Language Cluster (word fluency, sentence repetition, and answering questions). Second, on the Language Cluster, 21 out of 39 subjects showed a positive change in performance from two weeks to six months (mean 4.2 points) and only 4 subjects lost 1 or 2 points. However, even at six months, 25 subjects fell below the Language Cluster cut-off score based on one standard deviation below the mean.

Third, NPSI scores appeared much more sensitive to cognitive-based neurological dysfunction than did the Glasgow Outcome Performance Scales. At two weeks, 85% of subjects received the top rating of Good Cerebral Performance, yet only 20% obtained NPSI scores within the normal range. Similarly, at six months, 92% of subjects received top cerebral performance ratings, yet only 39% received normal range scores on the NPSI. It should be noted, however, that the best Cerebral Performance rating obtained by any subject during the first 24 hours post-arrest was highly predictive of Language Cluster performance at six months ($r = -.88$, $p < .001$).

Fourth, Language Cluster scores at two weeks showed moderate correlation ($r = +.50$, $p < .01$) with Language Cluster scores at six months. Finally, when subjects were sorted on the basis of arrest and CPR times, and on the presence or absence of retrograde and anterograde amnesia, Language Cluster performance at two weeks was found to be poorer if CPR times were longer and if anterograde amnesia persisted until six months. Language Cluster performance at six months was found to be poorer if Total Arrest Times were longer, if anterograde amnesia was reported at two weeks, and if retrograde amnesia persisted at six months.

Taken together, these findings permit several conclusions. The most important is that, in an anoxic encephalopathic subject population selected only for ability to respond to testing, language deficits are characteristic of the group as a whole. Despite the anticipated scatter of deficits, almost two-thirds of the six months survivors displayed less than optimal performance in this domain. Particularly sensitive areas appeared to be word fluency, sentence repetition, and answering questions. Since Language Cluster performance on the NPSI continued to improve from two weeks to six months, it is impossible to determine the long-term outcome with respect to language functioning. However, even mild linguistic deficits of six months duration are likely to have a profound impact on quality of life, particularly if coupled with other deficits in cognitive or emotional functioning.

Another important conclusion is that global neurological outcome measures frequently overestimated the degree of recovery in resuscitated cardiac arrest patients. Patients described as having normal cerebral functioning on the Glasgow Outcome Performance Scales still evidenced language deficits at six months. This observation does not negate the value of the Glasgow scales, since best Cerebral Performance achieved on this measure during the first 24 hours strongly predicted language performance at six months.

Data from this preliminary investigation provide clear support for the presence of language impairment in some resuscitated cardiac arrest patients. Coupled with findings from the work of Armengol/Moes (1986) and Kotila/Kajaste (1984), among others, the need for further focused linguistic research with individuals suffering diffuse brain disease of relatively acute onset is apparent.

5. Conclusions

Despite growing concerns about quality of life for the survivor of cardiac arrest and other conditions producing diffuse brain damage, it appears that few practitioners are aware of the likelihood that neuropsychological linguistic deficits in such patients may occur. Of particular concern are the group of individuals whom Kotila/Kajaste (1984) designate as "outwardly normal". Once the threat to life has been resolved and medical and neurological status is broadly stable, these individuals may return to their homes and families with the understanding that they have overcome their ordeal. Previously undetected deficits in cognitive and linguistic functions, as well as personality and emotional adjustment, may emerge at this time (c. f., Reich/Regestein/Murawski et al. 1983; Vlay/Fricchione 1985). Unfortunately, these behavioral changes may be sufficiently subtle to escape notice in routine medical follow-up. Evaluation and potentially beneficial treatment services for patients and families may be neglected.

The preceding brief review of relevant portions of the neuropsychological literature, coupled with recent data pertaining to post-arrest linguistic deficits in the BRCT II clinical trial population, provides sufficiently strong support to conclude that linguistic dysfunction does occur with some regularity in the anoxic encephalopathy population. The nature and extent of such deficits remains ill-defined, and further research concerning linguistic deficits in cardiac arrest survivors is needed. A comprehensive research protocol should include the following:

All resuscitated cardiac arrest patients should be administered a neuropsychological screening examination similar to the NPSI at two weeks, three months, six months, and one year. Patients should not be eliminated due to the presence of aphasic deficits or any other selection criteria. This process will provide much-needed basic epidemiological data concerning the frequency of occurrence of neuropsychological deficits and behavioral change over time. In addition, individuals can be targeted for further testing.

Patients identified during the screening process should receive further intensive neuropsychological testing, including a battery of tasks designed specifically to tap a variety of language functions. Functional communication and discourse assessment must be incorporated into this battery. A common test battery could be identified by a core group of researchers across multiple sites, and a data bank which would include neuroradiological and medical data should be developed. With sufficiently large numbers of subjects, distinct performance profiles could identified for differential diagnostic purposes. Follow-up testing for several years would also permit identification of prognostic variables influencing recovery.

A separate but parallel series of experimental investigations should probe more closely into the source of linguistic impairment – attempting to identify the contributions of attentional, memory, perceptual and other deficits to observed language dysfunction. Further, studies of the efficacy of different treatment protocols would shed further light on the underlying nature and causes of language deficit.

Selected cardiac arrest survivors and their families should be followed longitudinally in an attempt to determine the longterm impact of residual deficits upon quality of life, and the relative contribution of linguistic and communicative breakdown to reduced quality of life. This information would be crucial in counseling with patients and families and in designing family-oriented interventions.

In addition to the above-described research efforts, professionals in speech-language pathology, neuropsychology, and neurology should work to increase sensitivity to the need for cognitive and linguistic intervention in the cardiac arrest population. Without enhanced sensitivity and awareness, the knowledge base related to language consequences of anoxic encephalopathy will remain inadequate and the individual with diffuse brain damage of acute onset will continue to be underserved.

Acknowledgment: This work was supported by a grant (NS/5295) from the Natural Institutes of Health (USA).

6. References

Armengol, C. G. & Moes, E. J. (1986). Neuropsychological profiles of patients with anoxic encephalopathy. *Journal of Clinical and Experimental Psychology*, *8*, 120 (Abstract).

Bass, E. (1985). Cardiopulmonary arrest: Pathophysiology and neurologic complications. *Annals of Internal Medicine*, *103*, 920–927.

Bedell, S. E., Delbanco, T. L., Cook, E. F. & Epstein, F. H. (1983). Survival after cardiopulmonary resuscitation in the hospital. *New England Journal of Medicine*, *309*, (10), 569–575.

Bengtsson, M., Holmberg, S. & Jansson, B. (1969). A psychiatric-psychological investigation of patients who had survived circulatory arrest. *Acta Psychiatrica Scandinavica*, *45*, 327–346.

Bigler, E. D. & Alfano, M. (1988). Anoxic encephalopathy: Neuroradiological and neuropsychological findings. *Archives of Clinical Neuropsychology*, *3*, 383–394.

Brain Resuscitation Clinical Trial I Study Group (1986). Randomized clinical study of thiopental loading in comatose survivors of cardiac arrest. *New England Journal of Medicine*, *314* (7), 397–403.

Brain Resuscitation Clinical Trial II Study Group (1989). A randomized clinical trial of calcium entry blocker administration to comatose survivors of cardiac arrest: Design, methods, and patient characteristics. International Resuscitation Research Center, University of Pittsburgh, Pittsburgh, PA.

Caronna, J. J. & Finklestein, S. (1978). Neurological syndromes after cardiac arrest. *Stroke*, *9*, 517–520.

Cermak, L. S. (1976). Encoding capacity of a patient with amnesia due to encephalitis. *Neuropsychologia*, *14*, 311–326.

Cummings, J. L., Tomiyasu, U., Read, S. & Benson, D. F. (1984). Amnesia with hippo-campal lesions after cardiopulmonary arrest. *Neurology*, *34*, 679–681.

Kotila, M. & Kajaste, S. (1984). Neurological and neuropsychological symptoms after cardiac arrest. 25th Scandinavian Congress of Neurology: Cerebrovascular Diseases (1984, Bergen, Norway). *Acta Neurologica Scandinavica 69* (98), 337–338.

Krause, G. S., White, B. C., Aust, S. D., Nayini, N. R. & Kumar, K. (1988). Brain cell death following ischemia and reperfusion: A proposed biochemical sequence. *Critical Care Medicine*, *16*, 714–726.

Parkin, A. J., Miller, J. & Vincent, R. (1987). Multiple neuropsychological deficits due to anoxic encephalopathy: A case study. *Cortex*, *23*, 655–665.

Reich, P., Regestein, Q. R., Murawski, B. J., DeSilva, R. A. & Lown, B. (1983). Unrecognized organic mental disorders in survivors of cardiac arrest. *American Journal of Psychiatry*, *140*, 1194–1197.

Rose, F. C. & Symonds, C. P. (1960). Persistent memory defect following encephalitis. *Brain*, *83*, 199–211.

Safar, P. (1988). Resuscitation from clinical death: Pathophysiologic limits and therapeutic potentials. *Critical Care Medicine*, *16*, 923–941.

Shadden, B. B. & Holland, A. L. (1990). Neuropsychological outcomes in cardiac arrest survivors: Performance on the Neuropsychological Screening Instrument (NPSI). Unpublished manuscript.

Vlay, S. C. & Fricchione, G. L. (1985). Psychosocial aspects of surviving sudden cardiac death. *Clinical Cardiology*, *8*, 237–243.

Volpe, B. T. & Hirst, W. (1983). The characterization of an amnesic syndrome following hypoxic ischemic injury. *Archives of Neurology*, *40*, 436–440.

Volpe, B. T., Holtzman, J. D. & Hirst, W. (1986). Further characterization of patients with amnesia after cardiac arrest: Preserved recognition memory. *Neurology*, *36*, 408–411.

Willanger, R., Klee, A., Lindeneg, O. & Jorgensen, E. O. (1970). A neuropsychological study of cerebral anoxic sequelae of cardiac arrest. *Acta Neurologica Scandinavica*, Supp 43, 103–104.

Varnell, P. R. (1976). Neurological outcome of prolonged coma survivors of out-of-hospital cardiac arrest. *Stroke*, *7*, 279–282.

Audrey L. Holland, Tucson, Arizona (USA)/
Barbara B. Shadden, Fayetteville, Arkansas (USA)

III. Acquired Organic Pathologies of Language Behavior: Neurophonetic Disorders

37. Dynamical Systems and Speech

1. Introduction and Historical Perspective

The perception of phonological information is remarkably insensitive to acoustic variations introduced, for example, by changes in the rate at which an utterance is produced, the emphatic or syllabic stress level, or contextual effects. A primary concern of speech science and psychology from the late 1960's through most of the 1970's was to elucidate how the putatively invariant phonological information is encoded in the continuously varying acoustic signal. One early hypothesis was that the motor commands sent to the muscles would stand in one-to-one identity with an individual phonological segment, and that this invariance, although smeared in the acoustic signal, would be observable in electromyograms (Liberman/Cooper/Shankweiler/Studdert-Kennedy 1967). However, it was quickly demonstrated that electromyographic activity was itself strongly context-dependent (e. g., MacNeilage/DeClerk 1969). Shifting the focus of analysis to articulatory gestures also failed to reveal an invariant relationship between individual motor variables (e. g., displacement, velocity) and phonological segments (e. g., Butcher/Weiher 1976; Gay/Ushijima/Hirose/Cooper 1974; Kozhevnikov/Chistovich 1965; Kuehn/Moll 1976; Liberman/Cooper/Shankweiler/Studdert-Kennedy 1967; Lindblom 1963). In fact, the variability of individual articulatory gestures as a function of stress, rate, and contextual change is one of the few aspects of speech production on which most investigators agree (but see, for example, Kelso/Vatikiotis-Bateson/Saltzman/Kay 1985, for evidence of stable kinematic *relationships* in individual articulators across rate and stress; also Vatikiotis-Bateson 1988).

These studies underscore the qualitatively incommensurate nature of phonological segments (typically considered as discrete, static, and invariant across contexts) and the changing vocal tract shape which, like the resultant acoustic consequences, is both continuous and context-sensitive. It was thus necessary to postulate a mechanism for minimizing abrupt articulatory changes at segment boundaries. The general form of the proposed mechanism was to spread the individual features among neighboring segments, then translate the resulting feature bundles into commands to articulatory muscles for execution in sequence [see Fowler,Chapter 3; this volume; also Daniloff/Hammarberg 1973 for an example of production models of this type.]

The rules governing featural spread were often hotly debated (see Fowler, Chapter 3 this volume, for discussion of feature spreading, coproduction, etc.). Despite their differences, most theories assumed the final stage of translation of feature bundles into muscle commands. Our inadequate understanding of this stage began to be recognized, with a growing appreciation of the complexity of movement control and coordination as exemplified by the Soviet physiologist Nikolai Bernstein (1967). Although Bernstein's work was directed largely at understanding coordinated nonspeech limb and body movements, the concepts he identified also motivated empirical and theoretical work in speech production (Fowler/Rubin/Remez/Turvey 1980).

Bernstein's key insight was that the large number of potential degrees of freedom of the skeletomuscular system precludes the possibility that each is controlled individually at every point in time. He then proposed a scheme whereby many degrees of freedom could be regulated through the direct, executive control of very few. (Note that "executive" should not be considered here as solely a central or cortical function. For example, brainstem regions could play a putative "executive"role.) In this view, individual variables of the motor system are organized into larger groupings variously called 'linkages,' 'synergies,' 'collectives,' or 'coordinative structures' (Boylls 1975; Easton 1972; Gel'fand/Gurfinkel/Fomin/Tsetlin 1971; Turvey 1977). These groupings are generally thought to be functional, not hardwired, in that the same degrees of freedom may be constrained in different ways to achieve different purposes, and different degrees of freedom may be constrained to achieve the same goal. During a movement, the functional group can be controlled as if it had many fewer degrees of freedom than comprise its parts, thus reducing the number of control decisions required (e. g., Kelso/Southard/Goodman 1979). In what follows, direct evidence is presented for the speech articulators functioning cooperatively as a flexible task-specific unit. Also discussed are the stability and flexibility of the units and their actual dynamical description in terms of equations of motion. These dynamics refer to the 'coordination dynamics' of the central nervous system, not the physical mechanics of moving masses. Finally, the utility of a dynamical description of task-specific units in speech modelling and the relevance to speech disorders are considered.

2. Functional Constraints on Multiarticulator Coordination

2.1. Spatial Constraints

Examples of functional constraints on speech movement, coordinative structures, are evident in speakers' adjustments to static and dynamic disruptions of articulation. When speakers wear a 'biteblock,' a spacer that maintains a constant separation between the upper and lower jaw, they are nonetheless able to produce isolated vowels, and consonant-vowel-consonant syllables within the normal range of acoustic and kinematic variability (e. g., Lindblom/Sundberg 1971). Significantly, speakers do so even when the availability of acoustic, tactile, or proprioceptive feedback is drastically reduced (e. g., Kelso/Tuller 1983; Lindblom/Lubker/Gay 1979). A similar outcome is obtained when lip protrusion is impeded during production of rounded vowels. Compensation is achieved even on the first trial by lowering the larynx to a degree that preserves the vocal tract length characteristic of the vowel and produces acoustically normal vowels (Riordan 1977).

Unexpected dynamic pertubation of articulatory motions also fails to disrupt production. In one such experiment, the speaker produces the syllable/bæb/a number of times. On a few of the productions, the jaw motion is suddenly perturbed while moving toward the final /b/ closure. The upper lip actively compensates for the jaw disruption by increasing displacement so as to produce the bilabial closure for /b/, even on the first occurrence of the perturbation; no concurrent increase in tongue muscle activity is observed. These remote reactions in the upper lip are observed only when the jaw is perturbed during the closing phase of the motion, that is, when the reactions are necessary to preserve the identity of the utterance. When the upward jaw motion is perturbed during the transition to the final /z/ of /bæz/, no compensatory increase in displacement is observed in the lip motions, but the tongue activity increases, an appropriate compensation to achieve the tongue-palate approximation for fricative production. Thus, functionally-specific (phonetically-specific) near-immediate compensation to unexpected perturbation is observed in articulators remote from the locus of the perturbation, on the first occurrence of the perturbation. [Abbs/Gracco/Cole 1984; Kelso/Tuller/Vatikiotis-Bateson/Fowler 1984; Shaiman 1989, among many others].

The findings just described are not easily accounted for by traditional motor control models. For example, closed-loop (feedback-dependent) models can account for the accurate production of vowel sounds despite changes in initial position of the jaw (due to the biteblock), but they could not explain why production remains within the normal range when acoustic, tactile, and proprioceptive information is restricted. In theory, open-loop (feedback-independent) models could incorporate the results of restricted afferentation, but have difficulty explaining satisfactorily adjustments to unanticipated perturbations. Considering the degrees of freedom of the vocal tract as a 'constrained functional group' means that the system has an intrinsic goal which is attainable from any initial configuration by virtue of the system dynamics. That is, the system exhibits 'equifinality' (von Bertalanffy 1973).

One very simple example of a dynamical system that displays equifinality, is a mass-spring system. This system has been used as a model for understanding the adaptive behavior of the articulatory system in perturbed (biteblocks, disruptions of articulator movements) as well as unperturbed speech (variations in stress, speaking rate, contextual variations, etc. See for examples Ostry/Munhall 1985; Kelso/Vatikotis-Bateson/Saltzman/Kay 1985). A mass-spring system is simply a spring attached at one end to a fixed support and at the other end to a mass (cf. Fowler/Rubin/Remez/Turvey 1980). When the spring is stretched or compressed and then released, it always equilibrates at the same resting length regardless of the amount the mass is initially displaced. In most but not all cases, the mass-spring description is not meant to be a literal representation of the physiological speech system with springs and masses representing muscles and articulators. Rather, the mass-spring system is used as an abstract description of articulatory behavior. A mass-spring system belongs to a generic class of dynamical system with the simplest attractor type, a point attractor (or stable fixed point) to which all neighboring trajectories converge (see Section 3.2.). In an abstract description, the attractor may be conceived of as a limit set in a functionally-defined physiological space.

2.2. Temporal Constraints

Speech production depends not only on the spatial relationships among articulator positions but also on their temporal patterning and serial ordering (Lashley 1951). Examples of constraints on timing of multiple articulators are becoming increasingly common (e. g. Kent/Netsell 1971; Kent/Moll 1975; Kozhevnikov/Chistovich 1965; Löfqvist/Yoshioka 1981). Our own work has focussed on the relative timing of vowel-related, *V*, and consonant-related, *C*, events across changes in speech rate and syllable stress. Basically, we reported that across these suprasegmental changes the timing of medial consonant production in $CV_1 \# CV_2C$ utterances (e. g., */ba # wab/*) remains stable relative to the interval between events associated with the flanking vowels. The relationship between these articulatory event durations (the interval from V_1 to C and from V_1 to V_2) was described well by a linear function with a positive slope and nonzero intercept. This occurred whether 'segment-associated activity' was observed at the electromyographic (Tuller/Kelso/Harris 1982; 1983) or kinematic levels (Kelso/Saltzman/Tuller 1986; Tuller/Kelso 1984; Tuller/Kelso/Harris 1983). These 'relative timing' results hint at the presence of a functional constraint on movement timing whereby individual system elements are constrained within a particular temporal relationship, while metrical adjustment of the components affords flexibility.

The foregoing experiments motivated a flurry of activity among speech scientists, some of whom subsequently corroborated the basic result (Gentil/Harris/Horiguchi/Honda 1984; Linville 1982; Löfqvist 1986; Lubker 1983), and some of whom failed to do so (Munhall 1985; Nittrouer/Munhall/Kelso et al. 1988). In what follows, we argue that the interpretation of relative timing information depends crucially on the experimental paradigm and, more generally, on the distinction between invariance and stability in system behavior. The problem arises because different relative timing stability regimes exist as a function of the independent variable of interest (e. g., speaking rate).

3. Coordination Dynamics of Speech

3.1. Invariance vs. Stability

It is commonplace to assume that if a variable does not change much over a range of parameter values, it is an invariant. Schmidt (1982), for example, argues that the 'invariance' of proportions of time spent in various phases of the locomotion step cycle provides evidence for walking and jogging programs. Criteria for invariance are seldom specified, however, leading to much confusion (cf. Sternberg/Knoll/Turock 1990). One may ask: invariant with respect to what? Or, how much can the mean value of a variable change before one decides that the variable is not invariant?

An alternative approach is to show that a variable such as relative timing remains *stable*, not necessarily strictly invariant, over a range of parameter values, then shifts to a new value as a consequence of *loss of temporal stability*. Thus, pattern stability and change arise from the same underlying nonlinear dynamics. Whether loss of stability is observed depends crucially on the range of parameter values selected for study. An hypothesized collective variable, such as relative timing, may change little across a wide range of speaking rates. But the fact that relative timing undergoes a phase transition at some critical speaking rate may be more fundamental, undercutting the invariance concept by providing a metric for evaluating fluctuations in the mean value of a variable. Recent observations of phase transitions in speech movement (and perceptual) patterns demonstrates that the dynamical concept of stability (which incorporates stochastic features) is fundamental, it can be tightly coupled to experimental measures, and it better serves the understanding of speech and other forms of motor control than the rather vague use of the term 'invariance.' The latter term we reserve for describing symmetry under a group of transformations.

3.2. Theoretical Considerations

The dynamical approach to speech production originated from the study of bimanual movement coordination and is based upon theories of self organization and pattern formation in nonequilibrium systems, particularly Haken's (1975; 1983) synergetics (see for example Kelso/DelColle/Schöner 1990). The aim is to understand coordinated movement as a pattern formation process. In synergetics, when a certain parameter or combination of parameters (referred to as 'controls') reach a critical point, structure or change in structure occurs spontaneously. At so-called nonequilibrium phase transitions, the emerging patterns may be characterized by *collective variables* whose dynamics (equations of motion) are low-dimensional. Synergetics thus promotes a search for these collective variables (also called *order parameters*) in experimental model systems and the determination of control parameters that move the system through collective states.

The dynamics of collective variables may be determined by studying the stability and loss of stability of movement patterns. Specific empirical phenomena are predicted to occur jointly at transition points. One is the presence of enhanced fluctuations, in which the values of the collective variable undergo large fluctuations with no change in the mean state (cf. earlier remarks on invariance in Section 3.). Another predicted phenomenon is critical slowing down, whereby a system close to a transition point reacts more and more slowly to external perturbations than in other situations when it is far from criticality. Both features are characteristic of self-organization and both have been observed experimentally in movement systems (for recent reviews see Kelso/Schöner/Scholz/Haken 1987; Kelso/Schöner 1988; Schöner/Kelso 1988).

What are the collective variables and control parameters in the speech production system? There are many possible modifiers of articulation that might lead the system through different coordinative patterns and hence reveal the underlying coordination dynamics. These control parameters include, but are not limited to, stress, loudness, speaking rate and speaking style. If the nonspecific influence of a continuously varying control parameter results in a change of pattern, then one should be able to identify collective variables that correspond to the observed patterns and determine their dynamics through an analysis of stability.

The identification of relevant collective variables for a given behavior is not trivial and will be addressed further in Section 3.3. Assume, for the moment, that a set of collective variables has been found that characterizes the articulatory pattern for a given phonetic string and that can be expressed by a low-dimensional vector x. Underlying the dynamic view is the assumption that $\vec{x} = \vec{x}(t)$, where t is time, obeys a dynamical law on a macroscopic scale:

(1) $\dot{x}_t = f(x_t, \mathit{parameters, noise})$

where f is, in general, a nonlinear function of the typically high-dimensional state vector x_t. This function may also depend on a number of parameters representing, for example, the speaking style or rate, as well as random noise that reflects the many degrees of freedom acting on the system but which are unaccounted for in the state vector x_t. For a large class of functions f, special solutions of the equation (called 'attractors') exist. By definition, an attractor is (asymptotically) stable, that is, all neighboring solutions converge in time to the attractor solution. In the present formulation, phonological units may well correspond to stable collective states, or attractors, of the order parameter dynamics (cf. Schöner/Kelso 1988).

In Section 2.1., we described a simple dynamical system, a mass-spring system, that has been used to model speech production. A mass-spring system is a form of point attractor, the simplest attractor type. Recent work has explored systems that support richer dynamics, such as periodic attractors, as more appropriate for modelling speech production. Many more complicated attractor types exist, giving rise to very complex behavior of the solutions of Eq.1. In general, low-dimensional nonlinear dynamical systems can exhibit extremely rich behavior, including multistability, switching, bifurcations, intermittency, and even deterministic chaos. Many of these features have been observed in human movement coordination (see for review Kelso/DeGuzman/Holroyd 1991) and to a more limited extent in speech production and perception.

3.3. Empirical Evidence

A dynamical account of multiarticulator coordination that includes complicated attractor types holds promise for understanding the flexibility or change of articulatory patterns, thus allowing phonetically rich sequences. In many theories of speech, and of motor control in general, there is a tendency to account for the appearance of new patterns as resulting from the selection of a new motor program, or motor engram. An alternative strategy recognizes that in multidegree of freedom systems in which component interactions occur, new patterns of organization and behavior appear that are not easily predictable from the preceding ones. This 'symmetry breaking' occurs in physical systems, as well as biological and psychological ones and the new spatiotemporal patterns are sometimes referred to as 'emergent properties'.

There is already a hint in the literature that certain kinds of phonetic and syllabic change correspond directly to phase transitions among articulatory gestures (see Kelso/Saltzman/Tuller 1986) and hence may enable us to specify relevant collective variables. Consider an example provided by Stetson (1951; also Kelso/Munhall 1988), who observed that gradual increases in rate of producing a repetitive syllable string (such as *at, at, at ...)* causes a change in the phasing of component gestures and hence of the syllable affiliation of the consonant (*ta, ta, ta ...* is produced). Stetson thought that the need to simplify coordination caused the syllable-final consonant to become syllable-initial because the final consonant was "off-phase, out of step with the syllable movement (p. 96)." One interpretation of Stetson's data is that phasing among component gestures is the collective variable, or order parameter, underlying both stability and change in syllabic structure and that consonant-initial syllables are more stable than vowel-initial syllables, particularly at fast rates.

The relative stability of consonant-initial and vowel-initial syllables has been explicitly investigated in recent work by Tuller/Kelso (1990). The work exploits the abrupt change in interarticulator phasing observed by Stetson (1951) as a special entry point for understanding both the stability and change of articulatory patterns. The phenomena Stetson observed allow the necessary and nontrivial step of identifying the collective variables that characterize a given articulatory pattern (an enterprise closely affiliated with the ecological approach to perception and action, advocated by Gibson (1966; 1979) and his school, for example, Turvey/Shaw/Mace 1979). In addition, the dynamics of the collective variables can be determined through an analysis of stability. This involves a step beyond the phenomena, namely, a mapping onto a dynamical model which in turn generates predictions.

In the Tuller/Kelso (1990) study, subjects said /ip/ or /pi/ repetitively, at increasing speaking rates, while their acoustic speech signal and glottal and lip movements were recorded. For repetitive sequences of /pi/ across the range of speaking rates, the subject's peak glottal opening maintained a stable phase lag relative to minimum lip aperture. For repetitive sequences of /ip/, interarticulator relative phasing often changed markedly as speaking rate increased. At slow rates, peak glottal opening occurred temporally close to minimum lip aperture; at some critical value of rate an abrupt shift in relative phase value occurred to that observed for /pi/. In follow-up perceptual experiments, listeners perceived the consonant's syllable affiliation to change abruptly from syllable-final to syllable-initial on precisely the same syllable as the observed shift in interarticulator relative phase (Tuller/Kelso 1990; 1991).

The greater relative stability observed for consonant-initial syllables, as compared with vowel-initial syllables, is consistent with the linguistic descriptions of distributional frequency of syllable types (e.g., Jakobson 1966). The finding also suggests that at slower speaking rates several attractors with different basins of attraction coexist (a feature called multistability). As speaking rate increases, the change in available articulatory patterns arises solely as a result of the dynamics of the system (the patterns are self-organized). The finding also points to the importance of relative phase as a key collective variable for characterizing the articulatory pattern as a low-dimensional vector (see also Lisker/Abramson 1964; Löfqvist/Yoshioka 1981).

3.4. Modelling Approaches

Empirical analyses of speech production are complemented by modelling of the communicative process. For example, Lindblom/MacNeilage/Studdert-Kennedy (1983) explored whether phonological structure could be understood as an emergent property that arises from the interaction of subsystems. First, they defined a universal signal space with seven possible stop closures as beginnings, and nineteen possible vowel-like endpoints (133 resulting 'syllable' patterns). Thus the trajectories assumed as primitives were consistent with a consonant-initial syllable. Next, they postulated two talker-based constraints and two listener-based constraints on combinations of start- and endpoints that maximized perceptual effect and minimized articulatory cost. A computer program selected the twenty-four syllable subset that best satisfied the four constraints. Remarkably, the program quickly converged on a common set of syllables regardless of which item was used as the initial seed for the calculation. Moreover, the set contained many instances of 'minimal pairs', whose members differed only in initial closure position, or vowel end position, but not both. Note that neither the number of start and end combinations nor the constraints themselves in any way required the resulting segmental structuration. These striking results suggest that structuration of phonological universals such as segments and features may be an emergent property arising from the constrained interaction of system elements.

Various other modelling studies of speech production have successfully used a dynamical systems approach. Of particular interest is Jordan's (1986) connectionist model of speech patterning over time. At the lowest level of the model are output units that represent values of abstract phonetic features, such as voicing, nasality, and lip rounding. Unlike distinctive feature theory, the model allows values of the output units to vary continuously. At the highest level of the network are state units whose actions are defined by an equation of motion. In essence, the equation of motion defines an intrinsic temporal evolution for sequential speech motions in much the same way that the equation of motion defines the displacement-velocity relationship in a mass-spring system. The state units and output units are connected, using a nonlinear mapping, by a layer of hidden units. A second set of inputs to the hidden units is provided by plan units, which increase system flexibility by allowing the network to 'learn' a single set of weights for production of several different speech sequences.

The 'learning' procedure uses the 'back propagation' method, or 'generalized delta rule' of Rumelhart/Hinton/Williams (1986) in which error signals generated at the output units are projected back into the network, allowing the hidden units to change their weights in a manner proportional to the sum of the errors received. An engineer might refer to this as a sophisticated technique for system's identification. Jordan trained the network to produce sequences of phonemes, where each phoneme is defined as a bundle of context-independent target values for the features. After training, the network produced continuous trajectories for the feature values (not articulatory movement patterns). The feature trajectories showed context-dependent anticipatory and carryover coarticulation effects whose temporal extent fit remarkably well with empirical studies of acoustic and kinematic effects of coarticulation.

Jordan's simulation sheds light on a longstanding debate in the speech production literature on whether timing control in speech is intrinsic (e. g., Fowler 1977; 1980) or extrinsic (e. g., Kozhevnikov/Chistovich 1965; Lindblom 1983). Note that the temporal ordering among the output units of the model is not explicitly represented anywhere in the network; there is no extrinsic timing device. Rather, the temporal structure is an implicit consequence of the input-output relationship of the system elements, the pattern of connections among the elements, and the strengths of each connection. In this sense, the patterning over time of the output units (and thus the temporal extent of coarticulatory effects) is an emergent property of the intrinsic network dynamics (as proposed by Kelso/Tuller 1987).

Jordan's model relies on a list of abstract phonetic features as dimensions for the output units and thus is some distance removed from articulatory movement patterns. An approach to the modelling of speech patterns that is tied explicitly to articulatory gestures was proposed by Saltzman (1986) and Saltzman/Kelso (1987; see also Kelso/Saltzman/Tuller 1986). In their 'task-dynamic' model of speech production, articulatory patterns emerge from a dynamical system with functionally distinct but interacting levels. At one level, active gestural units organize the articulators temporarily and flexibly into functional groupings (coordinative structures) that accomplish particular gestural goals (such as the formation and release of constrictions). The influence of the gestural units on articulator trajectories waxes and wanes over time, thus introducing variability across segmental contexts and suprasegmental changes. The model's strength lies in capturing the essential features of interarticulatory coordination patterns observed during unperturbed and experimentally perturbed speech. A persistent shortcoming of the model has been its reliance on an explicit proscription of the activation intervals for gestural units. Recently, Saltzman/Munhall (1989) have proposed incorporating Jordan's serial network into the task-dynamic modelling. This provides the possibility for a dynamic model of speech production that is more closely tied to the articulatory gestures and allows sequential timing to evolve from the network structure and dynamics without an explicit temporal score.

4. Conclusions

Dynamical systems theory offers a powerful and theoretically unified account of articulatory patterns generated during speech. Empirical observations and computer simulations have converged on dynamical accounts of the temporal unfolding of articulatory patterns and their relative stability despite changing segmental context, speaking rate, speaking style, or stress. Dynamical approaches to modelling speech have also reproduced the experimentally-observed stability of the articulatory system in adjusting to unanticipated, externally-applied perturbations and its flexibility in switching from one configuration to another.

The concepts and tools of dynamical systems theory is likely to be of value for understanding speech disorders. In a model of stuttering that dovetails nicely with the dynamical approach, Nudelman/Herbrich/Hoyt/Rosenfield (1989) propose that when the phase lag increases between speech motor control systems with different characteristic time scales, the total system becomes unstable and speech dysfluencies result (see also Zimmerman/Brown/Kelso et al. 1988 for a related idea). Two aspects of their model particularly suggest the utility of dynamical systems theory for an understanding of stuttering. First, the relative phasing of the hypothesized speech motor control systems may vary continuously without producing dysfluencies. Instabilities (and hence dysfluencies) only occur when the control systems reach a critical value of relative phase. Second, the standard deviation of relative phase, not the mean value, is the best predictor of stuttering frequency. Stability is thus implicated as a more meaningful concept than invariance in understanding stuttering behavior (see Section 3). Our interpretation of these data is that the appearance of a dysfluency is indicative of a phase transition from a more to a less ordered state. In contrast, the shift from vowel-initial to consonant-initial syllables produced by fluent speakers as speaking rate increases is a transition between two ordered states. Demonstrations of nonlinear phase transitions are much more numerous in perception and production of nonspeech behaviors. Nevertheless, these initial forays into speech production and phonological structure have proven insightful and offer new ways to attack old problems.

5. References

Abbs, J. H., Gracco,V. L., & Cole, K. J. (1984). Control of multimovement coordination: Sensorimotor mechanisms in speech motor programming. *Journal of Motor Behavior,* 16, 195–232.

Bernstein, N. S. (1967). *The Coordination and Regulation of Movements.* Oxford: Pergammon.

Boylls, C. C. (1975). A theory of cerebellar function with applications to locomotion. II. The relation of anterior lobe climbing fiber function to locomotor behavior in the cat. *COINS Technical Report, 76–1.* Department of Computer and Information Science, University of Massachusetts.

Butcher, A. & Weiher, E. (1976). An electropalatographic investigation of coarticulation in VCV sequences. *Journal of Phonetics, 4,* 59–74.

Daniloff, R. & Hammarberg, R. (1973). On defining coarticulation. *Journal of Phonetics, 1,* 239–248.

Easton, T. A. (1972). On the normal use of reflexes. *American Scientist, 60,* 591–599.

Fowler, C. A. (1977). *Timing Control in Speech Production*. Bloomington, IN: Indiana University Linguistics Club.

Fowler, C. A. (1980). Coarticulation and theories of extrinsic timing control. *Journal of Phonetics, 8,* 113–133.

Fowler, C. A., Rubin, P., Remez, R. E., & Turvey, M. T. (1980). Implications for speech production of a general theory of action. In B. Butterworth (Ed.), *Language Production. 373–420.* New York: Academic.

Gay, T., Ushijima, T., Hirose, H., & Cooper, T. S. (1974). Effect of speaking rate on labial consonant-vowel articulation. *Journal of Phonetics, 2,* 46–63.

Gel'fand, I. M., Gurfinkel, V. S., Fomin, S. V., & Tsetlin, M. L. (1971). *Models of the structural-functional organization of certain biological systems.* Cambridge, MA: MIT Press.

Gentil, M., Harris, K. S., Horiguchi, S., & Honda, K. (1984). Temporal organization of muscle activity in simple disyllables. *Journal of the Acoustical Society of America, 75,* S23.

Gibson, J. J. (1966). *The Senses Considered as Perceptual Systems.* Boston: Houghton-Mifflin.

Gibson, J. J. (1979). *The Ecological Approach to Visual Perception.* Boston: Houghton-Mifflin.

Haken, H. (1975). Cooperative phenomena in systems far from thermal equilibrium and in non-physical systems. *Review of Modern Physics, 47,* 67–121.

Haken, H. (1983). *Synergetics, An Introduction: Non-equilibrium Phase Transitionsand Self-organization in Physics, Chemistry, and Biology.* Berlin: Springer.

Jakobson, R. (1966). Implications of language universals for linguistics. In J. H. Greenberg (Ed.), *Universals of Language* 263–278. Cambridge, MA: MIT Press.

Jordan, M. I. (1986). Serial order in behavior: A parallel distributed processing approach. *Technical Report 8604,* University of California, Institute for Cognitive Science, Dan Diego.

Kelso, J. A. S., DeGuzman, G. C., & Holroyd, T. (in press). Synergetic dynamics of biological coordination with special reference to phase attraction and intermittency. In H. Haken & H. P. Koepchen (Eds.), *Synergetics of Rhythms.* Berlin: Springer.

Kelso, J. A. S., DelColle, J. D., & Schöner, G. S. (1990). Action-perception as a pattern formation process. In M. Jeannerod (Ed.), *Attention and Performance XIII. 139–169.* Hillsdale, NJ: Erlbaum.

Kelso, J. A. S. & Munhall, K. G. (1988). *R. H. Stetson's Motor Phonetics: A Retrospective Edition.* San Diego: College Hill.

Kelso, J. A. S., Saltzman, E. L., & Tuller, B. (1986). The dynamical perspective on speech production: data and theory. *Journal of Phonetics, 14,* 29–60.

Kelso, J. A. S. & Schöner, G. S. (1988). Self-organization of coordinative movement patterns. *Human Movement Science, 7,* 27–46.

Kelso, J. A. S., Schöner, G. S., Scholz, J. P., & Haken, H. (1987). Phase-locked modes, phase transitions and component oscillators in biological motion. *Physica Scripta, 35,* 79–87.

Kelso, J. A. S., Southard, D., & Goodman, D. (1979). On the coordination of two-handed movements. *Journal of Experimental Psychology: Human Perception and Performance 5,* 229–238.

Kelso, J. A. S. & Tuller, B. (1983). Compensatory articulation under conditions of reduced afferent information: A dynamic formulation. *Journal of Speech and Hearing Research, 26,* 217–224.

Kelso, J. A. S. & Tuller, B. (1987). Intrinsic time in speech production: Theory, methodology, and preliminary observations. In E. Keller & M. Gopnik (Eds.), *Sensory and motor processes in language* 203–221. Hillsdale, NJ: Erlbaum.

Kelso, J. A. S. & Tuller, B., Vatikiotis-Bateson, E., & Fowler, C. A. (1984). Functionally specific articulatory cooperation following jaw perturbations during speech: Evidence for coordinative structures. *Journal of Experimental Psychology: Human Perception and Performance, 10,* 812–832.

Kelso, J. A. S., Vatikiotis-Bateson, E., Saltzman, E. L., & Kay, B. A. (1985). A qualitative dynamic analysis of reiterant speech production: Phase portraits, kinematics, and dynamic modeling. *Journal of the Acoustical Society of America, 77,* 266–280.

Kent, R. D. & Moll, K. L. (1975). Articulatory timing in selected consonant sequences. *Brain and Language, 2,* 304–323.

Kent, R. D. & Netsell, R. (1971). Effects of stress contrasts on certain articulatory parameters. *Phonetica, 24,* 23–44.

Kozhevnikov, V. A. & Chistovich, L. A. (1965). *Speech Articulation and Perception.* Joint Publications Research Service, Washington, DC.

Kuehn, D. P. & Moll, K. L. (1976). A cineradiographic study of VC and CV articulatory velocities. *Journal of Phonetics, 4,* 303–320.

Lashley, K. S. (1951). The problem of serial order in behavior. In L. A. Jeffress (Ed.), *Cerebral Mechanisms in Behavior: The Hixon Symposium. 112–136.* New York: John Wiley and Sons.

Liberman, A. M., Cooper, F. S., Shankweiler, D. P., & Studdert-Kennedy, M. (1967). Perception of the speech code. *Psychological Review, 74,* 431–461.

Lindblom, B. (1963). Spectrographic study of vowel reduction. *Journal of the Acoustical Society of America, 35,* 1773–1781.

Lindblom, B. (1983). Economy of speech production. In P. F. MacNeilage (Ed.), *The Production of Speech. 217–245.* New York: Springer-Verlag.

Lindblom, B., Lubker, J., & Gay, T. (1979). Formant frequencies of some fixed-mandible vowels and a model of speech motor programming by predictive simulation. *Journal of Phonetics, 7,* 147–161.

Lindblom, B., MacNeilage, P., & Studdert-Kennedy, M. (1983). Self-organizing processes and the explanation of phonological universals. In B. Butterworth, B. Comrie, & O. Dahl (Eds.), *Explanations of Linguistic Universals.* 181–203. The Hague: Mouton.

Lindblom, B. & Sundberg, J. (1971). Acoustical consequences of lip, tongue, jaw and larynx movement. *Journal of the Acoustical Society of America, 50,* 1166–1179.

Linville, R. (1982). *Temporal aspects of articulation: Some implications for speech motor control of stereotyped productions.* Unpublished Doctoral Dissertation. University of Iowa, Iowa City, Iowa.

Lisker, L. & Abramson, A. (1964). A cross-language study of voicing in initial stops: Acoustical measurements. *Word, 20,* 384–422.

Löfqvist, A. (1986). Stability and change. *Journal of Phonetics, 14,* 139–144.

Löfqvist, A. & Yoshioka, H. (1981). Interarticulator programming in obstruent production. *Phonetica, 38,* 31–34.

Lubker, J. (1983). Comment on 'Temporal invariance in the production of speech' by Harris, Tuller and Kelso. *Paper presented at Conference on invariance and variability in speech processes.* M.I.T. Cambridge, MA, U.S.A., October 1983

MacNeilage, P. F. & DeClerk, J. (1969). On the motor control of coarticulation in CVC monosyllables. *Journal of the Acoustical Society of America, 45,* 1217–1233.

Munhall, K. G. (1985). An examination of intra-articulator relative timing. *Journal of the Acoustical Society of America, 78,* 1548–1553.

Nittrouer, S., Munhall, K., Kelso, J. A. S., Tuller, B., & Harris, K. S. (1988). Patterns of interarticulator phasing and their relation to linguistic structure. *Journal of the Acoustical Society of America, 84,* 1653–1661.

Nudelman, H. B., Herbrich, K. E., Hoyt, B. D., & Rosenfield, D. B. (1989). A neuroscience model of stuttering. *Journal of Fluency Disorders, 14,* 399–427.

Ostry, D. J. & Munhall, K. (1985). Control of rate and duration in speech. *Journal of the Acoustical Society of America, 77,* 640–648.

Riordan, C. J. (1977). Control of vocal tract length in speech. *Journal of the Acoustical Society of America, 62,* 998–1002.

Rumelhart, D. E., Hinton, G. E., & Williams, R. J. (1986). Learning internal representations by error propagation. In D. E. Rumelhart & J. L. McClelland (Eds.), *Parallel Distributed Processing: Explorations in the microstructure of cognition, Vol. 1. Foundations* 318–362. Cambridge, MA: MIT Press.

Saltzman, E. L. (1986). Task dynamic coordination of the speech articulators: A preliminary model. *Experimental Brain Research, Ser. 15,* 129–144.

Saltzman, E. L. & Kelso, J. A. S. (1987). Skilled actions: A task-dynamic approach. *Psychological Review, 94,* 84–106.

Saltzman, E. L. & Munhall, K. G. (1989). A dynamical approach to gestural patterning in speech production. *Ecological Psychology, 1,* 333–382.

Schmidt, R. C. (1982) *Motor Control and Learning.* Illinois: Human Kinetics.

Schöner, G. S. & Kelso, J. A. S. (1988). Dynamic pattern generation in behavior and neural systems. *Science, 239,* 1513–1520.

Shaiman, S. (1989). Kinematic and electromyographic responses to perturbation of the jaw. *Journal of the Acoustical Society of America, 86,* 78–88.

Sternberg, S., Knoll, R. L., & Turock, D. L. (1990). Hierarchical control in the execution of action sequences: Tests of two invariance properties. In M. Jeannerod (Ed.), *Attention and Performance XIII. 1–56.* Hillsdale, NJ: Erlbaum.

Stetson, R. H. (1951). *Motor Phonetics: A Study of Speech Movements in Action.* Amsterdam: North-Holland.

Tuller, B. & Kelso, J. A. S. (1984). The timing of articulatory gestures: Evidence for relational invariants. *Journal of the Acoustical Society of America, 76,* 1030–1036.

Tuller, B. & Kelso, J. A. S. (1990). Phase transitions in speech production and their perceptual consequences. In M. Jeannerod (Ed.), *Attention and Performance XIII. 429–452.* Hillsdale, NJ: Erlbaum.

Tuller, B. & Kelso, J. A. S. (1991). The production and perception of syllable structure. *Journal of Speech and Hearing Research*, 34, 501–508.

Tuller, B., Kelso, J. A. S., & Harris, K. S. (1982). Interarticulator phasing as an index of temporal regularity in speech. *Journal of Experimental Psychology: Human Perception and Performance, 8,* 460–472.

Tuller, B., Kelso, J. A. S., & Harris, K. S. (1983). Converging evidence for the role of relative timing in speech. *Journal of Experimental Psychology: Human Perception and Performance, 9,* 829–833.

Turvey, M. T. (1977). Preliminaries to a theory of action with reference to vision. In R. Shaw & J. Bransford (Eds.), *Perceiving, Acting, and Knowing: Toward an Ecological Psychology. 211–266.* Hillsdale, NJ: Erlbaum.

Turvey, M. T., Shaw, R. E., & Mace, W. (1979). Issues in a theory of action: Degrees of freedom, coordinative structures and coalitions. In J. Requin

(Ed.). *Attention and Performance VII*. Hillsdale, NJ: Erlbaum.

Vatikiotis-Bateson, E. (1988). *Linguistic structure and articulatory dynamics: A cross-language study*. Unpublished Doctoral Dissertation, Indiana University, Indiana.

von Bertalanffy, L. (1973) *General System Theory*. London: Penguin.

Zimmerman, G., Brown, C., Kelso, J. A. S., Hurtig, R., & Forrest, K. (1988). The association between acoustic and articulatory events in a delayed auditory feedback paradigm. *Journal of Phonetics, 16*, 437–451.

[Work supported by NIDCD grant R29 DC00411, NIMH grant R01-MH-42900, and BRS grant S07-RR07258.]

Betty Tuller/J. A. Scott Kelso, Boca Raton, Florida (USA)

38. Pathophysiology of Disordered Articulation

1. Viewpoint

The present chapter provides an overview of neurologic speech disorders and some perspectives on how these problems can be evaluated, studied, and understood. In the last two decades, these disorders increasingly have been viewed as fundamental neurobiological impairments. Efforts in this direction, starting just about the time of the publication of the seminal work by Darley/Aronson/Brown (1969 a; b), reflect the perspective that while speech and language have behavioral, social, linguistic and ecological consequences, they are fundamentally biological actions. This emphasis was most strongly articulated by individuals with clinical or medical interests in disorders of speech. It has been suggested that if one is to diagnose, understand, and treat disorders of speech and take advantage of modern medical advances, it is necessary to consider explicitly the underlying nervous system functions and dysfunctions. – A medical approach to neurologically based speech disorders draws upon the principle that effective diagnosis and treatment are related to (1) the knowledge of underlying pathophysiology and (2) the extent to which reliable assessment procedures are devised to exploit that knowledge. In this respect, speech motor difficulties present special clinical problems because of the complexity of speech generation. If used in isolation, the classical means of assessment, largely consisting of listening to and classifying a patient's speech errors, are particularly limiting when it comes to identifying pathophysiology. – Basically, many observable speech events are not simple reflections of underlying neurobiological processes; surface analysis procedures (i. e., intelligibility measures, severity ratings, etc.) offer few perspectives regarding etiology or directions for possible treatment. For example, an observed speech error (say 'distortion') in a disordered speaker could be due to a multitude of factors including (1) anatomical properties of the vocal conduit (orofacial anomalies, tongue grooving or muscle tissue loss in motor neuron disease), (2) unsteady or weak muscle contraction (due to loss of motoneurons, neocortical pyramidal cells, cerebellar inputs), (3) disruption of reflex or long latency corrective adjustments (at medullar, pontine motor nuclei or neocortical somatic sensory-to-pyramidal cells), (4) aberrant prediction of upcoming movements by nervous system motor programming centers (cerebellum, basal ganglia, premotor or supplementary motor cortices), (5) inappropriate transmission of learned speech motor objectives (from cerebellar or parietal cortical centers), (6) unsuccessful corrections for speech element selection errors (posterior parietal or lateral precentral cortex – Brodmann's Area 44), (7) improper selection of proper linguistic features (posterior parietal), (8) faulty neural communication among these or several other levels of the speech motor control process, or (9) dozens of other, but yet different, motor control and coordination functions. – Extending this argument, consider the common problem in dysarthric subjects of unsteady or weak muscle contractions. Patients with amyotrophic lateral sclerosis, multiple sclerosis, cerebellar disease, upper motoneuron damage, and even Parkinson's disease display these problems; obviously while their underlying nervous system damage is quite different, the slowed and somewhat odd-sounding speech, due possibly to weakness and unsteadiness, is almost a universal and ubiquitous feature. – Obviously the mere presence or absence of a given speech sign, or its influence upon speech understanding, does not yield much clinical information. It is this realization that has provided motivation for a stronger focus upon the biological bases of motor speech disorders, and in turn upon the manner in which normal speech movements are generated.

2. Basic Speech Motor Actions

Speech motor functions are perhaps less well understood or appreciated than similar motor behaviors of like complexity, due in part to the fact that the multiple movements are not entirely visible, as in locomotion, for example. Fortunately, speech movements do not appear to be controlled differently than most other movements; there appears to be a fair amount of similarity in the basic neural control of speech motor actions and other related behaviors (i. e., locomotion, handwriting, typing, dance). As a first step in appreciating these neural control processes, it is illuminating to outline what it is that the nervous system is controlling. At the same time, considering these motor output requirements sets the proper stage for appreciating many disorders of speech described in other chapters in this volume. – Often, in introductory texts on speech three 'components of the speech production apparatus' are identified, the so-called respiratory, phonatory, and articulatory (upper airway) systems. While this is a step in the correct direction, the implied separation cannot be justified functionally. Interactions among respiratory, laryngeal, and upper airway neural control processes are well-described and of major importance. Related to this concern, it is useful to consider a more basic description. For generation of even a single vowel or consonant, approximately 70 muscles are involved. These muscles actively control (1) the respiratory movements of the rib cage, diaphragm, and abdomen, (2) laryngeal movements of the thyroid, cricoid, and arytenoid cartilages, and (3) the upper airway actions of the pharynx, tongue, soft palate, lips, and jaw. Many of these muscles contribute to both respiratory and laryngeal actions (extrinsic laryngeal muscles, adductors and abductors of the glottal opening) and likewise to laryngeal and upper airway gestures (mylohyoid, pharyngeal constrictors, anterior belly of diagastric). The interdependent neural control of these different muscle groups also is reflected in their ubiquitous brain stem interconnections. – These muscles contribute in generating movements with several functional consequences, including air volume/pressure manipulation, sound generation, and vocal tract resonances. Specifically, movements of the tongue not only act to change the shape of the upper air way for vowel-related resonances, but also reduce or enlarge the air volume for stop consonants and occlude air flow as part of sound generation for fricatives and for stop consonant release. – A major component of speech motor control involves the orchestration of all these muscles and movements as well as parceling their different contributions to the final acoustic output. Furthermore, because actions for a given element must follow and precede actions for adjacent elements, there is a major sequencing component as well. All of these considerations raise issues as to what might be the most fragile elements of this process, or conversely what aspects of control are most likely to be lost or impaired with damage to the nervous system. In a word, because multiple motor actions are involved both in parallel and sequentially, it is apparent that the most critical problem faced by the nervous system in the generation of speech is coordination. The brain must keep track of all of the parts, their status, intended changes to meet upcoming objectives, the degree to which those objectives are met, or are going to need correction, etc. All of these factors are interdependent. These considerations lead to the next component of this chapter, namely what kind of neuromotor control processes are involved in this rather remarkable effort. – In understanding speech motor disabilities associated with brain damage, it becomes important to have an understanding of how the parallel and sequential actions described above are generated. In this respect, a long standing issue in the brain's control of the complex movements for speech involves the degree to which the events described above are (1) each specified in advance and then played out subsequently, or rather (2) generated on-line and afresh each time production of a given speech event is repeated. If the muscle contraction patterns for each speech event are stored and then simply regurgitated each time that event is called for, outputs would be stereotypic and there would be no need for sensory input. However, as described in chapter 45, Feedback Impairments in Dysarthria, in recent years, studies from several different laboratories have shown that both the coordination among the multiple movements for speech and their sequencing are dependent, to a considerable degree, on sensory influences. For example, the coordination among the upper lip, lower lip, and jaw in control of oral opening and closing is flexibly manipulated via sensory monitoring of the positions of each of these articulators and moment-to-moment motor adjustments. – Critical to this issue is the importance of multi-movement coordination in speech. Most important features of speech (oral occlusions, vocal tract resonances, respiratory or upper airway volumes) are not generated by a single movement. Rather, combinations of jaw, lip, and tongue movements produce oral occlusions/constrictions, while rib cage, abdominal, and diaphragm movements combine to control respiratory volumes and hence air pressures. Regarding speech motor functions and dysfunctions, these observations indicate that the primary controlled outputs for speech production are not individual upper airway, laryngeal, or respiratory movements, but rather overall vocal tract or respiratory configurations. – While several studies support sensory-based coordination, it is apparent from simple consideration of speech. The orofacial system obviously serves multiple functions of chewing, swallowing, and breathing, superimposed upon and in parallel with speech. Less natural intrusions include a cigarette between the lips, a pipe between the teeth, etc. Because most or all of these activities can be performed simultaneously, without major interference or conscious adaptation, a nervous system capability for on-line adjustment among the multiple movements and muscle contracitons is most appealing. – The recent acknowledgement that individual muscle contractions and movements are adjusted via sensory input also is consistent with research on the primate nervous system indicating that all major brain centers classically associated with motor functions are likewise centers of sensorimotor integration. This is discussed further in chapter 45, Feedback Impairments in Dysarthria. In this respect, it is likely that many dysarthric symptoms and signs may well be as critically dependent upon problems of sensorimotor integration as they are upon problems of pure motor function.

3. Classification of the Motor Speech Disorders

Historically, the term dysarthria (or anarthria in its complete form) has referred solely to disturbed articulation, subsequent to neurologic impairment. Grewel (1957) is credited, however with the concept that dysarthria – or more precisely, the dysarthrias – are more complex than articulatory dysfunction and may, in fact, have localizing value. Canter (1967) first attempted to differentiate and classify the dysarthrias based on site of lesion using the terms peripheral dysarthria for those secondary to primary muscle, myoneural junction cell body and/or axon involvement and central dysarthria representing bilateral upper motor neuron, extrapyramidal and cerebellar system disease. He recognized also that dysarthria represented "a disturbance in the execution of motor patterns for speech due to paralysis, weakness or discoordination of the speech musculature" (Canter 1967, 660), and thus potentially involves not only articulation but the other subsystems of speech as well. These include phonation, respiration, resonation and speech prosody (e. g., rhythm, intonation, inflection, stress, etc.). Although Canter's work is noteworthy, his report was basically tutorial and descriptive in nature and thus suffered from an absence of data driven, quantified support. This matter was rectified, in part, by Darley/Aronson/Brown (1969 a; b) in their now classic studies concerning the perceptual characteristics of dysarthria, although the conceptual framework has been challenged. In their definition, dysarthria represents a group of speech disorders which was characterized by disturbances in speech muscular control due to paralysis, paresis, weakness, slowness, incoordination and/or altered tone that may encompass one or more of the basic motor speech subsystems mentioned previously. Subsequent research has stressed not only the perceptual/acoustic characteristics of the dysarthrias, but co-occurring neurophysiologic bases for the disorders as well. – Like Canter, Darley/Aronson/Brown recognized six dysarthria subtypes, four of which were associated with central lesions, one which implied lower motor neuron involvement and one which represented both central and peripheral impairment. Recently, Hartmann/Abbs (1989) quantified and described a seventh type of dysarthria felt to have localizing value. – Although each of the dysarthrias appear to have distinct perceptual/acoustic and neurophysiologic characteristics, the neuropathologic substrate underlying each of the dysarthrias is not as clear. The clinician, therefore, relies on cardinal motor speech symptoms and signs frequently in conjunction with other neurologic findings to achieve diagnoses. – Apraxia of speech has been described as a motor speech planning disorder. Whether it is a speech or language disorder or a combination thereof has been a point of controversy. This topic is dealt with elsewhere. – Table 38.1 presents site of lesion, typical conditions, primary neurologic manifestations, and dysarthric sequelae. The table is not intended to be all inclusive. Also, many of the conditions listed may present with more than one type of dysarthria. For example, while multiple sclerosis classically presents with symptoms and signs associated with cerebellar impairment, as the disease progresses cortical white matter involvement yields a mixed ataxic/spastic dysarthria. A brief commentary on each motor speech disorder is provided, as means of orientation.

3.1. Unilateral Upper motor neuron Dysarthria

Focal lesion of one corticobulbar tract produces different motor speech signs than noted for bilateral involvement. The one prospective study to date reported that diminished loudness, lack of pitch flexibility (monopitch), consonant imprecision, short phrases and decreased speaking rate entotal were unique for this particular dysarthria. Consonant imprecision may be an outstanding feature due, primarily, to involvement of contralateral facial and lingual musculature. However, unlike the spastic dysarthria, related pathologic reflexes are uncommon suggesting that bilateral pyramidal tract damage is necessary for disinhibition to occur on a central level.

3.2. Spastic Dysarthria

Bilateral damage to the corticobulbar tracts innervating the cranial motor nuclei V, VII, IX–XII at the cortical, subcortical or brain stem level produces a disinhibitory phenomenon along with weakness, hypertonicity and paresis of those muscles involved. Both laughing and crying as well as pathologic sucking, jaw-jerk, biting, palmomental and pharyngeal reflexes are evident. Speech is labored and slow, while voice quality is characterized by vocal straining and a quality not dissimilar from that heard in volitional crying. The respiratory support for speech is comparably diminished. Similarly, involvement of the velopharyngeal musculature may result in either continuous or intermittent abnormal resonance consisting of hypernasality with nasal air escape. The strain-strangle or wail-like quality, particularly in severe forms of the disorder is pathognomonic.

3.3. Apraxia of Speech

Apraxia of speech has been described as a motor planning (programming) disorder characterized by relatively unpredictable sound omission, substitution, and/or addition errors. These errors are influenced by articulatory complexity and include sound repetitions and prolongations, articulatory groping as the speaker seeks the accurate (intended) target and prosodic alterations including variable or slowed rate and stuttering (dysfluency). Co-occurring oral apraxia is not uncommon. The signs are not adequately explained on the basis of weakness, altered tone, or language impairment. Discoordinated movements are said to bear a resemblance to ataxic dysarthria as seen in cerebellar disease.

3.4. Ataxic Dysarthria

The dysrhythmic characteristics of cerebellar involvement are manifested in a dysarthria by variable articulatory imprecision with frequent omission and/or distortion of sounds, particularly at word, phrase or sentence endings; irregular prosodic pattern characterized by variations in stress without respect to context; and frequently a harsh voice quality. The intoxicated character of ataxic dysarthric speech is notable and conceivably represents generalized discoordination of motor speech control.

3.5. Hypokinetic Dysarthria

Selectice unilateral or bilateral lesions of the substantia nigra or its projections result in a diminution of movement frequently accompanied by a resting tremor. Dysarthric manifestations include limitations in pitch variability, decreased loudness, imprecise articulation, inappropriate silences or pausing within an utterance and short rushes of what

Site of Lesion	Typical Conditions·	Cardinal Neural Signs	Speech Disorder
Unilateral Upper Motoneuron (UUMN)	Cerebrovascular Disease	Contralateral Weakness, Spasticity	UUMN Dysarthria
Bilateral Upper Motoneuron	Cerebrovascular Disease	Spasticity, Brisk Reflexes Weakness, Disinhibition	Spastic Dysarthria
Broca's Area	Cerebrovascular Disease	None, if a focal lesion*	Apraxia of Speech
Cerebellum	Friedreich's Ataxia, Olivopontocerebellar Syndrome, Multiple Sclerosis	Discoordination, Intention Tremor, Hypotonia, Dysmetria	Ataxic Dysarthria
Basal Ganglia	Parkinsonism, Dystonia, Dyskinesias, Athetosis, Huntington's Disease, Tourette's Syndrome	Rigidity, Bradykinesia, Tremor, Abnormal Posturing, Tics, Adventitious Movement, Writhing	Hypo- or Hyperkinetic Dysarthria
Lower Motoneuron	Amyotrophic Lateral Sclerosis, Myotonic & Muscular Dystrophy, Myasthenia Gravis, Möbius Syndrome	Muscle Atrophy, Weakness, Absent/Reduced Reflexes, Abnormal EMG	Flaccid Dysarthria

* Typically presents with concurrent contralateral facial-limb weakness implying pyramidal tract involvement as well

Table 38.1: Disorders or articulation

might be perceived as rapid speech. The term hypokinetic dysarthria is broadly synonymous with parkinsonism of which paucity of movement is pathognomonic. Parkinsonian features including hypokinetic dysarthria, however, are frequently co-occurring manifestations of multisystem disease including multiple systems atrophy with dysautonomia (Shy-Drager syndrome) and progressive supranuclear palsy (Steele-Richardson-Olszewski syndrome) (see Hartman/Abbs 1988).

3.6. Hyperkinetic Dysarthria

Whereas hypokinetic dysarthria is characterized by limitation of movement, hyperkinetic dysarthria, which can be described in terms of slow, quick or tremor forms, is characterized by a preponderance or an exacerbation of movement that may or may not be involuntary (see Hartman/Abbs 1988). Although essentially true for all dysarthrias, the impact that hyperkinetic dysarthria has on speech production and intelligibility seems to be dependent more so on those speech subsystems directly involved in the movement disorder. Lesions of the striatum (putamen, caudate nucleus) and/or pallidum (globus pallidus) and/or their tracts appear responsible for these aberrations of movement.

3.6.1. Slow Forms include dystonia, (tardive) dyskinesia and athetosis. Certain forms of spastic (spasmodic) dysphonia may be form fruste of a more generalized widespread movement disorder or remain a focal sign of laryngeal involvement in some patients. The presence of adductory or abductory voice arrest or combinations thereof are cardinal signs of spastic dysphonia. Although they generally represent neurologic disease, in some patients they are manifestations of psychopathology thus warranting careful investigation and differential diagnosis. – Neuroleptic toxicity may produce adventitious mouthing, chewing, and tongue protruding. Conversely, parkinsonism with co-occurring oral motor manifestations may also result from protracted use of neuroleptics in some patients. Speech manifestations have been described as "stuttering" and altered prosody including audible inspiration and voice tremor. – Athetoid movements are frequently a component of congenital cerebral palsy or may be seen in conjunction with chorea. Motor speech signs include short sentences, articulatory imprecision due, in part, to inappropriate positioning of the tongue, prolonged transition time for articulatory movements and discoordinated velopharyngeal closure (Kent/Netsell 1978). Neilson/O'Dwyer (1981; 1984) have pointed out that the dysarthria of athetosis may be, in part, due to compensatory postures and thereby represent abnormal voluntary attempts at modification rather than variable involuntary muscle activity.

3.6.2. Quick Forms of hyperkinetic dysarthria include the speech changes that accompany Huntington's disease with imprecise consonant production, prolonged pause times, variable speaking rate, limited pitch variability, harsh voice quality and variable alterations in loudness or excess loudness. There is some question as to whether the dysarthric features demonstrated with Huntington's disease are a manifestation of degenerative changes within the basal ganglia or a consequence of the chorea itself (Caligiuri/Murray 1984; Ramig 1986). The motor and vocal tics associated with (Gilles de la) Tourette's syndrome include involuntary vocalization, coprolalia, palilalia and echolalia. Abnormal dopamine metabolism or dopamine hyperactivity is felt to be responsible for the aberrations of movement seen in Tourette's syndrome.

3.6.3. Tremor Forms. Regular and relatively rhythmic contractions of the soft palate, posterior pharyngeal wall, base of tongue and larynx at rest are pathognomonic of palatal-pharyngeal-laryngeal myoclonus (palatal myoclonus, palatal nystagmus). The cardinal features of this dysarthria are audible changes in volume between 2 and 4 hertz notable on prolongation of the neutral vowel *ah* that cooccur with musculature contractions of involved structures. Movements are present at rest. The signs of *palatal myoclonus* have been ascribed to lesions of the brain stem or cerebellum, particularly the dentato-rubro-olivary tracts. There is only one report concerning the dysarthria associated with action myoclonus (Aronson/O'Neill/Kelly 1984). – *Voice tremor*, as a manifestation of the essential tremor syndrome (including benign heredofamilial tremor) is characterized by relatively regular and rhythmic changes in phonation volume between 4 and 12 hertz. Unlike palatal myoclonus, however, movements are not present at rest. Certain forms of spastic dysphonia are a manifestation of essential tremor. Changes within the extrapyramidal system were proposed as the cause of essential tremor.

3.7. Flaccid Dysarthria

Involvement of one or more of the cranial or spinal nerves subserving motor speech control at the level of the nucleus, axon, myoneural junction or muscle results in lower motor neuron signs or flaccid dysarthria. Unlike the dysarthric types mentioned previously, flaccid dysarthria can result from isolated subsystem involvement. For example, a lesion of the recurrent laryngeal nerve produces vocal fold paralysis with resultant phonatory signs, e. g., hoarseness and breathiness, but with spared articulation and resonance. Conversely, multiple lower motoneuron involvement as in the case of myoneural junction disease, e. g., myasthenia gravis may present with compromised velopharyngeal function with resultant hypernasality; articulatory dysfunction with associated sound distortion and variably impaired intelligibility; laryngeal involvement with hoarseness and breathiness; respiratory involvement with resultant decreased support for speech and prosodic involvement with compromised rate and intonation patterns.

3.8. Mixed Dysarthria

Multisystem neurologic involvement is potentially capable of producing pyramidal, extrapyramidal, cerebellar and lower motor neuron signs concurrently. The manifestations of such signs depend on (1) the specific sites of involvement, and (2) when in the course of the disease the patient is examined. For example, amyotrophic lateral sclerosis commonly presents with primary bulbar involvement (e. g., progressive bulbar palsy) with resultant flaccid (lower motoneuron) dysarthria. As the disease progresses, upper motoneuron signs (corticobulbar tract) appear, resulting in a spastic component, thus flaccid-spastic dysarthria. Other conditions include Shy-Drager syndrome (multisystem atrophy with dysautonomia), with resultant hypokinetic-flaccid mixed dysarthria (which can include vocal fold paresis), Wilson's disease (hepatolenticular degeneration), with resultant ataxic-hypokinetic-spastic dysarthria, and Steele-Richardson-Olszewski syndrome (progressive supranuclear palsy) with hypokinetic-spastic-ataxic dysarthria. Olivopontocerebellar atrophy may be characterized by spastic-ataxic, flaccid-spastic (with stuttering) dysarthria.

4. Considerations for Classification of Motor Speech Disorders

The classical studies by the Mayo Clinic group provided the most systematic and comprehensive framework for identifying and classifying dysarthria and apraxia of speech. However, a comment on the nature of such classification and description is warranted. A very basic issue in this respect is the division of these disorders with respect to implied segregation of brain functions. Starting with dysarthria, this is a speech production system manifestation of a generalized problem of movement. Specifically, with damage or disease to various brain centers, motor functions of walking, manual manipulation, writing, balance, etc. are impaired along with those of speech. Damage of the cerebellum, basal ganglia, primary motor cortex, motoneurons, etc. all are agreed-upon etiologies for dysarthria. By contrast, it is commonly claimed that apraxia of speech is not a dysarthria, but due to "problem in programming or coordination of the movements of speech." Indeed, several recent studies of motor control in this latter population support those descriptions. Unfortunately, it is not clear that problems in "coordination and programming" are not also experienced by patients with dysarthria. For example, based upon extensive studies in nonhuman primates and in humans, impairments of the basal ganglia and the cerebellum are characteristic in manifesting 'motor programming' disorders. Likewise, the cerebellum, damage to which yields ataxic dysarthria, is commonly believed to be an primary center of movement coordination, with studies going back to the classic work of Gordon Holmes. – Similarly, if one argues that apraxia of speech results from brain damage to areas that are distinct from those yielding dysarthria, the distinction is further clouded. That is, if one accepts the argument that apraxia of speech is due to damage to Brodmann's Areas 44/45 (lateral precentral cortex), recent data indicate that the primary outputs of the deep cerebellar dentate nucleus associated with orofacial function project not to the motor cortex, but rather to regions of the cortex overlapping Area 44. Yet other studies indicate that Area 44 has some direct projections to motor nuclei of the tongue, lips, and jaw, presumably acting in parallel to projections from primary motor cortex. Given these considerations, it is not surprising that it is only the rare patient who presents with a 'pure' apraxia, without either motor signs (i. e., unilateral facial weakness, tongue deviation) and/or serious problems with language expression or comprehension. – Difficulties of understanding are likely if one attempts to impose inappropriate distinctions among motor control, linguistic, and cognitive deficits. Specifically, motor control is now recognized to involve phenomena such as anticipation, adaptation, set, attention, instruction, task goals, etc. Moreover, these factors appear to be operating via brain centers that were not classically considered to have cognitive functions, such as the basal ganglia, cerebellum, pre- and supplementary motor neo-cortices. For speech motor control, especially given its higher cortical nature, such cognitive factors must be intricately involved. Taking this argument to an obvious end, the demarcation between language and speech functions also is suspect. A number of linguistic factors influence the aspects of speech motor control, and conversely. Because language is manifest in the selection and sequencing of respiratory, laryngeal, and upper airway movements to generate acoustic signals carrying messages, one cannot separate that sequencing and selection from the neuromotor control of those movements. – Despite the aforementioned cautions, it is a matter of practical significance to categorize and evaluate the major features of the different forms of neurologic speech disorders. The continued challenge will be to develop increasingly biologically based criteria for such classification and have the flexibility to accept the elimination of some categories and merging of others.

5. References

Aronson, A. E., O'Neill, B. P. & Kelly, J. (1984). The dysarthria of action myoclonus. Presented at the Clinical Dysarthria Conference, Tucson, AZ, 1984.

Caligiuri, M. D. & Murray, T. (1984). Identification of a performance deficit in dysarthria associated with Huntington's disease. Presented at the Clinical Dysarthria Conference, Tucson, Arizona, 1984.

Canter, J. (1967). Neuromotor pathologies of speech. *American Journal of Physical Medicine, 46*, 659–666.

Darley, F. L., Aronson, A. E. & Brown, J. R. (1969 a). Differential diagnostic patterns of dysarthria. *Journal of Speech and Hearing Research, 12*, 246–269.

Darley, F. L., Aronson, A. E. & Brown, J. R. (1969 b). Clusters of deviant speech dimensions in the dysarthrias. *Journal of Speech and Hearing Research, 12*, 462–469.

Grewel, F. (1957). Classification of dysarthrias. *Acta Psychiatrica Scandinavica, 32*, 325–327.

Hartmann, D. E. & Abbs, J. H. (1988). Dysarthrias of movement disorders. In J. Jankovic & E. Tolosa (Eds.), *Advances in Neurology, Vol. 49: Facial Dyskinesias. 289–306*. New York: Raven Press.

Hartmann, D. E. & Abbs, J. H. (1989). Perceptual and physiologic characteristics of unilateral upper motor neuron (UUMN) dysarthria. Presented at the American Speech-Language-Hearing Association Meeting, St. Louis, Missouri, 1989.

Kent, R. & Netsell, R. (1978). Articulatory abnormalities in athetoid cerebral palsy. *Journal of Speech and Hearing Disorders*, *43*, 353–373.

Neilson, P. & O'Dwyer, N. (1981). The pathophysiology of dysarthria in cerebral palsy. *Journal of Neurology Neurosurgery and Psychiatry*, *44*, 1013–1019.

Neilson, P. & O'Dwyer, N. (1984). Reproducibility and variability of speech muscle activity in athetoid dysarthria of cerebral palsy. *Journal of Speech and Hearing Research*, *27*, 502–517.

Ramig, L. (1986). Acoustic analyses of phonation in patients with Huntington's disease. *Annals of Otology Rhinology and Laryngology*, *95*, 288–293.

James H. Abbs/David E. Hartman, Madison, Wisconsin (USA)

39. Assessment Methods in Neurophonetics: Speech Production

1. Introduction

Phonetics is the science of speech, – of the motor processes associated with its production, of its characteristics as an acoustic signal, and of the auditory-perceptual processes associated with the comprehension of speech. 'Neurophonetics' thus encompasses the study of disturbed speech production and perception in neurologic patients. According to this definition, neurophonetics spans a wide field, ranging from the pathophysiologic nature of disturbed speech processes to the phonetic aspects of the resulting communication problems. A correspondingly wide range of diagnostic methods is employed to study these questions, including techniques adopted from e. g. physiology, experimental psychology, or signal processing. – This article reviews methodological approaches in the study of neurologically disordered speech production, i. e. predominantly in motor speech disorders like dysarthria and apraxia of speech. The field may be delimited from non-linguistic approaches, e. g. in cranial nerve neurology and reflexology, although the findings of these disciplines clearly have a strong impact on the understanding of disturbed speech functions. A further delimitation must be drawn towards 'higher level' processes in the production of spoken language, but the precise location of this border, which is often characterized as separating motor speech functions from processes of language encoding, is controversial.

2. Assessment Techniques

In the assessment of speech disturbances of neurogenic origin, speech events may be captured at rather different levels of their manifestation. Neurophonetic assessment may start out at the neuromuscular level, drawing on the electric muscle potentials associated with muscular activity in the speech organs, the muscular forces, or the kinematic aspects of speech movements. Or, it may deal with the aerodynamic or acoustic effects of speech movements, and it may capture the perceptual features of disturbed speech. In this order of presentation, the different approaches roughly follow a hierarchy of decreasing pathophysiologic and increasing functional significance.

2.1. Movement Parameters

The most natural approach towards an understanding of the pathophysiology underlying the various neuromotor speech disorders would be to analyse the movement parameters generally used in studies of motor disorders, i. e. electrophysiologic, dynamic, and kinematic measures of movement. The recording of these parameters in the speech system, however, is impeded by the fact that most speech organs are concealed deep in the oral and pharyngeal cavity and difficult to access by instrumentation. Moreover, since speech is a highly adaptive motor activity even minimally obtrusive techniques might lead to alterations in the organization of the processes to be observed. For these reasons, the study of movement parameters in motor speech disorders is considerably less advanced than physiologic research in the motor functions of the extremities.

2.1.1. Muscle Action Potentials

In the execution of speech movements, the motor commands edited by the brain are transmitted to the motor units of the speech muscles involved, where electrical activation, i.e. muscle action potentials (MAPs), can be measured. Electromyographic measurements of MAPs are performed using either surface electrodes, needle electrodes, or hooked wire electrodes, the latter having the main advantage of being light, causing virtually no movement artifacts and staying in place even during rapid movements. – Electromyographic techniques have been applied in virtually all muscles relevant for speaking and have, for example, been used in investigations of the specific roles of different speech muscles or in the study of interarticulatory relations. EMG applications to speech pathology have been focussed on easily accessible systems, i.e. predominantly on labial and mandibular muscles, but electromyography of lingual or laryngeal muscles in neurologic patients is not uncommon (Shipp/Izdebski/Reed/Morrisey 1985). Clinical diagnostic applications are mainly concerned with the question of whether a particular muscle is, as a consequence of peripheral nerve involvement, insufficiently innervated (Hirano/Nozoe/Shin 1987). In research, EMG methods have been used, for instance, to assess resting and background activity and reciprocal suppression in the context of spasticity or rigidity, to compare tremorous activities in different structures, or to measure temporal relationships in the activation patterns of synergistic or antagonistic muscle groups (e.g., Neilson/O'Dwyer 1981; Hunker/Abbs 1990). – The methodological value of electromyography is characterized by its high pathophysiological significance. However, there are severe limitations to this method. A critical source of error is electrode placement (Gans/Gorniak 1980). Normally, 'calibration gestures' are used to verify correct placement of electrodes, but this technique may cause problems in patients with motor speech disorders. Further, the probability of inserting a pair of electrodes into a functionally homogeneous population of muscle fibers is rather low, meaning that EMG based assertions on e.g. co-contraction among antagonistic muscles are of limited validity (Blair/Smith 1986). This problem is even more severe when surface electrodes are used. Thorough investigations into the psychometric quality of electrode placement are therefore urgently needed (Tassinary/Caccioppo/Geen 1989).

2.1.2. Muscular Forces

The immediate effect of electrical muscle activity is the build-up of contractile muscular force. However, the pattern of muscular forces in the speech system reflects central processes much less directly than EMG patterns do, since muscle output force depends to a large extent on the mechanical properties of a muscle, i.e. its elasticity, velocity, and length. – The parameter of force is basic to important clinical conceptions of neuromotor disorders such as muscular weakness (e.g. in peripheral nerve involvement) or increased muscle tone (e.g. in spasticity). Nevertheless, instrumental force measurements are sparse and have been restricted to the lips, the tongue, and the jaw. Force measurements in these structures are traditionally made using strain gage force transducers sensitive to accelerations along a given spatial vector (Barlow/Abbs 1983). Relevant questions include maximum voluntary closing forces and fine force control, the latter being operationally defined as the skill of holding a given force as constant as possible. Applications in neurological patients have also focussed on these variables, with the question of differential subsystem impairment as an index of the role of muscle spindles in spasticity and Parkinsonian rigidity or of differential cranial nerve involvement in ALS (e.g. DePaul/Abbs/Caligiuri et al. 1988). – Closely related to the measures of active force control just described are measures of muscle stiffness, i.e. resistance of a muscle against passive displacement. The degree of muscle stiffness in the lower lip, operationally defined as the ratio of the force necessary to achieve lower lip displacement by a certain amount and the displacement amplitude, has been used as an index of labial rigidity in Parkinson's disease (Caligiuri 1987). – Like EMG, force measures are considered rather specific to the pathophysiology underlying a speech disorder. One should, however, bear in mind that force measurement techniques give no account of the contractile forces of single muscles, but rather of the effective forces resulting from contractions of various synergistic and antagonistic muscles in e. g. labial closure or tongue elevation. A second point to be made is that force measurements are exclusively related to nonspeech-tasks. This may, on the one hand, raise doubts as to their ecological validity and explain the lack of a correlation with measures of severity of dysarthric impairment (DePaul/Abbs/Caligiuri et al. 1988). On the other hand, nonspeech tasks may help to determine whether a deficit is one of elementary motor functions of the speech organs or if language plays a crucial role (McNeil/Weismer/Adams/Mulligan 1990).

2.1.3. Movement Kinematics

Descending from the levels of electrical muscle activity and muscular forces to the kinematic aspects of speech movements, i. e. measures of displacement and velocity, an increasing number of peripheral influences becomes effective. Speech movements are not only the result of a complex interplay of actively controlled synergistic and antagonistic muscle contractions, but are also influenced by passive recoil forces, inertia and aerodynamic processes. Nevertheless, kinematic measures of speech movements are considered a powerful inventory in the analysis and description of motor speech disorders. The techniques applied in studies of speech movement kinematics differ depending on which subsystem is to be observed.

Lips and jaw: The lips and the jaw are more easily accessible than the tongue, the velum, or the larynx, and have therefore been studied more often than the latter. The technique which has been most successful in labial and mandibular kinematics so far is based on strain gage movement transducers measuring inferior-superior movements of upper lip, lower lip, and jaw (Barlow/Cole/Abbs 1983). Lip and jaw movement data can also be obtained by radiographic or electromagnetic techniques, which are specifically devised for the recording of tongue movements. — Much of the work on labial and mandibular movement kinematics in normals has been devoted to questions of movement timing and coordination and to the search for motor invariants in the perioral system. In speech pathology, labial and mandibular kinematics have played a crucial role in studies of Parkinsonian dysarthria (e. g. Forrest/Weismer/Turner 1989), with the main objective of demonstrating hypokinesia and bradykinesia in the speech movements of Parkinsonian patients. The core parameters used in these studies are movement amplitude, peak velocity, and movement time. — A particular problem lies in the high variability in normals over different studies. This impedes the interpretation of some of the reported results and explains why the applied kinematic measures are usually uncorrelated with dysarthria severity.

Tongue: The recording of tongue movements is one of the major challenges in articulatory phonetics, since the tongue may be considered the most versatile subsystem in speech and, at the same time, an organ which is extremely difficult to observe. The many attempts to assess lingual kinematics can be classified in several ways, e. g. according to the underlying physical technique (radiography, electromagnetic induction, ultrasound imaging, contact detection), or according to the analysis plane (saggital vs. coronal). A further distinction can be made between point-tracking systems and imaging techniques. Each of the different measurement systems has its own advantages and limitations. — Two systems, which are similar in that they are based on point-tracking techniques and yield saggital views of the articulators, are the X-ray microbeam (XRMB) and the electromagnetic articulograph (EMA). The two systems provide X-ray beam or electromagnetic trackings of a set of pellets or coils attached to the articulators of the experimental subject (Abbs/Nadler/Fujimura 1988; Schönle/Gräbe/Wenig et al. 1987). Unlike earlier radiographic techniques the XRMB yields very low radiation exposures and offers negligible risk for both the experimental subject and the experimenter. The EMA system contrasts with the XRMB in that it is biologically entirely safe, lower-dimensioned, and considerably less expensive. Both systems are particularly suited for recordings of the anterior, medial, and dorsal part of the tongue. The midsaggital analysis plane allows investigation of horizontal and vertical tongue movements, whereas cross-sectional articulations of the medial and lateral surface cannot be assessed. The temporal and spatial resolution is sufficient for the study of lingual movements during speaking. Users of the systems mostly claim that tongue pellets would not interfere with articulation, but Stone (1990) holds that the tongue tip should be excluded from recording since XRMB pellets feel cumbersome. — A particular methodological problem with point-tracking measurements of lingual articulation lies in the separation of mandibular movement components from the observed pellet trajectories which contain information on both jaw- and tongue-related movements. According to Edwards/Harris (1990) the mandibular component of lingual movements should be modelled by a combined rotation and translation transform, which requires observation of two additional mandibular measurement points. – Applications of XRMB and EMA to normal aspects of lingual articulation are still sparse and much of our current knowledge e. g. on vowel articulation is still based on older cineradiographic techniques. One principal aim of this research is to build models which capture the many dimensions of tongue shape and the many degrees of freedom of lingual movements and thus may serve as a basis for future parametric investigations. – Studies of neuromotor impairments of lingual articulation have been restricted to a few individual cases so far. Qualitative descriptions of XRMB movement trajectories and some quantitative data on tongue dorsum velocities in rapid syllable repetitions of dysarthric individuals have been reviewed by Hirose (1986). – The scarcity of useful data concerning neuromotor disturbances of the tongue indicates that point tracking techniques of lingual assessment have not yet reached the point where they can be successfully handled in neurologic patients. Besides multiple technical problems, a major difficulty is in the complexity of tongue shape deformations during articulation which can be grasped but insufficiently by a small set of measurement points. – A method which does not rely on single point tracking is ultrasound imaging (Stone/Sonies/Shawker et al. 1983). Sonography has the disadvantage that important reference structures such as the hyoid bone and the hard palate are not visualized. Further, the tongue tip cannot be measured by ultrasound techniques since there is usually some air-filled space beneath it which causes ultrasound wave reflection. In contrast, an important advantage is that sonography may provide information on the tongue shape in either the cross-sectional or the saggital plane, which renders it useful in tongue modelling (Stone 1990). Keller/Ostry (1983) used a simpler sonographic technique which measures tongue height at a single dorsal point and is confined to a one-dimensional assessment of tongue backing movements. Similar to other tongue recording techniques, applications of sonography to motor speech disturbances are still restricted to very few single cases. – Information on cross-sectional tongue shape during articulation is also provided by electropalatography. In this method the subject wears an acrylic palate with a grid of sensors distributed over its surface. The contact pattern of the anterior part of the tongue with the hard palate during articulation is recorded and transmitted to a screen by wires led out through the corner of the mouth (Hardcastle/Jones/Knight et al. 1989). Due to the complexity of the signal which contains dynamic information on usually more than 60 electrodes it is important to apply suitable data reduction techniques (Hoole/Ziegler/Hartmann/Hardcastle 1989). Palatometry is limited by its restriction to anterior lingual consonants and has the disadvantage that each subject must be provided with his/her own tailored palate. Moreover, subjects have to become accustomed to the device during a training period, which may impose particular difficulties to patients with motor learning impairments. Nevertheless, a number of problems can be adequately addressed by palatometric techniques, as for instance the characterization of articulatory configurations in lingual consonants and the assessment of coarticulation patterns. Applications to neuromotor disorders of speech have focussed on spatial and temporal abnormalities of anterior lingual articulations in dysarthria and apraxia of speech (Hardcastle/Jones/Knight et al. 1989).

Velum: Unlike the tongue with its many degrees of freedom and its configurational versatility the velum is mostly described as a relatively simple 'valve-like' organ, with the essential function of controlling the airflow through the nasal cavity and thereby marking the distinction between oral and nasal sounds. The symptom of velopharyngeal incompetence found in several types of dysarthria is of high functional importance, since it usually results in severely distorted speech. – Direct observation of velar movements may be achieved by the XRMB or by video-endoscopy. Endoscopic views of the velum are inherently nonlinear, meaning that inferences regarding absolute displacement cannot be drawn, and between-subject comparisons of movement amplitude should be avoided. A less direct method of velar observation utilizes the transillumination technique to measure the amount of light passing through the velopharyngeal port when a fiberoptic light source is brought behind the velum and a photodetector is placed within one of the nostrils. While the photodetector signal is highly correlated with velar height it is also sensitive to lateral pharyngeal wall movements associated with velar closure and fails to discern velopharyngeal adaptations that may occur after closure (Zimmermann/Dalston/Brown et al. 1987). Similarly indirect measures of velar control are provided by aerodynamic techniques (cf. 2.2.). — Questions typically addressed by the described methods are mainly concerned with the speed and timing of velar movements. The issue of velar timing was raised by Itoh/Sasanuma (1984) in their analyses of aphasic and apraxic patients — a study which has had some impact on the discussion of the nature of aphasic speech errors (cf. 4.). — A problem which is particularly relevant in the case of velar movements concerns the functional significance of movement variables. It is known that normal speakers may differ in their patterns of lateral pharyngeal adaptation and velar elevation during velopharyngeal closure. Further, the velopharyngeal port need not be completely closed but may vary considerably in its size during the production of oral vowels and consonants. Examination of the velum alone therefore yields a rather poor prediction of the actual quality of speech and even estimates of velopharyngeal port size should be carefully interpreted if implications concerning for instance the degree of perceived nasality are to be drawn in dysarthric patients.

Vocal folds: The notion of vocal fold movement may be understood in two different ways: in the sense of active glottal ad- or abduction during running speech, predominantly used for distinguishing between voiced and voiceless sounds ('laryngeal articulation'), or in the sense of passive, quasi-periodic oscillation of the adducted vocal folds during the production of voiced sounds. While the former are produced voluntarily and, in this respect, may be compared to the articulatory movements discussed so far, the latter are the result of an aerodynamic and myoelastic process depending essentially on subglottal pressure, glottal width, and vocal fold stiffness and may therefore provide indirect information on the complex interplay between respiration, laryngeal function, and articulation. A methodologically relevant difference lies in the temporal characteristics of both movement types, with vocal fold oscillations typically ranging between approximately 100 and 250 cycles per second in adults, whereas voluntary repetitive laryngeal ad- and abduction is typically performed at a rate of ca. 5 per second. — Laryngeal behavior can be observed directly by telescopic or fiberoptic endoscopy. Endoscopic inspection of the larynx and the hypopharynx is clinically indispensible for the assessment of abnormal shapes or postures of laryngeal or hypopharyngeal structures, of abnormalities in the degree of adduction, or of involuntary laryngeal movements. If laryngeal articulations during speaking are to be assessed, transnasal endoscopy is required. Quantitative evaluation of laryngeal movements is impeded by the shortcomings associated with the non-linearity of endoscopic views. If vocal fold oscillations are to be assessed in some detail, ultra high-speed photography is required. As may be expected, evaluation of high-speed films requires a high expenditure in frame-by-frame analysis, if not automatic image processing techniques. — Part of the information contained in high-speed films may also be captured by electroglottography (EGG) or photoglottography (PGG) (Baer/Löfqvist/McGarr 1983). EGG uses a pair of electrodes placed bilaterally on the neck at the level of the thyroid prominence to measure the electrical impedance of the larynx, which is considered to vary reciprocally with the degree of vocal-fold contact. PGG ist based on the transillumination principle and may for instance utilize the light source of a nasal endoscope to measure the amount of light arriving at a phototransistor placed on the surface of the neck, below the cricoid cartilage. The method is susceptible to artifacts of various kinds, e. g. changes in light source or photodetector position or interposition of the epiglottis, and should therefore be controlled by parallel fiberoptic endoscopy. — EGG and PGG are considered to provide complementary information on the oscillatory cycle of the vocal folds, with EGG conveying information on the patterns of vocal fold contact and the PGG signal providing an index of peak glottal opening and glottal closure (Baer/Löfqvist/McGarr 1983). While EGG is predominantly used in phonation analyses, PGG has proven particularly useful in the analysis of laryngeal gestures during articulation. — In motor speech disorders, EGG and PGG methods have, for instance, been applied to study laryngeal dynamics in patients with spasmodic dysphonia (Ludlow/

Connor 1987). Application of EGG and PGG methods to study the vibratory cycle of vocal fold oscillations in dysarthria is strongly suggested by Ward/Hanson/Gerratt et al. (1989). However, Childers/Hicks/Moore et al. (1990) are doubtful as to the diagnostic potentials of electroglottography, since for one thing, relevant types of insufficient vocal fold contact remain undetected.

Respiratory organs: The term 'Respiratory kinematics' usually refers to the anteroposterior movements of the thoracal and abdominal walls, which are the result of a rather complex interplay of active contractions of the diaphragm and the intercostals, of aerodynamic processes, and of passive recoil forces of the chest wall (Weismer 1985). Kinematic parameters of speech breathing are assessed using either strain gage belt pneumographs or magnetometers to measure changes in the circumference or A-P-diameter of the rib cage and the abdomen (Murdoch/Chenery/Bowler/Ingram 1989; Hoit/Hixon/Watson/Morgan 1990). Volume calibration techniques are applied to estimate the relative contributions of thoracal and abdominal displacement to lung volume change (Reich/McHenry 1990). A large body of data has been collected to describe volume displacements of rib cage and abdomen in normal subjects, including populations varying in sex, age, or body type (cf. Hoit/Hixon/Watson/Morgan 1990). Up to now, examinations of neurologically impaired subjects have focussed on the detection of atypical or paradoxical patterns in charts describing abdominal versus thoracal displacement over time (Weismer 1985; Murdoch/Chenery/Bowler/Ingram 1989).

2.2. Aerodynamic Parameters

Whereas most of the parameters discussed above have their parallels in other motor systems, aerodynamic parameters like air pressure and volume velocity are peculiar to speech. They reflect respiratory, laryngeal, and articulatory maneuvers and as such may be used as an index of speech motor control. Yet, aerodynamic parameters are rather indirect correlates of the motor processes associated with speaking since they combine a blend of different influences which are difficult to discern. – Relevant parameters are lung volume changes, subglottal, oral, and nasal pressures, and oral and nasal airflow rates. Lung volume measures of speech breathing are considered to reflect thoracal and abdominal activities and can be estimated from kinematic parameters of chest wall movements (cf. 2.1.3.). Oral and nasal pressure and airflow are a function of pulmonary pressure and their mutual relation is dependent on the velopharyngeal port area (Laine/Warren/Dalston/Morr 1988). They can be measured using a differential pressure transducer with a catheter being inserted into the subject's oral cavity or nostril. Subglottal pressure depends on lung volume and expiratory control and may be regarded as a major determinant of vocal intensity and, together with glottal width and vocal fold stiffness, one of the factors influencing vocal fold vibration (Holmberg/Hillman/Perkell 1988). Its direct measurement would require sensors to be placed below the glottis level or within the esophagus, which is highly invasive. A clinically applicable method to derive subglottal pressure from intraoral pressures is based on pressure measurements during complete oral closure and simultaneous glottal opening, as in /p/ (Kitajima/Fujita 1990). When this procedure is applied in dysarthric patients, care must be taken that the lips are completely sealed and that air is prevented from passing through the nose. – Measures of airflow rates are usually obtained by a pneumotachometer attached to an air-tight face mask (Holmberg/Hillman/Perkell 1988). If nasal and oral flow rates are to be differentiated, a two channel mask must be used. – Aerodynamic parameters of speech disturbances of neurogenic origin have predominantly been applied to measure velopharyngeal function in dysarthria (Hoodin/Gilbert 1989). Aerodynamic measures of respiratory function have been assessed in Parkinsonian dysarthria and in ALS, yet with a strong focus on basic nonspeech pulmonary function (Murdoch/Chenery/Bowler/Ingram 1989).

2.3. Acoustic Parameters

The motor processes and associated aerodynamic events described so far ultimately result in a sound pressure wave which is radiated from the lips and the nose and is the physical carrier of the speech code. Since the acoustic signal is the end-product of respiratory, laryngeal, and articulatory movements, parameters extracted from it may be used to characterize the consequences of speech dysfunctions at different levels. Compared to physiologic and aerodynamic techniques the recording of the speech wave is uncomplicated since it is usually performed outside the vocal tract and does not interfere with speaking. To be sure, the ease of assessment is gained at the expense of physiologic significance, because the sound pressure wave integrates all motor activities associated with its production, and there is no straightforward way to single out the contribution of any of the different subsystems. However, this shortcoming can be partly compensated for at least by using appropriate speech tasks (cf. 3.1.). On the other hand, speech wave parameters may capture the functionally relevant aspects of a patient's speech impairment since they draw upon the signal by which the patient attempts to communicate. — The recording of the audio signal requires a high quality microphone and tape recorder and is usually performed in a sound-treated test booth. The extraction of acoustic parameters has long been based on analog devices like the sound spectrograph. In the meantime, these techniques have largely been substituted by digital signal processing methods, with microcomputer applications becoming increasingly important. — In principle, the speech signal can be analyzed in the temporal or the spectral domain, or by mathematical modelling techniques like linear predictive coding (LPC). Parameters of the temporal domain include, for instance, sound pressure level contours or durations of identifiable signal portions, whereas spectral analysis draws upon the distribution of signal energy over the frequency band up to about 10 kHz. LPC analysis over short signal portions yields considerable data reduction and allows, for instance, the fast computation of smoothed spectra. — Applications to normal speech have been based on a multitude of measures characterizing, for instance, consonants produced at different places or with different manners of articulation, or sound contrasts based on voicing or nasality. Further relevant issues are the analysis of phonatory parameters like fundamental frequency and the characterization of prosodic features. These investigations typically try to establish a correspondence between the acoustic parameter in question and some articulatory or perceptual correlate. — Acoustic descriptions of dysarthric or apraxic articulation have largely been based on the signal parameters known from acoustic phonetics, e. g. formant frequencies in vowel articulation (Ziegler/Hartmann/Hoole/Cramon 1990) or stop gap durations and voice onset times in plosive articulation (Caruso/Burton 1987). Measures of the variability of segment-, syllable- or word durations have been considered valuable in descriptions of ataxic dysarthria or of aphasic speech disturbances (cf. Baum/Blumstein/Naeser/Palumbo 1990). Many of the measures studied so far have the disadvantage of relying on the presence of certain 'landmarks' in the speech signal, e. g. a clearly discernible plosive burst as is characteristic of the release of stop consonants in normals. In severe dysarthria these landmarks may no longer be present so that alternative approaches towards temporal measures of dysarthric speech are needed (Ziegler/Hartmann/Hoole/Cramon 1990). — Acoustic analyses of dysphonia following lesions to the central nervous system are surprisingly rare when compared to voice disorders of peripheral origin. A differentiation between several perceptually determined voice types in patients with dysarthria of traumatic and cerebro-vascular origin has been performed by Hartmann/Cramon (1984). A number of studies was focussed on acoustic features of spasmodic dysphonia, such as voice tremor or the occurrence of phonatory aperiodicities and voice breaks (Ludlow/Connor 1987). — Finally, acoustic measures have been applied in the description of prosodic impairments, for instance in Parkinson's disease, in aphasia, or in right hemisphere lesions (cf. Behrens 1989). The parameters used in these studies typically include measures of prosodic variation of fundamental frequency, intensity, and duration.

2.4. Auditory Parameters

The goal of any kind of speech motor activity is the production of perceptually acceptable, intelligible speech. From the patient's perspective the perceived quality of his/her speech output is the most relevant aspect of his/her speech disorder. Likewise, perceptual features provide the most relevant criterion for the severity of a speech disorder. It thus seems natural that any kind of clinical diagnostics is primarily based on auditory evaluation. Yet, the perceived quality of disturbed speech reflects the underlying pathology even less directly than the acoustic signal does, since auditory parameters are mediated by the complex processes of auditory perception. — Attempts have been made to implement a standard inventory of terms to be used in the auditory assessment of dysarthric speech (Darley/Aronson/Brown 1975), but the diagnostic methods based on such inventories are probably not sufficiently reliable (Zyski/

Weisiger 1987). Moreover, such inventories are not founded on empiric perceptual investigations and many of the applied dimensions seem considerably unspecific or poorly defined (Sheard/Adams/Davis 1991). – The method traditionally used by phoneticians to describe the perceptual quality of speech is (narrow) phonetic transcription. This technique uses a standardized set of symbols, the 'International Phonetic Alphabet (IPA)', which serves to represent a wide range of sounds that can be produced by the human vocal apparatus. The IPA has been extended by diacritics which are specifically suitable for the transcription of disturbed speech (Duckworth/Allen/Hardcastle/Ball 1990). The method of phonetic transcription is widely accepted and a sufficiently high agreement can be obtained between trained transcribers. Transcription based analyses become increasingly important in the evaluation of aphasia and apraxia of speech (Odell/McNeil/Rosenbek/Hunter 1990). Yet, applications in dysarthria are rare (Vogel/Cramon 1983), probably since phonetic transcription is predominantly segment-oriented and requires high expenditure for assessing, segment-by-segment, the relatively constant features of dysarthric speech. – More recent approaches have tried to establish psychophysical scaling techniques for the judgment of e. g. voice quality or speech naturalness (cf. Toner/Emanuel/Parker 1990). The development of such scales is often based on synthetic or semi-synthetic stimuli or on voice samples from patients with peripheral lesions. Their reliabilty is known to improve with training (Bassich/Ludlow 1986). Apart from a few studies on speech quality in stuttering (Metz/Schiavetti/Sacco 1990), these methods have yet to be applied systematically to patients with neuromotor speech disorders. – A variable of considerable importance for evaluating the severity of a patient's speech impairment is intelligibility. Psychophysical scales may be used to rate intellegibility (Fucci/Ellis/Petrosino 1990). However, such ratings fail to yield an intelligibility 'profile' that would indicate which sound classes have the highest contribution to a patient's disturbance. This information, which is crucial from the point-of-view of clinical management, is provided by intelligibility tests based on multiple choice word identification tasks with phonetically balanced materials (Ziegler/Hartmann/Cramon 1988).

3. Assessment Paradigms

3.1. Variation of Tasks

Important in the investigation of motor dysfunctions are the appropriate choice and the systematic variation of motor tasks. In motor speech disorders, this variation is achieved by choosing among different modalities of speaking (e. g. repetition vs. spontaneous production), among speech materials of different length (e. g. single syllables vs. sentences) or different phonetic structure (e. g. labial sounds vs. lingual sounds), or by requiring maximum performance with respect to e. g. speed or effort. – The choice of the stimulus modality is guided by a number of considerations: Precise control over the target utterance to be produced is best achieved in repetition and reading tasks, but these tasks are poor models of 'natural' speech and are of only limited value in e. g. the assessment of prosodic deficits (Behrens 1989). – By choosing appropriate designs even indirect methods such as acoustic evaluation may yield rather specific results. So, for instance, the influence of labial articulation can be inferred approximately from the speech signal by varying systematically between vowels contrasting in the amount of lip rounding required for their production (Ziegler/Hartmann/Hoole/Cramon 1990). A high selectivity can be achieved by using minimal pairs, i. e. pairs of utterances differing in exactly one segment (Ziegler 1987). – Maximum performance tasks are usually applied with the aim of increasing the diagnostic sensitivity by driving the motor system to its limits. Examples are rapid syllable repetition, which imposes particular demands on articulatory motility and is generally considered as the speech equivalent of wrist diadochokinesis, or maximum vowel or fricative prolongation, which requires a high vital capacity, good expiratory control and skillful laryngeal or articulatory valving (Kent/Kent/Rosenbek 1987). A special case of maximum performance testing is the measurement of reaction time in the initiation of speech. Suitable variation of stimulus-response conditions in reaction-time testing may give insight into specific speech onset and motor programming problems. – A problem inherent to all kinds of maximum performance tasks in neurological patients is that the degree to which these patients can be motivated to optimum performance is influenced by various neuropsychological factors, and the results often cannot be explained solely in motor terms. Further, most of these tasks need a high number of repetitions, when stable measures are to be obtained (Kent/Kent/Rosenbek 1987).

3.2. Variation of Constraints

A further approach in the study of speech motor performance uses experimental manipulation of the motor constraints in speaking. This approach is motivated by questions concerning the integrity of motor programs or the processing of sensory information that would be necessary to control the implementation of a motor program under altered conditions. The paradigm which has been studied most thoroughly in normals encompasses the unpredicted perturbation of lip movements during closure (cf. Gracco/Abbs 1989). This research aims at an analysis of sensory-motor interaction in movement programming, with a particular focus on the issue of motor equivalence, i.e. the capability of the speech motor system to achieve a desired motor goal in several different ways. So, for instance, immediate adaptations of the upper lip and the jaw compensate for unpredicted lower lip perturbations to achieve the goal of bilabial closure for /b/ or /p/ (Gracco/Abbs 1989). — This kind of articulatory flexibility has stimulated hypotheses and investigations in neurophonetics. DePaul/Abbs/Caligiuri et al. (1988) reported on particular problems of their ALS patients to compensate for the altered conditions imposed by a bite-block. A systematic investigation of the effects of jaw-fixing on vowel articulation in Broca's aphasia was carried out by Sussman/Marquardt/Hutchinson/NacNeilage (1986). A similar issue was raised by Marshall/Gandour/Windsor (1988) in their report on a Broca's aphasic whose articulation deficit was profoundly influenced by application of an electronic artificial larynx, i. e. by a reduction of the degrees of freedom within the complex laryngeal-articulatory system. Variation of the conditions under which the speech apparatus works is further applied in studies of speech breathing, with examinations often being performed on subjects in both an upright and a supine body position.

4. Neurophonetic Assessment: Means and Ends

Each of the assessment techniques described in this chapter has its own strengths and weaknesses, and therefore any question to be answered in neurophonetics requires careful selection of the most appropriate assessment method. — The most straightforward way to study the pathophysiologic nature of neurogenic speech dysfunctions is certainly by physiologic examinations, i. e. EMG, force, or kinematic measurements. However, if other motor systems like the extremities are taken as a model in such research, a number of differences should be considered. Unlike the extremities, many of the speech organs are difficult to access and often only indirect measures of their movements can be obtained. Moreover, the single-joint movement model, which plays a major role in the extremities, is generally not applicable in the speech system. A most striking example is the tongue, which is not only difficult to observe but even more difficult to be grasped in a parametric model. Further, the calibration of measurement systems often requires active and skillful cooperation of the subject which cannot be taken for granted in neurologic patients. Still more fundamental than these difficulties, however, seems the problem of how to choose the movement parameters that are relevant in the description of speech motor control and its disturbances. Most of the kinematic parameters discussed in the literature demonstrate considerable within- and between-subject variability and the problem of movement invariants in speech is still open. Taking bilabial closure, for example, it is not only the case that the upper lip, the lower lip, and the jaw may be adjusted independently to realize closure with a high functional flexibility, but also that complete closure is not even absolutely necessary to achieve a perceptually acceptable bilabial stop consonant. The same is true for other subsystems, e. g. the velopharynx (cf. 2.1.3.). The spatial aspects of movements therefore seem to play fundamentally different roles in speech, with its acoustically defined goals, and in e. g. grasping, where motor goals are defined in terms of an external spatial metric. This may be one reason why kinematic measures of dysarthric speech have failed to be ecologically valid thus far (cf. 2.1.). At the same time, acoustic and perceptual methods obtain an important status in assessing whether a speech target has been realized adequately. — A special case of the issue of how speech motor goals are realized is encountered in questions concerning the nature of aphasic speech errors. In a traditional view the occurrence of phonemic paraphasias represents a failure at the level of 'phoneme selection', i. e. the selection of discrete and abstract motor goals. This view is supported by studies based on phonemic ('broad') transcription, which tends to neglect subtle deviations in the realization of a speech sound. More generally, perception-based analysis methods seem to foster a discrete model of sound substitution, due to the tendency of the auditory system to perceive categorically. However, investigations based on kinematic or acoustic measures have shown that both perceptually adequate and paraphasic speech sounds may demonstrate gradual aberrations from normal, which is generally interpreted as a failure in the implementation of motor goals (Ziegler/Hoole 1989). An important though controversial contribution to this issue comes from coarticulation studies investigating the transition between sounds and the anticipation of speech targets (Ziegler/Cramon 1986; Katz/Machetanz/Orth/Schönle 1990). The coarticulation paradigm seems particularly useful in differentiating between phoneme selection and implementation models. — Besides questions embarking on the nature of motor speech dysfunctions, a wide field of neurophonetic applications is concerned with the implications these dysfunctions may have for a patient's communicative abilities. From the point of view of neurologic rehabilitation, this issue is of primary relevance. As pointed out above, the movement parameters examined so far do not yield valid indices of a patient's overall speech impairment and may not be used as predictors of e. g. the 'naturalness' or the intelligibility of a patient's speech. In this domain, therefore, perception-based methods remain relevant and great efforts should be taken to improve their psychometric quality. In the future, considerable support can also be expected from speech acoustics, which may for instance be used in the modelling of intelligibility (Weismer/Kent/Hodge/Martin 1988). — A further important domain of neurophonetics are those assessment methods directly oriented at therapeutic applications. An example is the recording of speech parameters that may be used in feedback therapy. In principle, any acoustic, aerodynamic, or movement parameter may be applied, provided that it can be determined in realtime and is specific to the motor function to be trained. However, the fundamentals of feedback-based motor learning in neuromotor speech disorders and the details of therapeutic applications are still to be elaborated.

5. References

Abbs, J. H., Nadler, R. D. & Fujimura, O. (1988). X-ray microbeams track the shape of speech. *Soma*, 29—34.

Baer, T., Loefqvist, A. & McGarr, N. S. (1983). Laryngeal vibrations: A comparison between high-speed filming and glottographic techniques. *Journal of the Acoustical Society of America*, *73*, 283—291.

Barlow, S. M. & Abbs, J. H. (1983). Force transducers for the evaluation of labial, lingual, and mandibular motor impairments. *Journal of Speech and Hearing Research*, *26*, 616—621.

Barlow, S. M., Cole, K. J. & Abbs, J. H. (1983). A new head-mounted lip-jaw movement transduction system for the study of motor speech disorders. *Journal of Speech and Hearing Research*, *26*, 283—288.

Bassich, C. J. & Ludlow, C. L. (1986). The use of perceptual methods by new clinicians for assessing voice quality. *Journal of Speech and Hearing Disorders*, *51*, 125—133.

Baum, S. R., Blumstein, S. E., Naeser, M. A. & Palumbo, C. L. (1990). Temporal dimensions of consonant and vowel production: An acoustic and CT scan analysis of aphasic speech. *Brain and Language*, *39*, 33—56.

Behrens, S. J. (1989). Characterizing sentence intonation in a right hemisphere-damaged population. *Brain and Language*, *37*, 181—200.

Blair, C. & Smith, A. (1986). EMG recording in human lip muscles: Can single muscles be isolated? *Journal of Speech and Hearing Research*, *29*, 256—266.

Caligiuri, M. P. (1987). Labial kinematics during speech in patients with Parkinsonian rigidity. *Brain*, *110*, 1033—1044.

Caruso, A. J. & Burton, E. K. (1987). Temporal acoustic measures of dysarthria associated with amyotrophic lateral sclerosis. *Journal of Speech and Hearing Research*, *30*, 80—87.

Childers, D. G., Hicks, D. M., Moore, G. P., Eskenazi, L. & Lalwani, A. L. (1990). Electroglottography and vocal fold physiology. *Journal of Speech and Hearing Research*, *33*, 245—254.

Darley, F. L., Aronson, A. E. & Brown, J. R. (1975). *Motor Speech Disorders*. Philadelphia: W. B. Saunders Company.

DePaul, R., Abbs, J. H., Caligiuri, M., Gracco, V. L. & Brooks, B. R. (1988). Hypoglossal, trigeminal, and facial motoneuron involvement in amyotrophic lateral sclerosis. *Neurology*, *38*, 281—283.

Duckworth, M., Allen, G., Hardcastle, W. & Ball, M. (1990). Extensions to the International Phonetic Alphabet for the transcription of atypical speech. *Clinical Linguistics and Phonetics*, *4*, 273—280.

Edwards, J. & Harris, K. S. (1990). Rotation and translation fo the jaw during speech. *Journal of Speech and Hearing Research*, *33*, 550—562.

Forrest, K., Weismer, G. & Turner, G. (1989). Kinematic, acoustic, and perceptual analyses of connected speech produced by Parkinsonian and normal geriatric adults. *Journal of the Acoustical Society of America, 85*, 2608–2622.

Fucci, D., Ellis, L. & Petrosino, L. (1990). Speech clarity/intelligibility: test-retest reliability of magnitude-estimation scaling. *Perceptual and Motor Skills, 70*, 232–234.

Gans, C. & Gorniak, G. C. (1980). Electromyograms are repeatable: Precautions and limitations. *Science, 210*, 795–797.

Gracco, V. L. & Abbs, J. H. (1989). Sensorimotor characteristics of speech motor sequences. *Experimental Brain Research, 75*, 586–598.

Hardcastle, W., Jones, W., Knight, C., Trudgeon, A. & Calder, G. (1989). New developments in electropalatography: a state-of-the-art report. *Clinical Linguistics and Phonetics, 3*, 1–38.

Hartmann, E. & Cramon, D. von (1984). Acoustic measurement of voice quality in central dysphonia. *Journal of Communication Disorders, 17*, 425–440.

Hirano, M., Nozoe, I. & Shin, T. (1987). Electromyography for laryngeal paralysis. In M. Hirano, J. A. Kirchner & D. M. Bless (Eds.), *Neurolaryngology. 232–248*. Boston: College Hill.

Hirose, H. (1986). Pathophysiology of motor speech disorders (dysarthria). *Folia Phoniatrica, 38*, 61–88.

Hoit, J. D., Hixon, T. J., Watson, P. J. & Morgan, W. J. (1990). Speech breathing in children and adolescents. *Journal of Speech and Hearing Research, 33*, 51–69.

Holmberg, E. B., Hillman, R. E. & Perkell, J. S. (1988). Glottal airflow and transglottal air pressure measurements for male and female speakers in soft, normal, and loud voice. *Journal of the Acoustical Society of America, 84*, 511–529.

Hoodin, R. B. & Gilbert, H. R. (1989). Parkinsonian dysarthria: An aerodynamic and perceptual description of velopharyngeal closure for speech. *Folia Phoniatrica, 41*, 249–258.

Hoole, P., Ziegler, W., Hartmann, E. & Hardcastle, W. (1989). Parallel electropalatographic and acoustic measures of fricatives. *Clinical Linguistics and Phonetics, 3*, 59–69.

Hunker, C. J. & Abbs, J. H. (1990). Uniform frequency of Parkinsonian resting tremor in the lips, jaw, tongue, and index finger. *Movement Disorders, 71*, 71–77.

Itoh, M. & Sasanuma, S. (1984). Articulatory movements in apraxia of speech. In J. C. Rosenbek, M. R. McNeill & A. E. Aronson (Eds.), *Apraxia of Speech: Physiology, Acoustics, Linguistics, Management. 135–165*. San Diego: College-Hill Press.

Katz, W., Machetanz, J., Orth, U. & Schönle, P. (1990). A kinematic analysis of anticipatory coarticulation in the speech of anterior aphasic subjects using electromagnetic articulography. *Brain and Language, 38*, 555–575.

Keller, E. & Ostry, D. J. (1983). Computerized measurement of tongue dorsum movements with pulsed-echo ultrasound. *Journal of the Acoustical Society of America, 73*, 1309–1315.

Kent, R. D., Kent, J. F. & Rosenbek, J. C. (1987). Maximum performance tests of speech production. *Journal of Speech and Hearing Research, 52*, 367–387.

Kitajima, K. & Fujita, F. (1990). Estimation of subglottal pressure with intraoral pressure. *Acta Otolaryngologica (Stockholm), 109*, 473–478.

Laine, T., Warren, D. W., Dalston, R. M. & Morr, K. E. (1988). Screening of Velopharyngeal Closure Based on Nasal Airflow Rate Measurements. *Cleft Palate Journal, 25*, 220–225.

Ludlow, C. L. & Connor, N. P. (1987). Dynamic aspects of phonatory control in spasmodic dysphonia. *Journal of Speech and Hearing Research, 30*, 197–206.

Marshall, R. C., Gandour, J. & Windsor, J. (1988). Selective impairment of phonation: a case study. *Brain and Language, 35*, 313–339.

McNeil, M. R., Weismer, G., Adams, S. & Mulligan, M. (1990). Oral structure nonspeech motor control in normal, dysarthric, aphasic and apraxic speakers: isometric force and static position control. *Journal of Speech and Hearing Research, 33*, 255–268.

Metz, D. E., Schiavetti, N., Sacco, P. R. (1990). Acoustic and psychophysical dimensions of the perceived speech naturalness of nonstutterers and posttreatment stutterers. *Journal of Speech and Hearing Disorders, 55*, 516–525.

Murdoch, B. E., Chenery, H. J., Bowler, S. & Ingram, J. C. L. (1989). Respiratory function in Parkinson's subjects exhibiting a perceptible speech deficit: a kinematic and spirometric analysis. *Journal of Speech and Hearing Disorders, 54*, 610–626.

Neilson, P. D. & O'Dwyer, N. J. (1981). Pathophysiology of dysarthria in cerebral palsy. *Journal of Neurology, Neurosurgery, and Psychiatry, 44*, 1013–1019.

Odell, K., McNeil, M., Rosenbek, J. C. & Hunter, L. (1990). Perceptual characteristics of consonant production by apraxic speakers. *Journal of Speech and Hearing Disorders, 55*, 345–359.

Reich, A. R. & McHenry, M. A. (1990). Estimating respiratory volumes from rib cage and abdominal displacements during ventilatory and speech activities. *Journal of Speech and Hearing Research, 33*, 467–475.

Schönle, P. W., Gräbe, K., Wenig, P., Höhne, J., Schrader, J. & Conrad, B. (1987). Electromagnetic articulography: use of alternating magnetic fields for tracking movements of multiple points inside and outside the vocal tract. *Brain and Language, 31*, 26–35.

Sheard, C., Adams, R.D. & Davis, P.J. (1991). Reliability and agreement of ratings of ataxic dysarthric speech samples with varying intelligibility. *Journal of Speech and Hearing Research, 34,* 285–293.

Shipp, T., Izdebski, K., Reed, C. & Morrissey, P. (1985). Intrinsic laryngeal muscle activity in a spastic dysphonia patient. *Journal of Speech and Hearing Disorders, 50,* 54–59.

Stone, M. (1990). A three-dimensional model of tongue movement based on ultrasound and x-ray microbeam data. *Journal of the Acoustical Society of America, 87,* 2207–2217.

Stone, M., Sonies, B.C., Shawker, T.H., Weiss, G. & Nadel, L. (1983). Analysis of real-time ultrasound images of tongue configuration using a grid-digitizing system. *Journal of Phonetics, 11,* 207–218.

Sussman, H., Marquardt, T., Hutchinson, J. & NacNeilage, P. (1986). Compensatory articulation in Broca's aphasia. *Brain and Language, 27,* 56–74.

Tassinary, L.G., Cacioppo, J.T. & Geen, T.R. (1989). A psychometric study of surface electrode placements for facial electromyographic recording. I. The brow and cheek muscle regions. *Psychophysiology, 26,* 1–16.

Toner, M.A., Emanuel, F.W. & Parker, D. (1990). Relationship of spectral noise levels to psychophysical scaling of vowel roughness. *Journal of Speech and Hearing Research, 33,* 238–244.

Vogel, M. & Cramon, D. von (1983). Articulatory recovery after traumatic midbrain damage: A follow-up study. *Folia Phoniatrica, 35,* 294–309.

Ward, P.H., Hanson, D.G., Gerratt, B.R., Berke, G.S. (1989). Current and future horizons in laryngeal and voice research. *Annals of Otology Rhinology Laryngology, 98,* 145–152.

Weismer, G. (1985). Speech breathing: Contemporary views and findings. In R. Daniloff (Ed.), *Speech Science: Recent Advances. 47–72.* San Diego: College-Hill Press.

Weismer, G., Kent, R.D., Hodge, M. & Martin, R. (1988). The acoustic signature for intelligibility test words. *Journal of the Acoustical Society of America, 84,* 1281–1291.

Ziegler, W. (1987). Phonetic realization of phonological contrast in aphasic patients. In J.H. Ryalls (Ed.), *Phonetic Approaches to Speech Production in Aphasia and Related Disorders. 163–179.* Boston: Little, Brown and Company.

Ziegler, W. & Cramon, D. von (1986). Disturbed coarticulation in apraxia of speech: Acoustic evidence. *Brain and Language, 29,* 34–47.

Ziegler, W., Hartmann, E. & Cramon, D. von (1988). Word identification testing in the diagnostic evaluation of dysarthric speech. *Clinical Linguistics and Phonetics, 2,* 291–308.

Ziegler, W., Hartmann, E., Hoole, P. & Cramon, D. von (1990). *Akustische Dimensionen dysarthrischer Störungsmerkmale.* München: GSF.

Ziegler, W. & Hoole, P. (1989). A combined acoustic and perceptual analysis of the tense-lax opposition in aphasic vowel production. *Aphasiology, 2,* 449–463.

Zimmermann, G., Dalston, R.M., Brown, C., Folkins, J.W., Linville, R.N. & Seaver, E.J. (1987). Comparison of cineradiographic and photodetection techniques for assessing velopharyngeal function during speech. *Journal of Speech and Hearing Research, 30,* 564–569.

Zyski, B.J. & Weisiger, B.E. (1987). Identification of dysarthria types based on perceptual analysis. *Journal of Communication Disorders, 20,* 367–378.

Wolfram Ziegler, Munich (Germany)

40. Speech Apraxia

After decades of debate, speech apraxia has earned a place in the nosology of neurogenic speech-language disorders. This development may well owe less to strong arguments from true believers than to natural processes that guarantee all conflicts – regardless of right – eventually end. Opponents get tired and interests change. If the conflicts are among older practitioners, positions soften and mature. More and better data accumulate; best of all, doubts creep in. This chapter will be about selected arguments, data, and accords. It will also be about doubts.

1. Definition

Liepmann (1913) was among the first to identify a speech apraxia and differentiate it from aphasia. He said, "In 1900 I called the aphasia of my patient apraxia of the speech muscles" (97). It was from these and other historical materials that Darley (1969) built what has become, for many, the standard definition of speech apraxia, "An articulatory disorder resulting from impairment, as a result of brain damage, of the capacity to program the positioning of speech musculature and the sequencing of muscle movements for the volitional production of phonemes. No significant weakness, slowness, or incoordination in reflex and automatic acts. Prosodic alterations may be associated with the articulatory problem, perhaps in compensation for it" (Darley 1969, 2).

This definition of speech apraxia was complete enough to earn the disorder a place in the taxonomy of neurogenic speech-language disorders. However, the boundaries of that place, its actual location in relation to other conditions such as conduction aphasia and dysarthria, and even the label itself with its implications for underlying mechanisms have fostered decades of debate and much remains to be resolved. What goes undebated is recognition that brain-damaged speakers exist whose speech is more marred by articulatory substitutions, distortions, distorted substitutions, and dysprosody than their sensation, cognition, language, and strength and tone suggest it should be. Careful testing usually confirms the diagnosis of what will be called speech apraxia in this chapter.

2. Related Conditions

Speech apraxia has been called a synonym for a variety of other terms including aphemia, cortical dysarthria, anarthria, and phonetic disintegration (Johns/Darley 1970). Probably each of these terms, as used by at least one group of scholars, refers to a pattern of speech impairment identical to what is being called speech apraxia in this chapter. It is impossible to know for sure, however, until the sound of persons with each of these diagnoses is heard. Unfortunately, clinical scientists seem never to have committed to an exchange of tapes. That leaves published descriptions. Prior to Alajouanine/Ombredane/Durand (1939), published reports contained so little carefully collected speech-language data that modern readers are left to guess about the similarity of the writer's and their own use of terms. Compounding the difficulty is that even some modern reports contain insufficient speech-language and neurologic data for confident comparison of subject groups called by different names. However, one condition, Broca's aphasia, has been described frequently and completely enough to support the position that it is not a synonym for speech apraxia. To make the terms synonyms is damaging to the conceptual underpinnings of the nosology in neurogenic speech-language disorders. Broca's aphasia is a language disorder characterized by agrammatism; speech apraxia is not.

One related condition, oral apraxia, deserves special attention. Hughlings Jackson's description (1878) of a patient's inability to protrude his tongue upon request but ability to do so when eating and drinking is cited as one of the earliest written reports about the condition. Oral apraxia is usually differentiated from speech apraxia, although until recently, co-occurrence was assumed to be common and the two conditions were often described as representing nothing more than different severities of a common deficit in praxis. Data by DeRenzi/Pieczuro/Vignolo (1966) demonstrating that oral apraxia could occur in the absence of speech deficit and could accompany even fluent aphasia helped to change that assumption.

The contemporary conclusion seems to be that oral, nonspeech movements and speech movements may be under different patterns of neuromotor control and may be differentially involved.

3. History

Speech pathologists, neurologists, psychologists, and linguists (Head 1926; Critchley 1970; Lecours/Nespoulous/Pioger 1987; Lebrun 1976; Benton 1981) appear to have agreed that modern understanding of speech apraxia began with Broca's description of an expressive abnormality he called aphemia. Broca's contributions, it is traditionally argued, did not spring from barren soil unnourished by anything but his own clinical case studies, however. Buckingham (1981) describes the influence of the phrenologists and of practitioners such as Bouillaud. Darley's papers on apraxia of speech (1968; 1969) are another benchmark in speech apraxia's history. Not only did Darley write an enduring definition, he provided a durable description of the apraxic speaker's performance. This description included inconsistent 'phonemic' errors of substitution, distortion, omission, and addition accompanied by effortful, trial and error groping. For nearly two decades this description dominated clinical research and education.

The years between Broca and Darley were not an intellectual wasteland. Alajouanine/Ombredane/Durand's description (1939) of what they called the syndrome of phonetic disintegration is noteworthy because the experimenters controlled the testing materials and completed both auditory perceptual and acoustic analyses of speech. Bay (1962) used auditory perceptual evaluation and the glossogram, which measured changes in pressure of the tongue against the palate during a variety of nonspeech tasks, to study a motor speech deficit he called cortical dysarthria. Shankweiler/Harris (1966) published a carefully designed auditory perceptual analysis of speech by five patients with the syndrome of phonetic disintegration.

After Darley's papers, an unprecedented flood of studies and position papers, all of which have been reviewed extensively (Wertz/LaPointe/Rosenbek 1984), appeared. These years were also marked by mordant debates, usually fueled by at least a soupcon of data, between those who felt that speech apraxia was a motor disorder and those who felt it was a language disorder.

No publication marks the end of what can be called speech apraxia's history. No wall fell. No treaty of scientific cooperation was signed. No voice was raised that shifted the paradigm for conceptualizing, studying, and interpreting the data in speech apraxia. Instead what seems to have happened gradually is that the experimental soil began to be worked by fewer researchers and ones less interested in defending what was assumed to be true and more interested in discovering what might be true or at least replicable.

4. Signs of Speech Apraxia

The goal of this next section is to develop and evaluate a modern profile of speech apraxia. Signs of speech apraxia have been identified at three levels of analysis, the auditory perceptual, the acoustic, and the physiologic.

4.1. Auditory Perceptual Analysis

Auditory perceptual analysis takes the form of either broad or narrow phonetic transcription. Most of the data contained in the earliest modern descriptions of speech apraxia resulted from broad transcription and suggested that speech sound substitutions were the most frequent apraxic error type. Narrow phonetic transcriptions, while limited in number, are now increasingly common. One of the earliest (Square/Darley/Sommers 1982), revealed that distortions of both consonants and vowels were more frequent than substitutions. Odell/McNeil/Rosenbek/Hunter (1990) followed with a narrow phonetic transcription of consonant productions in words by four pure apraxic subjects. Distortions were the most frequent error type (25%), followed by omissions, substitutions, distorted substitutions, and additions. Odell/McNeil/Rosenbek/Hunter (1991) also reported the narrow phonetic transcription of vowels for the same four subjects. The mean error rate for vowels was 49% with considerable intra-subject variability. Distortions were the most frequent error type (65%) for three of the four subjects. In another report, Odell/McNeil/Rosenbek/Hunter (1991) had two judges rate three categories of prosodic deviation: abnormalities in syllabic stress, deviations in intraword temporal parameters, and what were called repeated production difficulties. Syllabic stress errors were frequent, as were difficulties in making transitions from one sound to the next and in initiating speech. Unfortunately, the data do not say anything about the degree to which prosodic disturbances are a primary part of apraxic symptomatology. A study adequate to the challenge of answering that question appears not to have been done.

The most significant finding to emerge from the auditory perceptual data is that speech sound distortions are a prominent part of apraxic symptomatology. Another finding for which there was some historical precedent (Lebrun/Buyssens/Henneaux 1973) is that vowels are as likely to be involved in some apraxic speakers as are consonants. Finally, the data add specificity to the description of prosodic disturbances.

4.2. Acoustic Analysis

Acoustic analysis has certain advantages in the study of speech apraxia. A major one is that many acoustic features have known relationships to both perceptual phenomena and physiologic events (Weismer 1984). Acoustic data, therefore, are important in speech apraxia research where increasingly the emphasis is on both description and explanation.

The most frequent acoustic analysis has been of voice onset time (VOT) (Blumstein/Cooper/Zurif/Caramazza 1977; Blumstein/Cooper/Goodglass et al. 1980; Shewan/Leeper/Booth 1984; Hoit/Murry/Knopp 1983; Itoh/Sasanuma/Tatsumi et al. 1982) despite controversy over how the data are to be interpreted (Tuller 1984; Ziegler 1984; Blumstein 1981). VOT errors identified in speakers labelled or assumed to be apraxic are usually interpreted as providing evidence of speech sound distortion resulting primarily from dyscoordination of laryngeal and oral-lingual movements (Freeman/Sands/Harris 1978).

A variety of other acoustic abnormalities have also been identified. These include: 1) abnormally long, but highly variable, speech sound durations (Duffy/Gawle 1984; Ryalls 1981); 2) abnormalities in intensity and fundamental frequency variation, especially the latter (Kent/Rosenbek 1983); 3) lingual-laryngeal, lingual-velar, and lingual-labial phrasing abnormalities (Ziegler/von Cramon 1986); 4) abnormally long intersegmental durations (Strand/McNeil 1987); 5) longer than normal transitions from sound to sound (Kent/Rosenbek 1983); 6) longer than normal verbal response times even with time to prepare (Strand 1987); and 7) difficulty adjusting speaking rate (Kent/McNeil 1987; McNeil/Liss/Tseng/Kent 1990) especially in increasing it.

4.3. Physiologic Analysis

Physiologic analyses, or analyses using instrumentation to measure movements, are beginning to appear in the speech apraxia literature. A substantial review of the physiologic data was prepared by McNeil/Kent (1990). They divide the studies into those of force and position control (McNeil/Weismer/Adams/Mulligan 1990); intraarticulator kinematics, including movement duration, velocity, and displacement (Itoh/Sasanuma 1987; Itoh/Sasanuma/Hirose et al. 1980; Robin/Bean/Folkins 1989; McNeil/Adams 1991; McNeil/Caligiuri/Rosenbek 1989; McNeil/Liss/Tseng/Kent 1990); interarticulator kinematics or timing and coordination (Itoh/Sasanuma/Ushijima 1979; Itoh/Sasanuma/Hirose et al. 1980; Hardcastle 1987); and electromyography (Shankweiler/Harris/Taylor 1968; Forrest/Adams/McNeil 1991; Hough/Klich 1987; Towne/Crary 1988; McNeil/Prescott/Lemme 1976).

The procedures and data in most of these studies are complex and best read in the original. Some tentative conclusions about the data are possible, however.

The physiologic data support the conclusions from other methods of analysis that distortion and variability are cardinal features of apraxic performance. They also begin laying the foundation for a more sophisticated understanding of why apraxic speech sounds the way it does. Dyscoordinated movements of the speech structures seem to be a critical influence. In addition, selected of the data suggest that the perceptual impression of apraxic slowness may have more to do with range than velocity of movement. An even stronger message from the data about the so-called slowness of apraxic speech is that its movement correlates are complex and still to be explored (Adams/McNeil/Weismer 1989). Indeed the relationship of all physiologic signs to auditory-perceptual signs in speech apraxia is yet to be established.

4.4. Caveats

It is easy to exaggerate the power of instruments. For several reasons speech apraxia research's march toward methods requiring the latest technology is not necessarily a march toward truth. Methods are being used with impaired speakers before sufficient normative data, especially from geriatric control subjects, have been collected. Intuition and informal extrapolation from limited normative data are frequently the shaky bases for conclusions about abnormal speech, including apraxic speech, and the pathophysiology underlying it. Forrest/Weismer/Adams (1990) discuss the dangers of such an approach. In the absence of sufficient normative data, researchers risk being trapped by the assumption that performance on some measure by one or more apraxic talkers is apraxic performance and that such performance somehow explains the accompanying speech signs. Probably some of the extant data from apraxic speakers will turn out to be signs of normal aging, some will turn out to reflect generalized effects of brain damage or of illness, and some will turn out to be unrelated to speech movement abnormalities. It may result that some of the physiologic data are less useful and more misleading than are the perceptual despite the greater 'subjectivity' of perceptual analysis.

Physiologic data, and indeed most of the data gathered from apraxic speakers, are threatened from another source as well. Munhall (1989) observes that very few studies have been designed to measure or control variability in speech apraxia. Munhall's notion is that all speech is variable, and he urges studies of apraxia designed specifically to reveal the variability that is apraxic. Among the few studies designed to separate normal from apraxic variability are those by LaPointe/Horner (1976) and Deal (1974). Until more studies designed with Munhall's caveat in mind appear, conclusions about speech apraxia's nature, and even about its signs, must be tentative indeed.

5. A Contemporary Portrait of Speech Apraxia

Apraxic speech is lawfully variable, is especially sensitive to phonetic influences such as response length and complexity, and is characterized by a mixture of speech sound distortions and substitutions with distortions and distorted substitutions predominating. Variations in fundamental frequency and intensity are abnormally reduced in some utterances. Apraxic speech is slow because of prolonged transitions, steady states, and intersyllabic pauses. Apraxic speakers have difficulty controlling rate and initiating speech even when they know the utterance to be produced. Movements underlying the perceptual and acoustic signs are variable but dyscoordination is prominent. A speaker with this pattern of speech and movement performance, if language and cognition including attention and memory, are near normal, can be hypothesized with a high degree of confidence to have a speech apraxia.

6. Subtypes of Speech Apraxia

It is traditional to divide apraxic limb and body movements into limb kinetic, ideomotor, and ideational types. Liepmann (1913), a major contributor to this division, says "There is a moment of fiction in the theoretical statement" differentiating types of apraxia, but the "division is a very helpful guide in an otherwise very dark sphere" (100). Speech scientists have used Liepmann's light to aid the search for types of speech apraxia (Luria 1970; Deutsch 1984). Square/Darley/Sommers (1982) studied four apraxic speakers, three with cortical lesions and one with a subcortical lesion. A unique error pattern may have emerged from the analysis of the subcortical speaker who was described as sounding "pseudo-foreign." Kertesz (1984) compared 10 cases with what he calls verbal apraxia resulting from lesions of the striatum with twelve patients having cortical lesions. He reported that individual subcortical cases may be different from the cortical group because of 'lower' rate, volume, and fluency and that some of the subcortical patients had severe dysgraphia, a combination also reported by Rosenbek/McNeil/Teetson et al. (1981).

It is critical to be cautious with assumptions about speech apraxia subtypes (Robin/Schienberg 1990). However, with increasingly sophisticated imaging techniques and experimental designs, the time is ripe to go looking for them. The clinical and research dividends may be considerable.

7. Localization

Mohr and his colleagues (Mohr/Pessin/Finkelstein et al. 1978) published what for many has become the classic reference on speech apraxia's localization. They identify two syndromes characterized by disproportionate difficulty with speech which they call little (probably a synonym for speech apraxia) and big Broca aphasia. In little Broca aphasia the lesion is limited to Area 44, or Broca's area, in the frontal operculum. Mutism which quickly evolves into 'effortful articulation' and rapidly resolving language deficit are the signs of little Broca aphasia. Big Broca aphasia, characterized by significant deficits across all language modalities and agrammatic speech, results from a larger lesion involving much of the frontal operculum, insula, and underlying white matter. This large lesion suggests involvement of the upper division of the left middle cerebral artery, while the lesion in little Broca aphasia suggests involvement of one branch of that division. It has also been posited that speech apraxia may result from parietal (Luria 1970) and subcortical, including basal ganglia (Square/Darley/Sommers 1982) and striatum (Kertesz 1984) lesions. All these reports antedate modern brain imaging methods such as positron emission computed tomography (PET) and magnetic resonance imaging (MRI).

Modern methods of imaging the brain, autopsy data, and phonetically and linguistically sophisticated motor speech and language testing will refine our understanding of the parietal lobe and basal ganglia's contributions to motor speech control. Even the extant data, however, support a series of testable hypotheses about the cortical-subcortical network responsible for speech performance. It can be hypothesized that a region shaped roughly like a pyramid and involving frontal and parietal opercula and the basal ganglia constitute a motor control mechanism. Damage to any part of this mechanism may cause speech apraxia.

8. Explanations

By calling a speech abnormality apraxia, the clinical scientist is specifying at least something about the disturbed mechanism underlying the signs and symptoms. Praxis refers to skilled movement and is the responsibility of what might be called a psychomotor level of motor control (Darley/Aronson/Brown 1975). In a hierarchical organization of the neural substrates supporting verbal expression, the psychomotor level resides between the executive and language processing levels. It corresponds in neurolinguistic terms to the third articulation (Lecours/Lhermitte 1969) or interface (Lesser 1978) where phonemic units interact with movement parameters.

Buckingham (1979) and Mlcoch/Noll (1980) have published perspicacious reviews of explanatory concepts in apraxia of speech. Buckingham evaluated the early centers and connections approaches to explanation in apraxia. A variety of other explanations, most of which can be called either primarily linguistic or primarily motoric, and debates about which was superior were also reported even in the earliest literature (Buckingham 1979), but were more common after Darley. One modern form of the controversery involving linguistic and motoric explanations, especially popular in the 1970's and 80's, was whether the errors in speech apraxia were phonemic/phonologic or phonetic. The phonemic/phonologic-phonetic distinction is increasingly unpopular (Abbs/Rosenbek 1985; Kent/Rosenbek 1983), however. One reason for the unpopularity is that the distinction is simplistic. Another is that making it requires the highly subjective interpretation of data. Both speech sound substitutions and distortions, for example, may be manifestations of either linguistic (phonemic/phonologic) or motor (phonetic) performance deficits. Another reason is that data supporting it are limited (Folkins/Bleile 1990).

The search for better explanations continues. Folkins/Bleile (1990) suggest new terminology, including the term phonomotor, and new research strategies as aids to explaining apraxic signs. They propose tasks which hold phonologic requirements stable while articulatory or motor requirements are being systematically altered. Having subjects perform the same utterance several times at different rates or with and without a bite block (Netsell 1985) to stabilize the jaw are examples. It can be hypothesized that a motor performance deficit would function differently under different conditions while an intact motor performance system would be relatively uninfluenced or no more influenced than the normal speaker's system.

Other neural scientists are also advocating different models and experimental paradigms to guide the next generation of research into the mechanisms underlying conditions such as speech apraxia. Despite some reservations (Reed 1982), the movement appears to be toward adapting models of motor control, many of which are constructed hierarchically and thereby capable of accommodating the now popularly recognized interactions of cognitive, linguistic, and motor systems. Rosenbek/Kent/LaPointe (1984) review a variety of these explanatory concepts. One of the most elaborate attempts to apply models to normal and apraxic movements belongs to Kent/McNeil (1987). They try to account for the influence of a host of cognitive, affective, linguistic, and motor variables on normal and apraxic speech performance. Their model, like the others previously alluded to, deserves to be studied in the original. They are introduced here primarily as support for the observation that the challenges to explain speech apraxia continue.

9. Diagnosis

Speech diagnosis requires creating and testing hypotheses about what a speaker has until the number of possibilities is as small as can be and confidence in one of those possibilities is as high as can be. Speech apraxia's signs frequently co-exist with the signs of other similar conditions. In addition, speech apraxia shares many signs, such as speech sound distortions, with other conditions, such as dysarthria. Therefore, diagnosis requires a battery of speech and oral motor tests and measures of language, cognition, and any other ability such as hearing, which, if impaired, could contribute to a speaker's sounding apraxic. It also requires considerable clinical acumen.

Wertz/LaPointe/Rosenbek (1984) describe an elaborate battery. They recommend formal language tests such as the Boston Diagnostic Aphasia Examination (Goodglass/Kaplan 1972) and the Aachen Aphasia Test (Huber/Poeck/Willmes 1984). Such tests of reading, writing, auditory and reading comprehension, and special skills are necessary especially to establish the presence and severity of aphasia. Wertz/LaPointe/Rosenbek (1984) also suggest a speech evaluation involving tasks to elicit spontaneous and imitiative speech, diadochokinesis, and measures of variability. These tasks provide controlled responses which the clinician can evaluate for signs of speech apraxia. Comparing spontaneous and imitative speech informs about the possibility of a conduction aphasia, because conduction aphasia and speech apraxia can sound similar in connected speech and different during imitation. Diadochokinetic testing can help rule out a dysarthria. Because all slowness or irregularity on such testing is not necessarily dysarthric, however, there is an additional need for a measure of variability such as having the speaker say the same utterance several times. Most dysarthric speakers will be reasonably consistent and most apraxic speakers will be reasonably variable on such a task.

Even this much testing may leave the diagnosis in doubt, however. Repeating the test battery, or portions of it, or using more sensitive tests of one or more ability may help. Kent/Kent (1988) created a flow chart that orders the special procedures that may increase a diagnostician's confidence about the diagnosis. They recommend four types of assessment. The first is the evaluation of prosody. The second is a collection of 'performance load tests' in which response length, rate, phonetic complexity, and other variables known to influence speech apraxia are systematically manipulated. The third is the traditional measurement of bulbar function during nonspeech tasks, including procedures contained in oral, nonverbal apraxia testing (DeRenzi/Pieczuro/Vignolo 1966). The fourth is maximum performance testing, including vowel prolongation and diadochokinesis with and without a bite block. All these procedures have their pitfalls (Kent/Kent/Rosenbek 1987), but all may help the insightful clinician make decisions.

In the acute stage the best diagnostic test may be treatment. Apraxic speakers respond to different treatments than do speakers with the forms of aphasia and dysarthria. Apraxic speakers hear and try to self-correct with no prompting from the clinician. Apraxic speakers anticipate and try to prevent errors. They are predictably variable and often move closer to targets if the clinician is alert to proper stimulus selection and cueing. Apraxic speakers retain and generalize the lessons of each session. Aphasic and dysarthric speakers may do some or all of these things, but often not to the same degree; hence the value of experience and acumen in sorting through all these responses and arriving at a confident diagnosis.

10. Conclusions

Speech apraxia has been called many things. Some labels seem never to pass across national boundaries, and even if a particular term does travel, the national enthusiasm for its appropriateness is often stopped at the border. Fortunately, neuroscience does not require one vocabulary, and a single enthusiasm would be its death knell. It does require thoughtful hypotheses, careful subject selection and description, exquisite experimental designs and procedures, and clear reporting. Speech apraxia is beginning to benefit from all four. Broca would probably be as pleased as Darley is.

11. References

Abbs, J. H. & Rosenbek, J. C. (1985). Some motor control perspectives on apraxia of speech and dysarthria. In J. Costello (Ed.), *Speech disorders in adults. 21–58.* San Diego: College-Hill Press, Inc.

Adams, J. G., McNeil, M. R. & Weismer, G. (1989, unpublished). Speech movement velocity profiles in neurogenic speech disorders. Paper presented to the American Speech and Hearing Association. St. Louis, Missouri.

Alajouanine, T., Ombredane, A. & Durand, M. (1939). *Le syndrome de disintegration phonetique dans l'aphasic.* Paris: Masson.

Bay, E. (1962). Aphasia and nonverbal disorders of language. *Brain, 85*, 411–426.

Benton, A. (1981). Aphasia: Historical perspectives. In M. T. Sarno (Ed.), *Acquired aphasia. 1–25.* New York: Academic Press, Inc.

Blumstein, S. (1981). Phonological aspects of aphasia. In M. T. Sarno (Ed.), *Acquired aphasia. 192–255.* New York: Academic Press, Inc.

Blumstein, S. E., Cooper, W. E., Goodglass, H., Statlender, S. & Gottlieb, J. (1980). Production deficits in aphasia: A voice-onset time analysis. *Brain and Language, 9*, 153–170.

Blumstein, S. E., Cooper, W. E., Zurif, E. B. & Caramazza, A. (1977). The perception and production of voice-onset time in aphasia. *Neuropsychologia, 15*, 371–383.

Buckingham, H. W. (1979). Explanation in apraxia with consequences for the concept of apraxia of speech. *Brain and Language, 8*, 202–226.

Buckingham, H. W. (1981). A pre-history of the problem of Broca's aphasia. In R. H. Brookshire (Ed.), *Clinical aphasiology: Conference proceedings, 1981. 3–16.* Minneapolis: BRK Publishers.

Critchley, M. (1970). *Aphasiology.* London: Edward Arnold.

Darley, F. L. (1968, unpublished). Apraxia of speech: 107 years of terminological confusion. Paper presented to the American speech and Hearing Association. Denver, Colorado.

Darley, F. L. (1969, unpublished). Input and output disturbances in speech and language processing. Paper presented to the American Speech and Hearing Association. Chicago, Illinois.

Darley, F. L., Aronson, A. E. & Brown, J. R. (1975). *Motor speech disorders.* Philadelphia: W. B. Saunders Company.

Deal, J. L. (1974). Consistency and adaptation in apraxia of speech. *Journal of Communication disorders, 7*, 135–140.

DeRenzi, E., Pieczuro, A. & Vignolo, L. A. (1966). Oral apraxia and aphasia. *Cortex, 2*, 50–73.

Deutsch, S. E. (1984). Prediction of site of lesion from speech apraxic error patterns. In J. C. Rosenbek, M. R. McNeil & A. E. Aronson (Eds.), *Apraxia of speech: Physiology-acoustics-linguistics-management. 113–134.* San Diego: College-Hill Press, Inc.

Duffy, J. R. & Gawle, C. A. (1984). Apraxic speakers' vowel duration in consonant-vowel-consonant syllables. In J. C. Rosenbek, M. R. McNeil & A. E. Aronson (Eds.), *Apraxia of Speech: Physiology-acoustics-linguistics-management. 167–196.* San Diego: College-Hill Press, Inc.

Folkins, J. W. & Bleile, K. M. (1990). Taxonomies in biology, phonetics, phonology, and speech motor control. *Journal of Speech and Hearing Disorders, 55*, 596–611.

Forrest, K., Adams, S. & McNeil, M. R. (1991). Perioral EMG activity in aphasic, apraxic, and dysarthric speakers. In C. Moore, D. Beukelman & K. Yorkston (Eds.), *Motor speech disorders: Management approaches.* 147–171. Austin: pro-ed.

Forrest, K., Weismer, G. & Adams, S. (1990). Statistical comparison of movement amplitudes from groupings of normal geriatric speakers. *Journal of Speech and Hearing Research, 33*, 286–389.

Freeman, F. J., Sands, E. S. & Harris, K. S. (1978). Temporal coordination of phonation and articulation in a case of verbal apraxia: A voice onset time study. *Brain and Language, 6*, 106–111.

Goodglass, H. & Kaplan, E. (1972). *The assessment of aphasia and related disorders.* Philadelphia: Lea and Febiger.

Hardcastle, W. J. (1987). Electropalatographic study of articulation disorders in verbal dyspraxia. In J. H. Ryalls (Ed.), *Phonetic approaches to speech production in aphasia and related disorders. 113–136.* Boston: A College-Hill Publication, Little, Brown and Company.

Head, H. (1926). *Aphasia and kindred disorders of speech. Volume 1.* London: Cambridge University Press.

Hoit, J., Murry, T. & Kopp, H. G. (1983). Voice onset time production and perception in apraxic subjects. *Brain and Language, 20*, 329–339.

Hough, M. S. & Klich, R. J. (1987). Effects of word length on lip EMG activity in apraxia of speech. In R. H. Brookshire (Ed.), *Clinical aphasiology, Volume 17. 271–276.* Minneapolis: BRK Publishers.

Huber, W., Poeck, K. & Willmes, K. (1984). The Aachen aphasia test. In F. C. Rose (Ed.), *Advances in neurology, volume 42, progress in aphasiology. 291–303.* New York: Raven Press.

Itoh, M. & Sasanuma, S. (1987). Articulatory velocities of aphasic patients. In J. H. Ryalls (Ed.), *Phonetic approaches to speech production in aphasia and related disorders. 137–161.* Boston: A College-Hill Production, Little, Brown and Company.

Itoh, M., Sasanuma, S., Hirose, H., Yoshioka, H. & Ushijima, T. (1980). Abnormal articulatory dynamics in a patient with apraxia of speech: X-ray microbeam observation. *Brain and Language, 11*, 66–75.

Itoh, M., Sasanuma, S., Tatsumi, I., Murakami, S., Fukusako, Y. & Suzuki, T. (1982). Voice onset time characteristics in apraxia of speech. *Brain and Language, 17*, 193–210.

Itoh, M., Sasanuma, S. & Ushijima, T. (1979). Valar movements during speech in a patient with apraxia of speech. *Brain and Language, 7*, 227–239.

Jackson, H. (1878). Remarks on non-protrusion of the tongue in some cases of aphasia. *Lancet, 1*, 716.

Johns, D. F. & Darley, F. L. (1970). Phonemic variability in apraxia of speech. *Journal of Speech and Hearing Research, 13*, 556–583.

Kent, R. D. & Kent, J. F. (1988). Motor speech disorders. In D. E. Yoder & R. D. Kent (Eds.), *Decision-making in speech-language pathology. 154–155.* Toronto: B. C. Decker, Inc.

Kent, R. D., Kent, J. F. & Rosenbek, J. C. (1987). Maximum performance tests of speech production. *Journal of Speech and Hearing Disorders, 52,* 367–387.

Kent, R. D. & McNeil, M. R. (1987). Relative timing of sentence repetition in apraxia of speech and conduction aphasia. In J. H. Ryalls (Ed.), *Phonetic approaches to speech production in aphasia and related disorders. 181–220.* Boston: A College-Hill Production, Little, Brown and Company.

Kent, R. D. & Rosenbek, J. C. (1983). Acoustic patterns of apraxia of speech. *Journal of Speech and Hearing Research, 26,* 231–249.

Kertesz, A. (1984). Subcortical lesions and verbal apraxia. In J. C. Rosenbek, M. R. McNeil & A. E. Aronson (Eds.), *Apraxia of speech: Physiology-acoustics-linguistics-management. 73–90.* San Diego: College-Hill Press, Inc.

LaPointe, L. L. & Horner, J. (1976). Repeated trials of words by patients with neurogenic phonological selection-sequencing impairment (apraxia of speech). In R. H. Brookshire (Ed.), *Clinical aphasiology: Conference proceedings. 261–277.* Minneapolis: BRK Publishers.

Lebrun, Y. (1976). Neurolinguistic models of language and speech. In H. Whitaker & H. A. Whitaker (Eds.), *Studies in neurolinguistics, Volume 1, 1–30.* New York: Academic Press.

Lebrun, Y., Buyssens, E. & Henneaux, J. (1973). Phonetic aspects of anarthria. *Cortex, 9,* 126–135.

Lecours, A. R. & Lhermitte, F. (1969). Phonemic paraphasias: Linguistic structures and tentative hypotheses. *Cortex, 5,* 193–228.

Lecours, A. R., Nespoulous, J. L. & Pioger, D. (1987). Jacques Lordat or the birth of cognitive neuropsychology. In E. Keller & M. Gopnik (Eds.), *Motor and sensory processes of language, 1–16.* New Jersey: Lawrence Erlbaum Associates, Publishers.

Lesser, R. (1978). *Linguistic investigations of aphasia.* London: Edward Arnold.

Liepmann, H. (1913). Motor aphasia, anarthria, and apraxia. *Translations of the 17th international congress of medicine (London). Section X1, Part 2,* 97–106.

Luria, A. R. (1970). *Traumatic aphasia: Its syndromes, psychology and treatment.* The Hague: Mouton.

McNeil, M. R. & Adams, S. (1991). A comparison of speech kinematics among apraxic, conduction aphasic, ataxic dysarthric and normal geriatric speakers. In T. E. Prescott (Ed.), *Clinical aphasiology, Volume 19.* 279–294. Austin: pro-ed.

McNeil, M. R., Caligiuri, M. & Rosenbek, J. C. (1989). A comparison of labio-mandibular kinematic durations, displacements, velocities and dysmetrias on apraxic and normal adults. In T. E. Prescott (Ed.), *Clinical aphasiology, Volume 18. 173–193.* Boston: A College-Hill Production, Little, Brown and Company.

McNeil, M. R. & Kent, R. (1990). Motoric characteristics of adult aphasic and apraxic speakers. In G. R. Hammond (Ed.), *Advances in psychology: cerebral control of speech and limb movements.* 349–386. New York: Elsevier/North Holland.

McNeil, M. R., Liss, J., Tseng, C.-H. & Kent, R. D. (1990). Effects of speech rate on the absolute and relative timing of apraxic, and conduction aphasic sentence production. *Brain and Language, 38,* 135–158.

McNeil, M. R., Prescott, T. E. & Lemme, M. L. (1976). An application of electromyographic biofeedback to aphasia/apraxia treatment. In R. H. Brookshire (Ed.), *Clinical aphasiology: Conference proceedings, 1976. 151–171.* Minneapolis: BRK Publishers.

McNeil, M. R., Weismer, G., Adams, S. & Mulligan, M. (1990). Oral structure nonspeech motor control in normal, dysarthric, aphasic and apraxic speakers: Isometric force and static position control. *Journal of Speech and Hearing Research, 33,* 255–268.

Mlcoch, A. G. & Noll, J. D. (1980). Speech production models as related to the concept of apraxia of speech. *Speech and Language, 4,* 201–238.

Mohr, J. P., Pessin, M. S., Finkelstein, S., Funkenstein, H. H., Duncan, G. W. & Davis, K. R. (1978). Broca aphasia: Pathologic and clinical. *Neurology, 28,* 311–324.

Munhall, K. G. (1989). Articulatory variability. In P. Square-Storer (Ed.), *Acquired apraxia of speech in aphasic adults. 64–83.* London: Taylor and Francis.

Netsell, R. (1985). Construction and use of a bite-block in evaluating and treating speech disorders. *Journal of Speech and Hearing Disorders, 50,* 103–106.

Odell, K., McNeil, M. R., Rosenbek, J. C. & Hunter, L. (1990). Perceptual characteristics of consonant productions by apraxic speakers. *Journal of Speech and Hearing Disorders, 55,* 345–359.

Odell, K., McNeil, M. R., Rosenbek, J. C. & Hunter, L. (1991). A perceptual comparison of prosodic features in apraxia of speech and conduction aphasia. In T. E. Prescott (Ed.), *Clinical aphasiology, Volume 19. 295–306.* Austin: pro-ed.

Odell, K., McNeil, M. R., Rosenbek, J. C. & Hunter, L. (1991). Perceptual characteristics of vowel and prosody production in apraxic, aphasic, and dysarthric speakers. *Journal of Speech and Hearing Research, 34,* 67–80.

Reed, E. S. (1982). An outline of a theory of action systems. *Journal of Motor Behavior, 14,* 98–134.

Robin, D. A., Bean, C. & Folkins, J. W. (1989). Lip movement in apraxia of speech. *Journal of Speech and Hearing Research, 32*, 512–523.

Robin, D. A. & Schienberg, S. (1990). Subcortical lesions and aphasia. *Journal of Speech and Hearing Disorders, 55*, 90–100.

Rosenbek, J. C., Kent, R. D. & LaPointe, L. L. (1984). Apraxia of speech: An overview and some perspectives. In J. C. Rosenbek, M. R. McNeil & A. E. Aronson (Eds.), *Apraxia of speech: Physiology-acoustics-linguistics-management. 1–72.* San Diego: College-Hill Press, Inc.

Rosenbek, J. C., McNeil, M., Teetson, M., Odell, K. & Collins, M. (1981). A syndrome of neuromotor speech deficit and dysphagia. In R. H. Brookshire (Ed.), *Clinical aphasiology: Conference proceedings, 1981. 309–315.* Minneapolis: BRK Publishers.

Ryalls, J. H. (1981). Motor aphasia: Acoustic correlates of phonetic disintegration in vowels. *Neuropsychologia, 19*, 365–374.

Shankweiler, D. & Harris, K. S. (1966). An experimental approach to the problem of articulation in aphasia. *Cortex, 2*, 277–297.

Shankweiler, D., Harris, K. S. & Taylor, M. L. (1968). Electromyographic studies of articulation in aphasia. *Archives of Physical Medicine and Rehabilitation, 49*, 1–8.

Shewan, C. M., Leeper, H. A. & Booth, J. C. (1984). An analysis of voice onset time (VOT) in aphasic and normal subjects. In J. C. Rosenbek, M. R. McNeil & A. E. Aronson (Eds.), *Apraxia of speech: Physiology-acoustics-linguistics-management. 197–220.* San Diego: College-Hill Press, Inc.

Square, P. A., Darley, F. L. & Sommers, R. K. (1982). An analysis of the productive errors made by pure apraxic speakers with differing loci of lesions. In R. H. Brookshire (Ed.), *Clinical aphasiology: Conference proceedings, 1982. 245–250.* Minneapolis: BRK Publishers.

Strand, E. A. (1987, unpublished). Acoustic and response time measures in utterance production: A comparison of apraxic and normal speakers. Doctoral dissertation, University of Wisconsin-Madison: Madison, Wisconsin.

Strand, E. A. & McNeil, M. R. (1987). Evidence for a motor performance deficit versus a misapplied rule system in the temporal organization of utterances in apraxia of speech. In R. H. Brookshire (Ed.), *Clinical aphasiology, Volume 17. 260–270.* Minneapolis: BRK Publishers.

Towne, R. L. & Crary, M. A. (1988). Verbal reaction time patterns in aphasic adults: Consideration for apraxia of speech. *Brain and Language, 35*, 138–153.

Tuller, B. (1984). On categorizing aphasic speech errors. *Neuropsychologia, 22*, 547–557.

Weismer, G. (1984). Acoustic descriptions of dysarthric speech: Perceptual correlates and physiological inferences. In J. C. Rosenbek (Ed.), *Current views of dysarthria. 293–314.* Seminars in speech and language. Volume 5, Number 4. New York: Thieme Inc.

Wertz, R. T., LaPonte, L. L. & Rosenbek, J. C. (1984). *Apraxia of speech in adults: The disorder and its management.* Orlando, Florida: Grune and Stratton.

Ziegler, W. (1984). What can the spectral characteristics of stop consonants tell us about the realization of place of articulation in Broca's Aphasia? A reply to Shinn and Blumstein. *Brain and Language, 23*, 167–170.

Ziegler, W. & von Cramon, D. (1986). Timing deficits in apraxia of speech. *European Archives of Psychiatry and Neurological Sciences, 236*, 44–49.

John C. Rosenbek, Madison, Wisconsin (USA)

41. Spastic Dysarthria

1. Introduction

Spastic dysarthria designates a speech disorder resulting from an inferred or demonstrated neurologic condition of spasticity, or upper motor neuron lesion. The description of the speech disorder therefore is twofold: analysis of the speech abnormalities, and consideration of the underlying pathophysiology in relation to the speech disturbances.

1.1. Terminology

Spasticity is a neurologic term that denotes a syndrome of hypertonus with exaggeration of stretch reflexes, resulting from lesions to the corticobulbar or corticospinal tracts. A frequently cited definition of spasticity is from

Lance (1980): spasticity is a motor disorder characterized by a velocity-dependent increase in tonic stretch reflexes ("muscle tone") with exaggerated tendon jerks, resulting from hyperexcitability of the stretch reflex, as one important component of the upper motor neuron syndrome. Clinically, spasticity is usually accompanied by paresis so that characterization of the motor impairment is twofold (Delwaide/Young 1985).

1.2. Relationship between Speech and Neurologic Impairment

First, it should be stressed that spasticity is a heterogeneous disorder, with the severity, distribution, and nature of clinical signs varying with the localization and combination of lesions as well as with the time between examination and insult (Delwaide/Young 1985). Not all individuals with spasticity have a speech disturbance. Unilateral damage often is associated with spastic hemiplegia, in which speech disturbances tend to be transient or mild, but bilateral damage, or pseudobulbar palsy, is more serious and can produce severe dysarthria (Edwards 1984; Love/Webb 1986). The unilateral form is less impairing to speech because the speech muscles generally receive bilateral innervation from the cranial nerves. The dysarthria associated with spasticity is variously termed spastic dysarthria, upper motor neuron dysarthria, or pseudobulbar dysarthria. The speech disturbances often result from impairments in the respiratory, laryngeal and upper airway (supraglottal) systems. Spastic dysarthria is distinguished from spastic (spasmodic) dysphonia which has different characteristics and perhaps a different etiology, or etiologies (Schaefer 1983).

2. Attributes of Spastic Dysarthria

The speech characteristics associated with spastic dysarthria have been reported for both acquired dysarthria (pseudobulbar palsy) and congenital dysarthria (the latter appearing in children with spastic cerebral palsy). Reports in the literature usually discuss these two forms of the disorder separately and this account will do likewise.

2.1. Pseudobulbar Dysarthria

In the classic description and classification of dysarthria, Darley/Aronson/Brown (1969 a, b; 1975) rated 38 auditory-perceptual dimensions of dysarthric speech and identified the most prominent clusters of dimensions for several types of dysarthria. Their data for acquired spastic dysarthria (pseudobulbar palsy) indicated the following ranked dimensions characteristic of the speech disorder: 1 – imprecise consonants; 2 – monopitch; 3 – reduced stress; 4 – harsh voice; 5 – monoloudness; 6 – pitch level; 7 – rate; 8 – hypernasal; 9 – strained-strangled voice; and 10 – short phrases. Several of these dimensions (imprecise consonants, monopitch, harsh voice, monoloudness, rate, hypernasal and short phrases) were commonly associated with other dysarthric types identified by Darley et al. The dimensions of pitch level, reduced stress and strained-strangled voice were more narrowly associated with spastic dysarthria. It is noteworthy that the deviant dimensions embrace a number of voice and resonance qualities.

Enderby's work (1983; 1986) paralleled that of Darley/Aronson/Brown in her attempts to identify distinguishing characteristics of dysarthric groups. With respect to spastic dysarthria, she reported the main characteristics to be: poor movement of the tongue in speech, slow rate of speech, poor phonation and intonation, poor intelligibility in conversation, reduced alternating movements of the tongue, poor lip movements in speech, reduced maintenance of palatal elevation, poor intelligibility of description, hypernasality and lack of control in volume. As in the case of the Darley/Aronson/Brown studies, Enderby's analyses point to several dimensions of speech and voice impairment.

Whereas perceptual rating is the predominant method used in clinical assessment, acoustic and physiologic methods are an increasing source of information in clinical practice and research. Acoustic measurements of diadochokinetic syllable repetition reported by Portnoy/Aronson (1982) showed that spastic patients were both slower and more variable than normal-speaking controls. X-ray observations of spastic dysarthria indicate that the speech movements are slow and of restricted range (Kent/Netsell/Bauer 1975; Hirose/Kiritani/Sawashima 1980). Ziegler/von Cramon (1986) concluded from an acoustic study that gross lingual movements were more impaired for the dorsum than for the blade. The acoustic measures also showed that spastic subjects, relative to normals, had increased word and syllable duration, centralized vowels and ineffectively articulated plosives. The spastic subjects tended to have a retracted tongue position, which was judged to contribute to their speech difficulties. Ziegler/von Cramon (1986) reported that spastic subjects often had considerable difficulty with the task of rapid diphthong repetition. Some subjects experienced an articulatory breakdown shortly after beginning the task, whereas others accomplished the task with slow, prolonged articulatory movements. The interpretation for this difficulty was that the spastic subjects were impaired in their ability to alter rapidly the synergistic-antagonist patterns of muscle activation.

These x-ray and acoustic data help to explain the high ratings for the dimension of imprecise consonants in the Darley/Aronson/Brown (1969 a) results for spastic dysarthria. They also help to identify sensitive tasks for speech assessment. For example, the Ziegler/von Cramon (1986) study suggests that rapid repetition of diphthongs is a sensitive speech task.

2.2. Dysarthria in Spastic Cerebral Palsy

Early reports on the dysarthria in spastic cerebral palsy in children were inconsistent in their description of speech characteristics. Many of these studies attempted with little success to define the differences in speech and voice between athetoid and spastic cerebral palsy (Byrne 1959; Hedges 1955; Irwin 1955; Leith 1954; Rutherford 1939; Shapiro 1960). More recently, Workinger/Kent (1991) reported that although the differences between the two types of dysarthria are subtle, the most characteristic dimensions of each were as follows: spastic – consistent hypernasality, breathy voice, and voice quality change; athetoid – reduced stress, inappropriate voice stoppage or release; and slow rate. The most characteristic dimensions for the children with spastic cerebral palsy pertained to resonance and voice quality, whereas the most characteristic dimensions for the athetoid group indicated difficulties with timing and coordination of movements. Workinger/Kent also reported that experienced listeners could distinguish spastic and athetoid speakers. Earlier research with inexperienced listeners failed to demonstrate a differentiation of the two types (Hedges 1955, Shapiro 1960).

2.3. Similarities between the Acquired and Congenital Dysarthrias

Some similarities can be seen between the results summarized above from the Workinger/Kent study of congenital spastic vs athetoid cerebral palsy and the results obtained by Darley/Aronson/Brown for the similar neurologic pairing of spastic (pseudobulbar) vs slow hyperkinesia (dystonia) dysarthria in adults. The uniquely characterizing features for the two groups studied by Darley/Aronson/Brown were: Spastic – low pitch; hypernasality, pitch breaks, breathy voice, and excess and equal stress; slow hyperkinesic – irregular articulatory breakdowns, inappropriate silences, prolonged intervals and phonemes, excessive loudness variation and voice stoppage. Common features between the congenital and acquired forms of spastic dysarthria are hypernasality, breathy voice, and change in voice quality or pitch. Common features between congenital athetoid and acquired dystonic dysarthria are voice stoppages and slow rate (the latter being equivalent to prolonged intervals and phonemes).

3. The Pathophysiology of Spasticity

The usual neurologic characterization of spasticity is in terms of increased limb tone (claspknife type of resistance to passive movement), exaggerated tendon jerks and clonus, Babinski responses in the lower extremities, and impairment of voluntary control of skeletal muscles. The pathophysiology has been described in terms of a twofold imbalance between excess excitation (such as increased phasic stretch reflexes) and deficient inhibition (such as suppression of the tonic vibration reflex, reflex irradiation and abnormal silent intervals in an electromyogram).

Myklebust/Gottlieb/Penn/Agarwal (1982) drew attention to another neurological feature in patients with spasticity resulting from perinatal suprasegmental insults. They determined from electromyographic recordings that these patients had a "reciprocal excitation," a phenomenon in which segmental stretch reflexes are simultaneously expressed in the agonist, stretched muscle and the antagonistic, shortening muscle. This pattern contrasts with the normal pattern of reciprocal inhibition. Myklebust/Gottlieb/Penn/Agarwal concluded that their results require an expansion of the classic definition of cerebral palsy as a disorder involving solely the brain. Their suggested redefinition includes damage to the "immature suprasegmental structure that imposes a secondary, developmental disorder on the spinal cord" (Myklebust/Gottlieb/Penn/Agarwal 1982, 373).

The nonspeech (feeding) movements of biting, sucking, swallowing and chewing were compared with speech articulation in a group of 60 cerebral-palsied subjects by Love/Hagerman/Taimi (1980). Although the nonspeech and speech performances were related, individual subjects did not necessarily exhibit the group pattern. For example, of 19 subjects who were rated as having no speech, two of them had adequate feeding skills. Love/Hagerman/Taimi also reported that there was no systematic relationship between speech ability and the presence of abnormal oral reflexes.

Barlow/Abbs (1984) investigated the ability of subjects with congenital spasticity to regulate fine forces in the lips, tongue and jaw. These three muscle systems differ in the density of muscle spindles and presence of monosynaptic reflexes. The lips apparently lack spindles, the tongue contains a modest number of spindles in some fibers, and the jaw is comparatively well endowed with spindles. If hyperactivity of muscle-spindle monosynaptic reflexes were a primary determinant of the motor impairment in spasticity, then it would be predicated that the three muscle systems would be impaired to different degrees. The results indicted that, generally, force control was poorest for the tongue and nearly equivalent for the lips and jaw. This result argues against the explanation of impaired orofacial movements in terms of hyperactivity of muscle-spindle monosynaptic reflexes. Although Barlow/Abbs reported that their spastic subjects had difficulties in fine force control, Ziegler/von Cramon (1986) observed relatively little impairment in the ability of their spastic subjects to sustain a fricative articulation (which was considered to be a task involving fine force control).

Neilson/O'Dwyer (1981) similarly concluded that hypertonus is a not a causal factor in the impaired speech movements of spastic subjects. In asking what does cause the dysarthria in cerebral palsy, they pointed to a possible motor learning deficit as proposed by Kent/Netsell (1978) for athetoid cerebral palsy. They explained that if "motor commands are generated on the basis of previously learned correlations between motor events and their sensory consequences ..., then impairment of sensory-motor integration processes involved in establishing such correlations should disrupt the ability to formulate appropriate motor commands" (Kent/Netsell 1978, 1018). In this connection, the results of Mykelbust/Gottlieb/Penn/Agarwal should be recalled: a developmental disorder may contribute to the motor impairment in spastic cerebral palsy. Evarts (1985) proposed that the negative symptoms following pyramidal tract lesions could be explained in terms of emergent features in the motor cortex. Specifically, he pointed to impairment of emergent properties of pyramidal tract neurons associated with short-latency, goal-oriented and set-dependent movements.

A direction for future research, then, is to identify the aspects of spasticity that are most closely associated with impaired movements. Recent research does not indicate that hypertonus is the only, or even the primary, cause of the movement disorder. Particularly with respect to speech movements, it may be necessary to consider the participation of the motor cortex in the regulation of the affected musculature.

4. Management of the Individual with Spastic Dysarthria

Medical management typically relies on chemotherapy for the spasticity (accompanying paralysis is not treatable by such means). The primary agents are benzodiazepines (especially diazepam), baclofen and dantrolene (Helme 1986). Physical therapy often is useful, especially to prevent contracture. Less frequently used managements include peripheral nerve blockade, electrical stimulation of the cerebellum, and intrathecal phenol injection.

Suggestions for speech management have been discussed by Aten (1983), who relied heavily on the Darley/Aronson/Brown (1969 a) rating system to identify the speech abnormalities and plan respective treatments. Aten recommended that treatment begin with the most deviant perceptual dimension. He suggested specific interventions aimed at the following objectives: facilitating air flow, improving intelligibility, reducing hyperadduction of the vocal folds, reducing length of utterance, and achieving muscular and emotional balance. Linebaugh/Wolfe (1984) noted that intelligibility and naturalness decreased as syllable duration increased in spastic speakers. This result may mean that reduction of word and syllable durations is a reasonable goal for speech management. However, there is no clear evidence to show that shortening of durations will of itself lead to improved intelligibility. Vogel/von Cramon (1983) described articulatory recovery in five patients with traumatic mutism, three of whom presented with spasticity. Recovery of articulatory ability was summarized in terms of four stages, which, with the exception of one patient, spanned an interval of three months or less.

5. References

Aten, J. L. (1983). Treatment of spastic dysarthria. In W. H. Perkins (Ed.), *Current Therapy of Communication Disorders. Dysarthria and Apraxia. 69–77.* New York: Thieme-Stratton.

Barlow, S. M. & Abbs, J. H. (1984). Orofacial fine motor control impairments in congenital spasticity: Evidence against hypertonus-related performance deficits. *Neurology, 34,* 145–150.

Byrne, M. (1959). Speech and language development of athetoid and spastic children. *Journal of Speech and Hearing Research, 24,* 231–240.

Darley, F. L., Aronson, A. E., & Brown, J. R. (1969 a). Differential diagnostic patterns of dysarthria. *Journal of Speech and Hearing Research, 12,* 246–269.

Darley, F. L., Aronson, A. E., & Brown, J. R. (1969 b). Clusters of deviant speech dimensions in the dysarthrias. *Journal of Speech and Hearing Research, 12,* 462–496.

Darley, F., Aronson, A., & Brown, J. (1975). *Motor Speech Disorders.* Philadelphia: W. B. Saunders.

Delwaide, P. J. & Young, R. R. (1985). *Clinical Neurophysiology in Spasticity.* Amsterdam: Elsevier.

Edwards, M. (1984). *Disorders of Articulation.* Wien: Springer-Verlag.

Enderby, P. (1983). *Frenchay Dysarthria Assessment.* San Diego: College-Hill.

Enderby, P. (1986). Relationships between dysarthric groups. *British Journal of Disorders of Communication, 21,* 189–197.

Evarts, E. V. (1985). Emergent features in motor cortex as keys to negative symptoms following pyramidal tract lesions. In P. J. & Delwaide R. R. Young (Eds.), *Clinical Neurophysiology in Spasticity. 13–25.* Amsterdam: Elsevier.

Hedges, T. A. (1955). The relationship between speech understandability and the diadochokinetic rates of certain speech musculatures among individuals with cerebral palsy. Unpublished doctoral dissertation, Ohio State University, Columbus, Ohio, U.S.A.

Helme, R. D. (1986). Movement disorders. In M. A. Samuels (Ed.), *Manual of Neurologic Therapeutics,* 3rd Ed. *316–334.* Boston: Little, Brown.

Hirose, H., Kiritani, S., & Sawashima, M. (1980). Patterns of dysarthric movements in patients with amyotrophic lateral sclerosis and pseudobulbar palsy. *Annual Bulletin of the Research Institute of Logopedics and Phoniatrics* (Tokyo) *14,* 263–272.

Irwin, O. C. (1955). Phonetic equipment of spastic and athetoid children. *Journal of Speech and Hearing Disorders, 20,* 54–57.

Kent, R. D. & Netsell, R. (1978). Articulatory abnormalities in athetoid cerebral palsy. *Journal of Speech and Hearing Disorders, 43,* 353–373.

Kent, R. D., Netsell, R., & Bauer, L. L. (1975). Cineradiographic assessment of articulatory mobility in the dysarthrias. *Journal of Speech and Hearing Disorders, 40,* 467–480.

Lance, J. W. (1980). Symposium synopsis. In R. G. Feldman, R. R. Young, & W. P. Keollo (Eds.), *Spasticity: Disordered Motor Control. 485–494.* Chicago: Year Book Publishers.

Leith, W. R. (1954). A comparison of judged speech characteristics of athetoids and spastics. Unpublished master's thesis, Purdue University, West Lafayette, Indiana, U.S.A.

Linebaugh, C. W. & Wolfe, V. E. (1984). Relationships between articulation rate, intelligibility, and naturalness in spastic and ataxic speakers. In M. R. McNeil, J. C. Rosenbek, & A. E. Aronson (Eds.), *The Dysarthrias: Physiology, Acoustics, Perception, Management. 197–205.* San Diego: College-Hill Press.

Love, R. J., Hagerman, E. L., & Taimi, E. G. (1980). Speech performance, dysphagia and oral reflexes in cerebral palsy. *Journal of Speech and Hearing Disorders, 45,* 59–75.

Love, R. J. & Webb, W. G. (1986). *Neurology for the Speech-Language Pathologist.* New York: Butterworths.

Myklebust, B. M., Gottlieb, G. L., Penn, R. D., & Agarwal, G. C. (1982). Reciprocal excitation of antagonistic muscles as a differentiating feature in spasticity. *Annals of Neurology, 12,* 367–374.

Neilson, P. D. & O'Dwyer, N. J. (1981). Pathophysiology of dysarthria in cerebral palsy. *Journal of Neurology, Neurosurgery and Psychiatry, 44,* 1013–1019.

Portnoy, R. A. & Aronson, A. E. (1982). Diadochokinetic syllable rate and regularity in normal and in spastic and ataxic dysarthric speakers. *Journal of Speech and Hearing Disorders, 47,* 324–328.

Rutherford, B. (1939). Frequency of articulation substitutions in children handicapped by cerebral palsy. *Journal of Speech and Hearing Disorders, 4,* 285–287.

Schaefer, S. (1983). Neuropathology of spasmodic dysphonia. *Laryngoscope, 93,* 1183–1204.

Shapiro, J. (1960). An investigation of the ability of auditors to assess athetoid and spastic cerebral palsy by listening to speech samples. Unpublished master's thesis, Syracuse University, Syracuse, New York, U.S.A.

Workinger, M. S. & Kent, R. D. (1991). Perceptual analysis of the dysarthrias in children with athetoid and spastic cerebral palsy. In C. Moore, K. Yorkston & D. Beukelman (Eds.), *Dysarthria and Apraxia of Speech: Perspectives on Management*. Baltimore, Maryland: Brookes Publishing Co.

Vogel, M. & Cramon, D. von (1983). Articulatory recovery after traumatic mutism. *Folia Phoniatrica, 35*, 294–309.

Ziegler, W. & Cramon, D. von (1986). Spastic dysarthria after acquired brain injury: An acoustic study. *The British Journal of Disorders of Communication, 21*, 173–187.

Raymond D. Kent, Madison, Wisconsin (USA)

42. Flaccid Dysarthria

1. Introduction

Flaccid dysarthria (also referred to as 'peripheral dysarthria', or 'lower motor neuron dysarthria') results from damage to the peripheral nervous system (PNS). The PNS can be affected by a wide variety of disease processes, and the damage to speech functions can be quite selective. This chapter, therefore, will present an overview of the peripheral neuromuscular structures involved in speech, and will look at those disorders of the PNS which lead to dysarthric speech symptoms. The structures involved include the brainstem nuclei of the cranial nerves mentioned below which carry motor and/or sensory information, the anterior horn cells and the peripheral nerves involved in breathing, the neuromuscular junction, and the muscles. The clinical results of lower motor neuron disease are most obvious when there is complete damage to the peripheral nerve as caused by trauma. The immediate effect is complete paralysis of dependent muscles, regional loss of sensation, and progressive atrophy of the muscles as a result of disuse; the degree of atrophy is proportional to the number of damaged nerve fibers. Reflexes are absent. The muscles also become lax (flaccid). Electromyographic investigation shows characteristic changes. In most neurogenic diseases the effects of denervation appear more slowly than in the case mentioned above. The resistance of muscles to passive movements is decreased, a condition known as hypotonia. Further clinical signs of neurogenic disorders are fasciculations (visible twitches of muscle), and fibrillations which are only detectable by electromyography. Fasciculations are typical for slowly progressing diseases and are uncommon in peripheral neuropathies.

2. Peripheral Neuromuscular Structures and Speech Characteristics Associated with Flaccid Dysarthria

More than any other type of dysarthria, flaccid dysarthria is far from being a uniform syndrome. The speech symptoms vary depending upon which particular nerve(s) and/or muscles are primarily affected. The neurology of flaccid dysarthria therefore necessitates a systematic evaluation of several components of the vocal tract, including respiratory, laryngeal, velopharyngeal and orofacial structures. A differentiated knowledge of neuromuscular structures and functions is essential for the clinician so that he/she can identify the overall pattern of motor speech dysfunction and can recognize subtle changes which occur in progressive diseases.

2.1. Respiration

The primary muscles of the respiratory system (inspiratory: diaphragma, external intercostals, and interchondral portion of the internal intercostals; expiratory: rectus abdominis, external and internal oblique abdominis, and transversus abdominis) are innervated by a system involving the multiple innervation patterns provided by the brachial and cervical plexus and direct spinal nerves. The sites of the cell bodies comprise the 3rd–5th cervical and 1st–12th thoracic and 1st lumbar segments of the spinal cord. Clinically significant symptoms of flaccid paralysis of respiratory function (varying depending on the site of motor neuron lesion) may be marked weakness of inspiratory and/or expiratory breathing, short or inadequate linguistic phrasing, decreased vital capacity, reduced loudness, and asymmetrical or abnormal breathing patterns (e. g. "reversed breathing" as defined by Davis 1987). (For details relating to methods of investigation of respiratory function as well as respiratory dysfunction in flaccid dysarthria see Hixon/Putnam/Sharp (1983).)

2.2. Phonation

Two branches of the vagus nerve (X) – the external branch of the superior laryngeal nerve and the recurrent laryngeal nerve are essential to phonatory functions. The intrinsic muscles of the larynx – except the crycothroid – are all supplied by the recurrent laryngeal nerve, a main branch of the cranial nerve X. The external branch of the superior laryngeal nerve carries motor axons to the cricothyroid muscle. – Sensory information from the mucous membrane of the larynx above the level of the vocal folds is carried by branches of the internal laryngeal nerve. The mucous membrane below the level of the vocal folds is supplied by the recurrent laryngeal nerve. Both, the internal and the recurrent laryngeal nerve carry afferent fibers from stretch receptors of the intrinsic laryngeal muscles. Flaccid dysphonia may result from damage to the vagus nerve at any point along its pathway from the nucleus ambiguus in the brainstem to the laryngeal musculature. A lesion above the bifurcation of the pharyngeal branches paralyzes the cricothyroid muscle and all other intrinsic laryngeal muscles on the side of the lesion. The unilateral paralysis or weakness produces breathy or hoarse voice quality, reduced range of pitch and loudness. The affected vocal fold is fixed in an abducted position. In the case of bilateral lesions only whispery voice (aphonia) is possible. If there is a lesion of the recurrent laryngeal nerve only, the vocal fold is fixed in a paramedian position, and voice quality is breathy or hoarse. Bilateral lesion would make breathing difficult. Superior and recurrent laryngeal nerves may be damaged simultaneously or selectively. Consequently, the functions of the intrinsic laryngeal musculature will be either spared or disturbed. Details on the effects of lesions on the vagus nerve as well as information regarding examination techniques and differential diagnosis are described in Aronson (1985, 79–98).

2.3. Articulation

The motor innervation of the articulators of speech is mainly provided by the cranial nerves V, VII, XI, and XII. The supralaryngeal mechanism serves not only as an acoustic resonator but also as a sound generator, with the velopharyngeal valve playing a major role. The principal motor innervation of velar muscles is derived from the cranial accessory nerve, which arises from the nucleus ambiguous in the medulla oblongata. It travels with the vagus nerve, and clinically, disorders of the cranial accessory are regarded as disorders of the vagus nerve. A unilateral lesion will normally cause slight hypernasality. Incomplete velopharyngeal closure caused by bilateral paralysis reduces intraoral pressure and consequently the sharpness of oral consonant production, reducing sound production to only nasal vowels and consonants in its most severe form. Insufficient velopharyngeal valving may also have a major impact on respiration (premature exhaustion of air support) and phonation (loss of voicing contrasts, compensatory hypertension of the vocal folds) as result of nasal air escape.

All intrinsic and extrinsic tongue muscles except the palatoglossus muscle receive their motor innervation from the hypoglossal nerve. It exits the brainstem between the pyramid and the inferior olive, leaving the cranium via the hypoglossal foramen and running caudally and anteriorly to the level of the hyoid bone. Along its route through the tongue it branches off to the extrinsic and intrinsic tongue muscles. In unilateral flaccid paralysis the tongue deviates to the paralyzed side, thus the place of articulation will be slightly shifted. This normally leads to only mild distortion of the lingual consonants. The client frequently judges the impairment to be more severe. Bilateral hypoglossal nerve lesions results in severe loss of the ability to elevate and protrude the tongue as well as to change the shape of the tongue. Depending upon the degree of paresis this condition will primarily affect the manner of articulation, and in cases of severe impairment, articulatory movements are only approximate blurring the differences between vowel and consonant articulation.

Motor innervation for the craniomandibular complex is provided by the mandibular division of the trigeminal nerve. The anterior division of the mandibular branch contains most of the motor nerves supplying the groups opening and closing the jaw. Unilateral trigeminal lesion does not disturb articulatory sound production. Bilateral lesions will, however, severely affect labial consonant and vowel production as well as tongue adduction movements. Labial movements are mainly controlled by the buccal and mandibular branches of the facial (VII) nerve. The facial nerve emerges from the lateral aspect of the brainstem at the lower border of the pons. According to Bernstein/Nelson (1984) the branches of the facial nerve show some variability in their pathway. The buccal branch innervates the orbicularis oris superior, levator labii, buccinator, and zygomaticus muscles, and the muscles of the side of the nose. The mandibular branch innervates the orbicularis oris inferior, depressor anguli oris, depressor labii, and mentalis muscles. Unilateral weakness of the lips following lesions of the facial nerves disturbes production of labial vowels and consonants, particularly clusters of several labial sounds. In bilateral flaccid paralysis, labial sounds are often unintelligible. Finally, it should be mentioned, that changes in the amount of saliva produced in the oral cavity due to damage of the superior salivatory nucleus or to the parasympathetic preganglionic of the facial nerve, will make articulation very labored. The afferent innervation of the articulators concerned with proprioception is complex. The supply of the articulatory apparatus with muscle spindles varies considerably, and cannot be discussed here in detail. Further research into the role of noncontractile element innervation of the speech apparatus would be of considerable value in understanding flaccid dysarthria more fully. For a comprehensive review of the neuroanatomy and neurophysiology of the speech mechanism, see Kuehn/Lemme/Baumgartner (1989).

The clinical characteristics of flaccid dysarthria established by Darley/Aronson/Brown (1969), Carrow/Rivera/Mauldin/Shamblin (1974), and Enderby (1986) refer mainly to those syndromes with multiple damage to lower motor neurons. The rank order of deviant speech dimensions in these studies differ considerably. As indicated earlier, occurrence and prominence of particular speech characteristics depend on which nerves and muscles are affected. Aside from this aspect, they have some prominent features in common, like imprecise consonants, breathiness, hypernasality, harsh voice, and short phrases.

3. Neurological Causes of Flaccid Dysarthria

The following is a brief overview of the major groups of neurologic diseases which may affect the lower motor neurons controlling the muscles used for speech, and the diseases of the muscles themselves. For details see Swash/Schwartz (1988), and Adams/Victor (1985).

3.1. Neurogenic Disorders

Neurogenic disorders are generally classified according to the site of the major pathological process involved.

3.1.1. Motor Neuron Disease

This is a progressive disorder often of unknown origin which may involve both lower and upper motor neurones. A subdivision of motor neuron disease is progressive bulbar palsy with progressive degeneration of the motor nuclei of the lower brainstem. The clinical signs are progressive wasting and weakness of the speech muscles; in later stages the weakness also affects the respiratory muscles. When weakness spreads to the hands, arms, and legs, this condition is then usually referred to as amyotrophic lateral sclerosis. – Prognosis depends on the severity of bulbar involvement; the duration of the disease is generally 2 – 5 years. Less frequent diseases with progressive bulbar weakness and atrophy are the spinal muscular atrophies where dysarthria and dysphagia may develop after several years. – Other rare anterior horn cell diseases with bulbar involvement are syringobulbia, herpes zoster, polyomyelitis or Creutzfeldt-Jakob disease.

3.1.2. Brainstem Lesions

Brainstem syndromes which involve caudal cranial nerves may be caused by vascular disturbances, e. g. occlusion of the vertebral or posterior inferior cerebellar artery leading to ipsilateral cranial nerve V, IX, X, and XI palsy (e. g. Wallenberg or other vascular syndromes). Other causes are tumors, encephalitic processes, or multiple sclerosis.

3.1.3. Damage to Cranial Nerves

Isolated or multiple injuries to the cranial nerves are of varying origins. The nerves may be damaged by intra- or extracranial tumors (e. g., acoustic neurinoma causing compression of the 7th cranial nerve) or meningeal carcinomatosis, aneurysm (e. g., compression of the left laryngeal nerve by an aortic arch aneurysm), trauma (e. g., extensive fractures of the skull), or iatrogenic damage (e. g., to the recurrent laryngeal nerve during thyroid surgery, or damage to the phrenical nerve during puncture of the jugular vein).

3.1.4. Polyneuropathies

Polyneuropathies may be caused by inflammation (viral, bacterial, allergic reactions), intoxication (medication, enviromental toxins), vascular diseases, deficiency diseases, or they may be of genetic origin. Speech may be affected as well as by paresis of particular respiratory muscles (e. g., paresis of the intercostal muscles as in post-diphteric polyneuropathy) and/or by muscles innervated by cranial nerves. The most frequently affected cranial nerves are the facial nerves followed by the glossopharyngeal and vagus nerves. One common acute form is idiopathic polyradiculoneuropathy or Guillain-Barré syndrome. Weakness develops more or less symmetrically in distal muscles over a period of a few days or weeks. Trunk, speech, and respiratory muscles are usually affected later, the facial nerves being more frequently affected than the caudal cranial nerves.

3.2. Disorders of the Neuromuscular Junction

The most common form of this type of disorder is myasthenia gravis. An autoimmune mechanism is thought to operate at the neuromuscular junctions. Repeated or persistent activity of a muscle group exhausts contractile power leading to a progressive paresis; rest may restore strength. Impairment of the muscles involved in speech is an early symptom in 30 % of cases.

3.3. Myopathies

In general, the term myopathy refers to all primary muscle disorders. In polymyositis weakness of facial, pharyngeal, and laryngeal muscles as well as of the respiratory muscles may occur. Muscular dystrophy is highly variable in its clinical symptoms. In some cases selective involvement of speech muscles is described, e. g. as laryngeal and pharyngeal weakness in oculopharyngeal dystrophy or in myotonic dystrophy. Metabolic or endocrine myopathies are rarely relevant.

4. Management

In some cases it may be necessary to focus initial intervention procedures on facilitating vital functions such as chewing or swallowing rather than on optimizing motor speech deficits. The evaluation and management of the patient with disordered oral feeding is discussed in Logeman (1983). — Patients, who are unable to communicate using speech may require a combination of approaches. In addition to dysphagia therapy the patient is provided with an alternative communication system (e. g. a simple alphabet board, or an electronic device). Excellent reviews are available that address this area (Beukelman/Yorkston/Dowden 1984). At a later stage the focus of therapy shifts to the specific treatment of the impaired motor speech.

In the acute stage of bulbar palsy, respiratory functions may also be severely affected due to paralysis of respiratory muscles or the vocal cords. Respiratory assistance or tracheostomy may be necessary. — As it is the case with management of all types of dysarthria, treatment must be based on an accurate evaluation of the speech motor apparatus. This applies particularly to flaccid dysarthria because, as mentioned previously, the different speech muscles may be selectively affected. Linebaugh (1983) recommends process-specific procedures. The choice of treatment focus depends on the relative involvement and the mutual speech process interdependencies. Efficient use of expiratory air flow can best be achieved by elimination of velopharyngeal incompetence by fitting a palatal lift prosthesis and then strengthening respiratory muscles. In Linebaugh's approach, strengthening exercises are assisted by biofeedback methods. — Patients may compensate for their poor respiratory support by using auxiliary respiratory muscles, as reported by Hixon/Putnam/Sharp (1983). Phonatory exercises focus on tension-producing maneuvers. Unilateral recurrent nerve paralysis may be compensated by means of adduction of the intact vocal fold across the midline. Surgical intervention like nerve transfer or Teflon injection may be successful (Crumley/Izdebski/McMiken 1988). In severe articulatory deficits as well as in selectively affected muscle control non-speech drills and tactile stimulation (pressure, stretching, tapping) might be most appropriate. Electrostimulation to restore innervation is not recommended because isometric muscle contraction is not possible. Patients with progressive disease are candidates for learning compensatory strategies, counseling can help to prevent maladaptive strategies or to optimize the 'communication environment'.

5. References

Adams, A. D. & Victor, M. (1985). *Principles of Neurology*. New York: MacGraw-Hill Book Company.

Aronson, A. E. (1985). *Clinical voice disorders*. 2 nd ed. New York/Stuttgart: Thieme.

Bernstein, L. & Nelson, R. (1984). Surgical anatomy of the extraparotid distribution of the facial nerve. *Archives of Otolaryngology, 110*, 177.

Beukelman, D. R., Yorkston, K. M., & Dowden, P. A. (1984). *Communication augmention: a casebook of clinical management*. San Diego: College-Hill Press.

Carrow, E., Rivera, V., Mauldin, M. & Shamblin, L. (1974). Deviant speech characteristics in motor neuron disease, *Archives of Otolaryngology, 100*, 212–218.

Crumley, R. L., Izdebski, K., & McMiken, B. (1988). Nerve transfer versus Teflon injection for vocal fold paralysis. *Laryngoscope, 98*, 1200–1204.

Darley, F. L., Aronson, A. E., & Brown, J. R. (1969). Differential diagnostic patterns of dysarthria. *Journal of Speech and Hearing Research, 12*, 246–269.

Davis, L. F. (1987). Respiration and Phonation in cerebral palsy: a developmental model. *Seminars in Speech and Language, 8*, 101–106.

Enderby, P. (1986). Relationships between dysarthric groups. *British Journal of disorders of Communication, 21*, 151–165.

Hixon, T. J., Putnam, A. H. B., & Sharp, J. P. (1983). Speech production with flaccid paralysis of the rib cage, diaphragm, and abdomen. *Journal of Speech and Hearing Disorders, 48*, 315–327.

Kuehn, D. P., Lemme, M. L., & Baumgartner, J. M. (1989). *Neural bases of speech, hearing, and language*. Boston/Toronto/London: College-Hill Press.

Linebaugh, C. W. (1983). *Treatment of flaccid dysarthria. in Current therapy of communication disorders: dysarthria and apraxia*. New York: Thieme-Stratton.

Logeman, J. A. (1983). *Evaluation and treatment of swallowing disorders*. San Diego: College-Hill Press.

Swash, M. & Schwartz, M. (1988). *Neuromuscular diseases*. Berlin/Heidelberg/New York: Springer.

Mathias Vogel, Munich (Germany)

43. Hypo- and Hyperkinetic Dysarthria

1. Types of Hypokinetic and Hyperkinetic Dysarthria

Hypokinetic dysarthria is characterized by reduced movement and occurs in patients with either Parkinson's disease, Multiple Systems atrophy (or Shy Drager Syndrome) or progressive supranuclear palsy (Steele Richardson Syndrome). Hypokinetic dysarthria is one subtype of akinesia, the inability to move, or speak, at will. The physiological abnormality which interferes with patients' abilities to move at will, has received considerable attention in both the speech and the movement disorders fields. Parkinson's disease is the form of hypokinetic dysarthria most often studied.

The hyperkinetic dysarthrias have received much less attention. Patients with these motor control disorders are unable to regulate their willed movements. In some types of hyperkinetic dysarthria, such as tardive dyskinesia and Huntington's chorea, an involuntary movement may interfere with the execution of the desired movement pattern. In other types, such as oral-mandibular dystonia and the spasmodic dysphonias, some component of the willed movement is excessive and interferes with the execution of the remainder of the movement pattern. The hyperkinetic dysarthrias are less well understood but have several intriguing characteristics which shed light on the organization of speech motor control in the central nervous system. Both the hypo- and hyperkinetic dysarthrias are thought to be the result of disease processes affecting the basal ganglia (Marsden 1982).

Although the hypokinetic and hyperkinetic dysarthrias differ in their speech production impairments, both represent a lack of control during speech execution. In this chapter, first, the characteristics of these disorder are reviewed regarding independent processing stages during speech execution such as: Speech planning, programming during movement execution, speech initiation, movement velocity range, and accuracy, and speech rate. Second, factors which modulate speech symptom occurrence/severity will be discussed and underlying pathophysiology. Finally, a review of these disorders suggests characteristics of the speech execution system.

2. Disorder Characteristics

2.1. Movement Abnormalities

Movement slowing can be manifested in two ways; by delayed movement onsets (akinesia) and by increased movement durations once movement has been initiated (bradykinesia).

2.1.1. Delayed Initiation Times

On limb movement tasks, Parkinson's disease (PD) patients are slower than controls on simple reaction time tasks but not on choice reaction time tasks (Sheridan/Flowers/Hurrell 1987). On simple reaction time tasks, the response type is known and advance planning can be performed before the 'go' signal while in choice reaction time paradigms, planning must be performed after the 'go' signal. Normal subjects are slower on choice than on simple reaction time tasks involving limb movements (Sheridan/Flowers/Hurrell 1987), possibly because movement planning must be performed after the 'go' signal. Because Parkinson patients have the same latency on both simple and choice reaction time tasks and are slower than normal primarily on simple reaction time tasks, their slow performance has been taken to indicate a movement planning disorder (Marsden 1982). On speech simple reaction time tasks, however, PD patients are not impaired in comparison with normal (Ludlow/Connor/Bassich 1987), suggesting that speech planning, and initiation, is not impaired in PD patients.

In hyperkinetic disorders such as spasmodic dysphonia (SD), speech initiation reaction times are slower than normal (Ludlow/Connor 1987), although in other types of hyperkinetic disorders, such as patients with Huntington's chorea, speech reaction times are normal (Ludlow/Connor/Bassich 1987). The increased speech reaction times in SD, however, are not due to a planning disorder because laryngeal movement onset after the 'go' signal was at the same time or earlier than normal, even though the speech onset was delayed (Ludlow/Connor 1987). These patient's delays, then, were due to an execution problem rather than motor planning deficits.

2.1.2. Reduced Movement Speed

In limb movements studies, PD patients have prolonged movement times and reduced movement velocities (Hallett/Khosbin 1980). In speech, however, jaw and lip movement durations are normal (Connor/Abbs/Cole/Gracco 1989) and word, phrase and sentence durations are not prolonged in PD patients (Ludlow/Bassich 1983; 1984; Ludlow/Connor/Bassich 1987). The differences in PD patients performance of limb and speech movement tasks was addressed by Connor/Abbs (1991). The same jaw movement was measured in patients and controls during visual tracking, production of a speech syllable and production of the syllable in a sentence. The PD patients differed from the controls only on the visual tracking task and not on the two speech tasks. The non-speech and speech production tasks differed in their degree of familiarity, complexity and reliance upon visual guidance. The results suggest that complexity is not important in determining the deficits of PD patients. Connor/Ludlow/Schulz (1989) found that acoustic mesaures of syllable production in isolated and repeated productions were similar, and not more impaired with increased task complexity or length. In fact, in the Connor/Abbs/Cole/Gracco (1989) study, the greatest movement amplitudes and velocities were found on the sequential speech task in comparison with the isolated syllable production task. Therefore, the differences in movement slowing between limb and speech tasks does not seem to be due to task complexity. The reason for these differences is as yet unclear. Most limb movement tasks are visually guided, while speech is not. Alternatively, learning is usually required for skilled performance of many limb movement tasks while speech is a previously learned and higly practiced motor skill in adults.

In hyperkinetic disorders, Huntington's disease (HD) patients have increased speech production times for sentences, slower syllable repetition rates, and increased pause lengths between phrases (Ludlow/Connor/Bassich 1987). Bradykinesia has also been reported in finger movement studies (Hefter/Hömberg/Lange/Freund 1987). In SD patients, sentence durations are increased from normal and are improved with treatment (Ludlow/Naunton/Sedory et al. 1989). In hyperkinetic speech disorders, however, it is not known whether the bradykinesia is due to slow voluntary movements or the intrusion of involuntary movements.

2.2. Loss of Control

2.2.1. Speaking Rate in PD

Clinically, PD patients give the impression that they are speaking at an uncontrollably fast rate, often referred to as 'speech rushes' (Darley/Aronson/Brown 1969 a; 1969 b). Some PD patients exhibit palilalia (LaPointe/Horner 1981; Kent/LaPointe 1982) which is uncontrolled repetition of syllable and words. The symptom is similar to acquired stuttering following brain injury (Ludlow/Rosenberg/Salazar et al. 1987).

Impaired speech performance with continued speech can be improved in both PD and palilalia by regulating speech rate either by external pacing either using a pacing board, or auditory cues such as a metronome or delayed auditory feedback (Hanson/Metter 1983; Downie/Low/Lindsay 1977).

Quantitative studies of speech rate have failed to substantiate these impressions (Ludlow/Bassich 1983; Caligiuri 1989). An acoustic study of reiterative palilalia demonstrated that the perceptual impression of an increasingly rapid rate of repetition was not substantiated; the final utterance of a repetition train was either longer in duration or equivalent to preceding productions (Kent/LaPointe 1982). Further, when the change in rate during syllable repetition was computed in PD, patient's rates demonstrated the opposite, greater slowing than normal over 5.5 seconds (Ludlow/Connor/Bassich 1987). The perceptual impression of increasing speech rate may be due to reductions in movement amplitude and accuracy with continued speech production (Caligiuri 1989). The reduced range is often referred to as rigidity in PD and may be unrelated to akinesia and bradykinesia. Although movement duration is not impaired during speech in PD patients, movement range for the upper lip and jaw is reduced and motor coordination may be affected (Connor/Abbs/Cole/Gracco 1989). In another study, formant transition rates were reduced in PD patients both in isolated and repeated syllables suggesting that movement accuracy is reduced (Connor/Ludlow/Schulz 1989). Caliguiri (1989) studied lip movement displacements in PD patients and controls at different speech rates. He found PD patient's reductions in movement amplitude from normal became more pronounced as the PD patients speech rate increased to a normal rate (Caliguiri 1989). The decreased movement accuracy during speech production may underlie the perceptual impression of uncontrolled rate in PD patients speech. Therefore, of the three movement abnormalities in PD, akinesia, bradykinesia and rigidity (reduced movement amplitude), rigidity seems to affect speech production to the greatest degree.

2.2.2. Involuntary Movements in Hyperkinetic Dysarthria

Involuntary movements occur in patients with tardive dyskinesia (TD), oral-mandibular dystonia (OMD), HD and SD. There are large differences however, in the characteristics of these intrusive movements. In tardive dyskinesia, continual grimacing, tongue writhing, lip smacking and teeth grinding usually occur at rest and are usually suppressed by speech or other voluntary movements. Therefore, although the involuntary movements are severe in these patients, often speech production is relatively spared.

In oral-mandibular dystonia (OMD), patients have involuntary abnormal sustained postures such as constant jaw opening, jaw closing, sustained tongue protrusion and grimacing. These postures are sustained while the patient is awake and interfere with voluntary movement such as speech. Quantitative studies are needed to address whether OMD is a constant hypertonia of some muscles interfering with the activation of muscle antagonists, or if the total pattern of muscle activation is disturbed. That is, if the non-hypertonic muscles, normally active for voluntary movement, are suppressed. If this is the case, the disorder may be more one of movement programming rather than execution. This might explain why injection of hypertonic muscles with botulinum toxin is not as beneficial in OMD as in other dystonias (Jankovic/Schwartz/Donovan 1990).

In SD, both spasmodic bursts and hypertonia of several of the laryngeal muscles interfere with movement. In adductor SD, uncontrolled spasmodic bursts occur in both the thyroarytenoid and cricothyroid muscles and both muscles evidence hyperactivation (Ludlow/Hallett/Sedory et al. 1990). In addition, the thyroarytenoid is increased over resting levels to a much greater percentage than the cricothyroid (Ludlow/Baker/Naunton/Hallett 1987; Ludlow/Naunton/Sedory et al. 1990). Therefore, the pattern of laryngeal muscle activation both at rest and during speech and swallow is abnormal, suggesting a movement programming disorder.

3. Symptom Modulation

3.1. Task Specificity

For many years, SD was thought to be a psychogenic disorder. The basis for this belief was the observation that adductor SD patients can usually cough, sing, and whisper and only have difficulty when they attempted to speak. Similarly, patients with abductor SD can normally perform throat clearing, coughing, laughter and crying but are breathy or have intermittent voice loss when speaking. More recently, this has become better understood as a characteristic of the focal dystonias (Rosenbaum/Jankovic 1988). The patients will develop abnormal posturing during one task but be clinically unaffected during another task using similar movements. This is also evident in OMD; often patients will be more impaired during speech than during chewing or vice versa (Paulson/Barnes 1988). This intriguing feature of the focal dystonias suggests that the neural substrates for different tasks can be independent in the central nervous system and that the pathways for one task can be affected while others controlling the same muscles are unaltered. Task specificity in SD is not dependent upon whether or not a task is a vegetative non-learned movement or a movement dependent upon a previously learned skill. These patients are often dramatically more impaired in speaking than in singing and whispering, which are all skilled tasks.

Task specificity may also be a feature of the hypokinetic dysarthrias. Differences in impairment for the same jaw movement whether it is used for a non-speech visually guided movement or used for isolated or embedded speech syllables were demonstrated in PD patients (Connor/Abbs 1991). However, as suggested earlier, these tasks differ in other respects; the use of visual guidance and the degree of previous skill. Certainly, task differences are not as clinically dramatic in PD as they are in the focal dystonias. Additional studies are needed to determine whether task specificity is a feature of PD.

3.2. Variations in Performance

Situational and temporal factors can alter speech performance in both the hypokinetic and hyperkinetic dysarthrias. Most hyperkinetic dysarthric patients are better early in the day. This is most likely due to the exacerbation of muscle hypertonia by muscle activation. Hypokinetic PD patients fluctuate widely during the day and variations in performance can be particularly dramatic in patients on medications (Nutt 1990). Usually patients are less rigid between one and two hours after dopamine medication and then rigidity will return within 3 to 4 hours after medication. Some patients develop dyskinesias and can have hyperkinetic dysarthria symptoms in one to two hours after their medication. Rapid swings between hypokinesia and hyperkinesia in PD patients being treated with dopamine is known as the 'on-off' phenomenon and develops after a patient has been treated for several years. Although not formally investigated, patients usually report their speech improved during dyskinesia over hypokinesia.

3.2.1. Exacerbated by Stress

Patients have daily fluctuations in their symptom severity and can usually report whether it is a good day or bad day for their disorder. Stress seems to exacerbate symptoms and can also be related to periods of waxing and waning in symptoms over several days or weeks. Often patients first notice their symptoms after a stressful event. High expectations of successful treatment often can depress symptoms, while depression and anxiety can exacerbate them. This can alter responses to treatment making the need for controlled studies of treatment effects necessary. Random assignment to a treatment and control group with some intervention in both groups or double blind placebo versus treatment are the designs which can provide accurate assessment of treatment effects in both the hyperkinetic and hypokinetic dysarthrias.

3.2.2. Improvements with Task Constraints

One of the most frustrating experiences in studying patients with motor control disorders, are the differences between their performance in everyday situations and their performance in a controlled testing environment. When the parameters of a task are significantly controlled, the patients' performance usually improves markedly. Therefore, a structured speech test with repetition of limited speech items or the elicitation of well defined speech items will not provide samples representative of a patient's dysarthria. Relatives observing such testing often remark how much better the patient performs during speech testing in the clinical setting than at home. This is the effect of constraining the performance parameters and directing the patient's attention to controlling particular behavioral factors.

3.3. Focal Disturbance

The most focal disturbances occur in the dystonias, such as spasmodic dysphonia and oral mandibular dystonia, where symptoms are confined to one component of the vocal tract such as the laryngeal musculature or the jaw and facial muscles. Although symptoms appear in one area, however, subclinical abnormalities may be present in other regions, such as abnormal blink reflexes in SD (Cohen/Ludlow/Warden et al. 1989).

In assessing the dysarthrias, Netsell (1986) proposed that functional components be examined independently for involvement. Evaluations of PD patients have consistently demonstrated that voicing control is often more disturbed that other aspects of speech on tests of speech articulation (Logemann/Fisher/Boshes/Blonsky 1977; Logemann/Fisher 1981). Darley/Aronson/Brown (1969) found that ratings reflecting voice quality such as breathiness, monopitch and monoloudness were included in the most affected characteristics of PD. Objective acoustic measures similarly found that measures of phonation were also most affected (Canter 1963; Ludlow/Bassich 1983; Weismer 1984). However, no physiological comparisons of muscle activation or movement reductions have been conducted across functional components. It could be that laryngeal control appears most affected because the speed demands on control of vocal fold position for speaking is more constrained for normalcy than other aspects of speech control. Voicing onset and offset must be accurate within a few milliseconds for distinctions between voiced and voiceless consonants. Therefore, hypokinesia may be more evident in laryngeal control because of the very precise timing required for voicing contrasts in speech. Tongue movement is usually much slower and labial control must only be rapid for the production of /p/.

The early and severe involvement of vocal fold movement in Shy Drager Syndrome (multiple systems atrophy) is an important feature of the disorder (Bassich/Ludlow/Polinsky 1984; Hanson/Ludlow/Bassich 1983). Few other dysarthrias have been investigated from a functional component approach examining for selective impairment of one component. However, studies of the basal ganglia and the basal forebrain pathways suggest a topographic organization (DeLong/Alexander/Mitchell/Richardson 1988; Koliatsos/Martin/Walker et al. 1988). Such an organization would certainly support selective focal involvement of one body part with relative sparing of another in basal ganglia disease.

4. Pathophysiology

Few formal studies have been conducted of the pathophysiology of the dysarthrias. Such studies have been conducted on patients with other movement control disorders to examine whether they have exaggerated responses to sensory stimuli. In studies of H reflex responses to stimulation of spindle afferents, patients with limb dystonia had reduced inhibition of responses in comparison with normal (Panizza/Lelli/Nilsson/Hallett 1990). This suggests that muscle activation feedback produces greater motoneuron activation than normal in dystonia. One study has been conducted in SD patients of blink reflex responses to stimulation of the supraorbital nerve. Reduced inhibition of the blink reflex in response to electrical stimulation was found in SD patients in comparison with normal. This suggests that inhibition is reduced in response to afferent stimuli to other cranial motoneurons in SD (Cohen/Ludlow/Warden et al. 1989).

The blink reflex is also heightened in PD patients (Estaban/Gimenez-Roldan 1975) as well as peroral responses to mechanical stimuli (Caligiuri/Abbs 1987). Therefore, in general, a loss of normal inhibition seems to be present in many of these disorders.

De Long (1990) has suggested that in hypokinesia excessive tonic and phasic inhibitory output from the basal ganglia to the thalamus results in reduced responsiveness of cortical mechanisms because of a reduction in thalamocortical activation. The findings of a more slowly rising bereitschaftspotential in PD would support this model (Dick/Rothwell/Day et al. 1989). Hyperkinetic disorders, on the other hand, may be the result of disinhibition of the thalamus due to a reduction in output from the motor globus pallidus. This makes the thalamocortical neurons increasingly responsive and more likely to discharge spontaneously. These models of the hypo- and hyperkinetic dysarthrias are in agreement with the fluctuating characteristics or these disorders. That is, the movement planning and programming for speech production is intact but movement regulation and control is not.

5. Characteristics of the Speech Execution System Based on the Hypo- and Hyperkinetic Dysarthrias

In addition to the need to better understand speech disorders for improved treatment, the study of speech production disorders can also improve our understanding of the speech motor control system. Some of the characteristics of the hypo- and hyperkinetic dysarthrias suggest the following characteristics.

(a) Speech production deficits may differ from limb movement deficits in basal ganglia disease.
(b) Reduced movement range may interfere with speech intelligibility to a greater degree than bradykinesia (movement slowing) or akinesia (movement initiation difficulties).
(c) Highly skilled over-learned motor control tasks may be less affected than new or visually guided tasks by basal ganglia disease.
(d) Alterations in movement accuracy can alter impressions of speaking rate on listeners.
(e) The motor control of vocal tract gestures for chewing and other activities is independent from that for speech.
(f) Speech performance can be improved by reducing the number of parameters which the speaker must control at one time.
(g) Individual vocal tract components can be independent in their neural control.
(h) The role of the basal ganglia in speech production is one of modulation of speech execution. Its function may alter the range and accuracy of speech movements but not the planning or programming of previously learned speech gestures.

6. References

Bassich, C. J., Ludlow, C. L., & Polinsky, R. J. (1984). Speech symptoms associated with early signs of Shy Drager syndrome. *Journal of Neurology, Neurosurgery, and Psychiatry, 47*, 995–1001.

Caligiuri, M. P. (1989). The influence of speaking rate on articulatory hypokinesia in parkinsonian dysarthria. *Brain and Language, 36*, 493–502.

Caligiuri, M. M. & Abbs, J. H. (1987). Response properties of the perioral reflex in Parkinson's disease. *Experimental Neurology, 98*, 563–577.

Canter, G. J. (1963). Speech characteristics of patients with Parkinson's disease: I. Intensity, pitch, and duration. *J. Speech Hear. Dis.*, 28: 221–229.

Cohen, L. G., Ludlow, C. L., Warden, B. S., Estegui, M. D., Agostino, R., Sedory, S. E., Holloway, E., Dambrosia, J., & Hallett, M., (1989). Blink reflex excitability recovery curves in patients with spasmodic dysphonia. *Neurology, 39*, 572–577.

Connor, N. P. & Abbs, J. H. (1991). Task-dependent variations in Parkinsonian motor impairments. *Brain, 114*, 321–332.

Connor, N. P., Abbs, J. H., Cole, K. J., & Gracco, V. L. (1989). Parkinsonian deficits in serial multiarticulate movements for speech. *Brain, 112*, 997–1009.

Connor, N. P., Ludlow, C. L., & Schulz, G. S. (1989). Stop consonant production in isolated and repeated syllables in Parkinson's disease. *Neuropsychologia, 27*, 829–838.

Darley, F., Aronson, A. E., & Brown, J. (1969 a). Differential diagnosis patterns of dysarthria. *Journal of Speech and Hearing Research, 12*, 246–269.

Darley, F. L., Aronson, A. E., Brown, J. R. (1969). Clusters of deviant speech dimensions in the dysarthrias. *J. Speech Hear. Res.*; *12*, 469–496.

DeLong, M. R. (1990). Primate models of movement disorders of basal ganglia origin. *Trends in Neuroscience, 13*, 281–285.

DeLong, M. R., Alexander, G. E., Mitchell, S. J., & Richardson, R. T. (1986). The contributions of basal ganglia to limb control. In H. J. Freund, U. Buttner, B. Cohen, & J. Noth (Eds.), *Progress in Brain Research. 161–174.* Amsterdam: Elsevier Science Publishers.

Dick, J. P. R., Rothwell, J. C., Day, B. L., Cantello, R., Buruma, O., Gioux, M., Benecke, R., Berardelli, A., Thompson, P. D., & Marsden, C. D. (1989). The bereitschaftspotential is abnormal in Parkinson's disease. *Brain, 112*, 233–244.

Downie, A. W., Low, J. M., & Lindsay, D. D. (1981). Speech disorders in Parkinsonism: Usefulness of delayed auditory feedback in selected cases. *Journal of Neurology, Neurosurgery, and Psychiatry, 44*, 852–853.

Estaban, A. & Gimenez-Roldan, S. (1975). Blink reflex in Huntington's chorea and in Parkinson's disease. *Acta Neurologica Scandinavia, 52,* 145–157.

Hallett, M. & Khoshbin, S. (1980). A physiological mechanism of bradykinesia. *Brain, 103,* 301–314.

Hanson, D. G. Ludlow, C. L., & Bassich, C. J. (1983). Vocal fold paresis in Shy-Drager syndrome. *Annals of Otology, Rhinology, and Laryngology, 92,* 85–90.

Hanson; W. R. & Metter, E. J. (1983). Speech rate modification in Parkinson's disease: A report of two cases. In W. R. Berry (Ed.), *Clinical Dysarthria. 231–251.* San Diego, CA: College-Hill Press.

Hefter, H., Hömberg, V., Lange, H. W., & Freund, H. J. (1987). Impairment of rapid movement in Huntington's disease. *Brain, 110,* 585–612.

Jankovic, J., Schwartz, K., Donovan, P. T. (1990). Botulinum toxia treatment of cranio-cervical dystonia, spasmodic dysphonia, other focal dystonias and hemifacial spasm. *Journal of Neurology Neurosurgery and Psychiatry,* 53, 633–639.

Kent, R. D. & LaPointe, L. L. (1982). Acoustic properties of pathologic reiterative utterances: a case study of palilalia. *Journal of Speech and Hearing Research, 25,* 95–99.

Koliatsos, V. E., Martin, L. J., Walker, L. C., Richardson, R. T., DeLong, M. R., & Price, D. L. (1988). Topographic, non-collateralized basal forebrain projections to amygdala, Hippocampus, and anterior cingulate cortex in the rhesus monkey. *Brain Research, 463,* 133–139.

LaPointe, L. L. & Horner, J. (1981). Palilalia: A descriptive study of pathological reiterative utterances. *Journal of Speech and Hearing Disorders, 46,* 34–38.

Logemann, J. A. & Fisher, H. B. (1981). Vocal tract control in Parkinson's disease: Phonetic feature analysis of misarticulations. *Journal of Speech and Hearing Disorders, 46,* 348–352.

Logemann, J. A., Fisher, H. B., Boshes, B., & Blonsky, R. (1977). Frequency and cooccurrences of vocal tract dysfunctions in the speech of a large sample of Parkinson patients. *Journal of Speech and Hearing Disorders, 42,* 47–57.

Ludlow, C. L., Baker, M., Naunton, R. F., & Hallett, M. (1987). Intrinsic laryngeal muscle activation in spasmodic dysphonia. In R. Benecke, B. Conrad, & C. D. Marsden (Eds.), *Motor Disturbances. 119–130.* Orlando: Academic Press.

Ludlow, C. L. & Bassich, C. J. (1983). The results of acoustic and perceptual assessment of two types of dysarthria. In W. Berry (Ed.), *Clinical dysarthria. 121–153.* San Diego: College-Hill.

Ludlow, C. L. & Bassich, C. J. (1984). Relationships between perceptual ratings and acoustic measures of hypokinetic speech. In M. R. McNeil, J. C. Rosenbek, & A. E. Aronson (Eds.), *The dysarthrias. 163–195.* San Diego: College-Hill.

Ludlow, C. L. & Connor, N. P. (1987). Dynamic aspects of phonatory control in spasmodic dysphonia. *Journal of Speech and Hearing Research, 30,* 197–206.

Ludlow, C. L., Connor, N. P., & Bassich, C. J. (1987). Speech timing in Parkinson's and Huntington's disease. *Brain and Language, 32,* 195–214.

Ludlow, C. L., Hallett, M., Sedory, S. E., Fujita, M., & Naunton, R. F. (1990). The pathophysiology of spasmodic dysphonia and its modification by botulinum toxin. In A. Beradelli, R. Benecke, M. Manfredi, & C. D. Marsden (Eds.), *Motor Disturbances. 274–288.* Orlando: Academic Press.

Ludlow, C. L., Naunton, R. F., Sedory, S. E., Schulz, G. S., & Hallett, M. (1989). Effects of botulinum toxin injection on speech in spasmodic dysphonia. *Neurology, 30,* 123–456.

Ludlow, C. L., Rosenberg, J., Salazar, A., Grafman, J., & Smutok, M. (1987). Site of penetrating brain lesions causing chronic acquired stuttering. *Annals of Neurology, 22,* 60–66.

Marsden, C. D. (1982). The mysterious motor function of the basal ganglia: The Robert Wartenberg lecture. *Neurology, 32,* 514–530.

Netsell, R. (1986). *A neurobiologic view of speech production and the dysarthrias,* San Diego, CA: College-Hill Press, 3–4.

Nutt, J. G. (1990). Levodopa-induced dyskinesia: Review, observations, and speculations. *Neurology, 40,* 340–345.

Panizza, M., Lelli, S., Nilsson, J., & Hallett, M. (1990). H-reflex recovery curve and reciprocal inhibition of H-reflex in different kinds of dystonia. *Neurology, 40,* 824–828.

Paulson, G. W. & Barnes, J. (1988). Oral facial dystonia triggered by speech. *Psychosomatics, 29,* 236–238.

Rosenbaum, F. & Jankovic, J. (1988). Task specific focal tremor and dystonia: Categorization of occupational movement disorders. *Neurology, 38,* 522–527.

Sheridan, M. R., Flowers, K. A., & Hurrell, J. (1987). Programming and execution of movement in parkinson's disease. *Brain, 110,* 1247–1271.

Weismer, G. (1984). Articulatory characteristics of Parkinsonian dysarthria: Segmental and phrase-level timing, spirantization, and glottal coordination. In M. R. McNeil, J. R. Rosenbek, & A. E. Aronson (Eds.), *The Dysarthrias: Physiology, Acoustics, Perception, Management. 101–130.* San Diego: College-Hill.

Christy L. Ludlow, Bethesda, Maryland (USA)

44. Cerebellar Dysarthria

1. Introduction

Cerebellar dysarthria results from damage to the cerebellum and/or its afferent or efferent connections due to structural or functional (e. g. alcohol intoxication) alterations. It comprises a somewhat inhomogeneous symptomatology which is a consequence of the functional complexity the cerebellum plays in motor control. Yet, the inhomogeneity has not been worked out to a syndromatic level comparable to the aphasic syndroms. Often, ataxic dysarthria is used as a synonymous term to label cerebellar speech deficits (Darley/Aronson/Brown 1975; Kent/Netsell/Abbs 1979).

The review will take into account the anatomical and functional aspects of the cerebellum, give a description of cerebellar breakdown of speech production at the perceptual, phonetic, acoustic, and kinematic levels.

1.1. Neuroanatomical, Neurophysiological and Clinical Aspects

The cerebellum contains complete sensory and motor representations of the body; yet lesions lead neither to muscle weakness nor to disorders of perception. However, the cerebellum controls the timing and the pattern of muscles activated during movement. Furthermore, the cerebellum modulates spinal cord and brain stem mechanism involved in postural control. Therefore, lesions of the cerebellum produce disturbances in the coordination of limb, eye, and orofacial movements as well as disorders of muscle tone and posture.

The neocerebellum (pontocerebellum), the evolutionary latest portion to develop after the archicerebellum (vestibulocerebellum) and the paleocerebellum (spinocerebellum), plays a major role in planning and initiation of movements (especially with its lateral parts of the cerebellar hemispheres) and is of primary interest to speech. Symptoms of damage to the lateral cerebellar hemispheres comprise 1) abnormalities in timing and build-up of force (intentional movements (grasping/pointing) are slower, delayed in initiation and termination resulting in overshoot, slowness of alternating movements (dysdiadochokinesis), 2) loss of fine tuning and irregular decomposition of voluntary movements with errors in direction, deviations of proper course, discontinuity, dysmetria (mostly overshoot), and tremor (increasing with proximity to target). The temporal composition of the exact time sequence of a complex program is deranged which involves multiple functional subunits of agonist-antagonist interactions composing a coordinate action (synergism, asynergia). This ataxic symptomatology — commonly seen in the limbs — has also been shown to occur in the orofacial motor system (Schönle 1988).

1.2. Hemisphericity and Localization of Speech in the Cerebellum

The predominantly contralaterality of the cerebrocerebellar connections suggests a right hemisphere dominance of the cerebellum for speech motor control. Premotor and motor cortical areas (Brodmann area 4 and 6) project through the cortico-pontocerebellar tract to the contralateral neocerebellar hemispheres and their output is conveyed back to these cerebrocortical areas via red nucleus and the thalamus. However, clinical observations are equivocal with respect to hemispheric lateralization and localization of speech functions. While Holmes (1917; 1922) localized speech functions to the vermis (cerebellar midline structure) Amici/Avancini/Pacini (1976) found cerebellar dysarthria most often with damage to the paravermal and lateral parts of the hemispheres. Disordered speech was uncommon with vermal destruction. In a review of 162 case histories collected over 30 years Lechtenberg/Gilman (1978) observed a significant association of dysarthria with left cerebellar hemisphere lesions in the superior paravermal segment. Consequently, left-sided dominance for cerebellar speech motor control was assumed by the authors. However, close look at the diagnostic categories reveals 141 tumor cases versus 6 infarctions only (3 right hemisphere patients (2 with dysarthrias) and 3 left hemisphere patients (3 with dysarthrias). Given the poor localizing value of tumors and given that CCT-information was available only in 65 cases the question of cerebellar speech dominance remained unsettled.

In the most thorough clinico-neuro-radiological MRI (magnetic resonance imaging) study of 12 patients with cerebellar infarction Ackermann/Vogel/Petersen/Poremba (1991) found the paravermal region of the superior portions of the cerebellum to be of critical importance for speech motor control. The 8 patients with infarctions in the territory of the posterior inferior cerebellar artery (PICA) (five on the left side) sparing the superior parts showed no speech deficits. Of the four patients with superior cerebellar artery infarcts three had right-sided lesions and one a bilateral infarct. These data – despite the small case number – question a left hemisphere dominance for speech in the cerebellum and leave the problem open for further MRI-investigations.

1.3. Diseases of the Cerebellum Affecting Speech

Although the cerebellar symptomatology is alike in most cerebellar diseases speech alterations appear to be more prominent in some affections of the cerebellum e. g. in infarctions of the paravermal region of the superior portions of the cerebellum or some degenerative diseases.

In hereditary cerebellar ataxia (Nonne-Pierre-Marie, manifestation age: app. 35 yrs.), a multi-system degenerative disease, a type of cerebellar dysarthria occurs which was clinically termed 'vox leontina' (lion's voice). Phonation becomes deeper, harsh and louder; articulation is slurred, slow, and explosive with overshooting innervation (speaking with excessive loss of air). Some hereditary cerebellar ataxias only involve degeneration of the cerebellum and allow for better clinicoanatomical correlations than most other cerebellar diseases (e. g. Ackermann/Ziegler 1991).

In the group of spino-ponto-cerebellar atrophies which also involve several neuronal systems, Friedreich's ataxia (manifestation age: app. 13 yrs.) dysarthria develops in the context of dysdiadochokinesia, intention tremor and nystagmus. Very often cerebellar dysarthria occurs in multiple sclerosis presenting with the triad of Charcot (nystagmus, intention tremor, and scanning speech). Alcoholic cerebellar degeneration, the most common acquired cerebellar degeneration, results in slurred speech only in an advanced stage. In contrast, acute alcohol intoxication leads to speech disturbances even at low blood levels (Schönle/Poser/Conrad 1988).

In idiopathic paroxysmal ataxia, cerebellar dysarthria occurs suddenly for seconds, reappearing over a variable time period together with other cerebellar symptoms (loss of balance, blurring of vision, nystagmus). Netsell/Kent (1976) reviewed 13 cases of paroxysmal ataxic dysarthria and found multiple sclerosis to be the most likely etiology. Olivo-ponto-cerebellar degeneration (OPCA) is characterized by progressive ataxia, beginning with a disorder of gait and dysarthria (mixed ataxic-spastic), later evolving into a severe disturbance of coordinated movements of all limbs. – Lesions of the dentate – red nucleus – central tegemental tract – ipsilateral olive circuit result in palatal myoclonus in which patients show a continuous tremor of facial and pharyngeal muscle with distortion of speech production. The multisystem nature of many of the cerebellar diseases make careful selection, investigation, and description of patient population a perequisite when studying purely cerebellar dysarthria.

2. Clinical Perceptual Attributes of Cerebellar Dysarthria

Since the early characterization of cerebellar speech disturbances (Bonhoeffer 1908; Charcot 1877) auditory perceptual descriptors of cerebellar dysarthria have become commonly accepted in clinical use including features like scanning, slow, slurring, staccato, explosive, intermittent, jerky, irregular, hesitant and garbled speech and altered accent (Brown/Darley/Aronson 1970). The sum of the difficulties with the regulation of speech in cerebellar diseases was called dysprosody by Holmes (1917). The most easily recognized feature, scanning speech, was first described by Charcot (1877) as a 'peculiar difficulty of enunciation' with speech production slowed and words 'measured or scanned'. – Darley and coworkers (Darley/Aronson/Brown 1969 a; b; 1975; Brown/Darley/Aronson 1970) designed a classification system for basic abnormalities of speech ('deviant dimensions') and investigated 30 patients with cerebellar lesions. They found 10 speech dimensions to be severely deviant (above 1.5 of their severity scale): imprecise consonants, excess and equalized stress, irregular articulatory breakdown, distorted vowels, harsh voice, prolonged phonemes, prolonged intervals, monotone pitch, monotony of loudness, and slow rate. Other deviant speech characteristics with lower ranking in severity occured in 14 out of the 30 patients: low pitch, excess loudness variations, hypernasality, strain-strangled sound, pitch breaks, and voice tremor. Unfortunately, diagnoses were not specified nor was the presence of other neurological symptoms commented upon and no information about lesion localization was provided. – However, Gilman/Kluin (1984), based on their clinical experience, questioned the findings of Darley/Aronson/Brown (1969 a; b; 1975) that cerebellar dysarthria includes continuously low pitch, monotony of pitch, monotony of loudness, and strain-strangled sounds. In a careful study they compared the speech output of patients with olivo-pontocerebellar atrophy (OPCA) and Friedreich's ataxia. While the OPCA-patients exhibit signs of upper neuron disease such as hyperactive gag reflex, enhanced jaw stretch reflex, limited range of facial movement (as seen in pseudobulbar palsy), the Friedreich's patients did not and, therefore, presented a more 'pure' cerebellar disorder without cortibulbar involvement. – Perceptual analysis of the speech production of the Friedreich's ataxia patients revealed 'pure' ataxic dysarthria with imprecise consonants, excess and equalized stress, irregular articulatory breakdowns, distorted vowels, harsh voice, prolonged phonemes, prolonged intervals and slow rate but without continuously low pitch, monotony of pitch, monotony of loudness, or strain-strangled sound. These signs were observed, however, in the OPCA patient group. While Darley/Aronson/Brown (1969 a; b; 1975) rated articulation as the most deviant dimension in cerebellar patients, Gilman/Kluin (1984) found the phonatory and prosodic dimensions to be the most aberrant in patients with ataxic dysarthria from Friedreich's disease. Strain-strangled sounds resulting from effortful squeezing of air through the glottis, or obstruction of the exhaled airstraim appears to be a sign of corticobulbar tract involvement seen in OPCA (in form of a mixed ataxic spastic dysarthria) or in pseudobulbar palsy and upper motor neuron involvement in amyotrophic lateral sclerosis.

The results of Gilman/Kluin were in accord with studies by DeJong (1979) and Joanette/Dudley (1980). DeJong described sudden pitch changes and ataxic, staccato and explosive elements as prominent speech disturbances in Friedreich's disease. In a study of 22 patients with Friedreich's disease Joanette/Dudley (1980) found two groups of speech characteristics, defining two distinct subgroups of patients: a) a general dysarthric factor and b) a pattern of phonatory stenosis. The former included imprecise consonants and prolonged phonemes as most prominent variables. These together with most of the variables in Darley's et al. clusters constitute ataxic dysarthria with explosive -hesitant and scanning speech. The second factor, phonatory stenosis, involved harshness and pitch breaks, but not monotony of pitch, monotony of loudness or strained-strangled sound. Transient harshness was also found in the Gilman/Kluin study (1984) but was linked to fluctuating pitch levels as harsh voice is generally associated with low pitch (Boon 1979).

Taken these studies together, 'pure' ataxic dysarthria (i. e. in patients without upper motor neuron involvement) is mainly characterized by prosodic/phonatory changes fluctuating pitch levels, 'explosive' transients, breathiness, alternating loudness, excess and equalized stress patterns and audible inspirations; other features such as slow and dysrythmic rate, prolonged phonemes and prolonged intervals, occasional imprecise consonants, irregular breakdown of articulation, mild hypernasality and harsh voice represent the spastic component of mixed spastic ataxic dysarthria.

3. Phonetic Attributes

In their study of speech deficits in patients with circumscribed cerebellar ischemic lesions Ackermann/Vogel/Petersen/Poremba (1991) assessed speech functions with a comprehensive phonetic test battery. Articulatory deficits were evaluated by phonetic analysis of speech samples drawn from spontaneous speech, repetition tasks (including all consonants and cardinal vowels), reading a short story and diadochokinetic tasks. For assessment of prosodic features patients had to realize stress contrasts and different intonation patterns; laryngeal functions, voice quality and stability, pitch, and loudness, were evaluated perceptually.

As the most prominent feature of ataxic dysarthria fluctuation and irregularity in speech production was identified by Ackermann/Vogel/Petersen/Poremba including irregular articulatory breakdown, fluctuations of pitch and loudness, and voice tremor. Articulatory precision was reduced with slurred pronunciation of single consonants and consonant clusters; occasionally, stop consonants were exaggerated due to lengthening. The articulatory deficits occurred inconsistently throughout all speech samples (irregular articulatory breakdown). Fluctuations of pitch and loudness were observed in the more impaired patients. Two patients revealed syllabic speech with segregation of words into syllables. Slowing of speech tempo was noted in all patients. Breathy voice, variable speech rate, audible inspirations, excess and equalized stress, and impaired intelligibility was not observed in contrast to the Gilman/Kluin (1984) and Darley/Aronson/Brown (1975) studies; this may be due to Ackermann/Vogel/Petersen/Poremba's small number of patients and their lower degree of severity. – As the principal outcome of Ackermann's study irregularity and fluctuation in speech production represent the core deficit in cerebellar dysarthria which can be considered to be the only deficit in circumscribed paravermal cortical lesions.

4. Acoustic Attributes

Kent/Netsell/Abbs (1979) performed an acoustic analysis of ataxic dysarthric speech from five patients with degenerative diseases of the cerebellum. As the most consistent and marked abnormalities they observed changes of the normal timing pattern with lengthening of a variety of segments, equalization of syllable duration and separation of syllables. Disproportional segment lengthening, particularly of unstressed vowels, resulted in a disruption of the normal stress and timing pattern of speech. In words with a consonant-vowel-consonant sequence the measures of vowel formant frequency were normal except for longer durations of syllables and formant transitions, and occasionally, voice onset times. With increasing severity the number of lengthened segments increased as well as the length of individual segments itself. Durational adjustments of the syllables in a word was inconsistent; when suffixes were added ataxic subjects made smaller reductions than normal speakers. Abnormal contours of fundamental frequency, particularly monotone and syllable-falling patterns, frequently accompanied disturbances of syllable timing. Equal duration and regular separation of syllables were found to constitute scanning speech. – The articulation rate of spastic and ataxic speakers was compared by Linebaugh/Wolfe (1984) using acoustic measurements. No significant differences were found for the two groups in contrast to the perceptual findings of Darley/Aronson/Brown (1969 a) whose spastic dysarthric patients were significantly slower than the ataxic group. Portnoy/Aronson (1982) also found no significant differences in mean syllable durations between their spastic and ataxic dysarthric subjects. This discrepancy has to remain unresolved as no information is provided about severity of dysarthria, patient selection criteria, neurological symptomatology or diagnoses.

5. Kinematic Attributes

With the development of new techniques (cineradiography (Kent 1972; Kent/Netsell/Bauer 1975; the X-ray microbeam system (Kiritani/Itoh/Fujimura 1975) and electromagnetic articulography (Schönle/Wenig/Schrader et al. 1983; Schönle/Gräbe/Wenig et al. 1987) attempts have been made to directly investigate movements in patients with speech motor disorders including cerebellar dysarthria.

In a cineradiographic study of an ataxic dysarthric patient with cerebellar degeneration Kent/Netsell 1975 observed abnormalities in speaking rate, stress patterns, articulatory placements for vowels and consonants. Velocities of movements were abnormally reduced and durations of vowel steady states and consonant constrictions abnormally lengthened. Some consonant constrictions were missed entirely, others were inappropriately formed. Range of movements was restricted not only for complex but even for 'simple' movements, e. g. during production of isolated vowels. – In a cineradiographic study of a patient with paroxysmal ataxic dysarthria Netsell/Kent (1976) found the same disturbances as in the above subject, in particular with regard to rate, range and direction of movements. – Using the X-ray microbeam system Hirose/Kiritani/Ushijima/Sawashima (1978) performed a kinematic analysis in a patient with ataxic dysarthria from spinocerebellar degeneration. They found inconsistencies in range and velocity of jaw and lip movements during repetition of the monosyllable /pa/. Alternation of movement direction was sluggish in comparison to normals. Velocities of lip displacement were extremely inconsistent in the ataxic, however, maximum velocities reached normal values. – Hunker/Bless/Weismer (1981) observed in a plethysmographic study of the respiratory system that circumferential size changes of the rib cage and abdomen were abnormal in the same ataxic speaker described by Kent/Netsell (1975). While in normal speakers rib cage and abdominal wall move in a coordinated way, they were moving in opposition (paradoxically) in the ataxic patient. As a consequence, this discoordination between the rib cage and the abdomen could have resulted in some interference with lung volume control and subglottal air pressure with the effect of uncontrolled phonatory changes. – In a kinematic analysis of ataxic dysarthria with electromagnetic articulography (Schönle 1988) interarticulatory temporal coordination and the kinematics of orofacial movements were investigated in 12 patients (eight patients with multiple sclerosis, three with cerebellar infarcts, one with Friedreich's heredoataxia) who showed marked cerebellar pathology on clinical testing, in particular cerebellar ataxia and dysarthria. Interarticulatory timing was evaluated for the coordination of jaw opening movements and laryngeal activities during repetitive production of 25 /pa/ syllables. While normal control subjects showed a highly correlated temporal relationship between jaw cycles and phonatory activities, opening movements for the /p/ and initiation of vocal cord vibration ran loose in the ataxic patients with a complete loss of the temporal coordination. The good correlation in the normal subjects was taken as evidence that the interarticulatory timing is precisely controlled during normal speaking while precise control of interarticulatory temporal coordination is impaired in cerebellar patients. Loss of coordinative structures (Turvey 1977) and functional synergies (Rondot/Bathien/Toma 1979) were concluded to be part of the pathophysiological mechanisms underlying cerebellar dysarthria.

With respect to orofacial kinematics the influence of aberrant articulatory movements on speech production due to cerebellar impairment was demonstrated for the first time (Schönle 1988, 86). Some representative data from this study are presented in figures 44.1 – 3. Fig. 44.1. demonstrates ataxic alterations of movement trajectories during jaw opening in four successive trials of repetitive production of /pa/. In contrast to the smooth, sinusoidal opening and closing movement of the jaw in a normal speaker the movements are segmented and jerky with untimely speed changes resulting in decomposed and dys-

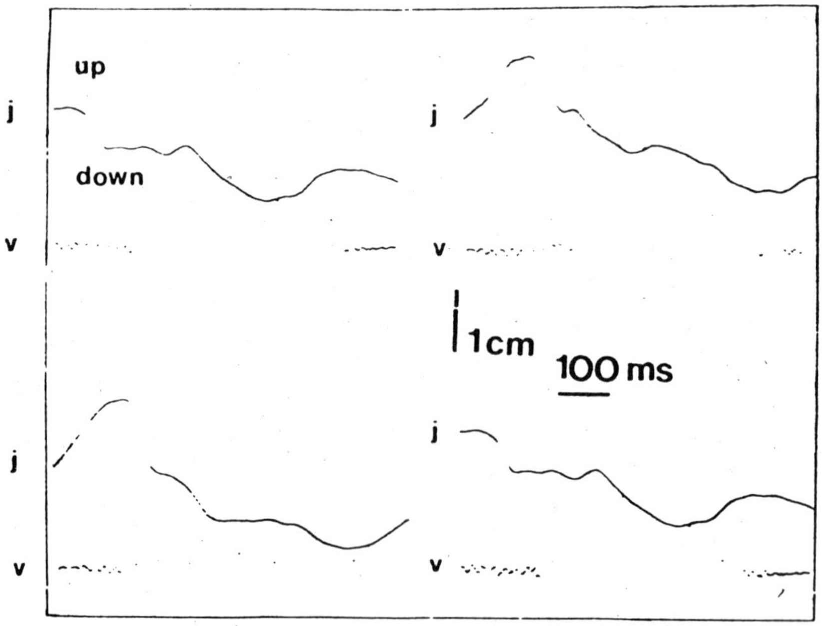

Fig. 44.1: Jaw opening trajectories in four successive trials of repetitive production of /pa/ (j: jaw, v: acoustic speech signal).

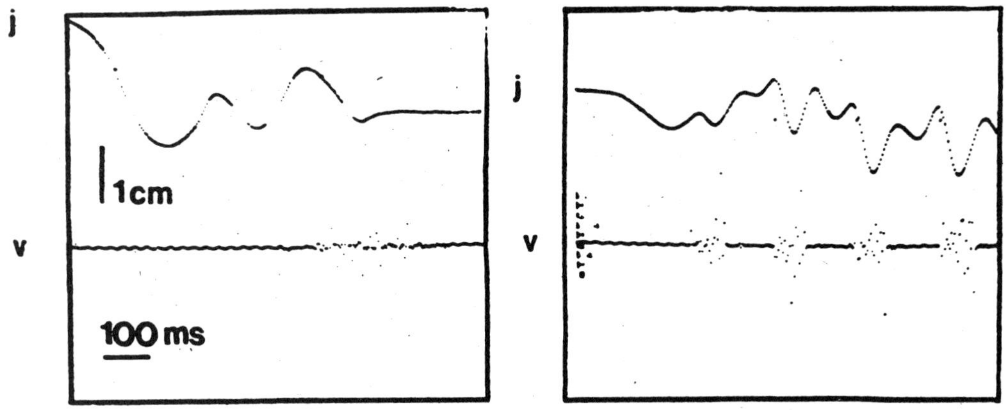

Fig. 44.2: Production of /pa/ at a spontaneous rate (left side); two oscillations of an intention tremor occur at the end of the jaw opening movement interfering with interarticulatory timing. Fast production of /pa/ (right side): note an instability of movement amplitudes from one utterance to the next.

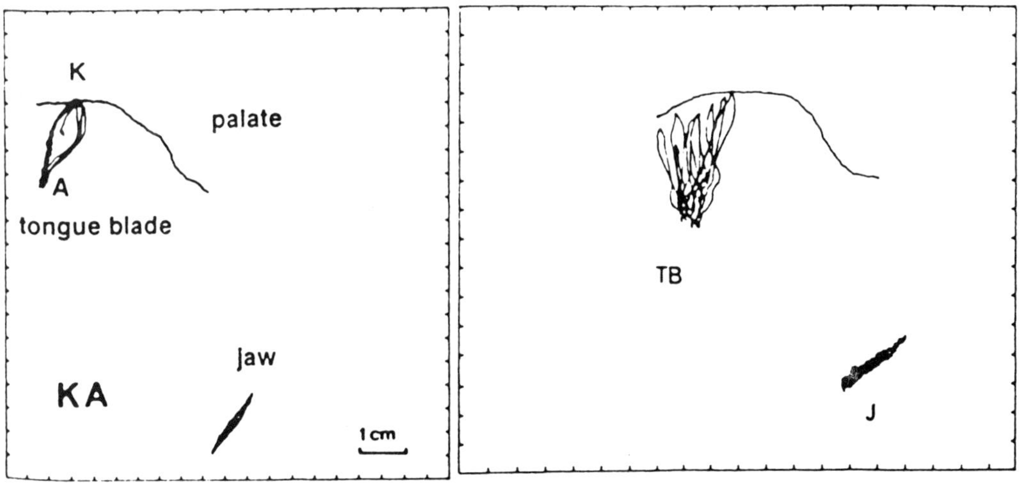

Fig. 44.3: Trajectories of tongue blade and jaw during repetitive utterance of /ka/ at a spontaneous rate (tongue pellet position 45 mm from the tongue tip); utterances of a normal speaker (left side) and of a patient with cerebellar impairment (right side).

metric trajectories. As a consequence, these intra-articulatory changes lead to an alteration of the geometry of the vocal tract from which a distortion of the acoustic of the speech output results.

Speech production may also be altered by intention tremor (fig. 44.2, left side), amplitude instability (fig. 44.2, right side), and loss of end-positional control (fig. 44.3). The occurrence of oscillatory movements in the final phase of the jaw opening (fig. 44.2) results in a disturbance of the temporal coordination of mandibular and phonatory movements, voicing onset is delayed until the end of the oscillatory activity of the jaw. As a consequence on the behavioral level the /pa/-production falls apart and is perceived as segmented. Inspection of the lingual movement (upper trace in fig. 44.2) reveals that the tongue does not perform oscillatory motions as would be the case if the tongue would passively follow the jaw movements. Obviously, the tongue is controlled well in advance to counteract and compensate for the mandibular oscillations in order to reach a stable target positioning for the /a/-production.

Fig. 44.3 shows tongue blade movement trajectories during repetitive utterance of /ka/

at a spontaneous rate. In the normal speaker (fig. 44.3. left side) the tongue movements form a highly consistent pattern with exact closure of the tongue at the palate for the /k/ and exact target positioning for the /a/. In contrast, when the patient in fig. 44.3. (right side) produces sequences of /ka/ both amplitudes and directions of the movements change from one production to the next. This impairment of end-positional control leads to changes in the configuration of the vocal tract which results in aberrant speech acoustics ranging from almost correct to highly abnormal speech sounds. — A loss of endpositional control and alterations in the control of temporal coordination between jaw movements and phonatory activity during repetitive production of /pa/ syllables was also observed in functional impairments of the cerebellum after alcohol ingestion even at low levels of blood alcohol (Schönle/Poser/Conrad 1988).

6. Pathophysiological Mechanisms in Cerebellar Dysarthria

The kinematic studies revealed detailed and rich information about the pathophysiological mechanisms underlying ataxic dysarthria. While speech gestures are appropriate in their overall gestalt they lack precision in their temporo-spatial metrics due to impaired motor control. Control variables such as force, velocity, amplitude, direction and timing appear to be affected in cerebellar dysarthria in much the same way as in cerebellar disturbances of limb and eye movements.

Loss of the ability to modulate force generation due to cerebellar hypotonia may be responsible for slowness of movements, prolongation of speech segments, and the tendency to equalize segment length as observed in scanning speech. Loss of exact timing between articulators with 'random coordination' underlies what is perceived at the behavioral level as irregular breakdown of the speech output and inconsistency in speech movements, be it in the articulatory, phonatory or respiratory subsystems.

7. Management of Patients with Cerebellar Dysarthria

No commonly used and generally accepted pharmacological therapeutic regimens exist currently for cerebellar ataxia.

While Rosenbeck/La Pointe (1978) stated that no specific treatment programs exist for the different types of dysarthria, Yorkston/Beukelman (1981) developed a treatment program which they specifically designed for four patients with ataxic dysarthria. The treatment sequences were based on intelligibility and prosodic considerations. Control of speaking rate was used to increase intelligibility. Normal prosodic patterning was not achieved due to the inability to learn precise coordination of fundamental frequency, loudness and timing adjustments for expression of stress. However, durational adjustments could be made and target words were stressed appropriately.

In a single case study Simmons (1983) applied acoustic analysis to monitor the treatment program in one ataxic speaker which was based on Yorkston/Beukelman (1981) approach. In a hierarchy of tasks four treatment phases were applied over a period of one year: 1) loudness and pitch variation to reduce monotone speech quality; 2) modification of word and sentence stress patterns: 3) shortening of overall syllable durations; 4) increase of naturalness to decrease exaggerated pitch and loudness variations and smoothing word transitions. The program led to compensated speech rather than to normal speech as was expected. Acoustic analysis could be shown to improve the efficiency of the therapeutic interventions. — Berry/Goshorn (1983) applied immediate visual feedback using a storage oscilloscope in the treatment of an ataxic patient who spoke too rapidly and loudly. The treatment goal was to slow the speaking rate and thus to improve intelligibility. Over a period of five weeks the patient learned to control loudness and to slow the rate of speech by prolonging pauses. Intelligibility improved not only in the experimental but also in natural settings.

Taken together, further research is necessary to develop new intervention strategies which focus on specific patho-physiological processing deficits and apply results from kinematic and acoustic analyses for remediation of dysarthric speech. Communicative effects should be controlled at the perceptual level by perceptual rating scales (e. g. Sheard/Adams/Davis 1991).

8. References

Ackermann, H., Vogel, M., Petersen, D., & Poremba, M. (1991). *Speech deficits in ischemic cerebellar lesions*. Unpublished manuscript.

Ackermann, H. & Ziegler, W. (1991). Cerebellar voice tremor: an acoustic analysis. *Journal of Neurology, Neurosurgery, & Psychiatry*, 54, 74–76.

Amici, R., Avancini, G., & Pacini, L. (1976). *Cerebellar Tumors. Monographs in Neural Sciences, Vol. IV.* Karger Basel 4.

Berry, W. R. & Goshorn, E. L. (1983). Immediate Visual Feedback in the Treatment of Ataxic Dysathria: A Case Study. In W. R. Berry (Ed.), *Clinical Dysarthria. 253–265.* College Hill Press, San Diego.

Bonhoeffer, K. (1908). Über den Einfluß des Zerebellums auf die Sprache. *Monatsschrift f. Psychiat. u. Neurol.*, 24, 88–92.

Boon, D. R. (1979). *The Voice & Voice Therapie.* Englewood Cliffs: Prentice-Hall.

Brown, J. R., Darley, F. L., & Aronson, A. E. (1968). Deviant Dimensions of Motor Speech in Cerebellar Ataxia. *Trans. Am. Neurol. Assoc.*, 93, 193–196.

Brown, J. R., Darley, F. L., & Aronson, A. E. (1970). Ataxic Dysarthria. *Internat J. Neurol.* 7, 302–316.

Charcot, J. M. (1877). *Lectures on the Diseases of the Nervous System. Vol. 1.* London: The New Sydenham Society.

Darley, F. L., Aronson, A. E., & Brown, J. R. (1969 a). Differential diagnostic patterns of dysarthria. *Journal of Speech and Hearing Research, 12, 246–249.*

Darley, F. L., Aronson, A. E., & Brown, J. R. (1969 b). Clusters of deviant speech dimensions in the dysarthrias. *Journal of Speech and Hearing Research*, 12, 462–296.

Darley, F., Aronson, A., & Brown, J. (1975). *Motor Speech Disorders.* W. B: Saunders Company. Philadelphia.

DeJong, R. N. (1979). *The Neurologic Examination.* 4th ed., Hagerstown: Harper & Row.

Delawaide, P. J. & Young, R. R. (1985). *Clinical Neurophysiology in Spasticity.* 13–25. Amsterdam: Elsevier.

Gilman, S. & Kluin, K. (1984). Perceptual Analysis of Speech Disorders in Friedreich Disease and Olivopontocerebellar Atrophy. in J. R. Bloedel, J. Dichgans, & W. Precht (Eds.), *Cerebellar Functions.* 148–163. Berlin: Springer.

Hirose, H., Kiritani, S., & Sawashima, M. (1980). Patterns of dysarthric movements in patients with amyotrophic lateral sclerosis & pseudobulbar palsy. *Annual Bulletin of the Research Institute of Logopedics and Phoniatrics* (Tokyo) 14, 263–272.

Hirose, H., Kiritani, S., Ushijima, T., & Sawashima, M. (1978). Analysis of Abnormal Articulatory Dynamics in two Dysarthric Patients. *Journal of Speech and Hearing Disorders*, 43, 96–105.

Holmes, G. (1917). The symptoms of acute cerebellar injuries due to gunshot injuries. *Brain* 40, 461–535.

Holmes, G. (1922). The Croonian Lectures on the Clinical Symptoms of Cerebellar disease and their interpretation. *Lancet* 1, 1177–1182, 1231–1237; 2, 59–65, 111–115.

Hunker, C., Bless, D., & Weismer, G. (1981). Respiratory Inductive Plethysmography: A Clinical Technique for Assuring Respiratory Function for Speech. Paper Presented at the Meeting of the American Speech-Language-Hearing Association Convention in Los Angeles. Cited from Abbs, J. H., Hunker, Ch. J., & Barlow, St. M. (1983). Differential Speech Motor Subsystem Impairments with suprabulbar lesions: Neurophysiological Framework and Supporting Data. In W. R. Berry (Ed.), *Clinical Dysarthria.* 21–56. San Diego: College Hill Press.

Joanette, Y. & Dudley, J. G. (1980). Dysarthric Symptomatology of Friedreich's Ataxia. *Brain and Language* 10, 39–50.

Kent, R. D. (1972). Some considerations in the cinefluorographic analysis of tongue movements during speech. *Phonetica*, 26, 16–32.

Kent, R. & Netsell, R. (1975). A case of an ataxic dysarthric: Cineradiographic and spectographic observations. *Journal of Speech and Hearing Disorders*, 40, 115–134.

Kent, R. D., Netsell, R., & Abbs, J. H. (1979). Acoustic characteristics of dysarthria associated with cerebellar disease. *Journal of Speech and Hearing Research*, 22, 627–648.

Kent, R. D., Netsell, R., & Bauer, L. L. (1975). Cineradiographic assessment of articulatory mobility in the dysarthrias. *Journal of Speech and Hearing Disorders*, 40, 467–480.

Kiritani, S., Itoh, K., & Fujimura, O. (1975). Tongue-Pellet Tracking by a Computer-Controlled X-Ray Micorbeam System. *Journal of the Acoustical Society of America*, 57, 1516–1520.

Lechtenberg, R. & Gilman, S. (1978). Speech Disorders in Cerebellar Disease. *Annals of Neurology*, Vol. 3, 285–290.

Linebaugh, C. W. & Wolfe, V. E. (1984). Relationships between articulation rate, intelligibility, and naturalness in spastic and ataxic speakers. In M. R. McNeil, J. C. Rosenbek & A. E. Aronson (Eds.), *The Dysarthrias: Physiology, Acoustics, Perception, Management.* 197–205. San Diego: College Hill Press.

Netsell, R. & Kent, R. D., (1976). Paroxysmal ataxic dysarthria, *Journal of Speech and Hearing Disorders*, 41, 93–109.

Portnoy, R. A. & Aronson, A. E. (1982). Diadochkinetic syllable rate and regularity in normal and in spastic and ataxic dysarthric speakers. *Journal of Speech and Hearing Disorders*, 47, 285–287.

Rondot, P., Bathien, N., & Toma, S. (1979). Physiopathology of cerebellar movement. In J. Massion, K. Sasaki (Eds.), *Cerebro-cerebellar interactions*. 203–230. Amsterdam: Elsevier.

Rosenbek, J. C. & LaPointe, L. L. (1978). The Dysarthrias: Description, Diagnosis, and Treatment. In Johns, D. F. (Ed.), *Clinical Management of Neurogenic Communication Disorders*. Boston: Little, Brown and Company.

Schönle, P. W. (1988). *Elektromagnetische Artikulographie. Ein neues Verfahren zur klinischen Untersuchung der Sprechmotorik*. Springer: Berlin, Heidelberg, New York.

Schönle, P. W., Gräbe, K., Wenig, P., Höhne, J., Schrader, J., & Conrad, B. (1987). Electromagnetic articulatory: use of alternating magnetic fields for tracking movements of multiple points inside and outside the vocal tract. *Brain and Language*, 31, 26–35.

Schönle, P. W., Poser, W. E., & Conrad, B. (1988). Änderungen der Sprechmotorik unter niedrigen Blutalkoholspiegeln. In W. Arnold, W. E. Poser, M. R. Möller (Eds.), *Suchtkrankheiten, Diagnose, Therapie und analytischer Nachweis*. 228–232. Berlin: Springer.

Schönle, P. W., Wenig, P., Schrader, J., Gräbe, K., Bröckmann, E., & Conrad, B. (1983). Ein elektromagnetisches Verfahren zur simultanen Registierung von Bewegungen im Bereich des Lippen-, Unterkiefer- und Zungensystems. *Biomed. Tech.* 28, 263–267.

Sheard, Ch., Adams, R. D., & Davis, P. J. (1991). Reliability and Agreement of Ratings of Ataxic Dysarthric Speech Samples With Varying Intelligibility. *Journal of Speech and Hearing Research*, 34, 285–293.

Simmons, N. N. (1983). Acoustic Analysis of Ataxic Dysarthria: An Approach to Monitoring Treatment. In W. R. Berry (Ed.), *Clinical Dysarthria*. College Hill Press, San Diego, 283–294.

Turvey, M. T. (1977). Preliminaries to a theory of action with reference to vision. In R. Shaw, J. Bransford (Eds.), *Perceiving, acting, and knowing: Toward an ecological psychology*. Hillsdale: Erlbaum.

Yorkston, K. & Beukelman, D. (1981). Ataxic Dysarthria: Treatment sequences based on intelligibility and prosodic considerations. *Journal of Speech and Hearing Disorders*, 46, 398–404.

Paul W. Schönle/Berthold Gröne, Allensbach (Germany)

45. Feedback Impairments in Dysarthria

1. Background

Theories regarding the role of sensory information in the control of speech production and deficits therein as potential etiologies for speech disorders have a very long history. Modern research on this issue began with the discovery in the post-WWII period that delay of the speech auditory signal caused severe disruption of speech. In the 1950s and 1960s, coincidental with popularization of cybernetics, investigators used a number of sensory disruption techniques to verify the exact role of sensory feedback in speech. Unfortuntely, most experiments addressing this hypothesis were directed toward a general either-or resolution, with little focus on specific mechanisms or the benefit of the concept that contributions of sensorimotor processes might vary with different articulators, different types of speech movements, or during different phases of a given movement. Due to this approach, until about 15 years ago, unequivocal experimental evidence to document the role of sensory information in the control of speech movements was basically lacking. Many of the early experiments involved overt disruption of sensory information, via auditory masking, delay of auditory feedback, or different regimen of topical or trigeminal nerve anesthesia. In most cases, there was substantial intersubject variability and measures very often were limited to the numbers and kinds of speech errors that could be detected by listeners. In retrospect, these studies appear to have suffered from a lack of full appreciation of the plasticity and adaption of the nervous system; specifically, subjects were able, more or less successfully, to utilize alternate sensory inputs to accomplish the same speech motor goals. As noted, "claiming that sensation is not essential for speech motor control, from those early data, is analogous to claiming that vision is not important to upright posture and equilibrium, simply because the blind can stand and balance themselves" (Abbs 1991, 133). In the last few years, a different experimental paradigm has been utilized that documents sensorimotor contributions to speech production. Specifically, the critical experiment involved disruption of the ongoing speech movements mechanically, without anticipation or prior knowledge by the subject, and observation of the extent to which those induced errors were corrected. Since 1975, a number of experiments have employed this technique and the results are quite decisive. Specifically, if one introduces an unanticipated mechanical disturbance on jaw elevation during the execution of lip closure for a bilabial stop sound [p], relatively short latency (< 100 msec.) articulatory adjustments are observed which effectively eliminate any speech manifestations of the induced error. Because these kinds of adjustments are observed in naive subjects the very first time a disruption is introduced, it has been surmised that the sensorimotor adjustments responsible are a natural part of the speech motor process (Abbs/Gracco 1984; Gracco/Abbs 1985; 1989; Shaiman 1989). Demonstration of an important role for sensory information in the control of speech is entirely consistent with results from parallel studies in the last decade on sensorimotor control of arm, hand, eye, head, and locomotion movements. With this background, questions naturally are raised regarding the possible contributions of sensory or feedback aberrations in the movement control deficits associated with many speech disorders.

2. Possible Sensory Impairments in Dysarthria

Perhaps the most convincing documentation of the sensory bases for so-called speech motor disorders is the wide-spread neuroanatomical coincidence between sensory and motor functions throughout the nervous system. Fortunately, modern techniques in neurophysiology and neuroanatomy have dramatically improved the data that address this overlap. Specifically, brain studies in non-human primates were for many years confined to recording and stimulation under deep anesthesia, revealing only a select set of sensory and motor connections. Recent techniques, pioneered by the late Ed Evarts, permitted microelectrode recording and stimulation in the central nervous system of awake animals, in many cases revealing sensory activity in association with motor task performance. These studies revealed a ubiquitous interconnection of sensory and motor processes, such that the latter is seldom manifest without the former, and conversely. The sections that follow provide a brief review of these interconnections and some indications as to how certain classes of motor speech disorders may involve both motor and sensory impairments.

2.1. Cerebral Cortex

The importance of sensory information in the control of movements has changed dramatically with the observation in awake primates that stimulation of the lips or tongue elicits short latency responses in pyramidal cells of primary motor cortex (Brodmann's area 4) and lateral regions of premotor cortex (Brodmann's area 6 and 44). This observation can only mean that those cortical cells, some with single synapse connections to lingual and labial motoneurons – the pyramidal cells, are directly responsive to powerful sensory input. Similar observations have been made regarding sensory inputs to other regions of cerebral cortex, with equally important implications. The classic view of the neocortex in the control of speech has been one of posterior cortical function in language components with transmission of information anteriorly for speech motor execution. While this perspective is not incorrect it is lacking the essential component of how sensory input influences these processes. Based upon research in waking primates and parallel observations in humans using improved imaging techniques, it appears that sensory information is involved at all levels of this process. For example, orofacial sensory inputs shown to project to the posterior parietal area have been argued to contribute to the monitoring of general overall vocal tract goals, as are associated with phonological elements (Abbs 1986; Abbs/Welt 1985). By contrast, sensory inputs to the primary motor cortex (Brodmann's area 4) and regions more lateral and anterior (Brodmann's areas 6 and 44) appear to have somewhat different functions. While the different influences of sensory input to different regions of the cerebral cortex associated with speech are outside the scope of this chapter, the implications for disorders of speech seem obvious. First, because of the ever-present overlap between sensory and motor functions on the cerebral cortex, damage to any of these areas is likely to yield both motor and sensory deficits. In fact it may not be possible, despite classic sensory-motor stratification of clinical nosology, to separate sensory from motor manifestations. This observation is borne out in certain studies of speech disordered populations with cerebral damage. For example, patients with so-called apraxia of speech long have manifested difficulty in processing orofacial sensory input (Rosenbek/Wertz/Darley 1973). Interestingly, it has been argued that apraxia of speech is a disorder of speech movement coordination – a motor function increasingly believed to require sensorimotor processes (Abbs/Connor 1989); to this point is the observation that sensory input to Broca's cortical speech area (Brodmann's area 44) converge from multiple orofacial sites, as would be necessary for motor control of such coordinative functions.

2.2. Cerebellar Functions

The cerebellum has been described as the head ganglion of the somatic sensory system. This statement reflects the dense projections to the cerebellum from tendon, joint, and skin receptors and muscle afferents that project to the cerebellum. The role of sensory projections to the cerebellum has been somewhat elusive; however, increasingly it has been hypothesized that the role of sensory inputs to the cerebellum is in integrating multiple movements that are a necessary aspect of most natural movements, including speech. In a general respect, the cerebellum has also been implicated in the on-line sensorimotor correction of potential movement errors, particularly longer latency corrections for errors that might be anticipated. Specifically, cerebellar output has been shown to be modified with experience such that the need for ongoing corrections might be anticipated and hence correction would be enhanced or expedited. Of particular importance to the motor control of speech is the fact that projections from the orofacial system, particularly skin and mucosal receptors, are particularly numerous. Conversely, lingual muscle spindle afferents, unlike muscle spindles from jaw and respiratory muscles, do not project to cerebellar sites. To the extent that muscle spindles are thought to play an important role in speech motor control, these data would argue for a different role for the cerebellum in control of tongue than in control of the jaw or respiratory system. To this point, while lip muscles lack muscle spindles, and hence also do not have spindle afferents that project to the cerebellum, there are dense cerebellar projections from mechanoreceptors in the facial skin and in the mucosal tissue of the lips and tongue. Damage to the cerebellum leads to ataxic dysarthria, a condition characterized by unsmooth, jerky movements (cf. Winstein/Muller/Abbs 1990) and some evidence of reduced muscle tone. While sensory impairments as contributing factors in this disorder are equivocal, investigators have reported specific problems in coordination among movements of the rib cage, abdomen and diaphragm – said to be due to inadequate modulation of motoneuron activity by spindle afferents – a modulation shown to be influenced by the cerebellum.

2.3. Basal Ganglia

Putative motor control functions assigned to the basal ganglia have often been a subject of controversy. It appears generally clear that this brain center is however important in speech motor control and motor control in general. In particular, based upon recording of single neurons in awake primates during the production of movement, the basal ganglia have been documented as a site for integration of sensory inputs with motor outputs. Indeed, recent studies have involved sensory mapping of orofacial and upper limb projections to the basal ganglia. In parallel with observations in the motor cortex, basal ganglia (pars reticulata and globus pallidus) neurons receiving sensory input from a given skin region also show discharge in association with spontaneous movement of that region. In parallel with the sensorimotor connections of the cerebral cortex and cerebellum, the basal ganglia have also been thought to contribute to sensorimotor error correction in movement control. The dysarthria associated with *Parkinson's disease* is the most common speech motor disturbance resulting from damage to the basal ganglia. Clearly these patients manifest an inability to self monitor their speech and manifest inappropriate control of loudness and rate, suggesting abnormal utilization of auditory information. Interestingly, Parkinson's patients appear to manifest different kinds of impairments in speech movements of the lips versus those of the jaw (Connor/Abbs/Cole/Gracco 1989), a difference quite possibly related to the presence of spindles in jaw muscles and their absence in the muscles of the lips. In this respect, Parkinson's patients show hyperactive trigeminal reflexes; stretching of the facial skin in normal subjects elicits no muscle responses, while Parkinson's patients manifest these abnormal reflexes quite readily (Caligiuri/Abbs 1987). These results have been interpreted to indicate that the basal ganglia have a role in gating of sensory information from the orofacial region; with damage, that gating is disturbed. While conclusive proof is lacking, the multiple speech problems in Parkinson's patients are as likely due to impaired sensory function as motor deficits, especially given the substantial interdependence of these two processes in normal speech motor control.

3. Clinical Assessment of Sensorimotor Integrity

Because many speech disorders appear to have underlying sensory as well as motor deficits, several researchers have attempted to devise techniques for testing orofacial somatic sensory integrity. Obviously the normal sensory inputs associated with orofacial motor function are due to muscle contraction forces and length changes, displacements and skin deformation produced by contraction, and air pressure variations in the vocal tract. One problem in testing whether these inputs are received and processed normally is devising mechanical stimuli that are natural. A second issue is in developing a means for determining the degree that such stimuli are processed normally; it is clear that most sensory input for control of motor actions is processed subliminally. Asking patients to give verbal reports regarding psychophysical properties of such stimuli is obviously an artificial process. Finally, classical psychophysical testing using even natural stimuli is very far removed from normal sensorimotor function and is dependent on the faulty premise that the brain is a passive sensory processor. The very aspect of function being ignored with discrete presentation of test stimuli to a passive subject – active processing of inputs related to ongoing motor tasks – may be the critical component that is impaired in patients with speech disorders. Based on these concerns, such testing, while properly motivated in a general respect, obviously must be conducted and interpreted very carefully.

4. Implications for Treatment

The recognition that some of the manifestations of so-called motor speech disorders may, in fact, be due to *sensori*motor difficulties does offer some insights for potentially new treatment techniques as well as explanations as to the success and failure of some existing treatments. For example, if speech movements are guided, corrected, and refined by moment-to-moment sensory input, loss or impairment of that input would require a greater rote learning of such movements. The effectiveness of treatments that stress articulation drill might be due to the need to generate these movements without such on-line correction and refinement – sort of like building up a set of fixed motor programs. Similarly, the value of delayed auditory feedback or masking noise with some dysarthric groups (such as Parkinson's patients) may require that they more consciously monitor articulatory output, hence improving their control. However, the most promising treatment for speech disorders with an etiology of impaired sensorimotor function would appear to be biofeedback. Specifically, with biofeedback treatment patients are provided with instrumentally-enhanced sensory information (usually visual) of an important motor output parameter; it is expected that they will utilize that information to regain control in non-instrumental settings. Some successes have been reported with this technique, largely in the form of case reports. However there are a number of variables that are said to contribute to success or failure. Speech is a complex motor behavior and consciously monitoring more than one or maybe two of the critical motor output parameters is not an easy task, especially for an individual with brain damage. As such, biofeedback successes in speech motor disorders have most generally occurred in training regimes focused on single dimensioned, static variables such as background muscle tone, overall strength (in non-speech tasks), or control of limited movements in articulators like the velum (cf. Rubow, 1984, for a review). Other complicating factors or issues that need to be resolved include the issue of whether training for a slow, non-speech control will have a positive transfer to control of more complex speech movements. In the 15 years since the advent of biofeedback as a treatment for speech disorders, many answers remain unresolved. Obviously, scientists and clinicians must work to practically address these complications before such treatment will be successfull for more than a few cases.

5. Conclusions

While sensory functions associated with the control of speech are inseparable from motor functions, using that knowledge in the assessment and treatment of speech disorders remains a difficult prospect. Nevertheless, full appreciation of such ubiquitous sensorimotor integration is a key element to research and practice on many speech disorders.

6. References

Abbs, J. H. (1986). Invariance and variability in speech production: A distinction between linguistic intent and its neuromotor implementation. In J. Perkell & D. H. Klatt (Eds.), *Invariance and Variability in Speech Processes. 202–219*. Hillsdale, NJ: Lawrence Erlbaum Associates.

Abbs, J. H. (1991). Evaluation of somatic sensory processes contributing to the production of speech: From the laboratory to the clinic. In *Assessment of Speech and Voice Production: Research and Clinical Applications*. NIDCD Monographs. 132–138, in press.

Abbs, J. H. & Connor, N. P. (1989) Motor coordination for functional human behaviors: Perspectives from a speech motor data base. In S. A. Wallace (Ed.), *Perspectives on the Coordination of Movement. 157–183*. New York: Elsevier Science Publishers.

Abbs, J. H. & Gracco, V. L. (1984). Control of complex motor gestures: Orofacial muscle responses to load perturbations of the lip during speech. *Journal of Neurophysiology, 51*, 705–723.

Abbs, J. H. & Welt, C. (1985). Structure and function of the lateral precentral cortex: Significance for speech motor control. In R. Daniloff (Ed.), *Recent Advances in Speech Science. 155–191*. San Diego: College Hill Press.

Caligiuri, M. P. & Abbs, J. H. (1987). Response properties of the perioral reflex in Parkinson's disease. *Experimental Neurology, 98*, 563–572.

Connor, N. P., Abbs, J. H., Cole, K. J., & Gracco, V. L. (1989). Parkinsonian deficits in serial multiarticulate movements for speech. *Brain, 112*, 997–1009.

Gracco, V. L. & Abbs, J. H. (1985). Dynamic control of the perioral system during speech: Kinematic analyses of autogenic and nonautogenic sensorimotor processes. *Journal of Neurophysiology*. 54, 418–432.

Gracco, V. L. & Abbs., J. H. (1989). Sensorimotor characteristics of speech motor sequences. *Experimental Brain Research*. 75, 586–598.

Rosenbek, J. C., Wertz, R. T., & Darley, F. L. (1973). Oral sensation and perception in apraxia of speech and aphasia. *Journal of Speech and Hearing Research, 16*, 22–36.

Rubow, R. (1984). Role of feedback, reinforcement, and compliance on training and transfer in biofeedback-based rehabilitation of motor speech disorders. In M. R. McNeil, J. C. Rosenbek, & A. Aronson (Eds.), *The Dysarthrias: Physiology-Acoustics-Perception-Management. 207–230*. San Diego: College Hill Press.

Shaiman, S. (1989). Kinematic and electromyographic responses to perturbation of the jaw. *Journal of Acoustical Society of America, 86*, 78–88.

Winstein, C. J. Muller, F., Abbs., J. H., Connor, N. P., Dichgans, J., & Diener, H. C. (1990). Discoordination of multiarticulate movements in patients with diffuse cerebellar atrophy: evidence from speech. *Movement Disorders, 5* (Supplement 1). 5.

James H. Abbs/Roxanne DePaul, Madison, Wisconsin (USA)

46. Therapy of Dysarthrias and Speech Apraxia

1. Definitions

The term 'dysarthria' is generally used in a rather broad sense to denote the effect of a movement disorder on respiratory, phonatory as well as articulatory functions involved in speech sound production. More accurately might be the designation 'dysarthrophonia', or even 'dysarthrophonopneumia', which have been proposed as terminological improvements (Netsell 1984).

Speech apraxia is less well defined: "... there is little consensus of opinion regarding underlying disrupted mechanisms and symptomatology, and no definitive guidelines for the selection of the most efficacious treatment procedures for individual verbally apractic patients ..." (Square-Storer 1989 a, XV).

There is an ongoing debate as to whether the deficit in speech apraxia is phonological, i. e. aphasic, or articulatory, i. e. motor, in nature (for a discussion, see Square-Storer/Roy, 1989). In the context of this chapter, speech apraxia will be regarded as a disturbance of the programming of the spatial and temporal coordinates of speech movements.

This contribution first presents some general guidelines for dysarthria therapy. It then goes on to discuss more specific treatment measures designed to alleviate the respiratory, phonatory and articulatory dysfunctions hindering speech production. The final section of the paper handles treatment methods for speech apraxia.

2. Therapy of the Dysarthrias

The dysarthrias have been broadly classified into the spastic (or central paretic), paretic, hypokinetic, hyperkinetic and ataxic varieties and dysarthria with feedback impairment. Although the underlying movement disorders of the spastic, paretic, and hypokinetic type are clearly distinct (central and peripheral paresis, extrapyramidal disease), the articulatory performance in these disorders, as evident in acoustic parameters, is usually quite similar (Darley/Aronson/Brown 1975). Imprecise consonants, monopitch and monoloudness are noted in all three varieties. Hypernasality and shortening of phrases occur in both central and peripheral paretic types.

According to Netsell/Rosenbek (1986) and Vogel/Ziegler/Morasch (1988), treatment is based upon a physiologically oriented speech analysis aiming at those pathophysiological mechanisms and interactions which cause anomalous movements and coordination. Netsell (1983) has stressed that evaluation must focus on how the perceived speech abnormalities relate to the integrity of each functional component of the speech system. These include the following anatomical structures: the diaphragm, the abdomen and the rib cage for respiration, the larynx for phonation, and the velopharynx, the tongue blade and tip, the lips and the jaw for articulation.

In treatment planning, a target symptom is usually selected which is critical for the patient's comprehensibility. A hypothesis concerning the pathophysiological and functional basis of this target symptom is then formed. Finally, this hypothesis is used to set a sequence of therapeutic goals. Such physiologically oriented diagnostic evaluation may reveal, e. g., that an imprecise consonant production is the result of inadequate intraoral air pressure and not a symptom of articulatory impairment (Kearns/Simmons 1988). This example demonstrates that a malfunction in one component may seriously influence perceptual characteristics associated with others.

Darley/Aronson/Brown (1975, 270–271) advanced the following underlying principles of dysarthria therapy:

- *Compensation* by functional utilization of those neuronal and muscular capacities that are retained following damage. The patient learns to "work around" the impairment that has altered his/her speech habits.
- *Purposeful activity:* The patient must now learn to do what he had been doing automatically before by means of conscious voluntary control and must become sensitive to the obstacles that interfere with the listener's understanding. The goal of being heard and understood replaces the former goals of being quick and expressive in a personal way.
- *Monitoring:* As he/she speaks, the patient must be self-critical and recognize and, if necessary, correct errors. He/she must learn from mistakes how to do better next time.
- *An early start of treatment.* With progressive diseases, therapy started early helps retard speech impairment, and with static lesions, maladaptive and inefficient speech habits may be prevented.
- *Motivation* is maintained by structuring the clinician-patient relationship so as to provide emotional support, concern and understanding and minimize feelings of panic, discouragement, and despair.

Briefly, treatment consists of improving what patients have and improving what patients do with what they have (Rosenbek/LaPointe 1985). The overall goal of treatment is rarely normal speech, but rather to establish maximal intelligibility (Rosenbek/LaPointe 1985), which may be obtained by:

- learning to improve the residual speech motor abilities
- learning to improve coping with the speech motor deficit

- reducing maladaptations
- acquiring functional compensatory behaviour
- adapting the structure of the articulatory system.

With respect to speech breathing, a direct improvement of residual abilities can frequently be achieved by training the transition from the resting respiratory pattern to the speech pattern, correction of posture and recruitment of both thoracic and abdominal respiration.

Coping with the speech motor deficit may be improved, e. g., by adapting phrase length to a reduced expiratory phase, by reducing speech rate or by developing a strategy of producing a phrase syllable by syllable.

Reduction of maladaptations may include the use of biofeedback to reduce movements or tonus of synergistic muscles.

A functional compensation for the production of phonemes that require isolated elevation of the tongue tip (e. g. /l/, /t/, /s/, /n/) may be achieved by elevating the tongue blade instead. Moreover, a palatal lift prothesis may be used as a substitute in such cases in which comprehensibility is severely compromised by paresis or malfunction of the soft palate (Netsell/Rosenbek 1986).

Most authors (e. g. Darley/Aronson/Brown 1975, Kearns/Simmons 1988, Vogel/Ziegler/Morasch 1988) agree that the therapy of the dysarthrias tends to be more symptom than syndrome specific. That is to say, the treatment of, e. g., spastic dysarthria is not necessarily different from that of hypokinetic dysarthria. The presentation of treatment methods will therefore be organized according to the anatomical components involved in speech production and not by syndromes or diseases. No consideration will be given to pharmacological therapy, although especially in the case of hypokinetic dysarthria in Parkinson's Disease, the optimal medication is the basis of speech therapy. In this condition, changes in medication may have a dramatic effect upon articulatory proficiency.

2.1. Treatment of Respiratory Dysfunction

Dysarthria treatment only rarely focusses on non-speech breathing (for methods, compare Vogel/Ziegler/Morasch 1988). On the other hand, many if not most dysarthric patients suffer from either a markedly decreased expiration phase during articulation (Ziegler/Hartmann/Hoole/von Cramon 1990), an inability to provide sufficient subglottal pressure (Netsell/Daniel 1979) or an inability to switch in a controlled way from the non-speech breathing pattern to a coordinated pattern of speech breathing. The non-speech breathing pattern is characterized by a similar duration of inspiration and expiration with blood gas levels as the regulated variable. In contrast, the pattern of breathing during speech consists of short inspiration and prolonged expiration with subglottal pressure as target parameter (Kim 1968, Hixon/Goldman/Mead 1973).

Both volume and force of expiration can be increased by changes in posture. Usually, various positions must be tried out and their corresponding effect upon speech analyzed (Kearns/Simmons 1988). Physiotherapy including sensory stimulation (Farber 1974; Tegart/Mitto 1987) can improve strength and tonus of the respiratory musculature, and the patient may learn to increase abdominal breathing and also make use of auxiliary breathing muscles. Aerodynamic biofeedback measuring subglottal pressure has been used successfully in dysarthria treatment (Netsell/Daniel 1979). There are various methods to increase expiration length and control that include phonatory and articulatory as well as isolated breathing tasks and strategies to adapt speech planning to reduced respiratory capacities. These approaches either focus on drill or on enhanced monitoring and control (for descriptions, see Kearns/Simmons 1988, Vogel/Ziegler/Morasch 1988).

2.2. Treatment of Phonatory Dysfunction

In cases of mutism, anarthria and aphonia two approaches, frequently in combination, are used to trigger phonation (Vogel/Ziegler/Morasch 1988):

- passive manipulation of the larynx, such as pressure upon or upward movement of the thyroid cartilage,
- sensory stimulation by vibration or massage.

Adequate control of respiration is a prerequisite for success. The same manipulations may be employed in training coordination between phonation and articulation.

Darley/Aronson/Brown (1975) stressed that most dysarthric patients produce excessively low pitch and therefore have access to only a limited pitch range. Feedback may be used to help these patients to perform at their optimum pitch level thus providing a greater range of variation. Frequently, pitch control is difficult to establish. Vogel/Ziegler/Morasch (1988) point out that prosodic contour may be more easily obtained by variations in volume. With the exception of Parkinson patients, dysarthric speakers tend to speak excessively loudly and, except for those with ataxic and hypokinetic dysarthria, do not vary loudness to a great degree. Feedback should train patients to reduce loudness to a level appropriate for conversation (Berry/Goshorn 1983). Collaterally, left on their own, these patients attempt to increase intelligibility by slowing the rate of speech, frequently producing one syllable at a time with equal stress and loudness. A therapy plan geared towards approximating normal speech would help the patient to train pitch and loudness variation, to vary vowel length and to increase the length of unpaused productions. Parkinson patients, on the other hand, may avoid a drop in loudness and intelligibility by learning to produce shorter phrases. Parkinson patients have proved able to reduce their speech rate by use of delayed auditory feedback (Hanson/Metter 1983).

The harsh voice quality of many dysarthric speakers may be amerliorated by postural adjustments. Further, relaxation techniques can help minimize phonatory effort. In more severe cases, phonation can begin with voiced sighing and gradually progress towards a sustained breathy phonation (Darley/Aronson/Brown 1975).

2.3. Treatment of Articulatory Dysfunction

Following Rosenbek/LaPointe (1985), we distinguish between the velopharyngeal and orofacial regions of articulation.

Hypernasality is the most common dysarthric symptom associated with velopharyngeal dysfunction. It is caused by central or peripheral paresis or hypokinesia of the soft palate. Among other things, treatment approaches can pinpoint nasal air emission as the target symptom. Feedback can be provided by holding a mirror under the nares or by electronically measuring nasal air flow (Kearns/Simmons 1988). Further treatment methods include sensory stimulation of the soft palate by massage, vibration, or ice application together with voluntary movement. Another strategy for diminishing nasal emission is increasing oral egress. In severe cases, application of a palatal lift prosthesis or palatal surgery may be required.

Isotonic and isometric exercises can be applied in the treatment of paresis and hypokinesia of the orofacial articulators (Rosenbek/LaPointe 1985). With severe, especially posttraumatic dysarthria, Vogel/Ziegler/Morasch (1988) propose focussing first upon restoring oral sensibility and modulating pathological reflexes by applying sensory stimuli which serve to either inhibit or facilitate these reflexes. They advocate using passive support of articulatory movements in order not to trigger off associated movements.

With nonverbal movements, the patient should learn to move articulators individually and differentially using adequate strength and speed to ultimately reach the correct target. Shaping of articulation then starts with vowels and those consonants that are produced in a steady state, i. e., those that require a constant position of articulators. Occasionally, biofeedback is used to reduce excess movement or muscle tone (Netsell/Cleeland 1979). In patients with oral sensory deficits, the phonetic placement technique (van Riper/Irwin 1958) may be used to improve movement control, or oral sensory awareness may specifically be trained. Phonemes are embedded in syllables as early as possible. Many patients will have to learn to overarticulate in order to overcome slurred speech. Special attention should be paid to medial and final consonants. Again, intelligibility and not normality of production is generally the central goal of treatment. If a patient proves unable to make contact between the tip of the tongue and the alveolar ridge or hard palate, he/she may be able to compensate by elevating the tongue blade. Bilabials may be approximated by contact between the upper teeth and the lower lip and consequent mandibular movement (Darley/Brown/Aronson 1975).
In cases of ataxic and hyperkinetic dysarthria, a bite block may be useful to stabilize the jaw during speech (Netsell 1985).

In milder cases or after some therapeutic success, the transfer of treatment gain into everyday communication may become a major problem. Many patients learn to articulate quite acceptably when they focus attention upon speech production. However, in real life communication, attention is usually distracted by the social surroundings, perception of information and to the content of the intended message. At this stage, communicative acts in patient groups or other settings become the primary target of therapy.

3. Treatment of Speech Apraxia

Most speech apraxic patients also suffer from aphasia. Only when the apraxic impairment becomes critical for speech production, will its treatment be the central goal of therapy.

Most approaches focus upon a key apraxic symptom (for a more detailed review and requirements for use of the different therapies, compare Square-Storer 1989 b):

1) In apraxic mutism and in severe speech apraxia, phonetic derivation of phonemes from non-speech sounds is attempted (van Riper/Irwin 1958).
2) When distorted production of phonemes is the central problem, the content network approach (Shewan 1980) is called for. Its goal is to develop voluntary access to articulation by using multimodal stimulation (auditory, visual, tactile and combinations) and to establish multiple means of feedback and control.
3) When the sequencing of speech sounds is the prominent deficit, the so-called speech sound sequencing intervention strategy (Dabul/Bollier 1976) may be applied. Its central feature is drilling the production of phoneme sequences of alternating place of articulation. Vogel/Ziegler/Morasch (1988) recommend guidance of the individual treatment by phonetic criteria, e. g. under consideration and systemic variation of place and mode of articulation.
4) In those cases, in which word initialization is the greatest obstacle, the key-word technique is often helpful (Irwin/Griffith 1973). This approach utilizes the patient's ability to produce some words constantly and with little effort. The patient is trained to produce these key words under volitional control and derive from them other words with the same initial. As an alternative, Willbold/Johannsen-Horbach/Wallesch (1984) have described a technique in which the intact praxis of the upper limb is employed as a trigger or as a motor model for articulation of the initial phoneme.
5) As the impairment tends to increase with effort, relaxation techniques with EMG-feedback have been administered with some success (Rosenbek/Kent/LaPointe 1984).
6) Vogel/Ziegler/Morasch (1988) also emphasize that fluency and comprehensibility, but not accuracy are the primary goals of treatment of speech apraxia. Therefore, the patient's attempts at self correction should only be encouraged, if his/her comprehensibility is impaired. In most patients, fluency is the communicatively more important aim.
7) The Melodic Intonation Therapy Program, which attempts to carry speech production by an accentuated prosodic contour (Sparks/Helm/Albert 1974) has also been reported to improve production in speech apraxics (Tonkovich/Marquardt 1977).

A more physiologically oriented strategy, Prompts for Restructuring Oral Muscular Phonetic Targets (PROMPT), has recently been described by Square-Storer/Hayden (1989). In this strategy, the patient is provided with an "enhanced and, initially, clinician-controlled somatosensory description of the postural fixators or articulatory end-points, velocities, and trajectories of movements, and the 'phasing' or temporal assembly of motor subroutines. The clinician acts as an 'external programmer'. After having mapped the program, he/she then ensures that the patient remains motorically but not sensorily passive. Immediately following, the patient is allowed motoric control while the clinician continues to provide somatosensory support for the constraints and patterns of movement. Eventually, the patient appears to internalize the program for each target and (...) begins to generate related programs ..." (Square-Storer/Hayden, 192). According to the authors, the underlying physiological rationale is that the programming of motor events is directly influenced and potentially guided step by step by somatosensory information. This guidance is thought to compensate for the defect in program generation in speech apraxia. The intact linguistic plan of the intended utterance may be utilized to facilitate stepwise motor program processing. PROMPT differs from the other approaches outlined above (with the exception of Melodic Intonation) in that it is applied predominantly at the phrase level. Square-Storer/Hayden (1989) obtained impressive results with this therapy program. Comparative studies with other treatment programs are being presently conducted.

4. References

Berry, W. R. & Goshorn, E. L. (1983). Immediate visual feedback in the treatment of ataxic dysarthria: a case study. In W. R. Berry (Ed.), *Clinical dysarthria. 253–265*. San Diego: College Hill.

Dabul, B. & Bollier, B. (1976). Therapeutic approaches to apraxia. *Journal of Speech and Hearing disorders, 41*, 268–276.

Darley, F. L., Aronson, A. E., & Brown, J. R. (1975). *Motor Speech Disorders*. Philadelphia: Saunders.

Farber, D. S. (1974). *Sensorimotor evaluation and treatment for allied health personnel*. Indianapolis: University of Indiana Foundation.

Hanson, W. R. & Metter, E. J. (1983). DAF speech rate modification in Parkinson's disease: a report on two cases. In W. R. Berry (Ed.), *Clinical dysarthria. 231–251*. San Diego: College Hill.

Hixon, T., Goldman, M., & Mead, J. (1973). Kinematics of the chest wall during speech production. *Journal of Speech and Hearing Research, 16*, 78–115.

Irwin, J. V. & Griffith, F. A. (1973). A theoretical and operational analysis of the paired stimuli technique. In W. D. Wolfe & D. J. Goulding (Eds.), *Articulation and Learning: New dimensions in research, diagnostics, and therapy. 156–194*. Springfield: Thomas.

Kearns, K. P. & Simmons, N. N. (1988). Motor speech disorders: The dysarthrias and apraxia of speech. In N. J. Lass, L. V. McReynolds, J. L. Northern, & D. E. Yoder (Eds.), *Handbook of Speech-Language Pathology and Audiology. 592–621*. Toronto: Decker.

Kim, R. (1968). The chronic residual respiratory disorder in post-encephalitic Parkinsonism. *Journal of Neurology, Neurosurgery and Psychiatry, 31*, 393–398.

Netsell, R. (1983). Speech motor control: theoretical issues with clinical impact. In W. R. Berry (Ed.), *Clinical dysarthria. 1–19*. San Diego: College Hill.

Netsell, R. (1984). A neurobiologic view of the dysarthrias. In M. R. McNeil, J. C. Rosenbek, & A. E. Aronson (Eds.), *The dysarthrias: physiology, acoustics, perception, management. 1–36*. San Diego: College Hill Press.

Netsell, R. (1985). Construction and use of a bite block for evaluating and treating speech disorders. *Journal of Speech and Hearing Disorders,* 50, 103–106.

Netsell, R. & Cleeland, C. (1979). Modification of lip hypertonia in dysarthria using EMG feedback. *Journal of Speech and Hearing Disorders,* 38, 131–141.

Netsell, R. & Daniel, B. (1979). Dysarthria in adults: physiological approach to rehabilitation. *Archives of Physical Medicine and Rehabilitation, 60*, 502–508.

Netsell, R. & Rosenbek, J. C. (1986). Treating the dysarthrias. In R. Netsell (Ed.), *A neurobiologic view of speech production and the dysarthrias. 123–152*. San Diego: College Hill Press.

Rosenbek, J. C., Kent, R. D. & LaPointe, L. L. (1984). Apraxia of speech: an overview and some perspectives. In J. C. Rosenbek, M. R. McNeil, & A. E. Aronson (Eds.), *Apraxia of speech: physiology, acoustics, linguistics, management. 1–72*. San Diego: College Hill Press.

Rosenbek, J. C. & LaPointe, L. L. (1985). The dysarthrias: description, diagnosis and treatment. In D. F. Johns (Ed.), *Clinical management of neurogenic communication disorders*. 97–129. Boston: Little, Brown.

Shewan, C. M. (1980). Verbal dyspraxia and its treatment. *Human Communication, 5*, 3–12.

Sparks, R., Helm, N., & Albert, M. (1974). Aphasia rehabilitation resulting from melodic intonation therapy. *Cortex, 10*, 303–316.

Square-Storer, P. (1989a). Preface. In P. Square-Storer (Ed.), *Acquired apraxia of speech in aphasic adults*. XV–XVII. London: Taylor & Francis.

Square-Storer, P. (1989b). Traditional therapies for apraxia of speech – reviewed and rationalized. In P. Square-Storer (Ed.), *Acquired apraxia of speech in aphasic adults. 145–161*. London: Taylor & Francis.

Square-Storer, P. & Hayden (Chumpelik), D. (1989). PROMPT Treatment. In P. Square-Storer (Ed.), *Acquired apraxia of speech in aphasic adults. 190–219*. London: Taylor & Francis.

Square-Storer, P. & Roy, E. A. (1989). The apraxias – commonalities and distinctions. In P. Square-Storer (Ed.), *Acquired apraxia of speech in aphasic adults. 20–63*. London: Taylor & Francis.

Tegart, L. & Mitto, H. (1987). Die Therapie der spastischen Dysarthrie. In L. Springer & G. Kattenbeck (Eds.), *Aktuelle Beiträge zur Dysarthrophonie und Dysprosodie. 25–58*. München: tuduv.

Tonkovich, J. D. & Marquardt, T. P. (1977). The effects of stress and melodic intonation on apraxia of speech. In R. H. Brookshire (Ed.), *Clinical aphasiology conference proceedings. 97–102*. Minneapolis: BRK.

Van Riper, C. & Irwin, J. (1958). *Voice and articulation*. Englewood Cliffs: Prentice Hall.

Vogel, M., Ziegler, W. & Morasch, H. (1988). Sprechen. In D. von Cramon & J. Zihl (Eds.), *Neurophysiologische Rehabilitation. 319–359*. Berlin: Springer.

Willbold, B., Johannsen-Horbach, H., & Wallesch, C. W. (1984). Zur Therapie der artikulatorischen Apraxie. *Sprache–Stimme–Gehör,* 8, 24–26.

Ziegler, W., Hartmann, E., Hoole, P., & von Cramon, D. (1990). *Entwicklung von diagnostischen Standards und von Therapieleitlinien für zentrale Stimm- und Sprechstörungen (Dysarthrophonien)*. München: Gesellschaft für Strahlen- und Umweltforschung.

Helga Johannsen-Horbach/Claus-W. Wallesch, Freiburg (Germany)

47. Effects of Anatomical Alterations on Fully Developed Articulation

1. Introduction

The cognitively intact adult with normal speech who suffers sudden loss of parts of the speech mechanism through ablative surgery constitutes an interesting research opportunity for linguists. What adjustments or maladjustments does the individual make in phonetic output and other linguistic behavior? Such individuals provide a research population for investigating the plasticity of the speech production mechanism, that is, for studying the minimum physical requirements for normal speech production or for exploring aberrant speech production which nevertheless recognizably realizes the phonological system. In addition, adjustments in speech production are influenced by idiosyncratic factors as well as by the particular ablative procedures and subsequent reconstructions, further challenging the linguist in teasing apart the role that each factor plays in speech. The purpose of this chapter is to orient the linguist to the area of orofacial ablative surgery with respect to opportunities for the analysis of the phonetic realization of phonological structures. Information is organized according to type of resection and, when appropriate, to effects of surgical or prosthetic treatment on speech production. Combination resections of multiple oral structures are common, but information on speech in such reports is often missing (e. g., Kavanagh/Hinkle 1987) and, if offered, is presented only in general terms.

2. Maxillary Resections

Articulation is imperiled by removal of normal dental, alveolar and palatal contacts; resonance is altered if the ablation destroys the normal separation between the oral and nasal cavities (Arndt/Shelton/Bradford 1965; Fletcher/Sooudi/Frost 1974; Majid/Weinberg/Chalian 1974). The consensus of clinical reports is that most patients regain intelligibility once fitted with appropriate prosthetic devices (Kipfmueller/Lang 1972; Majid/Weinberg/Chalian 1974; Plank/Weinberg/Chalian 1981). See Peterson-Falzone 1988, for summary.

3. Ablation of the Soft Palate

These resections are typically accompanied by partial or total maxillectomy, and result in loss of velopharyngeal closure, with the expected effects of nasal air loss on obstruent consonants and hypernasal resonance on vowels and vocalic segments. Correction of the physical defect may be approached surgically or prosthetically; few data are available delineating benefits of one approach over the other, probably due to individual factors affecting adjustments to prostheses (obturators for the velopharyngeal port) versus surgical approaches. Casey/Emrich (1988) reported development of 'compensatory' motion of the pharyngeal musculature (commonly called Passavant's ridge) in 83% of patients undergoing soft palatectomy, but had no data on presence or absence of such movement preoperatively. (Inward movement of pharyngeal musculature is known to be of significant benefit in prosthetic treatment of patients with clefts and other forms of velopharyngeal insufficiency [Karnell/Rosenstein/Fine 1987]). Minsley/Warren/Hinton (1988) reported that four patients with oronasal defects due to resection of the maxilla and/or soft palate increased respiratory volumes four-fold following the resections, thus maintaining supralaryngeal vocal tract air pressures within the normal range despite the reduction in vocal tract resistance. This compensation is similar to that evidenced by speakers with cleft palate. Significant differences were found in the respiratory volumes accompanying voiced and voiceless consonants; thus the linguistic contrast was retained even with the elevated volumes.

4. Mandibulectomy

Reports on speech after mandibulectomy are usually descriptions of cases involving partial or total ablation of the tongue (following section). Most articles focus on surgical technique and discuss speech only in terms of "intelligibility" after reconstruction (e. g., Jewer/Boyd/Manktelow et al. 1989; Weissler/Goldsmith/Martinkosky 1988). Hemimandibulectomy causes little disturbance in function if the bone resection does not pass the midline (Bloomer/Hawk 1973).

5. Glossectomy

A very large body of clinical data on the effects of partial or total glossectomy on speech is available, much of it difficult to interpret. Several reports have described the ability of some patients to develop intelligible speech without prosthetic or surgical reconstruction (Bloomer/Hawk 1973; Duguay 1964; Goldstein 1940; Herberman 1958). Goldstein (1940) even went so far as to conclude that the tongue was not an indispensable articulator. However, the descriptions given by these early authors are often lacking in details regarding individual phones, and even the definition of 'intelligible' is unspecified.

The literature on glossectomy indicates that impairment in function is not always proportional to the amount of tissue removed. Skelly/Spector/Donaldson et al. (1971) reported remarkably similar (and low) intelligibility for partial and total glossectomees. However, Rentschler/Mann (1980) reported a correlation of −.726 between extent of surgery and intelligibility. More important than the difference between partial or subtotal glossectomy and total glossectomy is the fact that most of these occur as part of combined ablations of the floor of the mouth, mandible, pharynx and even larynx. In an early report on a patient with a partial glossectomy (Lehman/Hulicka/Mehringer 1966), the "total lack of speech" was due to concomitant laryngectomy rather than to resection of lingual tissue.

Some reports on partial glossectomees describe articulatory adjustments developed either spontaneously or with training. Backus (1940) described a boy who substituted labial consonants for tongue-tip phonemes after anterolateral excision of one-third of the tongue. Bloomer/Hawk (1973) described a hemiglossectomee who substituted a lingual-alveolar constriction for midline lingual grooving on sibilants.

Skelly/Spector/Donaldson et al. 1971) described a therapy program, later elaborated by Skelly (1973), for teaching compensatory articulations to partial and total glossectomees. Intelligibility for the partial glossectomees increased from a pre-therapy rating of 6−24% to post-therapy values of 24−46%. For the total glossectomees, 0−8% intelligibility increased to 18−42%. The partial glossectomees were observed to make marked use of the residual stump rather than resorting to the more varied substitutions used by the total glossectomees, some examples of which were production of /z/ by bilabial tension obstruction of the airstream (also described by LaRiviere/Seilo/Dimmick 1975); production of /g/ by pharyngeal constriction, with slight bulging of the retroglossal pharyngeal wall; and production of /d/ by lower lip contact with the maxillary teeth, or in edentulous patients, with the maxillary alveolar ridge. Skelly/Donaldson/Schinsky (1972) emphasized consistency of phoneme substitution as critical in intelligibility, and stated that usable gains in compensatory articulation required 6 to 8 months in total glossectomees.

Duguay (1964) supplied a list of "acceptable acoustic approximations" drawn from his own observations and from a survey of the literature. These included production of tip-alveolars either by elevation of the floor of the mouth or by retraction and elevation of the lower lip to contact the upper incisors; substitution of labiodental for interdental consonants; production of sibilants by airflow through the teeth, lips protruded; substitution of glottal stops for the stop feature of affricates; production of linguavelar consonants by contact of buccinator muscles with the molars, or by 'movements approximating the palatal arches,' or replacement of /k/ and /g/ by glottal stops and /ng/ by nasalization of the preceding vowel; and replacement of /r/ by a 'laryngeal' or uvular articulation.

LaRiviere/Seilo/Dimmick (1975) described speech in a patient left with a small remnant of lingual tissue posterior to the faucial pillars. Bilabial and labiodental consonants were highly intelligible, as would be expected, but so were /t, s, n, l/ and the voiced affricate. Intelligibility of vowels ranged from 90% for /ae/ to 9% for vocalic /r/, with a mean of 45.8%. Sentence intelligibility was 88.8%. Listeners confused /t, p/ and /d, b/, and acoustic analysis revealed that the durations of these pairs had been reversed. However, /s/ and /f/ were also confused perceptually and their durational values were not similar. This suggests that durational differences cannot compensate for all ambiguous acoustic properties although they may add to the confusion if inappropriate. Linguadental stops and interdental fricatives were produced by movements normally associated with bilabial stops and labiodental fricatives. Sibilants were produced by blowing air through closed teeth. In general, the speaker preserved manner and voicing of consonants while necessarily sacrificing place of production.

Some information on effects of lingual ablation on vowel intelligibility is available (Ballard/Kerner/Tyson 1986; Gillis/Leonard 1983; Landahl/Karnell 1990; LaRiviere/Seilo/Dimmick 1975; Skelly 1973; Skelly/Donaldson/Fust/Townsend 1972). Skelly/Donaldson/Fust/Townsend (1972) noted that the value of F_1 extended over a wide range in less intelligible speakers, that is, exhibited a greater than normal bandwidth, and the intensity of F_2 was diminished. In line with the findings of psychoacoustic investigations on perception of vowels produced by normal speakers, intelligibility increased as F_1 decreased in bandwidth and F_2 became more defined. In the patient described by LaRiviere/Seilo/Dimmick (1975), vowels were neutralized both perceptually and acoustically, with F_1 more stable than F_2. Gillis/Leonard (1983) reported 48% vowel intelligibility in single words in their glossectomy speaker.

Georgian/Logemann/Fisher (1982) provided extensive perceptual and acoustic data on a patient following resection and reconstruction of the tongue and floor of the mouth. The speech samples were CVC syllables consisting of voiced and voiceless bilabial and tip-alveolar stops in various vowel contexts. The greatest perceptual misidentification was observed when both bilabials and tip-alveolars occurred in context with /i/. (Note that many glossectomy speakers described in the literature spontaneously substitute, or have been taught to substitute, labial consonants for tongue tip consonants.) Among the acoustic findings were absence of stop bursts, weakened F_3, and frequent convergence of F_2 towards F_1. Negatively sloped transitions, as opposed to normally positively sloped, were observed for all bilabial productions except /bi/. Landahl/Karnell (1990) also compared perceptual to acoustic data on two glossectomee speakers, one whose speech was rated as 80% intelligible and the other at 50% intelligible. They reported that, for the latter, removal of poorly identified vowel information enhanced listeners' identification of the consonants. For the less impaired speaker, full CV's were well identified while removal of vowel information diminished correct consonant identification. The authors concluded that, when onset spectra are ambiguous, the vowel transitions weight the onset spectrum to influence identification of the consonant place of articulation, in some instances away from the intended category.

Several reports have described patients undergoing glossectomy combined with partial mandibulectomy (Ballard/Kerner/Tyson et al. 1986; Cantor/Curtis/Shipp et al. 1969; Curtis/Cantor 1974; Knowles/Chalian/Shanks 1984; Wheeler/Logemann/Rosen 1980); two reports have described patients who have undergone glossectomy with total mandibulectomy. Shedd (1976) said his patient was 70 to 80% intelligible, but gave no details on articulatory compensations or treatment procedures. The patient described by Meyerson/Johnson/Weitzman (1980) lost the mandible together with the anterior one-half of the tongue with excision of the mylohyoid, hyoglossus, genioglossus and digastric muscles. After multiple surgical reconstructions, all consonants except /h/ were severely distorted. Bilabial consonants were affected due to lack of bony support for the lower lip. Intelligibility was zero at the initial evaluation, and 50% eighteen months later, before formal therapy was initiated. Speakers were taught to use pharyngeal constrictions to approximate velar stops. Linguoalveolar stops were approximated by contact between the lower lip and upper teeth. A slower rate of speech was encouraged to increase intelligibility, which was 80% by the conclusion of therapy. Acoustical analysis at this time showed the vowel space to be diminished in comparison to normal speakers, with the most limitation in the range of F_2.

Prosthetic approaches to rehabilitation have yielded interesting results recently, although many reports are poorly detailed. These consist of attempts (a) to provide a prosthetic tongue, and (b) to lower the palatal arch to facilitate articulatory contacts. Cantor/Curtis/Shipp et al. (1969) reported the latter devices to facilitate velar consonant production for patients with severe restrictions in lingual mobility but negative effects for those with modest restriction. Wheeler/Logemann/Rosen (1980) described a series of patients with 10 to 90% of the tongue excised whose speech intelligibility ranged from 72% to 81% (note that even the patient with 90% of the tongue extirpated had not lost more than 18% of his intelligibility). Without their "maxillary reshaping prostheses," no patient exceeded 90% intelligibility; with these devices, 6 of 10 reach this criterion. In 3 of 4 patients provided with "thickening of the maxillary denture" (Lauciello/Vergo/Schaaf/Zimmerman 1980), both articulation and resonance were reported to improve. A similar approach was used by Knowles/Chalian/Shanks (1984). Aramany/Downs/Beery/Aslan (1982) suggested palatal augmentation prostheses for partial glossectomees, mandibular tongue prostheses for total glossectomees. Palatography (mapping of articulatory contacts sensed by electrodes imbedded in a palatal plate) was suggested by both Christensen/Hutton/Hasegawa/Fletcher (1983) and McKinstry/Aramany/Beery/Sansone (1985) for optimal fitting of prostheses, but patient material was limited.

Mandibular tongue prostheses have been described in several reports (Ballard/Kerner/Tyson et al. 1986; Belsky 1978; deSouza/Martins 1975; Moore 1972; Gillis/Leonard 1983) offering somewhat mystifying descriptions of the devices and little specific information on speech. (There are multiple articles on surgical reconstruction attempting either to restore lingual function or to prepare the mandible and floor of the mouth to support a lingual prosthesis; unfortunately, these reports discuss recovery of function primarily in terms of deglutition rather than speech.) Moore (1972) fashioned a prosthesis with a "highly flexible tip" so that his patient could produce tongue-tip sounds, but there was not note of how the tip was controlled. Gillis/Leonhard (1983) designed several experimental prostheses for their patient, but did not describe in detail which design produced the best speech results, which were improvements in vowel intelligibility from 48% to 64% and consonant intelligibility from 82% to 90% in single words. Ballard/Kerner/Tyson et al. (1986) noted that their patient who had been fitted with a combination mandibular/tongue prosthesis shifted the anterior-to-posterior position of the mandible to achieve tip-alveolar and linguavelar consonants.

It is worth noting that the most comprehensive speech habilitation program for glossectomy patients is still the "compensatory physiologic phonetics" of Skelly and associates, despite the fact that the work is now nearly 20 years old (1971, 1972a, 1972b, 1973). In addition to the compensatory gestures taught in an effort to achieve approximations of normal consonants, Skelly and coworkers sought to improve intelligibility through manipulation of vowel duration, vocal intensity, pause length, habitual pitch, pitch range and variation in pitch patterns. No follow-up reports have appeared, but no other speech pathologists have replaced or significantly augmented Skelly's work. Clearly, improvements in therapeutic approaches will be dependent upon investigations which relate the physiology with acoustic output and the perceptual responses of listeners.

6. References

Aramany, M. A., Downs, J. A., Beery, Q. C., & Aslan, Y. (1982). Prosthodontic rehabilitation for glossectomy patients. *Journal of Prosthetic Dentistry, 48,* 78–81.

Arndt, W. B., Shelton, R. L., & Bradford, L. J. (1965). Articulation, voice, and obturation in persons with acquired and congenital palatal defects. *Cleft Palate Journal, 2,* 377–383.

Backus, O. (1940). Speech rehabilitation following excision of the tip of the tongue. *American Journal of the Disabled Child, 60,* 368–370.

Ballard, J. L., Kerner, E., Tyson, J., Ashford, J., & Rees, R. (1986). Adenocarcinoma of the tongue complicated by hemimandibulectomy: Soft tissue support for a tongue prosthesis in an edentulous glossectomy patient. *Journal of Prosthetic Dentistry, 56,* 470–473.

Belsky, M. W. (1978). Prosthetic reconstruction of mandibular tongue prostheses. *Journal of Prosthetic Dentistry, 39,* 650–653.

Bloomer, H. H. & Hawk, A. M. (1973). Speech considerations: Speech disorders associated with ablative surgery of the face, mouth and pharynx – ablative approaches to learning. ASHA Report No. 8: *Orofacial Anomalies: Clinical and Research Implications. 42–61.* Washington, D. C.: American Speech and Hearing Association.

Cantor, R., Curtis, T. A., Shipp, T., Beumer, J., & Vogel, B. S. (1969). Maxillary speech prostheses for mandibular surgical defects. *Journal of Prosthetic Dentistry, 22,* 253–260.

Casey, D. M. & Emrich, L. J. (1988). Passavant's ridge in patients with soft palatectomy. *Cleft Palate Journal, 25,* 72–77.

Christensen, J. M., Hutton, J. E., Hasegawa, A., & Fletcher, S. G. (1983). Evaluation of the effects of palatal augmentation on partial glossectomy speech. *Journal of Prosthetic Dentistry, 50,* 539–543.

Curtis, T. A. & Cantor, R. (1974). The forgotten patient in maxillofacial prosthetics. *Journal of Prosthetic Dentistry, 31,* 662–679.

DeSouza, L. J. & Martins, O. J. (1975). Swallowing and speech after radical total glossectomy with tongue prosthesis. *Oral Surgery, 39,* 356–360.

Duguay, M. J. (1964). Speech after glossectomy. *New York State Journal of Medicine, 64,* 1836–1838.

Fletcher, S. G., Sooudi, I., & Frost, S. D. (1974). Quantitative and graphic analysis of prosthetic treatment for "nasalance" in speech. *Journal of Prosthetic Dentistry, 32,* 284–291.

Georgian, D. A., Logemann, J. A. & Fisher, H. B. (1982). Compensatory articulation patterns of a surgically treated oral cancer patient. *Journal of Speech and Hearing Disorders, 47,* 154–159.

Gillis, R. E. & Leonard, R. J. (1983). Prosthetic treatment for speech and swallowing in patients with total glossectomy. *Journal of Prosthetic Dentistry, 50,* 808–814.

Goldstein, M. A. (1940). Speech without a tongue. *Journal of Speech Disorders, 5,* 65–69.

Herberman, M. A. (1958). Rehabilitation of patients following glossectomy. *Archives of Otolaryngology, 67,* 182–183.

Karnell, M. P., Rosenstein, H., & Fine, L. (1987). Nasal videoendoscopy in prosthetic management of palatopharyngeal dysfunction. *Journal of Prosthetic Dentistry, 58,* 479–484.

Kavanagh, K. T. & Hinkle, W. G. (1987). Reconstruction of the soft palate after jaw, tongue, neck dissection with subtotal palatectomy (velopharyngoplasty). *Laryngoscope, 97,* 1461–1463.

Kipfmueller, L. J. & Lang, B. R. (1972). Presurgical maxillary prosthesis: An analysis of speech intelligibility. *Journal of Prosthetic Dentistry, 28,* 620–625.

Knowles, J. C., Chalian, V. A. & Shanks, J. C. (1984). A functional speech impression used to fabricate a maxillary speech prosthesis for a partial glossectomy. *Journal of Prosthetic Dentistry, 51,* 232–237.

Landahl, K. L. & Karnell, M. P. (1990). Acoustic invariants in glossectomee speech. Manuscript in preparation.

LaRiviere, C., Seilo, M. T. & Dimmick, K. C. (1975). Report on the speech intelligibility of a glossectomee: Perceptual and acoustic observations. *Folia Phoniatrica, 27,* 201–214.

Lauciello, F. R., Vergo, T., Schaaf, H. G. & Zimmerman, R. (1980). Prosthodontic and speech rehabilitation after partial and complete glossectomy. *Journal of Prosthetic Dentistry, 43,* 204–211.

Lehman, W. L., Hulicka, I. M. & Mehringer, E. J. (1966). Prosthetic treatment following complete glossectomy. *Journal of Prosthetic Dentistry, 16,* 344–350.

Majid, A. A., Weinberg, B. & Chalian, V. A. (1974). Speech intelligibility following prosthetic obturation of surgical acquired maxillary defects. *Journal of Prosthetic Dentistry, 323,* 87–96.

McKinstry, R. E., Aramany, M. A., Beery, Q. C. & Sansone, F. (1985). Speech considerations in prosthodontic rehabilitation of the glossectomy patient. *Journal of Prosthetic Dentistry, 53,* 384–387.

Meyerson, M. D., Johnson, B. H. & Weitzman, R. S. (1980). Rehabilitation of a patient with complete mandibulectomy and partial glossectomy. *American Journal of Otolaryngology, 1,* 256–261.

Minsley, G. E., Warren, D. W. & Hinton, V. (1988). Maintenance of intraoral pressure during speech after maxillary resection. *Journal of the Acoustical Society of America, 83,* 820–824.

Moore, D. J. (1972). Glossectomy rehabilitation by mandibular tongue prosthesis. *Journal of Prosthetic Dentistry, 28,* 429–433.

Peterson-Falzone, S. J. (1988). Speech disorders related to craniofacial structural defects, Part I. In N. J. Lass, L. V. McReynolds, J. L. Northern & D. E. Yoder (Eds.), *Handbook of speech-language pathology and audiology. 442–476.* Toronto: B. C. Decker.

Plank, D. M., Weinberg, B. & Chalian, V. A. (1981). Evaluation of speech following prosthetic obturation of surgically acquired maxillary defects. *Journal of Prosthetic Dentistry, 45,* 626–638.

Rentschler, G. J. & Mann, M. B. (1980). The effects of glossectomy on intelligibility of speech and oral perceptual discrimination. *Journal of Oral Surgery, 38,* 348.

Shedd, D. (1976). Rehabilitation problems of head and neck cancer patients. *Journal of Surgical Oncology, 8,* 11–21.

Skelly, M., Donaldson, R. C. & Schinsky, L. (1972), Substitution consistency as a factor in glossectomee intelligibility. *Journal of the Missouri Speech and Hearing Association, 5,* 21–23.

Skelly, M., Donaldson, R. C., Fust, R. S. & Townsend, D. L. (1972). Changes in phonatory aspects of glossectomee intelligibility through vocal parameter manipulation. *Journal of Speech and Hearing Disorders, 37,* 379–389.

Skelly, M. (1973). *Glossectomee speech rehabilitation.* Springfield, II.: C. C. Thomas.

Skelly, M., Spector, D. J., Donaldson, R. C., Brodeur, A. & Paletta, F. X. (1971). Compensatory physiologic phonetics for the glossectomee. *Journal of Speech and Hearing Disorders, 36,* 101–114.

Weissler, M. C., Goldsmith, M. M. & Martinkosky, S. (1988). A method of closure after resection of anterior floor of mouth cancers. *Otolaryngology-Head and Neck Surgery, 99,* 315–320.

Wheeler, R. L., Logemann, J. A. & Rosen, M. S. (1980). Maxillary reshaping prostheses: Effectiveness in improving speech and swallowing of post-surgical oral cancer patients. *Journal of Prosthetic Dentistry, 43,* 313–319.

Sally J. Peterson-Falzone, San Francisco, California (USA)/Karen L. Landahl, Chicago, Illinois (USA)

48. Disorders of Phonation

1. Introduction

This article starts with a discussion of the voice with respect to its role in communication. Then the anatomic, physiological and pathological foundations of voice production will be introduced as a backdrop for the understanding of the relationships to be presented here. In view of the space available for the chapter on disorders of phonation in this handbook, only a very general overview of the various causes of phonation disorders can be given in favor of a more thorough treatment of the effects of craniocerebral injury and other brain diseases on the larynx and its functions. After that, the direct effects of these brain diseases on the center controlling laryngeal functions will be examined. Finally, we will look into those effects actually resulting from interventions, such as long-term intubation, that had been necessary in the acute phase of the illness.

The realization of communication demands precise coordination of respiration, phonation and articulation. The disturbance of a part of the system disrupts the whole and may even cause it to break down entirely. This contribution handles the voice and its disorders, well knowing that a voice disorder is often caused by an impediment in the coordination of the three different functions, and therefore signals a more encompassing disorder. In this case, the voice disorder may be the initial symptom of another illness which may progress and affect other functions. Or, the voice disorder may not occur until other disorders are apparent.

A normal voice tells more about its carrier than his or her speech. A person's voice often has quite individual and unmistakable sound properties, that vary within a certain range and depend on the speaker's physical and psychological state. The singularity of each voice is determined by the anatomic structures in the larynx and in the vocal tract. Interestingly, one can hardly voluntarily influence this set up to change one's special sound of voice. In fact, a normal speaker will even have difficulty attempting to alter learned speech behaviors, which have been partly influenced by 'vocal' role models, such as volume, pitch level, intonation and other parameters.

A person's voice will only be perceived as being appropriate, when its pitch level and sound characteristics reflect the appearance and the personality of the speaker and when its volume meets the demands of the situation. Even minor deviations from the modalities mentioned lead to a noticeable clash between the speaker and his or her voice, usually arousing negative emotions or downright rejection on the part of the hearer.

The human voice is produced in the larynx, which is situated at the top of the trachea, at the point where the trachea and the esophagus branch. The larynx consists of a cartilage box (Fig. 48.1), which is held together by ligaments, muscles and mucous membranes. The joint linking the cricoid cartilage to the 2 arytenoid cartilages is flexible enough to allow the larynx to carry out opposing functions. That is, the larynx must open for respiration and close for phonation (Fig. 48.2). Almost all of the muscles involved in voice production have an effect on these joints, to open or to close the glottis or to tense the vocal folds. These muscles receive their nervous impulses from two branches of the vagus nerve (X), the superior and inferior laryngal nerves (N. laryngicus superior et N. laryngicus inferior = N. recurrens), and regulate the position of the vocal folds and their tension. The vibrations of the vocal folds, which give rise to the primary sound production of the larynx, are caused by a breath stream coming from the trachea and flowing against the closed glottis. The air flow induces quite even, regular movements in both vocal folds (myoelastic-aerodynamic theory of voice production; van den Berg 1956; 1958).

Immediately after passing through the vibrating vocal cords, this primary sound of the larynx is but yet a still completely undifferentiated sound pattern with a lot of overtones. It must then be transformed into the diverse sounds of speech by means of free resonance in the vocal tract, that is in the entrance of the larynx, the low and middle pharynx, the oral and nasal cavity and the nose. (For further details about the anatomy

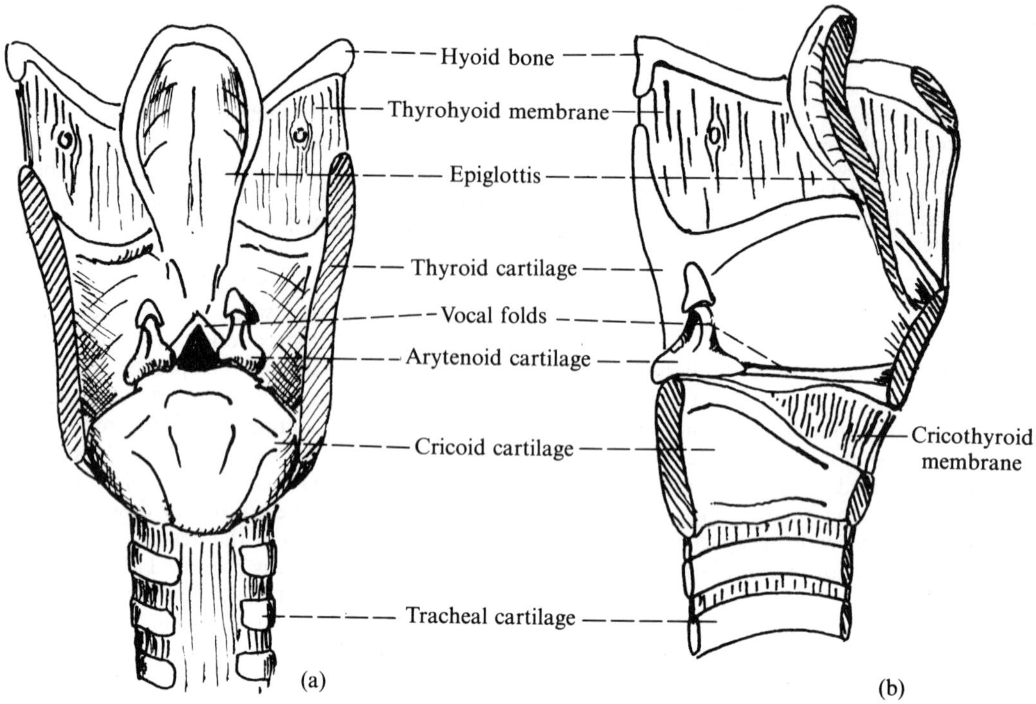

Fig. 48.1: Posterior (a) and lateral (b) views of the hyoid bone and the laryngeal and tracheal cartilages and their connecting membranes

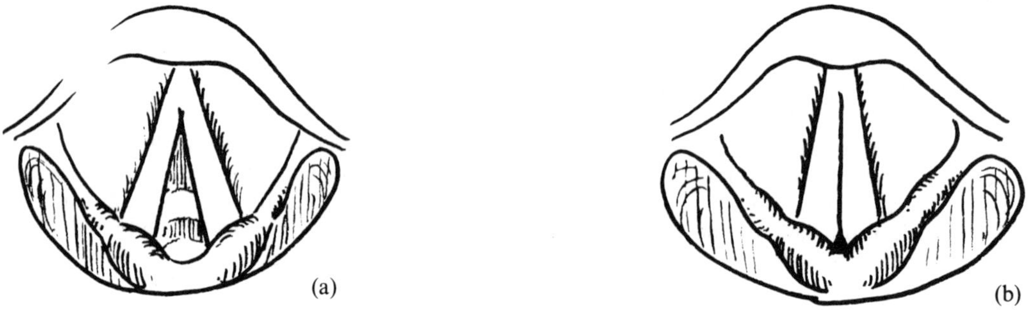

Fig. 48.2: Normal larynx in indirect laryngoscopy during respiration (a) and phonation (b)

and physiology of phonation, see Aronson's (1990) textbook on clinical voice disorders.)

Not only do the manifold functions of the normal voice just mentioned depend on intact centers, neurons and pathways from the motor control center to the larynx, not to mention the condition of the larynx itself, but they also depend on the emotional affective state of the speaker. With this in mind, the diversity of disorders that can affect voice function is no surprise.

Clinicians treating disorders of phonation are faced with certain hindrances. One difficulty is the lack of knowledge about premorbid idiosyncrasies or even possible disorders of phonation in the patients to be treated. A further difficulty is posed by the fact that several different factors can alter phonation in an individual patient. Thus primary and secondary effects on pitch are hard to differentiate. For example, many voice disorders, no matter whether they are organic, functional (in a narrow sense) or psychogenic in origin can cause the patient to compensate in such a manner that the illness inducing factors are masked.

Furthermore, certain voice disorders do not clearly fit into the categories mentioned. At the top of this list is adductor (spastic) dysphonia, which is probably a generic term for phonation disorders of different origins, these being neurological as well as psychological and having the same or similar vocal symptoms (Aronson 1990). Among other things, this uncertainty may have led to the fact that international researchers have not been able to agree on a standard classification of voice disorders. On the other hand, this lack of standardization, may also be a sign that the use of constantly refined diagnostic instruments has put us in a better position to create more and more closed and distinct subcategories for both centrally as well as peripherally-induced voice disorders. (For more detailed information on voice disorders, see the excellent articles by Habermann (1980) and Schultz-Coulon (1980) as well as the textbook by Aronson (1990).)

Well aware that a binding categorization cannot be undertaken here either, I will nevertheless dare to make a tentative one for the sake of providing an overview of all of the disorders of phonation. This will also allow me to classify the voice disorders arising after craniocerebral injury trauma (to be looked at more closely below), as well as those resulting from the therapy of such injuries. Finally, I will attempt to present these disorders in a comprehensive classification (Table 48.1; without claim to completeness). The table distinguishes between organic and functional voice disorders. An organic voice disorder can be brought about by an anatomic disease of the larynx itself. Alternatively, it may result from a general illness also affecting the larynx or an illness befalling the structures controlling the larynx. In contrast, a functional voice disorder is considered to be a disturbance of pitch and/or vocal performance without primary organic damage. A further division of functional voice disorders is based on that of Perelló's (1962). In his classification system, phonoponoses are considered to be the result of improper, uneconomical voice production or a constant strain on the organs of speech. Thus they are generally of mechanical origin. In contrast, phononeuroses are mainly attributed to psychological alterations. Indeed, this dualistic division into mechanical and psychological causes is subject to criticism. Despite the fact that it represents numerous overlapping and hybrid illnesses, it oversimplifies and distorts the typical multifactorial genesis of the functional dysphonias (Pascher 1982). In addition, it appears to be problematic to group every psychologically-induced voice disorder among the (phono)neuroses, a term which is not always appropriate. Clinical practice has repeatedly shown that individual cases can prove difficult to classify according to these two groups. This is usually the case, since there are no distinguishing criteria either in the symptoms or in the results of the voice and larynx examination.

2. Organic Voice Disorders

Whatever their pathogens, infections lead to alterations of the audible sounds produced by phonation to varying degrees. Infectious cells infiltrate the mucous membrane of the larynx and possibly even that of the vocal fold muscles. Here, they upset the periodic shift of the mucous membrane of the vocal folds on the tensed Mm. vocales to different degrees. If the infection persists, is repeated or progresses, permanent changes in the mucous membrane may occur, such as those in chronic laryngitis. The symptoms are worsened by toxic substances like cigarette smoke, alcohol or industrial fumes.

Tumors may also provoke changes in the voice production, in that they alter the mass of the oscillating vocal folds.

Aside from severe fractures of the cartilage supporting the larynx and endolaryngeal lesions following intubation, external mechanical influences can cause hemorrhaging, granulation, or ruptures in fibers. These reactions may end in permanent changes in the structure of the vocal folds and consequently in the clearness of the voice. Vocal fold paresis after long-term intubation will be discussed more thoroughly below.

The organic voice disorders stemming from neurological illnesses can be differentiated according to whether they involve vocal fold paralysation or more extensive neurological illnesses.

Paralysis of the vocal folds may have a wide variety of causes, because of the great length of the laryngal nerves and their connection to the base of the skull as well as to different throat and thorax organs (Tucker 1980). Vocal fold paresis is usually the result of paralysis of the recurrent laryngeal nerve, a main branch of the cranial nerve which transmits nervous impulses to all intrinsic

CLASSIFICATION OF VOICE DISORDERS

- Organic voice disorders
  - laryngeal diseases
    - inflammation of the larynx
      - acute laryngitis
      - chronic laryngitis
      - monochorditis vasomotorica
      - tuberculosis
    - beningnant and malignant tumors
      - polyps
      - oedema
      - granuloma
      - cysts
      - papilloma
      - carcinoma
    - trauma
    - lesions after intubation
      - granuloma
      - microtrauma
      - cricoarytenoidankylosis*
      - interarytenoidfibrosis*
      - luxation of the arytenoid* cartilage
  - neurologic diseases
    - vocal fold paresis
      - paresis of the recurrent nerve
      - paresis of the N. laryng. sup.
    - bulbar palsy
    - pseudobulbar palsy
    - cerebellar ataxia
    - chorea, parkinsonism, athetosis
    - craniocerebral injury
      - rigid dysarthrophonia*
      - spastic dysarthrophonia*
      - atactic dysarthrophonia*
      - mixed dysarthrophonia*
  - endocrine disorders
    - hyperthyreosis
    - hypothyreosis, myxedema
    - acromegaly
    - mutational voice disorders
  - malformations of the larynx
    - congenital laryngeal web
    - sulcus glottidis
    - laryngomalacia
- Functional voice disorders
  - Phonoponoses
    - vocal hyperfunction
      - secundary alterations
        - nodules
        - contact granuloma
    - vocal hypofunction
    - ventricular dysphonia
      - desirable form
      - undesirable form
  - Phononeuroses
    - hyperfunctional form of psychogenic dys- and aphonia
    - hypofunctional form of psychogenic dys- and aphonia
    - adductor spastic dysphonia

Table 48.1: Classification of voice disorders (*: see p. 495)

muscles of the larynx except for the m. cricothyroideus. The cricothyroid muscle is innervated by the external branch of the superior laryngeal nerve. Therefore, impairment of this nerve alone is not sufficient to cause any significant movement deficit in the vocal cords. However, impairment of the superior laryngeal nerve combined with recurrent laryngeal nerve paresis will indeed cause paralysis of the vocal folds.

Vocal folds paresis accompanied by hoarseness due to its corresponding position outside the median line of the vocal tract, is a symptom, not an illness in its own right. Therefore, in the case of an illnes in which the cause and effect cannot be easily determined, such as in strumectomy, for instance, additional neurological, medical, and radiological examinations are called for.

A voice disorder may occur as an initial symptom of an extensive neurological disorder. Usually, however, a voice disorder develops later, in conjunction with dysarthria (also referred to as dysarthrophonia) and disturbances in swallowing (dysphagia). The vocal changes occurring in dysarthrophonia after craniocerebral injury will be discussed in detail below.

Another cause of organic voice disorders are hormonal illnesses, which lead to fine tissue changes of the vocal folds and subsequently to alterations of the sound. Particularly evident is the dependence of the voice as a secondary sex characteristic on the sex hormones, such that all illnesses involving hyper- or hypogonadism in male and female patients often lead to quite typical voice disorders (Pascher/Johannsen 1975). However, not all mutational voice disorders are caused by hormones, but rather they may also stem from defective auditive control of phonation in non-musicality, or in a strong mother-son bond with inadequate separation.

3. Functional Voice Disorders

Above I made a distinction between phonoponoses, functional voice disorders in a narrow sense caused by strain, and phononeuroses, psychogenic voice disorders. The most common form of the phonoponoses is the hyperfunctional dysphonia, which is characterized by a non-physiological overfunctioning of the muscle systems involved in phonation, articulation and respiration, exceeding the boundaries of economic functioning. The major cause is a discrepancy between individual vocal performance and its demands on vocal function. In hypofunctional dysphonias, the tension and the function of the muscle systems are reduced, often coinciding with a consumptive illness. This disorder may also result after several years hyperfunction, when the muscle tonus can no longer be maintained. The ventricular dysphonia (= dysphonia plicae ventricularis) can be viewed as an extreme form of hyperfunctional dysphonia. In this disorder, phonation does not take place on the level of the vocal folds, but on the false or ventricular vocal folds. This may even be desirable, when one or both true vocal folds can no longer oscillate, for example after an operation removing a carcinogenic vocal fold. Conversely, voice production on the ventricular vocal fold level is undesirable, when it would otherwise be possible on the vocal fold level.

Psychological voice disorders clearly show what a finely-tuned indicator of the psychological state of the carrier, the human voice really is. All different kinds of acute and chronic disorders are expressed in the voice of the patient. The severity of the disorder, in hyper- as well as in hypofunctional form, can range from mild hoarseness to voicelessness (Kramer 1963). An extreme form of the psychogenic voice disorders are considered to be part of the adductor (spastic) dysphonias, whose etiology was mentioned above. Phonoponoses and phononeuroses are not mutually exclusive. A voice disorder can alternate between the two, not only because of multifactoral causes, but also in the course of the disease. The challenge this poses for the clinician is not to be underestimated.

In the following, central and possible peripheral voice disorders arising after craniocerebral injury will be presented in more detail. In the more extensive section on central voice disorders, I will discuss the dysarthrophonias, disorders affecting the three functional areas of respiration, phonation and articulation. The section on peripheral voice disorders looks at cases requiring artificial respiration with endotracheal intubation over a long period of time, possibly made necessary by trauma or respiratory depression in the acute phase of illness, marked by a * in Table 48.1. Special demands face the diagnostician, when a central voice disorder is complicated by an additional peripheral voice disorder by intubation.

4. Central Voice Disorders Following Craniocerebral Injury (CI)

After severe CI, patients' symptoms eventually stabilize allowing classification. But first, the symptoms of large portions of these patients develop in quite characteristic stages of recovery of speech and voice function (von Cramon 1981; Morasch/von Cramon 1984). The recovery stages proceed from an initial mute stage, to one of whispering and culminate in a stage of voiced phonation. This is especially the case following traumatic midbrain syndrome.

In the mute stage which coincides with complete anarthria, the patients are not capable of voluntarily moving their lips. In effect, they are voiceless. Sound utterances can only be stimulated by means of the cough and gag reflex. At this point of the illness, laryngoscopic examination of the larynx shows nothing unusual. The vocal folds are normally abduced. Respiration-dependent movements of the vocal folds are apparent. There is no change in reaction upon request to phonate. Von Cramon/Vogel (1981) believe the cause of this laryngeal akinesis to lie in a functional disturbance of supranuclear neurons in the oral brain stem.
In the ensuing whispering stage, which only lasts a few days, the adduction movements of the vocal folds increase as the patient attempts to phonate. The patient, however, cannot voluntarily perform a glottal stop.

In the subsequent stage of voiced phonations, the disturbance of the voluntary adduction movements of the vocal folds continues to improve. The voices of such patients still sound breathy, however, because the vocal folds are not yet closed (Ziegler/von Cramon 1987). An endoscopy of the larynx at this time would reveal signs of a rapidly developing spasm (Aronson 1990), which may favor one side depending on the localization of the lesion.

Not until the next stage do distinct groups of disorders appear. These include: the rigid, the spastic and the atactic dysarthrophonias (Hermann 1965) as well as the mixed dysarthrophonias (Ziegler/von Cramon 1987). This classification schema is based on that by Darley/Aronson/Brown (1975). Many researchers object to the application of the same disorder categories of the extremity motoric to the articulation and phonation movements. However, at present there is no better pathogenetic classification system to replace it.

4.1. Rigid Dysarthrophonia

The laryngoscopic finding in this form of dysarthrophonia is characterized by incomplete adduction of the tense and stretched vocal folds. The voice of these patients sounds harsh and breathy; pitch and volume remain constant.

4.2. Spastic Dysarthrophonia

These patients have a markedly squeezed and strained voice of rather low volume. As in rigid dysarthrophonia, pitch and volume vary minimally. Such voice quality characteristics correspond to the shortening and thickening of the vocal folds seen in hyperadduction.

4.3. Atactic Dysarthrophonia

The ring of the voice of these patients ranges from harsh to squeezed and strained. More peculiar to the atactic dysarthrophonias, however, are involuntary, sometimes erratic variations in pitch and volume, which consequently have a striking effect on prosody. These noticeable traits arise from constantly changing glottal size and vocal fold length as the larynx repeatedly attempts and fails to meet the demands of the target.

4.4. Mixed Dysarthrophonia

Approximately a third of the patients do not fall into any of the three categories mentioned above (Ziegler/von Cramon 1987). One reason for this is that symptoms belonging to different subgroups may be observed simultaneously. Or, the changes taking place in the various functional areas of phonation and articulation do not fit in the same subgroup. Furthermore, the patient's constellation of symptoms can be complicated by damage to the peripheral cranial nerves coming into play.

As far as the voice of such patients with CI is concerned, the presence of vocal function disturbances in addition to those of dysarthrophonia must be recognized. The frequent co-occurrence of centrally induced voice disorders with those disorders caused by peripheral voice disturbances, especially in those patients requiring long-term artificial respiration by means of intubation, has been indicated above. Under these conditions, it is easy to see how mucous membrane lesions such as edema, hemorrhages in one or both vocal folds or intubational granuloma can impede voice production. Results of long-term intubation even more important and more challenging for the diagnostician are those disorders related to a paresis of one or both vocal folds. Vocal folds paresis tends to be an exception, although it is still the most common diagnosis.

The diversity of the attempts to explain these kinds of pareses resulting from long-term intubation make the accuracy of such diagnoses seem doubtful, since they are extremely unlikely. And in view of the anatomic relationship between the larynx, the trachea and the N. recurrens (see Johannsen 1984), explanations such as "pressure arising from an overinflated cuff of the endotracheal tube" really are almost impossible (Lim/Chia/Ng 1987).

In fact, in the past 10 years several authors have indicated that direct damage to the larynx and thus the especially to one or both of the cricoarytaenoid joints is more logical and more likely (Berendes 1982; Johannsen 1984; Johannsen/Pirsig 1987; Gallivan/Dawson/Robbins 1989). There are 3 ways intubation can cause immobility of one or both vocal folds: Cricoarytaenoidankylosis, interarytaenoidfibrosis and luxation of the arytenoid cartilage. The latter can also occur after only brief intubation.

4.5. Cricoarytaenoidankylosis

After intubation lasting only 2 days, the pressure of the tube can lead to lesions of the mucous membrane or the cartilage in the area processus vocales of the arytenoid cartilages or the posterior plate of the cricoid cartilage (see Fig. 48.1). These lesions serve as an entrance way for germs causing infection. In this manner, the cricoarytaenoid joint can become infected with an ankylosis as a consequence (Johannsen 1984; Johannsen/Pirsig 1987).

Since there is usually a delay between the extubation of a patient and the ensuing laryngeal diagnosis, signs of acute infection are no longer apparent upon examination. Patients in the initial mute stage following traumatic mid-brain syndrome are clearly at risk for ankylosis, since in addition to intentional vocal fold mobility, reflectory mobility, as in coughing for example, is impaired. Therefore, cricoarytaenoidankylosis therapy must mobilize the joint by tearing scarred connective tissue or even shattering a cartilage buildup in the joint (Johannsen/Pirsig 1987).

4.6. Interarytaenoidfibrosis

Much rarer than ankylosis is the likelihood that an interarytaenoidfibrosis with its scar tissue will bind both arytenoid cartilages (Beck/Mann 1978; Schlöndorff/Elies 1985). The sheet of scar tissue on the ventral side of the posterior plate of the cricoid cartilage can hardly ever be seen in an indirect laryngoscopic or larynxendoscopic examination. This disorder can be clearly distinguished from the mute state of mid-brain syndrome: In fibrosis, the vocal folds remain near the medial line, so that some patients in the acute stage require a tracheotomy a few days after the extubation. In contrast, in patients in the mute stage, the vocal folds are in the normal respiration position. Moreover, in interarytaenoidfibrosis as well as in ankylosis, reflexive movements are no longer possible. The excision of the sheet of scar tissue is recommended, which may have to be repeated in some cases.

4.7. Luxation of the Arytenoid Cartilage

Compared to the large number of intubations, luxations of one or even both arytenoid cartilages are very rare (Quick/Merwin 1978; Rudert 1974). This fact is caused by the extensive passive flexibility of the cricoarytaenoid joints with its' extremely limp joint capsule. The luxation of the arytenoid cartilage occurs dorsally more often than ventrally. It is obviously the convex curvature of the distal third of the tube that is pressing against the arytenoid cartilage. The ensuing asymmetry of the larynx makes the diagnosis straightforward, that is, as long as this possibility is taken into account. The arytenoid cartilages can almost always be successfully repositioned.

The syndromes of voice disorders are presented here as part of the mostly more extensive disorders of the communicative ability of the patients with CIT. Although they appear to be quite distinct, in actuality, these constellations are much more diffuse. This places high demands on the diagnostician, requiring him or her to precisely calculate intricate findings. It also means that he or she must have extensive experience examining and treating such patients.

5. References

Aronson, A. E. (1990). *Clinical voice disorders*. 3rd ed. New York: Thieme.

Beck, C. & Mann, W. (1978). Das immobilisierte Aryhöckergelenk. *Archiv für Ohren-, Nasen- und Kehlkopfheilkunde, 219*, 494–495.

Berendes, J. (1982). Organisch bedingte Funktionsstörungen des Kehlkopfes. In J. Berendes, R.

Link & F. Zöllner (Eds.), *Hals-Nasen-Ohrenheilkunde in Praxis und Klinik. Bd. 4/1. 5.1–5.30.* Stuttgart: Thieme.

Darley, F. L., Aronson, A. E. & Brown, J. R. (1975). *Motor speech disorders.* Philadelphia, London, Toronto: W. B. Saunders.

Gallivan, G. J., Dawson, J. A. & Robbins, L. D. (1989). Videolaryngoscopy after endotracheal intubation: Implications for voice. *Journal of Voice, 3,* 76–80.

Habermann, G. (1980). Funktionelle Stimmstörungen und ihre Behandlung. *Archiv für Ohren-, Nasen- und Kehlkopfheilkunde, 227,* 171–345.

Hermann, K. (1965). Post-traumatic dysarthria. Proceedings of the 8th International Congress of Neurology. Wien: 1, 135–137.

Johannsen, H. S. (1984). Stimmlippenstillstand nach Intubation – neurogen oder durch Ankylose des Cricoarytaenoidgelenkes? *Laryngologie Rhinologie Otologie, 63,* 255–256.

Johannsen, H. S. & Pirsig, W. (1987). Therapie der Ankylose des Krikoarytaenoidgelenkes nach Intubation. *Laryngologie Rhinologie Otologie, 66,* 82–83.

Jürgens, U. (1986). The squirrel monkey as an experimental model in the study of cerebral organization of emotional vocal utterances. *European Archives of Psychiatry and Neurological Sciences, 236,* 40–43.

Kramer, E. (1963). Judgement of personal characteristics and emotions from nonverbal properties of speech. *Psychological Bulletin,* 60, 408–420.

Lim, E. K., Chia, K. S. & Ng, B. K. (1987). Recurrent laryngeal nerve palsy following endotracheal intubation. *Anaesthesia and Intensive Care, 15,* 342–345.

Morasch, H. & von Cramon, D. (1984). Laryngoskopische Befunde bei Dysphonie nach traumatischem Mittelhirnsyndrom. *HNO, 32,* 13–16.

Pascher, W. (1982). Funktionelle Krankheiten der Stimme. In J. Berendes, R. Link & F. Zöllner (Eds.), *Hals-Nasen-Ohrenheilkunde in Praxis und Klinik. Bd. 4/1. 7.1–7.45.* Stuttgart: Thieme.

Perelló, J. (1962) Dysphonies foncitonelles. *Folia phoniatrica (Basel) 14,* 150–205.

Pascher, W., Johannsen, H. S. (1975). Angewandte Phoniatrie. III. Juvenile Stimmstörungen, hormonelle Stimmstörungen. *HNO,* 23, 383–391.

Quick, C. A. & Merwin, G. E. (1978). Arytenoid dislocation. *Archives of Otolaryngology, 104,* 267–270.

Rudert, H. (1984). Über seltene Intubationsbedingte innere Kehlkopftraumen. *HNO, 32,* 393–398.

Schlöndorff, G. & Elies, W. (1985). Stimmbandstillstand mit Stridor infolge Interarytaenoidfibrose – eine Komplikation in der Intensivpflege. *Laryngologie Rhinologie Otologie, 64,* 403–404.

Schultz-Coulon, H.-J. (1980). Die Diagnostik der gestörten Stimmfunktion. *Archiv für Ohren-, Nasen- und Kehlkopfheilkunde, 227,* 1–169.

Tucker, H. M. (1980). Vocal cord paralysis 1979: etiology. *The Laryngoscope,* 90, 585–590.

Van den Berg, J. W. (1956). Physiology and physics of voice production. *Acta Physiologica et Pharmacologica Neerlandia, 5,* 40–55.

Van den Berg, J. W. (1958). Myoelastic-aerodynamic theory of voice production. *Journal of Speech and Hearing Research, 1,* 227–244.

Von Cramon, D. (1981). Traumatic mutism and the subsequent reorganization of speech functions. *Neuropsychologica, 19,* 801–805.

Von Cramon, D. & Vogel, M. (1981). Der traumatische Mutismus. *Nervenarzt, 52,* 664–668.

Ziegler, W. & von Cramon, D. (1987). Zentrale Stimmstörungen. In L. Springer & G. Kattenbeck (Eds.), *Aktuelle Beiträge zur Dysarthrophonie und Dysprosodie. 59–79.* München: tuduv Verlag.

Helge S. Johannsen, Ulm (Germany)

49. Pure Word Deafness (Verbal Auditory Agnosia)

1. Cortical Deafness

Since the late nineteenth century, various auditory disorders caused by cerebral lesions have been reported. The details of the clinicopathological correlations, however, remain unclear to this day. Bilateral cerebral lesions only exceptionally lead to severe hearing disturbance. This condition is generally called 'cortical deafness' (Earnest/Monroe/Yarnell 1977; Graham/Greenwood/Lecky 1980; Bahls/Chatrian/Mesher et al. 1988) since the primary auditory cortex (Heschl's gyrus) is involved bilaterally in most cases. Recent studies on humans and animals, however, have questioned whether bilateral lesions in the primary auditory cortex cause severe hearing loss at all. As Vignolo (1969) pointed out, cases have been reported in which only minimal hearing loss was detected by audiometry, despite complete destruction of the primary auditory cortex and/or its underlying white matter bilaterally. Abundant experimental evidence also shows that bilateral ablation of the primary auditory cortex in animals does not cause permanent deafness, although a transient decrease in acuity may be observed (Neff/Diamond/Casseday 1975). Furthermore, severe, persistent hearing loss has been reported to be caused by bilateral lesions in the white matter adjacent to the putamen (Clark/Russell 1938) or underlying the insular cortex and Heschl's gyrus (Hirano 1973; 1983), with sparing of Heschl's gyrus.

2. Auditory Agnosia

Besides cortical deafness, inability to interpret the meaning of sounds has been reported in the presence of otherwise adequate hearing as measured by standard audiometry. This condition is called 'auditory agnosia'. This term, however, has been used ambiguously (Albert/Sparks/von Stockert/Sax 1972; Bauer/Rubens 1985), generally describing two different clinical conditions. In a broad sense it has been used to refer to impaired capacity to recognize both verbal and nonverbal sounds, and in a narrow sense to refer to a selective deficit in the recognition of nonverbal sounds only. The latter, often called auditory sound agnosia, is far less common than the former, probably because patients with auditory sound agnosia are less likely to seek medical advice than those with a disorder of speech comprehension and also because nonspecific auditory complaints are often discounted when pure tone audiometric and speech discrimination thresholds are normal (Bauer/Rubens 1985). Auditory sound agnosia has been reported in relation to unilateral lesions of the right (Spreen/Benton/Fincham 1965; Fujii/Fukatsu/Watabe et al. 1990) or of the left hemisphere (Spinnler/Vignolo 1966; Faglioni/Spinnler/Vignolo 1969; Albert/Goldblum/Benson/Hécaen 1971), and bilateral temporoparietal lesions (Albert/Sparks/von Stockert/Sax 1972). Recently, Motomura/Yamadori/Mori/Tamaru (1986) reported a patient with typical auditory agnosia caused by bilateral subcortical lesions neighboring the medial geniculate body. Their case was unique in that the clinical picture began with generalized auditory agnosia and changed, over two months, to auditory sound agnosia. This case suggests that the auditory processing mechanisms for nonverbal and verbal sounds may be different, even at a subcortical level.

3. Pure Word Deafness

Selective impairment of verbal sound recognition has also been reported. This condition also can be regarded as an auditory agnosia; however, the term 'pure word deafness' has been widely employed (Brown 1974; Hécaen/Albert 1978; Benson 1979; Bauer/Rubens 1985), although some authors have preferred the term 'verbal auditory agnosia' or 'auditory agnosia for speech (Goldstein 1974) or linguistic material (Ulrich 1978)'. The neuroanatomic substrate of this disorder is better elucidated than those of other 'cortical' auditory disorders. Thus, the remainder of this article focuses on this impairment.

Patients with pure word deafness cannot comprehend spoken words, although they can read, write, and speak in an almost normal manner. Comprehension of nonverbal sounds is relatively retained. The syndrome is 'pure' only in the sense that internal language is intact (Nielsen 1946), although many of the reported cases show symptoms of Wernicke's aphasia (Brown 1974; Benson 1979; Bauer/Rubens 1985). The key characteristic of 'pure' word deafness is the extreme disproportionality of the impairment in auditory comprehension when compared to other language functions. The disorder was first described by Kussmaul (1877), who coined the term 'reine Worttaubheit' (pure word deafness) to describe a patient unable to comprehend spoken words with otherwise intact speech production and hearing. He attributed this to the destruction of the left first temporal gyrus. Lichtheim (1885) defined the disorder as "the inability to understand spoken words unaccompanied by disturbance of spontaneous speech and by severe disturbance in writing and understanding of the printed words". He called this syndrome 'isolierte Sprachtaubheit (isolated speech deafness)', and considered it to be the result of a disruption in the pathway from the auditory reception center to the auditory word impression center. Similarly, Bastian (1897) thought of the syndrome as arising from isolation of the auditory word center rather than its destruction.

3.1. Lesion Anatomy

There was once uncertainty about the concept that pure word deafness was a distinct disorder of cerebral function. Freud (1891) suspected that a peripheral hearing loss was necessary for the development of an isolated word deafness. On the basis of two cases with labyrinthine dysfunction, Freund (1895) concluded that the syndrome was primarily due to hearing loss. However, in a very carefully studied patient in whom ordinary deafness was clearly excluded, Liepmann (1898) showed that this syndrome could be produced by a left unilateral cerebral lesion. The pathology was described in fuller detail by Liepmann/Storch (1902). The lesion, located subcortically in the left temporal lobe, had destroyed the left auditory radiation as well as the callosal fibers from the right auditory region. The subsequent well-documented autopsy cases established the cerebral origin of the syndrome (Goldstein 1974). Freund himself later reported that one of his two patients clinically thought to have had word deafness due to bilateral labyrinthine dysfunction actually had a tumor in the left first temporal gyrus (Hemphill/Stengel 1940; Goldstein 1974). Geschwind (1965) in his review of the disconnection syndromes noted that most cases had bilateral, usually cortical-subcortical lesions in the anterior part of the superior temporal gyrus, leaving Heschl's gyri essentially intact; and that the less common unilateral cases involved subcortical lesions that interrupted auditory radiation fibers as well as callosal fibers from the contralateral auditory cortex. He concluded that the syndrome ultimately represented a disconnection of the auditory cortex from Wernicke's area.

Recently, pure word deafness caused by bilateral infarctions of the primary auditory cortex (Coslett/Brashear/Heilman 1984) or by bilateral damage to its underlying deep white matter (Brick/Frost/Schochet et al. 1985) has been reported. A patient with lesions similar to those described by Coslett/Brashear/Heilman (1984) has been reported previously by Kanshepolsky/Kelley/Waggener (1973). These indicate that, as Coslett/Brashear/Heilman (1984) suggested, comprehension of verbal sounds may be mediated by the pathway into and from Heschl's gyrus, and comprehension of nonverbal sounds may be mediated by other cerebral structures such as the auditory association cortex.

3.2. Auditory Processing Deficits

Some investigators have recently attempted to characterize the nature of the deficit of this syndrome from a functional point of view, and have emphasized the defects in auditory processing (Jerger/Weikers/Sharbrough/Jerger 1969; Kanshepolsky/Keller/Waggener 1973; Albert/Bear 1974; Auerbach/Allard/Naeser et al. 1982), temporal resolution (Albert/Bear 1974), phonemic discrimination (Chocholle/Chedru/Botte et al. 1975; Denes/Semenza 1975; Saffran/Marin/Yeni-Komshian 1976; von Stockert 1982), and prephonemic discrimination (Auerbach/Allard/Naeser et al. 1982). For instance, Jerger/Weikers/Sharbrough/Jerger (1969) presented extensive audiologic data obtained from a patient with presumed bilateral temporoparietal lesions. They demonstrated impairments in the ability to discriminate the loudness of stimuli, to localize sounds in space, to identify the order in which different auditory events occur in time, and to perceive brief sounds. Albert/Bear (1974) experienced a patient with probable left temporoparietal lesion in whom understanding of spoken language improved dramatically when the examiner spoke at an abnormally slow rate. To confirm this rate-dependent comprehension, they examined the ability of the patient to count the number of clicks presented for one second (click counting), and the threshold at which two clicks could be distinguished as separate (click fusion). Their patient performed poorly for rates greater than 2 per second, and was unable to discriminate two clicks separated by less than 15 msec, whereas normals counted 8 to 11 clicks per second, and distinguished two clicks at 1 to 3 msec intervals. From these observations, they emphasized that one of the important factors for the development of pure word deafness was a defect in temporal resolution of auditory stimuli rather than in specific phonetic impairment. Saffran/Marin/Yeni-Komshian (1976), on the other hand, showed that the auditory comprehension of their patient was facilitated significantly when the spoken words were drawn from a particular category and also when context was provided by placing the word at the end of a meaningful sentence (e.g., *boat* in the sentence, *The boy sailed a boat.*). Auerbach/Allard/Naeser et al. (1982) also observed a severe deficit in temporal resolution in a case of bilateral temporoparietal lesions, as in the case of Albert/Bear (1974). Based on their exceptionally detailed case study and a review of the literature, they regarded all the abnormalities in click fusion, click counting, and duration discrimination as 'temporal auditory acuity disorder' since all these measurements represent a function of time of the auditory system. They considered it 'prephonemic' if a phonemic discrimination disorder could be attributed to a disorder in acoustic processing such as temporal auditory acuity. From these considerations, they suggested that two distinct types of pure word deafness could be described. The first is a disorder of prephonemic temporal auditory acuity and has been associated with bilateral temporal lobe lesions. This type is characterized by (1) particular difficulty with rapid formant transitions, leaving vowel discrimination relatively preserved; (2) improved performance with an increase in the number of distinctive features distinguishing two target phonemes; (3) a particular vulnerability for the distinctive feature of place of articulation when compared to the feature of voicing. The second type of pure word deafness is a disorder in phonemic discrimination that cannot be attributed to a difficulty in temporal auditory acuity and has been associated with left unilateral temporal lesions (Denes/Semenza 1975; Saffran/Marin/Yeni-Komshian 1976). This type shows an inconsistent pattern in linguistic studies, that is, either a particular vulnerability for the feature of voicing compared to that of place of articulation (Saffran/Marin/Yeni-Komshian 1976) or no particucular pattern (Denes/Semenza 1975). Auerbach/Allard/Naeser et al. (1982) suggested that the first type is an apperceptive disorder secondary to pathology involving the auditory cortices whereas the second represents a higher disorder in phonemic discrimination, and may be considered a fragment of Wernicke's aphasia. This division follows the classification of Lissauer (1890), who attempted to distinguish between the ability to synthesize sensory information into an adequate perception (apperception) and the ability to analyze perception in relation to meaning and other perceptions (association) in discussing visual agnosia. More recently, Yaqub/Gascon/Alnosha/Whitaker (1988) also have reported a patient with bilateral temporal lesions who showed a pattern similar to the first type of Auerbach/Allard/Naeser et al. (1982), supporting the view of the latter.

We performed several sophisticated auditory tests in a case of pure word deafness caused by bilateral temporoparietal lesions (Tanaka/Yamadori/Mori 1987). Our patient also demonstrated extremely long auditory fusion threshold for clicks (300 msec) and markedly decreased ability to count the number of clicks (inaccurate for rates greater than 2 per second). These findings support the view of Albert/Bear (1974) who emphasized that the defect in auditory temporal resolution was an important factor for the development of word deafness. Our patient, however, presented a problem inexplicable by this hypothesis. We presented two tones with the same duration and intensity, and asked the patient to report whether one or two tones were heard as the interval between the two tones was varied. The duration of a tone ranged from 20 to 500 msec. For each duration, sensation level was set at 20 dB above the threshold which had been measured in the threshold-duration function test. Our patient demonstrated marked improvement in the ability to discriminate two tones as the duration of a tone was prolonged. However, the auditory comprehension did not improve at all, even if the patient was spoken to slowly enough. This indicates that there are other factors besides a defect in auditory temporal resolution for the poor recognition of spoken words in our case. Our patient had marked impairment in perception of brief sounds and in discrimination of loudness, pitch and tone duration. These elemental auditory disturbances, especially impairment in discriminating sound duration, may be responsible for the poor recognition of spoken words in our case. In linguistic investigation with natural speech stimuli, our patient was able to identify vowels at a better than chance level but failed in consonant-vowel (CV) discrimination, with no particular pattern of error, even if the number of distinguishing features increased. In natural speech, vowel durations usually average 100 to 150 msec but may last as long as 400 msec. In CV combinations, the consonant is characterized by rapid frequency changes within the first 40 msec of stimulus onset (Auerbach/Allard/Naeser et al. 1982). Our patient required a duration difference of 380 msec to discriminate a duration of two tones correctly, whereas normals required a duration difference of only 20 to 30 msec. Accordingly, complete inability to identify and discriminate CV combinations, but some retained capacity to discriminate vowels in our patient may be explained by severe impairment in discriminating sound duration. If this is true, our patient must have a temporal auditory acuity disorder, the first type proposed by Auerbach/Allard/Naeser et al. (1982). Thus, a detailed analysis of each patient with word deafness by means of sophisticated auditory tests probably sheds light on understanding of how speech sounds are processed by the human brain.

Our patient produced another intriguing result during rhythm discrimination testing: severe impairment in the recognition and reproduction of the simple rhythm patterns at a fast rate regardless of the modalities of perception, i. e., either audition, vision, or touch. This finding supports the view of Mavlov (1980) who demonstrated a supramodal defect only in the recognition and reproduction of rhythm patterns in a case of a professional musician following a vascular stroke in the left posterior parietal or parietotemporal region. However, in our patient, this condition improved significantly in all modalities when the rate was decreased, indicating that rhythm sense is essentially preserved. Since perception of rhythm requires registration of time intervals, this rate-dependent supramodal defect is attributable to a supramodal defect in temporal resolution. Indeed, our patient had a disturbance of temporal resolution in all the three sensory modalities tested, and the temporal resolution markedly improved in at least both audition and vision as the duration of the tone and the light increased. This finding has led us to speculate that there is a 'time-organizing system' which is both independent of and central to the sensory mechanism. Therefore, rhythm sense probably reflects one aspect of a 'time-organizing system' situated in the temporoparietal region, predominantly in the left hemisphere. Thus, a deficit of temporal resolution described by Albert/Bear (1974) appeared to be related to rhythm sense but not to auditory comprehension in our patient.

4. References

Albert, M. L., Goldblum, M.-C., Benson, D. F., & Hécaen, H. (1971). Mechanisms of auditory comprehension. II. Cerebral dominance. *Transactions of the American Neurological Association, 96,* 132–135.

Albert, M. L., Sparks, R., von Stockert, T., & Sax, D. (1972). A case study of auditory agnosia: linguistic and non-linguistic processing. *Cortex, 8,* 427–443.

Albert, M. L. & Bear, D. (1974). Time to understand: a case study of word deafness with reference to the role of time in auditory comprehension. *Brain, 97,* 373–384.

Auerbach, S. H., Allard, T., Naeser, M., Alexander, M. P., & Albert, M. L. (1982). Pure word deafness: analysis of a case with bilateral lesions and a defect at the prephonemic level. *Brain, 105,* 271–300.

Bahls, F. H., Chatrian, G. E., Mesher, R. A., Sumi, S. M., & Ruff, R. L. (1988). A case of persistent cortical deafness: clinical, neurophysiologic, and neuropathologic observations. *Neurology, Cleveland, 38,* 1490–1493.

Bastian, H. C. (1987). Some problems in connexion with aphasia and other speech defects. *Lancet i,* 933–942, 1005–1017, 1131–1137, 1187–1194.

Bauer, R. M. & Rubens, A. B. (1985). Agnosia. In K. M. Heilmann & E. Valenstein (Eds.), *Clinical Neuropsychology. 209–217.* New York: Oxford University Press.

Benson, D. F. (1979). Pure word deafness. In D. F. Benson (Ed.), *Aphasia, Alexia, and Agraphia. 133–134.* New York: Churchill Livingstone.

Brick, J. F., Frost, J. L., Schochet, Jr. S. S., Gutmann, L., & Crosby, T. W. (1985). Pure word deafness: CT localization of the pathology. *Neurology, Cleveland, 35,* 441–442.

Brown, J. (1974). *Aphasia, Apraxia and Agnosia: clinical and theoretical aspects.* 127–135. Springfield, Illinois: Charles C. Thomas.

Chocholle, R., Chedru, F., Botte, M. C., Chain, F., & Lhermitte, F. (1975). Étude psychoacoustique d'un cas de 'surdité corticale'. *Neuropsychologia, 13,* 163–172.

Clark, W. E. Le G. & Russell, W. R. (1938). Cortical deafness without aphasia. *Brain, 61,* 375–383.

Coslett, H. B., Brashear, H. R., & Heilman, K. M. (1984). Pure word deafness after bilateral primary auditory cortex infarcts. *Neurology, Cleveland, 34,* 347–352.

Denes, G. & Semenza, C. (1975). Auditory modality-specific anomia: evidence from a case of pure word deafness. *Cortex, 11,* 401–411.

Earnest, M. P., Monroe, P. A., & Yarnell, P. R. (1977). Cortical deafness: demonstration of the pathologic anatomy by Ct scan. *Neurology, Minneapolis, 27,* 1172–1175.

Faglioni, P., Spinnler, H., & Vignolo, L. A. (1969). Contrasting behavior of right and left hemisphere: damaged patients on a discriminative and a semantic task of auditory recognition. *Cortex, 5,* 366–389.

Fujii, T., Fukatsu, R., Watabe, S., Ohnuma, A., Teramura, K., Kimura, I., Sato, S., & Kogure, K. (1990). Auditory sound agnosia without aphasia following a right temporal love lesion. Cortex, 26, 263–268.

Freud, S. (1891). *Zur Auffassung der Aphasien: eine kritische Studie.* Vienna: Franz Deuticke.

Freund, C. S. (1895). *Labyrinthtaubheit und Sprachtaubheit*. Wiesbaden: Bergmann.

Geschwind, N. (1965). Disconnexion syndromes in animals and man. *Brain, 88*, 237–294.

Goldstein, M. N. (1974). Auditory agnosia for speech ('pure word deafness'): a historical review with current implications. *Brain and Language, 1*, 195–204.

Graham, J., Greenwood, R. & Lecky, B. (1980). Cortical deafness: a case report and review of the literature. *Journal of the Neurological Science, 48*, 35–49.

Hécaen, H. & Albert, M. L. (1978). *Human Neuropsychology*. 265–276. New York: John Wiley & Sons.

Hemphill, R. E. & Stengel, E. (1940). A study on pure word-deafness. *Journal of Neurology and Psychiatry, 3*, 251–262.

Hirano, M. (1973). On the 'So-called' cortical deafness. *Psychiatria et Neurologia Japonica, Tokyo, 75*, 94–138 (in Japanese).

Hirano, M. (1983). What is 'Cortical Deafness'?: review of literature. *Clinical Psychiatry, Tokyo, 25*, 337–343 (in Japanese).

Jerger, J., Weikers, N. J., Sharbrough, F. W., & Jerger, S. (1969). Bilateral lesions of the temporal lobe: a case study. *Acta Oto-Laryngologica, Supplement, 258*, 1–51.

Kanshepolsky, J., Kelley, J. J., & Waggener, J. D. (1973). A cortical auditory disorder: clinical, audiologic and pathologic aspects. *Neurology, Minneapolis, 23*, 699–705.

Kussmaul, A. (1877). Disturbances of speech. In H. von Ziemssen (Ed.), *Cyclopedia of the Practice of Medicine. Volume 14. 581–875*. New York: William Wood.

Lichtheim, L. (1885). On aphasia. *Brain, 7*, 433–484.

Liepmann, H. (1898). Ein Fall von reiner Sprachtaubheit. In C. Wernicke (Ed.), *Psychiatrische Abhandlungen*. Breslau: Schletter.

Liepmann, H. & Storch, E. (1902). Der mikroskopische Gehirnbefund bei dem Fall Gorstelle. *Monatsschrift für Psychiatrie und Neurologie, 11*, 115–120.

Lissauer, H. (1890). Ein Fall von Seelenblindheit nebst einem Beitrag zur Theorie derselben. *Archiv für Psychiatrie und Nervenkrankheit, 21*, 222–270.

Mavlov, L. (1980). Amusia due to rhythm agnosia in a musician with left hemisphere damage: a non-auditory supramodal defect. *Cortex, 16*, 331–338.

Motomura, N., Yamadori, A., Mori, E., & Tamaru, F., (1986). Auditory agnosia: analysis of a case with bilateral subcortical lesions. *Brain, 109*, 379–391.

Neff, W. D., Diamond, I. T., & Casseday, J. H. (1975). Behavioral studies of auditory discrimination: central nervous system. In W. D. Keidel & W. D. Neff (Eds.), *Handbook of Sensory Physiology, Volume 5, Part 2. 307–400*. Berlin: Springer.

Nielsen, J. M. (1946). *Agnosia, Apraxia, Aphasia. Their value in cerebral localization*. 2nd edition. New York: Hoeber Publishing.

Saffran, E. M., Marin, O. S. M., & Yeni-Komshian, G. H. (1976). An analysis of speech perception in word deafness. *Brain and Language, 3*, 209–228.

Spinnler, H. & Vignolo, L. A. (1966). Impaired recognition of meaningful sounds in aphasia. *Cortex*, 337–348.

Spreen, O., Benton, A. L., & Fincham, R. W. (1965). Auditory agnosia without aphasia. *Archives of Neurology, Chicago, 13*, 84–92.

Tanaka, Y., Yamadori, A., & Mori, E. (1987). Pure word deafness following bilateral lesions: a psychophysical analysis. *Brain, 110*, 381–403.

Ulrich, G. (1978). Interhemispheric functional relationships in auditory agnosia: an analysis of the preconditions and a conceptual model. *Brain and Language, 5*, 286–300.

Vignolo, L. A. (1969). Auditory agnosia: a review and report of recent evidence. In A. L. Benton (Ed.), *Contributions to Clinical Neuropsychology. 172–231*. Chicago: Aldine Publishing.

von Stockert, T. R. (1982). On the structure of word deafness and mechanisms underlying the fluctuation of disturbances of higher cortical functions. *Brain and Language, 16*, 133–146.

Yaqub, B. A., Gascon, G. G., Alnosha, M., & Whitaker, H. (1988). Pure word deafness (acquired verbal auditory agnosia) in an arabic speaking patient. *Brain, 111*, 457–466.

Yasufumi Tanaka, Tochigi (Japan)

50. Speech Tics in Tourette's Syndrome

1. Characteristics of Tourette's Syndrome

Tic behaviors in Gilles de la Tourette's syndrome (TS) include the random and stereotypic production of complex oral and laryngeal movements and sounds, sometimes syllables and phrases, which are referred to as vocal or speech tics. The diagnostic criteria for TS (Diagnostics and Statistical Manual of Mental Disorders 1987) include:

(a) both multiple and one or more vocal tics have been present at some time during the illness, although not necessarily concurrently;
(b) the tics occur many times a day (usually in bouts), nearly every day or intermittently throughout a period of more than one year;
(c) the anatomic location, number, frequency, complexity, and severity of the tics changed over time;
(d) onset was before age 21; and
(e) occurrence was not exclusively during psychoactive substance intoxication or known central nervous system disease.

The definition of whether a tic is simple or complex, motor or vocal, is important for identifying TS separate from simple tic disorder, or chronic multiple tic disorder. Complex motor tics are differentiated from simple motor tics. The former include motor patterns such as jumping, hitting and finger tapping. These must be differentiated from simple motor tics such as a shoulder shrug, eyeblink, head twitch, or facial grimace. Simple vocal tics include throat clearing, squeaks, sniffing and grunting while complex vocal tics include words, echolalia, palilalia (syllable repetition) and coprolalia (swearing). TS is differentiated from chronic multiple tic disorder which includes only vocal tics, or only motor tics, but not both.

TS occurs worldwide, is more frequent in caucasians than blacks or hispanics and all cases are now thought to have a genetic etiology. Prevalence is greater in males than females (3 : 1) and between .1 and .5 per thousand. Onset is usually well before 13 years of age and symptoms diminish or disappear in 70% before adulthood (Singer/Walkup 1991).

2. Characteristics of Tics in Tourette's Syndrome

Tics in TS are not the same as jerks or tremor in that they are complex motor patterns, sudden movements, gestures or utterances which mimic some aspect of the repertoire of normal behavoir. TS tics differ from movements in tardive dyskinesia which include repetitive continuous movements such as; bruxism, jaw opening and closing, licking or lip smacking. TS tics also differ from oromandibular dystonia where a continuously abnormal posture interferes with speaking, such as sustained and uncontrolled jaw opening or jaw clenching. Tics are sudden, rapid and sporadic and may occur often in bursts or bouts and then will be absent for a time. Such bouts of tics may include a rapid stream of a variety of tics. The exact order and combination of tics usually differs each time. Many persons with TS report they can suppress tics for a short interval (30 minutes) but then must release them. Most persons affected with this disorder report that they have premonitary feelings or urges to perform a tic. They are usually aware of their tics and are annoyed and embarrassed by them. However, more recently in family studies individuals have been identified with TS or chronic tics who are unaware of their disorder and have never sought medical assistance for their disorder (Kurlan 1989). Tics will wax and wane throughout the disorder and change over time. One type of tic, such as facial grimacing may predominate over 6 months to be replaced by shoulder shrugs and coprolalia for 8 months and then may be replaced by lip smacking and/or eyeblinks the next year. Coprolalia, repeated swearing, is the most troubling of the symptoms but does not occur in all cases. Many of the vocal tics are less obvious such as *oh boy*, *yup*, and *OK*.

2.1. Vocal Tic Types

In our studies of TS (Ludlow/Polinsky/Caine et al. 1982; Caine/Polinsky/Ludlow et al. 1982; Caine/Ludlow/Polinsky/Ebert 1984; Polinsky/Ebert/Caine et al. 1980), we divided tics into 10 categories with the following tic definitions:

(a) Laryngeal: throat clearing, coughing, humming, shriek, grunting, high pitched sounds, barks, squeaks, hooting, whistling.
(b) Lingual: slurping, hiss, clicks.
(c) Nasal: sniffing, snorting.
(d) Respiratory Exhalations: sighs, blowing, wheezing.
(e) Respiratory Inhalations: air gulping, gasps.
(f) Labial: smacking, spitting, raspberry noises, bronx cheers, kissing sounds.
(g) Words: stereotypic or hesitation phenomena, interjected words, echolalia.
(h) Palilalia: single or multiple strings.
(i) Jargon: single or multiple meaningless syllables.
(j) Coprolalia: swearing.

All of the tics we identified were normal behaviors, although usually inappropriate in the social context. None were produced with a struggle; all were produced without effort in a quick fluid fashion. Classification of tics into the above categories was somewhat arbitrary, but used to measure how behavior changed over time and with treatment. Four of these categories include behaviors that would be classified as speech or verbal, while the remainder were non-speech vocal tract gestures.

2.2. Frequency of Tic Types

The frequency with which TS patients exhibit these different categories of tics follows a somewhat regular pattern. In a study of 54 patients (Ludlow/Polinsky/Caine et al. 1982), the percentage of tics in each category was as follows: lingual 35.6%; laryngeal 23.5%; nasal 14.5%; respiratory inhalation 8.9%; respiratory exhalation 4.7%; labial 5.5%; jargon 4.1%; and coprolalia 2.8%. Therefore, the most frequent tic types were nonverbal categories and the least frequent were speech tics.

When TS patients and controls were compared on the numbers of tics in each group within each category (Ludlow/Polinsky/Caine et al. 1982), the TS groups produced laryngeal, nasal, inhalation, exhalation, labial, and coprolalia more frequently than the controls ($p \leq .03$). Surprisingly, the TS patient and controls did not differ in the frequency of lingual tics, suggesting that not only was this a normal behavior but that it was not more frequent than normal. The only tic category that did not occur in the controls was coprolalia, however, this was the least frequent category in TS. Therefore, TS tics could be viewed as normal behaviors, only increased in frequency and intensity.

2.3. Severity and Tic Types

Because differences appear in the frequency of tics in TS, the relationship between tic types was examined to determine if there is a progression across tic types in TS; that is, does one tic type appear in mild forms of the disorder, while other types only appear in more severe forms. We examined this issue in 13 TS patients. The mildest patient had lingual, laryngeal and exhalation tics; four more impaired patients had lingual, laryngeal, exhalation, and nasal tics; a further impaired patient had lingual, laryngeal, exhalation, and coprolalia; the next four more severe patients had lingual, laryngeal, exhalation, nasal, and coprolalia; a further impaired patient had lingual, laryngeal, exhalation, nasal, and labial tics, the next more severe patient had lingual, laryngeal, exhalation, nasal, coprolalia, and jargon while the most severely impaired patient had all tic types. This suggests that tic categories were added in a progressive order with increased severity of the disorder from lingual in the mildest forms, through laryngeal, exhalation, nasal, coprolalia, and labial, to jargon in the most severe cases.

In fact when psychiatrists' ratings of patient severity were related with a) the number of tic categories produced, and b) the total number of tics produced in 2 minutes, Spearman Rank Correlation Coefficients demonstrated a higher relationship with the number of tic categories ($R = .71$) than with tic frequency ($R = .57$). Therefore, the number of tic categories present might be a better measure of patient severity than the frequency of tics.

3. Effects of Speech Behavior on Tic Frequency

To examine how vocal tic production is modified by patients' ongoing behavior, the frequency and types of tics produced by TS patients while silent, during oral reading, and during speech conversation, was examined in 13 TS patients. The mean number of tics per minute in speech was 20.9, while it was 18.1/min during oral reading and 14.2/min when patients were resting or listening to the examiner. Therefore, vocal tics tended to be more frequent during speaking than at other times. To determine whether the 13 TS patients would have similar ratings of severity whether their tic frequency was measured at rest, while speaking or reading, they were rank ordered based on their mean rate of tic production across all three conditions and this rank was related to their rank in each of the conditions. The Spearman Rank Correlation Coefficients were 0.85 between speaking and the mean for all conditions, 0.76 for reading and 0.53 in silence. Therefore, measures made while speaking were most representative of patients severities of tic production. Tic production was studied when changes in speaking rate were effected using delayed auditory feedback and white noise. Although significant reductions in speaking rate were produced from 125 words/min to 80 words/min, no changes occurred in the rate of vocal tic production. Thus although tics are likely to occur more often during speech than at rest, they are not affected by speaking rate.

4. Position of Tics in Speech

Several studies have addressed whether tics are randomly produced during speech by TS patients. Martindale (Martindale 1976; 1977) analyzed the location of tics in speech in one subject and found that tics occurred at points of low information in speech such as during pauses and before conjunctions and pronouns. He also found that tics were more frequent in longer sentences than short sentences. He suggested that non-inhibited subcortical centers inject tics into the speech stream when cortically based speech centers are less active. Frank (1978) studied the position of tics in speech in 3 TS patients examining the position relative to speech clauses and reported that tics occurred most frequently just before the first word of a clause, somewhat less frequently immediately after the final word, and third in pauses between clauses. Tics occurred much less frequently however, between words within a clause. The same issue was examined in 13 TS patients in our clinic with similar results: 72% of tics occurred on speech initiation and only 28% occurred within speech; only 5% occurred within syllables.

In summary, then,

(a) vocal tics in TS are more frequent occurrences and socially inappropriate occurrences of normal behaviors;
(b) the types of tic categories a patient exhibits, rather than the frequency, will indicate the severity of his disease;
(c) more severely affected patients will have verbal or speech tics;
(d) vocal tics occur more frequently during speaking than during silence, but occur during interruptions in speech flow; and
(e) vocal tics occur at points of low information in speech.

5. Are Tics Voluntary or Involuntary?

Most TS patients report premonitary feelings or urges before they produce a tic. Obsessive compulsive thoughts are often associated with this disorder (Frankel/Cummings/Robertson et al. 1986) and some have characterized the production of tics as compulsions to perform motor acts. Lang (1991) examined patients' perceptions of symptom production systematically in 170 patients with various hyperkinesias and 60 tic disorder patients. Fifty-six of the sixty TS patients (95%) reported their tics were voluntary while 92.7% of the non-tic movement disorder patients reported their movements were involuntary. Although the TS patients reported that their tics were voluntary, they did feel that the intention to tic was involuntary, leading Lang to coin the phrase, "intentional unvoluntary" (Lang 1991, 227). Several patients have described their tic productions as intentional actions used to satisfy or eliminate unfulfilled sensations or urges. These observations emphasize that sensory experiences are a primary or dominant feature of the illness whereas the tics are considered only as responses to these sensory experiences (Lang 1991; Kurlan 1989).

6. Pathophysiology of Tic Behavior

The physiological basis for the TS syndrome is unknown but is thought to be due to striatal dopamine receptor supersensitivity. This hypothesis is based on significant tic reductions with dopamine receptor antagonists and tic increases with drugs that enhance dopaminergic neurotransmission (Caine/Ludlow/Polinsky/Ebert 1984; Kurlan 1989).

Little information is available concerning the pathophysiology of this disorder. A comparison of the presence of the readiness potential preceding simple tics and volitional imitation of the same tics, demonstrated an absence of the readiness potential preceding spontaneous simple tics (Obeso/Rothwell/Marsden 1981; 1982). Similar comparisons need to be made prior to spontaneous speech tics and patients' imitations of speech tics because speech tics are usually more complex. Such findings might suggest that tics are produced by different brain regions than normal speaking behavior. This possibility is suggested by the occurrence of tics during all stages of sleep (Glaze/Frost/Jankovic 1983) and also by the observation that 30% of TS patients may not be aware of their tic production (Kurlan 1989).

7. Associated Behaviors

During our studies of TS, we noted that an unexpectedly large percentage of our TS population had other speech and language deficits. Based on individual interviews of our TS patients, 45% reported a stuttering problem at some point in their lifetime, 45% reported language delay and 56% reported a reading disorder. We investigated this in a more formal manner in 54 TS patients and 54 age and sex matched controls (Ludlow/Polinsky/Caine et al. 1982) using the only language testing tool available at that time which would span the age range to be studied from 5 to 60 years of age; the Neurosensory Center Comprehensive Examination for Aphasia with Gaddes/Crockett (1975) norms for children from 5 to 13 years of age and the Spreen/Benton (1969) norms for those above 14 years. A similar pattern of language deficits was found across all age groups: significantly poorer scores than normal on language expression, written expression, writing to dictation and copying. The particular subtests with impaired performance included word fluency, sentence construction (in speaking and writing) reading names, writing names, and digit repetition. No significant relationship was found, however, between the number or frequency of tics and the degree of language deficit on these subtests, suggesting that these two functions were independent in TS. The language deficits were interpreted as demonstrating impaired language execution both in speaking and writing with normal speech repetition. Singer/Walkup (1991) have interpreted the neurophysiological deficits of TS patients as, "deficits in the executive function domain – the capacity to plan and sequence complex behaviors and to organize and sustain goal-directed activities" (Singer/Walkup 1991, 22).

8. Relationships with Other Deficits

Many behavioral and learning disorders frequently accompany TS such as obsessive compulsive disorder, attention deficit hyperactivity disorder, learning deficits, sleep abnormalities, dyslexia, phobias, depression and stuttering (Comings/Comings 1987a; 1987b; 1987c; Kurlan 1989; Singer/Walkup 1991). Considerable controversy exists in the field today on whether a) these associated disorders are different expressions of the same gene (Comings/Comings/Knell 1989) or that only obsessive compulsive disorder and chronic multiple tics are expressions of the TS gene (Pauls/Leckman 1986). Comings and his coworkers examined the pedigrees of over 1200 TS families with information on other disorders gathered through indirect interview and have suggested that TS is inherited in a semi-dominant semi-recessive fashion with variable expression ranging from minimal tics to many disorders including obsessive compulsive disorder, stuttering, depression, and dyslexia (Comings/Comings/Knell 1989). In contrast, Pauls and his coworkers conducted direct interviews and segregation analyses and suggested an autosomal dominant pattern with sex-specific and incomplete patterns (Pauls/Leckman 1986). Their examination of familial patterns of obsessive compulsive disorder, chronic tic disorders and TS demonstrated that obsessive compulsive disorder and chronic multiple tic disorder are alternate phenotypes of the TS gene with higher penetrance for males (.99) than for females (.70) (Pauls/Towbin/Leckman et al. 1986; Pauls/Pakstis/Kurlan et al. 1990). On the other hand, although attention deficit hyperactivity disorder has been found to have an increased frequency in families of TS patients, when a rigorous family study was conducted, the two traits segregated independently (Pauls/Hurst/Kruger et al. 1986). Further careful study is needed to determine whether there is a genetic relationship between TS and the other disorders reported to occur frequently in association with TS, such as anxiety, conduct disorders, depression, dyslexia, mania, panic attacks, phobias, and stuttering (Comings/Comings/Knell 1989).

9. Conclusions

Speech tics in TS are intriguing to those interested in speech pathology because of their similarities and dissimilarities with chronic developmental stuttering. Both disorders seem to have a genetic component and in fact may be related in some way (Comings/Comings/Knell 1989). More males are affected by both disorders, both wax and wave in severity, have a great deal of heterogeneity, remit spontaneously in late childhood and later adolescence in a significant proportion of cases, both are frequently associated with language learning difficulties, and both respond well to haloperidol, a dopaminergic antagonist. There are some other marked differences in their manifestation in speech however, stuttering is reduced at slower than normal speaking rates and occurs within speech while tics in TS precede speech and are unaffected by changes in rate. The new methods of studying the human genome and analyzing the locations and genetic materials responsible for these disorders may uncover biological mechanisms contributing to both disorders.

10. References

Caine, E. D., Ludlow, C. L., Polinsky, R. J., & Ebert, M. H. (1984). Provocative drug testing in tourette's syndrome: d- and l-Amphetamine and haloperidol. *Journal of the American Academy of Child Psychiatry, 23 : 2,* 147–152.

Caine, E. D., Polinsky, R. J., Ludlow, C. L., Ebert, M. H., & Nee, L. E. (1982). Heterogeneity and variability in Tourette Syndrome. In A. J. Friedhoff & T. N. Chase (Eds.), *Gilles de la Tourette Syndrome. 437–442.* New York: Raven Press.

Comings, D. E. & Comings, B. G. (1987a). A controlled study of Tourette syndrome: IV. Obsessions, compulsions, and schizoid behaviors. *American Journal of Human Genetics, 41,* 782–803.

Comings, D. E. & Comings, B. G. (1987b). A controlled study of Tourette syndrome: VI. Early development, sleep problems, allergies, and handedness. *American Journal of Human Genetics, 41,* 822–838.

Comings, D. E. & Comings, B. G. (1987c). A controlled study of Tourette syndrome: I. Attention deficit disorder, learning disorders and school problems. *American Journal of Human Genetics, 41,* 701–741.

Comings, D. E., Comings, B. G., & Knell, E. (1989). Hypothesis: Homozygosity in Tourette Syndrome. *American Journal of Medical Genetics, 34,* 413–421.

Diagnostic and Statistical Manual of Mental Disorders, Revised (1987). 3rd Ed.. Washington, D. C.: American Psychiatric Association.

Frank, S. M. (1978). Psycholinguistic findings in Gilles de la Tourette syndrome. *Journal of Communication Disorders, 11,* 349–363.

Frankel, M., Cummings, J. L., Robertson, M. M., Trimble, M. R., Hill, M. A., & Benson, D. F. (1986). Obsessions and compulsions in Gilles de la Tourette's syndrome. *Neurology, 36,* 378–382.

Gaddes, W. H. & Crockett, D. J. (1975). Spreen-Benton aphasia tests, normative data as a measure of normal language development. *Brain and Language, 2,* 257–280.

Glaze, D., Frost, J. D. Jr., & Jankovic, J. (1983). Sleep in Gilles de la Tourette's syndrome: disorder of arousal. *Neurology, 33,* 586–592.

Kurlan, R. (1989). Tourette's syndrome: Current concepts. *Neurology, 39,* 1625–1630.

Lang, A. (1991). Patient perception of tics and other movement disorders. *Neurology, 41,* 223–228.

Ludlow, C. L., Polinsky, R. J., Caine, E. D., Bassich, C. J., & Ebert, M. H. (1982). Language and speech abnormalities in Tourette Syndrome. In A. J. Friedhoff & T. N. Chase (Eds.), *Gilles de la Tourette Syndrome.* 351–361. New York: Raven Press.

Martindale, C. (1976). The grammar of the tic in Gilles de la Tourette's syndrome. *Language and Speech, 19,* 1–20.

Martindale, C. (1977). Syntactic and semantic correlates of verbal tics in Gilles de la Tourette's syndrome: A quantitative case study. *Brain and Language, 4,* 231–247.

Obeso, J. A., Rothwell, J. C., & Marsden, C. D. (1981). Simple tics in Gilles de la Tourette syndrome are not prefaced by a normal premovement potential. *Journal of Neurology, Neurosurgery and Psychiatry, 44,* 735–738.

Obeso, J. A., Rothwell, J. C., & Marsden, C. D. (1982). The neurophysiology of tourette syndrome. In A. J. Friedhoff & T. N. Chase (Eds.), *Gilles de la Tourette Syndrome.* 105–114. New York: Raven Press.

Pauls, D. L., Hurst, C. R., Kruger, S. D., Leckman, J. F., Kidd, K. K., & Cohen, D. J. (1986). Gilles de la Tourette's syndrome and attention deficit disorder with hyperactivity: Evidence against a genetic relationship. *Archives of General Psychiatry, 43,* 1177–1179.

Pauls, D. L. & Leckman, J. F. (1986). The inheritance of Gilles de la Tourette's syndrome and associated behaviors: Evidence for autosomal dominant transmission. *New England Journal of Medicine, 315,* 993–997.

Pauls, D. L., Pakstis, A. J., Kurlan, R., Kidd, K. K., Leckman, J. F., Cohen, D. J., Kidd, J. R., Como, P., & Sparkes, R. (1990). Segregation and linkage analysis of Tourette's syndrome and related disorders. *Journal of American Academy of Child and Adolescent Psychiatry, 29,* 195–203.

Pauls, D. L., Towbin, K. E., Leckman, J. F., Zahner, G. E. P., & Cohen, D. J. (1986). Gilles de la Tourette's syndrome and obsessive-compulsive disorder: Evidence supporting a genetic relationship. *Archives of General Psychiatry, 43,* 1180–1182.

Polinsky, R. J., Ebert, M. H., Caine, E. D., Ludlow, C., & Bassich, C. J. (1980). Cholinergic treatment in the tourette syndrome. *The New England Journal of Medicine, 302 : 23,* 1310–1311.

Singer, H. S. & Walkup, J. T. (1991). Tourette syndrome and other tic disorders: diagnosis pathophysiology, and treatment. *Medicine, 70,* 15–32.

Spreen, O., & Benton, A. L. (1969). *Neurosensory Center Comprehensive Examination for Aphasia,* Victoria, B. C.: University of Victoria.

Christy L. Ludlow, Bethesda, Maryland (USA)

IV. Pathologies of Language Use in Psychiatric Disorders

51. Language Behavior in Alexithymia

1. Neurosis and Psychosomatic Disease

As clues to individual psychological organization, stylistic properties of speech have been employed in medicine since the introduction of 'talking cures', particularly psychoanalysis. Verbal communication complemented traditional 'medical gaze' and emphasized dyadic and group interaction in diagnosis and treatment. — In psychoanalysis, the term 'neurosis' refers to a psychological organization developed in response to intense and partly repressed affects, especially anxiety and hostility. Language, one of the systems for dealing with such affects, may show relevant 'defense mechanisms'. The psychoanalytic methods have also been applied to somatic disorders, first explained by principles similar to those proposed for neurotic symptoms, mostly conversion. It became evident that a homogeneous model might be complemented with an heterogeneous one, implying different organization for neurosis and somatic illnes. Ruesch (1948) distinguished between 'arrested' development, leading to psychosomatic disorder, and 'pathological' development, resulting in neurosis. Others indicated that verbal communication differs in bearers of neurosis and psychosomatic disorders (Lolas/von Rad 1989). — The term 'neurosis' is not employed in the 'Diagnostic and Statistical Manual of the American Psychiatric Association' (DSM-III-R) and is included only as adjective in the 10th revision of the 'International Classification of Diseases' (ICD-10). 'Psychosomatic disease' is no longer used as a nosological entity, being replaced by "psychological factors affecting physical conditions" (DSM-III-R) and "behavioural syndromes and mental disorders associated with physiological dysfunction and hormonal disturbances" (ICD-10), categories replacing it within a multiaxial biopsychosocial framework. The group 'somatoform disorders', without organic basis or known pathophysiology, lies between 'purely psychological' and 'purely organic' disorders. — These comments highlight the problem of ascribing speech patterns to pathological entities without due regard to their true definition. What appeared in the past as 'fixed' or structural characteristics has often been reformulated as communication patterns or systemic attributes of dyads and groups.

2. Affect Verbalization and Alexithymia

Irrespective of the way they choose to describe them, psychotherapists have long been aware of patients not inclined to verbalize feelings. Ferenczi and Zilboorg described people unable to establish affective rapport with therapists, in whom somatic affect is discordant with verbal expression. These "difficult patients" (Shands 1975) appear dull, boring and impoverished by comparison to psychologically-minded neurotics, more prone to verbal expression. Among the features Ruesch (1948) included in his concept of "infantile personality" were inability to discharge tension through verbal or creative symbolism and tendency to employ somatic expression. These impair people to cope with frustration and affects and could lead to somatic illnesses. The pattern overlaps with Shands 'difficult patients' who, aside from difficulties to describe feelings, are unable to use the pronoun *I* in emotionally meaningful contexts. Among subjects likely to exhibit this cognitive, affective and relationship pattern are those afflicted by 'psychosomatic' conditions, alcoholism, drug dependence and post-traumatic stress (Krystal 1988). From a psychodynamic point of view, French psychoanalysts (Marty/de M'Uzan/David 1963) described a cognitive style adhering to concrete facts, reduced dreaming and fantasy and a particular type of relatedness to others, whereby these are seen as stereotyped images of oneself. Constriction of emotional functioning, impoverishment of fantasy life and tendency to use action instead of language to deal with conflict were included in the concept of alexithymia, proposed by Sifneos (1973) as a cluster of features prevalent in 'psychosomatic' patients (psychosomatic meaning the "holy seven" diseases of Alexander (1950), with tissue changes and psychological mediating links in etiology and/or pathogenesis). The contrast between alexithymic and neurotic styles has greatly influenced research. Although the core disturbance is inability to verbally express feelings ('a-lexithymia'), the concept was construed as a pervasive inhibition or block of self-caring and self-regulating functions and failure to identify and use emotionally meaningful nonverbal expressions as signals to the self. Somatization and regression to somatic forms of expression would result from an inability to cope verbally ('mentally') with stress and conflict. The behavior pattern was explained as dysconnection between cognition and affect, as inhibition of affect verbalization due to defenses or as sociocultural constraint. The relationship of alexithymia to bodily dysfunction, and its prevalence in otherwise normal populations, have been sources of debate and confusion.

3. Communication of Emotional Meaning

Alexithymia and its related theories uncovered the importance of communication and interaction in diagnosis, prognosis and therapy. 'Communication of emotional meaning' has become a dimension descriptive of persons, dyads, groups, or situations (Lolas/von Rad 1982 a; b). Under this systemic viewpoint empirical studies can be reevaluated. – Operationalization of alexithymia has taken different forms. Psychometric questionnaires, studies of elicited and spontaneous speech, and physiological measurements have been used. Data from non-propositional speech probes (questionnaires) have differentiated alexithymia from other psychopathological labels and explored its prevalence in different populations. For evaluating communication of emotional meaning studies of spontaneous natural speech seem appropriate, since the clinical dialogic situation was the primary observational setting of alexithymia.

4. Content Analysis and Emotional Meaning

Content analysis is a technique for making replicable inferences from a text to its context (cf. Koch/Schöfer (Eds.) 1986). The latter can refer to psychological, behavioral or situational features. Early studies emphasized structural aspects (i. e. number of words produced in an interview, number of times the pronoun *I* is used, number of verbs and adjectives per 1000 words, 'affectladen words'), showing that alexithymic individuals produce less textual markers related to affect than psychoneurotics during monologues and dialogues (von Rad/Lolas 1978; Taylor/Doody 1985). Psychoneurotic patients express more anxiety at the first psychoanalytical interview, particularly in relation to guilt and shame, and more hostility directed towards the self, employing grammatical clauses as coding units (Gottschalk/Lolas/Viney 1986). When similar samples of patients were compared during monologues, differences appeared only for mutilation anxiety, with higher scores for psychosomatic patients. This illustrates the influence of situational context on the differences and cast doubt on any static characterization of subjects by means of speech measures alone (Lolas/von Rad/Scheibler 1981). Other authors find similar results in monadic situations (Taylor/Doody 1985). Using interview data, affect patterning was investigated. While psychosomatic (alexithymic) subjects tend to associate hostility directed outwards with shame and anxiety, psychoneurotics show an association between hostility outwards and guilt anxiety. When both dyadic and monadic conditions are combined within the same session, differences between cardiac neurosis and ulcerative colitis patients do not appear during monologues (von Rad/Lolas 1982 a; b). Employing a form of content analysis based on single words and automatic processing, psychoneurotics were shown to agree more with interviewers, suggesting that alexithymia might be a dyadic feature depending upon thematic synchrony between patients and therapists (Lolas/von Rad 1982 a; b). Assuming a continuum along the dimension communication of emotional meaning, content analysis scores differentiated between generalized anxiety disorder, irritable bowel and peptic ulcer patients. The latter were the less expressive, with irritable bowel subjects in an intermediate position between them and anxious patients (Lolas/Heerlein 1986). Carefully planned studies conclude that the degree of association between alexithymia and other psychopathological features is not redundant (Taylor/Doody 1982). It has been suggested that expressive deficits are restricted to cognitive/functional and not to unconscious aspects (Ahrens 1985) and that it may affect more the expression of negative affects.

5. Concluding Remarks

Research on the distinction between psychoneurosis and psychosomatic disease, kindled by psychoanalytical theory, has drawn attention to verbal communication of affect and emotion as diagnostic dimension. Restricted expression of feelings through words (alexithymia) has been described as part of a syndrome characterized by limited fantasy life and tendency to bodily expression. Although dependent on situational context and limited by prevailing nosologies, this research suggests that language has an homeostatic function in psychosomatic organization. Its control and self-regulation functions in biopsychosocial health are expressed in the dimension 'communication of emotional meaning', which may serve as a useful descriptive and diagnostic tool. Several techniques of content and meaning analysis can be employed for this purpose. Clause-based methods have been successfully used for differentiating different clinical pictures (Schöfer/Müller/von Kerekjarto 1979; Oxman/Rosenberg/Schnurr/Tucker 1988). It should be kept in mind that a specific match between speech characteristics and clinical diagnoses depends to a great extent on prevailing nosologies and that the distinction between psychosomatic diseases and neuroses is in a state of revision. Caution should also be exercised when considering pauses, verbal productivity and other formal features of speech, as well as nonverbal behavior, as differentiating elements. As with language behavior, diagnostic usefulness of such sources of communication data depends on a critical balance between appropriate operationalization of relevant descriptive constructs and sound taxonomy of illnesses.

6. References

Alexander, F. (1950). *Psychosomatic medicine.* New York: Norton.

Ahrens, S. (1985). Alexithymia and affective verbal behaviour in three groups of patients. *Social Science and Medicine, 20,* 691–694.

Gottschalk, L., Lolas, F., & Viney, L. (1986). *Content analysis of verbal behaviour.* Berlin–Heidelberg: Springer.

Krystal, H. (1988). *Integration and selfhealing: Affects, trauma, and alexithymia.* Hillsdale, N. J.: Analytic Press.

Koch, U. & Schöfer, G. (Eds.) (1986). *Sprachinhaltsanalyse in der psychiatrischen und psychosomatischen Forschung.* Weinheim/München: PVU.

Lolas, F. & Heerlein, A. (1986). Content category analysis of affective expression in irritable bowel, duodenal ulcer and anxiety disorder patients. *Psychopathology, 19,* 309–316.

Lolas, F. & von Rad, M. (1982a). Communication of emotional meaning: a biopsychosocial dimension in psychosomatics. In S. B. Day (Ed.), *Life stress. 138–144.* New York: Van Nostrand-Reinhold.

Lolas, F. & von Rad, M. (1982b). Psychosomatic disease and neurosis: a study of dyadic verbal behaviour. *Comprehensive Psychiatry, 23,* 19–24.

Lolas, F. & von Rad, M. (1989). Alexithymia. In S. Cheren (Ed.), *Psychosomatic medicine. 189–237.* Madison, CT: International Universities Press.

Lolas, F., von Rad, M., & Scheibler, D. (1981). Situational influences on verbal affective expression of psychosomatic and psychoneurotic patients. *Journal of Nervous and Mental Disease, 169,* 619–623.

Marty, P., de M'Uzan, M., & David, C. (1963). *L'investigation psychosomatique.* Paris: Presses Universitaires de France.

Oxman, T. E., Rosenberg, S. D., Schnurr, P. P., & Tucker, G. J. (1988). Diagnostic classification through content analysis of patient's speech. *American Journal of Psychiatry, 145,* 464–468.

Ruesch, H. (1948). The infantile personality. *Psychosomatic Medicine, 10,* 134–144.

Schöfer, G., Müller, L., & von Kerekjarto, M. (1979). Die Differenzierung psychosomatischer Krankheitsgruppen mit der Gottschalk-Gleser-Sprachinhaltsanalyse. *Medizinische Psychologie, 5,* 24–38.

Shands, H. (1975). How are "psychosomatic" patients different from "psychoneurotic" patients? *Psychotherapy and Psychosomatics, 26,* 270–285.

Sifneos, P. (1973). The prevalence of "alexithymic" characteristics in psychosomatic patients. *Psychotherapy and Psychosomatics, 22,* 255–262.

Taylor, G., & Doody, K. (1982). Psychopathology and verbal expression in psychosomatic and psychoneurotic patients. *Psychotherapy and Psychosomatics, 38,* 121–127.

Taylor, G., & Doody, K. (1985). Verbal measures of alexithymia: What do they measure. *Psychotherapy and Psychosomatics, 43,* 32–37.

von Rad, M. & Lolas, F. (1978). Psychosomatische und psychoneurotische Patienten im Vergleich. Unterschiede des Sprechverhaltens. *Psyche, 32,* 956–973.

von Rad, M. & Lolas, F. (1982). Empirical evidence of alexithymia. *Psychotherapy and Psychosomatics, 38,* 91–102.

Fernando Lolas, Santiago (Chile)

52. Pathology of Language Behavior in Affective Psychoses

1. Introduction

A multitude of psychological symptoms can be assessed by analysis of language behavior; as one might expect, because of the complexity of the biological language system, cerebral pathology can alter speech and language behavior in any of a number of ways.

In contrast to language disorders like aphasia, the pathology of language and language behavior in depression and mania have been called language symptoms (Vetter 1969). The underlying abnormality may be, for example, a sign of disturbed emotionality or of tension. In such cases it is also possible to find signs of these disturbances in other domains like in gestures or the vegetative system. In other words the symptoms are not restricted to linguistic variables. It is very common to have the question, if a variable is affected by a thinking disorder, a pure language disorder or, for example, by a psychomotor disturbance.

Besides this distinction, which depends on the predominance of the disturbance in one or several subsystems, there is a further distinction between more or less pure linguistic and para-linguistic variables. Taxonomies for the para-linguistic variables have been attempted to establish e. g. by Newman/Mather (1938) and Mahl/Schulze (1964). Indeed, in some cases it is difficult to distinguish clearly between linguistic and para-linguistic disturbances.

Therefore it is important to identify those of pathogenetic factors in affective psychoses, which interfere with the function of subsystems of the language system. This task has been undertaken by some investigators in order to find objective parameters of relevant psychopathological variables.

The affective psychoses are subdivided into the unipolar major depressive disorder and the bipolar affective psychosis (see e. g. DSM III-R 1987), is a course of the illness characterized by depressive and manic phases. Many of the investigators did not report on the unipolar-bipolar distinction of their depressed patients and sometimes failed to report, whether the cases of depression were of a reactive (neurotic) or endogenous type (belonging to the affective psychoses). For this reason there is considerable inhomogeneity in most of the clinical samples of depression. In this chapter the symptoms regarding language and language behavior will be predominantly discussed for depression, since this disorder has been the object of the majority of investigations.

2. Speech Production

2.1. Articulation and Phonematic Variables

There is no clear evidence for defective articulation in either depression or mania. But ratings of the articulatory variables by trained phonetician do, in fact, demonstrate some abnormalities. For instance, Newman/Mather (1938) described articulation as lax and Darby (1981) noted imprecise consonants after antidepressive drug treatment, reflecting a possible medication induced effect. The articulation time for, e. g., counting has been found to be within the normal range in depression, and is not changing with the clinical improvement of the illness (Szabady/Bradshaw/Besson 1976; Greden/Carroll 1980; Nilsonne 1987; 1988). Contrary to these results Klos/Ellgring (1984) found a slightly prolonged articulation time.

Formal aphasia testing of depressed patients has not revealed phonematic difficulties in depression (Faber/Reichstein 1981; Emery/Breslau 1989; Newman/Sweet 1986). There are no reports of an increased frequency of slips of the tongue phonematic paraphasias or neologisms. Furthermore there is no disturbance in phoneme discrimination in depression (Kugler/Caudrey 1983).

It seems justified to conclude from the existing data, that in affective psychoses there are no specific problems with the phonematic aspects of language. Many of the alterations in articulation, which may occur, can be related to psychopharmacological effects.

2.2. Voice Quality and Prosody

2.2.1. Voice Quality and Loudness

Early studies characterized the quality of voice in depression (Newman/Mather 1938) as having a pharyngeal, sometimes nasal resonance with glottal rasping. In addition, a study involving speech deviation rating found signs of a hypokinetic extrapyramidal disturbance (Darby/Simmons/Berger 1984).

In most cases the fundamental frequency of the speech of depressed patients was found to be lower than that of controls, but there is considerable variation within the group of depressed patients (Hargreaves/Starkweather/Blacker 1965; Starkweather 1967). No significant group effect between depressed patients and normal controls was reported by Zuberbier (1957) and Nilsonne (1987; 1988). In contrast, Scherer (1979 b) found about a 10% increase in fundamental frequency after clinical improvement of depression. Several investigators noted medication effects (Smith 1982; Nevlund/Fann/Falk 1983; Helfrich/Standke/Scherer 1985; Weiß 1987), whereas Andreasen/Alpert/Marty (1981) did not found medication effects on acoustic parameters. A hoarse voice as a side effect of tricyclic antidepressaent medication was reported by Rhoades/Lowel/Hedgepeth (1979).

Depressed patients have been observed by clinicians to speak in a low or soft voice. The variable of loudnes has been measured by Whitman/Flicker (1966), Darby (1981) and Stassen/Kuny/Woggon/Angst (1989) and among others Hargreaves/Starkweather/Blacker (1965) noted considerable variablity. It must be stressed that there are severe problems in clinically measuring the sound pressure level in depressed patients (Andreasen/Alpert/Marty 1981).

In summary, acoustic parameters of the voice of depressed patients are obviously altered, but there is a considerable variation within the group of depressed patients.

2.2.2. Prosodic Variables

The dynamics of loudness have been found to be reduced in depressed patients by Zuberbier (1957). An early case study of depression, which analyzed both loudness and pitch, was performed by Zwirner (1930). Newman/Mather (1938) reported absent or rare emphatic accents, which include changes in loudness as well as changes in fundamental frequency. Clinical judgement of prosody as being monotonous is presumably caused by several factors, like changes in loudness and pitch – in syntax as well as in content (see below). Ratings by experienced phoneticians reflected several changes in the prosody of depressed patients (Newman/Mather 1938), i. e., narrow pitch range, and infrequent stepwise changes of perceived pitch. Moses (1954) stressed the observation of uniformity in the depressed voice with repetitions of a gliding down, (s. a. Darby/Hollien 1977).

After technically masking the semantic content (content filtering), raters percieved the speech of depressed patients as sad, regardless of the content of the story the patients were telling. At the same time, however, according to a reliable rating of the verbal transcript the stories were considered as sad, happy or angry. The expression of the affects sadness and anger was rated as inappropriate (Levin/Hall/Knight/Alpert 1985). If these findings can be replicated, they might direct the attention to the question, whether there is a more widespread disturbance of affective expression in depression, than has been previously presumed, which might go undetected because of the constant sadness in the behavior of the patients.

Depressed patients' variation of pitch (standard deviation of the pitch) was reported to be reduced by Zuberbier (1957), Leff/Aberton (1981) and Nilsonne (1987; 1988). But whereas Zuberbier (1957) found less downward deflection of the melodic line at the end of the utterance, no significant difference in the variable for this prosodic feature was observed in the study by Nilsonne (1988). Interestingly Hargreaves/Starkweather/Blacker

(1965) noted a high interindividual variability of the predominant melodic line of depressed patients. Nilsonne (1988) also reported lower values for two further variables in depression, namely the standard deviation of the rate of change and the average speed of the change.

It seems especially important to investigate, whether the monotonous voice of depressive patients is related to a general psychopathological symptom i. e., psychomotor retardation (Nilsonne 1988), or whether it is a normal expression of the emotional state of the patients. Andreasen/Alpert/Marty's (1981) finding, that acoustic parameters are more related to the designation of patients as being emotionally flat versus non-flat, independent of the clinical diagnosis of depression, mania or schizophrenia, might be interpreted as an argument against nosological significance of these variables. A further interpretation (Nilsonne 1988) is the involvement of the presumably lateralized systems which regulate the prosody in depression.

3. Syntax and Text

Investigations of the language production of depressed patients (Newman/Mather 1938) report little effort to elaborate phrases. The construction of sentences were described as loose and fragmentary and the syntactical devices as being mostly of the additive type (coordination and parallelism). The verbal responses in psychodiagnostic tests (Schafer 1948) were described as showing little spontaneous elaboration or qualification, and in association tests the language production seemed generally dull, stereotyped and blocked. Surprisingly, Andreasen/Pfohl (1976) found no significant differences in syntactic complexity of depressed and manic patients.

There have only been few quantitative investigations of specific syntactic parameters of depressed patients, which served mostly as psychiatric controls for schizophrenic patients. In one of these studies Pylyshyn (1970) found more negations and less qualifying subordinators in the language production of depressed patients. Moreover, he observed no significant differences for the type token ration of depressive patients, nor did Pinard/Roy/Tetreault (1972). In a different approach Weintraub/Aronson (1962; 1967) and Hinchcliffe/Lancashire/Roberts (1971) also reported more use of negation in depression. Andreasen/Pfohl (1976) established that, whereas the depressed patients used more qualifying adverbs and first person pronouns, manic patients used more adjectives. Contradicting these findings, Lorenz/Cobb (1952) and Lorenz (1953) reported, that in mania – in addition to an increased amount of language production – there is an increase in the use of verbs and pronouns and less use of adjectives and prepositions.

Text cohesion and text coherence was reported to be unimpaired in depression (Frommer/Tress 1989). Investigation of a 200-word sample with the cloze paradigm, which assesses the predictability of speech, reflected normal scores (0.55 in depression versus 0.55 in controls, Maher/Manschreck/Weisstein 1988) or even above normal scores (0.52 versus 0.47, Ragin/Oltmanns 1983). In contrast Maher/Manschreck/Weisstein (1988) found somewhat lower scores in their bipolar depressive patients.

It can be summarized that the quantitative analysis of language production of depressed patients demonstrates no abnormalities in syntactical variables or text parameters and thus fail to indicate a disturbance of the syntax system. The low elaboration of syntactical structures of utterances reported in the evaluation of spontaneous speech of depressed patients are paralleled by difficulties in reading comprehension at higher levels of complexity and as well as tasks of increased syntactical complexity (Emery/Breslau 1989), which may be discussed as complexity effects and not as symptoms of a disturbance of the language system.

In mania, on the contrary, a rich syntactic elaboration was reported, with diversified syntactic structures (Newman/Mather 1938). Quantitative linguistic investigations of manic patients have been done mostly in comparison with schizophrenic patients, which demonstrate more syntactical deviations (Andreasen/Grove 1979; Frommer/Tress 1989; Hoffman/Stopeck/Andreasen 1986; Wykes/Leff 1982).

4. Lexicon and Semantics

There are some studies which report reduced vocabulary scores, especially for older depressed patients, whereas vocabulary in normals actually increases with age (Savage/Britton/Bolton/Hall 1973; Kendrick/Gibson/Moses 1979; Reischies 1988).

In formal aphasia testing no naming disturbances were seen in depression, Faber/

Reichstein (1981), Emery/Breslau (1989). Bucci/Freedman (1981), however, found a deficit in 'referential activity function', which relies essentially on naming, in older depressed patients. They interpret their finding as a failure of integration of symbolic processing.

Word production with a speed component, like the word fluency tasks, e. g. finding words with a certain initial letter, are impaired in depression (Robertson/Taylor 1985; Reischies 1988; Reischies/von Spieß/Hedde 1990). But it has to be kept in mind that these tasks require a considerable effort, and it is likely that depressed patients fail in tasks which are effortful (Weingartner/Cohen/Murphy et al. 1982). In an untimed version of such a task Emery/Breslau (1989) also found word production deficits in depressed older patients, yet attributed them nevertheless to the task's high effort demand. It is possible that certain word retrieval problems contribute to the reduced quantity of language production of depressed patients and to the vagueness in the verbal expression, which was reported by Andreasen/Pfohl (1976).

Speech blockage has been reported as possible side effect of antidepressant medication (tricyclics, maprotiline and MAO-antagonists). It is characterized more often as "word blockage" in the sense of word finding problems (Schatzberg/Cole/Blumer 1978; Goldstein/Goldberg 1986), although articulation problems have also been observed (Sandyk 1986).

No disturbance in denotative versus connotative meaning has been found between depressed and manic patients in contrast to schizophrenic patients (Cutting/Murphy 1990). However, because there was no normal control group in this study, the result is difficult to interpret.

A memory bias in depressed patients favoring negative events has been found in some studies (Lloyd/Lishman 1975). This may possibly contribute to the preponderance of negation in their language production.

In summary, most of the abnormalities of depressed patients found for lexical or semantic variables appear to be related to effects of the general complexity or amount of effort required for the task. The question, if there is a semantic retrieval problem in depression, however, must be clarified in further studies.

5. Fluency and Speech Disruptions

Past descriptions of language in depression stressed the point that these patients talk rarely or say almost nothing at all, in contrast to manic patients (Wernicke 1906). Newman/Mather (1938) characterized the speech in depression as having a slow tempo, frequent pauses and hesitations, slow initiation of response and short length of the response. In contrast, the speech of manic patients differs in the initiation of the response, which is described as rapid, and in the length of the response, which is described as long (see also Lorenz/Cobb 1952).

The topic of fluency has been mentioned above in conjunction with word finding problems of depressed patients. Fillmore (1979) discusses fluency as one dimension of individual differences regarding competency in the use of one's language. The reduction of the basal amount of language production is seen by some researchers as a symptom of psychomotor retardation in depression. They therefore consider such factors as pause times, for example, to be quantification variables of retardation (s. below). The basal amount of language production may be considered – according to this approach – as an underlying variable, which can be assessed by many of the fluency parameters more or less reliably.

5.1. Basal Amount of Language Production

5.1.1. Elicited Language Samples

In speech of depressed patients the pauses between words seem to be prolonged. In view of this finding, researchers usually analyze sequences of automatic speech. Zuberbier (1957) for example, had her patients produce a series of *la, la* .... She noticed a slowing for the last 5 items. Furthermore there are several data about counting times in depression – the patients counting from 1 to 10 'at their own speed'. Table 52.1. shows the results for studies involving this paradigm. In most investigations only few patients have been studied. It has been found, that the pause time is almost twice as high in depression as compared to normal controls, as well as compared to patients in an euthymic state, that is, after recovery. However, this seems not to hold for bipolar patients in the depressed state (Hoffmann/Gonze/Mendlewicz 1985). It should be mentioned, that two of the studies tried to investigate manic patients as well, but it

Study	Depression Diagnosis-Criteria N Age Medicated	Pauses Depress.	Remission	Controls	Comment
Szabady 1976	4 22–56 yrs.	4.28 (1.49)	1.75 (0.54)	0.95 (0.71)	
Greden 1980	RDC 7 42–82 yrs. nonmed.	4.20 (3.14)	2.05 (0.80)		
Greden 1981	RDC Unipolar 24 57.2 yrs. Bipolar 12 52.3 yrs.	 3.44 (3.03) 3.13 (2.73)	 1.94 (1.05) 2.19 (1.48)	 1.87 (1.13)	
Godfrey 1984	DSM III 5	4.72	2.08	2.66	
Hardy 1984	DSM III 16 22–74 yrs. nonmed.	4.10 (1.48)	2.79 (1.11)		Corr. with retardation
Hoffmann 1985	RDC 6 unipolar 10 bipolar 21–71 yrs. nonmed.	 3.36 (1.21) 1.47 (0.79)		 1.74 (0.67)	 Corr. with simple react. time, and retardation
Nilsonne 1988	RDC 28 26–63 yrs.	3.1 (0.4)		2.9 (0.4)	

Table 52.1: Pause times in counting (Nine intervals from 1 to 10) (sd)

seemed to be almost impossible to have these patients perform this task properly (Greden/Carrol 1980; Godfrey/Knight 1984).

Correlational analyses have shown a relation of pause duration to measures of psychomotor retardation in the depressed state and also in the course of recovery. In addition, neuroleptics do not appear to alter pause times (Szabady/Bradshaw/Gazner 1980).

Reading times were found to be affected as well as the pause durations in depressed patients (Zuberbier 1957; Darby/Hollien 1977; Nilsonne 1987). Darby/Hollien (1977) and Newman/Mather (1938), found neither a strong relation between the state of the patients and the reading time nor specificity regarding the differentiation between psychiatric diagnostic groups. The effect of sedative drug effects on pauses in reading was noted by Hargreaves/Starkweather/Blacker (1965).

5.1.2. Language Production in an Interview Situation

The language production in an interview is dependent on many complex factors. In the language production of an interview, the proportion of speech of the depressed patient is reduced (Ellgring 1976; Rehm 1987, negative finding Rutter 1977). Monologue material from interview situations has been most often analysed for fluency parameters.

The word per minute count obtained in several studies is shown in Table 52.2. There are important differences regarding the exclusion of speech pauses. In the Klos/Ellgring study (1984), for example, only the time for the utterances was analysed, and dialogue material has been analysed, so that a slightly higher count results. Reischies (1988) found a significant correlation between the word per

Study	Sample	N Age	Depression	Remission	Control	Comment
Weintraub 1967	10 min	45	104.8 (30.8)		124.8 (35.5)	Exclus. longer pauses
Hichcliffe 1971	5 min	19 53 yrs.	101.6		123.4	
Klos 1984		16 55.6 yrs.	140.1 (38.8)	179.8 (33.9)		Exclus. pauses
Gottschalk 1986	5 min	29 37 yrs.	103.2		male 112.2 female 94.6	

Table 52.2: Words per minute in an interview situation (uninterrupted speech sample)

minute count for one minute to the global cerebral blood flow (r = 0.59). The corresponding counts of words per minute were in accordance with the reported data: 112.04 (sd 42.20) for the depressed state and 128.82 (sd 38.64, t = 1.98) for the remitted state of 28 patients, which have been investigated two times. As would expected, manic patients show an increased amount of language production (Newman/Mather 1938; Stoddard/Post/Bunney 1977), assessed as words per minute (Lorenz/Cobb 1952).

The amount of language production has been shown to be quite stable for an individual person (see Goldman-Eisler 1968) and to be related e. g. to personality factors like extraversion (Scherer 1979a). It varies, however, with the emotional state, especially anxiety, which is an common element of the depressive syndrome (Benton/Hartman/Sarason 1955; Pope/Blass/Siegman/Raher 1970; Murray 1971; Siegman 1978). Here the evaluation of the importance of the topic in the communicative situation may be mentioned. Manic patients usually feel as though they were contributing important topics to the conversation. It is even difficult to interrupt their speech (Newman/Mather 1938). In contrast, part of the psychopathology of depression is that the depressed patients think, they have nothing important to say. The possible role of cognitions like this in the explanation of the amount of language production seems to have not yet been systematically studied.

Because an imbalance of cholinergic and adrenergic effects in the brain of depressed patients has been postulated (Janowsky/El-Yousef/Davis/Serkerke 1972), the findings of decreased talkativeness after psychopharmacological interventions (e. g. the application of physostigmine, a central cholinergic drug, Bowers/Goodman/Sim 1964), and conversely increased talkativeness after an adrenergic stimulant amphetamine (Griffith/Stitzer/Corker 1977) are especially relevant. Furthermore frontal lobe damage can lead to less spontaneous language production (Stuss/Benson 1986), possibly in relation to an abolic state. The importance of such factors, which may influence verbal fluency, for the affective psychoses has not been studied in detail.

5.2. Speech Disruptions

There are grammatical and non-grammatical explanations for the discontinuation of speech (Miller 1973). Nongrammatical pauses are of more interest in the language behavior of depressed and manic patients. Reasons for non-grammatical pauses can be intrusions, stuttering, slips of the tongue, corrections and incompletion as well as omissions (Mahl 1956). The frequency of these classes of disruptions, which are related to affects like anxiety (Mahl 1956; Mahl/Schulze 1964; Glaister/Feldstein/Pollack 1980), seems to be not systematically investigated in conjunction with affective psychoses. Bouhuys/Mulder-Hajonides van der Meulen (1989) identified a factor of fragmentation of speech. The Pauses between speakers and the duration of vocal activity were included in this factor. The pauses between utterances have been found to be reduced in depression. Zuberbier (1957) reported a mean pause duration of 2.22 sec, versus 0.98 in controls, Klos/Ellgring (1984) 1.76 in depression and 1.05 sec. in the remitted state.

The latency from the end of an utterance of the interviewer to the utterance of the depressed patient is prolonged (Renford 1986; Nilsonne 1988), which might be an effect of a general increase in behavioral response latency, reported by Libet/Lewinson (1973).

Nongrammatical pauses can also be caused by cognitive activity, e. g. thinking about the continuation of the phrase (Miller 1973). Because depressed patients suffer from a disorder of decision (Corvin/Peselow/Feenan et al. 1990) with a tendency to decide more cautiously, a prolonged time for decisions may contribute to the fragmentation of speech and to the global reduction of language production. Since the reverse seems to be true for mania, the quick response of manic patients (Newman/Mather 1938) may be related to their altered decision behavior (Corvin/Peselow/Feenan et al. 1990).

6. Conclusion

As with all other disturbances of information processing in psychiatric diseases, there are several components or stages of the language system, which can be interfered with. This aspect would include the metabolic parameters of the disease, for example. On the other hand, there may be also a direct effect of an underlying dimension of psychopathology, like psychomotor retardation or the inability of depressed patients to invest effort for a task.

A third possibility is, that a language variable is altered as a physiological expression of an extreme affective state (like grief, anxiety). In this case, which may be true for some prosodic variables, it would be not justified to regard these aspects of the language behavior as abnormal. Further investigation of this problem is necessary. In depression as well as mania the interaction of disease factors with the language system seems mainly to occur at the possible multiple stages controlling fluency of language production.

7. References

Andreasen, N. C., Alpert, M., & Marty, M. (1981). Acoustic analyses: An objective measure of affective flattening. *Archives of General Psychiatry, 38,* 281–285.

Andreasen, N. C. & Grove, W. (1979). The relationship between schizophrenic language, manic language, and aphasia. In J. Gruzelier & P. Flor-Henry (Eds.), *Hemispheric asymmetries of function in psychopathology. 373–390.* Amsterdam: Elsevier.

Andreasen, N. C. & Pfohl, B. (1976). Linguistic analysis of speech in affective disorders. *Archives of General Psychiatry, 33,* 1361–1367.

Benton, A. L., Hartman, C. H., & Sarason J. G. (1955). Some relation between speech behavior and anxiety level. *Journal of Abnormal and Social Psychology, 51,* 295–301.

Bouhuys, A. L. & Mulder-Hajonides van der Meulen, W. R. (1984). Speech timing measures of severity, psychomotor retardation, and agitation in endogenously depressed patients. *Journal of Communication Disorders, 17,* 277–288.

Bowers, M. B., Goodman, E., & Sim, V. M. (1964). Some behavioral changes in man following anticholinesterase administration. *Journal of Nervous and Mental Disease, 138,* 383–389.

Bucci, W. & Freedman, N. (1981). The language of depression. *Bulletin of the Menniger Clinic, 45,* 334–358.

Corvin, J., Peselow, E., Feenan, K., Rotrosen, J., & Fieve, R. (1990). Disorders of decision in affective disease: An effect of ß-adrenergic dysfunction? *Biological Psychiatry, 27,* 813–833.

Cutting, J. & Murphy, D. (1990). Preference for denotative as opposed to connotative meanings in schizophrenics. *Brain and Language, 39,* 459–468.

Darby, J. K. (1981). Speech and voice studies in psychiatric populations. In J. K. Darby (Ed.), *Speech evaluation in psychiatry. 253–284.* New York: Grune/Stratton.

Darby, J. K. & Hollien, H. (1977). Vocal and speech patterns of depressive patients. *Folia Phoniatrica, 29,* 279–291.

Darby, J. K., Simmons, N., & Berger, P. A. (1984). Speech and voice parameters of depression: a pilot study. *Journal of Communication Disorders, 17,* 75–85.

Diagnostic and statistic manual of mental disorders, 3rd edition (revised) (1987). American Psychiatric Association, Washington.

Ellgring, J. H. (1976). Kommunikatives Verhalten im Verlauf depressiver Erkrankungen. In W. H. Tack (Ed.), *Bericht über den 30. Kongreß der DGfPs. 190–192.* Göttingen: Hogrefe.

Emery, O. B. & Breslau, L. D. (1989). Language deficits in depression: comparisons with SDAT and normal aging. *Journal of Gerontology, 44,* 85–92.

Faber, R. & Reichstein, M. B. (1981). Language dysfunction in schizophrenia. *British Journal of Psychiatry, 139,* 519–522.

Fillmore, C. J. (1979). On Fluency. In C. J. Fillmore, D. Kemper, & W. S.-Y. Wang (Eds.), *Individual differences in language ability and language behavior. 85–101.* New York: Academic Press.

Frommer, J. & Tress, W. (1989). Merkmale schizophrener Rede. Eine vergleichende Untersuchung von Dialogen mit Schizophrenen, Manikern, Depressiven und Hirnorganikern. *Fortschritte der Neurologie und Psychiatrie, 57,* 85–93.

Glaister, J., Feldstein, S., & Pollak, H. (1980). Chronographic speech patterns of acutely psychotic patients. *Journal of Nervous and Mental Disease, 168,* 219–223.

Godfrey, H. P. & Knight, R. G. (1984). The validity of actometer and speech activity measures in the assessment of depressed patients. *British Journal of Psychiatry, 145,* 159–163.

Goldman-Eisler, F. (1968). *Psycholinguistics – Experiments in spontaneous speech.* New York: Academic Press.

Goldstein, D. M. & Goldberg, R. L. (1986). Monoamine oxidase inhibitor-induced speech blockage. *American Journal of Psychiatry, 47,* 604.

Gottschalk, L. A. & Hoigaard-Martin, J. (1966). A depression scale applicable to verbal sample.s *Psychiatry Research, 17,* 213–227.

Greden, J. F., Albala, A. A., Smokler, I. A., Gardner, R., & Carroll, B. J. (1981). Speech pause time: A marker of psychomotor retardation among endogenous depressives. *Biological Psychiatry, 16,* 851–859.

Greden, J. F. & Carroll, B. J. (1980). Decrease in speech pause times with treatment of endogenous depression. *Biological Psychiatry, 15,* 575–587.

Griffiths, R., Stitzer, M., & Corker, K. (1977). Drug-produced changes in human social behavior: Facilitation by d-amphetamine. *Pharmacology, Biochemistry and Behavior, 7,* 365–372.

Hargreaves, W. A., Starkweather, J. A., & Blacker, K. H. (1965). Voice quality in depression. *Journal of Abnormal and Social Psychology, 70,* 218–220.

Helfrich, H., Standke, R., & Scherer, K. (1985). Vocal indicators of psychoactive drug effects. *Speech Communication, 3,* 245–252.

Hinchcliffe, M. K., Lancashire, M., & Roberts, F. J. (1971). Defense mechanisms in speech. *British Journal of Psychiatry, 118,* 471–472.

Hoffmann, G. M., Gonze, J. C., & Mendlewicz, J. (1985). Speech pause time as a method for the evaluation of psychomotor retardation in depressive illness. *British Journal of Psychiatry, 146,* 535–538.

Hoffman, R. E., Stopek, S., & Andreasen, N. C. (1986). A comparative study of manic vs. schizophrenic speech disorganisation. *Archives of General Psychiatry, 43,* 831–838.

Hutt, C. & Coxon, M. W. (1965). Systematic observation in clinical psychology. *Archives of General Psychiatry, 12,* 374–378.

Janowsky, D. S., El-Yousef, M. K., Davies, J. M., & Serkerke, H. J. (1972). A cholinergic-adrenergic hypothesis of mania and depression. *Lancet, 2,* 632–635.

Kendrick, D. C., Gibson, A. J., & Moses, I. C. A. (1979). The revised Kendrick battery: clinical studies. *British Journal of Social and Clinical Psychology, 18,* 329–340.

Klos, T. & Ellgring, J. H. (1984). Sprechgeschwindigkeit und Sprechpausen von Depressiven. In M. Hautzinger & R. Straub (Eds.), *Psychologische Aspekte depressiver Störungen. 4–26.* Regensburg: Roderer.

Kugler, B. T. & Caudrey, D. J. (1983). Phoneme discrimination in schizophrenia. *British Journal of Psychiatry, 142,* 53–59.

Lebovits, A. H. & Holland, J. C. (1983): Use of the Gottschalk-Gleser Verbal Content Analysis with medical ill patients. *Psychosomatic Medicine, 45,* 305–320.

Leff, J. & Abberton, E. (1981). Voice pitch measurements in schizophrenia and depression. *Psychological Medicine, 11,* 849–852.

Levin, S., Hall, J. A., Knight, R. A., & Alpert, M. (1985). Verbal and nonverbal expression of affect in speech of schizophrenic and depressed patients. *Journal of Abnormal Psychology, 94,* 487–497.

Libet, J. M. & Lewinson, M. (1973). Concept of social skill with special reference to the behavior of depressed persons. *Journal of Consulting and Clinical Psychology, 40,* 304–312.

Lloyd, G. G. & Lishman, W. A. (1975). Effect of depression on the speed of recall of pleasant and unpleasant experiences. *Psychological Medicine, 5,* 173–180.

Lorenz, M. (1953). Language as expressive behavior. *Archives of Neurology and Psychiatry, 70,* 277–285.

Lorenz, M. & Cobb, S. (1952). Language behavior in mania. *Archives of Neurology and Psychiatry, 69,* 763–770.

Maher, B. (1973). Language and Psychopathology. In G. A. Miller (Ed.), *Communication, language and meaning. 256–267.* New York: Basic Books.

Maher, B. A., Manschreck, T. C., & Weisstein, C. C. (1988). Cloze analysis in schizophrenic speech: scoring method and raters education. *Perceptual and Motor Skills, 67,* 911–918.

Mahl, G. F. (1956). Disturbances in silences in the patients' speech in psychopathology. *Journal of Abnormal and Social Psychology, 53,* 1–15.

Mahl, G. F. & Schulze, G. (1964). Psychological research in extralinguistic areas. In T. A. Sebeok, Hayes, M. C., & Bateson, M. C. (Eds.), *Approaches to semiotics. 51–143.* The Hague: Mouton.

Miller, G. A. (1973). Nonverbal communication. In G. A. Miller (Ed.), *Communication, language and meaning. 231–241.* New York: Basic Books.

Moses, P. J. (1954). *The voice of neurosis.* New York: Grune, Stratton.

Murray, D. C. (1971). Talk, silence, and anxiety. *Psychological Bulletin, 75,* 244–260.

Nevlund, G. N., Fann, W. E., & Falk, F. (1983). Acoustic parameters of voice and neuroleptic medication. *Biological Psychiatry, 18,* 1081–1084.

Newman, P. J. & Sweet, J. J. (1986). The effects of clinical depression on the Luria-Nebraska neuropsychological battery. *International Journal of Neuropsychology, 8,* 109–114.

Newman, S. S. & Mather, V. G. (1938). Analysis of spoken language of patients with affective disorders. *American Journal of Psychiatry, 94,* 913–942.

Nilsonne, A. (1987). Acoustic analysis of speech variables during depression and after improvement. *Acta Psychiatrica Scandinavica, 76,* 235–245.

Nilsonne, A. (1988). Speech characteristics as indicators of depressive illness. *Acta Psychiatrica Scandinavica, 77,* 253–263.

Pinard, G., Roy, J.-Y., & Tetreault, L. (1972). Etude du comportement verbal dans le dépression psychotique. *Revue de Psychologie Appliquée, 23,* 229–246.

Pope, B., Blass, T., Siegman, A. W., & Raher, J. (1970). Anxiety and depression in speech. *Journal of Consulting and Clinical Psychology, 35,* 128–133.

Pylyshyn, Z. W. (1970). Clinical correlates of some syntactic features of patients' speech. *Journal of Nervous and Mental Disease, 150,* 307–316.

Ragin, A. B. & Oltmanns, T. F. (1983). Predictability as an index of impaired verbal communication in schizophrenic and affective disorders. *British Journal of Psychiatry, 143,* 578–583.

Rehm, L. P. (1987). The measurement of behavioral aspects of depression. In A. J. Marsella, R. M. A. Hirschfeld, & M. M. Katz (Eds.), *The measurement of depression. 199–239.* Chichester: J. Wiley.

Reischies, F. M. (1988). Neuropsychologische Befunde bei der Depression im Involutionsalter und Senium und ihre Beziehung zur regionalen Hirndurchblutung. In G. Oepen (Ed.), *Psychiatrie des rechten und linken Gehirns. 187–197.* Köln: Deutscher Ärzte Verlag.

Reischies, F. M., v. Spieß, P., & Hedde, J.-P. (1990). Cognitive deterioration and dementia outcome in depression: the search for prognostic factors. In K. Maurer, P. Riederer, & H. Beckmann (Eds.), *Alzheimer's disease. 387–392.* Wien: Springer.

Renfordt, E. (1986). Quantitative analysis of speech behavior of depressed patients under a drug therapy. *Psychiatric developments, 4,* 135–146.

Rhoads, J., Lowel, S. H., & Hedgepeth, E. M. (1979). Hoarseness and aphonia as a side effect of tricylic antidepressants. *American Journal of Psychiatry, 136,* 1599.

Robertson, G. & Taylor, P. J. (1985). Some cognitive correlates of affective disorders. *Psychological Medicine, 15,* 297–309.

Rutter, D. R. (1977). Speech patterning in recently admitted and chronic long-stay schizophrenic patients. *British Journal of Social and Clinical Psychology, 16,* 47–56.

Sandyk, R. (1986). Speech blockage induced by maprotiline. *American Journal of Psychiatry, 143,* 391–392.

Savage, R. D., Britton, P. G., Bolton, N., & Hall, E. H. (1973). *Intellectual functioning in the aged.* London: Methuen.

Schafer, R. (1948). *The clinical application of psychological tests.* New York: International University Press.

Schatzberg, A. F., Cole, J. O., & Blumer, D. P. (1978). Speech blockage: A tricyclic side effect. *American Journal of Psychiatry, 135,* 600–601.

Scherer, K. R. (1979 a). Personality markers in speech. In K. R. Scherer & H. Giles (Eds.), *Social markers in speech. 147–209.* Cambridge: Cambridge University Press.

Scherer, K. R. (1979 b). Nonlinguistic vocal indicators of emotion and psychopathology. In C. E. Izard (Ed.), *Emotions in personality and psychopathology. 493–529.* New York: Plenum Press.

Sholomskas, A. J. (1978). Speech blockage in young patients taking tricyclics. *American Journal of Psychiatry, 135,* 1572.

Siegman, A. W. (1978). The meaning of silent pauses in the initial interview. *Journal of Nervous and Mental Disease, 166,* 642–654.

Smith, G. A. (1982). Voice analysis of the effects of benzodiazepine tranquillizers. *British Journal of Clinical Psychology, 21,* 141–142.

Starkweather, J. A. (1967). Vocal behavior as an information channel of speaker status. In K. Salzinger & S. Salzinger (Eds.), *Research in verbal behavior and some neurophysiological implications. 253–265.* New York: Academic Press.

Starkweather, J. A. & Hargreaves, W. A. (1964). The influence of sodium pentobarbital on vocal behavior. *Journal of Social Psychology, 69,* 123–126.

Stassen, H. H., Kuny, S., Woggon, B., & Angst, J. (1989). Affective state and voice: results of a pilot study. *Pharmacopsychiatry, 22 Suppl. 1,* 17–22.

Stoddard, F. J., Post, R. M., & Bunney, W. E. (1977). Slow and rapid psychobiological alterations in a manic-depressive patient: Clinical phenomenology. *British Journal of Psychiatry, 130,* 72–78.

Stuss, D. T. & Benson, D. F. (1986). *The frontal lobes.* New York: Raven.

Szabady, E., Bradshaw, C. M., & Besson, J. A. O. (1976). Elongation of pause-time in speech: A simple, objective measure of motor retardation in depression. *British Journal of Psychiatry, 129,* 592–597.

Szabady, E., Bradshaw, C. M., & Gazner, P. (1980). The comparison of the effects of DI-308, a potential new neuroleptic agent, and thioridazine on some psychological and physiological functions in healthy volunteers. *Psychopharmacology, 68,* 125–134.

Teasdale, J. D., Fogarty, S. J., & Williams, J. M. G. (1980). Speech rate as a measure of short-term variation in depression. *British Journal of Social and Clinical Psychology, 19,* 271–278.

Vetter, H. (1969). *Language behavior and psychopathology.* New York: Rand.

Weingartner, H., Cohen, R. M., Murphy, D. L., Martello, J. D. J., & Gerdt, C. (1982). Cognitive processes in depression. *Archives of General Psychiatry, 38,* 42–47.

Weintraub, W. & Aronson, H. (1962). The application of verbal behavior analysis to the study of psychological defense mechanisms. *Journal of Nervous and Mental Disease, 134,* 169–181.

Weintraub, W. & Aronson, H. (1967). The application of verbal behavior analysis to the study of psychological defence mechanisms IV. Speech pattern associated with depressive behavior. *Journal of Nervous and Mental Disease, 144,* 22–28.

Weiß, R. (1987). *Untersuchung über den Verlauf der beiden nonverbalen vokalen Sprachparameter Stimmlage und Stimmlagenmodulation bei stationären depressiven Patienten unter einer antidepressiven Therapie.* Dissertation, Psychiatrische Klinik, Freie Universität Berlin.

Wernicke, C. (1906). *Grundriß der Psychiatrie* (2nd Edition). Leipzig: Thieme.

Whitman, E. N. & Flicker, D. J. A. (1966). A potential new measurement of emotional state: A preliminary report. *Newark Beth-Israel Hospital, 17,* 167–172.

Wykes, T. & Leff, J. (1982). Disordered speech: Differences between manics and schizophrenics. *Brain and Language, 15,* 117–124.

Zuberbier, E. (1957). Zur Schreib- und Sprechmotorik der Depressiven. *Zeitschrift für Psychotherapie und Medizinische Psychologie, 7,* 239–249.

Zwirner, E. (1930). Beitrag zur Sprache der Depressiven. *Journal der Psychologie und Neurologie, 41,* 43–49.

Friedel M. Reischies, Berlin (Germany)

53. Thought Disorders and Language Behavior in Schizophrenia

1. Introduction

1.1. The Distinction between Language and Thought

The diagnosis of schizophrenia is significantly dependent upon the characteristics of the language utterances that the patient produces. It is by listening to the language utterances of the patient that the clinician concludes that the patient is delusional, that the coherence of his thought processes is disturbed, that his emotional experience is anomalous, that he is experiencing hallucinations, and so forth. However, the process of inferring disturbances of inner psychological states from overt utterances, spoken and written, is complicated by certain considerations.

We may present the problem succinctly by comparing the production of utterances as analogous to typing a manuscript from a text previously dictated onto an audio tape. If the finished typescript has significant deviations from normal patterns of utterance, there are several possible explanations:

- The typescript is a faithful transcript of a deviant text.
- The typing process is faulty, and has transformed a normal text into a deviant typescript.
- Both of the above have occurred in combination.

The problem that we face is created by the fact that we have access only to the typescript (i. e. the utterance); we cannot listen directly to the tape (i. e. the thought). Hence we are faced with the problem of differentiating between language disturbance and thought disturbance on the basis of a source text in which both may be compounded. At the heart of the matter is the question of whether or not language and thought may be conceptually and operationally differentiated from each other.

There is an additional complication to be considered. Thought disorder has been considered by many authorities to lie on a continuum with normal thinking. This was the case with Schneider, with Freud in his references to the "psychopathology of everyday life", with Beringer (1926) and with Kraepelin. It is not widely known that Kraepelin (1906) studied disturbances of language in dreams in order to understand the same phenomena as he encountered them in the clinic. He drew the material mainly from his own dreams, keeping a record of his own "dream-language" for a period of more than 20 years. Dream material has been a common source of inference about the possible nature of psychotic disorder. Later in this chapter we shall look at one of the few recent studies to use this in a laboratory study.

One of the implications of the view that thought disorder is best understood as an exaggeration and elaboration of normal thought processes is that it is thereby rendered less likely to be specific to a particular psychosis. Writing about thought disorder, Kurt Schneider commented

"... the thinking does not connect adequately with what has preceded it, so that for the investigator the various thoughts stand side by side as they are expressed, apparently unrelated. It is true that with schizophrenics this is a common fashion of speech and thought. Milder degrees of incoherence are not uncommon among normal people. There are those who are naturally scatterbrained and incoherent, and others who become so when in upsetting situations or when drunk and delirious. *However important these thought disorders may be for the theoretical definition of the nature of schizophrenia, they do not hold much weight in practice as diagnostic features.* The milder degrees which occur in ambiguous cases are far too difficult to pin down as unmistakable schizophrenic symptoms" (Schneider 1959, 99; our italics, translation slightly changed by the authors).

1.2. Strategies of Inference

As we cannot get at the thought of the patient in intelligible verbal form, we are compelled to turn to other strategies. Chief amongst these has been the comparison of characteristics of the language of schizophrenic patients with that of another diagnostic group. This approach is intended to establish that there are reliable phenomena associated with the presence of an entity labeled 'schizophrenia'. However, as the diagnosis of schizophrenia (as well as that of other psychiatric disorders) is heavily influenced by the verbal behavior of the patient, there is a dangerous element of circularity in this approach. The problem lies in the fact that such research may simply 'discover' differences that were used (consciously or not) by the clinician to determine the diagnosis in the first place. In this sense it may be telling us as much about the way that the clinician has been trained to diagnose as it does about the nature of the pathological phenomenon itself. While there is some value in the development of quantitative measures of the phenomena that the clinician had already assessed more loosely through clinical judgment, this value ultimately resides in its potential for research into the relationship of these measures to other nonverbal aspects of the patient's behavior.

Additional methodological issues should be mentioned here. Much credence is given to the view that schizophrenia is heterogeneous. That is to say, that there are subtypes of schizophrenia, each having unique features, and each sharing something in common with the other types. It is this common factor (whatever that may prove to be) that justifies our use of the single noun 'schizophrenia', at least for the time being. However, the selection of research subjects on the basis of a common diagnosis of schizophrenia necessarily entails the risk that samples of patients will not only be heterogeneous with regard to their clinical pictures, but also with regard to their performance on laboratory tests. This being the case, attempts to establish a common psychopathology in schizophrenia through the technique of comparison with non-schizophrenic samples is a blunt instrument. Unless the investigator has happened to have hit upon the common pathology, it is highly likely that some portion of a sample of schizophrenics will not exhibit the differences that have been hypothesized to distinguish them from non-schizophrenics. The ultimate solution to this problem lies in the conduct of large-scale comprehensive studies of schizophrenic samples, directed toward the discovery of clusters of symptoms and of laboratory responses that differentiate reliably and repeatedly within the population of schizophrenics generally.

Failing this, the next best tactic is to seek to relate differences within samples of schizophrenic patients on one set of measures with differences in another set of non-overlapping measures. The discovery that, for example, the average memory performance of a group of schizophrenics is lower than the average performance of other kinds of patient, is less informative than studies that relate individual differences within the schizophrenic sample to differences in memory efficacy.

In this article we shall review the state of current knowledge that is the outcome of this strategy. In order to set about this task, we must first consider the problem of the description and quantitative measurement of language utterances. With this done, we shall then turn to look at the relationships between these measures and measures of memory, motor behavior, attention and other non-verbal events. Each of these will be examined in the context of methods that have been employed in the study of normal behavior, and for which we have a reasonable understanding of the processes that are involved.

2. The Description and Quantitative Measurement of Schizophrenic Utterance

Bleuler (1950) gave emphasis to the significance of language as a reflection of the processes that he believed to be fundamental to the psychopathology of schizophrenia. He hypothesized that disturbances of the associational processes formed a crucial part of the inner core of the pathology. His clinical illustrations are, however, necessarily in the form of the overt utterances of the patient. Thus: *Olive oil is an Arabian liquor-sauce which the Afghans, Moors and Moslems use in ostrich farming. The Indian plantain tree is the whiskey of the Parsees and Arabs. The Parsee or Caucasian possesses as much influence over his elephant as does the Moor over his dromedary. The camel is the sport of Jews and Arabs Barley, rice and sugar cane called artichoke, grow remarkably well in India.* (Bleuler 1950, 15) Bleuler's own comment on this kind of example was: "Of the thousands of associative threads which guide our thinking, this disease seems to interrupt, quite haphazardly, sometimes single threads, sometimes a whole group, and sometimes even large segments of them. In this way, thinking becomes illogical and often bizarre". (1950, 14)

Bleuler, of course, employed vivid clinical instances to demonstrate his theoretical points. However, the progress of scientific understanding of clinical phenomena depends upon the development and application of objective quantitative measures to clinical material, and the construction of laboratory tests that make this approach possible.

Research investigations into the phenomena of schizophrenic utterance have typically employed two kinds of description and/or measurement – ratings and tabulated counts. They have also varied between seeking to describe an utterance by noting what is missing from it, versus seeking to describe and measure what is present in the utterance. Examples of the former include assessments of the 'incoherence', the 'lack of grammatical structure' or the 'unpredictability' of the utterances that are being examined. It will be at once apparent that this approach runs into significant conceptual difficulties. An utterance may be incoherent in many different ways. We find incoherence in the utterances of certain kinds of aphasic patient, utterances by normal individuals speaking in a language in which they are not fluent, utterances made by somebody who is speaking while trying to listen to somebody else speaking in the background and so on. Fine-grained analysis of the positive characteristics that are present in these various kinds of incoherence may reveal substantial differences between them; more to the point, these analyses may suggest hypotheses about the processes that produce them, processes that will be different in each case. Global judgments of attributes such as incoherence may be useful for certain kinds of crude initial clinical assessment (such as deviant versus normal), but are unlikely to be fruitful in suggesting the specific pathological processes that are at work in each case.

2.1. Descriptive Features of Schizophrenic Utterance

Descriptions of the anomalies of schizophrenic utterance have pointed to certain recurring characteristics. These characteristics are present in the utterances; their presence frequently gives rise to the global characteristic of reduced coherence that has been mentioned above. They have been summarized by one of us (Maher 1983) as follows:

(a) Repetition of Units: The repetition of words or phrases in ways that are not typically found in normal utterances. For example: *I fancy chocolate eclairs, chocolate eclairs donuts, I do want some syrup, a tin of golden syrup* ... (Critchley 1964, 361). Repetition may occur at the level of syllables as well as words or phrases. Thus the example: *Das ist vom Kaiserhaus, sie haben es von den Voreltern, von*

der Urwelt, Frankfurt-am-Main, das sind die Franken, Frankfurter Würstchen, Frankenthal, Frankenstein. (Mittenecker 1951, 366)
(b) Associative Intrusions: Schizophrenic utterances are sometimes marked by the inappropriate intrusion of words that are associated with some elements of the utterance, but that are out of place in the utterance itself. Examples: *My mother's name was Bill ... and coo?* (Chaika 1974); a patient of Bleuler, when listing her family members: *Father, son ... and Holy Ghost* (Bleuler 1950). These associations may be in the form of klang (rhyming) associations, punning associations or of associations that are connected to the utterance elements in a normal manner.
(c) Punning: Some intruding associations appear to be connected to an alternative meaning of one of the words in the utterance, thus giving the intrusion the semblance of a pun or play on words. Example: *To Wise and Company* [A department store] *If you think that you are being wise to send me a bill for money I have already paid I am nowise going to do so unless I get the whys and wherefores from you to me.* (Maher 1983, 8)
(d) Object chaining: In English-speaking patients there is a tendency to terminate sentences with a series of noun objects, many of these seeming to be chains of association. Example: *I have no way of knowing how much differences of opinion different editors, politicians, historians, sexologists, astrologers or theologians might have to say* ... (Maher 1983, 9)

As will be seen later on, the critical stimulus for the associative chain does not appear to be the noun object as such; rather it appears to be the component that occurs at the end of the sentence – a feature that is influenced by the normal patterns of the language in which the utterance is made.

2.2. Empirical Studies of Schizophrenic Utterance

We may now turn to reports of research in which the characteristics of schizophrenic utterance have been compared with those of other groups, using quantitative measures.

2.2.1. Repetition

Several investigators have studied the incidence of repetition in the utterances of schizophrenic patients. A thorough review of these studies is provided by Cozolino (1983). We may summarize and update the issue briefly here.

(a) The Type-Token Ratio: One measure of repetition uses the single whole word as the unit, computing the ratio of different words per segment of language as an index of repetition at the word level. Thus in the sentence immediately preceding this one there are thirty-one words. However, the word *as* appears twice, the word *of* appears three times, the word *word* appears twice, *the* four times, and *repetition* twice. Hence there are twenty-three different words. Division of this by thirty-one gives us a ratio of 0.74. This is the Type-Token Ratio (TTR). Token here means word, and Type means different word: The more repetitious the utterance, the lower the ratio. – While differences in patient samples and in the method of eliciting language utterance have complicated the interpretation of the literature, the general tenor of the fourteen studies reviewed by Cozolino is that schizophrenic patients have lower TTRs (i. e., are more repetitious) than controls. While the differences tend to be small, the direction of the findings is consistent. Schizophrenic patients without concurrent thought disorder (NTD) produce TTRs similar to those of control subjects, the lower values being found in patients with thought disorder (TD). Subsequent studies include work by Maher/Manschreck/Hoover/Weisstein (1987) and Manschreck/Maher/Celada et al. (1991) who report lower TTRs for TD schizophrenics than for other groups. In the first of these reports the investigators applied the concept of specifity/sensitivity developed by Anthony/LeResche/Niaz et al. (1982). Using a cut-off TTR of <0.64, the technique correctly identified 60% of the schizophrenics, correctly rejected 60% of the non-schizophrenics, but created 40% false positive and 40% false negatives respectively. These values are marginally improved when a TTR of <0.61 is used to distinguish TD schizophrenics from others. – These investigations make it clear that TD schizophrenics are reliably more repetitious than other schizophrenics or other types of psychiatric patient. However, the differences are insufficiently great to permit their use in the clinical assessment of individual cases.

(b) Syllable Repetition: Mittenecker (1951; 1953) investigated repetition in the speech of schizothymic and non-schizothymic normal German subjects. He counted the repetition of syllables rather than words, reporting that repetition was greater in the schizothymic sample. He proposed that the processes that give rise to repetitions are present in the potential patient before they become manifest in the morbid state. There do not appear to have been any replications of this rather interesting finding.

(c) Phrase Repetition: While units such as words or syllables may appear intuitively to be the components of chains of utterance, everyday observation suggests that phrases may act as units, and hence may be relevant to the investigation of repetitions. Maher/Manschreck/Hoover/Weisstein (1987) analyzed the distribution of two-word and three-word phrase repetitions in the utterances of their subjects. They found that schizophrenics differed very significantly from non-schizophrenic patients in their production of phrase repetitions of both kinds. They also reported that immediate sequential perseveration of single words in the utterances differed significantly between their comparison groups. Individual repetitions scores correlated significantly with certain kinds of thought disorder as assessed by the Schedule for Affective Disorders and Schizophrenia (SADS) of Spitzer/Endicott (1978). Specifically, rated scores on Derailment, Logic, Understandability and Poverty of Content were positively correlated with the various indices of repetition.

2.2.2. Object-Chaining

The appearance of chains of object nouns in the utterances of schizophrenic patients was first reported by Maher/McKean/McLaughlin (1966). Object chaining is measured by computing the ratio of object-nouns to subject nouns in each sentence. Thus in the example given in Paragraph 2.1. (d) above there is one subject-noun (*I*) and six object nouns, *editors, politicians, historians, sexologists, astrologers, theologians,* giving a ratio of 6.0 in that particular case. This measure was termed the OSR (object–subject ratio). In the Maher et al. (1966) study, TD schizophrenic patients produced a mean OSR of 1.40, while NTD schizophrenics produced a significantly lower mean OSR of 0.78. A replication by Manschreck/Maher/Celada et al. (1991) produced OSRs as follows: TD schizophrenics 1.26; NTD schizophrenics, 0.79; normal controls, 0.89. The first mean was significantly higher than the oher two. These data essentially replicate the original findings.

2.2.3. Predictability

Several techniques have been developed for the measurement of the predictability of the patient's utterance. The most common is the so-called 'Cloze' technique (Taylor 1953) in which portions of a transcript of the patient's utterance are eliminated systematically (every fifth word is a common standard). These mutilated texts are then given to a panel of normal readers, who are asked to fill in the omissions with their best estimate of the missing words. – A second technique, developed by Rutter/Draffan/Davies (1977), involves rearranging the order of the sentences spoken by the patient, normal readers then being asked to arrange them in the order in which they think that they were spoken. Both of these measures may be seen as measures of the coherence or internal organization of the utterance. They tell us what the text lacks, but do not give us a fine-grained analysis of the components of the text that make it incoherent.

3. Language and Motor Behavior

Relatively little effort has been put into the study of the relationship between motor anomalies and language behavior in schizophrenia, including the motor aspects of language utterances themselves. We begin with the latter question.

3.1. Motor Aspects of Schizophrenic Speech

Beattie/Butterworth (1979) report that in normal speech words of either low predictability in context (redundancy) or of low frequency in the language are preceded by longer pauses than are words of high redundancy or frequency. Low frequency words tend to be of low redundancy in most contexts, but statistical separation of their effects showed them to be independent. Maher/Manschreck/Molino (1983) investigated this relationship in schizophrenic patients. The redundancy of individual words was established via the Cloze procedure, word frequency from standard sources, and pause length by computerized measurement techniques. In this study NTD patients showed the normal relationship, but TD patients did not. Pause length seems to be related to the time taken for lexical access (related mainly to word frequency), and to the attentional load placed upon the listener by the occurrence of elements with high information load (low redundancy elements). Thus the pathological processes here may involve impairment in either or both of these factors.

Silverman (1972) performed an overall analysis of the pause-time to speech-time ratio in schizophrenic utterances and found greater pause times in chronic schizophrenics than in other patients. This ratio is closely related to simple speech rate. Some studies have failed to find significant difference between normal speech rates and those of schizophrenics. Hart/Payne (1973) did, however, report negative correlations between the severity of other symptoms and the speech rate of schizophrenics.

3.2. Motor Behavior

The clinical literature contains abundant descriptions of motor pathologies in schizophrenia. A good general review of these is to be found in Manschreck (1983). However, the quantitative laboratory study of motor behavior and its relationship to language pathology is relatively uncommon. This seems to be due in part to the difficulties that beset the measurement of voluntary motor behavior; it is also due to the absence of any coherent model of schizophrenic pathology from which the relations of language and motor behavior might be postulated.

Systematic work has, however, been recently reported by Manschreck, Maher and their colleagues. Manschreck (1983) provides a detailed review of these studies, the main elements of which can be summarized here. An initial study (Manschreck/Maher/Ader 1981) examined the relationship of the TTR, TD (measured by the SADS), and motor anomalies assessed clinically in different samples of psychiatric patients. A highly significant negative correlation (−0.59) between the TTR and motor anomalies was found. Motor anomaly scores for TD schizophrenics were significantly higher than for NTD patients. Relationships between specific TD elements and motor anomalies were also high. Thus: Poverty of Content 0.78; Impaired Understandability 0.71; Disturbed Logic 0.61. All coefficients were significant beyond the .01 level. – These studies demonstrated under reasonably well controlled conditions that clinically assessed motor anomalies in schizophrenia are correlated with clinically assessed thought disorder, and with quantitatively measured repetition in language utterance. While this research was promising, it was constrained by the limited reliabilities associated with clinical assessment. The need for quantitative measurement of all variables remained unfilled.

Accordingly, a subsequent investigation turned to the measurement of simple motor behavior. This required the patient to tap a key at the same rate as a series of audible clicks produced by an electronic signal generator. Several different rates were employed. Accuracy of the response at each rate was measured as (a) the actual mean interval produced by the patient, and, (b) the variability of the response as measured by the standard deviation around the mean interval. By these definitions a perfect score would be one in which the mean interval was the same as that of the auditory stimulus, with a standard deviation of zero. At rates between 40 beats per minute (bpm) and 80 bpm, there were marked differences between schizophrenic patients and normal and other psychiatric controls. Comparison of laboratory motor performance and clinical assessment of motor anomalies indicated a significant relationship, the correlation being −0.53, better performance being associated with fewer clinical anomalies. From this we may reasonably conclude that the two methods – laboratory and clinical assessment – are fundamentally reflecting the same disordered motor process. A third step in this investigative sequence turned to the association between quantitative measures of language and quantitative measures of motor behavior. Correlation of the TTR with motor tapping accuracy produced a significant coefficient of +0.35, i. e. lower rates of word repetition in speech are associated with greater accuracy in generating a rhythmic motor response.

At a later point in this paper we shall comment on the relevance of rhythmic motor movements for the understanding of schizophrenic pathology. Meanwhile it may be helpful to note that the generation of automatic responses of any kind depends upon the capacity to utilize predictabilities in sequences of environmental stimuli. As predictabilities are by definition redundancies, the role of impaired redundancy utilization may be of some interest to us.

4. Associational Processes

Bleuler, as we have seen, emphasized the loosening of "associative threads" in the discourse of schizophrenics. While the terminology is striking, the clinical phenomena of schizophrenic utterance suggest not so much that some "thread" has been "loosened", but that strongly linked associations have intruded into the thread of intended speech – this thread being ordinarily organized not in an associational manner, but in terms of an intended plan of utterance. Paradoxically, it is as if the threads of association are too strong and tight rather than weak and loose.

Contemporary cognitive science has found it useful to conceptualize associations as networks. Any given element in memory may be seen as the hub of a network of related stored elements. These elements may be in the form of words, visual icons, sounds, etc. Activation of an element by external stimulation produces activation of other elements in the network. The elements that are affected by spreading activation do not ordinarily enter consciousness, and appear to be rapidly inhibited by the sequential activations produced by serial stimulation from the environment.

Evidence for the activation of networks comes from several sources. One of the most important contemporary techniques used to detect activation is the method of lexical decision, or semantic priming. The subject faces a computer screen and is presented with a verbal stimulus – a single word – the 'prime'. After a brief exposure it is replaced with a second string of letters, the 'target'. These may constitute a word or a non-word, i. e. a random string of letters. The task of the subject is to decide whether or not the target is a word. This decision is signalled by pressing one of two keys as quickly as possible after recognition has taken place. The dependent measures are the accuracy of the identification and the speed with which this is made.

Many studies have established that when the prime and target are associated, recognition takes place more quickly than when they are not associated. This gain in speed of recognition is termed facilitation. Facilitation is interpreted as evidence that associates to the prime have been activated by the appearance of the prime, and that this leads to more rapid recognition because the task requires only an automatic matching of target with a limited number of activated network elements. Lack of association between prime and target, on the other hand, means that activated associations to the prime must be inhibited, and that recognition must involve searching a large lexicon of possible words for a match to the target. Clearly, individuals whose facilitation gains are larger than those of others may be regarded as having unusually high levels of activation of their associational networks. Given the general hypothesis that schizophrenic patients are subject to associational intrusion, it is reasonable to predict that they will produce superior facilitation to that of normal controls.

First reports of the use of this technique (Maher/Manschreck/Hoover/Weisstein 1987; Manschreck/Maher/Milavetz et al. 1988) report that TD schizophrenic patients showed facilitation that was superior to NTD schizophrenics, to unipolar depressed patients, and to normal controls. This is, of course, highly consistent with the proposition that thought disorder is a consequence of hyperactive associational processes. A replication by Kwapil/Hegley/Chapman et al. (1990) employed a somewhat different recognition technique. After the recognition threshold was calibrated for normal controls and schizophrenic patients, the target words to be recognized were presented in a degraded fashion by the random elimination of pixels from the screened representation of the words. Subjects could systematically restore portions of the word until they reached a level at which they could correctly identify the target. Associated words were recognized at lower thresholds than non-associated words. With this technique the investigators repeated the finding of superior facilitation in schizophrenics. As they did not divide their patient sample on the basis of thought disorder, it is not possible to replicate that particular component of the original reports.

In a study of normal subjects Spitzer/Mamelak/Stickgold et al. (1991) employed the lexical decision technique to test the hypothesis that REM sleep will be characterized by greater activation of associational processes. There is, of course, a long-standing history of comparisons between dreams and psychopathological states, notably schizophrenia. It would, of course, be a mistake to simply equate schizophrenic phenomena with those found in dream states. Nonetheless, the plausibility of the belief that associations are hyperactive in both suggests that facilitation in a lexical decision task given immediately upon being awakened from REM sleep should be greater than that found in the normal daily waking state.

In the study by Spitzer/Mamelak/Stickgold et al. (1991) subjects were presented with the lexical decision task under three conditions. Normal waking, awakened from non-REM sleep and awakened from REM sleep. The REM condition produced superior facilitation compared to the other two conditions.

These latter two conditions did not differ between themselves. As performance on the non-associated pairs was not different between conditions, it is clear that all of the effects may be properly ascribed to the facilitation produced by the associated condition. This study has the added value, in the context of the present chapter, of demonstrating the presence in normal subjects under special circumstances of a process that appears important in pathological subjects.

Two other aspects of these studies are important. The pairing of associated prime and target is done on the basis of word association norms, the assumption being that for most subjects the norms will adequately define the network of associations that will be activated. As this is only normatively likely, and will not be true for all individuals in the sample, the lexical decision technique probably underestimates the facilitation that might be gained were the prime-target pairings made on the basis of the previously established associations of the individual patients. A second more important consideration is the fact that the presence of a psychopathological impairment is here demonstrated by superior performance, rather than by the more common tactic of demonstration by deficient performance. Deficient performance may always be explained as due to lack of motivation, medication effects, fatigue or other non-specific factors, unless these are all carefully controlled – which is almost never the case. This makes it important to develop tasks in which what is usually an impairment becomes an advantage, thereby permitting the testing of hypotheses without the problem of non-specific disruptive factors. The lexical decision task presents many opportunities to advance our understanding of the associational processes of patients and normal subjects alike. We may expect to see increasing use of it for these purposes.

5. Memory and Language

The study of memory and language in schizophrenia is vulnerable to confounding due to the extensive reliance that is placed on verbal report in studies of memory. Verbal data that suggest a deficiency in memory may therefore simply reflect a deficiency in formulating the retrieved contents of memory into adequate verbal form. There are some solutions to this problem. One is to vary the conditions under which memory for verbal material is elicited, assuming that the disruptive effect of language disorder *per se* is constant across conditions. The other is to seek evidence of deficiency in performance on non-verbal memory tasks, and then to correlate this with measures of language disturbance. We shall confine ourselves to this kind of study in this chapter. General reviews of memory functioning in schizophrenia may be found in Koh (1978), Braff (1991), and Neufeld (1991).

5.1. Contextual Constraint and Memory in Schizophrenia

Miller/Selfridge (1950) demonstrated some years ago that items from lists of words would be recalled in increasing numbers as the lists increasingly resembled sentence-like sequences. The more the list approximated to a normal language sequence, the greater the number of words available to immediate recall. This effect has been shown to be robust across several languages (e. g. Maher/Skovengaard 1988): As word sequences in normal sentences have transitional probabilities between individual words greater than is the case for random word lists, it is assumed that these enhance the detection and storage of the elements of the list. The technique uses lists in which the words are of equal frequency, so that vocabulary knowledge does not affect recall.

Lewisohn/Elwood (1961) reported that schizophrenics were less able to recall language texts of low contextual constraint than were control comparisons. Maher/Manschreck/Rucklos (1980) employed the Miller-Selfridge technique to study the relationship between context effects in memory and language and thought disorder. Thought-disordered schizophrenics were significantly less able to profit in memory from increasing contextual constraint than were comparison groups of NTD schizophrenics, normals and depressed patients. This finding reminds us again of the difficulty that thought disordered patients have in any task in which performance is facilitated by redundancy.

5.2. Primacy and Recency Effects

Items in lists presented to be memorized tend to be learned, and to be available for recall before learning is complete, in a pattern in which items presented early in the list or late in the list are learned sooner than those in the middle of the list. These are referred to as the primacy effect and the recency effect respectively. Studies of these effects in schizophrenic patients have produced conflicting results. Some studies report no difference between schizophrenics and controls (Berg/Leventhal 1977; Mungas 1983). Other have reported reduced primacy (Oltmanns 1978; Frame/Oltmanns 1982), while one has reported reduced recency (Koh/Kayton 1974). The capacity to retain early items in a list suggests that the organization of verbal material into chunks is the underlying process. Grossberg (1982) suggests that this process is dependent upon stability of attentional input; it is likely therefore to be impaired in persons whose attentional processes are unstable.

With these considerations in mind, Manschreck/Maher/Celada et al. (1991) investigated primacy and recency effects in schizophrenics, depressed patients and normal controls, using the Miller-Selfridge lists. No difference in recency effects was discovered. However, substantially reduced primacy was found in the schizophrenic group, with less severe but significantly reduced performance in the middle segment of the list. Within the schizophrenic sample, reduced primacy was significantly related to inability to gain from context ($r = 0.44$). Reduced primacy was related to repetition in speech as measured by the TTR obtained from an independent sample of speech ($r = 0.54$). Comparison of a subset of drug-free patients with those on medication revealed no effect of medication on performance in these tasks. As this now brings to three the total number of reports of loss of primacy effects in schizophrenic memory, it seems reasonable to conclude that this is a reliable phenomenon.

5.3. Backward masking

The storage and retrieval of stimulus input involves a rather complex sequence of steps. One of the earliest of these is the process whereby an immediate input activates the peripheral receptor. Thus a visual stimulus activates the retina, an activation that decays over time. The retinal response creates a central event. Both the retinal and the central events continue for some time after the external stimulus has terminated. However, the input of another visual stimulus shortly after the onset of the first stimulus can mask the effect of the first. Thus the brief display of, for example, the letter *A*, followed rapidly by the letter *O* placed at the same focal point, can prevent the correct recognition of the *A*. Intervals of 50 msec. are effective in creating masking effects in about 50 percent of cases. In one of a series of important studies conducted by Saccuzzo and his associates, (Miller/Saccuzzo/Braff 1979) the data showed that masking effects were more pronounced in schizophrenic patients regardless of the presence or absence of thought disorder. This suggests that this defect in information processing is a trait rather than a fluctuating state. As language disorders in schizophrenic patients are related to thought disorder, and rise and fall in state-like fashion, it seems probable that excessive vulnerability to masking effects has little explanatory power in relation to the language deficits of schizophrenics. This conclusion is buttressed by reports that similar vulnerabilities have been found in bipolar and in unipolar psychotic patients. As it does not appear to be specific to schizophrenia, it seems to be of greatest interest in its potential relationships with either medication effects or with some general slowing of the information processing systems in psychosis.

6. A Model of Schizophrenic Utterance: The Association Activation Hypothesis

Any model designed to account for the phenomena of schizophrenic utterance must explain certain kinds of data. What must be explained are not only the bases of the utterance anomalies themselves. The findings from memory, lexical decision, motor activity and so forth must be plausibly connected together, at least in broad outline. Examination of the findings summarized here suggest that the model must encompass:

- The inability of the patient to benefit from predictabilities in sequences of events to which a response must be made. This includes the inability to generate predictabilities to improve response patterns that must be made by the patient.
- The range of specific language anomalies that are present to clinical observation.
- The many other kinds of anomaly that have been reported repeatedly in the clinical literature. These include distractibility, difficulties in filtering out external and internal stimulation when trying to focus on a limited field of conscious experience, difficulties in forming abstract categories or concepts.

In our view, it is useful to consider a broad general model along the following lines. We begin with the principle that adaptive behavior involves the utilization of predictabilities in sequences of events, i. e. redundancies. These must be exploited where this is useful, but must be ignored when circumstances require it. In simple terms this means that an organism surviving in a world of predators and prey must learn to recognize critical sequences in the environment. The shadow of the hawk that presages the attack that will follow must lead the sparrow to become motionless, Pavlov's dog must learn that the sound signal will be followed by food, if the adaptive salivary response is to be made in an effectively anticipatory fashion. In language, the formation of associations between commonly co-occurring words or phrases is a useful automatic mechanism. Associations are formed by repetitious pairing, a pairing that occurs naturally in the social habitat, but which is created systematically in the laboratory. Natural pairings give rise to transitional probabilities as they create a cumulative base upon which we may expect one element to be followed, predictably, by another. The priming effect that leads to the quicker recognition of an associated word may be seen as an advantageous process, one that makes the recognition of normal communication easier.

However, a counter-process of discrimination requires that the exploitation of redundancies be adjusted to the complex of circumstances (i. e. the context) in which the behavior is occurring. A simple response to a single element in the environment will be maladaptive if the context has not been inspected to determine whether a modified response is more appropriate. The process of discrimination sometimes requires the inhibition of the most common response in favor of a less common but more effective response. This principle has been beautifully demonstrated in the classic paper by Chapman/Chapman/Miller (1964) in which schizophrenic subjects exhibited an inability to inhibit high probabilities when the context called for the low probability response to be made.

From this point of view, the utterance of a coherent sentence requires that activated normal associations to each word be inhibited to prevent their disruptive intrusion into the planned utterance. They will be permitted to 'intrude' only if they are consistent with the plan of the utterance. These associations may intrude in various forms, including simple repetition of a previously uttered segment, the chaining of associations as in object chaining or enumeration, clang associations, tangential or derailed segments due to the simultaneous activation of association networks to both meanings of multiple meaning words – which produces the 'punning' effect already described, etc. The intrusion of these elements is hypothesized to be particularly likely at those points in an utterance at which the attentional demands of the speaking or writing task are minimal – as for example at clause and sentence boundaries. Object nouns tend to be placed most often at the end of sentences uttered in English, hence the phenomenon of associative chaining presents itself as object-chaining.

Associational intrusions do occur in normal speech with some frequency, but generally in ways that are congruent with the context and intent of the discourse; hence, they do not disrupt the plan of the utterance, but escape notice and do not create comprehension difficulties. Schizophrenic failure to be influenced effectively by the context of utterances, including their own, is assumed in this model to be not so much a positive failure of a mechanism responsible for adaptation to such influence but to reflect instead the overriding of this by an unusually strong degree of activation of associations. We have already examined the data from lexical decision studies, including data from normals awake and awakened from sleep, schizophrenics and depressed patients. These data support the notion that associational processes are activated more vigorously in patients with concurrent utterance anomalies than in other groups, and is thus consistent with the hypothesis.

The data from studies of memory and of motor behavior point again to impairment in the use of redundancies, and the relationship of this impairment to the presence of anomalies of language utterance – especially repetition. We have, as yet, no clear hypothesis as to the probable etiology of this impairment, other than to suggest strongly that the defect is neuropsychological in nature. Given the steady accumulation of evidence pointing to possible frontal lobe involvement in schizophrenia, it would not be surprising to find that language and other cognitive anomalies will prove to be associated with measured anomaly in frontal lobe structure and/or function. However, the data are only suggestive and this matter is still very much open.

Furthermore, the fluctuating nature of the language symptoms suggests that the most immediate underlying etiological factors are themselves of a fluctuating type. Finally, the probability of the heterogeneous nature of schizophrenic disorders suggests that assumptions of unitary etiologies and unitary patterns of language disturbance are unlikely to provide a comprehensive model for the understanding of empirical results.

In the immediate future, several questions for research can be identified. These are:

(1) The determination of the internal patterns of language disorder within the presumably heterogeneous group of schizophrenic patients who bear this diagnosis. Multivariate analysis of reliable, quantitative data seems to be the appropriate strategy here. Equally important is the determination of longitudinal patterns in these anomalies.
(2) The determination of the correlations between identifiable patterns of language disturbance, measurements of brain structure and function, and identifiable, quantitatively measured, patterns of disturbance in other non-verbal functions.
(3) The fine-grained analysis of the processes of associational activation in patients and controls. Specifically the determination of the duration of activation of associations, the role of transitional probabilities between words in limiting associational links in normal subjects, the effect of diurnal fluctuation and other threats to longitudinal stability in these measures.
(4) The study of verbal patterns in the utterances of family members of patient probands.
(5) The effect of neuroleptic treatments on the nature and duration of verbal disturbances.

We believe that progress in our knowledge of psychopathology will be made more rapidly by the use of reliable, ratio-scale quantitative measures of performance that are minimally dependent upon ratings made on the basis of clinical judgment. These latter approaches are suitable in the early stages of scientific research, but are severely limited in their usefulness in the investigation of the most significant questions that human abnormality poses to us.

7. References

Anthony, J. C., LeResche, L., Niaz, U., von Korff, M. R., & Folstein, M. F. (1979). Limits of the "Mini-Mental State" as a screening test for dementia and delirium among hospital patients. *Psychological Medicine, 12,* 397–408.

Beattie, G. W. & Butterworth, B. L. (1979). Contextual probability and word frequency as determinants of pauses and errors in spontaneous speech. *Language and Speech, 22,* 201–211.

Berg, P. A. & Leventhal, D. D. (1977). The effect of distractor strength against the rate of item presentation on retention in schizophrenia. *British Journal of Social and Clinical Psychology, 16,* 147–152.

Beringer, K. (1926). Denkstörungen und Sprache bei Schizophrenen. *Zeitschrift für Neurologie und Psychiatrie, 103,* 185–197.

Bleuler, E. (1950). *Dementia præcox or the group of schizophrenias.* (Originally published 1911), New York: International Universities Press.

Braff, D. L. (1991). Information processing and attentional abnormalities in schizophrenic disorders. In P. A. Magaro (Ed.), *Cognitive bases of mental disorders. 262–307.* New York: Sage Publications.

Chaika, E. (1974). A linguist looks at "schizophrenic" language. *Brain and Language, 1,* 113–118.

Chapman, L. J., Chapman, J. P., & Miller, G. A. (1964). A theory of verbal behavior in schizophrenia. In B. A. Maher (Ed.), *Progress in experimental personality research. Vol. 1. 49–77.* New York: Academic Press.

Cozolino, L. J. (1983). The oral and written productions of schizophrenic patients. In B. A. & W. B. Maher (Eds.), *Progress in experimental personality research. Vol. 12. 101–152.* New York: Academic Press.

Critchley, M. (1964). The neurology of psychotic speech. *British Journal of Psychiatry, 110,* 353–364.

Frame, C. & Oltmanns, T. F. (1982). Serial recall by schizophrenic and affective patients during and after psychotic episodes. *Journal of Abnormal Psychology, 91,* 311–318.

Grossberg, S. (1982). *Studies of mind and brain.* Holland/Boston: Reidel.

Hart, D. S. & Payne, R. W. (1973). Language structure and predictability in overinclusive patients. *British Journal of Psychiatry, 123,* 643–662.

Koh, S. D. (1978). Remembering verbal material by schizophrenic young adults. In S. Schwartz (Ed.), *Language and cognition in schizophrenia. 55–99.* Hillsdale, N. J.: Erlbaum.

Koh, S. D. & Kayton, L. (1974). Memorization of unrelated word strings by young non-psychotic schizophrenics. *Journal of Abnormal Psychology, 83,* 299–310.

Kraepelin, E. (1906). *Über Sprachstörungen im Traume.* [On disturbances of language in dreams]. Leipzig: Engelmann.

Kwapil, T. R., Hegley, D. C., Chapman, L. J., & Chapman, J. P. (1990). Facilitation of word recognition by semantic priming in schizophrenia. *Journal of Abnormal Psychology, 99,* 215–221.

Lewisohn, P. L. & Elwood, D. L. (1961). The role of contextual constraints in the learning of language samples in schizophrenia. *Journal of Nervous and Mental Diseases, 133,* 79–81.

Maher, B. A. (1983). A tentative theory of schizophrenic utterance. In B. A. Maher & W. B. Maher (Eds.), *Progress in experimental personality research. Vol. 12. 1–52.* New York: Academic Press.

Maher, B. A., McKean, K., & McLaughlin, B. (1966). Studies in psychotic language. In P. J. Stone, D. C. Dunphy, M. S. Smith, & D. M. Ogilvie (Eds.), *The General Inquirer.* Cambridge, Mass.: MIT Press.

Maher, B. A., Manschreck, T. C., Hoover, T. M., & Weisstein, C. C. (1987). Thought disorder and measured features of language production in schizophrenia. In P. Harvey & E. Walker (Eds.), *Positive and negative symptoms in psychosis: Description, research and future directions. 195–215.* Hillsdale, N. J.: Erlbaum.

Maher, B. A., Manschreck, T. C. & Molino, M. (1983). Redundancy, pause distributions and thought disorder in schizophrenia, *Language and Speech, 26,* 191–199.

Maher, B. A., Manschreck, T. C., & Rucklos, M. E. (1980). Contextual constraint and the recall of verbal material in schizophrenia: the effect of thought disorder. *British Journal of Psychiatry, 137,* 69–73.

Maher, B. A. & Skovengaard, J. (1988). Contexutual constraint: a Danish language replication of Miller-Selfridge with methodological improvements. *Scandinavian Journal of Psychology, 29,* 194–199.

Manschreck, T. C. (1983). Psychopathology of motor behavior in schizophrenia. In B. A. Maher & W. B. Maher (Eds.), *Progress in experimental personality research. Vol. 12. 53–99.* New York: Academic Press.

Manschreck, T. C., Maher, B. A., & Ader, D. N. (1981). Formal thought disorder, the type-token ratio and disturbed voluntary motor movement in schizophrenia. *British Journal of Psychiatry, 139,* 7–15.

Manschreck, T. C., Maher, B. A., Celada, M. T., Schneyer, M., & Fernandez, R. (1991). Object chaining and thought disordered speech. *Psychological Medicine, 21,* 443–446.

Manschreck, T. C., Maher, B. A., Milavetz, J. J., Ames, D., Weisstein, C. C., & Schneyer, M. L. (1988). Semantic priming in thought disordered schizophrenics. *Schizophrenia Research, 1,* 61–66.

Miller, S., Saccuzzo, D. P., & Braff, D. L. (1979). Information processing deficit in remitted schizophrenics. *Journal of Abnormal Psychology, 88,* 446–449.

Miller, G. & Selfridge, J. (1950). Verbal context and the recall of meaningful material. *American Journal of Psychology, 63,* 176–185.

Mittenecker, E. (1951). Eine neue quantitative Methode in der Sprachanalyse und ihre Anwendung bei Schizophrenen. *Monatsschrift für Psychiatrie und Neurologie, 121,* 364–375.

Mittenecker, E. (1953). Perseveration und Persönlichkeit. *Zeitschrift für Experimentelle und Angewandte Psychologie, 1,* 5–31.

Mungas, S. (1983). Differential clinical sensitivity of specific parameters with the Rey auditory verbal learning test. *Journal of Consulting and Clinical Psychology, 55,* 848–855.

Neufeld, R. W. J. (1991). Memory in paranoid schizophrenia. In P. A. Magaro (Ed.), *Cognitive bases of mental disorders. 231–261.* New York: Sage Publications.

Oltmanns, T. (1978). Selective attention in schizophrenic and manic psychosis: the effect of distraction on information processing. *Journal of Abnormal Psychology, 87,* 212–225.

Rutter, D. R., Draffan, J., & Davies, J. (1977). Thought disorder and the predictability of speech. *British Journal of Psychiatry, 131,* 67–68.

Schneider, K. (1959). *Clinical psychiatry* (transl. by M. W. Hamilton/E. W. Anderson). New York, London: Grune and Stratton.

Silverman, G. (1972). Redundancy, repetition and pausing in schizophrenic speech. *British Journal of Psychiatry, 122,* 407–413.

Spitzer, M., Mamelak, A., Stickgold, R., Williams, J., Koustaal, W., Rittenhouse, C., Maher, B. A., & Hobson, J. A. (1991). Semantic priming in a lexical decision task on awakenings from REM-sleep: Evidence for a disinhibited semantic network. *Sleep Research, 20,* 131.

Spitzer, R., & Endicott, J. (1978). *Schedule for Affective Disorders and Schizophrenia (SADS).* New York: Biometric Research, New York State Psychiatric Institute.

Taylor, W. L. (1953). "Cloze" procedure: A new tool for measuring readability. *Journalism Quarterly, 30,* 415–433.

Brendan A. Maher, Cambridge, Mass. (USA)/
Manfred Spitzer, Heidelberg (Germany)

54. Linguistic Aspects of Language Behavior in Schizophrenia

1. Linguistic Deviations in Schizophrenic Speech

1.1. Introduction

No domain of mental life is immune to schizophrenia. Thought, affect, perception and beliefs can all be altered, thereby challenging the very human essence of the person suffering from this disorder. Even with such a wide range of signs and symptoms, abnormalities of language behavior have long been considered the hallmark of schizophrenia (Bleuler/Perrault 1911/1950). These language alterations make it harder, and at times impossible, for the listener to discern the communicative intentions of the schizophrenic speaker (Hoffman/Kirstein/Stopeck/Cicchetti 1982). While the effects on the listener are fairly clear-cut, the nature of the language alterations themselves is much harder to determine. Certainly the content of what a schizophrenic has in mind to say may render the communicative intentions of the speaker more obscure; his thoughts, affects, perceptions and beliefs, are, at times, confused, complex, and bizarre, and may be difficult to express in words. The central question for this article, however, is the following: Are there specific 'linguistic deviations', defined as violations of linguistic rules and constraints, which obscure the comprehensibility of schizophrenic speech and are independent of the content, deviant or not, of what the speaker has in mind to say? This question has considerable empirical importance insofar as there is now evidence suggesting that at least some schizophrenics suffer from some sort of dominant hemisphere disturbance (Flor-Henry 1976; Morstyn/Duffy/McCarley 1983; Coffman/Andreasen/Nasrallah 1984; Crow/Ball/Bloom et al. 1989) which could impair linguistic abilities.

1.2. Typology of Linguistic Deviations

As is the case for many other classes of linguistically disturbed speakers, the irregularities produced by individuals suffering from schizophrenia are highly diverse in nature. Some schizophrenics produce words that do not belong to the conventional lexicon. This may reflect an alteration of a lexical morpheme, e. g.,

(1) *he is a grássical person* (Hoffman/Sledge 1983, 157),

or a deviation in phonetic construction:

(2) *he still had fooch with teykrimez, I'll be willing to betcha* (Chaika 1974, 261).

A more common type of lexical deviance occuring in schizophrenic speech corresponds to acceptable lexical morphemes inappropriately attached to an affix (Lecours/Vanier/Clément 1976). Examples of these construction, which are referred to as 'derived morphemic paraphasias' (Lecours/Vanier-Clément 1976), are:

(3) *attain vigoration and strength* (Hoffman/Sledge 1984, 150);

(4) *stated not necessarily factuated* (Vetter 1968, 5; quoting Maher 1966). –

In addition, some schizophrenics are prone to the inappropriate coupling of two lexical morphemes, a construction that has been referred to as 'composed morphemic paraphasias' (Lecours/Vanier-Clément 1976), e. g.,

(5) *lie-truths* (Bleuler/Perrault 1911/1950, 150). –

Schizophrenics can also demonstrate word-finding problems that result in inappropriate insertion of lexical elements in syntactic frames. A 'mild' example is:

(6) *He owns a store on Fifth Avenue, and that's never mentioned because that is his side-kick* (intended: *side-line*; Hoffman/Sledge 1988, 97).

A more 'severe' error in word selection produced by a schizophrenic patient inserts a noun into the verb slot of the sentence structure:

(7) *fish school in their own communities* (Hoffman/Sledge 1988, 97). –

Schizophrenic patients, moreover, also produce paragrammatical segments, i. e., utterances in which word order and/or word combinations deviate from acceptable syntactic forms. One example, which includes a derived morphemic paraphasia, at least approximates grammatical English:

(8) *That's why, you know, the fact there was no stigmatism* (sic) *attached to that clearly explained in the record why you were put back* (Hoffman/Sledge 1984, 154).

A much more deviant segment typifies what, in psychiatric terms, is referred to as 'word-salad':

(9) *The honest bring-back-to-life doctors agents much take John Black out through making up design meaning straight neutral underworld shadow tunnel* (Chaika 1977, 466; quoting Lorenz 1961). –

Finally, schizophrenics demonstrate difficulties in organizing and sequencing sentences to express a coherent message. I refer to these difficulties as 'pragmatic" insofar as: (i) they do not involve specific linguistic rules that govern sentence generation, and (ii) the degree of deviance experienced by the listener can be altered by changing the verbal and non-verbal context of the segment (cf. art. 53 and art. 56).

In summary, patients with schizophrenia demonstrate a wide spectrum of difficulties in word construction, selection, and sequencing which qualify as departures from conventional linguistic rules and constraints. Discovering the nature and significance of these linguistic abnormalities could yield important clues regarding the neurocognitive basis of schizophrenia.

1.3. Schizophasia as a Subtype of Schizophrenic Language Behavior

An important paper by Chaika (1974) discussed a particularly severe class of linguistic deviance produced by certain schizophrenics whereby the communicative intentions of the speaker are almost entirely hidden. She invokes the term "schizophasia" for this language behavior, and argues that this special subclass of schizophrenic utterances are very similar to jargonaphasia (cf. art. 55). Chaika suggests that schizophasia may therefore also be the product of some organic disturbance of the brain.

A reply to this position was provided by Lecours/Vanier-Clément (1976), who agreed that schizophasia does exist, that it can yield practically all manifestations ordinarily associated with jargonaphasia, but stressed that this syndrome is relatively rare among schizophrenic speakers. This was confirmed in a recent study by Hoffman/Sledge (1988), who examined randomly selected speech segments produced by eleven schizophrenics and only found one such speaker who produced segments whichin any approached the level of incomprehensibility described by Chaika. This particular patient produced example (7) (cf. above); the complete utterance containing this segment is as follows:

(7a) Interviewer: *Tell me about school?* (the question posed in the context of asking the patient about her childhood, the question therefore intending to refer to her experiences going to school)
Patient: *School? Well there are schools of play and schools of fish, mostly you see fish school, people edumacating* (sic) *themselves, you see, sea is one thing and education is another. Fish is school in their community, that's why the community of man stands in the way of the community of the sea, and once they see the light of sunny sunshine then they will let it be* (see also Hoffman 1986, 507).

Besides the paraphasic phonemic transformation, *edumacating,* (7a) demonstrates other features characteristic of schizophasia which were stressed by Chaika (1974) and, later, Lecours/Vanier-Clément (1976). These features include a preoccupation with too many semantic features of a particular word (re: the different uses of *school*), and production of words according to phonological features (*see, sea, be*) rather than according to topic. Lecours/Vanier-Clément (1976) argued that these forms of word play are not at all characteristic of jargonaphasia. When considered along with derived and composed morphemic paraphasias, which suggest intact though poorly regulated lexical generation abilities, word play in schizophasic speech raises the question of whether deviance is intentionally generated. Thus, Lecours/Vanier-Clément opposed Chaika's position by arguing that schizophasia reflects intact speech production abilities molded to deviant thought rather a primary impairment in language production per se.

It should be added that schizophasia occurs primarily in the more advanced stages of schizophrenic illness, and generally is associated with prolonged periods of social isolation and functional deterioration (Hoffman/Sledge 1984; Kirov 1985). Chronic social isolation, sustained alienation from other human beings, coupled with bizarre ideation, may, over time, cause the schizophrenic to volitionally disregard the constraints of ordinary language. Under these conditions, the interpersonal communicative goals of speech may be usurped by a kind of verbal game where language is molded to the bizarreness of the speaker's own ideas regardless of its communicative value to others. On the other hand, extremely chronic schizophrenic illness may be accompanied by the final stages of an as yet uncharacterized neurodegenerative process that could procedure a true aphasic syndrome. Moreover, just because schizophasia reflects word play that seems somehow willful by no means rules out the possibility that other types of linguistic deviance produced by the same speaker (e. g., certain paraphasias and paragrammatisms) are the unintended result of impaired speech production abilities. Thus the intentionality of schizophasic speech remains an open question.

1.4. Fromkin's Challenge

Besides the intentionality issue raised by Lecours/Vanier-Clément (1976), another noteworthy challenge to Chaika's hypothesis was provided by Fromkin (1975), who noted that the speech of normal individuals is often deviant as well (cf. art. 2 and art. 5). The following are typical examples of the kinds of slips of the tongue and other utterance irregularities that all of us, to some degree or other, are prone to:

(10) *soul hecond path* (intended: *whole second path;* Fromkin 1975);

(11) *in a manner of speakingly* (intended: *in a manner of speaking;* Fromkin 1975).

Chaika herself provides a representative sample of "nonproficient" writing by an "ostensibly normal college student":

(12) *Generalizations have no place in terms of different opinions insofar as the discussion of heros or any other topic ...* (Chaika 1977),

and the verbal excesses of political speechmaking:

(13) *In temperance due I don't see any reason why two men can't proceed as popular as ever both in themselves as a duocratic and as a demoncratic premise ...* (Chaika 1977; quoting Laffal 1965).

On the basis of segments such as these, Fromkin argued that the speech irregularities produced by schizophrenics are not specific to this disorder but reflect the imprecision of speech generation that all of us, to some degree or other, are vulnerable to. — Chaika (1977) responded to Fromkin by arguing that the deviance contained in schizophasic speech can be distinguished from the speech errors produced by normals insofar as the latter are readily decipherable in terms of communicative intent while the former are not. This position is questionable, however, because Chaika had already defined schizophasia so that it represents only the more extreme forms of deviance produced by schizophrenic speakers. It is likely that the most extreme forms of speech irregularities produced by normal speakers, even though extremely rare, could also be fairly incomprehensible.

There may, however, be another characteristic of speech irregularities produced by schizophrenics, besides degree of comprehensibility, that sets them apart from the speech irregularities produced by normal speakers. This is illustrated by deviant speech produced by a schizophrenic man (Hoffman/Sledge 1984). In spite of normal intelligence, he repeatedly generated quite distinctive speech errors, for instance:

(14) *the communists who have a class-struggle creation*

and a few seconds later:

(15) *a creation class-struggles.*

Examples (14) and (15) both reflected difficulties in generating the noun phrase, *creation of (a) class-struggle(s).* These errors can be understood as a failure to elaborate a particular type of grammatical structure via proper use of closed class words; here the term 'closed class' refers to the stable set of 'grammatical' words that each language contains. It is well known that normal speakers can drop closed class words yielding nongrammatical results (Butterworth/Howard 1987). What is unusual is that this particular type of speech error was repeated; this suggests that vulnerability to the speech error was sustained over a period of time. — Another example of a 'sustained' vulnerability to a certain type of error for this same patient was referred to earlier:

(8) *That's why, you know, the fact there was no stigmatism* (sic) *attached to that clearly explained in the record why you were put back* (Hoffman/Sledge 1984, 154).

Taken in context, this segment seems to discuss the consequences of being left back a grade in school. The target intention corresponds to something like the following (bracketed words need to be added to render the segment completely grammatical):

(8a) *[It] clearly explained in the record why you were put back ... that's why, you know, there was no [stigma] attached to the fact that I [was].*

Besides the erroneous attachment of an affix to *stigma,* the relationship between (8) and (8a) reflects the exchange and reordering of actual phrases. Of note is that this deviant segment was followed soon after by another:

(16) *It's a long term investment, insurance being one of your soundest investments, which now even you that's what those brings you know retirement policies and things, that'll pay you X amount of dollars.*

This segment can be 'unpacked' in a fashion very similar to segment (8), namely as exchanges of phrasal segments, thereby yielding the following, quite ordinary and non-bizarre speech intention:

(16a) *It's a long term investment, insurance being one of your soundest investments, which even now [will] pay you X amount of dollars, you know that's what those retirement policies and things bring.* –

These speech segments suggest that vulnerability to certain types of error, in particular, deficiencies in grammatical phrasing and exchanges in grammatical phrasing, can be sustained over time in schizophrenia (see also Chaika 1977). Slips of the tongue produced by normal speakers generally do not reproduce a particular structural problem within a matter of moments.

2. Systematic Studies of Naturally Occurring Schizophrenic Speech

2.1. Introduction

The above discussion, which primarily derives from case studies and analyses of isolated speech segments, highlights two important challenges that must be met in order to adequately evaluate and understand the nature of speech irregularities in schizophrenia. The first challenge is objectively determining the frequency of speech errors in schizophrenics as a group. The case study discussed by Hoffman/Sledge (1984) suggest that an important factor in differentiating normal and schizophrenic speech errors may be density of these errors within a corpus of speech. The second issue is the 'severity' of errors. Chaika defines schizophasia as utterances produced by schizophrenics which are relatively undecodable. However it is clear that errors produced by schizophrenics are often decodeable and correspond to relatively ordinary speech intentions. While these may not correspond to examples of traditionally defined schizophasia, in our experience they represent the majority of speech difficulties among schizophrenics. It may, however, be the case that gradations of error 'severity' rather than the simple dichotomy of decodeable vs undecodeable – still could shed light on the nature of schizophrenic speech irregularities.

2.2. Systematic Studies Examining Frequency of Errors

In a rigorously conducted study, Morice/Ingram (1982) examined the speech of 34 schizophrenics, 11 manics, and 18 normal control subjects. Manics are of considerable interest insofar as they represent another psychiatric disorder with severe symptomatology which also can lead to certain speech alterations (cf. art. 52). These are many so-called 'nonspecific factors' – e.g., preoccupation with bizarre or troubling thoughts, the effects of medication, and abnormal states of arousal – that can distrub the speech integrity of psychiatric patients. It is reasonable to assume that manics as well as schizophrenics respond to many of these same factors, especially when both of these patient groups are studied in an acutely decompensated state. – Approximately 1000 words of free speech for each subject were included in the Morice/Ingram study, which was then carefully transcribed and subjected to linguistic analysis. Schizophrenics were found to score low, relative to manics and normals, on the percentage of well-formed sentences. Replication studies by Morice/McNicol (1986) and Fraser/King/Thomas/Kendell (1986) found the total instances of speech errors to be considerably higher in schizophrenics than in manics and normals.

A challenge not taken up by these studies is the specification of the severity of instances of deviance. The idea that different errors differ in severity has an intuitive appeal, and is motivated by examples given above. Compare, once again, examples (6) and (7):

(6) *He owns a store on Fifth Avenue, and that's never mentioned because that is his side-kick* (intended: *side-line;* Hoffman/Sledge 1988, 97);

(7) *fish school in their own communities* (Hoffman/Sledge 1988, 97).

The problem in example (6) is that *side-kick* is a slang term that refers to an animate object, and *store* is decidely not aminate. The second error reflects the inappropriate use of the noun, *school*, in the verb syntactic slot. The first error seems somehow less 'pathological' than the second, though both reflect 'lexical selection' difficulties; the challenge is to find a way to operationalize this differentiation. One strategy for capturing this difference is to acknowledge that (6) has only one obvious correction, namely substituting *side-line* for *side-kick*. On the other hand, there are multiple alternative strategies for correcting (7). One correction might be

(7b) *communities of fishes form schools,*

Which corresponds to a major reworking of the syntax, while a second, though retaining the syntactic form, drops the word, *school*:

(7c) *fish swim in their own communities.*

This reasoning formed the basis for a later study by Hoffman/Sledge (1988) whereby speech errors were classified according to the relative ambiguity of what the target speech intention seemed to be. For the two examples reviewed above, (6) has only one plausible correction that is consistent with the rest of the segment, while (7) has two or more, some requiring alternations of the surface syntax of the sentence. Therefore (7) should be rated to be more severe than (6). – In this study, speech productions of eleven schizophrenics were compared to that of nine patients with psychiatric disorders other than schizophrenia. Both groups of patients had recently been hospitalized and therefore were acutely ill, and were well matched in terms of age, gender and educational level. Two of the responses were randomly selected for careful transcription and analysis of grammatical deviance. Slang and variations due to local dialect were not scored as deviant. All instances of dysfluency (word or phrase repetitions, word or phrase corrections, false starts) were eliminated from the error corpus. The fact that our control group consisted in other psychiatric patients controlled in part those 'non-specific' factors tending to produce speech errors, i. e., anxiety, stress, fatigue, etc. Speech analyses were conducted blind to diagnosis. – An important aspect of this study is that deviance was scored in a way to minimize the effects of ideational bizarreness of certain schizophrenic utterances. To illustrate how this was accomplished, consider the following segment (from Hoffman/Sledge 1988):

(17) *my family's sociology.*

One could assume that (17) is a simple lexical selection error, where the expressive intent of the utterance is something along the lines of *my family's social situation.* On the other hand, the phrase might be non-deviant if the speaker was referring to a particular set of behavioral rules governing the social interactions of his family. This ideationally offbeat notion could theoretically be within the realm of what the schizophrenic speaker was attempting to communicate. Consequently, our scoring system considered each putative error in all possible contexts, no matter how bizarre. Only instances of apparent deviance that were non-correctable by all contexts remained scored as errors. – After screening for the effects of ideational bizarreness, each remaining instance of grammatical deviance was classified in terms of whether it involved lexical selection or word order, and along the lines just discussed, the ambiguity of corresponding 'target' or intention for each instance of deviance was determined in order to assess error severity. – The major finding was, that schizophrenics produced grammatical deviance at a mean rate of .11 instances per clause while nonschizophrenics produced .045 instances per clause, a difference that was statistically significant at the .02 level. In terms of the type of error, there was a roughly equal number of inappropriate or poorly formed open-class words (nouns, verbs, adjectives, adverbs) among the two subject groups. However there was many more errors involving grammatical morphemes (prepositions, conjunctions, suffixes, etc.) among the schizophrenic patients. The following are two typical examples:

(18) *That was a decent things to do* (intended: *thing);*

(19) *We could be wheelchairs* (intended: *we could be in wheelchairs).*

Moreover there was a strong trend in the direction of more severe (i.e., ambiguous) syntactic or combinatorial deviance within the schizophrenic corpus, a difference that was statistically significant at the .05 level. Included among this group of errors was a relatively large number of syntactic blends. Here distinct syntactic structures are inappropriately combined. One such instance precipitated a paraphasia whose intended meaning can be guessed at from its context:

(20) *I guess we went upstate somewhere I don't know* w i r t h *white people* (the speaker, who was schizophrenic, was a black woman recounting a childood memory of attending a summer camp away from her native New York City; intended utterance seemed to be a blend of: *I guess we went upstate somewhere – don't know* w h e r e*/I guess we went upstate somewhere – I don't know –* w i t h *white people)*.

These data suggest that schizophrenics are prone to two types of difficulties when combining words into well-formed syntactic structures, the first reflecting difficulties in elaborating a particular syntactic frame (see examples [7] and [9]), and the second reflecting difficulties in selecting one syntactic frame over another (thereby producing syntactic blends as in example [20]; for more extensive discussion see Hoffman 1991). The frequency of these linguistic abnormalities in no way approached that of speakers who are classically 'aphasic.' Moreover, in practically all cases grammatical deviance was readily traceable to ordinary speech intentions, thereby not belonging to the class of schizophasia as defined by Chaika (1974). Although normal speakers can also produce syntactic errors of various sorts (Butterworth/Howard 1987; Morice/Ingram 1982; cf. art. 2 and art. 5), the abnormally high frequency of syntactic errors in the schizophrenic group seems to be a robust quantitative finding.

2.3. Studies of Syntactic Complexity in Schizophrenia

The importance of certain syntactic difficulties in schizophrenic speech is reinforced by studies of sentence structure. Analyses of trancribed spontaneously produced discourse by Morice/Ingram (1982), Morice/McNicol (1986), and Fraser/King/Thomas/Kendell (1986) have each demonstrated significant diminutions in syntactic complexity in schizophrenics compared to normals. Aspects of syntactic complexity that were relevant to differentiating schizophrenic and non-schizophrenic speakers included reductions in the number and depth of embedded clauses, the percentage of reduced relative clauses, and the precentage of dependent clauses with *wh*-pronouns. These findings suggest that the increased frequency of syntactic errors noted in schizophrenics may in fact reflect some impairment in combining words into complex syntactic structures.

2.4. Syntactic difficulties may alter speech performance at other levels

Perhaps a subgroup of lexical generation errors produced by schizophrenics also reflect disruptions at the level of syntactic or combinatorial processes. For instance, the context containing example (1) pertained to the educational pursuits of her boyfriend, suggesting that the underlying conversational intention of the speaker was something along the lines of:

(1a) *He is a person who studies/enjoys the Greek classics* (see also discussion in Hoffman/Sledge 1984).

It may be that the speaker was unable to elaborate this complex syntactic structure, but instead could only realize the simpler,

(1b) *He was a* (adjective) *person.*

In this case the nominal phrase, *Greek classics* would have to be pushed into the adjective position, resulting in

(1c) *He was a (Greek classical) person,*

which then becomes condensed into a single word:

(1) *He is a grassical person.*

In addition, example (20) demonstrates how a paraphasia can be induced by a syntactic blend. Thus the generation of certain non-words by schizophrenics may be triggered by a primary difficulty in elaborating complex syntactic structures. This hypothesized mechanism still requires the postulation of some impairment in self-monitoring of speech that permits the production of words that do not belong to the lexicon.

The hypothesis that difficulties in elaborating syntactic structures could reflexively alter language production at other linguistic levels is supported by another study (Hoffman/Hogben/Smith/Calhoun 1985). Twenty-four schizophrenics and 24 non-schizophrenics were given the Hunt test (Hunt 1970), a writing task which requires the subject to utilize complex sentential syntax to combine a set of simple propositions into a complex, extended narrative. An analysis of the rewritten paragraphs showed many more meaning errors in the schizophrenic group compared to the non-schizophrenic group. Relevant to the topic of this chapter is that schizophrenics were much more likely to produce meaning errors when the rewritten proposition assumed a more complex syntactic form, i. e., the passive. This finding held up even when the effects of message complexity was controlled for. We suggested that these data were evidence that syntactic processing was somehow more effortful in schizophrenics and the production of complex syntactic forms distracted the speaker from the meaning of his own speech and writing intentions.

3. Experimental Studies

The hypothesis that schizophrenia is associated with specific language processing defects has led to a range of psycholinguistic, cognitive, and neuropsychological investigations.

3.1. Sensitivity to Syntactic Structure

Two studies of psychiatric patients, one by Rochester/Harris/Seeman (1973) and the other by Carpenter (1976), examined the sensitivity to syntactic structure by embedded click paradigms. Schizophrenics tended to mislocate clicks at clausal boundaries to the same degree as normal subjects, suggesting that the ability to utilize syntactic structure to 'chunk' linguistic information into clausal units is intact in these patients. In addition, a study by Miller/Phelan (1980) compared the ability of schizophrenics and normal controls to determine the acceptablity of stimulus sentences which, to different degrees, were ungrammatical. No significant differences were found in the schizophrenics' ability to detect unacceptable syntax. These three studies thus appear to demonstrate that syntactic abilities during language comprehension remain intact in schizophrenia. While these findings are important, they do not rule out the possibility of deficits specifically in language production in schizophrenics.

3.2. Comparing Schizophrenic and Aphasic Language Abilities

Two studies have demonstrated that schizophrenics were superior to aphasic patients in terms of language ability. DiSimoni/Darley/Aronson (1977) administered a standard battery of tests to schizophrenics and compared their performance to previously collected data using aphasic subjects and other patients with 'organic' deficits. They concluded that schizophrenic patients did not demonstrate a classic 'aphasic' profile, though some impairments were noted in reading comprehension. Patients whose duration of illness was greater showed a general deterioration in performance, but the authors concluded that this pattern of deterioration most closely conformed with patients demonstrating a generalized intellectual impairment. While these findings are of interest, it should be noted that since a normal group of subjects were not included, one cannot conclude that the performance of schizophrenic subjects was actually in the normal range. Partially supporting the findings of the DiSimoni group is a study by Rausch/Prescott/DeWolfe (1980). In this study, subjects were requested to restore the order of sets of words derived from scrambled sentences. Aphasic patients performed more poorly than schizophrenics; however, it was noted that schizophrenics tended to produce somewhat more errors than normals, especially when sentences contained both direct and indirect objects.

In contrast, three systematically conducted studies have highlighted similarities between schizophrenics and aphasics. Kelter/Cohen/Engel et al. (1977) requested subjects to sort pictures of animals in order to assess the organization of semantic memory. The hierarchical patterns of sorting behavior were most diffuse for fluent aphasics and schizophrenics, and could be differentiated from the greater clarity of sorting behavior among nonfluent aphasics and normals. In a study by Faber/Reichstein (1981), schizophrenics, patients with affective disorder, and normals were administered the Boston Diagnostic Aphasia Examination. Schizophrenics who had 'formal thought disorder,' i. e., demonstrated diminished comprehensibility of their spontaneous speech, showed significant abnormalities compared to the other groups, particularly on the Token Test and the Phrase Repetition Test. These findings were interpreted as demonstrating that a subgroup of patients with the diagnosis of schizophrenia can show language performance deficits in the range of aphasic patients. Further support for this hypothesis was provided by a later study by Faber/Abrams/Taylor et al. (1983). Speech samples of 14 patients with schizophrenia with formal thought disorder were compared with the speech productions of 13 neurologically impaired patients with aphasia. Transcriptions were given to five 'specialists,' including a speech pathologist, two neurologists and two psychiatrists, who were requested to identify the diagnosis of the patient. Three of the five specialists performed better than chance but only one (the speech pathologist) achieved high discriminating ability. These findings were interpreted as indicating schizophrenics can share language abnormalities with aphasic patients, but do not exhibit a classic aphasic syndrome.

3.3. Cognitive Deficits vs Language Deficits

A wide range of studies have examined diverse parameters of cognitive functioning in schizophrenia, including selective attention, short-term memory, information filtering and context-sensitivity of perceptual processes; a review of this research as it pertains to language abnormalities in schizophrenia can be found in Schwartz (1982). Distracting ideas, preoccupation with certain words, or insensitivity to linguistic context could interfere with the speaker's ability to hold an appropriate syntactic structure in mind while speaking; this could theoretically lead to at least some of the syntactic problems described above for schizophrenics. On the other hand, it seems very hard to account for many of the paraphasias produced by schizophrenics in terms of a general cognitive defect. Certainly some of word finding problems described above could derive from excessive distractibility or impaired 'filtering' of candidate elements of the lexicon (see again example (6) and (7)). On the other hand, one is hard-pressed to propose a reasonable account, on the basis of general cognitive deficits, for the production of the types of nonwords in examples (1) – (5). With the exception of certain types of anticipation and transposition errors ordinarily produced by normal speakers (see again Garrett 1975; cf. also art. 5 and art. 7), it is hard to imagine how errors in matching phonetic strings to semantic entities and combining morphemes into words could derive from attentional problems or failures in context-sensitivity of cognitive outputs.

4. Conclusions

There is now considerable evidence that schizophrenic persons tend to produce abnormalities of speech corresponding to specific 'linguistic deviations' which are independent of the deviant content of what the speaker has in mind to say (see also a review recently published in German by Dittmann/Fehrenbach/Welsh 1989). The incidence of these speech abnormalities exceeds that of other psychiatric patients and probably normal speakers as well; many of these abnormalities, when considered individually, tend to be more 'pathological' than those produced by normal speakers or non-schizophrenic psychiatric patients, though nonetheless are relatively decodeable. On the other hand, these abnormalities, in general, are less 'severe' in terms of quantity and type when compared to aphasic speakers; they do not represent impaired 'linguistic competence' but do reflect episodic disruptions in the ability to produce well-formed speech. Moreover, a small subgroup of schizophrenics can produce very densely paraphasic and/or paragrammatical speech which is as disordered as aphasic speech; it is not clear if the cause of these more severe linguistic difficulties is some sort of organic lesion or is 'sociolinguistic' – i. e., an intentional disregard of the conversational maxim to speak clearly by upholding linguistic rules and conventions. On the other hand, it does seem clear that the more decodeable errors produced by schizophrenics represent episodic deficiencies in speech production which are not obviously creative or intentional. Disruptions in cognition not specific to language processes theoretically could account for some of the speech abnormalities produced by schizophrenics but not the more severe types of lexical difficulties.

The nature of brain dysfunction underlying these language difficulties is not known. Recent studies by this author and colleagues suggest that schizophrenics suffer from impairments in tranferring information between different cortical areas (Hoffman/Dobscha 1989; Hoffman/Buchsbaum/Escobar et al. 1991). If this applies to language production processes in schizophrenia, then their linguistic difficulties would reflect periodic breakdowns in the exchange of information between relatively intact language modules. We hope to directly test this hypothesis shortly.

5. References

Bleuler, J. F. & Perrault, C. R. (1911/1950). Dementia praecox or the group of schizophrenias. *Aschaffenberg's Handbuch*. International University Press.

Butterworth, B. & Howard, D. (1987). Paragrammatisms. *Cognition, 26,* 1–37.

Carpenter, M. D. (1976). Sensitivity to syntactic structure: Good versus poor premorbid schizophrenics. *Journal of Abnormal Psychology, 85,* 41–50.

Chaika, E. A. (1977). Schizophrenic speech, slips of the tongue, and jargonaphasia: A reply to Fromkin and to Lecours and Vanier-Clément. *Brain and Language, 4,* 464–475.

Chaika, E. A. (1974). A linguistic looks at "schizophrenic" language. *Brain and Language, 1,* 257–276.

Coffman, J. A., Andreasen, N. C., & Nasrallah, H. A. (1984). Left hemisphere density deficits in chronic schizophrenia. *Biological Psychiatry, 19,* 1237–1247.

Crow, T. J., Ball, K., Bloom, S. R., Brown, R., Bruton, C. J., Colter, N., Frith, C. D., Johnstone, E. C., Owens, D. G. C., & Roberts, G. W. (1989). Schizophrenia as an anomaly of development of cerebral asymmetry: A postmortem study and proposal concerning the genetic basis of the disease. *Archives of General Psychiatry, 46,* 1145–50.

Dittmann, J., Fehrenbach, R. A., & Welsh, C. (1989). Morphosyntaktische Abweichungen bei Schizophrenie. Ein Überblick über den Stand der Forschung. *Neurolinguistik, 2,* 145–173.

DiSimoni, F. G., Darley, F. L., & Aronson, A. E. (1977). Patterns of dysfunction in schizophrenic patients on an aphasia test battery. *Journal of Speech and Hearing Disorders, 41,* 498–513.

Faber, R. & Reichstein, M. B. (1981). Language dysfunction in schizophrenia. *British Journal of Psychiatry, 139,* 519–522.

Faber, R., Abrams, R., Taylor, M. A., Kasprison, A., Morris, C., & Weisz, R. (1983). Comparison of schizophrenic patients with formal thought disorder and neurologically impaired patients with aphasia. *American Journal of Psychiatry, 140,* 1348–1351.

Flor-Henry, P. (1976). Lateralized temporal-limbic dysfunction and psychopathology. *Annals of the New York Academy of Science, 280,* 77–797.

Fraser, W. I., King, K. M., Thomas, P., & Kendell, R. E. (1986). The diagnosis of schizophrenia by language analysis. *British Journal of Psychiatry, 148,* 275–278.

Fromkin, V. A. (1975). A linguist looks at "A linguist looks at schizophrenic language". *Brain and Language, 2,* 498–503.

Garrett, M. (1975). The analysis of sentence production. In G. Bower (Ed.), *The psychology of learning and motivation. Vol. 9. 133–177.* New York: Academic Pres.

Hoffman, R. E. (1986). Verbal hallucinations and language production processes in schizophrenia. *Behavioral and Brain Sciences, 9,* 503–548.

Hoffman, R. E. (1991). The microgenesis of schizophrenic symptoms. In Hanlon, R. (Ed.), *Microgenetic approaches to cognition: A neuropsychological perspective. 133–149.* Hillsdale: Lawrence Erlbaum Associates.

Hoffman, R. E., Buchsbaum, M. S., Escobar, M. D., Makuch, R. W., Nuechterlein, K. H., & Guich, S. M. (1991). EEG coherence of prefrontal areas in normal and schizophrenic males during perceptual activation. *Journal of Neuropsychiatry and Clinical Neurosciences, 3,* 169–175.

Hoffman, R. E. & Dobscha, S. (1989). Cortical pruning and the development of schizophrenia: A computer model. *Schizophrenia Bulletin, 15,* 477–490.

Hoffman, R. E., Hogben, G. L., Smith, H., & Calhoun, W. F. (1985). Message disruptions during syntactic processing in schizophrenia. *Journal of Communication Disorders, 18,* 183–202.

Hoffman, R. E., Kirstein, L., Stopek, S., Cicchetti D. V. (1982). Apprehending schizophrenic discourse: A structural analysis of the listener's task. *Brain and Language, 15,* 207–233.

Hoffman, R. E. & Sledge, W. (1984). A microgenetic model of paragrammatisms produced by a schizophenic speaker. *Brain and Language, 21,* 147–173.

Hoffman, R. E. & Sledge, W. (1988). An analysis of grammatical deviance occurring in spontaneous schizophrenic speech. *Journal of Neurolinguistics, 3,* 89–101.

Hunt, K. W. (1970). Syntactic maturity in schoolchildren and adults. *Monographs of the Society for Research in Child Development, 35,* 2–67.

Kelter, S., Cohen, R., Engel, D., List, G., & Strohner, H. (1977). The conceptual structure of aphasic and schizophrenic patients in a nonverbal sorting task. *Journal of Psycholinguistic Research, 6,* 279–303.

Kirov, K. (1985). Long-term study of schizophasic patients. *Psychopathology, 18,* 226–229.

Laffal, J. (1965). *Pathological and normal language.* New York: Atherton.

Lecours, A. R. & Vanier-Clément, M. V. (1976). Schizophrenia and jargonaphasia: comparative description with comments on Chaika's and Fromkin's respective looks at "schizophrenic" language. *Brain and Language, 3,* 516–565.

Lorenz, M. (1961). Problems posed by schizophrenic language. *Archives of General Psychiatry, 4,* 603–610.

Maher, B. A. (1966). *Principles of psychopathology.* New York: McGraw-Hill.

Miller, W. K. & Phelan, J. G. (1980). Comparison of adult schizophrenics with matched normal native speakers of English as to "acceptability" of English sentences. *Journal of Psycholinguistic Research, 9,* 579–592.

Morice, R. D. & Ingram, J. C. (1982). Language analysis in schizophrenia: Diagnostic implications. *Australian and New Zealand Journal of Psychiatry, 16,* 11–21.

Morice, R. D. & McNicol, D. (1986). Language changes in schizophrenia: A limited replication. *Schizophrenia Bulletin, 12,* 239–251.

Morstyn, R., Duffy, F. H., & McCarley, R. W., (1983). Altered P300 Topography in schizophrenic. *Archives of General Psychiatry, 40,* 729–734.

Rausch, M. A., Prescott, T. E., & DeWolfe, A. S. (1980). Schizophrenic and aphasic language: Discriminable or not? *Journal of Consulting and Clinical Psychology, 48,* 63–70.

Rochester, S. R., Harris, J., & Seeman, M. V. (1973). Sentence processing in schizophrenic listeners. *Journal of Abnormal Psychology, 82,* 350–356.

Schwartz, S. (1982). Is there a schizophrenic language? *The Behavioral and Brain Sciences, 5,* 579–626.

Vetter, H. (Ed.) (1968). *Language behavior in schizophrenia.* Springfield, Illinois: Thomas.

Ralph E. Hoffman, New Haven, Connecticut (USA)

55. Glossomania and Glossolalia in Schizophasia and their Linguistic Kinships to the Jargonaphasias

1. Schizophrenic Speech

In 1911, Eugen Bleuler combined the greek word for "split", "schizo", with the greek word for "mind", "phrenia", (also in "phrenology"). He needed this expression to refer to a form of dementia, a dreadful disorder of thought which first manifests itself relatively early in life ('dementia praecox'). Bleuler originally used the plural form of his new term. But, as the basic clinical manifestations of his "schizophrenias" were observed to remain constant irrespective of epochs and societies (Cancro 1983), and as evidence suggesting an organic substratum was repeatedly found (Weiner 1983), schizophrenia has come to be perceived as a single nosological entity. If only because of its 'hallucinatory' dimension, the mental status of schizophrenics causes repercussions throughout their behavior, overt speech included. Insofar as particular speech manners are thus inherent to schizophrenia, the notion of 'schizophrenic speech' is pertinent from the phenomenological point of view. As a matter of fact, clinicians do agree that episodes of unconventional speech-behavior represent an easily recognized sign of schizophrenia. Nonetheless, the linguistic characterization of schizophrenic speech remains imprecise; it has not yet been the object of explicit interpretations by psycholinguistic theories of cognition. Thus, although seemingly straight forward, diagnosing schizophrenia based on speech behavior continues to depend on largely overlapping, anecdotal, impressionistic clinical parsing. The unclarity as to exactly what makes up schizophrenic speech is reflected in the myriad of terms used to describe it: 'poverty of speech' ('laconic speech'), 'poverty of content of speech' ('poverty of thought', 'empty speech', 'alogia', 'verbigeration', 'negative formal thought'), 'pressure of speech', 'distractible speech', 'tangentiality', 'derailment' ('loose associations', 'paralogia', 'flight of ideas'), 'incoherence' ('word salad'), 'illogicality', 'clanging', 'neologisms', 'word approximations' ('metonyms'), 'circumstantiality', 'loss of goal', 'perseveration', 'echolalia', 'blocking', 'stilted speech', 'self-reference' (Andreasen 1979 a). Not unexpectedly given the richness and diversity of the above lexicon, the single nosological entity known as schizophrenia is said to encompass "18 subtypes of thought disorders" (Andreasen 1979 b, 1328). According to Andreasen (1979 a), the epitome of one of these subtypes, "poverty of content of speech", is the following quotation (1).

(1): "Many of the problems that I have ... are difficult for me to handle or to work on because I am not aware of them as problems which upset me personally. I have to get my feelers way out to see how it is ... I am, I think, becoming more aware that perhaps, on an analogy, the matter of some who understand or enjoy loud rages of anger ... The same thing can be true for other people and I have to kind of try to learn to see when that is true and what I can do about it."

From a clinical point of view, this type of behavior might be compared to that of brain-damaged subjects with *Einfallsleere* "lack of ideas" (Bay 1964); that is, with the particular form of verbal jargon occasionally observed – as illustrated in (2) – in patients with transcortical sensory aphasia (Lecours/Osborn/Travis et al. 1981).

(2): "C'est assez compliqué, hein. ... Ça devient assez compliqué de ... de tirer ça ... J'arrive à faire que le total arrive à faire un certain bien ... et qu'on arrive à arriver à ... à avoir des ... des marchandises." [It is quite complicated, eh. ... It becomes quite complicated to ... to draw that. ... I manage to do that the total manages to do something good ... and that we manage to manage to ... to have some ... some merchandises.]

2. Schizophasia

According to Porot (1975), Kraepelin coined the term 'schizophasia' at the turn of this century, to denote episodes of deviant speech behavior coexisting with conventional speech abilities. Furthermore, to the best of my knowledge, no convincing documents exist that might lead one to understand 'schizophasia' as being a synonym for 'schizophrenic speech'. On the contrary, cautiousness would rather lead one to consider schizophasia as specifying at least two forms of unconventional speech behavior, 'glossomanic schizophasia' and 'glossolalic schizophasia', which can be observed in certain psychotic subjects. Both can be utterly spectacular but nowadays neither can be said to represent a frequently observed clinical phenomenon (perhaps as the result of the addition of potent drugs to our current 'therapeutic' arsenal).

In glossomanic schizophasia the linguistic components of utterances – whether phonemes, words or more complex units – are selected and combined on the basis of phonological or semantic kinships rather than by docile compliance to a given topic. In contrast, glossolalic schizophasia can be defined as entirely or nearly entirely neologistic discourse-like speech.

2.1. Glossomanic Schizophasia

Glossomanic speech can be fluent and abundant. Like Wernicke's jargonaphasia, it can require only minimal participation from the interlocutor. Some first perceive its most striking characteristics to be at the level of word-like entities, although its essence, as I have just indicated, is probably best isolated at sentence level. In the present context, word-like entities will be referred to as 'neologisms' (Lecours 1982a) and discussed under three subheadings, 'derived morphemic deviations', 'composed morphemic deviations', and 'abstruse neologisms'. Attempts at a characterization of aberrations at the sentence level will be made under three further subheadings, 'full glossomaniac utterances', 'antonymic doublets', and 'virtuosity'.

2.1.1. Derived Morphemic Deviations

In this (morphologically constrained) type of glossomaniac production, the monolingual speaker associates legitimate roots and bound morphemes in line with the word derivation rules inherent to his or her native language, therefore creating, as in (3) to (6), neologisms with an obvious semic potential. (Except for (17), (25) and (26), all of the examples of glossomanic schizophasia quoted in this chapter were produced by the same psychotic subject in the course of a long interview made in Lausanne by Professor Gil Assal (Lecours/Nevert/Ross 1981).)

(3): prefix + ***'page'*** [page-boy] + suffix ⇒ ***"apagé"*** [one who is being made a page-boy], *idem* ⇒ ***"apageant"*** [one who makes someone else a page-boy], *idem* ⇒ ***"apagement"*** [the fact of being made a page-boy];
(4): prefix + ***'capitale*** [capital city] ⇒ ***"acapitale"*** [without a capital city];
(5): ***'douane'*** [custom] + suffix ⇒ ***"douanerie"*** [custom system];
(6): ***'logarithme'*** [logarithm] + suffix ⇒ ***"logarithmie"*** [logarithmic system].

Interestingly, one patient with Wernicke's jargonaphasia has been reported to produce – as illustrated in (7) – numerous deviations of this type (Lecours/Lhermitte 1972), although his lexical root selections were far more limited and the semic potential of his neologisms far less transparent than in the case quoted above.

(7): Root(s) + suffix(es) ⇒ *"C'est pas le* /**fɔrs-jal**/ *habituel. ... Je ne suis pas des* /**burs-jɛl**/ *personnels. ... les* /**prɔm-yr**/ *que j'ai promus. ... Mon* /**sɔld-aʒ**/ *s'emploie différemment."* [it is not the usual /**fɔrs-**

jal/. ... I am not from the personal /**burs-jɛl**/. ... the /**prɔm-yr**/ whom I promoted. My /**sɔld-aʒ**/ is to be employed differently.]

2.1.2. Composed Morphemic Deviations

In addition to combining morphemes in an unconventional way, the glossomanic speaker might also associate at least two legitimate open-class words in line with the word composition rules inherent to his or her language. In this way the speaker creates, as in (8) to (11), a second form of neologism with an obvious but usually perplexing semic potential:

(8): ***'quart'*** [quarter] + ***'cinquième'*** (fifth] ⇒ ***"quart-cinquième"*** [quarter-fifth];
(9): ***'été'*** [summer] + ***'hiver'*** [winter] ⇒ ***"été-hiver"*** [summer-winter];
(10): ***'jour'*** [day] + ***'nuit'*** [night] ⇒ ***"jour-nuit"*** [day-night];
(11): ***'ouvre'*** [open] + ***'ferme'*** [close] ⇒ ***"ouvre-ferme"*** [open-close].

To the best of my knowledge, this type of behavior is not congruent with the clinical picture of any type of jargonaphasia. It should be emphasized, however, that replacement of a word by a potential antonym is a form of 'semantic paraphasia' often observed in Wernicke's jargonaphasia.

2.1.3. Abstruse Neologisms

Whereas both derived and composed morphemic deviations have a recognizable semic potential, abstruse neologisms, phonologically constrained word-like entities, have no semic potential other than that which may perhaps be gleaned from the context. As (12) and (13) demonstrate, the abstruse neologisms of schizophasic glossomania can take part of their phonological components from previous utterances in the immediate context, and they can comprise morpheme-like components, especially affixes. These two features are also characteristic of the neologistic productions of a number of brain-damaged patients with Wernicke's jargonaphasia (Lecours/Osborn/Travis et al. 1981; cf. art. 16).

(12): *"Je fais mon classement des **'soudocheries'*** (/**sudɔʃri**/) *d'où je viens ... C'est pestilentiel, vous savez, cette **soude*** (/**sud**/) *... du **duché*** (/**dyʃe**/) *ou de communale ... "* [I make my classification of the /**sudɔʃri**/ from where I come ... It stinks, you know, this bicarbonate ... of the dukedom or commune ...]
(13): *"... en perdant la maîtrise de sa classification, en allant dire des **grossièretés**. ... C'est une espèce de maladie, de 'grossiomige'* (/**grosjomiʒ**/)*"*. [... by loosing the mastery of one's classification, by being **gross** in speech. ... It is a kind of disease, of /**grosjomiʒ**/.]

An essential difference between the abstruse neologisms of schizophasic glossomanics as opposed to those of Wernicke's jargonaphasics is that the former – but never the latter – will, as in (14) [where the speaker answers a question about the meaning of /grosjomiʒ/ (13)], are in no way anosognosic with regard to such utterances and will discuss and justify them if requested to do so. [This is in line with Bleuler's (1966) teachings about the neologisms of psychotics although it contradicts Chaika's (1974) assumptions.]

(14): [Concerning /**grosjomiʒ**/:] *"Oui, C'est une espèce de bête. Voilà! C'est un terme que j'ai créé, que j'ai fait, comme ça pour ... pour donner une petite base personelle, privée. Voilà!"* [Yes, it is a kind of beast. That's it! It is a term which I have coined, which I have created, just like that, in order to ... to provide a small personal, private basis. That's it!]

2.1.4. Full Glossomanic Utterances

As mentioned above, glossomanic characteristics can be observed not only at the phonological and lexical level, but also at the sentence level. Glossomanic schizophasia owes its name to a form of utterance that is apparently generated along more playful though rule-governed lines. As indicated above, such rules require sentence production to be guided, according to conventional syntactic constraints, by (paradigmatic) phonological similarities and/or potential semic kinships between individual words and word-like neologistic entities rather than by an intention to formulate an immediately sharable phrastic message. The 'game', which is not unlike one of Andreasen's (1979a) "18" subtypes of thought disorders [i.e., "clanging",], can be mostly phonological, as in (15) and (16), or mostly semantic, as in (17) [quoted from Chaika (1974)], but it usually is both, as in (18):

(15): *"C'est comme ça que les vieux faisaient les fondations. Ou bien de **cause*** (/**koz**/) : un /**kozam**/, *un* /**klozam**/, /**glozan**/. *Vous comprenez? Et, à ce casier, on a un savoir de **Lausanne*** (/**lozan**/)." [It is this way that the ancients built foundations. Or else of **cause**: a /**kozam**/, a /**klozam**/, /**glozan**/. You understand? And, in this bin, one has a knowledge from **Lausanne**];
(16): *"Et alors, il y a des **joues*** (/**ʒu**/), ***jours*** (/**ʒur**/), *des **j'ouvre*** (/**ʒuvr**/)*-ferme qui sont ..."* [And then, there are some **cheeks**, **days**, some '**I open**-close which are ...];

(17): "My mother's name was **Bill** ... and **coo**? St. Valentine's Day is the official startin' of the breedin' season of the **birds**. All **buzzards** can **coo**. I like to see it pronounced **buzzards** rightly. They work hard. So do **parakeets**";
(18): *"Mais oui, à cette organisation de travail, il y a donc des plans d'**heures** et un **calendrier** du plan de **secondes**, de **minutes**, d'**heures**, d'**horlogerie** et d'**orâge**. Vous appelez ça des **heures-âges**, d'où des **tonnes-âges** qui, de l'**âge** du **début** d'un certain **âge**, par rapport au **calendrier** ..."* [Yes indeed, to this organization of work, there are thus draughts of **hours** and a **calendar** of the draught of **seconds**, of **minutes**, of **hours**, of **clock-making** and of **gold-age**. You call that **hour-ages**, hence **ton-ages** which, from the **age** of the **beginning** of a certain **age**, by reference to the **calendar**...]

In exceptional cases, certain brain-damaged subjects with transcortical sensory aphasia occasionally produce, as in (19), sentences that would qualify as semantic glossomania. Likewise, as in (20), subjects with Wernicke's jargonaphasia may produce, within a same context, sequences of formally related abstruse neologisms. When viewed out of context, such neologisms are somehow remindful of phonological glossomania (Lecours/Vanier 1976).

(19): *"... on s'est aperçu que, partout ailleurs, ils ont mis des petits **colporteurs*** – literally: 'collar bearer' – *et ils ont pu, avec un **veston** ... avec un **manteau colporté** ..."* [... we realized that, everywhere else, they posted little **peddlars** and they were capable, with a **jacket** ... with a **peddled mantle** ...]
(20): "... *ces gens qui étaient à la /**kɔmi**/ ... au ... au /**glasrɔ**/ ... au /**kɔmorɔ**/ ... /**kɔrokɔmuit**/ ..."* [... those people who were at the /**kɔmi**/ ... at the ... at the /**glasɔ**/ ... at the /**kɔmorɔ**/ ... at the /**kɔrokɔmuit**/ ...]

2.1.5. Antonymic Doublets

The extreme and therefore 'pathognomic' (although probably not qualitatively different) form of 'full glossomanic utterance' on the sentence level, which cannot be grouped among any type of jargonaphasia resulting from focal brain damage, is the one simultaneously expressing a given notion and its opposite. This kind of utterance can be based on pairs of words, of phrases, or of more complex speech entities. The simplest way of creating an antonymy is by blending part of the phonemic components of two words with potentially opposite meanings [such as 'smig' for 'small + big' (fictious example)]. Two blends of this sort, which have the advantage of illustrating the fact that schizophasics will occasionally challenge phonological legality, a type of behavior so deliberate that it probably is incompatible with the very notion of aphasia are quoted in (21) below. Another way of building an antonymic doublet would be to attach antonymic affixes to the same root [as in 'unuseful' (fictious example)]. As in (9) to (11) above, as well as in the first part of (21) below, such 'self-contradicting' neologisms can also be created through composition, or else, as in (22) to (25), through more complex syntagmatic procedures, i. e., by incorporating antonymic words or phrases to the context of a same sentence:

(21). ***'froid'*** + ***'chaud'*** ⇒ ***"froid-chaud"*** /frwa-ʃo/ ⇒ "/**fʃowa**/" ⇒ "/**frʃowa**/": *"De **froid-chaud** ou de **chaud-froid**. De /**fʃowa**/. Ils ... Ils parlaient comme ça, les anciens. Ils disaient: Un /**frʃowa**/"*. [Of **cold-hot** or of **hot-cold**. Of **'chotld'**. They ... They talked like that, the ancients. (This assertion is strikingly in line with Freud's (1910) astonishing beliefs about the origins of language.) They said: a **'cohotld'**.]
(22): *"Et alors, je commence la première classification: ça me fait un homme **sain** et un homme **fou**."* [And then, I begin the first classification: this makes me a **healthy** man and a **crazy** man.]
(23): *"Lorsqu'on fait un siècle, il y a toujours un **début** et une **fin** ... Toujours, le **premier jour** du siècle correspond au **dernier jour de la fin** du siècle ... Le **vrai** calendrier est différent du **faux**."* [When one makes a century, there is always a **beginning** and there is an **end** ... Always, the **first day** of the century corresponds to the **last day of the end** of the century ... The **true** calendar is different from the **false** one.]
(24): *"Un **bureau ambulant**, un **cadavre vivant** ... où de la terre glaise a formé, de **dessus** aux bases classificatrices de **dessous**..."* [A **walking desk**, a **living cadaver** ... where clay has formed, from **above** to the classificatory bases of **under** ...]
(25): *"Je voudrais bien **avoir de nouveau un bon nombre d'années pour me retrouver dans l'âge de la jeunesse**."* [I really wish **I could be a great deal older anew** so that **I might find myself again in the age of youth**.] (From Schmidt/Perrot (1976)).

2.1.6. Virtuosity

Schizophasic speakers do not only combine opposing units of speech to form antonymic doublets, they will occasionally combine entire phrases and use them like single nouns, [for instance, see *"des j'ouvre-ferme"* (16)]. Indeed, production of this sort – which should obviously be considered syntactic virtuosity rather than dyssyntaxia – can, as illustrated in (26; the only example of 'schizographia' quoted in this chapter), become quite spectacular in cases such as the one reported by Levy-Valensi/Migault/Lacan (1931). Probably the most staggering glossomanic utterances are those in which – as in (27), (IPA transcriptions are provided in

Figure 55.1) – cascades of words and word-like entities stemming from a few paradigmatically associated roots are attached to antonymic affixes until nearly all possible combinations have been exploited within a single set of consecutive sentences (Figure 55.1).

(26): *"Je fais de* ***l'âme est lasse*** *à toujours vous servir. ... Si vous voulez faire le* ***tant l'aire est belle qu'il la faut majorer de faits****, c'est que vous êtes ... ... faire un beau* ***maitrisez-moi****."* [I make some **the-soul-is-weary** because I always serve you. ... If you wish to make the **so-beautiful-is-the-area-that-one-has-to-raise- it-up-with-facts**, it is because you are ... ... to make a beautiful **subdue-me**.]

(27): *"Pour prendre une* ***pierre****, ils l'appelèrent une* ***'pierre'*** *... la* ***lever*** *et la* ***poser****: ils* ***dépierrent*** *à* ***repierrer****, n'est-ce-pas? C'est juste: et on les appela* ***dépierra-repierra****. On les appela les* ***roches*** *de la* ***roche****, de définition. Et ils* ***arrochent*** *des* ***roches****. Vous comprenez? Et les deux* ***pierres*** *à deux* ***roches****, ça devient des* ***procha****. A classement de ... de généralité – n'est-ce pas? – transpositif de* ***pierra*** *es à* ***rocha****.* ***Rocha*** *est à ... est à deux* ***pierra*** *mais, à la synthèse des deux, c'est un* ***procha*** *de* ***pierra*** *ou de* ***rocha****."* [To take a **stone**, they named it **'stone'** ... to **lift it up** and to **put it down**: they **unstone** to **restone**, don't they?. It is adequate: and they were named **unstoned-restoned**. They were named the **rocks** of the **rock**, by definition. And they **arock** some **rocks**. You understand? And the two **stones** to two **rocks**, they become **strocka**. In a classification of ... of generality, right, transpositive of **stona** is to **rocka**. **Rocka** is to ... is to two **stona** but, at the synthesis of the two, it is a **strocka** of **stona** or of **rocka**.]

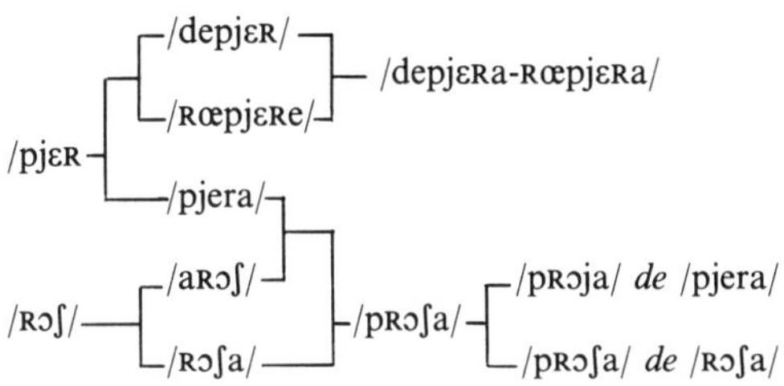

Figure 55.1

Clearly, the glossomanic schizophasic is one who should be taken at his or her word (rather than sentence). Although paradigmatic and syntagmatic constraints are respected throughout his or her enigmatic discourse, when they are not exaggerated, they somehow undermine their supposed intention, namely conventional sharing of ideas. Indeed, one retains the impression that glossomaniac behavior sometimes qualify as a variety of 'hyperphasia'.

2.2. Glossolalic Schizophasia

Just as some of the few who are believed to be episodically possessed by a devil, as well as otherwise healthy Pentecostal believers merely under the week-end influence of the Holy Ghost (Samarin 1972), certain psychotics will, on occasion, spew endless neologistic utterances (Cénac 1925). Bobon (1947), reported that such patients may resort to several different 'tongues'. This was the case of the psychotic subject whose 'English temperament' is quoted in (28).

(28) "/azumba bɛʀgɛs koʀᴏ bʀubjɛʀ paʀa bʀazja mnɛʀges keʀɔkoʀᴏ bʀubjɛʀ mizœ pʀiz aʀakaska ʀœkaʀœ bʀazjɛ mnɛʀgɛs keʀakɔʀᴏ. ... azaʀa kuʀu bʀubjɛr paʀa bʀasja minɛʀgɛs kɛʀœkuʀu bʀubjɛʀ mizœ pʀiz aʀakaska ʀœkaʀœ bʀasja minɛʀgɛs kaʀœkuʀu bʀubjɛʀ mizœ pʀiz aʀakaska ʀakaʀa bʀazja minɛʀgɛs kɛʀokoʀu bʀubjɛʀ mesi./"

Glossolalic schizophasia occurs in the form of asemantic although prosodically invested perseverative monologues in which (a) the tonic accent of the speaker's mother tongue can be replaced by another and (b) the speaker's regional accent can be attenuated. In the productions of the monolingual glossolalist, phonemes are those of the mother tongue but their relative frequency is grossly modified. The overall impression is that of a phonologically, lexically, and syntactically impoverished 'foreign' language (Lecours 1982 b).

Although such speech is very uncommon and thus far has been observed exclusively in polyglot elderlies (Lecours/Osborn/Travis et al. 1981; Perecman/Brown 1981), glossolalia can, as illustrated in (29), occur as a form of Wernicke's jargonaphasia. Both glossalic schizophasia and glossalic aphasia are not far from the segmental point of view but they differ in that the latter represents residual behavior, takes the form of a dialogue with an interlocutor and, to some extent, retains conversational prosody, whereas the glossolalia of schizophrenic subjects occurs episodically (that is, it coexists with a capacity for conventional speech production), takes the form of monologues, and assumes one form or another of stereotyped prosody (Lecours, 1982 b).

(29) "/sɛ̃ dikte di tʀɔ̃ dʀikɔ̃dedeʀe digœʀe dis tis tilavɛ kloʀe œ le dø tʀɔ̃ke ditibɛ dœʀe disœ te kotegoʀe dil kɔ̃deteʀe. ... a wi dœ vilɛbʀiʃ ʒe la lãbɛtɔʀi de dɛl lãtetɛʀœme di katedɔʀe e œ e ɛlzekute ɛlmœpurimakɔ̃te tã tutse dœgʀedœgʀɛ dis gy lateʀe digeloteʀe./"

3. Schizophrenic Speech, Schizophasia, and Jargonaphasia

As demonstrated above, schizophasia can have certain linguistic features in common with one form or another of fluent aphasia. However, whereas evidence of malfunction of at least one of the mechanisms of language production is always manifest in the former, it is evidence of exalted function, for instance, exaggerated but accurate use of word derivation or normalization rules, that one observes in the latter (Lecours/Vanier 1976). Whether or not schizophasia should be considered as a manifestation of schizophasia or of another form of psychosis remains an open question. At any rate, schizophasics, glossomanics in particular, can give proof of such mastery of rule-governed language that one can hardly conceive of their behavior as being a manifestation of focal brain damage involving the speech area [as suggested by Chaika (1974)]. On the other hand, I see no reason to exclude the possibility that a more subtle organic dysfunction, as in certain types of intoxication, might influence brain activities in a manner such that certain linguistic constraints are magnified to the detriment of the natural outcome of human language abilities, that is, conventional communication. As a matter of fact, the main difference between spectacular schizophasia and certain forms of literary creation (cf. art. 8) is that the former appears to be exclusively founded on formal and/or semic kinships between words and/or word-like entities, whereas the latter is both founded on such kinships and topic-guided (sharable).

Author's note: The author's research is funded by the "Conseil de la recherche médicale du Canada" and by the "Fonds de la recherche en santé du Québec".

4. References

Andreasen, N. J. C. (1979 a). Thought, language and communication disorders: I. Clinical assessment, definition of terms, and evaluation of their reliability. *Archives of General Psychiatry, 36,* 1315–1321.

Andreasen, N. J. C. (1979 b). Thought, language and communication disorders: II. Diagnostic significance. *Archives of General Psychiatry, 36,* 1325–1330.

Bay, E. (1964). Principles of classification and their influence on our concepts of aphasia. In A.V.S. de Reuck & M. O'Connor (Eds.), *Disorders of Language. 122–142.* London: Churchill.

Bleuler, E. (1966; translation from the 1911 German edition). *Dementia Praecox or the Group of Schizophrenias.* New York: International Universities Press.

Bobon, J. (1947). Trois langues artificielles d'origine ludique chez un paraphrénique hypomaniaque. *Journal belge de neurologie, 47,* 327–395.

Cancro, R. (1983). History and overview of schizophrenia. In H. I. Kaplan & B. J. Sadock (Eds.), *Comprehensive Textbook of Psychiatry (Volume I). 631–643.* Baltimore: Williams & Wilkins.

Cénac, M. (1925). *De certains langages créés par les aliénés: Contribution à l'étude des glossolalies.* Thèse de doctorat (Médecine), Paris: Université de Paris.

Chaika, E. O. (1974). A linguistic looks at schizophrenic language. *Brain and Language, 1,* 257–276.

Freud, S. (1910; 1964 translation). The antithetical meaning of primal words. In J. Strachey (Ed.), *The Standard Edition of the Complete Psychological Works of Sigmund Freud, Volume XI. 155–161.* London: Hogarth.

Lecours, A. R. (1982 a). On neologisms. In J. Mehler, E. C. T. Walker, & M. Garrett (Eds.), *Perspectives on Mental Representations. 217–247.* Hillsdale: Erlbaum.

Lecours, A. R. (1982 b). Simulation of speech production without a computer. In M. Arbib, J. Marshall, & D. Caplan (Eds.), *Neural Models of Language Processes. 345–367.* New York: Academic Press.

Lecours, A. R. & Lhermitte, F. (1972). Recherches sur le langage des aphasiques: Analyse d'un corpus de néologismes (notion de paraphasie monémique). *L'encéphale, 61,* 295–315.

Lecours, A. R., Nevert, M., & Ross, A. (1981). Langage et pensée du schizophase. *Confrontations psychiatriques, 19,* 109–144.

Lecours, A. R., Osborn, E., Travis, L., Rouillon, F., & Lavallée-Huynh, G. (1981). Jargons. In J. Brown (Ed.), *Jargonaphasia. 9–38.* New York: Academic Press.

Lecours, A. R. & Vanier, M. (1976). Schizophasia and jargonaphasia: A comparative description with comments on Chaika's and Fromkin's respective looks at schizophrenic language. *Brain and Language, 3,* 516–565.

Levy-Valensi, J., Migault, P., & Lacan, J. (1931). Ecrits inspirés: schizographie. *Annales médico-psychologiques, 89,* 1–26.

Perecman, E. & Brown, J. (1981). Phonemic jargon. A case report. In J. W. Brown (Ed.), *Jargonaphasia. 177–257.* New York: Academic Press.

Porot, A. (1975). *Manuel alphabétique de psychiatrie.* Paris: Presses Universitaires de France.

Samarin, W. J. (1972). *Tongues of Men and Angels*. New York: MacMillan.

Schmidt, P. & Perrot, M. (1976). A propos d'observation de troubles du langage dans la schizophrénie. *Annales médico-psychologiques*, *134*, 708–714.

Weiner, H. (1983). Schizophrenia: Etiology. In H. I. Kaplan & B. J. Sadock (Eds.), *Comprehensive Textbook of Psychiatry (Volume I)*. *650–680*. Baltimore: William & Wilkins.

André Roch Lecours, Montréal, Québec (Canada)

56. Communicative Behavior in Schizophrenia

1. Introduction

In analyses of schizophrenic speech, different concepts of 'communication' are often used. The target of this article are approaches which view communication as an actual communicative exchange aimed at achieving mutual understanding. There is general consent that at least with some schizophrenics the actual communicative exchange is at times difficult (Rühmke 1941; Wyrsch 1946), and that the cause of this 'mis-communications' must be examined. In tackling the problem the majority of investigations focuses on the schizophrenic's contribution to communication. That is, difficulties of communicative exchange are construed as being generated either by the schizophrenic's difficulty to produce understandable utterances or by his/her difficulty to correctly understand the adequate utterances of his/her healthy partners. It is assumed that the difficulty in understanding schizophrenic utterances is brought about by inherent features of content (Faria/Figueira 1989; Rosenberg/Tucker 1979) and/or form (van Belle 1987; Chaika 1982; Cohen 1978; Cohen/Camhi 1976; Cohen/Nachmani/Rosenberg 1974; De Decker/Van Campe 1989; Hoffman/Kirstein/Stopek/Cicchetti 1982; Penn 1987; Rochester/Martin/Thurstone 1977). Conversely, a schizophrenic recipient's difficulty in understanding his/her partner is based on the schizophrenic's deficient speech perception (Lawson/McGhie/Chapman 1964). In contrast, very few investigations focus on components of the communicative exchange itself, nor do they conceive of difficulties as at least dyadic problems of mutual understanding (Blakar 1984; van de Craen 1989). – Obviously, one must first pinpoint the key constituents of successful communication before one can locate the source of miscommunication in schizophrenic discourse and/or actual communicative exchange. With regard to the investigations under review successful communication on the one hand is narrowly conceived of as a contextfree understanding and of making oneself understood as a product of an individual achievement, and, on the other hand a conception of a mutually satisfactory process of interpretation which is determined by communicative intentions relevant to the given situation (Dittmann 1991; Fischer 1987; Leodolter 1975; Wróbel 1990, 21 ff). In the following an attempt is made to show with regard to each of these perspectives (a) how the basic communicative difficulties are described as specific deviances, and (b) what is known about the conditions under which they occur in which type of (schizophrenic) person.

2. Description of Deviances

2.1. Difficulties in Speech Production

In an empirical approach (Rutter 1979) raters' achievements in reconstructing the original discourse structure from a randomized set of clauses are quantified. Performance which is based on intuitions about language rather than on explicitly defined features of utterances is worse when raters are confronted with clauses from a schizophrenic's (vs a healthy person's) text. – In other approaches the analyses are based on explicitly described linguistic (Faria/Figueira 1989; Harvey 1983; Jones 1977; Rochester/Martin/Thurstone 1977; Schmidt-Knaebel 1983; Tress/Pfaffenberger/Frommer 1984; Wróbel 1990), specifically pragmatic (van Belle 1987; De Decker/van Campe, 1989), and logical (Hoffman/Kirstein/Stopek/Chicchetti 1982; Lincourt 1981; Nöth 1976; Werner/Levis-Matichek/Litowitz 1975) devices for the construction of meaning in discourse. Forms of deviation are determined against these types of backgrounds. — Qualitative and quantitative aspects of the well-defined devices of cohesion and reference (Halliday/Hasan 1976) are determined by trained analysts. These aspects lead to the finding that compared to healthy persons schizophrenics, especially those with a thought-disorder (TD) produce discourse which is characterized by cohesive weakness and unclear reference (Rochester/Martin/Thurstone 1977; Rochester/Martin 1979). Relations between propositions (Hoffman/Kirstein/Stopek et. al. 1982), and of semantic recurrence between units (e. g. paragraph, theme, topic) which hierarchically structure a text (Nöth 1976) are modelled in a global fashion by determining an individual degree of acceptability (Nöth 1976) or a score of deviation (Hoffman/Kirstein/Stopek et al. 1982). The findings that schizophrenics' scores of deviation systematically differ from the scores of non-schizophrenic psychotics (Hoffman/Kirstein/Stopek/Cicchetti 1982) and of manics (Hoffman/Stopek/Andreasen 1986) have to be judged against critical evaluations of the algorithm of description (Beveridge/Brown 1985; Käsermann 1989). The approaches mentioned so far describe aspects of the understandability of schizophrenics' discourses originating from an actual dialogue (usually a partially-structured interview with a staff member). It is noteworthy, however, that the descriptions do not encompass the healthy partner's actual achievement in understanding his/her schizophrenic interlocutor. — In experimental investigations of the specifically referential communication (Cohen 1978; Cohen/Camhi 1976; Cohen/Nachmani/Rosenberg 1974) a (schizophrenic) speaker is instructed to produce a clue which allows a hearer to identify the referent (one of the objects or words, usually synonyms, of a pair of stimuli). Comprehension is defined as proportion of a hearer's correct selections of the intended referent and is usually determined outside of an actual situation of communication. Compared to healthy persons schizophrenics show a reduced performance as communicators but not as recipients. The significance of this paradigm with regard to an understanding of schizophrenia is disputed (Neale/Oltmanns/Harvey 1985). — The given approaches describe the understandability of schizophrenics' discourse with regard to its objective informational effectiveness. An alternative view is the conception of verbal oddities as having the function of metacommunicative commentaries about the actual communicative situation (von Block 1979; Dieckmann/Dittmann 1989; Schmidt-Knaebel 1983; Werner/Levis-Matichek/Litowitz 1975): Hiding this function by not being clearly marked as such or entailing contradictory messages makes these utterances hard to understand (Käsermann 1988; Nöth 1976).

2.2. Difficulties in Speech Perception

Schizophrenics' difficulties in understanding utterances of their healthy partners is known from first person accounts (Chapman 1966; Freedman 1974; McGhie/Chapman 1961). While the schizophrenic's problem of producing understandable utterances is thought to stem from his/her failure at providing information necessary for the reconstruction of meaning, his/her difficulty in understanding is equated with his/her not being able to use information given in utterances. One type of information mediating meaning in discourse is the predictability within clauses (modelled by different word order approximations; Miller/Selfridge 1950) which schizophrenic listerners cannot use fully according to results of an experimental investigation (Lawson/McGhie/Chapman 1964). However, it can be shown (Rochester 1973; Rochester/Harris 1973) that schizophrenics' reduced performance as listeners is not primarily based on a disability in processing syntactic information but rather on an impaired processing of primary sensory data. — The analyses reviewed in sections 2.1. and 2.2. are characterized by the assumption that the difficulties experienced in communicative interaction with schizophrenics are based on the latters' deficient productive and perceptive treatment of syntactic, semantic, referential, propositional, and pragmatic (van Belle 1987; De Decker/van Campe 1989) aspects of language. Findings are interpreted mainly as an expression of the schizophrenic individual's problems with language and/or information-processing, and seldom as an expression of a schizophrenic individual's problems with communication. In comparison the communicative exchange as such is not a target of investigation (with the exception of Schmidt-Knaebel 1983). However, it is certainly topicalised theoretically either by proposing an algorithm used for describing speech oddities as a model of the (healthy) listener's interpretive difficulties (Hoffman/Kirstein/Stopek 1982), or by reflecting the possibility of speech oddities as being dependent on an interpersonal failure (Andreasen 1979; Nöth, 1976; Rochester/Martin/Thurstone 1977). However, at least the latter has been rejected as quite improbable (Rochester 1978) on the basis of results concerning paraverbal aspects of schizophrenics' linguistic performance (Rochester/Thurstone/Rupp 1977). – The controversy is unlikely to be solved within a framework capturing a primarily communicative phenomenon in terms of individual achievements and deficits. Even those findings about the schizophrenic individual's ability to decenter or to take another's perspective based on anecdotic (Wróbel 1990) or experimental evidence (Harrow/Lanin-Kettering/Miller 1989; Kreitler/Schwartz/Kreitler 1987; Strober 1979) gathered outside an actual communicative context, are of limited value in testifying for or against the interpersonal-failure-thesis, because in these settings the interpersonal situation as a variable itself is neglected.

2.3. Failures of Communicative Exchange

Investigations of problems of communicative exchange with schizophrenic persons are aimed either at aspects of enduring patterns of communication (Doane/Goldstein/Rodnick 1981; Vaughn/Leff 1976) or at features of the actual communicative interaction. – The attempt to locate difficulties of communicative exchange with schizophrenics in an ongoing conversational situation is based on the assumption that an adequate and satisfactory communicative process between interlocutors presupposes shared meaning or a contract, respectively (Rommetveit 1974; Swartz/Swartz 1987), processes of convergency (Alberti/Käsermann 1983), a cooperative endeavor (Grice 1975) in general (Buckingham jr. 1982; De Decker/van de Craen 1987; Käsermann 1983; Leodolter 1975), and, a cooperative endeavor aimed at organizing turn-taking (Schlatter/Käsermann 1991), respectively. Blakar (1973) proposes a method for investigating communicative interaction between interlocutors proceeding from presuppositions which by experimental induction are made to differ between participants. It can be shown, that parents with a schizophrenic offspring when conversing with each other (Blakar/Paulsen/Solvberg 1978; Blakar/Valdimarsdottir 1981) as well as when conversing with the schizophrenic communicate less efficiently and more egocentric about a given problem than do healthy dyades or triades (Mossige/Pettersen/Blakar 1979). Leodolter (1975) examined the characteristics of informations given in answering questions and distinguishes four types of dialogues with schizophrenics. Käsermann (1983; 1986; 1987) analysed adjacency pairs (Sacks/Schegloff/Jefferson 1974) and tried to determine the effect of the expected or non-expected request-reply exchange on the course of conversation. She proposed two types of algorithms to grasp expected and non-expected courses of interaction (Käsermann 1983; 1987). With regard to a schizophrenic's contribution to conversation the latter allows for discriminating types of deviations from a cooperative communicative behavior. This method of description can also be expanded to encompass the quality of the healthy partners' cooperation (Käsermann/Altorfer 1989). Within the framework of single case studies, it can be shown that differences in cooperation between healthy and schizophrenic interlocutors cannot be interpreted meaningfully without taking into account variables like overall goals of conversation and distribution of knowledge (Käsermann 1991). – The analysis of signals used to organize turn-taking (Duncan/Fiske 1977; Schlatter/Hänni 1989) show that a substantial proportion of so-called incoherences (Andreasen 1979) in a schizophrenic's utterances occur as a function of the healthy partner's refusal to take over the speaker's role (Schlatter/Käsermann 1991). This approach expands the description unit from two- to three-turn sequences. This allows for a type of analysis which systematically corroborates the impression (Schmidt-Knaebel 1983) that the healthy partner's backchannels or hearer signals acting as a substitute for an adequate substantial utterance may lead to oddities in the schizophrenic's communicative behaviour. These findings contrast with evidence from a two-turn-sequence analysis where the healthy partner's backchannels are interpreted as strategically adequate to keep conversion going (van Bijsterveld 1987). – With possible exceptions (Doane/West/Goldstein et al. 1981; Miklowitz/Strachan/Goldstein et al. 1986; Goldstein 1987) investigations of enduring patterns of communication do not focus on features of actual communicative interaction with a schizophrenic person but look at communicative styles of his/her relatives. Occurrence and frequency of specific message types (critical, hostile or positive remarks, emotional overinvolvement, warmth: Vaughn/Leff 1976; Leff/Vaughn 1985; criticism, intrusiveness, guilt induction, support: Doane/West/Goldstein et al. 1981) are registered. It is shown that a familial style of communication characterized by negative message types (e. g. criticism; emotional overinvolvement) is systematically related to occurrence (Doane/West/Goldstein et al. 1981) and course (esp. risque of relapse) of the schizophrenic condition (Vaughn/Leff 1976). — The manner of construing aberrations has major methodological implications. Aberrations constituted inductively by comparing the achievements of schizophrenics and (healthy) controls are not independent from specific features (of the situation, of the investigated persons) and limitations on sampling procedures of that investigation. As a consequence replications of given results are very rare. In contrast, the use of categories which define oddities as deviations from implicit (Dawson/Bartolucci/Blum 1980) or explicit standards (Swartz/Swartz 1987), especially the standards of linguistic or logic correctness (e. g. Rochester/Martin/Thurstone 1977; Rochester/Martin 1979) create descriptions which are independent of features of the actual situation. This independence forms an indispensable prerequisite for answering the following question (Chaika 1981; Lakoff 1981; Lecours/Vanier-Clément 1976).

3. Conditions of the Occurrence of Deviances

Generally speaking the conditions determining speech deviances cannot be isolated conclusively, neither by investigations proceeding without well-defined types of deviance, nor by single cases studies, not by investigations operating with unspecified samples of schizophrenics and controls.

3.1. Features of the (Schizophrenic) Subjects under Investigation

The question as to which schizophrenics show a given speech production deviance has been investigated with regard to the distinctions between process vs reactive (Putterman 1975), acute vs chronic (King/Fraser/Thomas/Kendell 1990; Thomas/King/Fraser/Kendell 1990), and, thought-disordered (TD) vs non-thought-disordered (NTD) conditions. The results suggest that within schizophrenia subgroups may be distinguished on the base of their respective productive achievements. It is a matter of controversy, however, whether cohesive weakness found in TD schizophrenics is specific for that subgroup or can also be found in TD manics (Harvey 1983; Harvey/Brault 1986; Schonauer/Buchkremer 1987; Villegas i Besora 1989; Wykes/Leff 1982), and NTD schizophrenics compared to NTD manics (Bartolucci/Fine 1987). Basic problems connected with a non-tautological definition of the TD-NTD distinction have been discussed by Andreasen (1979), Chaika, (1982), Dittmann (1991), and Rochester/Martin (1979); (cf. art. 53). It seems likely that deviances specific for schizophrenia or for one of its subgroups can only be found if sampling procedures take into account additional non-linguistic criteria (Andreasen/Tsuang/Canter 1974; Hoffman/Stopek/Andreasen 1986; Küfferle/Lenz/Schanda 1985), or if deviances are described more precisely on a morphosyntactic level (Dittmann/Fehrenbach/Welsh 1989; Fraser/King/Thomas 1986; King/Fraser/Thomas/Kendell 1990; Morice/Ingram 1982; Thomas/King/Fraser/Kendell 1990; cf. art. 54). In the reviewed investigations of difficulties in speech perception distinctions of subgroups are not made, and controls are healthy persons. — Investigations of failures of communicative exchange make clear that the communicative style found in families with a schizophrenic offspring prone to relapse (Doane/Goldstein/Rodnick 1981) is also present in families with a bipolar manic (Miklowitz/Goldstein/Nuechterlein et al. 1988), and, therefore is not specific for schizophrenia.

3.2. Features of Communicative Situation

The important fact that specific deviances can only be observed intermittently is sometimes not acknowledged at all (Tress/Pfaffenberger/Frommer 1984) or it is interpreted as a direct expression of the phasic nature of linguistic (Chaika 1982) and/or information-processing impairments in schizophrenics (Rochester 1978). By drawing attention to the infrequent occurrence of the specific variety of cohesive weakness found even for TD schizophrenics, however, a perspective biased towards interpreting observed deviances in terms of schizophrenic individuals' deficits may be a point of discussion (Rosenbaum/Sonne 1983). With regard to speech production it can be shown that all, TD, NTD, and healthy persons react to a variation of speech contexts (cartoon description, narrative, interview) with a differential use of types of cohesive devices (Rochester/Martin 1979; Villegas i Besora 1989). – No investigations of conditions determining the occurrence of deviances of speech perception exist. – Most of the investigations of situational conditions leading to deviances are in some way or other related to focussing on failures of communicative exchange. As these analyses often operate with deviances that have not been properly defined or stem from few case results, they have, at best, an exploratory character. The actual occurrence of deviances as a function of topic and/or style of conversation is described in the form of an anecdote (Leodolter 1975; Seeman/Cole 1977) or systematically investigated (Käsermann 1986; Rutter 1977; Shimkunas 1972; Spring/Briggs/Cozolino/Mannuzza 1982). There is evidence that deviances occur more frequently in interviews where topics distressful for the schizophrenic are pursued (Käsermann 1986; Shimkunas 1972; Spring/Briggs/Cosolino/Mannuzza 1982) and where the schizophrenic's interlocutor behaves in a conversationally invasive manner (Käsermann 1986). When the schizophrenic does not react in this manner then the selection of topics must not have disturbed him/her (Rutter 1977). – An important though not easily tangible condition of the occurrence of deviances seems to be the (restricted) quality of interpretation of the schizophrenic's (metacommunicative) conversational contribution (Schmidt-Knaebel 1983). – The actual effect of a specific communication style on the on-going conversation is investigated with regard to families with either a schizophrenic or a manic offspring: While both diagnostic groups show similar nonverbal signs of stress they can be discriminated on the base of their verbal coping strategies (Altorfer/Goldstein/Nuechterlein et al. 1990). – The set of variables which certainly play a role but as a rule are not controlled in studies dealing with schizophrenics' impaired production and perception may be conceived of as instances of emotionally distressful conditions of conversation. In recent models of schizophrenia (Gjerde 1983; Zubin/Spring 1977) schizophrenics' vulnerability to emotional stress manifested in speech deviances is construed as exclusively determined by the individual's disease. Alternatively, it has been proposed that higher-order communication variables like asymmetric and dominant characteristics of exchange may be introduced as interactionally effective mediating factors (Käsermann 1988; 1990; Szasz 1974). – Deviances cannot only be conceived of as reactions to specific conditions but also as instruments used by the schizophrenic in a goal-directed manner. The instrumental use of oddities is known from investigation of impression-management (Braginsky/Braginsky 1967; More/Malony 1982). In a single case study it has been shown that the frequency of some types of deviances changes as a function of the schizophrenic's partner being diverted from pursuing a distressful topic by their occurrence (Käsermann 1986). – Therapeutic endeavors make use of both the dependence of the occurrence of deviances on specific conditions as well as their instrumental use by trying to modify existing contingencies through communicative interventions during actual communicative exchange (Cohen/Florin/Grusche et al. 1973; Florin/Cohen/Meyer-Osterkamp 1973; Liberman/Teigen/Patterson/Baker 1973; Mace/Webb/Sharkey et al. 1988; Swift/Magaro/Antonitis 1977).

4. Summary

The review emphasizes the fact that difficulties of communicative exchange with a schizophrenic person are approached from two different angles, namely the monologic, and the dialogic one (Foppa 1987). The seeming disparity between these two perspectives (Dittmann 1991) may vanish readily if one considers (a) that the methodological core of each investigation should be created by a precise and replicable description of oddities as deviations from linguistic, logical, and/or conversational standards, and, (b) that such descriptions are the necessary prerequisite of probing into conditions which control the occurrence of a well defined phenomenon. A valid explanation of deviances presumes that their occurrence may be predicted on the base of knowledge about their relevant determinants.

5. References

Alberti, L. & Käsermann, M. L. (1983). Funktion des Sprachcodewechsels bei einem chronisch schizophrenen Patienten. *Sprache und Kognition, 3,* 148–154.

Altorfer, A., Goldstein, M. J., Nuechterlein, K. H., Miklowitz, D. J. & Käsermann, M. L. (1990). The patient's nonverbal activity in family interaction:

Altorfer, A., Goldstein, M. J., Nuechterlein, K. H., Miklowitz, D. J. & Käsermann, M. L. (1990). The patient's nonverbal activity in family interaction: Its relevance as an indicator of emotional stress (negative affective style AS) and its stability depending on the patient's reaction to emotional stress. Manuscript.

Andreasen, N. C. (1979). Thought, language, and communication disorders: I. Clinical assessment, definition of terms, and evaluation of their reliability. *Archives of General Psychiatry, 36,* 1315–1321.

Andreasen, N. C., Tsuang, M. T., & Canter, A. (1974). The significance of thought disorder in diagnostic evaluations. *Comprehensive Psychiatry, 15 (1),* 27–34.

Bartolucci, G. & Fine, J. (1987). The frequency of cohesion weakness in psychiatric syndromes. *Applied Psycholinguistics, 8,* 67–74.

van Belle, W. (1987). Assertive speech acts in psychotic discourse. In R. Wodak & P. van de Craen (Eds.), *Neurotic and psychotic language behaviour. 332–342.* Clevedon: Multilingual Matters Ltd.

Beveridge, A. W. & Brown, K. (1985). A critique of Hoffman's analysis of schizophrenic speech. *Brain and Language, 24,* 174–181.

van Bijsterveld, D. (1987). On the problem of accessibility in conversations with schizophrenic people. In R. Wodak & P. van de Crean (Eds.), *Neurotic and psychotic language behaviour. 304–331.* Clevedon: Multilingual Matters Ltd.

Blakar, R. M. (1973). An experimental method for inquiring into communication. *European Journal of Social Psychology, 3 (4),* 415–425.

Blakar, R. M. (1984). *Communication: A social perspective on clinical issues.* Oslo: Universitetsforlaget.

Blakar, R. M., Paulsen, O. G., & Solvberg, H. A. (1978). Schizophrenia and communication efficiency. A modified replication taking ecological variation into consideration. *Acta Psychiatrica Scandinavica, 58,* 315–326.

Blakar, R. M. & Valdimarsdottir, A. (1981). Schizophrenia and communication efficiency: A series of studies taking ecological variations into consideration. *Psychiatry and Social Science,* (Band) 43–52.

von Block, S. (1979). Dialogangebote in der Kommunikation Schizophrener. In W. Heindrichs & G. Rump (Eds.), *Dialoge: Beiträge zur Interaktions- und Diskursanalyse. 116–133.* Hildesheim: Gerstenberg.

Braginsky, B. M. & Braginsky, D. D. (1967). Schizophrenic patients in the psychatric interwiev: An experimental study of their effectiveness at manipulation. *Journal of Consulting Psychology, 31(6),* 543–547.

Buckingham jr., H. W. (1982). Can listeners draw an implicature from schizophrenics? Commentary to St. Schwartz: Is there a schizophrenic language? *Behavioral and Brain Sciences, 5,* 579–626; 592–594.

Chaika, E. (1981). How shall a discourse be understood? *Discourse Processes, 4,* 71–88.

Chaika, E. (1982). A unified explanation for the diverse structural deviations reported for adult schizophrenics with disrupted speech. *Journal of Communication Disorders, 15,* 167–189.

Chapman, J. (1966). The early symptoms of schizophrenia. *British Journal of Psychiatry, 112,* 225–251.

Cohen, B. (1978). Self-editing deficits in schizophrenia. *Journal of Psychiatric Research, 14,* 267–273.

Cohen, B. D. & Camhi, J. (1976). Schizophrenic performance in a word-communication task. *Journal of Abnormal Psychology, 72(3),* 240–246.

Cohen, B. D., Nachmani, G., & Rosenberg, S. (1974). Referent communication disturbances in acute schizophrenia. *Journal of Abnormal Psychology, 83(1),* 1–13.

Cohen, R., Florin, I., Grusche, A., Meyer-Osterkamp, S. & Sell, H. (1973). Dreijährige Erfahrung mit einem Münzsystem auf einer Station für extrem inaktive, chronisch schizophrene Patienten. *Zeitschrift für Klinische Psychologie, 2(4).* 243–277.

van de Craen, P. (1989). Communication, cognition, and schizophrenia. An introduction. *Communication & Cognition, 22(2),* 125–127.

Dawson, D. F. L., Bartolucci, G., & Blum, H. M. (1980). Language and schizophrenia: Towards a synthesis. *Comprehensive Psychiatry, 21(1),* 81–90.

De Decker, B. & van Campe, J. (1989). Delusional thinking in schizophrenia: A linguistic analysis. *Communication & Cognition, 22(2),* 145–156.

De Decker, B. & van de Craen, P. (1987). Towards an interpersonal theory of schizophrenia. In R. Wodak & P. van de Craen (Eds.), *Neurotic and psychotic language behaviour. 249–265.* Clevedon: Multilingual Matters Ltd.

Dieckmann, C. & Dittmann, J. (1989). Eine Fabel als Dialogangebot. Fallstudie zum Problem der Kommunikation mit Schizophrenen. In V. M. Roth (Ed.), *Kommunikation trotz gestörter Sprache. Aphasie-Demenz-Schizophrenie. 168–172.* Tübingen: Narr.

Dittmann, J., Fehrenbach, R. A., & Welsh, C. (1989). Morphosyntaktische Abweichungen bei Schizophrenie. Ein Überblick über den Stand der Forschung. *Neurolinguistik, Zeitschrift für Aphasieforschung und -therapie, 3(2),* 145–173.

Dittmann, J. (1991). Gesprächssituation und Situationsinterpretation. Normale und pathologische Prozesse. In J. Dittmann, H. Kästner, & J. Schwitalla (Eds.), *Erscheinungsformen der deutschen Sprache. Festschrift für H. Steger. 223–236.* Berlin: Schmidt.

Doane, J. A., Goldstein, M. J., & Rodnick, E. H. (1981). Parental patterns of affective style and the development of schizophrenia spectrum disorders. *Family Process, 20,* 337–349.

Doane, J. A., West, K. L., Goldstein, M. J., Rodnick, E. H., & Jones, J. E. (1981). Parental communication deviance and affective style. *Archives of General Psychiatry, 38,* 679–685.

Duncan, S. & Fiske, D. W. (1977). *Face-to-face interaction.* New York: Wiley.

Faria, H. I. & Figueira, M. L. (1989). Mental models about the self in paranoid schizophrenic discourse: an analysis of clinical interviews. *Communication & Cognition, 22(2),* 135–144.

Fischer, H. R. (1987). 'Grammar' and 'language-game' as concepts for the analysis of schizophrenic communication. In R. Wodak & P. van de Craen (Eds.), *Neurotic and psychotic language behaviour. 165–199.* Clevedon: Multilingual Matters Ltd.

Florin, I., Cohen, R., & Meyer-Osterkamp, S. (1973). Eine Untersuchung zum operanten Konditionieren sozialen Verhaltens bei chronischen Schizophrenen. *Zeitschrift für Klinische Psychologie, Beiheft 1,* 5–76.

Foppa, K. (1987). Dialogsteuerung. *Schweizerische Zeitschrift für Psychologie, 46,* 251–257.

Fraser, W. I., King, K., Thomas, P., & Kendell, R. E. (1986). The diagnosis of schizophrenia by language analysis. *British Journal of Psychiatry, 148,* 275–278.

Freedman, B. J. (1974). The subjective experience of perceptual and cognitive disturbances in schizophrenia. *Archives of General Psychiatry, 30,* 333–340.

Gjerde, P. F. (1983). Attentional capacity dysfunction and arousal in schizophrenia. *Psychological Bulletin, 93,* 57–72.

Goldstein, M. J. (1987). Family interaction patterns that antedate the onset of schizophrenia and related disorders: A further analysis of data from a longitudinal prospective study. In K. Hahlweg (Ed.), *Understanding major mental disorder: The contribution of family interaction research. 11–32.* New York: Family Process Press.

Grice, H. P. (1975). Logic and conversation. In: P. Cole & J. L. Morgan (Eds.), *Syntax and semantics, Vol. 3: Speech acts. 41–58.* New York: Academic Press.

Halliday, M. A. K. & Hasan, R. (1976). *Cohesion in English.* London: Longman.

Harrow, M., Lanin-Kettering, I., & Miller, J. G. (1989). Impaired perspective and thought pathology in schizophrenic and psychotic disorders. *Schizophrenia Bulletin, 15(4),* 605–622.

Harvey, P. D. (1983). Speech competence in manic and schizophrenic psychoses: The association between clinically rated thought disorder and cohesion and reference performance. *Journal of Abnormal Psychology, 92(3),* 368–377.

Harvey, P. D. & Brault, J. (1986). Speech performance in mania and schizophrenia: The association of positive and negative thought disorders and reference failures. *Journal of Communication Disorders, 19,* 161–173.

Hoffman, R. E., Kirstein, L., Stopek, S., & Cicchetti, D. V. (1982). Apprehending schizophrenic disourse: A structural analysis of the listener's task. *Brain and Language, 15,* 207–233.

Hoffman, R. E., Stopek, S., & Andreasen, N. C. (1986). A comparative study of manic vs schizophrenic speech disorganization. *Archives of General Psychiatry,* 43, 831–838.

Jones, J. E. (1977). Patterns of transactional style deviance in the TAT's of parents of schizophrenics. *Family Process, 16,* 327–337.

Käsermann, M. L. (1983). Form und Funktion schizophrener Sprachstörungen. *Sprache und Kognition, 2,* 132–147.

Käsermann, M. L. (1986). Das Phänomen der sprachlichen Inkohärenz in Dialogen mit einem Schizophrenen. *Sprache und Kognition, 5,* 111–126.

Käsermann, M. L. (1987). The analysis of dialogues with a schizophrenic patient. In R. Wodak & P. van de Craen (Eds.), *Neurotic and psychotic language behaviour. 277–303.* Clevedon: Multilingual Matters Ltd.

Käsermann, M. L. (1988). Schizophrenie: Zwei Umgangsweisen mit einer Beschreibung des Wahnsinns. *LiLi. Zeitschrift für Literaturwissenschaft und Linguistik, 69,* 21–40.

Käsermann, M. L. (1989). The assumption of functionality of communicative acts as tool for investigating cognition in schizophrenia. *Communication & Cognition, 22(2),* 157–168.

Käsermann, M. L. (1991). Obstruction and dominance: Uncooperative moves and their effect on the course of conversation. In: I Markova & K. Foppa (Eds.), *Asymmetries in dialogue. 101–123.* New York: Harvester Wheatsheaf.

Käsermann, M. L. & Altorfer, A. (1989). Obstruction in conversation: A triadic case study. *Journal of Language and Social Psychology, 8(1),* 49–58.

King, K., Fraser, I. W., Thomas, P., & Kendell, R. W. (1990). Re-examination of the language of psychotic subjects. *British Journal of Psychiatry, 156,* 211–215.

Kreitler, S., Schwartz, R., & Kreitler, H. (1987). The cognitive orientation of expressed communicability in schizophrenics and normals. *Journal of Communication Disorders, 20,* 73–91.

Küfferle, B., Lenz, G., & Schanda, H. (1985). Clinical evaluation of language and thought disorders in patients with schizophrenic and affective psychoses. *Psychopathology, 18,* 126–132.

Lakoff, R. T. (1981). Schizophrenia as communication. *Semiotica, 34(3/4),* 355–374.

Lecours, A. R. & Vanier-Clément, M. (1976). Schizophasia and jargonaphasia: A comparative description with comments on Chaika's and Fromkin's respective looks at "schizophrenic language". *Brain and Language, 3,* 516–565.

Leff, J. & Vaugn, C. (1985). *Expressed emotion in families. Its significance for mental illness.* New York. The Guilford Press.

Leodolter, R. (1975). Gestörte Sprache oder Privatsprache: Kommunikation bei Schizophrenen. *Wiener Linguistische Gazette, 10/11,* 75–95.

Liberman, R. P., Teigen, J., Patterson, R., & Baker, V. (1973). Reducing delusional speech in chronic, paranoid schizophrenics. *Journal of Applied Behavior Analysis, 6,* 57–64.

Lincourt, J. M. (1981). Schizophrenese as semiosis. *Ars Semiotica, IV(2),* 107–126.

Mace, F. C., Webb, M. E., Sharkey, R. W., Mattson, D. M., & Rosen, H. D. (1988). Functional analysis and treatment of bizzare speech. *Journal of Behavior Therapy & Experimental Psychiatry, 19(4),* 289–296.

McGhie, A. & Chapman, J. (1961). Disorders of attention and perception in early schizophrenia. *British Journal of Medical Psychology, 34,* 103–116.

Miklowitz, D. J., Goldstein, M. J., Nuechterlein, K. H., Snyder, K. S., & Mintz, J. (1988). Family factors and the course of bipolar affective disorder. *Archives of General Psychiatry, 45,* 225–231.

Miklowitz, D., Strachen, A. M., Goldstein, M. J., Doane, J. A., Snyder, K. S., Hogarty, G. E., & Falloon, I. R. H. (1986). Expressed emotion and communicative deviance in the families of schizophrenics. *Journal of Abnormal Psychology, 95(1),* 60–66.

Miller, G. A. & Selfridge, J. A. (1950). Verbal context and the recall of meaningful material. *American Journal of Psychology, 63,* 176–185.

More, S. T. & Malony, H. N. (1982). Games hospitalized mental patients play: Impression management in cooperative and uncooperative psychiatric patients. *Journal of Psychiatric Treatment and Evaluation, 4,* 7–15.

Morice, R. D. & Ingram, J. C. L. (1982). Language analysis in schizophrenia: diagnostic implications. *Australian and New Zeeland Journal of Psychiatry, 16,* 11–21.

Mossige, S., Pettersen, R. B., & Blakar, R. M. (1979). Egocentrism and inefficiency in the communication of families containing schizophrenic members. *Family Process, 18,* 405–425.

Neale, J. M., Oltmanns, T. F., & Harvey, P. H. (1985). The need to relate cognitive deficits to specific behavioral referents of schizophrenia. *Schizophrenia Bulletin, 11(2),* 286–290.

Nöth, W. (1976). Textkohärenz und Schizophrenie. *LiLi. Zeitschrift für Literaturwissenschaft und Linguistik, 6(23/24),* 175–194.

Penn, C. (1987). Pragmatic profiling of adult language pathology: An exercise in clinical linguistics. *African Studies, 46(2),* 307–327.

Putterman, A. H. (1975). Referential speaker processes in male and femal process-reactive schizophrenics. *Journal of Nervous and Mental Disease, 160(6),* 354–358.

Rochester, S. R. (1973). The role of information processing in the sentence decoding of schizophrenic listeners. *Journal of Nervous and Mental Disease, 137(3),* 217–223.

Rochester, S. R. (1978). Are language disorders in acute schizophrenia actually information processing problems? *Journal of Psychiatric Research, 14,* 275–283.

Rochester, S. R. & Harris, J. (1973). Sentence processing in schizophrenic listeners. *Journal of Abnormal Psychology, 82(2),* 350–356.

Rochester, S. R., Martin, J. R., & Thurston, S. (1977). Thought-process disorder in schizophrenia: The listener's task. *Brain and Language, 4,* 95–114.

Rochester, S. R., Thurston, S., & Rupp, J. (1977). Hesitations as clues to failures in coherence: A study of the thought-disordered speaker. In Rosenberg, S. (Ed.), *Sentence production: Development in research and theory. 65–87.* Hillsdale, N. J.: Erlbaum.

Rochester, S. & Martin, J. R. (1979). *Crazy talk. A study of the discourse of schizophrenic speakers.* New York: Plenum Press.

Rommetveit, R. (1974). *On message structure.* London: Wiley.

Rosenbaum, B. & Sonne, H. (1983). Crazy talk – A study of the discourse of schizophrenic speakers. *Journal of Pragmatics, 7,* 207–217.

Rosenberg, S. D. & Tucker, G. J. (1979). Verbal behavior in schizophrenia. *Archives of General Psychiatry, 36,* 1331–1337.

Rühmke, H. C. (1941). Het Kernsymtoom der Schizophrenie en het "Praecoxgevoel". *Nederlandsch Tijdschrift voor Geneskunde, IV,* 4516–4525.

Rutter, D. R. (1979). The reconstruction of schizophrenic speech. *British Journal of Psychiatry, 134,* 356–359.

Rutter, D. R. (1977). Visual interaction and speech patterning in remitted and acute schizophrenic patients. *British Journal of Social and Clinical Psychology, 16,* 357–361.

Sacks, H., Schegloff, E. A., & Jefferson, G. (1974). A simplest systematics for the organization of turn-taking in conversation. *Language, 50,* 696–735.

Schlatter, T. & Hänni, R. (1989). Zur Steuerung des Sprecherwechsels in einem Arzt-Patient-Gespräch. Eine Einzelfalluntersuchung. *Archiv für Psychologie, 141(4),* 273–286.

Schlatter, T. & Käsermann, M. L. (1991). Inkohärenz als Interaktionsphänomen. *Zeitschrift für Kli-*

nische Psychologie, Psychopathologie und Psychotherapie, 39(1), 89–98.

Schmidt-Knaebel, S. (1983). *Schizophrene Sprache in Monolog und Dialog. Psycholinguistischer Beitrag zu einer Charakteristik psychotischer Sprechakte mit Vorschlägen für das Gespräch in Klinik und Psychotherapie.* Hamburg: Helmut Buske Verlag.

Schonauer, K. & Buchkremer, G. (1987). Some effects of supportive psychotherapy on texts written by schizophrenics. In R. Wodak & P. van de Craen (Eds.), *Neurotic and psychotic language behaviour. 266–276.* Clevedon: Multilingual Matters Ltd.

Seeman, M. V. & Cole, H. J. (1977). The effect of increasing personal contact in schizophrenia. *Comprehensive Psychiatry, 18(3)*, 283–293.

Shimkunas, A. M. (1972). Demand for intimate self-disclosure and pathological verbalizations in schizhophrenia. *Journal of Abnormal Psychology, 80(2)*, 197–205.

Spring, B., Briggs, D., Cozolino, L., & Mannuzza, S. (1982) Predictability of schizophrenic speech about stressful and neutral topics. *Paper presented at the meeting of the American Psychological Association*, Washington, DC.

Strober, M. (1979). The structuring of interpersonal relations in schizophrenic adolescents: A decentering analysis of Thematic Apperception Test stories. *Journal of Abnormal Child Psychology, 7(3)*, 309–306.

Swartz, S. & Swartz, L. (1987). Talk about talk: Metacommentary and context in the analysis of psychotic discourse. *Culture, Medicine and Psychology, 11*, 395–416.

Swift, L. H., Magaro, P. A., & Antonitis, J. J. (1977). Use of aversive stimulation to elicit vocalization in mute schizophrenics. *Psychological Reports, 41*, 575–580.

Szasz, T. S. (1974). Language and humanism. *The Humanist, 34*, 25–30.

Thomas, P., King, K., Fraser, W. I., & Kendell, R. E. (1990). Linguistic performance in schizophrenia: A comparison of acute and chronic patients. *British Journal of Psychiatry, 156*, 204–210.

Tress, W., Pfaffenberger, U., & Frommer, J. (1984). Zur Patholinguistik schizophrener Texte. *Der Nervenarzt, 55*, 488–495.

Vaughn, Ch. & Leff, J. (1976). The measurement of expressed emotion in the families of psychiatric patients. *British Journal of Social and Clinical Psychology, 15*, 157–165.

Villegas i Besora, M. (1989). The failure of communication in schizophrenic thought disorder. *Communication and Cognition, 22(2)*, 191–202.

Werner, O., Levis-Matichek, G., & Litowitz, B. (1975). An ethnoscience view of schizophrenic speech. In M. Sanchez & B. Blount (Eds.), *Sociocultural dimensions of language use. 349–380.* N. Y.: Academic Press.

Wróbel, J. (1990). *Language and schizophrenia.* Amsterdam: John Benjamins Publishing Company.

Wykes, T. & Leff, J. (1982). Disordered speech: Differences between manics and schizophrenics. *Brain and Language, 15*, 117–124.

Wyrsch, J. (1946). Ueber die Intuition bei der Erkennung des Schizophrenen. *Schweizerische Medizinische Wochenschrift, 46*, 1173–1176.

Zubin, J. & Spring, B. (1977). Vulnerability – A new view of schizophrenia. *Journal of Abnormal Psychology, 86*, 103–126.

Marie-Louise Käsermann, Bern (Switzerland)

V. Pathologies and Disorders of Language Development

57. Landmarks in Children's Language Development

1. Introduction

The speed and course of normal language development are enormously variable, yet there are certain landmarks that all children pass on their way to becoming competent speakers of their native languages. The purpose of this chapter is to describe those landmarks and to provide an approximate timetable for their achievement. The goal is to describe 'what' children acquire and 'when' they do so. Issues of 'how' children acquire what they do fall outside the scope of this chapter. Thus this chapter is not a review of theories of language development, although some discussion of theoretical issues is necessary where the appropriate description of what the child has acquired is at issue. The first and largest section of this chapter describes the course of the development of linguistic competence with separate treatments of phonological, lexical, and grammatical development. Semantic development is not discussed as a separate topic, but the meanings of children's words and sentences are discussed in the sections on lexical and grammatical development, respectively. The second section adds to this account of children's mastery of their language, brief summaries of the development of the ability to communicate intentions and the development of the discourse skills required to use language for communication.

2. The Development of Linguistic Competence

2.1. Phonological Development

2.1.1. Production

2.1.1.1. Prespeech Phonological Development

The first perceptible landmark in the development of speech sounds occurs at around 6 to 8 weeks of age when the infant starts to coo. Before that the infant's vocal repertoire consists of cries, burps, sneezes, and other vegetative sounds which, like speech, require the vocal cord to vibrate and air flow to be stopped and started, but which bear no obvious resemblance to the sounds of speech. The coos that 8 week old infants produce sound like long, single-segment vowels, although careful analysis reveals the presence of some consonantal elements as well. Infants coo when they appear contented and, particularly, when they are engaged in social interaction. Between approximately 2 and 8 months of age, the vocal repertoire of the infant expands and the infant gains increasing control over the use of that repertoire. Cooing noises are concatenated in long, multi-segment series, laughter appears, the variety of vowel and consonantal sounds produced increases, and finally – toward the end of this period – these emerging features are produced together in increasingly long and complex combinations sometimes termed marginal babbling. Squealing, growling, and a variety of 'friction noises' are also characteristic of infant vocalizations during this period (see Stark 1986 for a more complete summary of early phonological development).

The second major landmark in phonological development is the appearance of canonical babbling, which occurs sometime between 6 and 9 months of age. Canonical babbling is distinguished from the vocalizations that preceded it by the presence of true syllables.

The definition of canonical babbling is highly technical (i.e., in terms of multiple acoustic parameters such as frequency resonance, intensity, rate of formant transition, and others (Oller 1986)), but the appearance of canonical babbling is obvious to the listener because of the clear syllabic quality of the infant's sounds, typically produced in reduplicated series of the same consonant-vowel combination such as [dada] or [nɜ nɜ nɜ]. Canonical babbling is not produced by deaf infants, and thus this landmark appears to be the first development that distinguishes the vocal development of hearing children from that of deaf children (Oller 1986).

The appearance of canonical babbling is followed by a period of variegated babbling in which new consonants and vowels are added to infants' repertoires, and consonant-vowel and consonant-vowel-consonant syllables are combined in series. Although some prosodic features may be present in infants' productions from the time of marginal babbling, if not earlier (Crystal 1986), once prosody is added to these strings of non-reduplicated babbles infants sound as though they were speaking – until close attention reveals that what is being produced is the melody of language, but not the words. By 8 months the prosodic contours of babbling sequences may begin to show the specific influence of the prosodic characteristics of the target language (Crystal 1986, de Boysson-Bardies/Sagart/Durand 1984), but the consonant and vowel repertoires of children at this stage seem consistent across children acquiring different languages (Vihman 1988). Children seem to vary in both the extent to which they produce these word-less intonation patterns and how long they persist at this. Some children spend months in this expressive jargon phase, and many children continue to produce long strings of jargon after producing their first words.

Next, and more so for some children than others, there is a transitional phase between babbling and the appearance of the first identifiable word. During this period children produce sound sequences, or sound plus gesture sequences, which seem to have consistent meanings for the child, but the meanings of these sequences are not derived in any obvious way from the target language. These sequences have been variously labelled protowords (Bates 1976), sensori-motor morphemes (Carter 1979), quasi-words (Stoel-Gammon/Cooper 1984) and phonetically consistent forms (Dore/Franklin/Miller/Ramer 1976). Their use tends to be tightly bound to particular contexts and/or pragmatic functions. Studies of the phonetic characteristics of vocalizations during this transitional period suggest that there are commonalities among children acquiring the same language and also that children's sound repertoires have been influenced by the phonological properties of the target language (Vihman 1988). In the vocalizations of children acquiring English, single syllables are most common, and some disyllabic units are produced. Among consonants, stops (e.g., [b] and [d]) are the most frequent, nasals (e.g., [m] and [n]) and fricatives (e.g., [f] and [đ]) are present but rarer, consonant clusters are infrequent. Central vowels (e.g., [ʌ], [ɜ], [æ]) are more frequent than high vowels (e.g., [i], [u]). (See Vihman 1988 for a more complete description).

2.1.1.2. Phonological Development During Early Language Development

Sometime within a few months before or after their first birthdays, children reach the landmark that ends the period of prespeech phonological development – they produce their first words. These first words make use of the same sound repertoires that were evidenced in children's late babbling and transitional forms. Even at the 50-word vocabularly mark (around 18 months) sounds that appeared in early babble are among the more frequently used, and many sounds are not yet produced. In children acquiring English, for example, [m], [b], and [d] are consistently present as initial consonants in their 50-word vocabularies, and [θ], [đ], [l], and [r] are consistently absent (Leonard/Newhoff/Meselam 1980). However, there is also considerable variety across children in the phonemes in their first 50 words.

Normative inventories of the phonemes in the speech of American children at different ages have been collected by Templin (1957) and Sander (1972). However, several factors limit the usefulness of such norms as descriptions of phonological development (Menyuk/Menn 1979). First, the likelihood that a sound will be articulated depends on the sound's position in the word and on the neighboring sounds in the word, and these factors affect different sounds differently. For example, fricatives tend to be produced first in word-final position; stops tend to be first produced in word-initial position. Second, there are individual differences in the course of phonological development, although the nature and extent of these differences is a matter of some controversy (Stoel-Gammon/Cooper 1984, Ferguson/Farwell 1975, Goad/Ingram 1987). And third, there is good evidence of cross-linguistic variability in the course of phonological development. According to Pye/Ingram/List (1987) children acquire first those distinctions which are most relevant in their language, and relevance in the target language is the most important determinant of the order of acquisition of phonemes.

A more useful way to try to describe phonological development is in terms of the kind of understanding of the phonological system children appear to have at different points in development, although there is not agreement on what this description should look like. The most widely held view is that children initially use the whole word as a single, unanalyzed phonological entity (Ferguson/Farwell 1975). Analysis into small units that can be recombined (i. e., phonemes or features) occurs later. The evidence for this is that there is a lack of phonological consistency across different words in children's early productive vocabularies and also that sometimes children initially articulate words well, and then the phonological quality of their productions later declines. This apparent regression is seen as evidence that the child's whole-word approach has been supplanted by a phonological system that is not yet adultlike. An alternative view of phonological development is that children's phonological systems operate over distinctive features from the start and that development consists of learning the contrasts relevant in the target language (Ingram 1988). The argument for this view is the claim that, when looked for properly, there is phonological systematicity to be found in children's early productions. Hence, the disagreement hinges on methodological considerations involved in arriving at children's phonological inventories.

Both these views of phonological development converge in identifying 18 months or the achievement of a 50-word productive vocabulary as a major landmark in phonological development. Some significant change in children's phonological systems seems to occur at this point that allows children to learn new words much more quickly than before and that therefore contributes to – if not fully explains – the spurt in children's vocabularies which occurs at this time. As described by Menyuk/Menn/Silber (1986) the change that occurs is the development of a system that maps phonemes in the target language to sounds within the child's more limited repertoire, thus allowing the child to approximate most one or two syllable words after only a few hearings. Many of these mapping rules (often termed processes or patterns) are common across children (at least within a language). These common patterns give young children's speech characteristic features such as reduplication (e. g., *bottle* – [baba]), substitution of stops for fricatives and cluster reduction (e. g., *sandwich* – [taewis], and substitution of glides for liquids (e. g., *rabbit* – [wæbɪt]) (Dale 1976). (See Ingram (1986) for a comprehensive discussion of the common phonological processes in children acquiring English).

In addition to the patterns that are common across children, there are also individual differences and even marked idiosyncracies in the patterns that children develop (Fey/Gandour 1982). And there are strategies other than the application of patterns that children may adopt when confronted with a new word in the target language. Children may avoid acquiring new words that use sounds that are not in their repertoires (Schwartz/Leonard 1982), or they may assimilate a new word to either another similar-sounding word in their lexicons or to a preexisting whole-word sound pattern (termed a canonical form). Some children seem to modify all new words to fit a small set of canonical forms, and for others the use of a few canonical forms coexists with a more elaborate system of phonological patterns. These individual differences and exceptions notwithstanding, the development of these patterns is a major change in children's phonological systems and their emergence is the last major landmark in phonological development. The rest of normal phonological development consists of the gradual lessening of reliance on these patterns as children's articulatory abilities develop. By the age of 4 years children's phonological systems are usually close to that of adults with only a few sounds still causing trouble. Normally, children sound adult-like by the age of 6 to 7 years.

2.1.2. Phonological Development in Perception and Comprehension

It is well established that prelinguistic infants are able to discriminate between sounds which differ in terms of features that mark phonemic contrasts in many of the world's languages. In experimental tasks in which discrimination is assessed using changes in infants' heart rates, sucking, or attention, infants as young as 1 to 4 months have shown discrimination of consonants based on differences in voice onset time and place of articulation, discrimination among several vowel contrasts, and discrimination of glides and liquids (Eilers 1980). Infants also show sensitivity to intonation and stress cues (Eilers 1980). Some of these discriminatory capabilities appear to be innate, but there also appears to be some learning taking place during the prelinguistic period as evidenced by effects of the target language on speech sound perception in infants as young as 6 to 8 months (Eilers/Gavin/Oller 1982), although there is controversy surrounding this claim (Jusczyk/Shea/Aslin 1984, Eilers/Oller/Bull/Gavin 1984).

The fact that two sounds are discriminable to infants does not mean that two words that differ in that feature will be understood by children to be two different words with different meanings. Children as old as 24 months fail to treat as phonemic, contrasts that are perceptible to prelinguistic infants (Barton 1978, Menyuk/Menn/Silber 1986). The particulars of when different phonemic contrasts are acquired in word perception are subject to disagreement over the appropriate method for testing their acquisition (Barton 1975, Garnica 1973). Even the relationship between the development of comprehension and production is unclear. Ingram (1989) has suggested that the course of phonological development in production depends on preceding developments in comprehension, and some production errors seem due to perceptual difficulties. On the other hand, some production errors seem to be more the result of motor difficulties (Vihman 1988), and certainly there is good evidence that comprehension of a contrast in the speech of others does not guarantee accurate production of that same contrast (Butler 1920/1980). Children seem to have mastered the phonemic contrasts in their language by 4 years (Menyuk/Menn/Silber 1986), but metaphonological knowledge and skills such as those involved in counting the number of segments in a word, in rhyming, and in appreciating puns develop after the age of 4 (Grunwell 1986).

2.2. Lexical Development

2.2.1. Production

2.2.1.1. Early Lexical Development

Sometime around their first birthdays most children produce their first recognizable word. This event is a major landmark in language development, but it does not seem to represent any discontinuity in children's internal representations of language. Like the protowords that preceded them, children's first words tend to be context bound. For example, *more* might be used only as a request and not to comment on recurrence and *no* might be used only to indicate refusal (Gopnik 1988). This sort of word use suggests that the child's mental representation of the word is that it is what one says to accomplish particular pragmatic ends, rather than that it is a label for a referent or a symbol for a more abstract meaning (Bates/Benigni/Bretherton et al. 1979, Dromi 1990, Gopnik 1988). Labels for people and things typically appear after the first context-bound words, but they tend to be less frequently used or less numerous in children's early vocabularies. However, there are individual differences in this, with some children producing more object labels from the start (Nelson 1973). A third word type, which typically appears later than either context-bound words or labels and which probably depends on cognitive developments that are not necessary for the use of these other two word types, are words with relational meanings such as *gone* – used to indicate disappearance, or *no* – used to indicate failure. Initially, for most children, the rate of vocabulary acquisition is relatively slow. Reported average rates of vocabulary acquisition between the first word and the achievement of the 50-word mark vocabulary range from 8 to 11 words per month (Benedict 1979, Goldfield/Reznick 1990, Nelson 1973). Also, during this early period of lexical development newly-learned words are not necessarily permanent additions to children's productive vocabularies.

Sometime around 18 months, but ranging from 15 to 24 months, children achieve a productive vocabulary of 50 words (Benedict 1979, Goldfield/Reznick 1990, Nelson 1973). Reaching this point in lexical development or reaching the age of 18 months – it is not clear whether age or productive vocabulary is the best indicator – represents the second major landmark in lexical development and does seem to reflect some underlying change in children's linguistic systems. At this point many children show a marked increase in the rate at which they acquire new words — to an average rate of 22 to 37 words per month (Benedict 1979, Goldfield/Reznick 1990) — and words acquired after this point tend to be permanent additions to children's vocabularies. An average difference in ease of word learning between children who are on either side of the 50-word vocabulary mark or 18 months of age has also been demonstrated experimentally (Lucariello 1987, Oviatt 1982). What appears to change lexical development at this point is a newly-developed ability to learn names for things. The word spurt is not a spurt in the acquisition of all kinds of words, rather it is a spurt in the acquisition of object labels (Goldfield/Reznick 1990). The occurrence of this spurt seems to depend on the convergence of several factors. As already suggested (see 2.1.1.2.), phonological development may play a part. There are also several proposals of cognitive prerequisites to the naming explosion including the development of the notion that things are members of categories (Gopnik/Meltzoff 1987), the development of the cognitive ability to break events down into nameable components (Nelson/Lucariello 1985) and the achievement of the insight that things have labels (Dore/Franklin/Miller/Ramer 1976, Stern/Stern 1907). In addition, having a mother who plays labelling games may be helpful if not necessary (Goldfield/Reznick 1990).

At the 50-word point in lexical development, children's vocabularies are typically described as consisting primarily of nouns or object labels, with verbs or actions words constituting a smaller proportion of children's vocabularies; modifiers and words which express affective states or serve social functions make up the remainder (Benedict 1979, Gentner 1978, Snyder/Bates/Bretherton 1981). First nouns typically include words for food, clothing, animals, body parts, household items involved in children's daily routines, and people (Clark 1979). Several sources, however, call into question the view that nouns predominate in early vocabularies. Children learning languages in which the verb is more salient in the surface structure of sentences than it is in English have been reported to acquire verbs at an earlier age than do children learning English (Clancy 1985, Gopnik/Choi 1990). Also, the extent to which nouns dominate at the 50-word vocabulary mark varies across children as a function of the individual differences in the early tendency to acquire labels vs. social function words. And Lieven (1990) has suggested that nouns dominate early vocabularies when children have mothers who play labelling games with them. (Lieven, E. V. M. (1990). Remarks made in the workshop "Non-referential children: slow or different?" Fifth International Congress for the Study of Child Language. Budapest.) Thus the current view of what is normative may be biased by the predominance of first-born, middle class children as subjects of child language research.

A separate question from what sort of words young children have in their productive vocabularies is what sort of meanings children have for the words that they use. Even once words no longer have the limited context-bound meaning of children's very first words, the meaning representations that children have may be different from the meanings of those words in adults' lexicons. Narrower meanings are reflected in the underextension of words — such as using *water* only to refer to water in a glass. Broader meanings are reflected in overextensions — such as using the word *dog* to refer to any four-legged animal or using the word *Daddy* to refer to any adult male. Although such overextensions are commonly reported, the phenomenon of overextension may be more salient to the listener than it is pervasive in children's word use. Most of children's early words are not overextended. Rescorla (1980) reported on the basis of 6 children whom she followed from 12 to 18 months that 33% of word uses were overextended but that only a few different words accounted for a disproportionate share of those overextensions. The bases of overextensions seem to be many, including perceptual similarity to the original word referent (e. g. *dog* for wolf), functional similarity (e. g., *hat* for a shirt stuck on someone's head) and contextual association (e. g., a child pointing to his father's briefcase and saying *Daddy*). Where overextensions occur, there is disagreement concerning the extent to which these overextended uses reveal children's overgeneral representations of word meanings or reflect a communicative strategy that is forced by the child's limited vocabulary (Huttenlocher/Smiley 1987, Hudson/Nelson 1984). As children acquire more differentiated vocabularies, for example words for animals other than *dog*, overextensions decline (Rescorla 1980).

2.2.1.2. Later Lexical Development

Less research attention has been given to the course of productive lexical development after the age of two years, although it is clear that changes take place in the size of children's vocabularies, the content of children's vocabularies, and possibly the ease with which new words are acquired. In terms of size, Templin (1957) estimated that children have vocabularies of approximately 8,000 words by 6 years and approximately 18,000 words at 8 years. In terms of content, children acquire new types of words that encode meanings and/or serve syntactic functions that are absent in the speech of younger children. For example, children add adverbs, syntactic connectives, and terms that indicate temporal and causal relations to their vocabularies (Bloom/Lahey/Hood et al. 1980, French/Nelson 1985, Scott 1984). In terms of the process of acquisition, Rice (1990) has suggested that starting at age 3 years, and increasingly thereafter, children become better at picking up new words (particularly object labels) from incidental exposure in context. There are also late-appearing errors in children's word use such as the production of novel verbs (e. g. *unstraighten* meaning to bend) or verbs used in novel ways (e. g., *Don't comb me baldheaded*) that appear to reflect that lexical development consists of changes in children's understanding of lexical principles – not just the acquisition of increasing numbers of lexical items (Bowerman 1985).

2.2.2. Comprehension

Children understand words in their language before they produce any, and it seems to take children less time to learn new words for the purpose of comprehension than to learn new words that are used in production. There are anecdotal reports of children as young as 5 months selectively responding to words (Vihman 1988). In her longitudinal study of eight children, Benedict (1979) found that children attained comprehension vocabularies of 20 words at ages ranging from 10 to 16 months. The average rate of growth in comprehension vocabulary during this period was 22 words per month. Comparison of these figures to comparable figures for the development of productive vocabulary reveals that comprehension vocabulary not only precedes productive vocabulary but also develops more rapidly even after productive language begins.

In addition to the differences in the times of onset and rates of lexical development in comprehension and in production, there are several other asymmetries between children's comprehension vocabularies and the vocabularies they use in productive language. The most obvious asymmetry is in size. Children's comprehension vocabularies are larger than their productive vocabularies at every age tested (Benedict 1979, Goldin-Meadow/Seligman/Gelman 1976). Comprehension and production vocabularies also differ in content. Benedict (1979) and Goldin-Meadow et al. found that there were proportionately more verbs in children's comprehension vocabularies than in their production vocabularies, perhaps, as Gentner (1978) has suggested, because communication works adequately with a minimal verb vocabulary. As noted before, however, the cross-linguistic generality of the later acquisition of verbs is suspect. Overextensions of word meanings, which is one of the most noted characteristics of early word use, occurs little, if at all, in comprehension (Kay/Anglin 1982, Chapman/Thompson 1980, Fregmen/Fay 1980, Huttenlocher 1974). Thus, the picture of early vocabulary development is one of greater competence in comprehension than in production, although occasionally children have underextended representations of word meanings or use words only in specific situations thereby appearing more competent than they really are.

The relation between comprehension and production for later-acquired terms is different. That picture is captured well in French/Nelson's (1985) treatment of the development of words that indicate relational meanings. Terms that express relations between propositions, such as *if, or, but,* and so forth, were correctly used in children's spontaneous speech as early as age 3, despite the fact that children failed to show full command of all the contrastive meanings of these terms in experimental tests of comprehension even years later (e. g., French 1988). Bassano/Champaud (1989) report similar findings for the French connective *même*.

One possible explanation for the discrepancy between the production and comprehension data is that children can use not-fully-acquired terms correctly by using them in memorized routines that are imitated from adult speech, such as *brush your teeth before you go to bed.* However, most of the utterances in French and Nelson's data base seem more likely to be children's own productions because they are things adults are unlikely ever to have said. Utterances that are factually incorrect are perhaps the clearest examples of utterances that are unlikely to be imitations (e.g., ... *a waiter comes, and if he sees us, he tells us what I, what I, what us, what what I want here.*) French and Nelson's explanation for children's ability to produce relational terms before they demonstrate full competence in comprehending relational terms is that young children can display competencies in the supportive context of describing familiar events that they are unable to display in typical experimental settings.

2.3. Grammatical Development

2.3.1. Production

2.3.1.1. The Emergence of Grammatical Structure in Children's Speech

The first time children combine two words or a single word plus a bound morpheme (such as adding a plural *-s* to a noun) in one utterance, they have reached a major landmark in their productive speech – the beginning of grammar. This landmark is typically reached around 18 to 24 months and only after children spend several months talking in single word utterances. Although the beginning of grammar is a significant landmark, it is not always an obvious one. Some children – typically those who produce long strings of jargon – produce utterances longer than one word by inserting one clear word into what is otherwise an incomprehensible babble sequence. Most children have at least some multiword phrases in their repertoires that have been memorized as unanalyzed wholes and that therefore do not reflect the development of the ability to combine words (Peters 1986). (*Iwant* and *Idon'tknow* are examples of unanalyzed wholes that are common in children's early language.) To further complicate matters, all these phenomena may exist simultaneously so that one child's 2-word utterances may include some rote-learned wholes, some filler + word combinations, and some truly productive word combinations. Some children seem to make heavy use of rote learned phrases, and the distinction between a word-by-word, analytic approach to language acquisition and a wholistic, gestalt approach to language acquisition is a major dimension of individual difference (Peters 1983). For some children grammatical development begins with a clear 2-word stage that may last for several months, and for other children the 2-word stage is brief and barely identifiable as a separate stage preceding the next landmark – the production of utterances with 3 or more words.

The first 2-, 3-, and 4-word utterances that children produce can be characterized as word-order correct (typically declarative form) sequences of words from the major grammatical categories of nouns, verbs, and adjectives, with few grammatical functors such as articles, prepositions, auxiliaries, and noun and verb inflections. Pronouns are frequent in the early word combinations of some children and rare in the speech of other children (Bloom/Lightbown/Hood 1975). Children's first sentences are frequently described as telegraphic because of their similarity to the style adopted by adults when writing telegrams in which each additional word carries a cost. Only the high information bearing words are included; inflections and words whose main functions is to mark grammatical structure are omitted (Brown/Fraser 1963). (This similarity to adults' telegrams is limited to the grammatical structure of utterances. The content of children's early multiword utterances, unlike that of telegrams, tends to be context bound.) The telegraphic quality of children's early word combinations has been reported in studies of children acquiring a variety of languages. However, children seem to acquire inflectional systems earlier in the course of language development if their language has a rich and regular inflectional system (Berman 1986). And children acquiring Turkish, which has a highly regular, rich, and perceptually salient inflectional system, have been reported to produce inflected forms prior to combining words (Aksu-Koc/Slobin 1985).

The appearance of 3-word utterances in children's speech is a major landmark in the course of grammatical development because it is at about this point that most children begin to add grammatical morphemes to their sentences. Children appear to follow relatively similar courses of early morphological development – albeit at varying rates. In his widely-known longitudinal study of Adam, Eve, and Sarah, Brown (1973) found that the orders of acquisition of some of the grammatical morphemes of English were very similar in the development of these three children, and the general sequence that he found was largely replicated in a cross-sectional study of children's spontaneous speech (de Villiers/de Villiers 1973a). These sources suggest, for example, that the present progressive verb inflection *(-ing)*, the plural noun inflection *(-*

s), and the prepositions *in* and *on* are among the first-acquired grammatical morphemes. Auxiliaries (i. e., the *is* in *is going* and the *have* in *have been*) are the latest acquired. In these studies, a grammatical morpheme was considered to have been "acquired" when it was used in 90% of obligatory contexts. However, when grammatical morphemes first appear they may not be used equally across all syntactic contexts, but instead their use may be limited by semantic factors. For example, when *-ing* first appears it is not used with all verbs but only with verbs that describe durative, non-completive action, and this sort of semantic constraint on the use of verb inflections has been found in children acquiring languages other than English (Bloom/Lifter/Hafitz 1980).

Another syntactic development, which typically begins around the time the first grammatical morphemes appear, is the development of the linguistic means for marking negation and asking questions. As Tager-Flusberg (1989) describes, children tend to first express negatives in utterances like *Not sit down* and to express questions in forms like *Where Daddy go?* Later, children use more advanced, but still not adult-like, forms such as *I no want book* and *What she is playing?* Children use adult forms of negatives and questions fairly late in syntactic development – at least in English – because these sentence forms depend on the acquisition of auxiliaries, and auxiliaries are among the last grammatical functors to be acquired.

After the development of grammatical morphemes and the development of different sentence forms is well under way, the next grammatical development is the appearence of sentences that contain more than one clause. The order of appearance of complex constructions in spontaneous speech (based on Bowerman 1979, Brown 1973, Limber 1973) appears to be first object complement constructions (e. g., *I see you sit down*), followed by wh- embedded clauses (e. g., *Can I do it when we go home*?), followed by coordinating and subordinating clause structures. Children produce complex sentences with *and* as the coordinating conjunction first (e. g., *You play with this one and I play with this*). Subordinate clause structures, such as clauses introduced with *before, after, because,* and so on, appear later with the order of appearance of particular conjunctions depending in part on the complexity of the concepts that they encode (Bloom/Lahey/Hood et al. 1980). Complex sentences first appear in children's speech around the age of 2½, and children use most of the major types of complex constructions by the age of 4 (Bowerman 1979, Limber 1973).

Probably for this reason, it is frequently asserted that children have essentially mastered the grammar of their language by the time they are 4 years old. However, there is good evidence that a further landmark is reached at 5 years when children begin to use grammatical devices to organize cohesive text. According to Karmiloff-Smith (1986), what changes at 5 years is not so much the forms children produce, but the way in which the forms are used and the internal linguistic representation of these forms. For example, pronouns are present in the speech of 2 and 3 year olds, but at that age the function of pronouns is only deictic, that is, to refer to a particular extralinguistic referent. For 2- to 3-year-old children, each utterance is a unit unto itself – its content and structure constrained only by the need to make the utterance match its nonlinguistic referent. It is only at age 5 that children start to connect sentences in discourse. Therefore, only at this time do pronouns come to be used anaphorically, that is, to refer to a referent in a prior utterance.

2.3.1.2. Meanings Expressed in Early Grammatical Speech

The semantic content of children's early multi-morphemic utterances is limited. In their early speech children talk almost exclusively about the here-and-now, and even at 3 years mention of absent or imaginary events is rare (Sachs 1983). In addition, children express a limited number of relational meanings in their first word combinations. Brown (1973) proposed a list of 8 semantic relations that he claimed accounted for the majority of meanings that children acquiring a variety of languages express in their first 2-word utterances. That list included relations between agents and actions (e. g., *Daddy sit*), actions and objects (e. g., *Drive car*), agents and objects (e. g., *Mommy sock*), actions and locations (e. g., *sit chair*), entities and locations (e. g., *toy floor*), possessors and possessions (e. g., *my teddy*), entities and attributes (e. g., *crayon big*), and demonstratives with entities (e. g., *this telephone*). (See also Bloom/Lightbown/Hood 1975 for a description of the semantic/syntactic relations in early combinatorial speech). When children begin to produce 3- and 4-word utterances, according to Brown, their utterances consist of combinations of these 2-term relations – with the redundant term mentioned only once (e. g., agent and action combined with action and locative yields an utterance such as *Daddy sit chair*). As children's syntax develops there is an increase in the proportion of their utterances that express 3- and 4-term relations.

2.3.1.3. Measuring Grammatical Development

As children acquire the grammar of their language, their utterances become increasingly complex, and this complexity results in the utterances becoming increasingly long. Because children seem to follow similar courses in adding complexity, the average length of children's utterances (counted in morphemes) has been widely used as a measure of syntactic development. Children with similar mean utterance lengths (MLUs) have been found to be similar to each other in other grammatical properties of their speech including the grammatical morphemes used and the phrasal and clausal structures used – up to an MLU of 3.0 (Rondal/Ghiotto/Bredart/Bachelet 1987). According to Brown (1973), MLU is a better predictor of the grammatical properties of children's speech than is age, and a timetable of grammatical development described in terms of MLU is more accurate than one described in terms of age. Brown used MLU as the basis for defining five stages of syntactic development. That stage terminology, somewhat modified subsequent to Brown's original proposal by Brown and others (de Villiers/de Villiers 1973 b, Miller/Chapman 1981) is widely used in the child language literature. The stages and their associated MLU intervals (based on Miller/Chapman 1981) are as follows: Early Stage I MLU = 1.0 – 1.5, Late Stage I MLU = 1.5 – 2.0; Stage II MLU = 2.0 – 2.5, Stage III MLU = 2.5 – 3.0, Early Stage IV MLU = 3.0 – 3.5, Late Stage IV and Early Stage V MLU = 3.5 – 4.0, Late Stage V MLU = 4.0 – 4.5. The major accomplishment of Stage I is the beginning of combinatorial speech, and the major accomplishment of Stage II is the beginning of morphological development. Sentence modalities (i. e., negative and question forms) begin to develop during Stage III, and complex sentences begin to emerge at Stage IV and continue to develop during Stage V. Based on Miller/Chapman's (1981) analysis of normally-developing American middle-class children, the age ranges during which approximately two thirds of children can be expected to reach these stages are as follows: Early Stage I, 16 – 26 months; Late Stage I, 18 – 31 months; Stage II, 21 – 35 months; Stage III, 24 – 41 months; Early Stage IV, 28 – 45 months, and Late Stage IV to Early Stage V, 31 – 50 months. However, the usefulness of MLU as a general index of grammatical development has been challenged by empirical findings that the power of MLU to differentiate among children at different levels of grammatical development is limited (Klee/Fitzgerald 1985), and the premise underlying the use of MLU as an index of grammatical development does not apply to children whose multi-morphemic utterances consist largely of a repertoire of rote-learned wholes.

2.3.2. Comprehension

The relation between comprehension and production in grammatical development echoes the relation between comprehension and production that was found for lexical development. That is, early developments occur receptively before they appear in production, but complex constructions first appear in children's spontaneous speech years before children demonstrate solid mastery in comprehension. In a task in which very young children can demonstrate sentence comprehension merely by looking longer at a videotaped event that matches a sentence than at a carefully controlled, but mismatched event, Hirsh-Pasek/Golinkoff (in press) have demonstrated that 17-month-old one-word speakers are sensitive to meaning carried by word order (e. g., they discriminate between *Cookie Monster's tickling Big Bird* and *Big Bird's tickling Cookie Monster*) and that 28-month-olds are sensitive to the distinction between the transitive and intransitive meanings of verbs (e. g., they discriminate between *Big Bird is turning Cookie Monster* and *Big Bird is turning with Cookie Monster*). Using more conventional methods, other researchers have also found that one-word speakers understand the meanings in multiword utterances, although in these cases there was no controlled test of meaning distinctions marked solely by syntax (Huttenlocher 1974, Sachs/Truswell 1978). Children who were just beginning to combine words have shown evidence of understanding word-order marked meanings (de Villiers/de Villiers 1973b), and telegraphic speakers have been found to be more responsive to commands that included grammatical morphemes than to commands that were more like the speech the children were producing themselves (Shipley/Smith/Gleitman 1969). In some circumstances 17-month-old girls, but not boys, have demonstrated understanding of the common-proper noun distinction marked only by the presence or absence of an article (e. g., *a biff* to indicate one of a class of items vs. *Biff* to indicate a particular item) (Katz/Baker/Macnamara 1974).

This picture of early comprehension of basic aspects of grammar before those grammatical devices appear in spontaneous speech contrasts with the results of studies of the comprehension of later-appearing grammatical structures. With respect to comprehension of complex sentences, the literature presents a complicated and not always consistent picture of children's abilities (Bowerman 1979). Two conclusions seem relatively clear: First, children employ a variety of strategies for interpreting complex sentences before children are capable of full analysis of the linguistic structures. For example, children interpret the order in which events are mentioned in a sentence to indicate the order in which those events occurred. This works for interpreting sentences such as *John played before Mary sang*, but it yields misinterpretations of sentences such as *John played after Mary sang* or *Before Mary sang, John played.* Second, how children interpret complex sentences is highly dependent on the nature of the experimental tasks that are employed. Reviewing studies of the comprehension of a variety of complex forms in different languages, Karmiloff-Smith (1986) concluded that children reach another landmark in language development at the age of 8 when their performance on comprehension tasks becomes consistent and unshakable, no matter how unnatural and contrived the experimental task. Karmiloff-Smith describes this landmark as the achievement of the capacity to cope with language abstractly. At that point children can process sentences without the support of the normally-present extralinguistic and discourse contexts.

3. The Development of Communicative Competence

3.1. Overview

Children who have acquired the sound system, the vocabulary, and the grammar of their language have acquired a system for expressing meaning in a sequence of uttered sounds. The most obvious manifestation of this accomplishment is that children communicate with other people by talking. In the last section of this chapter we briefly discuss the course of the development of the communicative functions to which language is put and the development of the discourse skills involved in talking to others.

3.2. The Development of Communicative Functions

Children produce vocalizations and other behaviors that have the effect of communicating before children acquire language. The cries and coos that infants produce can be interpreted by adults as signals of infants' internal states. However, these signals – at least initially – are reflexive, and their communicative value depends on adults' inclination to interpret these signals. A landmark in communicative development appears to be reached at 8 to 10 months when children start to use combinations of vocalizations, eye gaze, and sometimes touch for the purpose of gaining help in obtaining objects (Harding/Golinkoff 1979, Sugarman-Bell 1978). Exactly what sort of intentions these behaviors indicate is a matter of some dispute. Shatz (1983) and Shatz/Watson O'Reilly (1990) have argued that these prelinguistic behaviors and even the seemingly communicative behaviors of 1- and 2-year-olds are evidence only that children know that they can fulfill their own goals via others. Children do not have truly communicative intentions, that is, intentions to share ideas, until they have developed an understanding of the mental states of others – typically not before 3 years. However, a less restrictive definition of communication is more common, and those adopting a more liberal stance with respect to attributing communicative intent to young children have identified multiple communicative functions served by children's prespeech vocalizations and gestures and by children's early speech.

Chapman (1981) has surveyed the many systems that have been proposed for categorizing children's communicative intents, and her summary suggests the following description of the course of communicative development: At 8 to 10 months infants use gesture to request objects or activity, to reject, and to comment. Between 9 and 15 months vocalization is added to and eventually replaces gesture as a means for communicating these same intentions. During this period from 8 to 15 months the first words typically appear, yet, despite the availability of this means of reference, children's communicative intentions always pertain to something in the physical context. Between 16 and 22 months, as children's linguistic skills develop, children start also to express intentions that refer to the discourse itself – they request information, answer questions, and acknowledge prior speech. At approximately 24 months children begin to use language to refer to absent objects and events and to use language imaginatively, as in pretend play. Most descriptions of changes in the functions of child speech after 2 years focus on changes in the discourse functions of speech – for example children learn to query, to answer questions appropriately, to request clarification, and so on. An exception to this is Tough's (1977) system, which identifies four major meaning-defined functions of language in the speech of 3- to 7-year-old children: Language is used to direct the behavior of self and others, to interpret experience and to reason, to project (i. e. to refer to future events, other peoples' internal states, and imaginary contexts) and to mediate social relations. Tough's work focuses more on social class differences in the use of language than on developmental changes. Her controversial proposal is that children from more advantaged backgrounds use language for interpreting and projecting more frequently than do children from less advantaged backgrounds. (See Wells (1977) for a contrary view).

3.3. The Development of Discourse Skill

In Western culture, adults interact with infants in formats that have the rough structure of conversation from the time the infant is born (Snow 1977). Very young babies contribute to these interactions by looking at their mothers when the mothers vocalize. However, the turn-taking structure of the early interactions appears to depend on mothers building a conversational structure around their children's behavior, and it does not reflect interactive skill on the part of infants (Shatz 1983). There is no clear landmark that signifies the child's entry into conversational participation. Rather, the relative burdens carried by the adult and the child in sustaining conversation gradually become more equal as children develop an understanding that they have responsibilities as conversational participants, as they learn what is required of them to fulfill these responsibilities in different linguistic contexts, and as they master the linguistic devices for meeting those requirements (Shatz 1983).

One-year-old children demonstrate that they know that another speaker's utterance calls for some sort of response. An early strategy is to respond with action. This strategy is effective in allowing young children to respond appropriately to much of what is typically said to them such as *Why don't you play in the sandbox?* and *Where are your shoes?* However, the unsophisticated basis of such responding is revealed when an experimenter asks a 2-year-old *Why don't you wear shoes on your head?* and the child complies rather than answers verbally (Shatz 1978). Although children continue to rely on this action strategy in some circumstances, by 18 months children begin to more reliably respond to talk with talk, particularly in response to *where* or *what* questions (Chapman 1981). Before they reach 2 years children also respond differently to different types of utterances. They respond more frequently to questions than to non-questions (Bloom/Rocissano/Hood 1976, Hoff-Ginsberg 1990), and they respond to different forms of question with appropriately different forms of reply (Shatz 1983).

Thus 2-year-old children show a rudimentary ability to participate in conversation, but children improve considerably in that ability over the next few years. One salient change is an increase in the length of conversation that children are able to sustain. Brown (1980) estimated that the number of topically-related utterances children can produce in sequence (related either to their own prior utterance or to intervening utterances by adults) changed from an average of less than 1 utterance at MLU = 1.0 to an average of over 20 related utterances at MLU = 3.0 (This range in MLU, and the correlated variability in discourse skill, was found in a sample of 21 children all of whom were 30 months old.) Probably contributing to this increase in the length of conversations children can sustain are increases in children's abilities both to initiate topics and to produce utterances relevant to the topic under discussion (Bloom/Rocissano/Hood 1976, Foster 1986, Hoff-Ginsberg 1987). The most marked change in children's discourse that Bloom et al. found during the period from Stage I to Stage V was an increase in the proportion of children's responses that added new information that was relevant to the topic of the prior speaker's utterance. There is also development after 2 years of age in children's sensitivity to the discourse requirements of different types of utterances as evidenced by increases in the appropriateness of their replies. For example, 2-year-olds commonly respond to *why* questions as though they were *what* questions; 3- and 4-years-olds do so less frequently (Shatz/McCloskey 1984). Another developmental change in children's conversation is the emergence of new linguistic devices for maintaining discourse cohesion. For example, anaphoric use of pronouns to refer to a noun introduced earlier in discourse begins with the use of *I* at Stage II, and *you* appears at Stage IV. Auxiliary ellipsis appears at Stage IV or V (e. g., *Ellen did.* in response to *Who came?*) (Ervin-Tripp 1978).

Thus far we have been describing the developmental changes in how children fill their roles in conversation with an adult. Children also converse with peers from a farily early age. Keenan/Klein (1975), reporting on the early morning crib conversations of a pair of twin boys aged 2 ½, provide evidence that the children attended to each other's utterances and produced related responses. However, many of these related responses were not topically related but rather relied on repetition and sound play to maintain discourse cohesion. More truly social conversation among peers seems to emerge around the age of 3, and children improve at sustaining conversation through the school years (Dorval/Eckerman 1984, Garvey/Hogan 1973, Mueller/Bleier/Krakow et al. 1977). For example, Garvey/Hogan (1973) found in the free play interactions of previously unacquainted 3 ½- to 5-year-old children that children were able to sustain sequences of talk between 4 and 12 or more exchanges long and that between 21% and 77% of the children's utterances were contingent on the verbal or nonverbal behavior of others. Why preschoolers are sometimes social in their conversations but sometimes produce talk unrelated to what has preceded it may have in part to do with whether the children share background knowledge. Nelson/Gruendel (1979) have suggested that true dialogue between preschoolers is facilitated when shared knowledge of routines such as planning a meal or going shopping provides a script for their conversation. (See McTear (1985) for a comprehensive description of the development of conversation). Another conversational skill that children have is the ability to monitor the conversations of others and to take advantage of opportunities to gain the floor for themselves. The rudiments of this ability can be seen in 2-year-olds' intrusions into the conversations between their mothers and older siblings (Dunn/Shatz 1989), and that skill continues to develop through the preschool years (Forrester 1988).

4. Some Closing Words

The goal of this chapter was to paint in broad strokes a picture of the course of normal language development. Of necessity, much that is interesting and important was left out. Nothing was said about language development past the age of 8 years, although the exposure to reading, to writing, and to peer influences that come with entry to school affect all the aspects of linguistic and communicative development that were discussed in this chapter. The discussion of the development of discourse skills concentrated on conversation and ignored the burgeoning research on children's development of narrative skills. Perhaps the most serious omission for a chapter in a handbook on pathologies of language development is the omission of a full discussion of the range of individual differences in the course of early language development that nonetheless culminate in normal language acquisition. The chapter provided age ranges for the achievement of the landmarks it described, and those ranges can serve as a guide to the range of differences in language development rate that is observed in normal populations. However, normally-developing children differ in more than their rates of language development. Children present varied complexes of language capabilities.

A metaphor for language development that has been used by several authors is that it is a rope composed of multiple independent but interwoven strands (Peters 1986, Snow 1988, Tager-Flusberg 1988). The aspects of language development that were reviewed in this chapter – phonological development, lexical development, grammatical development, and the developments of communicative intentions and conversational skills – are major strands in that rope. The evidence suggests that children follow relatively consistent orders of development along each strand, but that children vary in the rates at which they progress – not only overall, but on each separate strand. Each individual child's language level at any given point in development is a composite of his or her levels of development on different strands. Using this metaphor, then, individual differences among children result from asynchronies of development along the various strands. I end this chapter with this metaphor in the hope that it helps to bridge the gap between the simplified picture of normative language development that this chapter has provided and the more complex and unique courses of development that individual children follow.

Author's note: I am grateful to JoAnn Buhr, Lucia French, Wendy Leeds-Hurwitz, and Amy Weiss for their thoughtful comments on an earlier version of this chapter.

5. References

Aksu-Koc, A. A. & Slobin, D. I. (1985). The acquisition of Turkish. In D. I. Slobin (Ed.), *The crosslinguistic study of language acquisition, volume 1: the data. 839–880.* Hillsdale, NJ: Erlbaum.

Barton, D. (1975). Statistical significance in phonemic perception experiments. *Journal of Child Language, 2,* 297–298.

Barton, D. (1978). The discrimination of minimally-different pairs of real words by children aged 2;3 to 2;11. In N. Waterson & C. Snow (Eds.), *The development of communication. 255–261.* New York: John Wiley.

Bassano, D. & Champaud, C. (1989). The argumentative connective *même* in French: an experimental study in eight-to ten-year-old children. *Journal of Child Language, 16,* 643–664.

Bates, E. (1976). *Language and context: the acquisition of pragmatics.* New York: Academic Press.

Bates, E., Benigni, L., Bretherton, I., Camaioni, L., & Volterra, V. (1979). *The emergence of symbols: cognition and communication in infancy.* New York: Academic Press.

Benedict, H. (1979). Early lexical development: comprehension and production. *Journal of Child Language, 6,* 183–200.

Berman, R. A. (1986). A crosslinguistic perspective: morphology and syntax. In P. Fletcher & M. Garman (Eds.), *Language acquistion, 2nd edition. 429–447.* Cambridge: Cambridge University Press.

Bloom, L., Lahey, M., Hood, L., Lifter, K., & Fiess, K. (1980). Complex sentences: acquisition of syntactic connectives and the semantic relations they encode. *Journal of Child Language, 7,* 235–261.

Bloom, L., Lifter, K., & Hafitz, J. (1980). Semantics of verbs and the development of verb inflections in child language. *Language, 56,* 386–412.

Bloom, L., Lightbown, P., & Hood, L. (1975). Structure and variation in child language. *Monographs of the Society for Research in Child Development, 40* (2, Serial no. 160).

Bloom, L., Rocissano, L., & Hood, L. (1976). Adult-child discourse: developmental interaction between information processing and linguistic knowledge. *Cognitive Psychology, 8,* 521–552.

Bowerman, M. (1979). The acquisition of complex sentences. In P. Fletcher & M. Garman (Eds.), *Language acquisition. 285–306.* Cambridge: Cambridge University Press.

Bowerman, M. (1985). Beyond communicative adequacy: From piecemeal knowledge to an intergrated system in the child's acquisition of language. In K. E. Nelson (Ed.), *Children's language, vol. 5. 369–398.* Hillsdale, NJ: Erlbaum.

Brown, R. (1973). *A first language: the early stages.* Cambridge, MA: Harvard University Press.

Brown, R. (1980). The maintenance of conversation. In D. R. Olson (Ed.), *The social foundations of language and thought. 187–210.* New York: W. W. Norton.

Brown, R. & Fraser, C. (1963). The acquisition of syntax. In C. N. Cofer & B. Musgrave (Eds.), *Verbal behavior and learning: problems and processes. 158–209.* New York: McGraw-Hill.

Butler, S. (1920). *The way of all flesh.* New York: E. P. Dutton & Co. Reprinted as "The tum phenomenon" in the *Journal of Child Language,* 1980, *7,* 428–429.

Carter, A. L. (1979). Prespeech meaning relations: an outline of one infant's sensorimotor morpheme development. In P. Fletcher & M. Garman (Eds.), *Language acquisition. 71–92.* Cambridge: Cambridge University Press.

Chapman, R. S. (1981). Exploring children's communicative intents. In J. F. Miller (Ed.), *Assessing language production in children. 111–136.* Austin, TX: Pro-Ed.

Chapman, R. S. & Thompson, J. (1980). What is the source of overextension errors in comprehension testing of two-year-olds? A response to Fregmen and Fay. *Journal of Child Language, 7,* 575–578.

Clancy, P. (1985). Acquisition of Japanese. In D. I. Slobin (Ed.), *The crosslinguistic study of language acquisition, volume 1: the data. 373–524.* Hillsdale, NJ: Erlbaum.

Clark, E. V. (1979). Building a vocabulary: words for objects, actions, and relations. In P. Fletcher & M. Garman (Eds.), *Language acquisition. 149–160.* Cambridge: Cambridge University Press.

Crystal, D. (1986). Prosodic development. In P. Fletcher & M. Garman (Eds.), *Language acquisition, 2nd edition. 174–197.* Cambridge: Cambridge University Press.

Dale, P. S. (1976). *Language development: structure and function, 2nd edition.* Chicago, IL: Holt, Reinhart & Winston.

de Boysson-Bardies, B., Sagart, L., & Durand, C. (1984). Discernible differences in the babbling of infants according to target language. *Journal of Child Language, 11,* 1–15.

de Villiers, J. & de Villiers, P. (1973a). A cross-sectional study of the acquisition of grammatical morphemes in child speech. *Journal of Psycholinguistic Research, 2,* 267–278.

de Villiers, J. & de Villiers, P. (1973b). Development of the use of word order in comprehension. *Journal of Psycholinguistic Research, 2,* 331–341.

Dore, J., Franklin, M. B., Miller, R., & Ramer, A. L. H. (1976). Transitional phenomena in early language acquisition. *Journal of Child Language, 3,* 13–28.

Dorval, B. & Eckerman, C. O. (1984). Developmental trends in the quality of conversation achieved by small groups of acquainted peers. *Monographs of the Society for Research in Child Development.* (*49,* Serial no. 206).

Dromi, E. (1990). Word-meaning acquisition in the one word stage: a reply to Nelson's review. *First Language, 10,* 75–82.

Dunn, J. & Shatz, M. (1989). Becoming a conversationalist despite (or because of) having an older sibling. *Child Development, 60,* 399–410.

Eilers, R. (1980). Infant speech perception: history and mystery. In G. Yeni-Komshian, J. F. Kavanagh, & C. A. Ferguson (Eds.), *Child phonology: Vol. 2 perception. 23–39.* New York: Academic Press.

Eilers, R. E., Gavin, W. J., & Oller, K. K. (1982). Cross-linguistic perception in infancy: early effects of linguistic experience. *Journal of Child Language, 9,* 289–302.

Eilers, R., Oller, D. K., Bull, D., & Gavin, W. (1984). Linguistic experience and infant perception: a reply to Jusczyk, Shea & Aslin (1984). *Journal of Child Language, 11,* 467–475.

Ervin-Tripp, S. (1978). Some features of early child-adult dialogues. *Language in Society, 7,* 357–373.

Ferguson, C. A. & Farwell, C. B. (1975). Words and sounds in early language acquisition. *Language, 51,* 439–491.

Fey, M. & Gandour, J. (1982). Rule discovery in early phonology acquisition. *Journal of Child Language, 9,* 71–82.

Forrester, M. A. (1988). Young children's polyadic conversation monitoring skills. *First Language, 8,* 201–226.

Foster, S. H. (1986). Learning discourse topic management in the preschool years. *Journal of Child Language, 13,* 231–250.

Fregmen, A. & Fay, D. (1980). Overextensions in production and comprehension: a methodological clarification. *Journal of Child Language, 7,* 205–211.

French, L. A. (1988). The development of children's understanding of "because" and "so." *Journal of Experimental Child Psychology, 45,* 262–279.

French, L. A. & Nelson, K. (1985). *Young children's knowledge of relational terms: some ifs, ors and buts.* New York: Springer-Verlag.

Garnica, O. (1973). The development of phonemic speech perception. In T. E. Moore (Ed.), *Cognitive development and the acquisition of language. 215–222.* New York: Academic Press.

Garvey, C. & Hogan, R. (1973). Social speech and social interaction: egocentrism revisited. *Child Development, 44,* 562–568.

Gentner, D. (1978). On relational meaning: the acquisition of verb meaning. *Child Development, 49,* 988–998.

Goad, H. & Ingram, D. (1987). Individual variation and its relevance to a theory of phonological acquisition. *Journal of Child Language, 14,* 419–432.

Goldfield, B. A. & Reznick, J. S. (1990). Early lexical acquisition: rate, content, and the vocabulary spurt. *Journal of Child Language, 17,* 171–184.

Goldin-Meadow, S., Seligman, M. E. P., & Gelman, R. (1976). Language in the two-year-old. *Cognition, 4,* 189–202.

Gopnik, A. (1988). Three types of early word: the emergence of social words, names and cognitive relational words in the one-word stage and their relation to cognitive development. *First Language, 8,* 49–70.

Gopnik, A. & Choi, S. (1990). Do linguistic differences lead to cognitive differences? A crosslinguistic study of semantic and cognitive development. *First Language, 10,* 199–215.

Gopnik, A. & Meltzoff, A. N. (1987). The development of categorization in the second year and its relation to other cognitive and linguistic developments. *Child Development, 58,* 1523–1531.

Grunwell, P. (1986). Aspects of phonological development in later childhood. In K. Durkin (Ed.), *Language development in the school years. 34–56.* Cambridge, MA: Brookline Books.

Harding, C. G. & Golinkoff, R. M. (1979). The origins of intentional vocalizations in prelinguistic infants. *Child Development, 50,* 33–40.

Hirsh-Pasek, K. & Golinkoff, R. M. (1991). Language comprehension: a new look at some old themes. In N. A. Krasnegor, D. M. Rumbaugh, R. L. Schiefelbusch & M. Studdert-Kennedy (Eds.), *Biological and behavioral determinants of language development. 301–320.* Hillsdale, NJ: Erlbaum.

Hoff-Ginsberg, E. (1987). Topic relations in mother-child conversation. *First Language, 7,* 145–158.

Hoff-Ginsberg, E. (1990). Maternal speech and the child's development of syntax: a further look. *Journal of Child Language. 17,* 337–346.

Hudson, J. & Nelson, K. (1984). Play with language: overextensions as analogies. *Journal of Child Language, 11,* 337–346.

Huttenlocher, J. (1974). The origins of language comprehension. In R. Solso (Ed.), *Theories in cognitive psychology. 331–368.* New York: Erlbaum.

Huttenlocher, J. & Smiley, P. (1987). Early word meanings: the case of object names. *Cognitive Psychology, 19,* 63–89.

Ingram, D. (1986). Phonological development: production. In P. Fletcher & M. Garman (Eds.), *Language acquisition, 2nd edition. 223–239.* Cambridge: Cambridge University Press.

Ingram, D. (1988, June). Toward a theory of phonological acquisition. Paper presented at the Symposium on Research in Child Language Disorders, Madison, WI.

Ingram, D. (1989). *First language acquisition: method, description, and explanation.* Cambridge: Cambridge University Press.

Jusczyk, P. W., Shea, S. L., & Aslin, R. N. (1984). Linguistic experience and infant speech perception: a reexamination of Eilers, Gavin & Oller (1982). *Journal of Child Language, 11,* 453–466.

Karmiloff-Smith, A. (1986). Some fundamental aspects of language development after age 5. In P. Fletcher & M. Garman (Eds.), *Language acquisition, 2nd edition. 455–474.* Cambridge: Cambridge University Press.

Katz, N., Baker, E., & Macnamara, J. (1974). What's in a name? A study of how children learn common and proper names. *Child Development, 50,* 1–13.

Kay, D. A. & Anglin, J. M. (1982). Overextension and underextension in the child's expressive and receptive speech. *Journal of Child Language, 9,* 83–98.

Keenan, E. O. & Klein, E. (1975). Coherency in children's discourse. *Journal of Psycholinguistic Research, 4,* 365–380.

Klee, T. & Fitzgerald, M. D. (1985). The relation between grammatical development and mean length of utterance in morphemes. *Journal of Child Language, 12,* 251–270.

Leonard, L. B., Newhoff, M., & Meselam, L. (1980). Individual differences in early child phonology. *Applied Psycholinguistics, 1,* 7–30.

Limber, J. (1973). The genesis of complex sentences. In T. Moore (Ed.), *Cognitive development and the acquisition of language. 169–186.* New York: Academic Press.

Lucariello, J. (1987). Concept formation and its relation to word learning and use in the second year. *Journal of Child Language, 14,* 309–332.

McTear, M. (1985). *Children's conversation.* Oxford: Basil Blackwell.

Menyuk, P. & Menn, L. (1979). Early strategies for the perception and production of words and sounds. In P. Fletcher & M. Garman (Eds.), *Language acquisition. 49–70.* Cambridge: Cambridge University Press.

Menyuk, P., Menn, L., & Silber, R. (1986). Early strategies for the perception and production of words and sounds. In P. Fletcher & M. Garman (Eds.), *Language acquisition, 2nd edition. 198–222.* Cambridge: Cambridge University Press.

Miller, J. P. & Chapman, R. S. (1981). The relations between age and mean length of utterance. *Journal of Speech and Hearing Research, 24,* 154–161.

Mueller, E., Bleier, M., Krakow, J., Hegedus, K., & Cournoyer, P. (1977). The development of peer verbal interaction among two-year-old boys. *Child Development, 48,* 284–287.

Nelson, K. (1973). Structure and strategy in learning to talk. *Monographs of the Society for Research in Child Development,* 1978, *38* (1 and 2, Serial No. 149).

Nelson, K. & Gruendel, J. M. (1979). At morning it's lunchtime: A scriptal view of children's dialogues. *Discourse Processes, 2,* 73–94.

Nelson, K. & Lucariello, J. (1985). The development of meaning in first words. In M. Barrett (Ed.), *Children's single-word speech. 59–86.* New York: John Wiley.

Oller, D. K. (1986). Metaphonology and infant vocalizations. In B. Lindbloom & R. Zetterstrom (Eds.), *Precursors of early speech. 21–35.* Stockton Press.

Oviatt, S. L. (1982). Inferring what words mean: early development in infants' comprehension of common object names. *Child Development, 53,* 274–277.

Peters, A. M. (1983). *The units of language acquisition.* Cambridge: Cambridge University Press.

Peters, A. M. (1986). Early syntax. In P. Fletcher & M. Garman (Eds.), *Language acquisition, 2nd edition. 307–325.* Cambridge: Cambridge University Press.

Pye, C., Ingram, D., & List, H. (1987). A comparison of initial consonant acquisition in English and Quiche. In K. E. Nelson & A. van Kleeck (Eds.), *Children's language, vol. 6. 175–190.* Hillsdale, NJ: Erlbaum.

Rescorla, L. A. (1980). Overextension in early language development. *Journal of Child Language, 7,* 321–335.

Rescorla, L. A. (1981). Category development in early language. *Journal of Child Language, 8,* 225–238.

Rice, M. L. (1990). Preschooler's QUIL: Quick incidental learning of words. In G. Conti-Ramsden

& C. E. Snow (Eds.), *Children's language, vol. 7. 171–196.* Hillsdale, NJ: Erlbaum.

Rondal, J. A., Ghiotto, M., Bredart, S., & Bachelet, J-F. (1987). Age-relation, reliability and grammatical validity of measures of utterance length. *Journal of Child Language, 14,* 433–446.

Sachs, J. (1983). Talking about there and then: the emergence of displaced reference in parent-child discourse. In K. E. Nelson (Ed.), *Children's language, vol. 4. 1–28.* Hillsdale, NJ: Erlbaum.

Sachs, J. & Truswell, L. (1978). Comprehension of 2-word instructions by children in the 1-word stage. *Journal of Child Language, 5,* 17–24.

Sander, E. K. (1972). When are speech sounds learned? *Journal of Speech and Hearing Disorders, 37,* 55–63.

Schwartz, R. & Leonard, L. (1982). Do children pick and choose? An examination of phonological selection and avoidance in early acquisition. *Journal of Child Language, 9,* 319–336.

Scott, C. M. (1984). Adverbial connectivity in conversations of children 6 to 12. *Journal of Child Language, 11,* 423–452.

Shatz, M. (1978). On the development of communicative understandings: an early strategy for interpreting and responding to messages. *Cognitive Psychology, 10,* 271–301.

Shatz, M. (1983). Communication. In P. H. Mussen (Ed.), *Handbook of child psychology. 841–889.* New York: Wiley.

Shatz, M. & McCloskey, L. (1984). Answering appropriately: A developmental perspective on conversational knowledge. In S. Kuczaj (Ed.), *Discourse development. 19–36.* New York: Springer-Verlag.

Shatz, M. & Watson O'Reilly, A. (1990). Conversational or communicative skill? A reassessment of two year olds' behaviour in miscommunication episodes. *Journal of Child Language, 17,* 131–146.

Shipley, E. F., Smith, C. S., & Gleitman, L. (1969). A study in the acquisition of language: free responses to commands. *Language, 45,* 322–342.

Snow, C. E. (1977). The development of conversation between mothers and babies. *Journal of Child Language, 4,* 1–22.

Snow, C. E. (1988). The last word: questions about the emerging lexicon. In M. D. Smith & J. L. Locke (Eds.), *The emergent lexicon: the child's development of a linguistic vocabulary. 341–353.* San Diego: Academic Press.

Snyder, L., Bates, E., & Bretherton, I. (1981). Content and context in early lexical development. *Journal of Child Language, 8,* 565–582.

Stark, R. E. (1986). Prespeech segmental feature development. In P. Fletcher & M. Garman (Eds.), *Language acquisition, 2nd, edition. 149–173.* Cambridge: Cambridge University Press.

Stern, C. & Stern, W. (1907). *Die Kindersprache.* Leipzig: Barth.

Stoel-Gammon, C. & Cooper, J. (1984). Patterns of early lexical and phonological development. *Journal of Child Language, 11,* 247–271.

Sugarman-Bell, S. (1978). Some organizational aspects of pre-verbal communication. In I. Markova (Ed.), *The social context of language. 49–66.* New York: Wiley.

Tager-Flusberg, H. (1988). On the nature of a language acquisition disorder: the example of autism. In F. S. Kessel (Ed.), *The development of language and language researchers. 249–268.* Hillsdale, NJ: Erlbaum.

Tager-Flusberg, H. (1989). Putting words together: morphology and syntax in the preschool years. In J. Berko Gleason (Ed.), *The development of language, 2nd edition. 135–166.* Columbus, OH: Merrill Publishing Co.

Templin, M. (1957). *Certain language skills in children.* University of Minnesota Institute of Child Welfare Monograph Series 26. Minneapolis: University of Minnesota Press.

Tough, J. (1977). *The development of meaning.* London: Unwin Education Books.

Vihman, M. M. (1988). Early phonological development. In J. Bernthal & N. Bambson, (Eds.), *Articulation and phonological disorders, 2nd edition. 60–109.* NY: Prentice Hall.

Wells, G. (1977). Language use and educational success: an empirical response to Joan Tough's 'The Development of Meaning' (1977). *Research in Education, 18,* 9–34.

Erika Hoff-Ginsberg, Kenosha, Wisconsin (USA)

58. Definition and Diagnosis of Language Development Disorders

1. Introduction

The human mind is biologically prepared to learn language — at a predicable age, without formal instruction, and with remarkable rapidity and case. Children begin to combine words into phrases by age two. By age three, they are producing full sentences and learning nine words a day; by age six, they are fluent conversationalists and are using language to think about hypothetical events and absent worlds. This human faculty for language learning is normally robust, but a small group of children, some 3—5% of the population (Stevenson/Richman 1976; Beitchman/Nair/Clegg/Patel 1986), present a different picture. They are late to talk, have restricted vocabularies, struggle with oral grammar, and are frequently unsuccessful in using language as the tool of thought. Such language problems are seen in children with mental retardation, autism or hearing impairment and are presumed secondary to the neurological and/or metabolic states which underlie these syndromes. Language delays may also occur in the virtual absence of other symptoms of disorder. This condition is known as 'developmental dysphasia' or 'specific language impairment' (SLI) and is discussed in detail in subchapters 61—63, 75. The purpose of this subchapter is to provide an orientation to the broader spectrum of developmental language disorders, focussing in particular on issues related to assessment.

2. Decline of the Medical Model

2.1. The Model and Clinical Practice

Developmental language disorders have been studied for almost two centuries (Weiner 1984) with a consequent evolution in diagnostic categories and method. For much of this period, however, the primary investigators were physicians, e. g. the Berlin Sprachärzte Treitel and Liebmann, and the frameworks used to study the disorders were consistently drawn from the medical sciences. In such 'medical models', emphasis is placed on differential diagnosis and classification by etiology with the ultimate goal of identifying and describing the underlying condition so that a cure may be found.

As practiced in North America, application of the medical model to the diagnosis of language development disorders has meant determining (a) whether a child's language behavior meets chronological age expectations, and if not, (b) whether the language delay is the result of mental retardation, autism, hearing loss, or specific language impairment. Other conditions, e. g. elective mutism, cerebral palsy, or low vision, are recognized as having implications for language development but are not routinely considered in the diagnostic argument.

Standardized language measures are the current most reliable means for answering the first diagnostic question. In order to decide whether a child's language behavior meets age expectations, the clinician must have normative data on the language performance of children at various ages. At best, these data should come from ecologically valid tasks, administered to large, well-described and representative groups of children. The data should also reflect language knowledge of diverse sorts, have proven predictive value, and be organized so as to indicate variance as well as central tendency. Since the development of normative instruments requires considerable time and expense, it is not surprising that only a few of them meet many of these criteria (McCauley/Swisher 1984). Psychometric weaknesses clearly compromise the decisions made from normative data. Even when quantitative criteria are met, clinicians must frequently choose reliability and representativeness over ecological validity. Normative data from spontaneous language samples may eventually remedy that situation, but as yet such data come from modest sized samples (e. g. Miller/Chapman 1981; Rescorla 1989), limited population sectors (Lee 1974), and/or earlier times (Templin 1957). Despite these problems, in all but the most extreme cases, only standardized language measures can confirm the presence of a delay in language development and determine the extent of that delay.

Having concluded that a language delay exists, the clinician operating from within the medical model continues on to make decisions about the condition which underlies this delay. Audiometric testing is used to establish hearing acuity; neurological examination to establish motoric function; intelligence tests, particularly those requiring little or no language, to measure mental abilities; and psychiatric interviews and/or observations to determine the normalcy of the child's socio-emotional development. Informed by these additional data, the clinician assigns the child to one or another diagnostic category. Children with subnormal nonverbal intelligence, normal hearing, and no signs of affective disturbance are diagnosed as 'mentally retarded'; children with poor auditory acuity are diagnosed as 'hearing impaired'; children with an early lack of social responsiveness, or inappropriate affect and rigidity are diagnosed as 'autistic'; children with normal nonverbal intelligence, normal hearing, and normal social relations are diagnosed as having 'specific language impairment (developmental dysphasia)'. In practice, of course, the decisions are seldom so straightforward. Clinicians frequently find themselves debating the proper category for a child whose language seems poorer than would be expected for the extent of a hearing loss, or whose level of nonverbal intellectual development is lower than age expectations but higher than language levels. It is also increasingly unclear how the child with frank neurological impairment fits into this scheme. Until recently, specific language impairments were presumed to imply neurological dysfunction (Proceedings, 1962). Proof of that dysfunction was useful, but was not considered necessary to the diagnosis given the absence of all other etiological factors and the presence of the language delay itself. This, of course, led to groups of children with widely varying degrees of neurological involvement. Perhaps to minimize this diversity, some researchers now define 'specific language impairment' so as to exclude children with known neurological dysfunctions (Stark/Tallal 1981). Incorporation of this shift into clinical practice would require some subdivision of the SLI category.

In short, working within the tradition of the medical model, clinicians and scientists have established the major parameters of diagnosis for developmental language disorders and have generated large literatures on topics such as 'specific language impairment', 'language in the retarded', 'language in autism', etc. There are now, however, growing signs that the conventional categorical approach to developmental language disorders may no longer be productive (Lahey 1988; Marge 1972).

2.2. Shortcomings of the Medical Model

2.2.1. Lack of Empirical Validity

Only one group of researchers to date has reported a validation study for the categorical labels that are traditionally assigned to language disordered children. At Stanford University, Rosenthal/Eisenson/Luckau (1972) used cluster analysis techniques to group 82 language disordered children who had been examined at a suburban medical centre. Thirty two variables derived from medical examinations, EEG, psychological testing, and language testing were involved in the analysis. The researchers' goal was to compare the resultant clusters with the groupings created by the diagnostic judgements of the centre's staff, i. e. dysphasic, hearing impaired, apraxic, disarthric, retarded, autistic, maturational lag (organic). In fact, the statistical analysis yielded only two clusters of children, those originally designated as retarded or autistic, and those designated as hearing impaired, dysphasic, or maturational lag (organic). Within these two groupings, children were not reliably different; between the groupings, differences were primarily related to nonverbal intellectual functions, children in the first cluster functioning at lower levels. A further attempt at analysis used a reduced number of variables, two from psychological tests, two from observations of emotional health, and twelve from the medical examination. When applied to data from 138 children, this matrix yielded only one cluster, the retarded/autistic cluster (N = 71) identified previously. Each of the remaining children merged as a 'group' of one. Rosenthal and his colleagues conclude that "the original diagnostic categories ... are neither unique nor homogeneous with respect to measurements routinely collected in the course of clinical evaluation" (1972, 135).

Since the time of the Stanford study, there have been important refinements in the clinical taxonomy. Autistic children are now routinely designated as 'high functioning', i. e. with normal range nonverbal intelligence, or 'low functioning'. The criteria for autism have also broadened (DSMIII 1980) so as to include children with more diverse and milder disturbances, children who might once have been classified as 'autistic-like' or 'language impaired with affective problems'. Children with mental retardation are now more frequently subcategorized by etiology, e. g. organic versus familial (Zigler/Hodapp 1986), and by behavioral profiles, e. g. without or without specific language impairment (Miller 1988).

These refinements may make it possible to validate the traditional clinical categories. A very large scale effort to do so is underway. Researchers at six university centres, under the current direction of I. Rapin, have been administering a comprehensive battery of psychological, psychiatric, medical and language examinations to some 500 children with autism, mental retardation, or specific language impairment. The children are being seen longitudinally at both preschool and school ages, with electrophysiological and magnetic resonance imagery data collected at the latter point. There is no doubt that this project will provide rich data on the psychosocial functioning of children with language disorders. Whether it meets its own goal of creating an "empirically based common nosology of higher cortical disorders of childhood" (Rapin 1990) remains to be seen. In the meantime, there is little empirical foundation for use of the medical model in studying language disorders. If children labelled as mentally retarded, for example, are not reliably different in behavior than those labelled as autistic, describing the medical condition of retardation or autism is not likely to explain the behavior, linguistic or otherwise.

2.2.2. Behavioral Syndromes Without Cause

Even if clinical categories had sharper boundaries, the traditional framework would still prove disappointing in its failure to address true etiologies. Although the medical model is oriented towards causal conditions, the taxonomy that is commonly applied to children with language disorders refers only to behavioral syndromes, hearing impairment being the major exception. If all goes well, behavioral syndromes are early heuristic tools that lead researchers to discover causal states and their cures. In the case of language disorders, however, it seems that the clinical categories have obscured more than they have revealed. Mental retardation is now known to result from a large and heterogenous collection of conditions that are metabolic (e. g. PKU), neurological (e. g. anoxia), physiological (e. g. lead poisoning), or genetic (e. g. Fragile X) in character. With such diversity, the single fact that a child's language delay is associated with retardation can imply neither cause nor cure. The likelihood of heterogeneity is also a theme in the current literature on autism (Wing/Attwood 1987), but efforts to establish the organic roots of this syndrome have not yet borne fruit (Prior 1987). Appeals to the condition of autism as an explanation for language delays remain empty. Finally, consider the inclusion of specific language impairment or developmental dysphasia as a diagnostic category within the medical model. As noted in 2.1, the diagnostic criteria for this category have evolved so as to systematically exclude most of the possible etiological factors, i. e. intellectual deficit, affective disorder, sensory or motor impairment, frank neurological insult. We are thus left with the paradox of an 'etiological' category which is defined by the absence of causal indices. One recent paper has gone so far as to suggest that the condition has no cause other than the normal distribution of language abilities among individuals (Leonard 1987). In the context of that argument, the promise of the medical model seems particularly hollow. As things now stand, the categories applied in the traditional diagnosis of developmental language disorders seldom refer to single conditions with known etiologies that can be identified and/or treated.

2.2.3. Absence of Unique Treatments

A third shortcoming of the medical model can be found in reports of language intervention with children. A wide variety of treatment programs are in current use by speech-language pathologists and educators in North America. They differ in the degree to which they rely on behavioral modification techniques, respond to the child's spontaneous activity, focus on pre-selected goals, or incorporate family members. They also employ different types of linguistic interaction, from imitative drill to free conversation. Many of the intervention programs have been subjected to controlled tests of effectiveness, and a recent meta-analysis indicates that "the average language disabled child involved in language intervention can be expected to perform better than 85% of [those] ... not receiving language intervention" (Nye/Foster/Seaman 1987, 350). However, the literature gives no indication that one type of treatment is more effective than another for children in a particular diagnostic category. Instead, master clinicians argue that the same principles of intervention apply regardless of diagnosis (Fey 1986; Lahey 1988).

2.3. Contributions of the Model

The shortcomings of the medical model indicate that alternate frameworks are needed for the study and treatment of children with language disorders. In developing such frameworks it will be important to maintain the strengths of the traditional approach. These contributions lie in two areas. First, the medical model treated language behavior as a symptom of some underlying disturbance. Longitudinal studies of children with specific language impairment attest to the wisdom of that stance. Even when these children learn to speak in ways that seem age appropriate, they continue to have trouble with academic tasks such as reading and mathematics (e. g. Aram/Ekelman/Nation 1984; Scarborough/Dobrich 1990; Stark/Bernstein/Condino/et. al 1984). By one interpretation, these data indicate some continuing, if hidden, specific impairment in language functions. It is also possible, however, that the impaired learning mechanisms that underlay the language delay in the first place remain operative and cause later difficulties with analogous tasks. A second contribution of the medical model has been to orient us to the general nature of such mechanisms. At the foundation of the traditional classification scheme is a set of psychological constructs such as intelligence, emotion, social relationship, and perceptual ability. These global parameters do not suffice to create unique classificatory groups: children with diagnoses of specific language impairment, mental retardation, or autism may all have intellectual impairments; children with diagnoses of autism, specific language impairment, hearing impairment, or mental retardation may all evidence emotional disturbance, and so forth. Nevertheless, these global parameters do draw our attention to the sorts of factors which determine language acquisition and use.

2.4. Conclusions

It is time to rethink our commitment to the use of the medical model in studying and treating children with language development disorders. The traditional diagnostic categories have little empirical support, little explanatory value, and little connection with treatment possibilities or practice. A more useful framework might be one that emphasized psychological states and mechanisms rather than physical conditions, that focused on individuals rather than groups, that stressed description rather than diagnosis, and that aimed towards effective intervention rather than cures. Steps in this direction have been taken by a number of researchers and clinicians over the past two decades. These scholars draw on contemporary linguistic and psychological theories to explain the language behavior of disordered children and to develop therapeutic regimen. At the same time, they use groups of language disordered children as natural experiments for the testing and validation of these theories. The products of this symbiosis will be reviewed in the following sections, again emphasizing issues related to assessment.

3. The Psychology of Language Development Disorder

This ambitious heading suggests more than will be delivered. It may also offend those who would prefer to see linguistics mentioned explicitly. However, if we take the term 'psychology' in its general sense to include psycholinguistic models, the phrase Psychology of Language Development Disorder captures much of the emergent alternative to a medical model. Clinicians and researchers who work from within contemporary, non-medical frameworks purpose a somewhat different assessment task than the traditional practitioner. They also use a wider range of assessment procedures and hence have come to new understandings of the nature of atypical language acquisition.

3.1. Assessment Tasks and Procedures

The first assessment task within non-medical models is still to decide whether or not a child's language performance is in accord with chronological age. The second goal is not, however, to determine which condition has caused the delay, but to describe the child's current language knowledge and the resources he or she will bring to the language learning task. This description is seen as the key to effective intervention (Crystal 1984; Fey 1986; Lahey 1988; Lund/Duchan 1988).

Standardized measures remain necessary to establish language and/or intellectual delays. They may even be necessary to establish relative levels of proficiency in various linguistic and/or cognitive domains. However, informal procedures, including the collection and analysis of spontaneous language samples, are the preferred tools for description (Fletcher 1991). Standardized measures provide reliable performance comparisons, but they usually demand metalinguistic/metacognitive skills, and a close adherence to established task procedures. Moreover, with most normative instruments, children are not free to pursue their own interests or speak their own communicative intents. [Schemes such as Lee's (1974) Developmental Sentence Analysis are the rare exception to this rule.] For these reasons, tests frequently underestimate the knowledge implicit in a young child's everyday language usage (e. g. Prutting/Gallagher/Mulac 1975). Yet it is exactly this knowledge which is central to intervention planning. What the child already knows about language influences his or her interpretation of new exemplars and hence determines what will or can be learned (e. g. Clark 1987; MacWhinney 1987; Peters 1983; Pinker 1989). No procedure captures this knowledge better than the systematic observation of spontaneous communication. The scope of this informal analysis will be guided by the clinician or researcher's theory of language, particularly in regard to the range of pertinent subsystems and their key features. Most investigators will, however, include analyses of the lexicon, sentence patterns (semantic relations, phrase structures, or predicate-argument structures), phonology, morphology, and patterns of use (e. g. speech acts, adherence to conversational postulates, discourse schemes).

The descriptive task must also be guided by broader theories of mind and person, since the resources a child brings to language learning include a variety of nonverbal, even nonintellectual, functions and schemes. Standardized tests may be useful, but informed observation of spontaneous play can again reveal much about a child's real-life conceptual repertoire, attention span, problem solving abilities and social relatedness. Here the nonmedically oriented investigator tries to determine those states and mechanisms which will facilitate or hinder further development.

What has been learned in these efforts to study language development disorders from within contemporary, non-medical models of language psychology? Without pretending to be comprehensive, and skirting many of the current theoretical debates, the following examples will serve to illustrate the value of this approach. Each section will begin with a brief statement of the basic psychological principle which informed the clinical investigations.

3.2. New Perspectives on Language Disordered Children

3.2.1. Language Knowledge is Abstract and Categorical

Psycholinguists are currently debating the nature of the processes which lead to the mental representation of language categories such as Subject. Some prefer to speak of hypothesis testing and rules, some of parameter setting, and others of the emergence of hidden nodes in neural networks. No one seems to be arguing, however, that language schemes are simple records of past behavioral events. Chomsky's maxim that language knowledge must be abstract to account for the speaker's productivity is still the consensus view.

This principle has influenced our understanding of language development disorders in at least two ways. First, it illuminates the 'rote' language seen in certain autistic, retarded or language impaired children. Fay/Schuler (1980, 78), for example, report a child who said *sea scallops to eat* whenever he saw a particular type of automobile tail light. Traditional views of such expressions have treated them as bizarre metaphors. However, the contemporary investigator, informed by an understanding of language knowledge as abstract and productive, tells a more interesting story. Children who use expressions of this sort seem to be learning unanalyzed phrases as single lexemes. This hinders their integration into larger systems of categorical rules, and leads to particularistic use (Prizant 1983). A predominance of such forms would greatly restrict abstraction and productivity. The importance of these expressions thus lies not in their lack of conventionality, but in their implications for the developing language system.

A second clinical lesson from this principle concerns the phenomena of generalization. Interventionists frequently report that children with language disorders learn new language patterns in therapy but fail to use these patterns outside the lesson. Traditional views would hold that language disordered children somehow fail to generalize their linguistic knowledge. Contemporary investigators, informed by the principle of abstraction, suggest a different interpretation. Such children may not have learned an abstract language pattern at all, or at least not one of the expected breadth (Johnston 1988a). Clinicians may help a child to say *cow eat, dog eat, baby eat,* etc. and believe they are teaching the Noun + Verb pattern, when in reality the child is only learning a local rule for the activity predicate EAT. In such cases, if the child later fails to say things such as *doggy run*, this behavior would indicate a lack of categorical knowledge rather than some failure to use known forms in new situations.

Now that the possibility of under-analysis and lexically-bound 'rules' is clear, clinicians are learning to assess productivity before assuming that a disordered child knows a particular language pattern. For example, distributional analysis of various lexemes in spontaneous speech can help determine the extent to which a given word occurs in a variety of linguistic contexts. Such analyses are increasingly possible with the advent of language sample analysis software such as SALT (Miller/Chapman 1985).

3.2.2. Language Knowledge is Multiplex

Scholars may disagree over the structuring, autonomy or origins of various linguistic subsystems, but there is no disagreement over the fact that language is comprised of diverse and systematized domains of knowledge. This principle has led to the solution of at least one clinical enigma and the setting of a major research and clinical agenda.

The enigma arose out of the literature on children with specific language impairment. Throughout the 1970s, a series of research studies reported that these children learned grammatical morphemes, phrase structure rules and certain lexical families in a surprisingly normal fashion. Acquisition of these forms was 'delayed', but the order in which they were learned and the developmental errors which occurred were highly similar to the patterns seen in normal children. Many clinicians, however, continued to hold the traditional view that children with specific language impairment used 'deviant' language. A resolution to this conflict began to emerge when investigators, informed by the multiplexity principle, proposed that various subsystems of language might be developing with a lack of normal synchrony (e. g. Johnston 1982; Kemp 1983). Subsequent research data confirmed this hypothesis. Earlier studies had focused on separate subsystems and thus indicated normalcy, but when several domains were viewed simultaneously, the total language system was revealed to be developing in an asynchronous fashion (Clahsen 1989; Johnston/Kamhi 1984; Liles/Watt 1984; Moore/Johnston in preparation).

The likelihood of asynchronous language development in disordered children makes the 'linguistic profile' a clinical and research necessity. Bloom/Lahey (1978; Lahey 1988) have long argued for broad stroke profiles that contrast a child's command of language form, content and use. It now seems additionally important to elaborate such profiles within the formal domain, contrasting competencies in, for instance, morphology, sentence patterns and the lexicon. (See Crystal 1982; Johnston/Ammon/Kamhi 1988; Miller 1982 for illustrative analysis systems.) Given asynchronous development, no single language measure can represent a child's current knowledge and provide a basis for intervention plans. Moreover, if we assume that 'dips' in a linguistic profile reflect some specific deficiency in the underlying learning mechanism, single measures will obscure psychosocial differences among disordered children that could be important for treatment or research. On the other hand, descriptive analyses of language competence in several domains can represent the child's verbal strengths and weaknesses, and can alert the practitioner to important experiential, perceptual, social and/or intellectual constraints on further learning. In short, recognition of the multiplex nature of language knowledge and subsequent evidence of asynchrony have added linguistic profiles to the assessment agenda.

3.2.3. Language Acquisition is Orderly

Detailed accounts of acquisition patterns have revealed an impressive orderliness in the way in which language knowledge develops, both within and across languages. Fine grained analyses have sometimes revealed alternative paths from one knowledge state to the next, but major deviations from the common sequence of surface patterns have proven rare. Researchers differ in their explanations for this orderliness, some emphasizing constraints within the language system, others emphasizing perceptual and cognitive factors or input variables. The normally predictable course of acquisition for a given language most probably reflects an interplay of all of these causal vectors.

Armed with knowledge of the common patterns, researchers have been able to describe the language acquisition of disordered children in considerable depth. What is most remarkable about these data is the degree to which language 'disordered' children have been revealed to be 'normal'. Mentally retarded children (Abbeduto/Rosenberg 1987), autistic children (Paul 1987), and children with specific language disorders (Johnston 1988b; but see also Grimm 1987) seem to learn language patterns in much the normal order, albeit late and more slowly. Where there is evidence of subsystem asynchronies, e. g. morphological problems for SLI children, vocabulary peaks for retarded children, or pragmatic gaps for autistic children, the normal causal influences can still be seen to be at work. For example, Rom/Leonard (1990) use Hebrew and English data to argue that basic perceptual mechanisms may be at the root of failure to master unstressed grammatical morphemes. These researchers also recognize the role of functionality, i. e. the relative importance of morphology in expressing semantic intent, as do Lindner/Johnston (in press) arguing from German and English data. Analogous arguments pointing to the influence of life experience in vocabulary learning and the influence of sociability in illocationary choices are made by Fazio/Johnston/Brandl (in press) and Johnston (1985b). Even the truly odd language behavior of some disordered children has assumed a degree of normalcy when viewed through the frameworks of language psychology. Echolalia is a good case in point. Immediate imitation of utterances used to be cited as proof of the bizarre, superficial nature of autistic language. However, such imitation is now know to be linked to language level (Caparulo/Cohen 1983; Howlin 1982), selective (e. g. Paccia/Curcio 1982), often functional (Prizant/Duchan 1981; Tager-Flusberg/Calkins 1990), and associated with more positive outcomes (Caparulo/Cohen 1983; Howlin 1982). Moreover, it frequently occurs at rates which fall within the range observed for young normal children (e. g. Cantwell/Baker/Rutter 1978). Imitative language in some autistic children persists longer than is normal, and it may have unusual phonetic veridicality, but it is not generally rote or meaningless.

The overwhelming normalcy of language development in disordered populations has revolutionized clinical practice in many countries. Disordered children are now routinely assessed by reference to normal 'stages' of acquisition (e. g. Crystal/Fletcher/Garman 1976; Johnston/Ammon/Kamhi 1988; Lahey 1988; Miller 1982), and normal data provide the basis for intervention programs in virtually all theoretical camps (Fey 1986, 101 – 8), the notable exception to this rule being the North American 'special education' establishment responsible for schooling. Greater sophistication in applying the normal data will be needed as we learn more about the extent and causes of developmental asynchrony. There may be, after all, no particular merit in replicating normal acquisition patterns if a given disordered child has resources which would allow him/her to forge ahead in particular areas of language competence. Psychological models of language development should continue to provide guidance in this regard.

3.2.4. Acquisition Depends on the Analysis of Exemplars

Children learn the language they hear. As they interact with care-givers and peers, children are provided with a stream of utterances which illustrate how to express various intents. Researchers argue as to whether specific features of this 'linguistic input' are keys to learning. How important is it for care-givers to talk about events which have already captured the child's attention? Or to repeat portions of what the child has just said, in a more grammatical fashion? Researchers also argue about the way in which the input data lead to changes in knowledge. Do children store exemplars for pattern induction? Do they compare exemplars to their own inner version of the same utterance? Do they do anything at all? This, of course, is language psychology's version of the nature-nurture debate and there is little chance of a single outcome. Even in the absence of conclusions, however, this literature has had a clinical impact by drawing attention to the role of language input.

One line of investigation has focused on the nature of the language used by parents of disordered children. As an extension of the folk wisdom which holds that late-talkers merely lack a reason to speak, researchers have wondered whether language disordered children receive normal input. The answer, thus far, appears to be yes. Investigations of parental speech to mentally retarded children (e. g. Rondal 1978), autistic children (Howlin/Rutter 1989), and children with specific language disorders (Grimm/Weinert 1990; Leonard 1987) have produced scant evidence to support the view that these children fail to learn because of the language they hear. Instead, parents of such children seem to speak to them in ways which are largely normal for their levels of language competence.

The language environment of disordered children does not seem to explain their language delays, but it may nevertheless play a key role in facilitating acquisition. The key to this paradox is the notion of 'supra-normal' input. Using psychological reports on 'motherese' and cognitive processing, some theorists now argue that language disordered children are ill-equipped to analyze regularities in the utterances they hear and thus require specially crafted input (e. g. Fey 1986, 21, 168–189). In the words of Lahey, "what may be an effective linguistic environment for the child learning language without difficulty may not be effective enough to facilitate language learning in the language disordered child". (Lahey 1988, 356). Caregivers, teachers and practitioners can assist poor language learners by presenting exemplar utterances at high proportional frequencies, in contexts which clarify meaning. Prosody and discourse can also be manipulated so as to highlight forms that may otherwise go unnoticed, and to illustrate just those linguistic patterns which correspond to the child's language level and communication needs (Johnston 1985c). Such techniques seem to provide unusually accessible data from which to learn, and have led to accelerated language growth in both normal and disordered children (e. g. Campbell/McNeil 1985; Hoff-Ginsberg/Shatz 1982; Johnston 1988a; Leonard 1975; Nelson 1976; Schwartz/Chapman/Terrell et al. 1985). Caregivers will differ, however, in their facility with the on-line metalinguistic analyses that are required by some of these procedures. This creates a new focus for collaborative assessment as clinicians and caregivers cooperate in determining how and when the language of the home should be altered.

3.2.5. Acquisition is Bound to Cognitive Development

This is surely the most controversial of the principles discussed in this chapter, and a point at which psychologists and linguists are likely to diverge. In part, the disagreements are theory based and concern the degree to which language is modularized. However, the debates also stem from a failure to recognize that the relationships between language and cognition vary with developmental level and with the aspect of language or cognition being considered (Johnston 1985a). Even for committed cognitivists, the literature in language psychology suggests four different sorts of developmental linkage between language and non-verbal cognition. First, early intellectual development seems to pave the way for language as the infant builds social relationships and learns to think instrumentally. At later ages, cognition can be seen to provide the general mechanisms for language analysis, and the components of meaning for verbal symbols. Finally, language, once learned, seems to be a powerful tool for reflection and problem solving. The first and last of these hypothesized relationships have had particular impact on our understanding of language disordered children.

Piagetian accounts of infancy have fuelled numerous studies of the connection between sensori-motor intelligence and language learning. The usual research question has focused on whether or not a particular level or product of intellect is prerequisite to language. To date, the strongest evidence points to the importance of Stage V intelligence: children who have not at least attained the means/ends reasoning, imitation skill, and object-related actions which are characteristic of this Stage do not seem to produce referential speech (e. g. Bates/Benigni/Bretherton et al. 1979; Ingram 1978; Snyder 1978). Research with the mentally retarded indicates that this constraint holds true even at older ages (Kahn 1975). The clinical implications of these findings seem quite clear. Some nonverbal retarded children or low functioning autistic children may not yet be cognitively prepared for language. Others may have achieved a general cognitive level which would support verbal communication, but have specific learning disorders which impede their analysis of the language system. Clinicians familiar with the frameworks of language psychology are now including cognitive assessments to try to distinguish between these two groups of nonverbal children.

A second, and quite different, sort of hypothesized relationship between language and cognition has influenced our understanding of specific language impairment. Insights in this case have come from the recognition that language is normally one of the major tools of representational thought (Olson 1975). Studies of visual imagery (e. g. Kosslyn 1980), as well as studies of deaf and SLI children

(e. g. Furth 1966; Inhelder 1966) have made it clear that language is not the sole path to reflective problem-solving. Language does, however, provide unique resources for propositional reasoning, and it thus seems unlikely that a person with limited language facility would be fully capable of normal intellectual achievement. How then are we to understand children with specific language impairment? Do they disprove the psychological theory, or have we over-estimated their mental abilities? Research in the last decade supports the latter conclusion. In spite of their normal-range nonverbal IQ, children with SLI have performed less well than their age peers on a wide range of nonverbal cognitive tasks. (See Johnston 1988b for a review.) The exact nature of these deficits is not yet known, but they may stem, at least in part, from limitations in attentional capacity. Johnston/Smith (1988) found that language impaired preschoolers had difficulty with verbal problem solving even when they could demonstrate knowledge of all of the elements required by the problem space. What they seemed unable to do was to use these resources simultaneously in the service of a particular reasoning task.

Data of this sort suggest that the focus in clinical assessment must broaden to include language performance as well as language competence. To succeed in language tasks, whether communication or thought, children must know the language system and be able to draw on this knowledge in a reliable and economical fashion. Extending Fletcher's argument, clinical assessments must gather evidence "not so much from syntax, but from syntax deployed in the language-production process" (Fletcher 1991, 186). This may require new techniques designed to measure a child's relative degree of mastery with familiar language patterns.

3.3. Summary and Conclusions

The renaissance of language psychology in this half of the twentieth century has had a profound impact on our approach to developmental language disorders. Some researchers and clinicians continue to search for first-causes and cures; they make use of traditional diagnostic categories in the hope that these groupings will point the way to an underlying causal condition. Other researchers and clinicians, however, have abandoned such medical models, and have built a new framework out of the principles of contemporary psycholinguistics. To greater and lesser degrees, they have moved beyond diagnosis to description. They have become less interested in conditions and more interested in characterizing the child's current knowledge state and learning mechanisms. When they invoke the traditional categories of developmental language disorder, they do so merely as a convenient shorthand for constellations of psycho-social variables.

The purpose of the present chapter has been to explain this shift in orientation, and to illustrate the sorts of assessment questions which have emerged from the frameworks of language psychology:

- Is this child intellectually and socially prepared to learn language?
- What does this child know about language? and what is he or she likely to learn next?
- Which aspects of this child's language are productive?
- How fully does this child control familiar language schemes?
- Are there aspects of language which are relatively easy or difficult for this child to learn?
- Does this child have intellectual, social or environmental resources which will make it possible to ignore the common acquisition sequences when selecting learning goals?
- How and where can language input be altered to facilitate this child's learning?

These questions are no easier to answer than the questions of differential diagnosis, but they seem to have a more direct application to the practice of language intervention. As we learn to answer them, we immediately improve our ability to help language disordered children become effective language users. This is an admittedly practical stance, one in which hopes for a cure have been tempered by the reality of persistent learning deficits. But it is also a visionary stance, one that insists on language as a human birthright.

4. References

Abbeduto, L. & Rosenberg, S. (1987). Linguistic communication and mental retardation. In S. Rosenberg (Ed.), *Advances in applied psycholinguistics, Vol. 1. 76–125.* Cambridge: Cambridge University.

Aram, D., Ekelman, B., & Nation, J. (1984). Preschoolers with language disorders: 10 years later. *Journal of Speech and Hearing Research, 27,* 232–244.

Bates, E., Benigni, L., Bretherton, I., Camaioni, L., & Volterra, V. (1979). *The emergence of symbols: Cognition and communication in infancy.* New York: Academic.

Beitchman, J., Nair, R., Clegg, M., & Patel, P. (1986). Prevalence of speech and language disorders in 5 year old kindergarten children in Ottawa-Carleton region. *Journal of Speech and Hearing Disorders, 51,* 98–110.

Bloom, L. & Lahey, M. (1978), *Language development and language disorders.* New York: John Wiley.

Campbell, T. & McNeil, M. (1985). Effects of presentation rate and divided attention on auditory comprehension in children with an acquired language disorder. *Journal of Speech and Hearing Research, 28,* 513–520.

Cantwell, D., Baker, L., & Rutter, M. (1978). A comparative study of infantile autism and specific developmental receptive language disorder – IV: Analysis of syntax and language function. *Journal of Child Psychology and Psychiatry, 19,* 351–362.

Caparulo, B. & Cohen, D. (1983). Developmental language studies in the neuropsychiatric disorders of childhood. In K. E. Nelson (Ed.), *Children's language, 423–463.* New York: Gardner.

Clahsen, H. (1989). The grammatical characterization of developmental aphasia. *Linguistics, 27,* 897–920.

Clark, E. (1987). The principle of contrast: a constraint on language acquisition. In B. MacWhinney (Ed.), *Mechanisms of language acquisition. 1–34.* Hillsdale, NJ: Lawrence Erlbaum.

Crystal, D. (1982), *Profiling linguistic disability.* London: Edward Arnold.

Crystal, D. (1984), *Linguistic encounters with language handicap.* Oxford: Basil Blackwell.

Crystal, D., Fletcher, P., & Garman, M. (1976). *The grammatical analysis of language disability.* New York: Elsevier.

DSM III (1980). *Diagnostic and statistical manual of mental disorders (Third Edition).* American Psychiatric Association, Washington, D. C.

Fay, W. & Schuler, A. (1980). *Emerging language in autistic children.* Baltimore: University Park.

Fazio, B., Johnston, J., & Brandl, L. (in press). Relationship between mental age and the development of vocabulary consisting of labels versus relational terms among mildly mentally handicapped children. *American Journal of Mental Deficiency.*

Fey, M. (1986). Language intervention with young children. San Diego: College Hill.

Fletcher, P. (1991). Evidence from syntax for language impairment. In J. Miller (Ed.), *Research on child language disorders: a decade of progress. 169–187.* Austin: Pro-Ed.

Furth, H. (1966). *Thinking without language.* New York: The Free Press.

Grimm, H. (1987). Developmental dysphasia: New theoretical perspectives and empirical results. *The German Journal of Psychology, 11(1),* 8–22.

Grimm, H. & Weinert, S. (1990). Is the syntax development of dysphasic children deviant and why? New findings to an old question. *Journal of Speech and Hearing Research, 33,* 220–228.

Hoff-Ginsberg, E. & Shatz, M. (1982). Linguistic input and the child's acquisition of language. *Psychological Bulletin, 82,* 3–26.

Howlin, P. (1982). Echolalic and spontaneous phrase speech in autistic children. *Journal of Child Psychology and Psychiatry, 23,* 281–293.

Howlin, P. & Rutter, M. (1989). Mother's speech to autistic children: a preliminary causal analysis. *Journal of Child Psychology and Psychiatry, 30,* 819–843.

Ingram, D. (1978). Sensorimotor intelligence and language development. In A. Lock (Ed.), *Action, gesture and symbol: The emergence of language. 261–290.* New York: Academic.

Inhelder, B. (1966). Cognitive development and its contribution to the diagnosis of some phenomena of mental deficiency. *Merrill-Palmer Quarterly, 12,* 299–319.

Johnston, J. (1982). The language disordered child. In N. Lass, L. McReynolds, J. Northern, & D. Yoder (Eds.), *Speech, language, and hearing, Vol. II. 780–801.* Philadelphia: W. B. Saunders.

Johnston, J. (1985a). Cognitive prerequisites: The evidence from children learning English. In Slobin (Ed.), *The crosslinguistic study of language acquisition, Vol. 2. 961–1004.* Hillsdale, NJ: Lawrence Erlbaum.

Johnston, J. (1985b). The discourse symptoms of developmental disorders. In T. Van Dijk (Ed.), *Handbook of discourse analysis, Vol. 3. 79–93.* London: Academic.

Johnston, J. (1985c). Fit, focus and functionality: An essay on early language intervention. *Child Language Teaching and Therapy, 1,* 125–134.

Johnston, J. (1988a). Generalization: The nature of change. *Language, Speech, and Hearing Services in Schools, 19,* 314–329.

Johnston, J. (1988b). Specific language disorders in the child. In N. Lass, L. McReynolds, J. Northern, & D. Yoder (Eds.), *Handbook of speech-language pathology and audiology. 685–715.* Philadelphia: B. C. Decker.

Johnston, J., Ammon, M., & Kamhi, A. (1988). Appendix: Language development chart. In

Kamhi, A., Early syntactic development, *Topics in Language Disorders, 8,* 26–43.

Johnston, J. & Kamhi, A. (1984). The same can be less: Syntactic and semantic aspects of the utterances of language impaired children. *Merrill-Palmer Quarterly, 30,* 65–86.

Johnston, J. & Smith, L. (1988). Six ways to skin a cat: Communication strategies used by language impaired preschoolers. Paper presented at the Symposium on Research in Child Language Disorders, University of Wisconsin, Madison, June.

Kahn, J. (1975). Relationship of Piaget's sensorimotor period to language acquisition of profoundly retarded children. *American Journal of Mental Deficiency, 79,* 640–643.

Kemp, J. (1983). The timing of language intervention for the pediatric population. In J. Miller, D. Yoder, & R. Schiefelbusch (Eds.), *Contemporary issues in language intervention, ASHA Reports No. 12. 183–196.* Rockville, MD: American Speech-Language-Hearing Association.

Kosslyn, S. (1980). *Image and mind.* Cambridge: Harvard University.

Lahey, M. (1988). *Language disorders and language development.* New York: MacMillan.

Lee, L. (1974). *Developmental sentence analysis.* Evanston: Northwestern University.

Leonard, L. (1975). The role of non-linguistic stimuli and semantic relations in children's acquisition of grammatical utterances. *Journal of Experimental Child Psychology, 19,* 346–357.

Leonard, L. (1987). Is specific language impairment a useful construct? In S. Rosenberg (Ed.), *Advances in applied psycholinguistics, Volume 1. 1–39.* Cambridge: Cambridge University.

Liles, B. & Watt, J. (1984). On the meaning of 'language delay'. *Folia Phoniatrica, 36,* 40–48.

Lindner, K. & Johnston, J. (in press). Grammatical morphology in language-impaired children acquiring English or German as their first language. A functional perspective. *Journal of Applied Psycholinguistics.*

Lund, N. & Duchan, J. (1988). Assessing children's language in naturalistic contexts. Englewood Cliffs, NJ: Prentice-Hall.

Marge, M. (1972). The general problem of language disabilities in children. In M. Marge & J. Irwin (Eds.), *Principles of childhood language disabilities. 82–94.* NY: Appleton Century Crofts.

McCauley, R. & Swisher, L. (1984). Psychometric review of language and articulation tests for preschool children. *Journal of Speech and Hearing Disorders, 49,* 34–42.

MacWhinney, B. (1987). The competition model. In B. MacWhinney (Ed.), *Mechanisms of language acquisition. 249–308.* Hillsdale, NJ: Lawrence Erlbaum.

Miller, J. (1982). *Assessing language production in children.* Baltimore: University Park.

Miller, J. (1988). The developmental asynchrony of language development in children with Down Syndrome. In L. Nadel (Ed.), *The psychobiology of Down Syndrome. 167–198.* Cambridge, MA: Bradford Books.

Miller, J. & Chapman, R. (1981). The relation between age and mean length of utterance in morphemes. *Journal of Speech and Hearing Research, 24,* 154–161.

Miller, J. & Chapman, R. (1985). *SALT: Systematic analysis of language transcripts.* Language Analysis Laboratory, Waisman Center, University of Wisconsin, Madison.

Moore, M. E. & Johnston, J. (in preparation). Expression of past time by normal and language impaired children. Unpublished manuscript, Illinois State University, Bloomington.

Nelson, K. E. (1976). Facilitating children's syntax acquisition. *Developmental Psychology, 13.* 101–107.

Nye, C., Foster, S., & Seaman, D. (1987). Effectiveness of language intervention with the language/learning disabled. *Journal of Speech and Hearing Disorders, 52,* 348–357.

Olson, D. (1975). On the relations between spatial and linguistic processes. In J. Eliot & N. Salkind (Eds.), *Children's spatial development. 67–110.* Springfield, IL: Charles, C. Thomas.

Paccia, J. & Curcio, F. (1982). Language processing and forms of immediate echolalia in autistic children. *Journal of Speech and Hearing Research, 25,* 42–47.

Paul, R. (1987), Communication. In D. Cohen & A. Donnellan (Eds.), *Handbook of autism and pervasive developmental disorders. 61–84.* New York: Wiley.

Peters, A. (1983). *The units of language acquisition.* Cambridge: Cambridge University.

Pinker, S. (1989). *Learnability and cognition: the acquisition of argument structure.* Cambridge, MA: MIT.

Prior, M. (1987). Biological and neuropsychological approaches to childhood autism. *British Journal of Psychiatry, 150,* 8–17.

Prizant, B. (1983). Language acquisition and communicative behavior in autism: Toward an understanding of the "whole" of it. *Journal of Speech and Hearing Disorders, 48,* 296–307.

Prizant, B. & Duchan, J. (1981). The functions of immediate echolalia in autistic children. *Journal of Speech and Hearing Disorders, 46,* 241–249.

Proceedings of the Institute on Childhood Aphasia (1962). California Society for Crippled Children and Adults and Stanford University School of Medicine.

Prutting, C., Gallagher, T., & Mulac, A. (1975). The expressive portion of the NSST compared to a spontaneous language sample. *Journal of Speech and Hearing Disorders, 40,* 40–48.

Rapin, I. (1990). Medical and neurological findings in 542 preschool children with communication disorders, autism or mental deficiency. Paper presented to the Child Neurology Society, October, Atlanta.

Rescorla, L. (1989). The language development survey: a screening tool for delayed language in toddlers. *Journal of Speech and Hearing Disorders, 54,* 587–599.

Rom, A. & Leonard, L. (1990). Interpreting deficits in grammatical morphology in specifically language-impaired children: preliminary evidence from Hebrew. *Clinical Linguistics and Phonetics, 4,* 93–105.

Rondal, J. (1978). Maternal speech to normal and Down's syndrome children matched for mean length of utterance. In C. Meyers (Ed.), *Quality of life in severely and profoundly mentally retarded people: Research foundations for improvement, 193–265.* Washington, DC: American Association on Mental Deficiency.

Rosenthal, W., Eisenson, J., & Luckau, J. (1972). A statistical test of the validity of diagnostic categories used in childhood language disorders: Implications for assessment procedures. *Papers and Reports on Child Language Development, 4,* 121–143. Stanford University.

Scarborough, H. & Dobrich, W. (1990). Development of children with early language delay. *Journal of Speech and Hearing Research, 33,* 70–83.

Schwartz, R., Chapman, K., Terrell, B., Prelock, P., & Rowan, L. (1985). Facilitating word combination in language-impaired children through discourse structure. *Journal of Speech and Hearing Disorders, 50,* 31–39.

Snyder, L. (1978). Communicative and cognitive abilities and disabilities in the sensorimotor period. *Merrill-Palmer Quarterly, 24,* 161–180.

Stark, R., Bernstein, L., Condino, R., Bender, M., Tallal, P., & Catts, H. (1984). Four-year follow-up study of language impaired children. *Annals of Dyslexia, 34,* 49–68.

Stark, R. & Tallal, P. (1981). Selection of children with specific language deficits. *Journal of Speech and Hearing Disorders, 46,* 114–122.

Stevenson, J. & Richman, N. (1976). The prevalence of language delay in a population of three year old children and its association with general retardation. *Developmental Medicine and Child Neurology, 18,* 431–441.

Tager-Flusberg, H. & Calkins, S. (1990). Does imitation facilitate the acquisition of grammar? Evidence from a study of autistic, Down syndrome and normal children. *Journal of Child Language, 17,* 591–606.

Templin, M. (1957). Certain language skills in children: Their development and interrelationships. *Child Welfare Monographs, No. 26.* Minneapolis: University of Minnesota.

Weiner, P. (1984). The study of childhood language disorders in the nineteenth century. *Asha, 26,* 35–38.

Wing, L. & Attwood, A. (1987). Syndromes of autism and atypical development. In D. Cohen & A. Donnellan (Eds.), *Handbook of autism and pervasive developmental disorders. 3–19.* New York: Wiley.

Zigler, E. & Hodapp, R. (1986). *Understanding mental retardation.* Cambridge: Cambridge University.

Judith R. Johnston, Vancouver (Canada)

59. Neurological Aspects of Language Development Disorders

1. Introduction

The allegedly unique potential of humans to develop language is based on the coordinated activity of their cerebral and thalamic/basal ganglia circuitry. The subcortical nuclei are involved in adopting verbal mental set, the task-specific activation of the cortical language areas (Cambier/Elghozi/Strube 1979, Ojemann 1975) and transducing verbal thought into speech. The cerebrum assumes the major role in language processing. Therefore the neurology of language development is primarily cerebral neurology. It subdivides into the normative and the clinical: How the language area and its connections differentiate in the course of normal brain maturation, and how pathology of early onset – structural, genetic and metabolic disease – compromises this aspect of brain maturation.

Conceivably, environmental variables (deprivation, stimulation) also affect the differentiation of language circuitry (Bertenthal/Campos 1987).

Spurred by claims for a unique 'language acquisition device' in the human brain, much effort has been expended on inquiry into the nature of the neural substrate for language. Neurolinguistics have sought support for the view that language represents a discontinuity, not only in the evolution of communicative systems, but also in the underlying neural hardware. Is the language area a focal dedicated ('modular') neural system, and one that cannot be replaced by other areas of brain, at least after an initial 'plastic' period, during which true language, transcending mere indexical utterance, is still emerging? Or is a continuity view more defensible; that language cortex is quite variable in location between individuals and readily if not fully replaceable at any age?

Neither macroscopically nor microscopically are there any attributes of neuronal morphology, or of neuronal connectedness, that uniquely characterize those areas of cortex that implement language function. This inability to verify modularity of language at the neuronal level may be because wide areas of cortex harbor language potential, and no distinctive language neurohistology exists. Alternatively, what in fact differentiates language from general cognitive cortex has so far eluded observation. In either case, it becomes necessary to adopt indirect means to locate language cortex. One way to do so is through observing the effects of brain damage.

Inferences about the neurological substrate of language development can be based on the effects of early damage of the language area. As in adults, given enough cases, it might become apparent which locations when damaged result in impaired language function, and which do not. Such effects can be obscured, however, by the compensatory potential of brain areas that would not in the normal course of events subserve language. This comes to light when the classical language area is damaged early on. In children, language compensation may be complete (Alajouanine/Lhermitte 1965), so that unless the language status is assessed acutely, immediately after the damage is done (which may not be practicable) no deficit is observed. Alternatively, language compensation may be incomplete (St. James Roberts 1981), either because the undamaged parts of the brain that compensate were not fully suited to assume language control, or because those that could have were also damaged by the insult.

Evidence from pathology derives from cases in which the abnormality preponderantly impacts on language development. It excludes generalized mental retardation. However, certain genetic mental redardation syndromes do have a disproportionate effect on language (Down syndrome, fragile X, Williams syndrome). The chromosomal basis of specific developmental language disorders is discussed by Netley (1983). Yet there is no independent evidence that these pathologies target the classical language area. This may be because, if damage is purely local, it would normally be substantially compensated by the developing brain. Specific developmental language disabilities similarly do not afford evidence of frank left hemisphere damage. These cases often give evidence of genetic transmission, in the form of pedigrees in which language problems are prominent (Ingram 1959). 24 % of his 75 probands had a least one parent with language difficulty as did 23 % of their siblings. Similar conclusions were reached by Bishop/Edmundson (1986) and Tallal/Ross/Curtiss (1989). A genetic causation for delayed language development leaves it open whether what is transmitted is a tendency toward rather subtle miswiring, or a risk factor for experiencing insults that induce neuronal dysgenesis at some stage during fetal existence.

In normally developing righthanders the left hemisphere is responsible for all aspects of language, except perhaps intonation (prosody) and some higher levels of verbal comprehension, including humor. But in the majority of nonrighthanders, language is bilaterally represented, apparently without loss of efficiency. How does left lateralization of language develop, and what is its functional significance?

Evidence on the development of language lateralization can be organized in relation to two competing hypotheses – progressive lateralization (Lenneberg 1967) and invariant lateralization (Kinsbourne 1975). The former conforms to a broad perspective on the emergence of the brain basis of higher mental functions, that exalts both the 'language acquisition device' and its lateralization as uniquely human. This is that greater lateralization of the brain basis corresponds to more sophisticated function, of the behavior that is represented, both in phylogeny and in ontogeny (Lenneberg 1967). As presented, progressive lateralization generally encourages a 'discontinuity' view, granting language special status. No corollary suggestion is made that nonverbal functions, such as those subserved by the right hemisphere, also emerge from a bilateralized base. Such a view would anticipate that lateralization is most marked for the neural representation of the highest level of behavioral control, in the brains of the behaviorally most sophisticated species, and, within a species, in those subgroups and individuals whose brains are most mature and whose behavioral control is most effective. The progressive lateralization hypothesis has spawned a multitude of hypotheses, according to which one would expect incomplete or absent lateralization in nonhuman species, in very young children, in mentally retarded, language impaired, learning deficient and even stuttering humans. Even gender differences among humans have been rationalized under the aegis of this sweeping hypothesis. Correspondingly, it also predicts that any group that deviates from the norm in including a greater proportion of ill-lateralized individuals (notably lefthanders) should evidence a relative language or other cognitive inferiority. New predicitons along these lines continue to be made, even though convincing support has not been forthcoming for this line of reasoning.

Progressive lateralization offers theorists a hypothetical process, the shift of language control from both hemispheres into the language 'dominant' hemisphere. This process might not yet have evolved in animals that have no language capability and might be unavailable to totally nonverbal humans. It may be delayed in those whose language development lags behind the norm. It may arrest prematurely in those whose language development arrests at a subnormal level. And, of practical importance, if it is slow to develop, or if it has prematurely arrested, then perhaps maneuvers can be devised which would get the lateralization process going again. This would enable the language therapist to bypass the demanding and often thankless task of remediating the language function by working on it directly. This tantalizing prospect contributes intensity to the continuing interest in the progressive lateralization model.

In contrast, according to the invariant lateralization hypothesis the origins of language rely on the same general area of brain that ultimately controls it in the fully mature individual. Usually this is the left hemisphere, but it can be the right hemisphere, or both hemispheres. In neither minority case does it follow that, in the absence of accompanying brain damage, any inferiority of language function would be expected. If one were to discover that in some language-deficient group, language lateralization is anomalous, this would not, according to the invariant lateralization hypothesis, serve to explain the language deficiency.

Progressive lateralization predicts that asymmetries of brain organization should become increasingly evident in those species whose behavioral control is relatively advanced. This expectation conflicts with a wealth of recently acquired information about lateralization of function in mammals (reviewed by Corballis 1989). Asymmetries abound, even in species as behaviorally limited as the rat, and no single organizing principle seems capable of predicting which function will be symmetrically and which asymmetrically represented. In nonhuman primates lateralization exists but has proven relatively hard to demonstrate. Whether lateralization develops in animals according to the progressive or the invariant model appears not yet to have been studied.

Potential sources of evidence in humans on the timing and location of the process whereby one hemisphere (almost always the left) assumes control over emerging language function include the following: Structural specializations of the language area or language hemisphere, asymmetries in apparent precursors of language, behavioral and/or psychophysiological asymmetries observable while language is developing, and the relative incidence of language impairment (aphasia) after left versus right cerebral damage.

2. Hemisphere Structure

Neither direct nor microscopic inspection of the normally developing cerebral hemispheres reveals the site of emerging language. Language-specific neuronal architectonics have not been characterized. The suggestion that the 'language hemisphere' has a distinctive shape, in particular a larger temporal planum (Geschwind/Levitsky 1968), led to examinations of the brains of newborns available at autopsy. Both Witelson/Pallie (1973) and Wada/Clarke/Hamm (1975) found significantly more asymmetries favoring the left planum temporale. If the larger planum truly marks the language hemisphere, then these findings are consistent with invariant lateralization, given the early stage at which they could be recognized. A test is the nonright-hander, who is often less or even conversely lateralized for language. Obviously such a test cannot be applied to the newborn children studied at autopsy, as they had no opportunity to demonstrate their hand preference. But even among adults, it is not clear that neuroanatomic asymmetries discriminate at a useful level of significance between right and left handers. Asymmetries in question include different slopes of the left and right Sylvian fissures and the right frontal and left occipital prominences that are found in most people (Le May 1976) and are already present in the fetus (Le May 1984).

If the above asymmetries are truly related to the language function, one might expect them to be observably modified in cases of language impairment. In general, group differences in the expected direction have been found (e. g. Roberts/Varney/Reinatz/Parkins 1988), though with too many individual exceptions to be of diagnostic use. In some language impaired individuals, language is lateralized to the smaller hemisphere (Pieniadz/Naeser/Koff/Levine 1983, Ratcliff/Dila/Taylor/Milner 1980). An interesting group difference is a tendency for the temporal plana to be more symmetrical than expected. But rather than implying a diminished and ill-developed left planum, as Geschwind and Levitsky thought, Galaburda/Corsiglia/Rosen/Sherman (1978) have suggested that it is the right planum that is overly large when the plana are symmetrical, perhaps on account of inadequate neural pruning, leading to miswiring of neurons with detrimental effects on function. Jernigan/Hesselink/Tallal (1987) reported a larger right than left posterior region in six of ten language-impaired children on magnetic resonance imaging.

In contrast to the weakly circumstantial evidence that derives from gross morphological asymmetries is the very specific evidence gathered from an admittedly limited number of autopsied cases. Landau/Goldstein/Kleffner (1960) reported a patient with developmental language disorder who had old bilateral infarctions of the Sylvian region and severe retrograde degeneration of both medial geniculate nuclei. This supports the view that bilateral damage is necessary, not only to impair language function but also to preclude contralateral compensation. But Cohen/Campbell/Yaghmai (1989) in their single case of developmental language disorder found only the expected lack of temporal planum asymmetry and a dysgenetic microgyrus in the left insula. The vast majority of language impaired children probably does not suffer from such gross pathology. But microscopic abnormalities have not been ruled out. A limited but growing data base of neurohistological abnormalities derives from cases of developmental dyslexia, a condition which, reading being based largely on access to oral language knowledge (Bertelson 1986) can be considered a subtype of language disorder (Vellutino 1979). Consistent with an early case report by Drake (1968), Galaburda and colleagues have published detailed accounts of microscopic foci of neuronal dysgenesis variably distributed across cerebral cortex of autopsied dyslexics, with a left-sided preponderance of lesions sometimes concentrated in the classical language area (Galaburda/Sherman/Rosen et al. (1987), and leftsided thalamus (Galaburda/Eidelberg 1982). Because this work is so labor-intensive, normal control studies are not yet available, so that there is no assurance of the specificity of this finding. Nonetheless, it is the first available anatomical confirmation of the general conviction that these cases of dyslexia are brain-based, and suggest an origin in mid-trimester, because this is when the affected neurons would normally have migrated to their proper locations. The widespread distribution of the lesions is unexpected were dyslexia a 'pure' or highly selective deficit in reading. Instead, it supports studies that highlight the wide range of cognitive deficits that can be discovered in these patients if they are thoroughly studied (e. g. Kavale/Nye 1991, Kinsbourne/Rufo/Gamzu et al. 1991, Vellutino 1979).

A study of regional cerebral blood flow of adult developmental dyslexics had a generally compatible outcome (Rumsey/Berman/Denckla et al. 1987). On a verbal task, patients exhibited more hemisphere asymmetry than controls. This could be interpreted as reflecting the greater effort they had to invest in the task. But on a line orientation task, generally considered right hemispheric, they also deviated from controls, in exhibiting a reduced anteroposterior gradient in richness of blood flow. This was interpreted as reflecting "a deficit in the ability of frontal systems to respond adequately to cognitive demands" (Rumsey/Berman/Denckla et al. 1987, 1144).

3. Associated Neurological Abnormalities

A relatively widespread distribution of neuronal abnormalities may help explain not only the lack of compensation for dysgenesis of the language area, but also the frequent though variable associated presence of miscellaneous nonspecific minor neurological findings. Certainly, dyslexia is not a clearcut deficiency in an anatomically circumscribed cerebral module. An increased incidence of clumsiness has been noted (Sheridan 1973) and perhaps vestibulocerebellar deficiencies (Horek/Shumway-Cook/Crowe/Black 1988). Johnston/Stark/Mellits/Tallal (1981) found that performance in finger recognition, left-right discrimination, rapid and involuntary movements discriminated their language impaired group from controls. Temporal processing impairment has been documented both in language impaired (Tallal/Piercy 1973, 1974) and dyslexic (Tallal 1980) samples. Kinsbourne/Rufo/Gamzu et al. (1991) not only found that neuromotor and temporal order judgement difficulties continue to distinguish dyslexics from controls in adulthood, but that some of these performances are quite highly discriminating. Electroencephalographic abnormalities are also relatively frequent in these children (Goldstein/Landau/Kleffner 1958).

3.1 Behavioral Laterality

When individuals listen to speech, speak, or think in words, certain associated behaviors, and certain associated physiological changes can be observed. The observable associated behaviors subdivide into (i) asymmetry in gaze and gesture (output laterality), (ii) asymmetry in the ability to identify verbal material presented by voice, vision or touch depending on whether the message originates to the right or left of the person (perceptual laterality tests), and (iii) asymmetry in the amount of interference between verbal and sensorimotor performance when both are performed simultaneously (dual task paradigms). Also observable are event-related asymmetries in electrophysiological and in metabolic cerebral activity while people are using language. Many behavioral and psychophysiological studies have monitored the laterality of emerging language in the infant and child. A few instances are given below.

3.2. Infant Laterality Studies

The more directly relevant evidence from infants derives from their behavior when exposed to speech. Entus (1977) found that infants aged 22 to 140 days could detect transitions from one consonant-vowel word to another more readily at the right than the left ear. Entus used a non-nutritive sucking disinhibition paradigm. Glanville/Best/Levenson (1977) reported similar results using cardiac dishabituation to input to the right ear compared to the left ear. Mac Kain/Studdert-Kennedy/Spieker/Stern (1983) observed that six month old infants could detect correspondence between voice and lip movements when orienting right but not when orienting left. Segalowitz/Chapman (1980) reported a right-sided 'stilling' of the limbs of premature infants of average age 36 weeks when they were exposed to speech, but leftsided stilling when they were exposed to music. The preferred direction of head turning is also affected by the categorical nature of the stimulus. Newborns turned more to the left during musical than during verbal stimulation (Young/Gascon 1990). Less directly, the long recognized rightward bias of infants' spontaneous head and eye turning lends itself to theories that relate laterality of speech control to preferred direction of orienting (Kinsbourne/Lempert 1980). In support of this point of view, Bates/O'Connell/Vaid et al. (1986) reported that pointing coordinated with emerging verbal utterance is predominantly righthanded. They suggest that there are 'cycles' in the manifestations of hand preference that are determined by competition for left hemisphere resources of the manual and the verbal performance. According to Archer/Campbell/Segalowitz (1988) hand preference, which tends to stabilize between ages 18 and 30 months, bears an indirect relationship to expressive language ability (mean length of utterance), qualified by gender. Electrophysiological evidence further supports the presence of this early asymmetry. For instance, Molfese/Freeman/Palermo (1975) reported higher amplitude evoked potentials in infants to speech sounds from the right, but to music from the left. Gardiner/Walter (1977) found differently lateralized changes in six months old infants' E. E. G. power spectra depending on whether they were exposed to speech or music.

Infant asymmetries such as the above controvert the notion of strict symmetry in the neural provisions for prospective language.

Because cerebral circuitry is largely immature at this age, they are most readily ascribed to asymmetrical hardwired activating projections from subcortical regions triggered by speech (or some stimulus parameters contained within speech). The asymmetries are inherent in the provisions for the use of cortex for language, not in the language cortex itself.

3.3. Childhood Laterality: Longitudinal Studies

The two models make critically different predictions about the effect of age on verbal laterality in childhood. According to the progressive lateralization model, there should be an interaction between age and degree of rightward bias on the laterality test used, because language function is increasingly left hemispheric as the children grow older. According to invariant lateralization, age should not affect the degree of asymmetry, because such verbal behavior as the child is capable of is left lateralized from the start.

By the age of three years laterality tests can be administered with meaningful results. It is therefore possible to test not only Lenneberg's (1967) concept of progressive lateralization in this way, but also Krashen's (1973) more restricted concept. In accord with Hiscock/Kinsbourne's (1977) initial study, numerous longitudinal designs have been used with children aged three and over (e. g. Geffen 1978, Hiscock/Kinsbourne 1978, 1980 a, 1980 b, Piazza 1977, White/Kinsbourne 1980). Earlier work had discovered right ear advantages in verbal laterality for still younger children (Ingram 1975, Lokker/Morais 1985, Nagafuchi 1970). Subsequent work is comprehensively reviewed by Hiscock (1988). The general finding that magnitude of asymmetry remains constant with increasing age is upheld, even for the preschool years, which Krashen had nominated for progressive lateralization in his weakened form of Lenneberg's hypothesis.

3.4. Hemisphere Equipotentiality

When one hemisphere is damaged before, during or soon after birth, the consequences for language function and further language acquisition provide additional information on language lateralization. Contrary to early impressions summarized by Lenneberg (1967), aphasia in children is usually caused by left hemisphere lesions (Woods/Teuber 1978) just as in adults. Of 15 known right handers who became aphasic as a result of their unilateral lesions, only one was damaged on the right. Several studies indicate that after early left hemisphere damage, language functions may shift to the right hemisphere (Bingley 1958, Penfield/Roberts 1959, Rasmussen/Milner 1977). Such language compensation would be most dramatic when the lesion inactivates the whole hemisphere, rendering within-hemisphere compensation impossible. However, studies of posthemispherectomy patients who have normal intelligence are few, and the conclusion drawn from them that the right hemisphere may support normal verbal intelligence (Aram/Ekelman 1986), but not normal syntactical function (Kohn 1980, Vargha-Khadem/Isaacs/Papalelondi et al. 1991), although appealing, are not always confirmed (Ogden 1988) and are subject to numerous confounds and artefacts (Bishop 1988). Group studies of children with less complete early hemispheric lesions do support the view that left sided lesions cause more compromise in verbal learning, reading and spelling than right (Aram/Whitaker 1988), but the large number of individual cases that behave otherwise remains to be explained. Some of the left hemidecorticates studied by Dennis and her colleagues performed syntactical tasks as well as the right hemidecorticates. The hypothesis that the newborn cerebral hemispheres are equipotential for the representation of language cannot at this time be rejected (Bishop 1988).

If the hemispheres are equipotential for language in infancy, what nominates the left hemisphere for language processing in most people? According to Lenneberg, it is progressive lateralization. The infant data already reviewed, and the evidence for invariant lateralization, suggest a different answer. In infancy, dedicated cerebrum cannot play a part because most cerebral areas are still immature at this early stage. Yet preverbal laterality exists in infants, and bears a predictable relationship to subsequent language lateralization. This suggests the alternative model that hemisphere lateralization is a consequence of asymmetric activation coupled with verbal input and the adoption of verbal mental set (Kinsbourne/Lempert 1980). The consistently activated area of cortex becomes the language area. The predominantly bilateral organisation of language circuitry in non-righthanders is thereby explained as due to little or no asymmetry in the relevant ascending activation (Kinsbourne 1980). As long as the activation is topographically consistent, deficient language preformance is not expected, even if the language area is quite differently located from the norm. Thus nonrighthanders as a group are not significantly deficient in language or other aspects of cognition (Hardyck/Petrinovitch 1977). Perinatal asphyxia abolishes the newborn's rightward turning tendency (Turkewitz/Moreau/Birch 1968). Whether this is permanent is not known. But if for any reason ascending activation is diffuse or variable, this might retard the differentiation of language circuitry and result in inferior language function. Inconsistent dichotic and verbal-manual interference patterns observed by Parlow/Kinsbourne (submitted) in severely mentally retarded patients with and without Down syndrome might indicate that these poor language performers do not consistently activate a given cerebral territory when they are verbally active.

Even if language does emerge in the same hemisphere as that in which it becomes permanently established, is its organisation within that hemisphere as differentiated initially as in the adult? Satz/Strauss/Whitaker (1990) have reminded us that that invariant lateralization does not imply invariant localization within a hemisphere. Indeed, given the greatly different myelogenetic cycles of different parts of the hemisphere, it would be surprising if the neural substrate of language in the left hemisphere did not change with increasing age. However, clinical evidence of developmental differences in the anatomical basis of the different syndromes of aphasia remains sparse. Ojemann's (1983) recent findings have cast serious doubt on the classical diagram of posterior-anterior verbal information flow. But one can at least ask whether the broad correspondence between fluent versus nonfluent aphasia and posterior versus anterior left hemisphere lesion holds for children. Fluent aphasia is, for unknown reasons, rare in children. But in four such cases, Van Dongen/Loonen/Van Dongen (1985) did document mid or posterior temporal lesions, rather than the more customary frontally localised lesions in nonfluent aphasia. Much more clinical evidence is needed before a definitive answer to this question can be offered.

4. A Critical Period for Language Acquisition?

Animal experimentation offers instances in which deprivation of the customary environment or experience impairs the emergence of perceptual capabilities if the deprivation is implemented early enough, within a 'critical period'. The theoretical position that treats emerging language as neurologically comparable to other biologically preprogrammed capabilities (Lenneberg 1967) is inclined to view the apparent ability of young children but not adults to acquire language without explicitly effortful learning as evidence for the concept of a critical period for language acquisition. Thus up to puberty, according to Lenneberg, or at least till five years of age, according to Krashen (1973), children should have an exceptional facility for learning languages. However, learning a first language and learning additional languages are sufficiently different for the comparison between children and adults to be hopelessly confounded. It is not at all clear that children are better language learners than adults under comparable conditions. When children and adults learned a second language, adults performed better (Snow/Hoefnagel-Hohle 1978), even with respect to acquiring the foreign pronunciation (Snow/Hoefnagel-Hohle 1977), an ability which has been claimed to be restricted to children within the 'critical period' (Scovel 1969). If, as has often been argued, infants do have a superior ability to utter as well as discriminate phonemes that are not used in the particular language into which they are growing, that early phenomenon is not congruent in timing with progressive lateralization and the alleged critical period. Additional evidence derives from individuals who, on account of abnormal rearing conditions, were precluded from hearing or using language for the initial years of their life. The most thoroughly studied such case, Genie (Fromkin/Krashen/Curtiss et al. 1974), did, when finally introduced into a linguistic environment, exhibit some drastic limitations on the type and extent of language learning she could accomplish. A possibility was raised that her left hemisphere was no longer able to subserve emerging language, and a more limited right hemisphere mechanism had taken over. However, it is not at all clear that the right hemisphere is necessarily a limited language learning device, even in the mature nervous system of the adult. Not only is there substantial evidence that the right hemisphere is capable of compensating for language impairment (i. e. aphasia) due to left-sided stroke (Czopf 1972, Kinsbourne 1971), but several individual case reports suggest that this compensation may be effectively complete (Nielsen 1946). Additional evidence for the 'lateral shift hypothesis' for the brain basis of aphasic speech is reviewed by Code (1987). The increasing evidence for relatively effective right hemisphere compensation for aphasia is in accord with doubts about the assumption that 'plasticity' (the recruitment of other areas of cortex to the programming of behavior impaired by a focal cerebral lesion) is greater in the immature nervous system, that is, in children as compared to adults (Robinson 1981). The question as to the extent, if any, to which right hemisphere compensation in language function is limited by the nature of its neuronal hardware awaits the development of a reliable means of diagnosing right hemisphere language in the individual case of aphasia, which can then be appropriately studied. In the meantime, there is still no neurological support for the existence of the allegedly unique and dedicated left hemisphere language acquisition device.

5. References

Alajouanine, T. H. & Lhermitte, F. (1965). Acquired aphasia in children. *Brain, 88*, 653–662.

Aram, D. M. & Ekelman, B. L. (1986). Cognitive profiles of children with early onset of unilateral lesions. *Developmental Neuropsychology, 2*, 155–172.

Aram, D. M. & Whitaker, H. A. (1988). Cognitive sequelae of unilateral lesions acquired in early childhood. In D. L. Molfese & S. J. Segalowitz (Eds.), *Brain lateralization in children. 417–436.* New York: Guilford.

Archer, L. A., Campbell, D., & Segalowitz, S. J. (1988). A prospective study of hand preference and language development in 18- to 30-month olds: II. Relations between hand preference and language development. *Developmental Neuropsychology, 4*, 93–102.

Bates, E., O'Connell, B., Vaid, J., Sledge, P., & Oakes, L. (1986), Language and hand preference in early development. *Developmental Neuropsychology, 2*, 1–15.

Bertelson, P. (1986). The onset of literacy: liminal remarks. *Cognition, 24*, 1–30.

Bertenthal, B. I. & Campos, J. J. (1987). New directions in the study of early experience. *Child Development, 58*, 560–567.

Bingley, T. (1958). Mental symptoms in temporal lobe epilepsy and temporal lobe gliomas. *Acta Psychiatrica et Neurologia, 33*, Supp 120.

Bishop, D. M. V. (1988). Can the right hemisphere mediate language as well as the left? A critical review of recent research. *Cognitive Neuropsychology, 5*, 353–367.

Bishop, D. M. V. & Edmunson, A. (1986). Is otitis media a major cause of specific developmental language disorders? *British Journal of Disorders of Communication, 21*, 321–338.

Cambier, J., Elghozi, D., & Strube, E. (1979). Haemorrhage of the head of the left caudate nucleus: Disorganization of speech and graphic expression and disturbances in gesture. *Revue Neurologique, 135*, 763–774.

Code, C. (1987). *Language, aphasia and the right hemisphere*, New York: Wiley.

Cohen, M., Campbell, R., & Yaghmai, F. (1989). Neuropathological abnormalities in developmental dysphasia. *Annals of Neurology, 25*, 567–570.

Corballis, M. C. (1989). Laterality and human evolution. *Psychological Review, 96*, 492–505.

Czopf, J. (1972). Über die Rolle der nicht dominanten Hemisphäre in der Restitution der Sprache des Aphasikers. *Archiv für Psychiatrie und Nervenkrankheiten, 216*, 162–171.

Dennis, M. (1980). Capacity and strategy for syntactic comprehension after left or right decortication. *Brain and Language, 10*, 287–307.

Drake, W. E. (1968). Clinical and pathological findings in a child with a developmental learning disability. *Journal of Learning Disabilities, 1*, 486–502.

Entus, A. K. (1977). Hemispheric asymmetry in processing of dichotically presented speech and non-speech stimuli by infants. In S. J. Segalowitz & F. A. Gruber (Eds.), *Language development and neurological theory, 64–73.* New York: Academic Press.

Fromkin, V., Krashen S., Curtiss, S., Rigler, D., & Rigler, M. (1974). The development of language in Genie: a case of language acquisition beyond the "critical period". *Brain and Language, 1*, 81–107.

Galaburda, A. M., Corsiglia, J., Rosen, G. D., & Sherman, G. F. (1978). Planum temporale asymmetry, reappraisal since Geschwind and Levitsky. *Neuropsychologia, 25*, 853–868.

Galaburda, A. M. & Eidelberg, D. (1982). Symmetry and asymmetry in the human posterior thalamus. II Thalamic lesions in a case of developmental dyslexia. *Archives of Neurology, 39*, 333–336.

Galaburda, A. M., Sherman, G. F., Rosen, G. D., Aboitiz, F., & Geschwind, N. (1987). Developmental dyslexia: Four consecutive patients with cortical anomalies. *Annals of Neurology, 18*, 222–233.

Gardiner, M. F. & Walter, D. O. (1977). Evidence of hemispheric specialization from infant E. E. G. In S. Harnad, R. W. Doty, J. Goldstein, J. Jaynes, & G. Krauthamer (Eds.), *Lateralization in the nervous system. 481–500.* New York: Academic Press.

Geffen, G. (1978). The development of the right ear advantage in dichotic listening with focussed attention. *Cortex, 14*, 169–177.

Geschwind, N. & Levitzky, W. (1968). Human brain: Left-right asymmetries in temporal speech region. *Science, 161*, 186–187.

Glanville, B. B., Best, C. T., & Levenson, R. A. (1977). Cardiac measure of cerebral asymmetries in infant auditory perception. *Developmental Psychology, 13*, 55–59.

Goldstein, R., Landau, W. M., & Kleffner, F. R. (1958). Neurological assessment of some deaf and aphasic children. *Transactions of the American Otological Society, 46*, 122–136.

Hardyck, C. & Petrinovitch, L. F. (1977). Left-handedness. *Psychological Bulletin, 84*, 405–411.

Hecaen, H. (1983). Acquired aphasia in children: revisited. *Neuropsychologia, 21*, 581–587.

Hiscock, M. (1988). Behavioral asymmetries in young children. In D. L. Molfese & S. J. Segalowitz (Eds.), *Brain lateralization in children. 85–169.* New York: Guilford Press.

Hiscock, M. & Kinsbourne, M. (1977). Selective listening asymmetry in preschool children. *Developmental Psychology, 13*, 217–224.

Hiscock, M. & Kinsbourne, M. (1978). Ontogeny of cerebral dominance: Evidence from time-sharing asymmetry in children. *Developmental Psychology, 14*, 321–329.

Hiscock, M. & Kinsbourne, M. (1980a). Asymmetries of selective listening and attention switching in children. *Developmental Psychology, 16*, 70–82.

Hiscock, M. & Kinsbourne, M. (1980b). Asymmetry of verbal-manual time-sharing in children: A follow-up study. *Neuropsychologia, 18*, 151–162.

Horek, F. B., Shumway-Cook, A., Crowe, T. K., & Black, F. O. (1988). Vestibular function and motor proficiency of children with impaired hearing or with learning disability and motor impairments. *Developmental Medicine and Child Neurology, 30*, 64–79.

Ingram, D. (1975). Cerebral speech lateralization in young children. *Neuropsychologia, 13*, 103–105.

Ingram, T. T. S. (1959). Specific developmental disorders of speech in childhood. *Brain, 82*, 450–467.

Jernigan, T. L., Hesselink, J., & Tallal. P. (1987). Cerebral morphology on magnetic resonance imaging in developmental dysphasia. *Society of Neuroscience Abstracts, 13*, 1, 651.

Johnston, R. B., Stark, R. E., Mellits, E. D., & Tallal, P. (1981). Neurological status of language-impaired and normal children. *Annals of Neurology, 10*, 159–163.

Kavale, K. A. & Nye, C. (1991). The structure of learning disabilities. *Exceptionality, 2*, 141–156.

Kinsbourne, M. (1971). The minor cerebral hemisphere as a source of aphasic speech. *Archives of Neurology, 25*, 302–306.

Kinsbourne, M. (1975). The ontology of cerebral dominance. In D. R. Aaronson & R. W. Rieber (Eds.), *Developmental psycholinguistics and communication disorders. 244–250.* New York: Academic Press.

Kinsbourne, M. (1980). A model for the ontogeny of cerebral organisation in non-right-handers. In J. Herron (Ed.), *Neuropsychology of left handedness. 177–185.* New York: Academic Press.

Kinsbourne, M. & Lempert, H. (1980). Does left brain lateralization of speech arise from right-biased orienting to salient percepts? *Human Development, 22*, 270–276.

Kinsbourne, M., Rufo, D., Gamzu, E., Palmer, R., & Berliner, A. (1991). Neuropsychological deficits in adults with dyslexia. *Developmental Medicine and Child Neurology, 33*, 763–775.

Kohn, B. (1980). Right hemisphere speech representation and syntax comprehension after left cerebral injury. *Brain and Language, 9*, 350–361.

Krashen, S. (1973). Lateralization, language learning and the critical period: some new evidence. *Language Learning, 23*, 63–74.

Landau, W. M., Goldstein, R., & Kleffner, F. R. (1960). Congenital aphasia: a clinicopathological study. *Neurology, 10*, 915–921.

Le May, M. (1976). Morphological cerebral asymmetries of modern man, fossil man and nonhuman primate. *Annals of the New York Academy of Sciences, 280*, 349–366.

Le May, M. (1984). Radiological, developmental and fossil asymmetries. In N. Geschwind & A. M. Galaburda (Eds.), *Cerebral dominance: The biological foundations.* Cambridge, MA: Harvard University Press.

Lenneberg, E. H. (1967). *Biological foundations of language.* New York: Wiley.

Lokker, R. & Morais, J. (1985). Ear differences in children at two years of age. *Neuropsychologia, 23*, 127–129.

Mac Kain, K., Studdert-Kennedy, M., Spieker, S. & Stern, D. (1983). Infant intermodal speech perception as a left hemisphere function. *Science, 219*, 1347–1349.

Molfese, D. L., Freeman, R. B., & Palermo, D. (1975). The ontogeny of brain lateralization for speech and non-speech stimuli. *Brain and Language, 2*, 356–368.

Nagafuchi, M. (1970). Development of dichotic and monaural hearing abilities in young children. *Acta Otolaryngologica, 69*, 409–414.

Netley, C. (1983). Sex chromosome abnormalities and the development of verbal and nonverbal abilities. In C. A. Ludlow & J. A. Cooper (Eds.), *Genetic aspects of speech and language disorders, 179–196*, New York: Academic Press.

Nielsen, J. M. (1946). *Agnosia, apraxia, aphasia: Their value in cerebral localization.* New York: Hoeber.

Ogden, J. A. (1988). Language and memory functions after long recovery periods in left-hemispherectomized subjects. *Neuropsychologia, 26*, 645–659.

Ojemann, G. (1975). Language and the thalamus: Object naming and recall during and after thalamic stimulation. *Brain and Language, 2*, 101–120.

Ojemann, G. (1983). Brain organisation for language from the perspective of electrical stimulation mapping. *Behavioral and Brain Sciences, 6*, 189–230.

Parlow, S. & Kinsbourne, M. (submitted). Consistency of laterality findings in Down and non Down mentally retarded subjects.

Penfield, W. & Roberts, L. (1959). *Speech and brain mechanisms*. Princeton: Princeton University Press.

Piazza, D. M. (1977), Cerebral lateralization in young children as measured by dichotic listening and finger tapping tasks. *Neuropsychologia, 15*, 417–425.

Pieniadz, J. M., Naeser, M. A., Koff, E. & Levine, H. L. (1983). CT scan cerebral hemispheric asymmetry measurements in stroke cases with global aphasia: atypical asymmetries associated with improved recovery. *Cortex, 19*, 371–391.

Rasmussen, T. & Milner, B. (1977). The role of early left brain injury in determining lateralization of cerebral speech functions. *Annals of the New York Academie of Sciences, 299*, 355–369.

Ratcliff, G., Dila, C., Taylor, L., & Milner, B. (1980). The morphological asymmetries of the hemispheres and cerebral dominance: a possible relationship. *Brain and Language, 11*, 87–98.

Roberts, R. J., Varney, N. R., Reinarz, S. J., & Parkins, R. A. (1988). CT asymmetries in developmentally dyslexic adults. *Developmental Neuropsychology, 4*, 231–237.

Robinson, R. O. (1981). Equal recovery in child and adult brain. *Developmental Medicine and Child Neurology, 23*, 379–383.

Rumsey, J. M., Berman, K. F., Denckla, M. B., Hamburger, S. D., Kruesi, M. J., & Weinberger, D. R. (1987). Regional cerebral blood flow in severe developmental dyslexia. *Archives of Neurology, 44*, 1144–1150.

Satz, P., Strauss, E., & Whitaker, H. (1990). The ontogeny of hemispheric specialization: Some old hypotheses revisited. *Brain and Language, 38*, 596–614.

Scovel, T. (1969). Foreign accents, language acquisition and cerebral dominance. *Language Learning, 19*, 245–253.

Segalowitz, S. J. & Chapman, J. S. (1980). Cerebral asymmetry for speech in neonates: A behavioral measure. *Brain and Language, 9*, 281–288.

Sheridan, M. (1973). Children of seven years with marked speech defects. *British Journal of Disorders of Communication, 8*, 9–15.

Snow, C. E. & Hoefnagel-Hohle, M. (1977). Age differences in the pronunciation of foreign sounds. *Language and Speech, 20*, 357–365.

Snow, C. E. & Hoefnagel-Hohle, M. (1978). The critical period for language acquisition: Evidence from second language learning. *Child Development, 49*, 1114–1128.

St. James-Roberts, I. (1981). A reinterpretation of hemispherectomy data without functional plasticity of the brain: 1. Intellectual function. *Brain and Language, 13*, 31–53.

Tallal, P. (1980). Auditory temporal perception, phonics and reading disabilities in children. *Brain and Language, 9*, 182–198.

Tallal, P. & Piercy, M. (1973). Defects of nonverbal auditory perception in children with developmental aphasia. *Nature, 241*, 468–469.

Tallal, P. & Piercy, M. (1974). Developmental aphasia: rate of auditory processing and selective impairment of consonant perception. *Neuropsychologia, 12*, 83–93.

Tallal, P., Ross, R., & Curtiss, S. (1989). Familial aggregation in specific language impairment. *Journal of Speech and Hearing Disorders, 54*, 167–173.

Turkewitz, G., Moreau, T., & Birch, H. G. (1968). Relation between birth condition and neuro-behavioral organization in the newborn. *Pediatric Research, 2*, 243–249.

Vargha-Khadem, F., Isaacs, E. B., Papalelondi, H., Polkey, C. E., & Wilson, J. (1991). Development of language in six hemispherectomized patients. *Brain, 114*, 473–495.

Van Dongen, H. R., Loonen, M. C. B., & Van Dongen, K. J. (1985). Anatomical basis for acquired fluent aphasia in children. *Annals of Neurology, 17*, 306–309.

Vellutino, F. R. (1979). *Dyslexia: Theory and research*. Cambridge, MA: MIT Press.

Wada, J., Clarke, J., & Hamm, A. (1975). Cerebral hemispheric asymmetry in humans. *Archives of Neurology, 32*, 239–246.

White, N. & Kinsbourne, M. (1980). Does speech output control lateralize over time? Evidence from verbal-manual time-sharing tasks. *Brain and Language, 10*, 215–223.

Witelson, S. F. & Pallie, W. (1973). Left hemisphere specialization for language in the newborn: Neuroanatomical evidence of brain asymmetry. *Brain, 96*, 641–646.

Woods, B. T. & Teuber, H-L. (1978). Changing patterns of childhood aphasia. *Annals of Neurology, 32*, 239–246.

Young, G. & Gascon, M. (1990). Neonatal laterality, birth stress, familial sinistrality and left brain inhibition. *Developmental Neuropsychology, 6*, 127–150.

Marcel Kinsbourne, Boston, Massachusetts (USA)

60. Psychiatric and Psychological Aspects of Language Development Disorders

1. Introduction

A growing body of research exists now to indicate that a variety of psychological factors can interfere with the process of normal language development. The factors which have been implicated range from exogenous influences such as maternal input to endogenous factors like temperament. Other variables which may be relevant, including gender, birth order and twinning are a particularly inextricable mix of exogenous and endogenous factors and these have been referred to by some authors as 'biosocial' variables. A great deal of controversy exists about the extent to which psychological and environmental factors can lead to a clinically significant language delay, as well as about the precise circumstances under which this may occur. Certainly some of these factors seem to affect rates of language development but they may not necessarily lead to variations outside the normal range. This article aims to discuss firstly whether the language acquisition process is vulnerable to external influences at all, and if it is what the effects of specific factors might be. The second main focus of this article is on the psychosocial sequelae of language disorders since it is now well-established that a child with a language development disorder will be at increased risk of educational retardation and/or behavioral or psychiatric abnormalities. A review of relevant research is presented together with a consideration of methodological issues and possible causative mechanisms.

2. Influences on Normal Language Development

The first question to ask is why language development should be vulnerable to any of these factors. Certainly if language-learning involves an unfolding series of robust programmed processes then it might be assumed to be immune from other influences, but such a completely biologically-determined explanation seems unlikely. What seems more probable is that both inborn and external factors have a role to play but there is heated debate about the relative contribution made by each side of the equation. The behaviorist viewpoint, for example, asserts that all knowledge derives from the environment and with respect to the language-learning task the child hears speech, imitates it and then acquires it through a process of selective reinforcement (Skinner 1957, 29 f). Whilst this approach gives support to the idea that language development is susceptible to external influences it is now generally accepted that processes such as imitation, reinforcement and generalization cannot alone account for all the linguistic changes which occur as children acquire language, although they may well be of value in explaining certain aspects of the process. The nativists, on the other hand, claim that certain linguistic features are innate, providing schemata which the child can apply to the particular language he is exposed to (e. g. Chomsky 1964). Whilst making a valid contribution to the debate, this approach is generally seen now as being rather restricted and the more satisfactory accounts are those such as the epigenetic-interactionist viewpoint (Cromer 1981). This aims to provide better incorporation of the roles of inner determinants with environmental factors and asserts that inherent in the human species are a number of unfolding developmental phenomena, some of which may be specifically linguistic, that interact with environmental variables. This approach differs from the nativist viewpoint in claiming not that children are born in possession of particular structures, but rather that structures are built up from an interaction of innate potential with environmental factors.

The disputes between linguists and psycholinguists who support the existence of innate language functions and psychologists who do not, have raged for a number of years now and seem likely to continue for some time. Although there is little consensus of opinion about the degree to which external factors can influence language development there is on balance, support for the basic idea that language development can indeed be susceptible to influence from environmental factors.

The precise nature of the relations between environment and development deserves closer examination, however. Some of the early work in this field took a unidimensional approach asserting that 'good environments' facilitate all aspects of development whilst 'bad environments' have the opposite effect. The issues are clearly not this simple and for the most part it is now well-established that relations between environment and development are highly specific in two respects. Firstly 'environmental specificity', i. e. different aspects of the environment, do seem to differentially influence specific aspects of development (Wachs/Chan 1986), and secondly 'organismic specificity' which predicts that the impact of the environment will be mediated by the individual characteristics of the individual child. The child and the environment will exert a dynamic influence on each other and consequently two children may be exposed to similar environmental stimulation but individual characteristics such as sex, temperament and biological vulnerability will contribute to a different outcome for each child.

It is vital that the whole issue of effects on language development is considered from a developmental perspective. A child of 3 years, for example, will perceive and assimilate stimuli in a quite different way from an infant of 12 months, and it is because of these changing circumstances that longitudinal research is of particular value in assessing influences on language development.

2.1. Exogenous Factors

Turning to the effects of specific factors, one of the basic external influences which human beings are subject to is interaction with other humans and there has been a great deal of interest in the extent to which qualitative and quantitative variations in the child's social environment can produce measurable differences in linguistic output. Much of this attention has focussed on the effect of maternal input and this topic is considered elsewhere in this volume, but other important bodies of information have been built up from studying children who have experienced a variety of linguistic backdrops, e. g. children who have been maltreated or institutionalized, those with depressed mothers and also hearing children of deaf parents. The most extreme form of these 'natural experiments' however are the well-documented reports of children who have been brought up in circumstances of extreme isolation where they have been deprived of social contact. These cases are horrific and fortunately rare but they do serve to highlight the important role that social interaction plays in language development. Skuse (1984) documents the cases of nine children who were raised in conditions of extreme social deprivation for periods from 2.5 to 12 years. Many of these children had been completely deprived of any contact with other people or with normal language and several had been physically restrained. A number of important findings emerge from the horrific experiences of these unfortunate children. First, it appears clear that severe environmental privation can lead to devastating cognitive and language impairments since these grossly isolated children were without useful language and functioned in the severely retarded range at the time they were rescued. Second, in most cases there was very substantial recovery within a matter of months of the children being placed in a normal environment, clearly demonstrating that the impairments were not due to congenital deficits. That being said, however, there were several children described in the case reports who did not recover after rescue and although it is plausible that unusually severe social isolation can on its own lead to a permanent and irreversible language handicap, it does seem very likely that the children in question may have had additional biological handicaps which complicated their recovery. A related issue, however, is whether the ultimate degree of recovery is influenced by protective factors during the period of isolation (e. g. twins described in one of the case reports had each other for company) or by particular remedial measures afterwards, but as yet there is little data on their importance. What may be of relevance is the suggestion that if language acquisition is to proceed normally then it must be acquired during the first 12 years of life (Curtiss 1981; Lenneberg 1967, 158).

Gross deprivation represents one extreme of the quantitative dimension of social interaction but there is evidence that the quality of attention that children receive, particularly from their principal caregivers, also plays an important role in cognitive development (Matas/Arend/Sroufe 1978; Slade 1987). Werner/Kaplan (1963, 42 ff) claim that the motivation to engage in symbolic activity emanates from the desire to share experiences with a social partner and Bruner (1975) takes a similar view arguing that through dyadic interactions with the caregiver the child develops linguistic knowledge. This view seems intuitively reasonable and implies that children who lack a responsive social partner will be disadvantaged in their language development. Maltreated children present a useful case for study here since a number of studies have found maltreating mothers to be unresponsive and not encouraging of the sorts of communicative exchanges described as being ideal for promoting language development. In general, neglecting mothers have been found to interact with their children far less than non-neglecting mothers (Burgess/Conger 1978), to provide less verbal instruction about the environment (Bousha/Twentyman 1984) and to use more controlling language. (Aragona/Eyberg 1981). They have also been found less likely than control mothers to initiate play interchanges (Wasserman/Green/Allen 1983). To investigate whether this impoverished communicative environment does actually affect linguistic development Gersten/Coster/Schneider-Rosen et al. (1986) studied two groups of lower socio-economic status toddlers – 20 who had been legally maltreated and 20 who had not. The children were observed at 25 months in both structured and unstructured play sessions with their mothers, and coders who were blind to the maltreatment status of the children rated their linguistic performance and communicative behavior. Perhaps surprisingly this study found that at 25 months there were no significant differences between the two groups for communicative behavior, although when attachment security was taken into account differences were apparent with the more securely attached toddlers talking more and consistently demonstrating a more elaborate vocabulary and complex use of syntax. The findings of this study imply that maltreatment in itself need not affect language development, although the mother-child relationship as expressed by attachment may well have an influence on rates of development. As discussed earlier, however, it is vital to consider environmental influences in the developmental context. Consequently the same group of researchers repeated the format of the earlier study but with children aged 31 months (Coster/Gersten/Beeghly/Cichetti 1989). These findings were interesting since in contrast to the situation with the younger children there were by 31 months significant differences in the linguistic behavior of the maltreated and nonmaltreated children. There were no differences in receptive language, nor in the total number of utterances, but the maltreated children used less complex syntax and a smaller range of words. They also used fewer descriptive utterances. These studies suggest that maltreatment may interfere with the processes of normal language development, but it is not clear whether the effects show merely in rates of development or whether clinically significant language delays can result.

Another factor likely to affect the quality and amount of attention received by a child is the mother's emotional state. Cox/Puckering/Pound/Mills (1987) found that depression can impair a parent's ability to interact responsively with his/her child and a number of other studies attest that depressed mothers interact with their children in ways which may prove disadvantageous to their children (Bettes 1988; Davenport/Zahn-Waxler/Adland/Mayfield 1984; Egeland/Sroufe 1981). In general, maternal mental disorder seems more likely to cause disturbances of behavior and socio-emotional functioning than to cause any form of cognitive impairment (Rutter 1985 a, b), but there have nonetheless been clinical reports of language delay in young children with depressed mothers. Richman/Stevenson/Graham (1982, 183), for example, found that maternal depression when children were aged three years was associated with somewhat lower language and reading scores at eight years even when the maternal IQ, social class and current depression were taken into account. Turning to the age of the child when the mother experiences depression this is likely to be influential and research by Coghill/Caplan/Alexandra et al. (1986) suggests that children may be particularly vulnerable to effect during their first year. Children whose mothers had been depressed before they were one year showed cognitive deficits at 4 years whilst concurrent depression had no effect.

The mechanisms through which maternal depression can influence cognitive development are unclear and there are probably several mechanisms in operation (Rutter 1990). First, the negative mood experienced by the mothers may lead to more negative affect being expressed towards their infants and they may also be less sensitive and responsive to their children's needs and cues. Second, it is not clear whether maternal depression in itself is what constitutes a risk factor for cognitive impairment or whether it is the associated factors such as social disadvantage and marital distress which so often co-exist with it (Gotlib/Hooley 1988; Rutter/Quinton 1984), and more research is needed to elucidate on this issue.

It has already been seen from the descriptions of the children raised in conditions of extreme privation that exposure to some sort of language is necessary for language to develop and further data on what happens when children have a restricted linguistic input is provided by studying hearing children raised by deaf parents. The findings are mixed and there has been little recent research but several studies have identified a range of speech/language problems in such children including articulation and syntactic deficits (Sachs/Bard/Johnson 1981; Schiff/Ventry 1976). Other writers, however, have concluded, perhaps unexpectedly, that such children have few or no speech or language deficits (Lenneberg 1967, 137; Vernon 1974). The information that is needed to interpret these findings relates to whether there are protective factors which allow some children to escape unscathed. An above average IQ is probably one of these but it is unclear how others such as the quality of the mother-child relationship may contribute.

All the cases to here concern variations in the quality of the relationship between the child and his/her mother but obviously not all children are brought up within a family, and many are raised in institutions. In the past, high rates of cognitive and language delay were found amongst institutionalised children (Burlingham/Freud 1943, 13 f; Goldfarb 1945), but thankfully improvements in the quality of residential nurseries have resulted in these delays no longer being characteristic of institution-reared children (Tizard/Cooperman/Joseph/Tizard 1972; Tizard/Rees 1974) carrying the implication that whilst interaction with adults is crucial to language development this need not necessarily take place with the mother. The quality of the institution does appear to be important, however, and in particular variables such as the amount of verbal interaction between staff and children and whether children's question are answered have been shown by Tizard/Cooperman/Joseph/Tizard (1972) to be systematically associated with variations in the progress of language development.

2.2. 'Biosocial' Variables

A number of 'biosocial' factors have been implicated as having an effect on rates of language development and in some instances on the development of language disorders, although it can be difficult to draw conclusions and distinguish between causal mechanisms which have their roots in variations within the social environment and those where a pure biological cause is in action. Gender is an example of such a biosocial factor and many studies of the pathological dimension have found language delay to be about twice as common in boys as in girls (Morley 1965, 54; Silva 1980; Stevenson/Richman 1976). This sex bias is not apparent in all types of language disorder, however, and Bartak/Rutter/Cox (1975) for example found no significant sex difference in children with severe receptive language difficulties. Observations of language development in the normal sphere, rather than from a clinical viewpoint (e. g. Bloom/Lightbown/Hood 1975) have led to suggestions that there is a gender-associated difference in early grammatical style with girls tending to use the referential style (a high proportion of common object names) as described by Nelson (1973) and boys more frequently employing an expressive style (heterogeneous vocabularies containing items from a variety of form classes). Several studies have found the referential style to correlate positively with rates of language development (Nelson 1973; Ramer 1976) but the suggestion of a sex bias in grammatical style is by no means widely accepted and indeed some studies of early language development have failed to find any evidence of gender-related differences in rates of development (e. g. Bates/Bretherton/Snyder 1988, 233; Macaulay 1978). This issue continues to be unresolved. One biological explanation for the sex bias in ultimate pathology may be very early undetected brain damage which for some reason affects the sexes differently, possibly involving testosterone (Geschwind/Galaburda 1985). It may also reflect some sort of genetic mediation and there is evidence that developmental language delays do indeed have a familial loading (Robinson 1987; Tallal/Ross/Curtiss 1989). The genetic hypothesis remains unproven as yet, however.

There have also been suggestions that birth order has an effect on language development with first-born and only children having an advantage in verbal intelligence (Douglas/Ross/Simpson 1968, 129 f) and reading attainment (Davies/Butler/Goldstein 1972, 176 ff; Record/Mc Keown/Edwards 1969). These differences are only small, however, and seem unlikely to result in clinically significant language disorder, although in combination with other factors they may play some role.

A particularly interesting area of research has been the language development of twins and results are consistent in confirming that on average twins are disadvantaged in their language development when compared with singletons (Conway/Lytton/Pysh 1980; Hay/Prior/Collet/Williams 1987). Mittler (1970) found that 4-year-old twins showed an average retardation of six months in their language development and evidence that the disadvantages of the twin situation can have longer-lasting effects comes from research by Johnston/Prior/Hay (1984) who found that older twins are more likely than singletons to be delayed in reading skills. In childhood twins have been shown to have a slightly lower verbal IQ than singletons (Record/Mc Keown/Edwards 1970; Mittler 1970; Johnston/Prior/Hay 1984) and there is an indication that some deficit is still present in the older age groups.

Rutter/Redshaw (1991) review the possible causes of the language deficit in twins and highlight factors in the social environment. The parents of twins, for example, in common with the parents of large families are faced with a dilemma of having to divide their attention between more than one child with the result that mothers of twins tend to speak to them less and to use less complex utterances when compared with mothers of singletons (Conway/Lytton/Pysh 1980; Lytton/Conway 1977). The possible influences of maternal mental disorder on language development have already been highlighted in this article and mothers of twins have been found to have higher levels of emotional distress than mothers of singletons (Thorpe/Golding/Mc Gillivray, submitted) with these stresses continuing beyond the twins' infancy years and still being apparent at 5 years. Several possible contributory factors to the observed verbal deficit in twins have therefore been identified and important evidence that this deficit may well be a consequence of factors in the postnatal environment is presented by Record/Mc Keown/Edwards (1970). They found that twins whose co-twin had died at birth or during the neonatal period had a measured IQ at the age of 11 years that was similar to that of singletons whereas those who had a living co-twin scored significantly lower. Aside from the possible social/environmental causes there is the possibility that biological factors are implicated since twins suffer from a higher rate of obstetric and perinatal complications (Watts/Lytton 1981). This possibility warrants further investigation although it should be said that in general obstetric and perinatal factors do not seem to play a major role in language delay (Mittler 1970).

The final factor which will be considered under this heading is social class. The whole issue of social class and its influence on language development is a very vexed one but some relationship does appear to exist (Davies/Butler/Goldstein 1972, 92; Douglas 1964, 152) with the main effect being seen in patterns of language usage (Bernstein 1971, 61 f; Robinson 1980), although there do seem to be some differences in language competence too (Tizard/Hughes/Carmichael/Pinkerton 1983). Social class, however, is a very broad term and it is not clear precisely which specific aspects of social class are relevant. Silva/Fergusson (1980) found that maternal general mental ability, maternal education and training in child development were all associated with the language level of 3-year-olds and these factors may represent some of the relevant factors associated within the term 'social class' but there is a clear need for further investigation.

2.3. Endogenous Factors

A number of factors from the external environment may impinge on the child's language development as has been seen already, but it is also important to consider what the child brings to the language-learning process. One aspect of this is temperament. Bates/Bretherton/Snyder (1988) suggest that sociability may be a significant factor in affecting language-learning style so that a child whose primary theme is to be with and be like other human beings is more likely to rely on rote processes in language-learning whilst a child for whom this is less of a primary theme is more likely to take an analytic approach. There is, however, very little research which links temperamental differences with variations in language development and no evidence as yet to suggest that temperamental differences can result in language pathology per se. The possibility remains nonetheless that temperamental differences when combined with other factors may increase the likelihood of a particular child developing a clinically significant language deficit. It should be borne in mind when considering the effect of any environmental factor that the interaction between the child and the environment will be bidirectional with each influencing the other. The difficulty lies in uncovering the interrelated mechanisms. To what extent, for example, is the mother influencing the child's response and conversely does the child have an inherent preference which encourages the mother to respond in a particular way.

Many of the findings presented so far are controversial, but there is nonetheless a strong thread running through the research on language development which suggests that interaction with adults is important in facilitating the growth of children's language. Clearly other factors must contribute to this process, however, and it should not be forgotten that there is a close relationship between language and intelligence and between language delay and low intelligence (Silva 1981).

3. Psychosocial Sequelae

As well as certain psychological factors being implicated in the development of language disorders it is now well-established that once children have developed a language disorder they are at an increased risk of other psychosocial problems such as educational retardation, behavioral difficulties and psychiatric symptoms. Although there has been a great deal of research in this area it has been difficult to compare studies and often researchers have obtained contradictory results because of methodological differences (Rutter/Mawhood 1991). There are six main methodological problems which bedevil this field of research. First, the groups studied have been quite heterogeneous in both type and severity of speech/language disorder. Second, the investigations have varied widely in the level of detail on individual diagnosis and the extent to which children with associated handicaps have been excluded. Third, some studies concern clinic samples with unknown referral biases whereas others are epidemiologically based. Fourth, investigations vary in the extent to which data on psychosocial sequelae have been both standardized and detailed. Fifth, studies differ in the degree to which longitudinal data have been available and statistically utilized in an effective manner. The consequence is that few studies separate the effects of transient language delay from those of persistent language impairment. Sixth, only some of the projects have used control groups or have had general population data that allow estimation of the degree to which the level of psychosocial disorder in the developmental language disorder is truly significantly raised.

The initial studies which looked at the associations between language development disorders and psychosocial difficulties were cross-sectional in design. More recently, however, there has been an increasing awareness that the psychosocial sequelae of language development disorders can be long-term and a number of studies have attempted to investigate the relationships between early language functioning and later psychosocial outcome.

3.1. Educational Retardation

Taking educational retardation first, numerous studies have documented the finding that children with developmental language disorders have a substantially increased risk for later reading difficulties (e. g. Aram/Nation 1980; Garvey/Gordon 1973; Griffiths 1969; Silva/Mc Gee/Williams 1983). There are six main issues which arise from this finding; (1) whether the scholastic risk is mainly a function of general intellectual impairment or a specific language deficit; (2) whether the risk is specifically for reading difficulties or more generally for a broad range of scholastic problems; (3) which types of speech/language deficit lead to the greatest scholastic risk; (4) whether the scholastic risk associated with a specific language disorder differs in degree or pattern from that associated with developmental disorders of non-language functions (such as motor or perceptual skills); (5) related to the last point, whether the risk stems from the fact that language as such is impaired or from neurodevelopmental or cognitive deficits that may underlie the language disorder; and (6) whether the risk applies only when there is continuing language impairment or whether it applies also to transient language difficulties.

Taking the first issue, it has been shown that much of the scholastic risk stems from general intellectual impairment, but that nonetheless reading difficulties arise with an increased frequency even when intellectual level has been taken into account (e. g. Debray-Ritzen/Mattinger/Chapuis 1976; Silva/Mc Gee/Williams 1983). Turning to the issue of whether the scholastic difficulties extend further than reading Aram/Ekelman/Nation

(1984) found that of 16 children with language delay and an IQ in the normal range, two thirds had required special tutoring or had repeated one or more school grades by adolescence and of the 11 with an initial IQ of at least 90, 5 were in the lowest decile for at least one subject out of reading, spelling and mathematics. It is of note that the scholastic difficulties were as evident in mathematics as in the other two areas and there is some evidence to suggest that any reading deficits may apply more to reading comprehension than to reading accuracy (Bishop/Adams 1990). Furthermore there are suggestions that these difficulties can continue into adult life. In a follow-up into adult life of boys with a developmental disorder of receptive language, and initially normal IQ, Mawhood/Rutter/Howlin (in preparation) found that the majority, as well as having deficits in reading and spelling also had poor mathematical abilities.

For the most part research findings indicate that articulation-impaired children are less likely than language-delayed children to experience serious educational problems (Bishop/Adams 1990; Debray-Ritzen/Mattinger/Chapuis 1976; Hall/Tomblin 1978). Some contradictory findings do exist, however, and Crookes/Green (1963) found that reading difficulties were similarly affected in language-impaired children and in those with pure articulation problems although arithmetical difficulties were greater in the former group.

There appears to be no research which has directly compared language disorders with other non-language developmental disorders and it is therefore not known whether the degree and pattern of scholastic risk associated with language disorders is specifically related to language functioning. Nonetheless this seems possible and a relevant finding comes from the Rourke/Strang (1983) study of learning disabled children, which showed that those with reading difficulties tended to have verbal deficits whereas those with mathematical difficulties were more likely to have visuo-spatial deficits.

One important issue which many follow-up studies have not controlled for is whether the language delay is resolved by the time the child starts school. Bishop/Adams (1990), however, in a well-planned study of 8-year-olds found that reading difficulties at age 8 were evident in children where there was a persistent language impairment but not in a comparison group who had also shown a clinically significant language deficit at age 4, but in whom the deficit had recovered by the age of 8.

3.2. Socio-Emotional Behavioral Disorders

Taking psychopathological problems next, there are numerous studies which have found significantly higher rates of behavioral problems in children who have developmental disorders of speech and language (e. g. Jenkins/Bax/Hart 1980; Prizant/Audet/Burke et al. 1990; Silva/Justin/McGee/Williams 1984; Stevenson/Richman/Graham 1985). In a Canadian study Beitchman/Nair/Clegg et al. (1986) found that amongst 1655 5-year olds 11 % had a speech/language disorder and on clinical examination 48.7 % of these showed some psychiatric disorder, particularly attention deficit disorders and emotional disturbances. The most comprehensive investigations, however, have been the Los Angeles series of studies (e. g. Baker/Cantwell 1982; Cantwell/Baker/Mattison 1979). The investigators took consecutive cases referred to a clinic for speech and language disorders and then carried out a full psychometric and psychiatric evaluation on them. Of the first 100 children to be investigated in this way 53 received at least one psychiatric diagnosis including attention deficit disorder, oppositional disorder and anxiety disorders.

An important methodological issue affecting comparison between studies is that they have varied greatly not only in their definitions of speech/language disorder but also in their measures of psychopathology and in whether the data is collected by observational or interview method. Nonetheless, taking all the available data into account the main associations between language development disorders and psychopathology seem to be in the domains of anxiety, social relationships and attention-deficit problems rather than in conduct disturbance or antisocial behavior (Rutter/Mawhood 1991). There are few adequate follow-up studies but those available suggest that psychopathological problems tend to increase rather than diminish as children grow older. Baker/Cantwell (1987) in their follow-up of a clinic-based sample found that the proportion with psychiatric disorder rose from 44 % to 60 %. Whilst a quarter of the sample were without identifiable disorder at the time of initial appraisal and developed disorder subsequently, only 8 % of the sample had a disorder when young which resolved during the follow-up period. Mawhood/Rutter/Howlin (in preparation) in one of the rare follow-ups into adulthood found that amongst boys who had experienced receptive developmental language disorder 70 % showed impaired social functioning in adulthood whereas only 35 % had shown poor peer relations in early childhood (Bartak/Rutter/Cox 1975) and 50 % in middle childhood (Cantwell/Baker/Rutter et al. 1989).

Turning more specifically to the factors which may affect psychosocial outcome, several studies have found that psychopathological problems are more frequent if language delay is accompanied by lower than average intelligence (Baker/Cantwell 1987; Beitchman/Hood/Rochun/Peterson 1989; Silva/Justin/Mc Gee/Williams 1984). The findings on whether the type of speech/language deficit affects psychosocial outcome are contradictory, but it seems that if children with a pure phonological problem are at any increased risk this is more likely to result in emotional problems rather than attention deficit disorders (Cantwell/Baker 1977).

It has been suggested by Tallal/Dukette/Curtiss (1989) that the raised incidence of behavioral difficulties in language-impaired children largely reflects neurodevelopmental impairment. They found that at age 4 years descriptions such as 'clumsy', 'confused' and 'can't concentrate' differentiated language-impaired children from controls. However in males, 'cries too much' and 'clings to adults', and in girls 'withdrawn', 'secretive' and 'compulsions' also did so. This is an interesting idea but on balance, and bearing in mind the findings that anxiety and poor peer relations also increase with age it is extremely unlikely that the socio-emotional difficulties consistently found to be raised in individuals with speech/language impairment are simply reflecting direct manifestations of neurodevelopmental impairment. Whether or not the socio-emotional difficulties stem specifically from speech/language impairment per se or more generally from neurodevelopmental or cognitive deficits that may underlie the language delay, however, is another matter. Systematic comparisons with other types of specific developmental disorder are lacking and are much needed. Without them it cannot be known whether the psychopathological risk with language delay differs in severity or type with that associated with, say, the clumsy child syndrome.

The reports to here have focused on common psychopathological problems but there is evidence that at least severe disorders of receptive language are also associated with risks for serious social abnormalities and for later psychoses. Cases of children with developmental disorders of language who show schizophrenic-like psychoses in early childhood have been observed (Mawhood/Rutter/Howlin in preparation) as have others showing autistic-like social abnormalities (Paul/Cohen 1984). It is well recognized that some cases of schizophrenia are preceded by developmental problems although these are not specifically in language alone (Rutter/Garmezy 1983), but difficulties arise in classifying both the early language disorder and the psychosis. There are probably diagnostic subgroups amongst language-disordered children, but at present little is known about how to identify them. Some promising work was done in this area by Lewis/Mezey (1985), who presented six case reports of individuals who were found on CAT-scanning to have a cavum septum pellucidum together with an unusual combination of developmental abnormalities including language delay in early childhood and the emergence of a paranoid psychosis in late adolescence or early adulthood. This research provided a puzzling but promising lead. Nonetheless, despite the interest it caused, it has yet to be replicated.

It is clear from the findings presented here that there are strong associations between developmental speech and language disorders and a variety of adverse psychosocial sequelae. These problems have been demonstrated in adolescence and one of the few follow-ups into adulthood has revealed a common picture of social isolation, a lack of sexual relationships and frequent job changes (Mawhood/Rutter/Howlin in preparation). What is much less well understood however, are the mechanisms which result in these sequelae. There is little research to help in answering this question but Howlin/Rutter (1987) suggest several possibilities which need consideration. It may be assumed that no one mechanism is likely to explain all the psychopathological associations but each may offer an answer for different varieties of language disorder. First, it is possible that in some cases there are common antecedents which can account for both the language delay and the associated psychopathology. Many of these factors have already been discussed in the first section of this article and include temperamental difficulty, neurodevelopmental impairment, family disadvantage, psychosocial deprivation and low IQ. It is plausible that some of the attention deficit disorders seen in language impaired children stem from an underlying neurodevelopmental disorder rather than from language difficulties as such. If this is the case, then they should be equally common in non-language disorders. A second potential mechanism is that speech/language disability may predispose to social or emotional problems because of the child's difficulties in communication or because language oddities increase the risk of social rejection. It could be hypothesized that the stressful social outcome of language impairment may lead to the raised incidence of anxiety disorders found as sequelae. Third, the scholastic problems that frequently follow language delay may create their own risks as a result of the stresses associated with educational failure (Yule/Rutter 1985). Fourth, the social impairments found in early childhood (Siegel/Cunningham/van der Spuy 1985) may constitute an intrinsic part of the language disorder, with both the language delay and the social impairment stemming from some underlying specific cognitive deficit. This mechanism may be useful in explaining why severe disorders of receptive language can show highly persistent social deficits. Finally, the language delay and the later psychopathology may be different manifestations of the same constitutional liability. This may be the case, for example, in the links between early developmental delay and the emergence of schizophrenia in late adolescence or early adult life. Adequate data to test these competing alternative explanations is lacking, and if the necessary progress is to be made, future research needs to be carefully designed to allow for some comparability between studies. In particular, prospective longitudinal research would be of immense value (see Rutter/Mawhood 1991 for review). The most urgent needs for future research in this field are to identify which children are most at risk of developing adverse psychosocial sequelae, and also to clarify which factors, if any, can protect them against this process. Perhaps the most basic question is whether the psychosocial outcome of these children is due to inescapable factors within themselves, or whether it can be accounted for by the intervention of external variables.

4. References

Aragona, J. A. & Eyberg, S. M. (1981). Neglected children: Mothers' report of child behavior problems and observed verbal behaviors. *Child Development, 52*, 596–602.

Aram, D. & Nation, J. (1980). Pre-school language disorders and subsequent language and academic difficulties. *Journal of Communication Disorders, 13*, 159–198.

Aram, D., Ekelman, B., & Nation, J. (1984). Preschoolers with language disorders 10 years later. *Journal of Speech and Hearing Research, 27*, 232–244.

Baker, L. & Cantwell, D. (1982). Psychiatric disorder in children with different types of communication disorders. *Journal of Communication Disorders, 15*, 113–126.

Baker, L. & Cantwell, D. (1987). A prospective psychiatric follow-up of children with speech/language disorders. *Journal of the American Academy of Child and Adolescent Psychiatry, 26*, 546–553.

Bartak, L., Rutter, M., & Cox, A. (1975). A comparative study of infantile autism and specific developmental receptive language disorder. I: The children. *British Journal of Psychiatry, 126*, 127–145.

Bates, E., Bretherton, I., & Snyder, L. (1988). *From first words to grammar: individual differences and dissociable mechanisms.* Cambridge: Cambridge University Press.

Beitchman, J., Hood, J., Rochun, J., & Peterson, M. (1989). Empirical classification of speech/language impairment in children, II. Behavioral characteristics. *Journal of the American Academy of Child and Adolescent Psychiatry, 28*, 118–123.

Beitchman, J., Nair, R., Clegg, M. Ferguson, B., & Patel, P. (1986). Prevalence of psychiatric disorders in children with speech and language disorders. *Journal of the American Academy of Child Psychiatry, 25*, 528–535.

Bernstein, B. (1971). *Class, codes and control. Vol. 1.* London: Routledge.

Bettes, B. A., (1988). Maternal depression and motherese: Temporal and intonational features. *Child Development, 59*, 1089–1096.

Bishop, D. & Adams, C. (1990). A prospective study of the relationship between specific language impairment, phonological disorders and reading retardation. *Journal of Child Psychology and Psychiatry, 31*, 1027–1050.

Bloom, L., Lightbown, P., & Hood, L. (1975). Structure and variation in child language. *Monographs of the Society for Research in Child Development, 40* (2), 1–97.

Bousha, D. M. & Twentyman, C. T. (1984). Mother-child interactional style in abuse, neglect, and control groups: Naturalistic observations in the home. *Journal of Abnormal Psychology, 93*, 106–114.

Bruner, J. S. (1975). The ontogenesis of speech acts. *Journal of Child Language, 2*, 1–19.

Burgess, R. & Conger, R. (1978). Family interaction in abusive, neglectful and normal families. *Child Development, 19*, 1163–1173.

Burlingham, D. & Freud, A. (1943). *Infants without families*. London: Allen & Unwin.

Cantwell, D. & Baker, L. (1977). Psychiatric disorder in children with speech and language retardation: a critical review. *Archives of General Psychiatry, 34*, 583–591.

Cantwell, D., Baker, L., & Mattison, R. (1979). The prevalence of psychiatric disorder in children with speech and language disorder. An epidemiologic study. *Journal of the American Academy of Child Psychiatry, 18*, 450–461.

Cantwell, D., Baker, L., Rutter, M., & Mawhood, L. (1989). Infantile autism and developmental receptive dysphasia: A comparative follow-up into middle childhood. *Journal of Autism and Developmental Disorders, 19*, 19–32.

Chomsky, N. (1964). Current issues in linguistic theory. In J. Fodor & J. Katz (Eds.), *The structure of language. 50–118*. New Jersey: Prentice-Hall.

Coghill, S. R., Caplan, H. L., Alexandra, H., Robson, K. M., & Kumar, R. (1986). Impact of maternal depression on cognitive depression of young children. *British Medical Journal, 292*, 1165–1167.

Conway, D., Lytton, H., & Pysh, F. (1980). Twin-singleton language differences. *Canadian Journal of Behavioral Science, 12*, 264–271.

Coster, W., Gersten, M., Beeghly, M., & Cichetti, D. (1989). Communicative functioning in maltreated toddlers. *Developmental Psychology, 25*, 1020–1029.

Cox, A. D., Puckering, C., Pound, A., & Mills, M. (1987). The impact of maternal depression on young children. *Journal of Child Psychology and Psychiatry, 28*, 917–928.

Cromer, R. (1981). Reconceptualizing language acquisition and cognitive development. In R. Schiefelbusch & D. Bricker (Eds.), *Early language: acquisition and intervention. 51–137*. Baltimore: University Park Press.

Crookes, T. & Green, M. (1963). Some characteristics of children with two types of speech disorder. *British Journal of Educational Psychology, 33*, 31–37.

Curtiss, S. (1981). Dissociations between language and cognition: cases and implications. *Journal of Autism and Developmental Disorders,11*, 15–30.

Davenport, Y. B., Zahn-Waxler, C., Adland, M. C. & Mayfield, J. (1984). Early child-rearing practices in families with a manic-depressive parent. *American Journal of Psychiatry, 141*, 230–235.

Davies, R., Butler, N., & Goldstein, H. (1972). *From birth to seven: A report of the National Child Development Study*. London: Longman.

Debray-Ritzen, P., Mattinger, M., & Chapuis, C. (1976). Étude statistique du devenir lexique des enfants présentant un retard de language. *Revue Neurologique (Paris), 132*, 651–655.

Douglas, J. (1964). *The home and the school*. London: MacGibbon and Kee.

Douglas, J., Ross, J., & Simpson, H. (1968). *All our future: a longitudinal study of secondary education*. London: Peter Davies.

Egeland, B. & Sroufe, L. (1981). Developmental sequelae of maltreatment in infancy. *New Directions in Child Development, 11*, 77–92.

Garvey, M. & Gordon, N. (1973). A follow-up study of children with disorders of speech development. *British Journal of Disorders of Communication, 8*, 17–28.

Gersten, M., Coster, W., Schneider-Rosen, K., Carlson, V. & Cichetti, D. (1986). The socio-emotional bases of communicative functioning: Quality of attachment, language development and early maltreatment. In M. E. Lamb, A. L. Brown, & B. Rogoff (Eds.), *Advances in developmental psychology, Vol. 4. 105–151*. Hillsdale, NJ: Erlbaum.

Geschwind, N. & Galaburda, A. (1985). Cerebral lateralization: Biological mechanism, associations and pathology: I. a hypothesis and a program for research. *Archives of Neurology, 42*, 428–459.

Goldfarb, W. (1945). Effects of psychological deprivation in infancy and subsequent stimulation. *American Journal of Psychiatry, 102*, 18–33.

Gotlib, I. & Hooley, J. M. (1988). Depression and marital distress: Current status and future directions. In S. Duck (Ed.), *Handbook of personal relationships. 543–570*. Chichester, England: Wiley.

Griffiths, C. (1969). A follow-up study of disorders of speech. *British Journal of Disorders of Communication, 4*, 46–56.

Hall, P. & Tomblin, J. (1978). A follow-up study of children with articulation and language disorders. *Journal of Speech and Hearing Disorders, 43*, 227–241.

Hay, D., Prior, M., Collett, S., & Williams, M. (1987). Speech and language development in preschool twins. *Acta Geneticae Medicae et Gemollologicae, 36*, 213–222.

Howlin, P. & Rutter, M. (1987). The consequences of language delay for other aspects of development. In W. Yule & M. Rutter (Eds.), *Language development and disorders. 271–294*. Oxford: Mac Keith Press.

Jenkins, S., Bax, M., & Hart, H. (1980). Behavioural problems in pre-school children. *Journal of Child Psychology and Psychiatry, 21*, 5–17.

Johnston, C., Prior, M., & Hay, D. (1984). Prediction of reading disability in twin boys. *Developmental Medicine and Child Neurology, 26*, 588–595.

Lenneberg, E. (1967). *Biological foundations of language*. New York: John Wiley.

Lewis, M. & Mezey, G. (1985). Clinical correlates of septum pellucidum cavities; an unusual association with psychosis. *Psychological Medicine, 15*, 43–54.

Lytton, H. & Conway, D. (1977). The impact of twinship on parent-child interaction. *Journal of Personality and Social Psychology, 35*, 97–107.

Macaulay, R. (1978). The myth of female superiority in language. *Journal of Child Language, 5*, 353–363.

Matas, L., Arend, R., & Sroufe, L. A. (1978). Continuity in adaptation in the second year: The relationship between quality of attachment and later competence. *Child Development, 49*, 547–556.

Mawhood, L., Rutter, M., & Howlin, P. (in preparation). A follow-up comparison of autism and specific developmental language disorder.

Mittler, P. (1970). Biological and social aspects of language development in twins. *Developmental Medicine and Child Neurology, 12*, 741–757.

Morley, E. (1965). *The development and disorders of speech in childhood.* Edinburgh: E. & S. Livingstone.

Nelson, K. (1973). Structure and strategy in learning to talk. *Monographs of the Society for Research in Child Development, 38*, (1), 1–135.

Paul, R. & Cohen, D. (1984). Outcomes of severe disorders of language acquisition. *Journal of Autism and Developmental Disorders, 14*, 405–422.

Prizant, B., Audet, L., Burke, G., Hummel, L., Maher, S., & Theadore, G. (1990). Communication disorders and emotional/behavioral disorders in children and adults. *Journal of Speech and Hearing Disorders, 55*, 179–192.

Ramer, A. (1976) Syntactic styles in emerging language. *Journal of Child Language, 3*, 49–62.

Record, R. G., Mc Keown, T., & Edwards, J. H. (1969). The relation of measured intelligence to birth order and maternal age. *Annals of Human Genetics, 33*, 61–69.

Record, R. G., Mc Keown, T., & Edwards, J. H. (1970). An investigation of the difference in measured intelligence between twins and single births. *Annals of Human Genetics, 34*, 11–20.

Richman, N., Stevenson, J., & Graham, P. J. (1982). *Preschool to school – a behavioral study.* London: Academic Press.

Robinson, R. J. (1987). The causes of language disorder: Introduction and overview. In *Proceedings of the First International Symposium on Specific Speech and Language Disorders in Children. 1–19.* London: AFASIC.

Robinson, W. P. (1980). Language management. In L. A. Hersov, M. Berger, & A. Nicol, (Eds.), *Language and language disorders in childhood. 23–48.* Oxford: Pergamon Press.

Rourke, B. & Strang, J. (1983). Subtypes of reading and arithmetical disabilities: a neuropsychological analysis. In M. Rutter (Ed.), *Developmental neuropsychiatry. 473–488.* New York: Guildford Press.

Rutter, M. (1985 a). Family and school influences on behavioural development. *Journal of Child Psychology and Psychiatry, 26*, 349–368.

Rutter, M. (1985 b). Family and school influences on cognitive development. *Journal of Child Psychology and Psychiatry, 26*, 683–704.

Rutter, M. (1990). Commentary: Some focus and process considerations regarding effects of parental depression on children. *Developmental Psychology, 26*, 60–67.

Rutter, M. & Garmezy, N. (1983). Developmental psychopathology. In E. Hetherington (Ed.), *Handbook of child psychology, Vol. 4: Socialisation, personality and social development. 4 th edn. 775–911.* New York: John Wiley.

Rutter, M. & Mawhood L. (1991). The long-term psychosocial sequelae of specific developmental disorders of speech and language. In M. Rutter & P. Casaer (Eds.), *Biological risk factors for psychological disorders.* Cambridge: Cambridge University Press.

Rutter, M. & Quinton, D. (1984). Parental psychiatric disorder: effects on the children. *Psychological Medicine, 14*, 853–880.

Rutter, M. & Redshaw, J. (1991). Growing up as a twin: Twin-singleton differences in psychological development. *Journal of Child Psychology and Psychiatry, 32*, 885–896.

Sachs, J., Bard, B., & Johnson, M. L. (1981). Language learning with restricted input: case studies of two hearing children of deaf parents. *Applied Psycholinguistics, 2*, 33–54.

Schiff, N. B. & Ventry, I. M. (1976). Communication problems in hearing children of deaf parents. *Journal of Speech and Hearing Disorders, 41*, 348–358.

Siegel, L., Cunningham, C., & van der Spuy, H. (1985). Interactions of language – delayed and normal preschool boys with their peers. *Journal of Child Psychology and Psychiatry, 26*, 77–83.

Silva, P. A. (1980). The prevalence, stability and significance of developmental language delay in preschool children. *Developmental Medicine and Child Neurology, 22*, 768–777.

Silva, P. A. (1981). The predictive validity of a simple two item developmental screening test for three year olds. *New Zealand Medical Journal, 93*, 39–41.

Silva, P. & Fergusson, D. (1980). Some factors contributing to language development in three year old children. *British Journal of Disorders of Communication, 15*, 205–214.

Silva, P., Justin, C., Mc Gee, R., & Williams, S. (1984). Some developmental and behavioral characteristics of seven-year old children with delayed speech development. *British Journal of Disorders of Communication, 19*, 107–154.

Silva, P., McGee, R., & Williams, S. (1983). Developmental language delay from 3 to 7 years and its significance for low intelligence and reading difficulties at age seven. *Developmental Medicine and Child Neurology, 28*, 783–793.

Skinner, B. F. (1975). *Verbal behaviour*. New York: Appleton-Century-Crofts.

Skuse, D. (1984). Extreme deprivation in early childhood: theoretical issues and a comparative review. *Journal of Child Psychology and Psychiatry, 25*, 543–572.

Slade, A. (1987). A longitudinal study of maternal involvement and symbolic play during the toddler period. *Child Development, 58*, 367–373.

Stevenson, J. & Richman, N. (1976). The prevalence of language delay in a population of three-year old children and its association with general retardation. *Developmental Medicine and Child Neurology, 18*, 431–441.

Stevenson, J., Richman, N. & Graham, P. (1985). Behavior problems and language abilities at 3 years and behavioral deviance at 8 years. *Journal of Child Psychology and Psychiatry, 26*, 215–230.

Tallal, P., Dukette, D., & Curtiss, S. (1989). Behavioral/emotional profiles of preschool language-impaired children. *Development and Psychopathology, 1*, 51–67.

Tallal, P., Ross, R., & Curtiss, S. (1989). Familial aggregation in specific language impairment. *Journal of Speech and Hearing Disorders, 54*, 167–173.

Thorpe, K., Golding, J., & MacGillivray, I. (submitted). Depression in mothers of twins.

Tizard, B., Cooperman, O., Joseph, A., & Tizard, J. (1972). Environmental effects on language development: a study of young children in long stay nurseries. *Child Development, 43*, 337–358.

Tizard, B., Hughes, M., Carmichael, H., & Pinkerton, G. (1983). Language deprivation and social class: is verbal deprivation a myth? *Journal of Child Psychology and Psychiatry, 24*, 533–542.

Tizard, B. & Rees, J. (1974). A comparison of the effects of adoption, restoration to the natural mother, and continued institutionalization on the cognitive development of 4-year old children. *Child Development, 45*, 92–99.

Vernon, M. (1974). Effects of parents' deafness on hearing children. In P. J. Fine (Ed.), *Deafness in infancy and early childhood. 219–224*. Baltimore: Williams and Wilkins.

Wachs, T. D. & Chan, A. (1986). Specificity of environmental action, as seen in environmental correlates of infants' communication performance. *Child Development, 57*, 1464–1474.

Wasserman, G., Green, A., & Allen, R. (1983). Going beyond abuse: Maladaptive patterns of interaction in abusing mother-infant pairs. *Journal of the American Academy of Child Psychiatry, 22*, 245–252.

Watts, D. & Lytton, H. (1981). Twinship as handicap: Fact or fiction? In L. Gedda, P. Parisi, & W. Nance (Eds.), *Twin research 3: Intelligence, personality and development. 283–286*. New York: Alan R. Liss.

Werner, H. & Kaplan, B. (1963). *Symbol formation: An organismic-developmental approach to language and the expression of thought*. New York: Wiley.

Yule, W. & Rutter, M. (1985). Reading and other learning difficulties. In M. Rutter & L. Hersov (Eds.), *Child and adolescent psychiatry, 2nd edn. 444–464*. Oxford: Blackwell.

Lynn Mawhood, London (United Kingdom)

61. Children with Specific Language Impairment (Developmental Dysphasia): Linguistic Aspects

1. Introduction

In this chapter I will discuss what characteristics I think distinguish dysphasic or specifically language impaired from normally developing children and other children with language disorders, what their language behaviors appear to be, and the relation between these children's oral language behaviors and the various processing difficulties they have. Although it had long been held that dysphasic children have no cognitive impairment, more recent research indicates that they have information processing difficulties of various kinds (for example, Johnston/Weismer 1983;

Menyuk 1978). It is from this point of view that the cognitive behaviors of these children will be briefly discussed.

Before the chapter begins, a brief discussion of how this author will use the term 'specific language impairment' or 'dysphasic children' is required. There have been a number of terms applied to the children I will be discussing. Over the past five decades, these children have been called functionally impaired, language disordered, language delayed, language learning disordered, language deficient, language deviant, specifically language impaired as well as dysphasic. I think that these varying terms have been applied to that group of children who have marked language problems but no other evident problems. Thus, children within the group are very loosely alike. The primary causes for the differences in the labels given these children may be first, the variability in their language behavior, and, second, the fact that there are probably distinctly different groups of children to which these labels have been applied despite their surface similarity. There are, also, children in this group who are at the very slow end of the continuum of the rate at which normally developing children acquire language, as well as children who show differences from normally developing children in their pattern of development.

2. Characteristics of Dysphasic Children

The best explanation of who dysphasic children are remains, at present, unattainable. By definition they are children who have suffered CNS lesion either pre-natally, natally or post-natally. This is a logical conclusion rather than one based on hard evidence in most instances. The exceptions, who will not be discussed in this chapter, are dysphasic children who have suffered stroke or brain injury from accident. In these instances it is clear that lesion of the CNS is present. Without such hard evidence, the only reason to suggest that such lesion exists is that there is no other explanation available. There is no evidence of any other physical difficulty. They do not appear to be mentally retarded or hearing impaired but their language development does deviate from the norm. These children come from a wide variety of socio-economic and socio-cultural groups. Thus, there is no reason to believe that their non-normal language development is the result of environmental factors. In summary, these children seem to be like other normally developing children except for their language impairment, and, therefore, it seems reasonable to conclude that this impairment is due to CNS lesion.

Outside of known or suspected CNS lesion, dysphasic children are uncharacterizable as a group. That is, there is a vast amount of individual variation in the language behaviors that are manifested by these children. That there is such great variation in their language behavior seems best explained by the possibility (we cannot claim fact) that their behavior is due to a particular type of lesion or structural difference in the CNS. Different dysphasic children have probably suffered different lesions and/or structural differences. Again, these lesions or structural differences do not appear to markedly affect other aspects of development outside of language, but they may do so in a subtle manner.

Some of the differences in the language behaviors of these children are quite similar to the differences seen in adult dysphasics. Dysphasic children may have primarily linguistic output difficulties or input difficulties, reminiscent of Broca's and Wernicke's adult aphasics. One factor, then, that varies among these children is whether they have a production or comprehension deficit or both. Other dysphasic children show subtle and minimal differences from that of normally developing children, and are, therefore, very different from adult aphasics. Other dysphasic children have great difficulty in processing and producing language in the way that normally developing children do, and these differences are quite marked. Another factor, then, that varies amongst these children is degree of involvement. As stated, some of these children are severely involved and others are minimally involved.

Still another factor that appears to lead to large differences among these children is the age at which the purported lesion occurs. Although there is a great deal of argumentation about what the duration of the so-called 'critical period' is, there is agreement that age of lesion is a very important factor in outcome. Thus lesion suffered before age two (pre-natal and natal injury are included in this period) or before age five years or pre-puberty (there are varying views about what is the 'critical period'), apparently affects the degree to which the behavior manifested resembles that of adult aphasics (Wittelson 1977), and, in fact, whether symptoms of language disorder are severe or not. By definition, all the children in the group to be discussed have, presumably, suffered pre-natal or natal lesion. Therefore, many of them should have only subtle signs of language problems. The fact that some have very evident language disorders indicates that very early lesion, depending on timing in fetal development, site and extent, can nevertheless have a marked and also lasting effect. Still another factor which might bring about variation within this group of children is the experiential one. As stated, these children come from various SES and socio-cultural groups, and may, therefore, have received different kinds of treatment.

In summary, dysphasic children are those who are not mentally retarded or hearing impaired. They have apparent, not overt, CNS lesion in areas which affect language development. However, there are several factors which lead to variation in the language behaviors of the children. These are: 1) lesion site or type which affects comprehension or production of language or both with varying degrees of severity, 2) (compounded by) the fetal age at which lesions were suffered, and 3) (influenced by) SES, socio-cultural background and treatment.

The above discussion should indicate how difficult it is to diagnose a child as being dysphasic until other aspects of development have been examined. Those aspects are peripheral hearing and general intellectual ability. Further, in instances of subtle manifestation of language disability, and given our current assessment capabilities, it is almost impossible to diagnose a child as being dysphasic under age three. This is due to the fact that children who are developing language normally may manifest different language development milestones at widely different ages. For example, most children are primarily holophrastic at 18 months and have a small repertoire of productive words (about 50) while some few others are producing two and three word combinations and have well over one hundred and fifty words in their lexicons. Still other children produce very few babbled utterances at 9 to 12 months and do not produce any word approximations by 18 months. These three groups of children are taking markedly different paths in early language development. However, it is not clear that one of these markedly different paths will lead to language disorder, and researchers are struggling to determine which early behaviors do, in fact, do so. Further, it is only long-term developmental research which will determine which patterns of early language development are, in fact, predictive of later language problems. Such research has yet to be carried out with sizeable numbers of these children.

It is clear that one must accept the fact that there are marked differences in the language behavior and patterns of language development among dysphasic children. However, one is left with the problem of describing the nature of these language behaviors and patterns which identify them as being that of dysphasics. An attempt will be made to describe the range of behaviors and patterns of language development from a linguistic perspective that appear to exist in this population of children that seem best described as language disordered.

3. Patterns of Language Behavior and Development

Traditionally, the language behavior of children with language disorders has been described in terms of comprehension and production difficulties. A larger proportion of dysphasic children have been found to have a language production rather than a comprehension problem. A recent definition of children with specific language impairment is that these children exhibit delays of one year or more in language production and one of six months or more in language comprehension on a set of standard tests of these behaviors (Stark/Tallal 1981). This definition and others seem to suggest across the board delay in the development of all aspects of language comprehension and production. Another possibility exists. It may be the case that particular aspects of components of language are affected to varying degrees in some dysphasic children whereas other aspects are not. To explore this possibility, the results of research examining the language behavior of dysphasic children within specific components of language will be reviewed. Researchers have explored the phonological, lexical, semantactic and discourse behavior and development of dysphasic children.

3.1. Phonology

Over the past fifty years there have been many studies of the speech sound production and perception of dysphasic children (for a summary of early studies see Powers 1957). Views of these children's phonological abilities were largely based on the results of experiments that sampled the children's speech only one time or assessed their production and perception on standard tests. Children with articulation and perception problems without any apparent organic cause were said to have 'functional disorders'. There have been comparatively few naturalistic studies of these children's phonological development (for example, Magnusson 1983; Schwartz/Leonard/Folger/Wilcox 1980). As might be expected, the results of the two types of studies are different. The former find differences between normally developing and dysphasic children in speech sound production, and sometimes perception, at the segmental level, within specific lexical items (after all the experiments and tests examined this behavior). Using speech samples obtained with varying amounts of frequency and over varying amounts of time, the naturalistic studies have found similarities between the two groups of children in the phonological processes that can be observed during development. These processes include weak syllable deletion, consonant cluster reduction, backward and forward assimilation, stopping of continuants, vowel and consonant harmony (syllable repetition) plus idiosyncratic realizations chosen by particular children. Although these processes describe the early phonological production of lexical items by both normally developing and language disordered children, they appear later and persist longer in children who are considered language disordered. These differences in findings between the two types of studies may be due to three factors: differences in the manner in which the data were obtained (already pointed to), differences in the ages of the children examined, and differences within the children themselves. As was pointed out earlier, it is difficult to diagnose a child as dysphasic under the age of three. Therefore, some naturalistic studies may have examined some children under age three who are delayed rather than dysphasic. Further, both naturalistic studies and studies using standard tests have found variation among older language disordered children in their speech sound realizations of target sounds, and in the phonological processes used.

Some possible and observed patterns of early (below age 5) phonological development in relation to lexical development among these children have been described (Stoel-Gammon 1991). Three patterns are suggested. One pattern is delay in both lexical and phonological domains. Another pattern is delay only in ways in which phonological realizations are mapped onto lexical items that are age appropriate. A large number of words are collapsed into a small number of realizations. A third pattern is one of an age appropriate lexicon but of unique phonological realizations of lexical items. Still another possibility is that these realizations vary depending on the linguistic and situational context in which a lexical item is targeted. A study of older dysphasic children (over 5) found that these children's realizations of speech sounds were very much affected by the contexts in which they were realized (Menyuk 1983). That is, the predictability of the target together with the motivation to succeed in reaching the target had an effect on how closely the child approximated the standard phonological realization of a lexical item.

It is apparent that no generalizations about all dysphasic children can be made about their phonological development. The naturalistic studies indicate that phonological development in children thought to be dysphasic at ages two and three years looks very like that of normally developing children only delayed. Interestingly, these same results have been found in studies of children with persistent otitis media during the first three years of life (Paden/Novak/Beiter 1987). This might suggest that the children have less accurate hearing, as is the case with children who have had frequent episodes of otitis media. However, analysis of the segmental errors made by children with early otitis as compared to children with specific language impairment indicates that a greater percentage of children with histories of otitis delete initial consonants, substitute /h/ or glottal stop for consonants, and denasalize, stop and change the place of nasal sounds (Shriberg/Smith 1983).

These phonological studies of very young dysphasic children may be concerned with children who are at the extreme end of normal development in terms of language, possibly because of some dampening of their hearing ability. With children over three years of age, who have been identified as being dysphasic, using the criteria described in the previous section, there are very marked differences in their phonological production (Menyuk/Looney 1972) and in their phonological perception (Tallal/Stark 1983). There are also differences among dysphasic children in their pattern of phonological production, ranging from those who produce speech sounds that are so different from the normal patterns that they are unintelligible, to children who produce consistent substitutions in their speech sound realizations that listeners can use to determine what they mean.

These children's perceptual difficulties may be based on the rate at which they can perceive speech sound differences that are of very short duration. Thus, their principal difficulty may be to distinguish between stop sounds. However, these children have also been found to have some difficulty in perceiving the differences between sounds that have their energy at high frequencies, and recent research points to more extensive differences among them in terms of fine-grained speech sound distinction abilities (Elliott/Hannen/Scholl 1989). Within a group containing both language impaired and normally developing children, the language impaired children were correctly identified 80 % of the time at ages 6 to 7, and 65 % of the time at ages 8 to 11 based on their ability to find just notable differences between /ba/ and /pa/ and among /ba/, /da/ and /ga/.

It may be the case that all dyphasic children's speech perception and production abilities are affected, and that these differences in abilities is the cause of the difficulties these children have in lexical, morphological, and syntactic development. Suggestions of this kind have been made by a number of researchers. It is also possible, however, that some of these children have specific difficulties with lexicon because of phonological difficulties, and others because of semantic difficulty. Some may have problems with syntax because of phonological difficulties and others because of semantactic problems. Some may have problems with connected discourse because of semantactic difficulties and others because of perceptual difficulties. These possibilities will be explored in further sections of this chapter.

Some of these children's morphological difficulties seem to be clearly related to their phonological difficulties. For example, they have been found to be somewhat delayed or extremely delayed in their ability to mark tense on the verb phrase and to mark number and possession on nouns. It has been suggested that the surface information of the morphological markers are an important factor in their causing so much difficulty (Leonard 1990). This is why there are differences between English and Italian speaking dysphasic children in which morphological markers are omitted. Markers that English speaking children have difficulty in acquiring, such as plural, are not omitted by Italian speaking children because in Italian they are marked by a vowel syllable (frequently /o/ or /a/) rather than a bound strident sound (frequently /z/ or /s/). Difficulty with morphological markers may be a product of processing problems not lack of linguistic knowledge. Some markers are more learnable than others because of the ease with which they can be isolated from the word and categorized. Markers that are separate syllables and are composed of comparatively more easily identified speech sound categories (are more perceptually salient) are the markers that are more easily acquired by both dysphasic and normally speaking children. Again, there is difficulty in distinguishing between very slow developers and dysphasic children in their pattern of development of morphological markers, since the bound morphemes that have little phonological information are composed of just those speech sound distinctions that create particular productive and perceptual problems for normally developing as well as dysphasic children, and for children with hearing problems. In a study comparing the reproduction of lexical items in sentences that are and are not composed of stems and bound morphemes (for example, friend versus planned), it was found that children with early histories of otitis repeated the word stems significantly more frequently than the morphological markers on the word stems (Teele/Klein/Chase et al. 1990). Again, the possibility of differences in hearing may account for the morphophonological problems of some dysphasic children.

Findings similar to those in phonological development have been found in studies of the morphological development of very young children with specific language problems. During the period at which both normally speaking children and the language disordered children are primarily producing one to three word sentences both groups of children have similar morphological problems (Lahey/Liebergott/Chesnick et al. 1990) and it is difficult to distinguish between the two groups. When the MLU of both groups of children increases, then more differences between them, in which morphological markers are acquried, can be observed. This may indicate that the dysphasic children have a problem in the amount of memory space they can allocate to the realization of all aspects of utterances, especially if they are having difficulty in encoding some aspects. Under these circumstances morphological markers may be sacrificed for lexical stems.

In summary, there appear to be at least two types of phonological problems that can be found among dysphasic children. The first is one of marked delay in the development of the phonological system (perhaps accompanied by delay in lexical development). Thus, phonological processes that are found in the speech of normally developing children can be found in the speech of these children but they appear at a later age and persist over a longer time. Some of these processes are concerned with segmental realization and others with syllabic structure, but in terms of both types of processes, the patterns found are in the speech of both so-called language impaired and normally developing children (Ingram 1989). It is possible that these delays may in part be due to a surface level auditory or speech sound perception problem. This may also be the case for some language impaired children who do not exhibit a lexical but only a phonological delay.

There is still another group of children who are much more variable in their speech sound realizations, and markedly differ from normally developing children in the consistency with which they realize sounds and in how far they depart from the target sounds within lexical items in terms of features of segments (Menyuk 1983). Some examples of these differences are the following imitations or spontaneous generations:

1. Imitates *See the ship* as /uh uh uh/
2. Generates *paper* as /maber/
3. Identifies *umbrella* as /pel/

It is possible that the basis for these phonological difficulties is a deeper problem having to do with how they process and then organize the acoustic information they receive, or how they map these organizations into speech sound movements. That is, there are children who have only a problem in planning speech sound realizations, and others who have both a perceptual organization and speech sound planning output problem. There is still, at least, one further possibility of variation in the phonological development of children labelled as language disordered. It is possible that the phonological errors made by some children are due to difficulties in mapping out target segments and sequences. These children, apparently, have no perceptual problem, only an end organ productive problem. They literally have difficulty in achieving the articulatory targets that they have planned. The assumption is that their underlying phonological representations for both perception and production are quite similar to those of normally developing children. Their phonological behavior has been likened to that of adult dyspraxics. Their speech can be highly unintelligible. Therefore, they are labeled as language disordered.

CAUSES	PRODUCTS
Group I-Very Slow Developers	
	Delayed Phonology
Dampened Perception	
	Delayed Lexicon
Group II-Slow Developers	
	Delayed Phonology
Dampened Perception	
Group III-Dysphasic children	
	Variable Phonology
Unstable Representations	
	Delayed Lexicon
Group IV Dyspraxic Children	
Motor Problems	
	Different Phonology

Fig. 61.1: Representation of causes of phonological problems and products in groups of language impaired children

Figure 61.1 above attempts to capture the possible differences between the four groups of children in terms of the causes for their phonological problems and the products of these problems. In Group I, very slow developers, the problem is one of less accurate perceptual abilities than in normally developing children which affects both phonology and lexicon. In Group II, only phonology is affected by the less accurate perception. In Group III, it is postulated, there are different representations of phonological categories which affects both phonology and lexicon. In Group IV only articulatory movements to achieve phonological targets are affected.

3.2. Semantactic Problems

It was hypothesized some years ago that online comprehension and production of utterances involves parallel processing of the categories and relations from each component of the grammar. Thus, each component contributes constant 'updates' on the information needed in the sequence being generated or comprehended. If this were the case, then, it was hypothesized, the phonological and semantactic components of the language should be affected to the same degree in language disordered children (Menyuk/Looney 1972). It was found that the children with the most severe phonological problems were also those with the most severe syntactic problems. In more recent studies variations in these findings have been observed.

In one study it has been found that in 30 speech delayed children, only two thirds of them also display an overall syntactic delay, and only one half display some limitations in their use of phonetically complex morphemes (Shriberg/Paul 1982). In a study employing sentence repetition to assess syntactic and phonological processing, however, it was found that the phonological complexity of the target lexical items disrupted the accuracy of repetition of syntactic structures. Both syllabic complexity and clause embedding contributed to the errors made by the children (Panagos/Prelock 1982). Thus, apparently, some language disordered children exhibit delays or problems with both syntax and phonology, and others have either only phonological problems or only syntactic problems. Yet to be determined is whether or not there is independence between the phonological and semantactic levels of the language in the language production of language disordered children. Such a determination has interesting implications for language processing in general.

A possible explanation for the differences in the findings concerning the relation between the two components of the language in language disordered children might lie in the differences among the children in the causes of their phonological and syntactic problems. Children who have difficulty in developing phonological representations of lexical items might also have difficulty in developing the semantactic structures that are governed by these lexical items and exhibit delay in both domains as well as in lexical development. Children who have only speech generation problems need not have difficulties in syntax comprehension, and, therefore, exhibit no delays in these developments. Children who have difficulties in formulating more sophisticated syntactic categories and relations need not have difficulties in phonological representations of lexical items, and only exhibit their problems at a later age. These are all suppositions. There have been very few studies of the simultaneous morphophonological, lexical and semantactic problems that language disordered children may have.

A number of studies have found that dysphasic children have both delays and some differences in their semantactic development. These findings have been based on analyses of language samples obtained from these children at different ages, and on results of experiments that have asked these children to engage in various semantactic tasks such as imitation, acting out commands that have been given orally, generating utterances from observed actions and pictures, generating utterances from a set of words, etc., as well as from standardized tests. The variety of means by which these children's semantactic production and comprehension have been assessed raise questions about the generalizability of the findings in any particular study. Therefore, the fact that there are similarities in findings is not only surprising but, also, suggests that there are particular semantactic behaviors which can be found in at least some children in this group of children.

For example, it has been found that dysphasic children stay at particular stages of the development of this aspect of language that mark reorganizations of semantactic knowledge (Menyuk 1978). Thus, younger dysphasic children are producing SVO sentences without expansion of the noun phrase or the verb phrase for a much longer time than their normally developing peers. They appear to plateau at this stage of development for a number of years. Older dysphasic children are producing simply expanded subject plus predicate sentences, and non-coordinated or embedded sentences for a much longer time than their normally developing peers. They, again, appear to reach a plateau but this plateau may exist for an even longer time than the previous one. Dysphasic children use much fewer different sentence patterns than their age peers, and, also, more frequently produce sentences with syntactic errors (Grimm 1987). Utterances with errors of commission appear after errors of omission. Despite producing sentences of the same length as MLU matched normally developing children, dysphasic children produce fewer propositions per utterance and make more syntactic errors in these utterances (Johnston/Kamhi 1984).

Some of these results indicate delays in general and marked delays during certain periods of development. These periods are those during which one can see significant changes in semantactic structures in, at least, the utterances produced by the child. Thus, the difference between normally developing and dysphasic children in semantactic development seems to be, on the surface at least, the rate at which some productive semantactic structures are acquired. However, there are differences as well.

The semantactic errors made by dysphasic children lend support to the notion that there are differences as well as delays in dysphasic children's development of this aspect of language. First, syntactic errors are a much more frequent occurrence in the sentences produced by three year old and older language disordered children than in those produced by normally developing children of a much younger age. Second, the errors made by the two groups of children appear to be different. For example, Grimm (1987) found that dysphasic German speaking children produce utterances such as the following, whereas normally developing children never do: *ein Boot Wasser nehmt ham* (a boat water taken have); *eine Brust ich sehen hab* (a breast I seen have).

The way in which these children order elements in phrases, as in the examples above, suggests that the underlying representations for these phrases are different. Fletcher (1991) presents some examples of what he calls formulation errors in the utterances produced by a group of 15 language impaired children in England and Scotland, and they are similar in kind to the German examples above: *here they got eyes to me; my mum was take me a picture.*

Fletcher characterized the syntactic problems of these language impaired children as being in four areas: 1) comprehension (as measured by standard tests), 2) output problems as indicated by maze generation (reformulations and repetitions, and formulation errors), 3) grammatical errors (omission of determiners, auxiliary and copula verbs, agreement errors, and morphological errors) and 4) problems in expansion of verb phrases, phrases and sentences (coordinated and embedded sentences). Semantactic problems such as those described by Grimm and Fletcher have been found in many studies of dysphasic children (Menyuk 1988). Variability in semantactic behaviors has also been found. Thus, some language disordered children largely strip their sentences of components other than the subject verb and object, whereas others commit the kinds of errors that normally developing children never commit.

Fletcher points to four sub-groups with differing types of combinations of problems and strengths in semantactic production and comprehension in this small group of children. Each group in the Fletcher study is obviously composed of a very small number of children, and 6 of the 15 children (40 %) are not exactly groupable, although 4 of these 6 are similar to established groups. All of the children on whom there are comprehension data have comprehension problems except two. Some studies have found children with only sentence production problems, others have found children with severe production problems and minor comprehension problems, and still others have found that some of these children, although they are comparatively fewer in number, may have more severe comprehension than production problems (Liebergott/Menyuk/Chesnik/Korngold 1988).

Three of the four different groups pointed to by Fletcher seem to represent somewhat different levels of input and output processing problems. If one examines the data presented from this point of view, the first group shows difficulties in all the areas of sentence generation described above. A second group shows difficulties in output (mazes and formulation errors) but in no other areas. Group three has output problems and, also, doesn't expand sentences. If we consider sentence expansion as requiring different abilities than phrase expansion then group 1 has difficulties in developing semantactic categories and mapping these categories into output sequences for both SVO and expanded SVO sentences. Group 2 only has difficulties in mapping categories into output sequences, and group 3 is similar to 2 except that they have additional difficulty in developing the categories for expanded SVO sentences. Thus, some children have difficulty in basic category development and in retrieving these categories (an encoding problem), while others primarily have difficulties in programming out these categories (a retrieval problem). Basic category development is different for single versus expanded sentences, and is probably different for different types of coordination and expansion.

That there are similarities within subgroups of these children and differences among subgroups is not surprising, given the initial hypothesis that these children suffer lesion of the CNS but suffer different types of lesions and/or structural differences. There is also the developmental factor. That is, children cannot display difficulty with an aspect of language until they have acquired that aspect of language. Thus, studies of dysphasic children when they are aged 3 or 5 years might show only delay, and a similar kind of delay. At later ages, when some of the children have acquired basic categories, and are having difficulty in programming them out than differences might appear. It may also be the case that among the children that have been classified as language impaired are children who are simply at the extreme end of slow language developers but who are developing normally. This same possibility was discussed in the section on phonological development.

As stated, studies of language impaired children show both similarities and differences in language behaviors among them. Some similarities among them are the data pointed to initially: the slow start, the plateaus in development at the point at which there are new categories to be developed and old categories expanded. Differences among them are, at least, the rate at which they acquire categories and whether or not they have severe production and mild comprehension problems, or a mixture of the two, or mild comprehension and severe output problems, or only output problems. Differences are usually observed in these children after age five to six years and similarities before this age.

Studies of these children's comprehension of semantactic structures in utterances is quite consistent with the findings concerning production similarities. That is, they have difficulty in acting out sentences that have more than one proposition when they are aged 3 to 5 years (Levy/Menyuk 1975). This seems to be an example of reaching a plateau in comprehension of sentence expansion as well as in production of these expansions. When they are around age 8 they continue to have semantactic comprehension problems (Menyuk/Chesnick/Liebergott et al. 1991). They have difficulties in answering questions about sentences that mark time (before and after) or dependent relations (WH clauses and complements) and have more than one proposition. They have difficulty in judging and correcting sentences that contain semantactic errors, both of phrase and clause construction and of morphological markers. They have great difficulty in filling in missing nouns, verbs and adjectives in simple sentences.

Task	Mean Correct Responses Dysphasic	Mean Correct Responses Low Average	p value
Answer Questions	7.32	9.43	.01
Judge & Correct	27.48	36.26	.002
Fill in Parts	11.07	16.14	.001

Table 61.1: Semantactic comprehension performance of dysphasic and average normal children on various tasks

Table 61.1 compares these children's and low average children's performance on these tasks. The low average children in this study were significantly different from normally developing children in their rate of developing language, but were not performing as poorly as specifically language impaired children on standard tests of language performance as well as on the tasks described above. An interesting paper suggests that these children might be classified as "low verbal normal" (Snyder 1987) or, as we have termed them here, at the very slow end of normal development of language.

A number of researchers who have examined the development of semantactic metalinguistic abilities in normally developing children (for example, Bialystok 1986; Karmiloff-Smith 1986; Menyuk 1983) have hypothesized that acquisition of language knowledge takes place in a number of steps. Roughly, the first step might be intuitive knowledge, then awareness of what is known, and finally automatic application of what is known. The state of knowledge of any particular aspect of language changes over these steps. Intuitive knowledge of a structure is 'fragile' or not well established knowledge. Bringing this structure to the level of conscious awareness more firmly establishes knowledge of this structure and makes more rapid retrieval possible. The most mature state of knowledge of this structure is automatic use under all appropriate conditions. This is achieved when retrieval of the structure takes place at an optimal rate. In addition to positing a semantactic input processing problem, and/or an output processing problem, it has been hypothesized that these children have a problem in meta-processing semantactic categories and relations in the language (Menyuk 1991). Thus, their knowledge of semantactic categories and relations and morpho-phonological categories and relations remains fragile for a much longer period of time than in normally developing children. The reason for these children having difficulty in becoming aware of what they know about language may be due to the ways in which they store representations of their knowledge. Lexical-semantic grammars suggest that lexical items, in particular verbs, and the syntactic structures they can find themselves in are stored simultaneously. Language impaired children may be unable to deal with this kind of storage requirement.

When discussing the increasing difficulty that language impaired children have in retrieving morphological markers in increasingly longer sentences, it was suggested that they have limitations on how much they can program out in a single utterance. In discussing their metalinguistic problems it was suggested that they have difficulty in storing certain kinds of representations. In discussing the kinds of errors that were labelled formulation errors, it was suggested that these children's underlying representations of phrases and clauses might be different. The first two suggestions are concerned with how these children process language information, but the last is concerned with the grammars of language they develop. There is a very real difference in these two types of explanations. Except for the formulation errors pointed to, most of the evidence points to processing differences rather than underlying grammar differences.

Various hypotheses have been presented to account for the particular kinds of difficulty and delays dysphasic children have in semantactic competence. These explanations include differences in the learning strategies they use, memorial problems, cognitive differences, and as discussed earlier, phonological problems. In addition to putting forth main causes for semantactic problems, some researchers have suggested that there are various subtypes of semantactic problems that these children have, and that these subtypes are due to different causes for the problem. These possibilities along with others will be discussed in the final section of this chapter.

3.3. Lexical Development

Given the findings of both phonological and semantactic delay and difference in dysphasic children, it would seem highly likely that these children would have problems in lexical acquisition. Their difficulties in preception and production of phonological segments and sequences would make acquisition of stable phonological representations of lexical items a problem. There is now data which indicates that this is substantively the case (Schwartz/Leonard/Frome Loeb/Swanson 1987). It has been found that when language impaired children are in the process of acquiring new lexical items, they appear not to take advantage of the phonological segments that are already in the lexical items they have acquired to add new lexical items containing these segments. To account for this finding, the researchers hypothesize that the children have either a motor output mapping problem or a difficulty in formulating stable phonological representations.

Lexical meanings are often derived from the linguistic and situational contexts in which they are used. If a child has difficulties in semantactic processing, these should lead to problems in development of lexical meanings as well. However, the bases for problems in lexical acquisition would be quite different in kind from those suffered by children with phonological representation and retrieval problems, and this difference should be exhibited in both spontaneous speech studies and in confrontation naming experiments. That is, phonological errors should occur in the first instance and hesitations and substitutions should occur in the second instance.

There have been comparatively fewer studies of the lexical development of these children than there have been of other aspects of language. The studies that have examined lexical problems and development in dysphasic children have come up with findings that are similar to those in studies of phonology and syntax. There are a group of studies which indicate that lexical development in language disordered children is much like that of normally developing children and others that have found differences.

For example, one study found that the inappropriate word extensions found in the speech of language disordered children were quite comparable to those found in the speech of normally developing children at the same linguistic level (Chapman/Leonard/Rowan/Weiss 1983). This finding suggests that language impaired children are acquiring and structuring their productive lexicons in ways that are similar to those of normally developing children. The language disordered children in this study were aged 2;8 to 3;4 years.

When the spontaneous speech of older language disordered children is examined, differences rather than similarities are found. The spontaneous speech samples of 7 to 12 year old language disordered children were compared to those of normally developing children, and it was found that there were a significantly greater number of reformulations and word substitutions (German 1982).

It, again, may be the case that at least two different populations were being assessed in the studies cited above. The language disordered children in the first study may be at the very delayed end of normal development while the children in the second study might, indeed, be language disordered. The other possibility is that the children in the first study were too young to manifest differences as well as delays in language development.

Difference has been a consistent finding in the studies that have examined the ability of language disordered children, as compared to normally developing children, to rapidly retrieve lexical items under the conditions of confrontation naming. The question that arises is whether or not these children have difficulty in acquiring lexical items as well as retrieving them. The answer to the question appears to be that they do when the data from confrontation naming studies is examined. In one such study (Fried-Oken 1987), it was found that language disordered children produced significantly more errors that were unrelated to the pictured items than did normally developing children. This was the case when both first and second responses were examined. This indicated that there was a significant difference between the two groups in the number of pictured items that could be named. The language disordered children simply had a smaller lexicon.

Outside of suggesting that there may be two groups of children in studies of dysphasic children's acquisition of lexicon, as stated above, language disordered children may, initially, have an encoding problem because of their inability to accurately encode the phonological representation of a lexical item. Later, they may have a lexical acquisition problem because they may have limited access to semantic properties (Menyuk 1988). In contradiction to this notion, there is reason to think that there are, indeed, different subtypes of lexical encoding problems in this population initially, as was stated at first. When the spontaneous speech samples of 7 to 12 year old dysphasic children were examined, two groups could be found. One group was significantly different from normally developing children in the number of different words produced. The researcher suggested they had a "productivity" problem. The other group was significantly different in terms of the number of reformulations and substitutions produced (German 1987).

If the second group of children had difficulty in encoding the semantic properties of lexical items rather than in acquiring lexical items, then they would exhibit difficulties in retrieval that reflect semantic errors. This is what they did rather than exhibiting gaps or errors unrelated to target items. It is this kind of evidence which supports the notion that there are two different kinds of lexical problems that dysphasic children exhibit, delay and difference.

A number of studies have examined the rapid autonomic naming of language learning disabled children or those with reading problems (Wolf 1984). In these kinds of studies behaviors similar to those of language disordered children in confrontation naming tasks and in studies of their spontaneous speech have been found. There are differences in the latency, accuracy and types of responses produced by these two groups of children as compared to the responses of normally developing children. The two types of errors most frequently produced by normally developing children are semantic field errors (for example, *knife* for *fork*) and semantic/perceptual errors (for example, *skirt* for *dress*). The most frequent errors produced by language disordered children are 1) circumlocutions (for example, *it's to dig with* for *shovel*), 2) comments unrelated to the pictured items or 3) no response at all. The latter two findings simply suggest that the language disordered children have fewer lexical items. The frequent circumlocutions these children respond with under all conditions (in spontaneous speech as well as confrontation naming and rapid autonomic naming) suggest that the semantic features of the lexical items that are acquired by language disordered children may be organized in a manner that is different from that of normally developing children. Functional features specific to a lexical item rather than generalizable perceptual features may be the primary organizers for the language disordered children. This could mark both a delay and a difference in the acquisition of semantic features for lexical items. It has been concluded that functional features, which are, however, used to generalize, are acquired first by normally developing children. There is a great deal of argument about whether or not this is the case, with some researchers presenting evidence that it is, and other researchers presenting contradictory evidence (Menyuk 1988). The differences between normally developing and language disordered children in acquisition of semantic features for lexical items may lie in the normally developing children acquiring a much greater variety of feature types for different lexical items, and in their ability to make a greater number of generalizations using these features. It is interesting to note, along these speculative lines, that syntactic class of lexical items has a more marked effect on the lexical acquisition of normally developing children than on language impaired children. In a study comparing the lexical learning of young (aged 2;8 to 4;2) children it was found that normally developing children learned object words better than action words. This was markedly less the case for language impaired children (Leonard/Schwartz/Chapman et al. 1982 b).

Finally, patterns of lexical development in these children may be similar to patterns of semantactic development. There may be plateaus reached in lexical development when the nature of the next set of lexical items to be acquired is more complex, just as plateaus in semantactic development occur when the next stage involves a serious complication in the structures to be acquired. There are few data to support such an hypothesis. These few data indicate the following. First, word frequency does play a role in the lexical retrieval problems of language disordered children. Less frequent words are more difficult for them to retrieve than more frequent ones (Liebergott/Menyuk/Chesnick et al. 1988). Of course, this is true of normally developing children as well but with dysphasic children the problem is more marked and lasts a longer time. For example, in the study cited above (Liebergott et al. 1988) it was found that letter and number naming was significantly less accurate than object naming for language impaired, low average and average children. However, there were significant differences between the language impaired children and the other two groups of children that persisted over the three years of the study. The rate of naming letters by the three groups of children over the period of the study is shown in Fig. 61.2 below.

As can be seen, the mean rate of naming score increased for most of the children over the period of the study because more of the

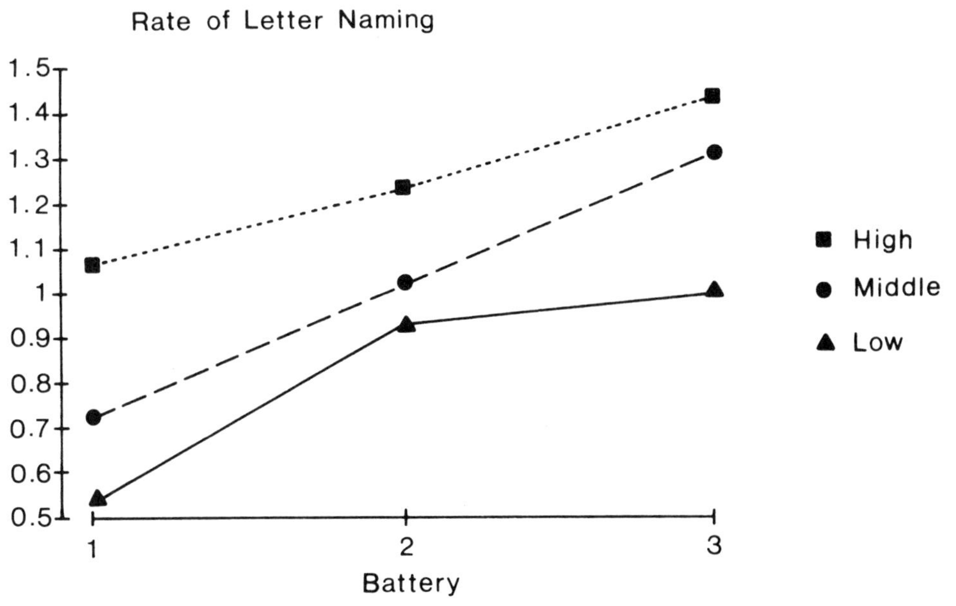

Fig. 61.2: Differences in rate of letter naming by language impaired (low), low average (middle) and average (high) children at three points in time

letters were being named by the low average and average children. This was not true for the language impaired children who seemed to reach a plateau in their letter naming ability.

This notion that lexical development becomes markedly slower as more complex words are to be acquired is further supported by the fact that lexical development continues to be slow in language impaired children over the school years. One of the most stable measures of lexical comprehension difficulties in language impaired children are word comprehension tests. Differences between language impaired and normally developing children on these measure can usually be observed from 3 to at least 18 years. The second kind of data to support this hypothesis is that language impaired children have particular difficulty with lexical items and phrases that have more than one meaning. There has been at least one study which indicated that interpretation of metaphor is different in pre-adolescent children with histories of early language difficulties as compared to those without such histories. In these children only differences in metaphorical interpretation can be observed. There are no differences between them and normally developing children on a standard test of literal lexical comprehension (Nippold/Fey 1983).

In summary, the studies of lexical acquisition in dysphasic children indicate that there may be at least two patterns of lexical acquisition within the groups of children called language impaired. One pattern appears to be very similar to that observed in lexical acquisition in normally developing children, only delayed. It was hypothesized that the primary cause of the lexical delay in these children may be their inability to form stable phonological representations for lexical items. This slows down their rate of acquisition of new lexical items but the way in which the semantic properties of these items are encoded does not seem markedly different.

Another group of children are also slow in lexical acquisition but their difficulties seem to stem from an inability to organize semantic features of lexical items in a categorical way, and in the limitations of the feature types acquired. In spontaneous speech and in confrontation and rapid autonomic naming tasks these children circumlocute and use substitute lexical items such as *thing* or *that*. Often these circumlocutions contain references to the functions of the target item. This seems to suggest that these children more easily store the functional features of lexical items, and then have difficulty in adding perceptual, syntactic and associative features. Their retrieval difficulties may stem from the limited number and types of semantic features they have for lexical items. If the speed of lexical accessing is a function of the number of different routes that have been laid down for reaching a lexical item, then the longer latency of their responses in spontaneous speech and in experimental tasks might be accounted for.

3.4. Pragmatics

Over the past decade there has been a heightened interest in the pragmatic development of dysphasic children. This was partially a function of heightened interest on the part of linguists in this aspect of language. However, it was primarily due to the fact that those concerned with the language behavior of these children came to the conclusion that communication, not sentence processing, should be the focus of their attention. There have been three principal strands in the recent research in this area. One of the strands is examination of the language disordered child's ability to tell or retell stories. Another strand has been examination of these children's ability to generate different types of speech acts and engage in communicative interaction with various partners. A third and less frequently examined strand has been these children's concepts of the conditions for communicative interaction. There is yet another strand, how parents communicate with their language impaired children, but much of this research sheds little light on the nature of the interactions. The emphasis is on input.

Pragmatic knowledge involves knowing what language to use under which circumstances. Thus, both knowledge of the communicative rules of one's culture and the rules of the language is required. Simultaneous processing of the situation (social and physical) and of the language that is being exchanged is required in using pragmatic knowledge. Thus, there should be a sizeable amount of strain imposed on the dysphasic child in communicative interaction situations as compared to sentence, lexical and phonological processing situations. However, unlike structural processing situations, there is a great deal of contextual support (visual and affective) which should help the language disordered child.

There are several factors that might play a role in whether or not dysphasic children have pragmatic problems. A primary factor appears to be whether or not the dysphasic children in the study do or do not have a comprehension problem. Another factor is the complexity of the communicative act that is being examined. A third factor is the conditions under which communication is being examined at what age. For example, if one looks at early speech acts such as commands and compares MLU matched language impaired and normally developing children, one might find no differences, since commands can be generated with single words marked with the appropriate intonation. Thus the complexity of the communicative act should play a role in studies examining this knowledge in language disordered children.

The results of the research are varied not only in terms of which strand was examined in a particular study, but also which aspects of each strand have been examined. The research carried out thus far, as in the case of lexical development, has been quite limited in terms of amount and the broadness of the questions asked.

There have been a few studies of the development of speech acts in language impaired children. In one study of young language disordered children (approximately 3 years) and normally developing children (approximately 2 years), the functions of utterances in a speech sample were examined. It was found that the language impaired children were similar to normally developing children in terms of the frequency of utterances serving most functions (Leonard/Camarata/Rowan 1982 a). Naming was more frequent in the normally developing children, and answering in the language impaired children. The two groups were the same in terms of the different lexical items that were used to serve the communicative functions of language at this young age.

Performative and presuppositional skills of these two groups of children was examined in another study. Again the children were young (the normally developing children were 1;4 to 2;1 years and the language impaired 2;8 to 4;2), and again speech samples were used. It was found that the two groups were similar in their use of imperative and declarative performative use, and similar in their tendency to encode changing versus static situational elements (Rowan/Leonard/Chapman et al. 1983). Thus, their use of speech acts, and what they selected to talk about (topics) were similar.

The findings are somewhat different when the ability of language impaired and normally developing children to comprehend and produce requests are examined. These abilities in language disordered children aged 3½ to 9 years were examined in role play and free play situations in a paradigm similar to that used with normally developing children (Prinz/Ferrier 1983). It was found that in role play direct requests predominated and indirect requests only increased slightly in older children. The researchers suggest that the language impaired children were at a pragmatic level in requesting that was 2 or more years behind their normally developing peers. It was not until 5½ to 6½ years that the children could discriminate between requests on the basis of politeness. These results indicate that more complex speech acts might impose greater strain on language impaired children. The form of indirect or more polite request in English is usually auxiliary or modal permuted questions (*Can you give me that one*?).

In another study the ability of language learning disabled and normally developing children, in grades 1 through 4, to deliver bad news was compared (Pearl/Donahue/Bryan 1985). In such a situation, both the speech acts used and how they are used (taking into account the perspective of the other) are involved in being tactful. As might be expected, the younger children (grades 1 and 2) were rated as being less tactful than the older children. The language learning disabled children were rated as being less tactful than the normally developing children. The experimenters raise the question of why this was the case. It was not clear from the results of the study whether the language learning disabled children were having problems in generating the linguistic structures necessary to convey tact or whether they were unable to take the perspective of the other. In another study of the ability of these children in grades 2, 4, 6 and 8 to engage in referential communication, these same experimenters conclude that language learning disabled children have syntactic deficits that limit their ability to engage in successful communications.

Although the latter two studies had as subjects language learning disabled children rather than dysphasic children, one might hypothesize that the syntactic problems of the orally language impaired children would be even more prominent. The results of studies of young language impaired children suggest similarity, albeit delay, in speech act development. The study of indirect requests and the studies of language learning disabled children suggest that very real barriers exist in these children's abilities to comprehend and produce speech acts that require semantactic structures that are more complex. There is little evidence to suggest that these children have impoverished notions of what communication is all about and are incapable of taking the perspective of the other.

This latter conclusion is reinforced by the findings of a study examining the conversational performance of language impaired and normally developing children who are the same age and younger than the language impaired children (Fey/Leonard 1984). In this study, the language impaired children and their normally developing age peers were aged 4½ to 6 years. The younger normally developing children were aged 2;11 to 3;5 years. The children engaged in conversation with an adult, a peer and a younger child. It was found that the language impaired children were similar to normally developing children in all aspects of their conversational interaction except that they generated fewer internal state questions, had shorter MLUs and shorter mean pre-verb lengths. They were better than the younger children in the normally developing group in adapting their language to the age of their conversational partner. These data reinforce the notion that the communication problems of dysphasic children are probably due to their semantactic difficulties and not problems about the requirements of communication interaction.

However, in a study of somewhat older language disordered children (between the ages of 5;6 and 6 years, the findings were very different. The language disordered children ignored and responded inappropriately to requests more frequently than normally developing children. Their responses were, occassionally, contrary to facts or unrelated to expected information (Brinton/Fujiki 1982). These findings suggest that language disordered children do have difficulties in acquiring the requirements of conversational exchange. However, the contradictory findings might be due to all the factors discussed in the review of studies of other aspects of language. Namely, 1) there might be true differences in the nature of the problems in pragmatics that different dysphasic or language disordered children have, due to underlying neurological differences, or 2) they might experience difficulties in the acquisition of the kinds of knowledge required in the more sophisticated components of an aspect of language and, thus, exhibit a plateau in development. Unfortunately, the longitudinal and across components of language data needed to determine whether one or two is the case are missing.

Evidence from other studies of the conversational interaction of dysphasic as compared to normally developing children, however, support the notion that there are at least two groups of children within the population in terms of the development of competence in communicative interaction. The ability of language disordered children of varying ages (4;0 to 6;2 years) to mark new versus old information in conversation was examined. It was found that over half of the language disordered children pronominalized more often than control children of ages 1;11 to 2;10 years. These language disordered children also demonstrated a proportionately different combination of language features for their MLU (Skarakis/Greenfield 1982). These findings suggest that there is a group of language disordered children who develop more sophisticated ways of marking new and old information in conversation despite the fact that their MLU remains the same as much younger normally developing children, and a group who do not. The former group of children appear to have an output problem. The latter might have an input problem. Another study (Craig/Evans 1989) examined the turn exchange characteristics of the conversations between language impaired children and adults, and age and MLU matched normally developing children. The language impaired children in this study were aged 8;8 to 13;11 years. Since there were only five language impaired children in the study, the behavior of individual children was examined closely. It was found that there were qualitative differences in terms of turn errors, interruptions, interactive attention, responsiveness and turn switch times among the SLI children. Children with reduced receptive skills had more difficulties. These data suggest that children who have problems in encoding information in conversational exchanges have more difficulties in responding and in responding appropriately than children who have retrieval problems. This, of course, makes sense.

There have been, by now, many studies of the narrative generation and, more frequently, recall abilities of dysphasic children. Most of the dysphasic children in these studies range in age from about 7 to 14 years. Therefore, unlike research in other aspects of language, only older language disordered children are included. For the most part, these studies indicate that language disordered children generate and recall fewer propositions and even episodes than normally developing children but, on the whole, maintain the structure of the narrative. There are, however, some differences in narrative processing that some researchers have found, and they are interesting. The language disordered children do not differ in factual recall but do so in terms of relations linking the critical parts of the story together (Merrit/Liles 1987). The language disordered children exhibit poorer use of cohesive conjunctions (Liles 1987). There are some language disordered children who show temporal inversions and transformations in their recall of stories, and their patterns of recall and story construction are atypical of children of that age (Johnston 1982 b). With these latter children the suggestion was made that they were having comprehension difficulties. Their narrative organization is poorer, and they are poorer in their use of cohesive categories and personal reference. They are equal in their responses to verbatim questions but differ from normally developing children in their ability to answer questions about the structure of the narrative (Liles 1985). Even when they recall a story, they have more problems with inferential questions (Crais/Chapman 1987).

The data on story recall and generation indicate that there are, again, possible differences within the population of dysphasic children in this ability. There are those who order story episodes in the manner of normally developing children and those who do not. Those who do not, apparently, have comprehension problems. Thus, there are children in the population who generate less and recall less than normally developing children and others who do the latter, and, also, generate and recall in a different manner than normally developing children. These difficulties in recall are probably related to the differences observed in the ability of language disordered children to answer inferential as compared to verbatim questions and to recall linking structures across the story. There have been differences observed in these children's ability to generate a variety of conjunctions and cohesive devises which is, presumably, unrelated to semantactic abilities. This suggests that at least some of these children have not acquired the sophisticated structures necessary to make discourse connected. This might be considered a particular pragmatic disability. Finally, in a study of these children's judgement of the adequacy of communicators it was found that they behaved like younger children, and could not accurately judge who was at fault in a poor communication situation (Meline/Brackin 1987).

In summary, some dysphasic children have difficulty in recall of discourse in terms of the amount to be recalled but not in the structure of recall, while others have difficulty in both. They converse in many ways like their peers when they are young but then have greater difficulties in adequate communication when they are older. They behave like their younger normally developing peers when metacognizing about the adequacy of the communication situation. They are, again, both delayed and different in their pragmatic development just as they are both delayed and different in other aspects of language development. Whether they appear to be delayed or different depends on the age at which their behavior is sampled and the conditions under which they are sampled. There appears to be a relation between comprehension difficulties and differences as well as delays in pragmatic development.

4. Information Processing Problems

The question that has arisen most frequently about dysphasic children and adults has been whether or not their language problem is due to some cognitive deficit or a specific language impairment. With dysphasic children the question has been asked in varying ways: 1) are they behind their age peers on Piagetian tasks?, 2) do they have a perceptual or conceptual problem? and 3) what is the nature of their memory problems? The answers that have been obtained to these questions do shed some light on possible relations between these children's information processing difficulties and their language problems.

The answer to the first question is, as usual, mixed. When comparing language disordered children with their MLU and age matched peers on haptic recognition, water level and classification tasks, it was found that they were better than their MLU peers on all tasks and worse than their age peers on one task, the haptic recognition task (Kamhi 1981). When comparing these same groups of children at a younger age on symbolic play, it was found that the language disordered children were more advanced than their MLU matched group in terms of the number of their play schemes but below age expectations. These data do not clarify the question but do cause serious doubt as to whether disabilities on Piagetian tasks cause disabilities in language development. The findings vis-a-vis haptic recognition might be related to oral motor problems in some dysphasic children but it is clear that not all dysphasic children have such problems.

The answer to the second question is also, apparently, mixed. As indicated in the section on phonology studies, the claim has been made that the auditory perpectual problems of these children are the bases for these children's developmental language problems. A group of language disordered and normally developing children's profiles on the Leiter scale were compared (Johnston 1982 a). Both groups of children did better on the perceptual tasks than on the conceptual. However, among the 16 language disordered children, 2 showed marked disparity between performance on the two types of tasks with performance on the perceptual always better. Four did better on the conceptual tasks than the perceptual. Still another study found no differences between the non-linguistic concept formation abilities of mental age matched language disordered and normally developing children's abilities (Kamhi/Catts/Koenig/Lewis 1984).

There are a number of studies that have found differences between language disordered children and their normally developing peers in terms of the rate at which they can encode and then retrieve information (Menyuk 1988). These problems in the rate at which information can be encoded may not be limited to auditory or linguistic information. For example, it has been found that language impaired children can decide whether two geometric arrays are similarly ordered when they are parallel and when they are rotated. There were no differences between them and their normally developing mental age peers in the accuracy of their performance or in the training needed to learn the task. The only significant difference was the mean response time of the groups. The accuracy of the identification of visual, auditory and crossmodal stimuli by language impaired and normally developing children was examined (Tallal/Stark/Kallman/Mellits 1981). The stimuli were presented in varying amounts and rates, and the children were aged 5 to 9 years. It was found that the language impaired children made significantly more errors than normally developing children when more than 2 item sequences were presented, or the stimuli were presented rapidly regardless of modality. The older language impaired children made twice as many errors with auditory than with visual stimuli. For the younger language impaired children the modality made no difference in error rate. These data suggest that language impaired children have a limit in the rate at which they can process all types of stimuli. The fast fading nature of auditory stimuli make such stimuli a particular problem for these children.

The rate at which information can be encoded and then retrieved may be a function of the strategies used to process information. These children appear to have less effective strategies than normally developing children, or do not use the strategies they have under stressful conditions such as information overload. Both capacity and strategy differences may bring about the behaviors observed. It is possible that children who show a delay in development are those who have the strategy but cannot use it under all the required circumstances. Children who showed differences in the pattern of their development may be those who have not developed the strategies necessary to encode the information as it increases in complexity.

Throughout the discussion of these children's development of the varying aspects of language two things have been emphasized. The first is that a number of these children are apparently at the very delayed end of normal development while others appear to have particular problems in learning new aspects of language that present a marked change in the complexity of stuctures, and still others exhibit differences in their pattern of language behavior and development. It is possible that the first group of children has difficulty in encoding auditory information accurately or rapidly anough to categorize it. The second group of children may have difficulty in developing the categories into which various classes and relations belong once those categories and relations reach a certain level of complexity. The third group of children may have difficulties in developing categories and relations at any level. The three groups of children have information processing problems but the nature of their problems varies.

There is certainly the possibility that there are other causes that might account for these children's language difficulties than those outlined above. There may also be differences among them in their patterns of language development and use not pointed to in this discussion. Future research may determine these causes and differences. However, unless this research includes long term developmental studies of all components of language in the same dysphasic children it is doubtful that more complete answers about causes and differences will be obtained.

5. References

Bialystok, E. (1986). Factors in growth of linguistic awareness. *Child Development, 57*, 498–510.

Brinton, B. & Fujiki, M. (1982). A comparison of request-response sequences in the discourse of normal and language disordered children. *Journal of Speech and Hearing Disorders, 47*, 57–62.

Chapman, K., Leonard, L., Rowan, L., & Weiss, A. (1983). Inappropriate word extensions in the speech of young language disordered children. *Journal of Speech and Hearing Disorders, 48*, 55–61.

Craig, H. & Evans, J. (1989). Turn exchange characteristics of SLI children's simultaneous and non-simultaneous speech. *Journal of Speech and Hearing Disorders, 54*, 334–347.

Crais, E. & Chapman, R. (1987). Story recall and inferencing skills in language learning-disabled and non-disabled children. *Journal of Speech and Hearing Disorders, 52*, 50–55.

Elliott, L., Hannen, M., & Scholl, M. (1989). Fine-grained auditory discrimination in normal children and children with language learning problems. *Journal of Speech and Hearing Research, 32*, 112–119.

Fey, M. & Leonard, L. (1984). Partner age as a variable in the conversational performance of specifically language-impaired normal-language children. *Journal of Speech and Hearing Research, 27*, 413–423.

Fletcher, P. (1991). Evidence from syntax for language impairment. In J. Miller (Ed.), *Research on child language disorders: A decade of progress. 169–188*. Austin, TX.: Pro-Ed.

Fried-Oken, M. (1987). Qualitative examination of children's naming skills through test adaptations. *Language, Speech, and Hearing Services in Schools, 18*, 206–216.

German, D. (1982). Word-finding substitutions in children with learning disabilities. *Language, Speech and Hearing Services in Schools, 13*, 223–230.

German, D. (1987). Spontaneous language profiles of children with word-finding problems. *Language, Speech, and Hearing Services in Schools, 18*, 217–230.

Grimm, H. (1987). Developmental dysphasia: New theoretical perspectives and empirical results. *The German Journal of Psychology, 11*, 8–22.

Ingram, D. (1989). *Phonological disability in children, 2nd ed.* London: Cole & Whurr.

Johnston, J. (1982a). Interpreting the Leiter I. Q.: Performance profiles of young normal and language disordered children. *Journal of Speech and Hearing Research, 25*, 291–296.

Johnston, J. (1982b) Narratives: A new look at communication problems in older language-disordered children. *Language, Speech and Hearing Services in Schools, 13*, 144–156.

Johnston, J. & Kamhi, A. (1984). Syntactic and semantic aspects of utterances of language impaired children: The same can be less. *Merrill Palmer Quarterly, 30*, 65–86.

Johnston, J. & Weismer, S. (1983). Mental rotation abilities in language disordered children. *Journal of Speech and Hearing Research, 26*, 397–403.

Kamhi, A. (1981). Non language symbolic and conceptual abilities of language impaired and normally developing children. *Journal of Speech and Hearing Research, 24*, 446–453.

Kamhi, A., Catts, H., Koenig, L., & Lewis, B. (1984). Hypothesis testing and nonlinguistic symbolic abilities in language-impaired children. *Journal of Speech and Hearing Disorders, 49*, 169–176.

Karmiloff-Smith, A. (1986). From meta-process to conscious access: Evidence from children's metalinguistic and repair data. *Cognition, 35*, 95–147.

Lahey, E., Liebergott, J., Chesnick, M., Menyuk, P., & Adams, J. (in press 1990). Variability in the use of grammatical morphemes: Implications for understanding language impairment. *Applied Psycholinguistics.*

Leonard, L. (1990). Some rival accounts of morphological deficits in specific language impairment: A crosslinguistic study. Paper presented at the Fifteenth Annual Boston University Child Language Conference, Boston, October.

Leonard, L., Camarata, S., Rowan, L., & Chapman, K. (1982a). The communicative functions of lexical usage by language impaired children. *Applied Psycholinguistics, 3*, 109–125.

Leonard, L. Schwartz, R., Chapman, K., Rowan, L., Prelock, P., Terrell, B., Weiss, A., & C. Messick (1982b). Early lexical acquisition in children with specific language impairment. *Journal of Speech and Hearing Research, 25*, 554–564.

Levy, C. & Menyuk, P. (1975). Cognitive and linguistic skills of children with normal and deviant language development. Paper presented at the American Speech, Language and Hearing Association Annual Convention, November, Washington, D. C.

Liebergott, J., Menyuk, P., Chesnick, M., & Korngold B. (1988). Language processing abilities and reading achievement in children. Mini-seminar presented at the Annual Convention of the American Speech, Language and Hearing Association, November, Boston.

Liles, B. (1985). Cohesion in the narratives of normal and language disordered children. *Journal of Speech and Hearing Research, 28*, 123–133.

Liles, B. (1987). Episode organization and cohesive conjunctives in narratives of children with and without language disorder. *Journal of Speech and Hearing Research, 30*, 185–196.

Magnusson, E. (1983). *The phonology of language disordered children: Production, perception and awareness*. Travaux de L'institut de Linguistique de Lund, C W K Glerup.

Meline, T. & Brackin, S. (1987). Language impaired children's awareness of inadequate messages. *Journal of Speech and Hearing Disorders, 52*, 263–270.

Menyuk, P. (1978). Linguistic problems in children with developmental dysphasia. In M. Wyke (Ed.), *Developmental dysphasia. 135–158*. London: Academic Press.

Menyuk, P. (1983). The role of context in misarticulations. In G. Yeni-Komshian, J. Kavanaugh, & C. Ferguson (Eds.), *Child phonology, Vol. 1. 211–228*. N. Y.: Academic Press.

Menyuk, P. (1988). *Language development: Knowledge and use*. Glenview, Il.: Scott Foresman/Little Brown College Division.

Menyuk, P. (1991). Metalinguistic abilities and language disorder. In J. Miller (Ed.), *Research on child language disorders: A decade of progress. 387–398*. Austin, TX.: Pro-Ed.

Menyuk, P., Chesnick, M., Liebergott, J., Korngold, B., D'Agostino, R., & Belanger, A. (1991). Predicting reading problems in at risk children. *Journal of Speech and Hearing Research, 34*, 893–901.

Menyuk, P. & Looney, P. (1972). Relationships among components of the grammar in language disorder. *Journal of Speech and Hearing Research, 15*, 395–406.

Merrit, D. & Liles, B. (1987). Story grammar ability in children with and without language disorder: Story generation, story retelling and story comprehension. *Journal of Speech and Hearing Research, 30*, 539–552.

Nippold, M. & Fey, S., (1983). Metaphoric understanding in preadolescents having a history of language acquisition difficulties. *Language, Speech, and Hearing Services in Schools, 14*, 171–180.

Paden, E., Novak, M., & Beiter, A. (1987). Predictors of phonologic inadequacy in young children prone to otitis media. *Journal of Speech and Hearing Disorders, 52*, 232–242.

Panagos, J. & Prelock, P. (1982). Phonological constraints in the sentence production of language disordered children. *Journal of Speech and Hearing Research, 25*, 171–177.

Pearl, R., Donahue, M., & Bryan, T. (1985). The development of tact: Children's strategies for delivering bad news. *Journal of Applied Developmental Psychology, 6*, 141–149.

Powers, M. (1957). Functional disorders of articulation-symptomatology and etiology. In L. Travis (Ed.) *Handbook of speech pathology. 707–768*. N. Y.: Appleton-Century-Crofts.

Prinz, P. & Ferrier, L. (1983). Can you give me that one?: The comprehension, production and judgement of directives in language impaired children. *Journal of Speech and Hearing Disorders, 48*, 44–54.

Rowan, L., Leonard, L., Chapman, K., & Weiss, A. (1983). Performative and presuppositional skills in language disordered and normal children. *Journal of Speech and Hearing Research, 26*, 97–106.

Schwartz, R., Leonard, L., Folger, M., & Wilcox, M. (1980). Early phonological behavior in normal speaking and language disordered children: Evidence for a synergistic view. *Journal of Speech and Hearing Disorders, 45*, 357–377.

Schwartz, R., Leonard, L., Frome Loeb, D., & Swanson, L. (1987). Attempted sounds are sometimes not: An expanded view of phonological selection and avoidance. *Journal of Child Language, 14*, 411–418.

Shriberg, L. & Paul, R. (1982). Associations between phonology and syntax in speech delayed children. *Journal of Speech and Hearing Research, 25*, 536–547.

Shriberg, L. & Smith, A. (1983). Phonological correlates of middle ear involvement in speech delayed children: A methodological note. *Journal of Speech and Hearing Research, 26*, 293–297.

Skarakis, S. & Greenfield, P. (1982). The role of old and new information in the verbal expression of language disordered children. *Journal of Speech and Hearing Research, 25*, 462–472.

Snyder, L. (1987). Defining language disordered children: Disordered or just "low verbal" normal. University of Denver, Denver, Colorado. Unpublished manuscript.

Stark, R. & Tallal, P. (1981). Selection of children with specific language deficit. *Journal of Speech and Hearing Disorders, 46*, 114–122.

Stoel-Gammon, C. (1991). Issues in phonological development and disorder. In J. Miller (Ed.) *Research on child language disorders: A decade of progress. 255–266*. Austin, TX.: Pro-Ed.

Tallal, P. & Stark, R. (1983). Speech perception of language delayed children. In G. Yeni-Komshian, J. Kavanaugh, & C. Ferguson (Ed.), *Child phonology, Vol. 2. 155–172*. N. Y.: Academic Press.

Tallal, P., Stark, R., Kallman, C., & Mellits, D. (1981). A reexamination of some nonverbal perceptual abilities of language impaired and normal children as a function of age and sensory modality. *Journal of Speech and Hearing Research, 24*, 351–357.

Teele, D., Klein, J., Chase, C., Menyuk, P., & Rosner, B. (1990). Otitis media in infancy and development of intellectual ability, school achievement, and speech and language at age seven years. *Journal of Infectious Diseases, 162*, 685–694.

Witelson, S. (1977). Early hemisphere specialization and interhemisphere plasticity: An empirical and theoretical review. In S. Segalowitz & F. Gruber (Eds.), *Language development and neurological theory. 303–319.* N. Y.: Academic Press.

Wolf, M. (1984). Naming, reading, and the dyslexias: A longitudinal overview. *Annals of Dyslexia, 34*, 87–115.

Paula Menyuk, Boston, Massachusetts (USA)

62. Children with Specific Language Impairment (Developmental Dysphasia): Perceptual and Cognitive Aspects

1. Introduction

Language is arguably the most complex of all human behaviors. Normal language development involves the integration of sensory and physical mechanisms; perceptual, cognitive, and linguistic processes; and social, motivational, and psychological factors. Deficiencies in one or more of these components will place a child at risk for delayed language development. Language disorders that can be directly attributed to one or more of these predisposing peripheral or central impairments are often considered to be resulting symptoms of a more pervasive disorder. Such disorders include mental retardation, hearing impairment, severe emotional disturbance, and frank neurological dysfunction (Tallal 1988). Mentally retarded children, for example, are not considered to be primarily language impaired.

Children with specific language impairments have significant difficulty acquiring language that cannot be attributed to any of the obvious causes mentioned above. Variously referred to as developmentally aphasic, dysphasic, language impaired, or language disordered, these children acquire language more slowly than their peers and often continue to have difficulty with spoken and written language throughout the developmental period into adulthood. The existence of a pure or uncontaminated group of language disordered children has intrigued theorists and researchers. Why should children with normal intelligence, intact speech and hearing mechanisms, and a supportive language learning environment have difficulty acquiring language?

Four accounts of the bases of specific language impairment or developmental dysphasia have received considerable attention during the past 25 years. The four accounts have attempted to link language delays with deficiencies in (a) auditory processing, (b) a conceptual/representational processes, (c) neurological functions, and (d) the child's communicative environment. Other chapters in this volume will discuss the neurological aspects of language disorders (cf. art. 59) and patterns of interaction and communication involving children with specific language impairments (cf. art. 68). The present chapter will focus on perceptual and conceptual/representational aspects of language disorders.

2. Perceptual Aspects

Normal language learning and conceptual processing requires the effective functioning of a variety of perceptual mechanisms. These mechanisms include not only those that are bound to specific senses, such as vision and audition, but also attentional and memory processes that span the senses. A large body of literature has examined auditory processing abilities in children with developmental dysphasia or specific language impairment (SLI). During the 1960's and 1970's, there were a number of claims that auditory processing deficits accounted for SLI children's difficulty learning language (e. g., Eisenson 1966; Lowe/Campbell 1965). As Leonard (1987) has pointed out, the meaning of the term 'auditory processing' varied from investigator to investigator. Studies included any one or more of the following abilities: auditory discrimination, sequencing, memory, and synthesis. SLI children often performed more poorly on these tasks than same-age normal-language children.

Lowe/Campbell (1965) are generally credited as being the first investigators to examine auditory temporal processes in SLI children. They compared eight SLI children who ranged in age from 7 to 14 years to a group of age-matched normal language (NL) children on two tasks: a 'succession' task which required the child to decide whether the stimuli presented were one or two sounds and a temporal order task which required the child to judge which of two sounds were presented first. The stimuli were two different 15 ms pure tones, 400 and 2200 Hz. In the succession task, the SLI children judge that the two sounds were one at an average inter-stimulus-interval (ISI) of 35.8 ms compared to 18.5 ms for the NO group. This difference was not statistically significant. On the temporal order task, however, the SLI children needed an average of 357 ms (range 55 – 700 ms) compared to 36.1 ms (range 15 – 80 ms) for the NL children to achieve the same average level of performance (75% correct). This dicrepancy was highly significant, leading Lowe and Campbell to conclude that impaired temporal ordering ability might be a major contributing factor to the language impairment in SLI children.

Rees (1973) pointed out three serious problems with Lowe and Campbell's study and other sequencing experiments conducted up to this point. First, she argued that the conclusions from these studies assumed that pure tones were processed in the same manner as speech sounds. Second, she noted that the use of verbal stimuli to assess perceptual abilities presented a possible confound of low-level auditory processing abilities and higher-level linguistic abilities. The impairment in temporal processing abilities might be one manifestation of the higher-level language impairment. Rees' final point was that no attempt had been made in these studies to establish a positive correlation between the extent of the auditory sequencing disorder and the degree of language impairment.

2.1. The Work of Tallal and Colleagues

The work of Tallal and her colleagues over the past 20 years has provided considerable data that directly addressed Rees' concerns. In the initial studies by Tallal/Piercy (1973 a, b), the first two concerns were addressed. Instead of using pure tones, nonverbal acoustic stimuli were synthetically generated to match the acoustic properties of steady-state speech sounds. These sounds did not match the acoustic spectrum of any specific phoneme. The experimental paradigm, referred to as the repetition method, used minimal verbal instructions and incorporated a training procedure to insure that children understood the task.

In the first study (Tallal/Piercy 1973 a), 12 SLI children (ages 6;9 to 9;3) were compared to same age NL peers. The children were presented two different 75 ms tones (100 and 305 Hz, ISI = 428 ms) and taught to respond to each tone separately by pushing one of two panels for one tone and the other panel for the other tone. The children were then taught to respond to each of the four two-tone sequences presented (1 – 2, 2 – 1, 1 – 1, 2 – 2) by pushing the panels in the appropriate order. After being trained in this manner, the children were tested on the same two-tone sequences using 12 different ISIs ranging from 8 ms to 4,062 ms.

The NL children performed significantly better than chance level for all 12 ISIs. SLI children did not perform better than chance at ISIs less than 305 ms. Similar findings were obtained when the task was changed to a same/different format in which children had to push one panel when the two tones were the same and the other panel when the two tones were different.

In a second experiment with the same subjects, Tallal/Piercy (1973 b) varied the duration of the tones and the modality of stimulus presentation. Seven different ISIs were used ranging from 8 ms to 428 ms. Four durations were examined: 75, 125, 175, and 250 ms. The SLI children performed below the level of NL children for all ISIs below 150 ms for the 75 and 125 durations. When the tone duration was 175 ms, the SLI children performed more poorly than the NL children only when ISIs were less than 15 ms. No group differences were found for the 250 ms tone.

The same procedures were used next to compare each group's ability to process visual stimuli consisting of light flashes of two different shades of green. Children were tested at several ISIs ranging from 30 ms to 428 ms. No significant group differences were found for any of the ISIs.

Based on the findings from these two studies, Tallal and Piercy suggested that SLI children have difficulty processing auditory information that is presented at a rapid rate. The time available for processing appeared to be critical for adequate performance.

In a subsequent series of studies with a different sample of children, Tallal/Stark/Kallman/Mellits (1980, 1981) sought to validate and extend the findings from the initial studies. Subjects in these studies were 36 SLI children from 5 to 9 years of age and 38 age matched peers. The auditory stimuli were the same 75 ms tones used in Tallal/Piercy (1973 a). The visual stimuli were changed from the earlier study. Slides of two nonsense letters were presented as light flashes 75 ms in duration. ISIs of 10, 70, and 500 ms were used in all tasks.

Both groups performed similarly on the discrimination task. On the sequencing task, the NL children performed better than the SLI children at all ISIs in both modalities. The poor performance of the SLI children for the visual modality was inconsistent with previous findings (Tallal/Piercy 1973 b). Tallal et al. (1981) suggested that age differences in the subject populations may explain the differences. Only the younger SLI children (5- and 6-years olds) performed poorly on the visual tasks. The other children, who were approximately the same age as the children in the previous study, performed poorly only in the auditory modality.

Tallal/Stark (1981) examined the ability of the same children to discriminate other types of verbal stimuli (e. g., [da] – [ta], [dab] – [dæb], [sa] – [sta]). For each contrast, the children heard a random list of syllables and had to press a response panel when one of the syllables was heard. No response was required for the other syllable. The SLI children performed more poorly than the NL children on three stimulus pairs: [ba] – [da], [da] – [ta], and [da] – [ʃa]. As Leonard notes (1987, 16), what is interesting about this finding is that brevity of acoustic cues did not have the same effect for all stimuli. The SLI children were able to distinguish between [ɛ] and [æ] even though they were only 40 ms in duration. These findings led Tallal/Stark/Kallmann/Mellits to conclude that the rate specific deficit in processing auditory information includes the processing of linguistically meaningful stimuli when these stimuli contain brief acoustic cues that are followed in rapid succession by other acoustic cues.

Bernstein/Stark (1985) reported the results of a four-year follow-up study of the children who participated in the 1980/81 studies. Fourteen NL and 29 SLI children were retested. The children now ranged in age from 8 to 12 years. The tasks (discrimination, sequencing, and serial memory) and stimuli ([ba] and [da]) were the same ones used in the earlier studies by Tallal/Piercy (1973 a, b). Both groups of children performed at the same levels on the various tasks. Only one SLI child failed to meet the $p < .001$ criterion for sequencing with the longest ISI. The findings from this study clearly indicated that SLI children's perceptual abilities improved with age. However, the extent of development was unclear because the tasks were too easy for both groups of children. The ceiling effects on the tasks made it impossible to consider the relationship between perceptual abilities and language impairment in older SLI children. The SLI children might perform below age level on more advanced perceptual tasks. Importantly, the data support the conclusion that early perceptual deficits do not preclude subsequent language development.

2.2. Relating Perceptual Skills to Measures of Speech and Language

The studies discussed thus far have addressed two of the three concerns raised by Rees (1973, 1981). Her third concern was that researchers had not established a positive relationship between the extent of the auditory processing deficit and the nature or extent of the language impairment. Tallal/Stark/Curtiss (1976) addressed this concern by comparing the speech production abilities of the SLI and NL children in the Tallal and Piercy studies. Speech proficiency was evaluated by having these children name pictures of objects and nonsense syllables. The SLI children were found to make many more errors on stop consonants and consonant clusters than on vowel and nasal sounds. Because the SLI children had the most difficulty on sounds containing rapid acoustic changes, Tallal/Stark/Curtiss concluded that auditory processing limitations were responsible for the speech errors.

In a more recent study, Curtiss/Tallal (1991) examined the relationship of higher-level language abilities to performance on the auditory processing tasks. Subjects were 67 SLI children, 57 age-matched peers, and 32 language-matched peers who were followed for five years beginning at age four. Measures of language included the receptive and elicited production tests from the CYCLE (Curtiss/Yamada 1988). The receptive tests consisted largely of sentence-picture matching items. The production task used a sentence-completion format. To examine the relationship between nonlinguistic sequencing impairments (poor performance on the temporal processing task) and language acquisition, items from the CYCLE were organized into two separate clusters: a + sequentially-cued (+ sc) cluster in which word order uniquely signalled grammatic and thematic role and a − sequentially-cued (− sc) cluster in which 'key formatives' cued roles and relations. The + cluster consisted of reversible SVO sentences, such as *The girl is pushing the boy* vs. *The boy is pushing the girl.* In these sentences, word order provides the only cue to the relationship between the noun phrases and the verb. The − sc cluster included attributive, stative, and negative sentences, such as *The ball is big* vs. *The ball is little* and *Here the boy is pulling the wagon but here the boy is not pulling the wagon.*

The key finding was that the SLI children performed significantly worse on the + sc cluster than on the − sc cluster. The age-matched normals consistently performed better than the SLI children and showed no difference in performance levels for the two clusters. Performance on the nonverbal sequencing tasks and the + sc cluster was moderately correlated at years 2 (.49) and 3 (.39) of the study. Based on these findings, Curtiss and Tallal suggest that a nonlinguistic sequencing impairment may impact directly on the processing of linguistic structures when the sequential order of linguistic elements uniquely signals important grammatical or semantic information.

2.3. Other Research on SLI Children's Perceptual Abilities

Tallal and her colleagues have not been the only investigators who have examined the perceptual abilities of SLI children. In this section, selected studies from other researchers are reviewed.

Tomblin/Quinn (1983) questioned whether SLI children's poor performance on the rapid processing tasks might be the result of factors other than an inherent deficit in temporal resolution ability. In their study, 10 NL children (ages 5 ; 8 to 6 ; 9) were administered the repetition task five times over a 5−7 day period. As expected, the children performed better on stimuli with longer ISIs. However, the children also performed better across the session. The finding that temporal processing abilities improve with experience led Tomblin and Quinn to suggest that poor performance on the task may be caused by limited experience, attention, or the inability to use appropriate processing strategies.

Some recent studies by Elliott and her colleagues have been more successful than Bernstein/Stark (1985) were in identifying perceptual problems in older SLI children. In a longitudinal study, Elliott/Hammer (1988) presented a set of finegrained auditory discrimination tasks to 21 SLI and 21 NL children over a three-year period. At the beginning of the study, the children averaged 7 years of age. The SLI children were all enrolled in a classroom for language-learning problems. Over the three years of the study, the SLI children consistently performed more poorly than the NL children on the Peabody Picture Vocabulary Test (Dunn/Dunn 1981), The Token Test for Children (DiSimoni 1978), and the Templin-Darley Screening Test of Speech Articulation (Templin/Darley 1969). No other information was given about the specific nature of the children's language problem. All the children were reported to have normal intelligence.

The stimuli were two continua of CV stimuli [ba − pa] and [ba − da − ga]. For [ba − pa], a five formant, eight item continuum that varied in VOT from 0 − 35 ms was created. For [ba − da − ga], 13 items were created, each having five formants. With these stimuli, it was possible to determine the smallest acoustic differences ('just noticeably differences' JNDs) that could be discriminated. On every trial, two syllables were presented sequentially with a 500 ms ISI. Subjects had to make same-different judgments by pushing one of two response buttons.

The JNDs for the SLI children were nearly always larger than those for the NL listeners in each year of testing. The differences tended to be statistically significant for the VOT continuum, but not for the place-of-articulation continuum. Based on these findings, Elliott and Hammer concluded that SLI children continue to have auditory discrimination problems past the pre-school years and also continue to exhibit speech and language problems.

Leonard (1989) has recently used cross-linguistic comparisons of Italian, Hebrew, and English speaking SLI children to support the relationship between rapid auditory processing deficiencies and specific linguistic deficiencies. He begins by noting that the most striking aspect of SLI children's language is their extraordinary difficulties with grammatical morphemes (e. g., Johnston/Kamhi 1984; Johnston/Schery 1976). These morphemes include inflected forms, such as the past tense, possessive, and plural, and function words such as articles and auxiliaries. Although SLI children consistently have trouble with grammatical morphemes, some morphemes cause less problems than others. The irregular past tense and present progressive -ing emerge only slightly below MLU expectations.

Using Pinker's (1984) learnability theory, Leonard suggests that SLI children have difficulty acquiring grammatical morphemes that have low 'phonetic substance' and do not have difficulty with grammatical morphemes that do not have low phonetic substance. Low phonetic substance is defined as "monosyllabic consonant segments and unstressed syllables, characterized by shorter duration than adjacent morphemes, and, often, lower fundamental frequency and amplitude" (Leonard 1989, 186). Leonard goes on to argue that the perceptual characteristics of low phonetic substance morphemes closely resemble the characteristics of acoustic stimuli that SLI children have difficulty processing.

Leonard also martials evidence from the speech production literature. He argues that final consonant deletion and weak syllable deletion that are common in the speech of SLI children also support the low phonetic substance explanation.

Leonard next attempts to show how Pinker's theory can explain the difficulty SLI children have with other language forms and structures. He suggests that the difficulty SLI children have with morphemes may impede their ability to parse sentences and thus develop new phrase structure rules. Leonard acknowledges, however, that this explanation is weak. He also notes that the definition of low-phonetic substance is simplistic because once a certain absolute duration is reached, relative duration may not be important (193).

2.4. Evaluation

The large body of literature documenting the below age-level performance of SLI children on rapid processing tasks is compelling. The studies by Tallal and her colleagues as well as other investigators have shown that compared to age-matched peers, SLI children have difficulty perceiving and producing information rapidly in time. The poor performance of the SLI children on visual tasks suggests that the processing deficit is not specific to auditory input (see Elliott/Hammer/Scholl 1990, for the alternative view). The "neural timing deficit," as Tallal (1988, 164) recently refers to it, accurately predicts (a) performance on the nonverbal and verbal serial memory tasks, (b) the pattern and type of speech production and perception errors, (c) the degree of receptive language impairment, and (d) classification of specific language impairment.

Despite the overwhelming evidence suggesting that a timing deficit provides a sufficient explanation for a specific language impairment, many remain unconvinced that such a deficit can account for the extent and nature of the specific language impairment (Johnston 1988; Leonard 1987; Rees 1981; Tomblin 1984). The problem lies not in the data or methodology of the studies, but with the bottom-up information processing or specific abilities models that provide the theoretical backdrop for most of the studies discussed in this section. An assumption that underlies these studies is that there are fundamental perceptual and memory processes that are necessary for, but independent of, language learning (Tomblin 1984). That is, language usage and learning depends on a set of component auditory perceptual abilities that are arranged in some serial, bottom-up, fashion. The perception and processing of sensory information is viewed as passive and unaffected by situational factors, knowledge states, and previous experiences of the individual.

The counterclaim is that perceptual and memory processes do not function independently of knowledge states and other conceptual processes. Several contemporary theories of language processing emphasize the complex interactions that occur among structural mechanisms, cognitive processes, knowledge states, and environmental forces (see Bohannon/Warren-Leubecker 1988). Piagetian (constructionist) notions that emphasize the active role the child plays in organizing and making sense of the world have become an important component of current accounts of language learning (e. g., Ingram 1989). There is a rich experimental literature demonstrating the effects higher-level language abilities have on speech perception (Pisoni 1978; Rees 1981). In the same vein, short-term memory abilities are known to increase when the individual is able to relate the information to previous knowledge or experiences (e. g., Chi 1976; Huttenlocher/Burke 1976).

There are at least two other significant problems with perceptual explanations of specific language impairment. The first stems from the fact that normally developing children younger than 4;6 cannot perform the Tallal tasks (Tallal 1976). Four and half-year-old NL children, however, have quite sophisticated language abilities. By this age, they produce many complex sentence structures and use a wide range of grammatical morphemes (Ingram 1989). Given that young NL children have sophisticated language abilities and cannot perform the processing tasks, one must seriously question what successful performance on Tallal's tasks means for language learning. The perceptual processing abilities of young NL children are apparently sufficient to comprehend and produce quite sophisticated language forms.

The second problem directly follows. In Leonard's words: "... we cannot lose sight of the fact that, although normal children improve across time in their performance on auditory processing tasks, there has been no serious attempt to explain language development on the basis of developing auditory skills" (Leonard 1987, 22). Leonard's point here is that in order to draw causal connections between perceptual deficiencies and language impairment, there needs to be some theorizing about how particular developments in auditory skills impact on the acquisition of specific linguistic forms and structures. Such theorizing would make specific predictions, for example, about what kinds of perceptual developments precede the acquisition of first words, word combinations, canonical word ordering (SVO), complex sentences, and so forth.

Interestingly, as discussed earlier in this section, since Leonard wrote these words, he has made a serious attempt to relate SLI children's problems with grammatical morphemes to the acoustic characteristics (i. e., low phonetic substance) of these forms. Some of the problems with the 'low phonetic substance' hypothesis have already been discussed. The most serious problem, as pointed out by Leonard himself, is that the hypothesis does not account well for SLI children's problems with other language forms and structures. The hypothesis also does not account well for the continued difficulty older SLI children have with these forms. Despite having heard these forms millions of times and being able to recognize them in reading, older SLI individuals still use them inconsistently in their speech (Tomblin 1990).

In light of these concerns, the most optimistic interpretation of the data is that perceptual limitations account for protracted acquisition of selected language forms such as grammatical morphemes. However, the perceptual deficit does not account well for continued problems with these language forms (e. g., through childhood and adolescence) nor does it account well for other language problems. The most pessimistic interpretation of the data is to argue that all the findings merely establish a strong correlation between rapid perceptual processing and a specific language impairment. The relationship between these perceptual skills and language is not unidirectional (i. e., from perception to language), but interactive and reciprocal, with a language deficit rather than a perceptual deficit being the primary or initial problem. That is, the higher-level language deficit causes poor performance on certain perceptual processing tasks. Although the perceptual deficit is secondary to the language deficit, it can adversely affect subsequent language development.

3. Conceptual and Representational Aspects

By definition, SLI children exhibit a significant discrepancy between language abilities and nonverbal performance scales of intelligence, such as the Leiter International Performance Scales (Arthur 1952), the WISC, and the Columbia Mental Maturity Scale (Burgemeister/Blum/Lorge 1972). SLI children's age-level performance on nonverbal intelligence tests initially discouraged investigations of cognitive abilities in areas not tapped by the intelligence tests. The assumption was that SLI children would show age-level performance in other cognitive measures, as long as the verbal component was minimized. Dissatisfaction, however, with perceptually-based explanations of specific language impairment led researchers to look for cognitive-based explanations for the impairment. Two articles first published in 1973, one by Rees and the other by Morehead and Ingram, were the first to suggest that SLI children might suffer from a more general cognitive impairment. Rees (1973) did not speculate what the nature of the cognitive deficit might be, but Morehead/Ingram (1973) suggested that SLI children might be deficient in symbolic representational abilities.

The theoretical justification for Morehead and Ingram's suggestion is found in Piagetian views of language development. According to Piaget (e. g., 1952), language emerges as part of a more general symbolic function – a function defined as the ability to represent symbolically an external event or object in its absence. This view led researchers to look for parallels in the development of language and other symbolic behaviors in NL and SLI children. Early studies with NL children (e. g., Bates/Benigni/Bretherton et al. 1979; Nicolich 1977) found relationships between developments in language and nonlinguistic symbolic behaviors such as means-ends relations and symbolic play. Subsequent studies involving SLI children (e. g., Johnston/Ellis Weismer 1983; Kamhi 1981; Roth/Clark 1987; Savich 1984; Terrell/Schwartz/Prelock/Messick 1984) have found that SLI children do not perform as well as NL peers on measures of symbolic play and mental imagery. The SLI children generally performed better than language-age matched peers on these measures. In the sections to follow, representative studies in these two areas will be reviewed.

3.1. Symbolic Play

Lovell/Hoyle/Siddall (1968) are generally credited as being the first researchers to investigate symbolic play abilities in SLI children. They compared 10 SLI and 10 children (ages 3;4 to 4;8) using Lunzer's (1959) adaptation and interaction play scales. No differences in symbolic play were found in the 3-year-old children. The play activities of the 4-year-old SLI children were more concrete, less cooperative, and less organized than the age-matched NL children. A significant positive relationship was also found between SLI children's MLU and the amount of time they spent in symbolic play.

Terrell/Schwarz/Prelock/Messick (1984) gave the Symbolic Play Test (Lowe/Costello 1976) to 15 SLI (ages 2;8 to 4;1) and 15 NL children (ages 1;4 to 1;10) matched for language age. Both groups were at the single-word level. The SLI children exhibited significantly higher symbolic play skills than the younger NL children.

Roth/Clark (1987) compared the symbolic play and social participation of six SLI (ages 5;1 to 7;10) to eight NL children (ages 2;8 to 3;0) matched for MLU (M = 3.3 morphemes). Play behaviors were assessed using three measures: (a) the Scale of Social Participation in Play, (b) the Symbolic Play Test, and (c) a modification of Lunzer's Play Scale. Compared to the NL children, the SLI children showed significant deficits in symbolic, adaptive, and integrative play behaviors. The SLI children also exhibited significantly more nonplay and less solitary and parallel play than their NL peers.

3.2. Mental Imagery

The earliest reports of a connection between mental imagery and language came from Piaget's colleagues Inhelder (1966) and de Ajuriaguerra (1966; cited in de Ajuriaguerra/Jaeggi/Guigard et al. 1976). De Ajuriaguerra et al. found that 17 SLI children (ages 4;3 to 10;10) had difficulty with imagery tasks that involved analyzing the movement of a projected shadow.

Kamhi (1981) compared the performance of 10 SLI children (mean age 4;11, mean MLU 4.82) on six Piagetian tasks to groups matched for MA and MLU. On five of the tasks, the SLI children performed comparably to the MA-matched group. On the sixth task, Haptic Recognition, the SLI children performed significantly worse than the MA-matched group, but significantly better than the MLU-matched children. Not coincidentally, this task, which involves blindly feeling geometric forms and then pointing to the corresponding shape from a visual array, was the only one that clearly required mental imagery.

Johnston/Ellis Weismer (1983) used a mental rotation task to investigate mental imagery abilities. Subjects were shown drawings of pairs of linear arrays of geometric forms and asked to push one of two buttons corresponding to same or different. Arrays were presented parallel or with the right hand array rotated either 45, 90, or 135 degrees. Subjects were six first-grade and six third-grade SLI children and age-matched controls. A significant linear relationship between degree of rotation and reaction time was taken as evidence that children in all groups used imagistic processes. SLI children did not differ from NL children in accuracy of judgment and the number of training trials required, but they did respond more slowly. These findings led Johnston and Ellis Weismer to conclude that SLI children have difficulty generating, maintaining, and/or interpreting mental images rather than difficulty transforming images.

Savich (1984) compared the performance of 18 SLI and age-matched NL peers (ages 7;6 to 9;6) on five imagery tasks. The SLI children were less successful than their age peers on all five tasks. For example, they had difficulty predicting the position of a 'snail' on a circular path, the position of fold lines on paper squares, and the configuration that best represented the assembly of a set of shapes.

3.2.1. Evaluation

As Johnston (1988) noted in her summary of the symbolic play and mental imagery research, the search for an underlying symbolic representational deficit seems to have paid off. SLI children consistently perform more poorly than NL peers on symbolic play and mental imagery measures. Correlations between performance on these tasks and measures of language (particularly receptive measures) generally have been moderate and significant (Savich 1984). In addition, Johnston pointed out that relative performance levels of verbal and nonverbal symbolic abilities are exactly in line with what would be expected for two cognitive systems that share a common symbolic feature, but differ in other aspects. In other words, verbal abilities have been reported to be better than nonverbal symbolic abilities (Roth/Clark 1987), equivalent to them (Terrell/Schwartz 1983), and worse than them (Kamhi 1981; Savich 1984). The data are thus consistent with the view that the linguistic impairment in SLI children reflects a more general deficit in symbolic representation.

Although the data support the symbolic representation hypothesis, the explanatory adequacy of this view has been questioned in recent years. Johnston (1988) raises the possibility that SLI children's symbolic deficits may reflect a more pervasive cognitive limitation that affects both symbolic and nonsymbolic aspects of mental activity. In other words, there are other cognitive limitations that may provide better explanations for the data. Johnston did not speculate what the nature of these limitations might be, but several possibilities will be considered in subsequent sections of this chapter.

A related problem with the symbolic deficit view is that it implies that there is one symbolic representational process. Many cognitive processes are involved in symbolic tasks, however, including, encoding, storing, integrating, interpreting, and retrieving information. To say that a child has a deficient symbolic function fails to specify where the actual breakdown may occur. Concluding that a general symbolic deficit underlies a specific language impairment thus has little explanatory adequacy.

A final problem with the symbolic deficit view is that the degree of symbolic deficit found in SLI children does not account well for the extent and type of linguistic deficiencies demonstrated by SLI children (Kamhi 1981). This is because on most symbolic tasks, SLI children perform more poorly than age-matched peers, but better than younger normal children with comparable language abilities. Clear structural parallels between nonlinguistic symbolic skills and SLI children's language problems also have rarely been shown. For example, what is the relationship between language and the ability to anticipate mentally the future position of a snail? Although some would argue that claims were never made about structural parallels, the lack of such parallels further detracts from the explanatory adequacy of the view.

3.3. Hierarchical Planning

One alternative explanation for SLI children's difficulty with verbal and certain nonverbal tasks has been offered by Cromer (1981, 1983). He suggests that a central planning mechanism is necessary in order to convert thoughts and intentions that are not temporally ordered into events that occur in real time. He refers to this as a hierarchical planning ability and suggests that this ability may be crucial both for the organization of incoming stimuli in perception and for the production of behavior (1983, 145).

Cromer (1983) cites research on SLI children's sense of rhythm to support his view. Kracke (1975), for example, found that 12 years-old receptively disordered SLI children performed significantly worse than NL or deaf peers identifying rhythmic sequences presented verbally and tactilely. In contrast to the NL and deaf children who processed the patterns in a Gestalt manner as wholes, the SLI children processed the rhythms element by element. Cromer suggests that an impairment of a more basic hierarchical planning ability may underlie SLI children's rhythmic problems.

In Cromer's (1983) study, he studied hierarchical planning using a construction task adapted from Greenfield/Schneider (1977). In the first task, children were shown a line drawing of a symmetrical tree structure and asked to copy the figure. In the second task, children were shown a completed 3-dimensional mobile built from plastic straws and asked to duplicate it. Subjects were five severely receptively impaired children (ages 9;6 to 16;4) diagnosed as having acquired aphasia with convulsive disorder, seven children diagnosed as having a primary expressive language impairment (ages 8;5 to 12;10), 12 profoundly deaf children, and 12 NL children matched for age to the disordered children. All the subjects performed within normal limits on a performance IQ test.

On both tasks, the performance of the two groups of SLI children were treated as one group because task performance was comparable. The measure of hierarchical planning was the number of shifts in construction from one subunit to another. Shifts that involved crossing from one side of the figure to the other were given a double weighting. A chain or sequential strategy resulted in a zero score. The most interrupted strategy – shifting every time – resulted in a score of 25. On both tasks, the SLI children obtained significantly lower scores than both their deaf and NL peers.

Although Cromer is careful to make no claims about a direct parallel between language and action, he does argue that it is difficult to imagine how a severe deficit in hierarchical planning could fail to affect language. Unfortunately, Cromer fails to specify the nature of the language deficits one would expect to result from such a disability. One might speculate that individuals with a hierarchical planning deficit would exhibit some difficulty producing well-organized spoken and written narratives, event descriptions, and related discourse forms.

3.3.1. Evaluation

Cromer's notion of a hierarchical planning deficit is provocative, despite its lack of specificity. The finding that many SLI children had difficulty on the two tasks clearly indicates that something is amiss. Why is it that these children could not create a hierarchically organized representation of the drawing and the mobile? The difficulty may not be in planning, which Cromer defines as the conversion of sequential events into real time events. Rather, the difficulty may lie in the actual construction of a hierarchically organized representation. SLI children's representational systems may be organized more sequentially than those of NL children.

Although Cromer makes it a point to disclaim direct parallels between language and action, the specific impact a hierarchical planning deficit would have on language needs to be addressed. Future studies are needed that attempt to find parallels between such a deficit and particular linguistic deficiencies.

3.4. Hypothesis Testing

Current views of language acquisition suggest that children learn language through a process of formulating and testing hypotheses about specific conceptual domains and linguistic rules (e. g., Slobin 1979). Deficient hypothesis-testing abilities, therefore, might play some role in explaining developmental language disorders. Researchers have examined this possibility by observing SLI children's performance on various concept formation and discrimination-learning paradigms. In a typical experiment, children view a series of cards each displaying two geometric shapes. One of the forms contains the correct hypothesis (e. g., large, small, circle, or square). On each trial, children point to the form containing their current solution to the problem. Periodic feedback allows the children to evaluate and modify their hypotheses. 'Blank-trial probes', in which no feedback is provided, enable the experimenter to determine the child's hypothesis, the assumption being that the child will maintain a hypothesis if no feedback is provided. Children could use simple object hypotheses (problem solutions are always of this type), alternation hypotheses (left/right, right/left), position hypotheses (left or right), or no hypothesis.

Four studies of this general type have been conducted with mixed results (Ellis Weismer 1991; Hoskins 1979; Kamhi/Nelson/Lee/Gholson 1985; Nelson/Kamhi/Apel 1987). Despite the methodological differences across these studies (e. g., age of subjects and feedback given), the data tend to show that SLI children have difficulty solving discrimination learning problems. This difficulty does not, however, appear to be caused by an inability to generate or test hypotheses (Kamhi et al. 1985). SLI children generated the same proportion of simple object hypotheses as NL age peers. The two most recent studies by Nelson et al. (1987) and Ellis Weismer (1991) raised some questions about the short-term memory demands of the tasks. Clearly, solving discrimination learning tasks taps many different cognitive processes, not simply hypothesis-testing abilities. The conflicting findings of the two most recent studies indicate that the difficulty SLI children have solving discrimination learning problems has yet to be adequately explained.

Another issue concerns the relationship between the explicit, conscious hypothesis-testing abilities employed in discrimination learning problems and the implicit, largely unconscious comparison processes involved in language learning. We might be comparing apples and oranges here; that is, the hypothesis-testing processes involved in discrimination learning problems and language learning might be qualitatively different (Johnston 1988). This indeed seems to be the case. Preschool and young school-age normally developing children, whose language is quite sophisticated, are unable to solve the orthogonal problems presented (Kamhi/Nelson/Lee/Gholson 1985). One would be hard-pressed to make claims for a direct relationship between hypothesis-testing abilities and language learning. SLI children's deficient problem solving abilities at best reflect some basic cognitive processing inefficiency that affects language learning as well as nonverbal task performance.

3.5. Analogical Reasoning

Within the past few years, there has been increasing interest in the development of analogical reasoning in young children. Such reasoning is assumed to represent a central mechanism in learning, transfer, and discovery (e. g., Brown 1989; Sternberg 1985). Analogical reasoning involves applying or transferring existing knowledge (a familiar concept) from a known situation to a novel one, even if the two situations are superficially dissimilar. Analogical reasoning also has a rich history in theories of language acquisition. For example, according to Bloomfield (1933/1961), a grammar is a description of the analogies that hold for a language. More recently, MacWhinney (1978) includes analogy as one of the three central constructs underlying language acquisition.

Traditionally, analogical reasoning has been examined by having subjects respond to proportional analogies of the form *A is to B as C is to D* (e. g., Nippold/Erskine/Freed 1988; Sternberg/Nigro 1980). An example of a proportional analogy is *Meaning is to semantics as sound is to?* Performance on proportional analogies, however, provides little information about the factors that influence analogical reasoning and the processes involved in reasoning analogically. These processes involve (a) learning the solution to the original problem, (b) noticing the correspondence between the known solution and the target problem, (c) retrieving the solution in terms of its general structure, and (d) applying the solution to the target problem (see Gholson/Eymard/Morgan/Kamhi 1987).

Only two studies have examined analogical reasoning abilities in SLI children. Nippold et al. (1988) found that 6- to 8-year-old SLI children performed more poorly than NL age peers on three analogical reasoning tasks. However, when differences in nonverbal intelligence were statistically controlled, the group differences on each task disappeared. The tasks used were two proportional analogies and a story problem adapted from Holyoak/Junn/Billmann (1984). In the story problem task, transfer performance in both groups of children was not good because only one analog was presented. Only one SLI children and two NL children solved the transfer problem without hints.

Kamhi/Gentry/Mauer/Gholson (1990) used the trial-by-trial acquisition procedures developed by Gholson et al. (1987) to compare analogical reasoning processes of 16 SLI children (ages 6;4 to 8;9) and 16 NL children matched for nonverbal MA. All children received two analogs of the Farmer's Dilemma (Wickelgren 1974), that required a specific sequence of seven moves to solve. In this problem, the subject must find a way to get a fox, goose, and corn across a river without anything being eaten. However, only one thing can be taken across the river at a time and the fox will eat the goose and the goose will eat the corn if either pair is left alone. The key move in solving the problem is taking the goose back across the river after it has already been taken across. Two analogs of this problem were created: one involving a lion, pony, and oats and the other a wolf, rabbit, and carrots. The constraints and goal structure of all the problems were similar.

Half of the children viewed physical demonstrations of the problems while they heard the verbal presentations of the problems. The remaining children heard only verbal presentations of each problem. Data consisted of (a) number of trials to reach the acquisition criterion, (b) the number of moves in the transfer task, and (c) trial-by-trial analyses of the proposition represented in the recall protocols.

For the acquisition data, the SLI children in the verbal-only condition needed significantly more trials (M = 15) to reach criterion than the other SLI children and the NL children in both conditions (M = 5 trials). No significant differences were found on the transfer task. The analyses of the recall data found that SLI children in the verbal-only condition were less likely to include the key back-up proposition in their recall protocols.

3.5.1. Evaluation

The age-level performance of the SLI children in the 'modeling' condition can be taken as evidence that analogical reasoning abilities are intact in SLI children. The difficulty they have learning language thus is not likely due to deficient analogical reasoning skills. However, the way in which the problems were presented had a significant impact on SLI children's problem solving abilities. SLI children's problem solving abilities decreased considerably when the story analogs were verbally presented without accompanying physical demonstrations. Although the findings are consistent with the notion that SLI children suffer from a verbal processing deficit, the perceptual studies reviewed earlier suggest that it was not the nature of the input (verbal or nonverbal) that determined performance, but the extent to which the input placed demands on SLI children's processing system (Stark/Tallal 1988). Input that occurs rapidly in time, such as speech, places particularly high demands on processing resources, resulting in a decrease in the quality of memory codes and the likelihood that these memory codes will decay rapidly over time. Of significance here is that SLI children will be at a disadvantage whenever a problem-solving task is presented verbally without accompanying visual support or when a time factor is involved.

4. The Search for Causal Factors: Conclusions and Future Directions

Reading or writing a review of SLI children's perceptual and cognitive strengths and weaknesses is bound to leave one feeling somewhat unsatisfied. This is because no single factor (perceptual or cognitive) or obvious combination of factors can explain the extent and nature of a specific language impairment. Failure to find the primary causal factor(s) has led some researchers and clinicians to question the value of continued research and clinical efforts that address causal issues.

Leonard (1987) has made the most compelling arguments to-date about the inadequacy of causal research. In the final section of his critical review of causal research, he noted that "accounts of specific language impairment fall short not only because they fail to identify the proper cause of this condition, but also because they assume that the condition is one for which a tangible cause must exist" (Leonard 1987, 30). At one level, all of the studies reviewed in this chapter have attempted to identify a contributing factor or possible cause of specific language impairment. Although some factors seem to have more explanatory adequacy than others, no factor by itself can explain the extent and nature of SLI children's language impairment. This leads most writers to speculate that SLI is caused by a variety of factors.

Leonard, however, views the cause of SLI children's language limitations as "simply the product of the same types of variations in genetic and environmental factors that lead some children to be clumsy, others to be amusical, and still others to have little insight into their own feelings" (Leonard 1987, 31). Leonard's view draws on Gardner's (1983) theory of multiple intelligences in which seven different kinds of intelligence are proposed. If the language delay is viewed as normal variation rather than a disorder or deficit, one effectively eliminates the need to search for a cause. In other words, there can be no cause for the disorder if there is no disorder. This view leads Leonard to the logical conclusion that research efforts in search of causal factors will not be high-yield enterprises.

There is a certain appeal to Leonard's view: By embracing it, we prevent future researchers from expending large amounts of time and resources searching for underlying causes that do not exist. There is, however, a more optimistic view of the causally-oriented research reviewed in this chapter. Johnston (1991), for example, points out that the claim that most SLI children are normal is not the same as the claim that the condition has no cause. Just because there is normal variation in an ability does not mean the cause of the variation is of no interest. Some researchers are presumably interested in the neurological correlates of exceptional musical ability. The same holds true for language variation. As Johnston notes, even if we agree with Leonard that the primary cause of specific language impairment is variations in genetic and environmental factors, we can still wonder about the causes of these variations. Why do these children have difficulty learning to talk?

Aram (1991) proposes four reasons why it is important to know about why SLI children have difficulty learning language. First, there is the level of science to which we want our profession to aspire. Without explanatory power, she argues, ours is a dead-end science, with the risk that we might become a dead-end profession. Second, there is our clinical responsibility to parents of SLI children. Most parents want to know why their child has a language impairment. Aram asks, "How long can a profession continue to say *We don't know* to the questions that prompt their consultation?" (Aram 1991, 86).

Aram's third reason is that the identification of causal factors has major implications for intervention programs. Finally, there is the issue of prevention. Aram argues that only through understanding 'why' can we have an impact on preventing specific language impairments. If we act as if causation does not matter, is unknowable, or is simply the inevitable result of a normal distribution, we will be unable to prevent future generations of children from having specific language impairments.

Aram concludes her short paper by noting that we do know something about the causes of specific language impairment. Johnston (1991) makes a similar point in arguing that we should abandon 'etiological' jargon because it has connotations of pathology and primary cause, and attempt to identify the mental processes and mechanisms that influence success in the language acquisition task. If the research on SLI children's perceptual and cognitive abilities is viewed in this light, we can reason that language learning requires (a) the ability to perceive and produce rapidly presented information, (b) the ability to generate, maintain, and interpret symbols, (c) the ability to organize information hierarchically, and (d) a variety of reasoning processes.

Although these claims are by no means earth-shattering, they do represent progress. The weakness of the work, according to Johnston, is not in the direction it takes, but in its infancy. Johnston finds no fault with the general research strategy that (a) compares the performance of SLI and NL children on various linguistic and nonlinguistic tasks, and (b) makes inferences about the mental abilities that are causally linked to language learning based on the patterns of performance found.

What all researchers seem to agree about, however, is that the basic research strategy needs to be refined. Aram (1991) sees particular promise in using sophisticated neuroimaging techniques, such as MRI and PET to determine whether there are subtle differences in brain morphology and/or activity in SLI children. Another promising avenue of research addresses the genetic bases of specific language impairment (e. g., Lewis/Ekelman/Aram 1989; Tomblin 1989).

Johnston (1991) suggests three refinements in future research efforts. First, we need to explore more complex patterns of association. Most research, she notes, has primarily tried to link language learning to another single mental ability, such as the symbolic function or perception of rapidly presented events. But simple causation models, as Hubbell (1981) has pointed out, do not adequately capture the complex biological and environmental interactions that underlie developments in language throughout the developmental period. Future studies need to examine the reciprocal causation effects that occur among maturing perceptual, cognitive, linguistic, and social abilities throughout the developmental period.

Second, we need to figure out how to formalize and operationalize promising mental constructs. For example, there should be other ways to measure hierarchical planning ability than using 3-dimensional mobiles. Or, as Johnston notes, there is currently no experimental task to evaluate the construct of 'extracting regularities', which has been suggested as a possible weakness in SLI children.

Johnston's third refinement is that we need to break down familiar constructs, such as language, into their component parts. Instead of looking for associations between generic notions such as language learning ability and other mental functions, we need to look for associations between discrete language subskills and nonverbal competencies. Leonard's cross-linguistic research discussed earlier is an example of the kind of research needed.

Another promising avenue of research is to compare SLI children's processing abilities to those of children with different developmental disabilities. For example, Ludlow/Cudahy/Bassich/Brown (1983) evaluated perceptual processing abilities in SLI children and children with attentional deficits who had no history of language learning problems. She found that the children with attentional deficits also had difficulty perceiving rapidly presented information, suggesting that poor auditory perception might cause language delays only when it is accompanied by other specific cognitive deficiencies.

Another example is research my colleagues and I have conducted with young school-age SLI children and reading disabled children without a history of language impairment (Kamhi/Catts 1986; Kamhi/Catts/Mauer et al. 1988). In these studies, we compared the performance of these two groups of children on measures of visual imagery, short-term memory, rapid naming, word repetition, and phonological awareness. Our objective in this research was to determine whether SLI and reading disabled children demonstrated similar processing limitations. The findings from these studies revealed more similarities between the children than we expected, suggesting that the spoken language problems in school-age SLI children cannot be explained by limitations in the processes underlying mental imagery, short-term memory, and phonological awareness tasks. If these process limitations were causally linked to the spoken language deficit, the reading disabled children should have had similar spoken language deficiencies.

It should be clear from the points made in this chapter that the causal underpinnings of spoken and written language disorders are far too complex to be sorted out by cross-sectional studies in which a particular perceptual or conceptual ability is evaluated. But these studies have served an important function in illuminating the kinds of perceptual and cognitive abilities associated with delayed rates of language learning. As our future research endeavors begin to reflect the refinements discussed in the previous paragraphs, we will develop a better understanding of how perceptual and cognitive abilities affect language learning throughout the developmental period.

5. References

Aram, D. (1991). Specific language impairment as a clinical category. *Language, Speech, and Hearing Services in Schools, 22,* 84–88.

Arthur, G. (1952). *The Arthur Adaptation of the Leiter International Scale.* Chicago: Stoelting.

Bates, E., Benigni, L., Bretherton, I., Camaioni, L., & Volterra, V. (1979). *The emergence of symbols.* New York: Academic Press.

Bernstein, L. & Stark, R. (1985). Speech perception development in language-impaired children: A 4-year follow-up study. *Journal of Speech and Hearing Disorders, 50,* 21–30.

Bloomfield, L. (1933/1961). *Language.* New York: Henry Holt.

Bohannon, J. & Warren-Leubecker, A. (1988). Theoretical approaches to language acquisition. In J. Berko Gleason (Ed.), *The development of language* (2nd ed.). *167–225.* Colombus, OH: Merrill.

Brown, A. (1989). Analogical learning and transfer: What develops? In S. Vosniadou & A. Ortony (Eds.), *Similarity and analogical reasoning. 368–412.* Cambridge, England: Cambridge University Press.

Burgemeister, B., Blum, L., & Lorge, I. (1972). *Columbia Mental Maturity Scale* (3rd ed.). New York: Harcourt Brace Jovanovich.

Chi, M. (1976). Short-term memory limitations in children: Capacity or processing deficits? *Memory and Cognition, 4,* 559–572.

Cromer, R. (1981). Reconceptualizing language acquisition and cognitive development. In R. Schiefelbusch & D. Bricker (Eds.), *Early language: Acquisition and intervention. 51–138.* Baltimore: University Park Press.

Cromer, R. (1983). Hierarchical planning disability in the drawings and constructions of a special group of severely aphasic children. *Brain and Cognition, 2,* 144–164.

Curtiss, S. & Tallal, P. (1991). On the nature of the impairment in language impaired children. In J. Miller (Ed.), *Research on child language disorders: A decade of progress. 189–211.* Austin, TX: Pro-Ed.

Curtiss, S. & Yamada, J. (1988). *The Curtiss-Yamada Comprehensive Language Evaluation* (CY-CLE).

de Ajuriaguerra, J., Jaeggi, A., Guignard, F., Kocher, F., Manquard, M., Roth, S., & Schmid, E. (1976). The development and prognosis of dysphasia in children. In D. Morehead & Morehead (Eds.), *Normal and deficient child language. 345–385.* Baltimore: University Park.

DiSimoni, F. (1978). *The Token Test for Children.* Boston: Teaching Resources Corporation.

Dunn, L. & Dunn, L. (1981). *Peabody Picture Vocabulary Test-Revised.* Circle Pines, MN: American Guidance Service.

Eisenson, J. (1966). Perceptual disturbances in children with central nervous system dysfunction and implications for language development. *British Journal of Disorders of Communication, 1,* 21–32.

Elliott, L. & Hammer, M. (1988). Longitudinal changes in auditory discrimination in normal children and children with language learning problems. *Journal of Speech and Hearing Disorders, 53,* 467–474.

Elliott, L., Hammer, M., & Scholl, M. E. (1990). Response to Tallal. *Journal of Speech and Hearing Research, 33,* 617–618.

Ellis Weismer, S. (1991). Hypothesis testing abilities of language impaired children. *Journal of Speech and Hearing Research, 34,* 1329–1338.

Gardner, H. (1983). *Frames of mind.* New York: Basic Books.

Gholson, B., Eymard, L., Morgan, D., & Kamhi, A. (1987). Problem solving, recall, and isomorphic transfer among third-grade and sixth-grade children. *Journal of Experimental Child Psychology. 43,* 227–243.

Greenfield, P. & Schneider, L. (1977). Building a tree structure: The development of hierarchical complexity and interrupted strategies in children's construction activity. *Developmental Psychology, 13,* 299–313.

Holyoak, K., Junn, E., & Billmann, D. (1984). Development of analogical problem-solving skill. *Child Development, 55,* 2042–2055.

Hoskins, B. (1979). *A study of hypothesis testing behavior in language disordered children.* Paper presented at the Annual Convention of the American Speech-Language-Hearing Association, Atlanta.

Hubbell, R. (1981). *Children's language disorders.* Englewood Cliffs, NJ: Prentice-Hall.

Huttenlocher, J. & Burke, D. (1976). Why does memory span increase with age? *Cognitive Psychology, 8,* 1–32.

Ingram, D. (1989). *First language acquisition: Method, description and explanation.* Cambridge: Cambridge University Press.

Inhelder, B. (1966). Cognitive development and its contribution to the diagnosis of some phenomena of mental deficiency. *Merrill-Palmer Quarterly, 12,* 299–319.

Johnston, J. (1988). Specific language disorders in the child. In N. Lass, L. McReynolds, J. Northern, & D. Yoder (Eds.), *Handbook of speech-language pathology and audiology. 685–715.* Philadelphia: B. C. Decker, Inc.

Johnston, J. (1991). The continuing relevance of cause: A reply to Leonard's 'specific language, impairment as a clinical category'. *Language, Speech, and Hearing Services in Schools, 22,* 75–80.

Johnston, J. & Ellis Weismer, S. (1983). Mental rotation abilities in language disordered children. *Journal Speech and Hearing Research, 26,* 397–403.

Johnston, J. & Kamhi, A. (1984). Syntactic and semantic aspects of the utterances of language-impaired children: The same can be less. *Merrill-Palmer Quarterly, 30,* 65–85.

Johnston, J. & Schery, T. (1976). The use of grammatical morphemes by children with communication disorders. In D. Morehead & A. Morehead (Eds.), *Normal and deficient child language. 239–259.* Baltimore: University Park Press.

Kamhi, A. (1981). Nonlinguistic symbolic and conceptual abilities of language impaired and normally developing children. *Journal of Speech and Hearing Research, 24,* 446–453.

Kamhi, A. & Catts, H. (1986). Toward an understanding of developmental language and reading disorders. *Journal of Speech and Hearing Disorders, 51,* 337–347.

Kamhi, A., Catts, H., Mauer, D., Apel, K., & Gentry, B. (1988). Phonological and spatial processing abilities in language- and reading-impaired children. *Journal of Speech and Hearing Disorders, 53,* 316–327.

Kamhi, A., Gentry, B., Mauer, D., & Gholson, B. (1990). Analogical learning and transfer in language-impaired children. *Journal of Speech and Hearing Disorders, 55,* 140–148.

Kamhi, A., Nelson, L., Lee, R., & Gholson, B. (1985). The ability of language disordered children to use and modify hypotheses in discrimination learning. *Applied Psycholinguistics, 6,* 435–451.

Kracke, I. (1975). Perception of rhythmic sequences by receptive aphasic and deaf children. *British Journal of Disordered Communication, 10,* 43–51.

Leonard, L. (1987). Is specific language impairment a useful construct? In S. Rosenberg (Ed.), *Advances in applied psycholinguistics, Volume I: Disorders of first-language development. 1–39.* NY: Cambridge University Press.

Leonard, L. (1989). Language learnability and specific language impairment in children. *Applied Psycholinguistics, 10,* 179–202.

Lewis, B., Ekelman, B., & Aram, D. (1989). A familial study of severe phonological disorders. *Journal of Speech and Hearing Research, 32,* 713–724.

Lovell, K., Hoyle, H., & Siddall, M. (1968). A study of some aspects of the play and language of young children with delayed speech. *Journal of Child Psychology, Psychiatry, and Allied Disciplines, 9,* 41–50.

Lowe, A. & Campbell, R. (1965). Temporal discrimination in aphasoid and normal children. *Journal of Experimental Child Psychology, 18,* 201–212.

Lowe, M. & Costello, A. (1976). *Manual for Symbolic Play Test.* London: National Foundation of Educational Research.

Ludlow, C., Cudahy, E., Bassich, C., & Brown, G. (1983). The auditory processing skills of hyperactive, language impaired and reading disabled boys.

In J. Katz & E. Lasky (Eds.), *Central auditory processing disorders: Problems of speech, language, and learning. 163–185.* Baltimore: University Park Press.

Lunzer, E. (1959). Intellectual development in play of young children. *Educational Review, 11,* 205–224.

MacWhinney, B. (1978). The acquisition of morphophonology. *Monographs of the Society for Research in Child Development, 43,* (No. 1).

Morehead, D. & Ingram, D. (1973). The development of base syntax in normal and linguistically deviant children. *Journal of Speech and Hearing Research, 16,* 330–352.

Nelson, L., Kamhi, A., & Apel, K. (1987). Cognitive strengths and weaknesses in language impaired children: One more look. *Journal of Speech and Hearing Disorders, 52,* 36–43.

Nicolich, L. (1977). Beyond sensorimotor intelligence: Assessment of symbolic maturity through analysis of pretend play. *Merrill-Palmer Quarterly, 23,* 89–99.

Nippold, M., Erskine, B., & Freed, D. (1988). Proportional and analogical reasoning in normal and language-impaired children. *Journal of Speech and Hearing Disorders, 53,* 440–449.

Piaget, J. (1952). *The origins of intelligence of children,* trans. M. Cook. NY: International Universities Press.

Pinker, S. (1984). *Language learnability and language development.* Cambridge, MA: Harvard University Press.

Pisoni, D. (1978). Speech perception. In W. Kates (Ed.), *Handbook of learning and cognitive processes* (Volume 6). *171–203.* Hillsdale, NJ: Erlbaum.

Rees, N. (1973). Auditory processing factors in language disorders: The view from Procrustes' bed. *Journal of Speech and Hearing Disorders, 38,* 304–315.

Rees, N. (1981). Saying more than we know: Is auditory processing disorder a meaningful concept? In R. Keith (Ed.), *Central auditory and language disorders in children. 94–120.* San Diego, CA: College Hill Press.

Roth, F. & Clark, D. (1987). Symbolic play and social participation abilities of language-impaired and normally-developing children. *Journal of Speech and Hearing Disorders, 52,* 17–29.

Savich, P. (1984). Anticipatory imagery in normal and language disabled children. *Journal of Speech and Hearing Research, 27,* 494–501.

Slobin, D. (1979). *Psycholinguistics* (2nd Ed.). Glenview, IL, Scott-Foresman.

Stark, B. & Tallal, P. (1988). *Language, speech, and reading disorders in children: Neurophysiological studies.* Austin, TX: Pro-Ed.

Sternberg, R. (1985). *Beyond IQ: A triarchic theory of human intelligence.* New York: Cambridge University Press.

Sternberg, R. & Nigro, G. (1980). Developmental patterns in the solution of verbal analogies. *Child Development, 51,* 27–38.

Tallal, P. (1976). Rapid auditory processing in normal and disordered language development. *Journal of Speech and Hearing Research, 19,* 561–579.

Tallal, P. (1988). Developmental language disorders. In J. Kavanagh & T. Truss, Jr. (Eds.), *Learning disabilities: Proceedings of the national conference. 181–272.* Parkton, MD: York Press.

Tallal, P. & Piercy, M. (1973 a). Defects of nonverbal auditory perception in children with developmental aphasia. *Nature, 241,* 468–469.

Tallal, P. & Piercy, M. (1973 b). Developmental aphasia: Impaired rate of non-verbal processing as a function of sensory modality. *Neuropsychologia, 11,* 389–98.

Tallal, P. & Stark, R. (1981). Speech acoustic-cue discrimination abilities of normally developing and language-impaired children. *Journal of the Acoustical Society of America, 69,* 568–574.

Tallal, P., Stark, R., & Curtiss, B. (1976). Relation between speech perception and speech production impairment in children with developmental dysphasia. *Brain and Language, 3,* 305–317.

Tallal, P., Stark, R., Kallman, C., & Mellits, D. (1980). Perceptual constancy for phonemic categories: A developmental study with normal and language impaired children. *Applied Psycholinguistics, 1,* 49–64.

Tallal, P., Stark, R., Kallman, C., & Mellits, D. (1981). A reexamination of some nonverbal perceptual abilities of language-impaired and normal children as a function of age and sensory modality. *Journal of Speech and Hearing Research, 24,* 351–357.

Templin, M. & Darley, F. (1969). *The Templin-Darley Tests of Articulation* (2nd edition). Iowa City, IA: Bureau of Educational Research and Services.

Terrell, B. & Schwartz, R. (1983). Object transformation: The linguistic aspect of symbolic play? *Proceedings of the Symposium on Research in Child Language Disorders, 4,* 127–136.

Terrell, B., Schwartz, R., Prelock, P., & Messick, C. (1984). Symbolic play in normal and language disordered children. *Journal of Speech and Hearing Research, 27,* 424–429.

Tomblin, J. (1984). Specific abilities approach: An evaluation and alternative method. In W. Perkins (Ed.), *Language handicaps in children. 27–41.* New York: Thieme-Stratton.

Tomblin, J. (1989). Familial concentration of developmental language impairment. *Journal of Speech and Hearing Disorders, 54,* 287–295.

Tomblin, J. (1990). *Language cognition and social characteristics of young adults with histories of developmental language disorder.* Paper presented at the Symposium for Research on Child Language Disorders, Madison, WI.

Tomblin, J. & Quinn, M. (1983). The contribution of perceptual learning to performance on a repetition task. *Journal of Speech and Hearing Research, 26,* 369–372.

Wickelgren, W. (1974). *How to solve problems.* San Francisco: Freeman.

Alan G. Kamhi, Memphis, Tennessee (USA)

63. Children with Specific Language Impairment (Developmental Dysphasia): Treatment

1. Introduction

Among the groups of children who exhibit language-learning difficulties is a group that shows normal hearing, normal motor and emotional functioning, and age-appropriate scores on nonverbal tests of intelligence. Currently, the most commonly used clinical term for this group (at least in the U.S.) is 'specific language impairment', though the term 'developmental dysphasia' is also employed. Although the former will be adopted here, the two terms are basically interchangeable.

In the decade since Leonard (1981) reviewed the available literature on language intervention with specifically-language-impaired (SLI) children, this area of work has received increasing attention. The purpose of this section is to provide a summary of these recent developments. To facilitate interpretation of the recent work, the section shall be organized as in the earlier review, with subsections added to highlight prominent changes. Although the studies reviewed here should prove to be representative of the work in this area, the relative emphasis placed on certain issues reflects the present author's own biases. For a review with a somewhat different look, the reader might consult Olswang/Bain (in press).

As in Leonard (1981), the focus shall be on language production (which still constitutes the bulk of the literature on treatment), excluding phonology. The studies included here provided documentation of oral language deficits in the children under investigation. Thus, investigations of learning disabled children, for example, were included only if it could be determined that problems in spoken language constituted part of their handicap. Finally, the review was restricted to studies in which gains coúld be attributed to treatment with some degree of confidence. Investigations of this type included: (1) the use of a no-treatment control group or a comparison group that received treatment unrelated to the linguistic features of interest; (2) the use of a single-subject design in which experimental control can be demonstrated, such as a multiple baseline or alternating treatments design; (3) the use of statistical estimation to evaluate observed gains relative to those expected from maturation; and (4) the use of a nonsense form whose acquisition could not be due to extra-experimental sources.

2. The Effectiveness of Language Treatment

As the authors of the other sections of this chapter have made clear, children with specific language impairment constitute a heterogeneous population. Even though all of these children display normal hearing, unremarkable emotional development, and age-appropriate scores on nonverbal intelligence tests, they differ from one another in the severity of their language deficit, and in the specific areas of language in which this deficit is most apparent. Unfortunately, a very large percentage of these children continue to have linguistic difficulties throughout childhood and beyond, and are at risk for academic difficulties. Clearly, language intervention is important for these children. However, it must be determined that such treatment is in fact effective.

If effectiveness is defined as a demonstrable gain in language performance, then clearly language intervention with SLI children is effective. A host of treatment approaches have produced gains of this type. These are discussed below.

2.1. Approaches to Treatment

Until the mid 1970s, the dominant treatment approach for SLI children was one that made significant use of elicited imitation. That is, the clinician produces the exact sentence or phrase required of the child, and the child is asked to repeat it. Although imitation-based approaches have consistently resulted in clear language gains by the children, such approaches have not been adopted as frequently in recent years. Olswang/Bain/Dunn/Cooper (1983) made use of elicited imitation to teach new lexical items to SLI children. Other investigators have incorporated imitation into comprehensive intervention programs that include a variety of techniques. For example, Warren/Kaiser (1986) successfully taught SLI children the use of two- and three-word utterances (e. g. *boy eat cake*) in a program that included picture pointing (e. g. "Show me *boy eat cake*"), performing the requested action (e. g. "Susan, eat cake"), imitating the target utterance (e. g. "Say *boy eat cake*"), describing pictures (e. g. "Tell me about this picture"), and describing the actions of others (e. g. "What's Jane doing?"). Though used less frequently, imitation-based approaches remain an effective alternative for clinicians.

A second type of approach involves the use of modeling. The child observes someone (the model) produce examples of utterances containing the linguistic form serving as the focus of training. The child is not asked to imitate the modeled utterances. However, he or she is instructed that the model will be talking in a special way. At this point, specific modeling approaches differ. In some approaches, the child observes only; in others, the child is asked to take turns producing examples of the target pattern once the observation period is over.

The majority of earlier studies that employed modeling showed clear gains in language production. More recent studies corroborate these findings. Examples of successful training through some variation of modeling have been reported by Bedrosian/Willis (1987), Johnston/Blatchley/Olness (1990), Skarakis-Doyle/Woodall (1988), and Weismer/Murray-Branch (1989), among others.

Another type of treatment approach is called 'incidental language teaching'. This approach resembles the above approaches in that the language targets used for training are preselected by the clinician. However, incidental language teaching is quite different in other respects. It is conducted in a more naturalistic setting, such as free play. The clinician arranges the setting to increase the likelihood that the child will initiate some form of communication. When the child indicates interest in the activity or object in question, the clinician shows attention and, as necessary, provides the child with increasingly specific cues for production of the target form. Natural contingencies are applied to the child's production of the target. For example, immediately following the child's successful production of the utterance *I want block*, the clinician gives the child the requested object.

Although numerous studies employing incidental language teaching can be found in the clinical literature, only a few have focused on SLI children. However, the results of these investigations leave no doubt that this approach can be effective with these children as well. Examples of studies reporting successful treatment with some variation of incidental language teaching include the works of Olswang/Kriegsmann/Mastergeorge (1982) and Warren/McQuarter/Rogers-Warren (1984).

Another approach that requires the child to be the initiator is expansion. This approach has its origins in the literature on normal language development, in which it was reported that mothers often responded to their young children's telegraphic utterances (e. g. *Abby daddy*) with a more complete and grammatical rendition (e. g. "yes, Abby is going with daddy"). Relatively few studies have employed the expansion approach with SLI children, and reported language gains have been minimal (Leonard 1981). However, an adaptation of expansion was found to be successful in an investigation by Schwartz/Chapman/Terrell et al. (1985). In this adaptation, the clinician, rather than the child initiated the communication. For example, in teaching one SLI child locative word combinations, the following interaction was representative:

Clinician:	*What's this?*
Child:	*block*
Clinician:	*What's the block in?*
Child:	*truck*
Clinician:	*The block is in the truck*

There are many treatment approaches that differ from one another in certain details but are similar in that they provide the child with concentrated exposure to particular linguistic forms. Leonard (1981) termed such approaches 'focused stimulation' approaches. Perhaps the most straightforward example can be seen in lexical training studies (e. g. Leonard/Schwartz/Chapman et al. 1982) in which the clinician introduces a new object during play and says its name several times per session.

In other types of focused stimulation approaches, the clinician tells the child a story that contains numerous examples of the target form (e. g. questions containing *why*), and the clinician and child then act out the story, each taking the role of one of the characters. Brooks/Benjamin (1989) found such a procedure to be quite effective in teaching specific grammatical forms. Other successful uses of focused stimulation can be found in the studies of Culatta/Horn (1982), Leonard/Schwartz/Allen et al. (1989), McGregor/Leonard (1989), Olswang/Bain/Rosendahl et al. (1986), Schwartz/Leonard/Messick/Chapman (1987), Schwartz (1988), and Wing (1990).

Many SLI children are enrolled in preschools or classrooms that emphasize language learning. Although special attention is sometimes placed on specific language features that are especially problematic for the child, the goals in settings such as these are usually much broader. Consequently, the language gains made in these settings are often assessed by means of comprehensive tests of language and related abilities. Programs of this type have been shown to be beneficial for SLI children (e. g. Rice/Sell/Hadley 1990, Ripley 1986).

2.2. Direct Comparisons of Treatment Approaches

Although several different approaches appear to be effective with SLI children, it is not clear that a single approach will emerge as the procedure of choice across all linguistic features. A meta-analysis conducted by Nye/Foster/Seaman (1987) seems to support this assumption. These investigators found a large mean effect size for treatment collapsed across type of approach. However, although the mean effect size for certain specific approaches seemed quite high (e. g. modeling), no one approach differed significantly from any other.

Nevertheless, it is reasonable to assume that certain approaches might be more effective than others in teaching specific language material. A number of studies of this type can be found in the literature. For example, Connell (1987) compared the effectiveness of an imitation-based approach and a modeling approach in teaching the use of an invented bound morpheme. Children were taught to add the form *-a* to nouns to express the notion "part of" (e. g. *cata* meant "part of a cat"). Connell found that the imitation-based approach was more successful with the SLI children. (Interestingly, the modeling approach was more effective with a group of normally-developing children). Other studies that have compared different approaches for teaching specific language targets include Hughes/Carpenter (1989), McGregor/Leonard (1989), Olswang/Coggins (1984), and Wing (1990).

Still another type of comparison pits one variation of a specific approach against another. For example, Weismer/Murray-Branch (1989) compared two types of modeling in teaching forms such as auxiliary *is* and *are*, and the nominative case pronoun *he*. In one version of modeling, no responses from the child were required during the observation period. In the other, the child was given intermittent opportunities to produce examples of the target form. Both procedures proved effective, but the variation that permitted active responding by the child resulted in a slightly more stable pattern of acquisition. Other studies that have compared variations of the same general approach include Olswang/Bain/Dunn/Cooper (1983) and Olswang/Bain/Rosendahl et al. (1986).

Just as one might expect certain approaches to be especially effective for teaching particular language targets, one might also assume that certain approaches would be especially well-suited for particular types of SLI children. In fact, earlier work suggested that imitation-based approaches might be the method of choice for SLI children of low ability. However, more recent work by Cole/Dale (1986) casts doubt on this interpretation. These investigators compared an imitation-based approach and a variation of incidental language teaching. Both approaches resulted in significant language gains, but neither proved superior for SLI children with lower (or higher) ability.

2.3. Generalization and Maintenance

Effective language treatment implies more than use of a linguistic feature in a narrowly-defined context. The child must also demonstrate the ability to use the feature in new ways. Most investigators do not regard treatment as successful unless, at a minimum, the child is able to use the feature in untrained sentences in a task that resembles the one(s) used during treatment. However, a number of researchers have made the requirement stiffer: The child must use the feature in new sentences during conversational speech. Most studies employing this type of generalization measure have reported positive results (e. g. Connell 1986 a, 1986 b; Olswang/Bain/Rosendahl et al. 1986; Warren/Kaiser 1986; Warren/McQuarter/Rogers-Warren 1984). The study by Hughes/Carpenter (1989) appears to be an exception.

Gains made during treatment do not mean very much if they are short-lived, so a number of investigators have made efforts to determine whether the higher levels of performance are maintained. The results are encouraging. For example, in three very different types of intervention studies, Dollaghan/Kaston (1986), McGregor/Leonard (1989), and Warren/McQuarter/Rogers-Warren (1984) all found that SLI children's performance one month after treatment remained higher than pre-treatment levels.

The issue of maintenance is a tricky one for researchers in the area of language treatment because once a language ability becomes relatively well-established, it eludes experimental control. For example, in a study by Hargrove/Holmberg/Zeigler (1986), the children serving as subjects appeared to maintain or even show an increase in the gains made during treatment two months earlier. However, when treatment resumed, followed by an additional maintenance phase, it became clear that the children's performance was no longer under experimental control. Periods of improvement and no improvement were not closely tied to whether treatment was being provided at the time. Given the seemingly permanent property of language behavior once it is established, researchers wishing to document that gains are attributable to treatment may only be able to do so early in the intervention process.

2.4. Catching Up or Not Losing Ground?

The fact that SLI children make gains in treatment that exceed those made without treatment does not necessarily mean than within a few months or years they will be on par with their normally-developing peers. Longitudinal and follow-up studies have demonstrated not only that linguistic features emerge at a later age in the speech of SLI children, but the period from emerge to mastery of these features is also protracted. Consequently, without treatment, these children fall even further behind their peers across time. Thus, treatment may actually permit SLI children to catch up, or it may have the more modest effect of allowing the children to begin to progress at a normal rate, so as not to fall further behind over time.

Of these two possibilities, the truth seems to fall somewhere in between. On the one hand, studies that make use of standardized tests to assess progress frequently report gains in standard scores and language quotients that are closer to the norm than before treatment began. Such large post-test gains do not appear attributable to a regression toward the mean because they are seen for tests on which the SLI children's pre-test scores approached or were at the norm, as well as for tests on which the children performed very poorly. Examples of SLI children closing the gap can be seen in the work of Cole/Dale (1986), Rice/Sell/Hadley (1990), and Warren/Kaiser (1986).

The acceleration of SLI children's learning through treatment notwithstanding, it appears that many children never reach a level of language ability that can be regarded as socially or educationally adequate. Two recent studies illustrate this point. Ripley (1986) reported on 120 children attending a school for SLI children; 90 of these children exhibited problems that extended beyond phonology. Many of these children had attended the school since the age of 7 or 8 years. The children showed very clear gains in verbal IQ scores, with typical increases in the order of 15 to 30 points. However, almost half of these children remained at this special school until the statutory school-leaving age, and the average verbal IQ for the 90 children at exit remained at least one standard deviation below the norm.

The second relevant study was conducted by Huntley/Holt/Butterfill/Latham (1988). These researchers examined the abilities of children five years after they had completed a two-year period of language treatment. A small decrease in the children's verbal IQs was noted following the termination of treatment, but these scores were nevertheless higher than those seen prior to intervention. However, approximately 40% of the children did not yet qualify for normal school placement, or were briefly in a regular school setting but did not succeed. A very real concern for clinicians is to ensure that the gains made by SLI children in treatment include improvement in aspects of language that are important for later functioning (see Damico 1988).

3. The Focus of Treatment

The last decade has witnessed a significant increase in both the diversity of linguistic features serving as the focus of treatment and in the sophistication with which some of these features have been taught. The former is important because it provides clinicians with a more varied database for serving the heterogeneous population of SLI children. The latter is important because it increases the likelihood that treatment will be directed toward features that play a pivotal role in the child's language problem rather than on features that are secondary consequences of this problem. Each of these will be discussed below.

3.1. Features of Language

Through the 1970s, the great majority of treatment studies dealt with syntax and morphology. These types of features continue to receive attention in the literature, and for good reason: They are perhaps the most vulnerable in the speech of SLI children. Some of the recent studies with this focus include Brooks/Benjamin (1989), Culatta/Horn (1982), Hughes/Carpenter (1989), Thal/Goldenberg (1981), and Weismer/Murray-Branch (1989).

Yet, the difficulties that SLI children often face in other areas of language warranted treatment research that went beyond the formal aspects of grammar. During the 1980s, work appeared that emphasized the semantic roles served by word combinations (Connell 1986 a; Olswang/Coggins 1984; Schwartz/Chapman/Terrell et al. 1985). However, the most striking developments have occurred in the area of the lexicon (words and their meanings) and in pragmatics (the social use of language).

Treatment studies focusing on SLI children's learning of new lexical items can be divided into two types. The first type is concerned with the goal of increasing the size of the child's lexicon. Emphasis is placed on establishing an association between the word and its referent, and progress is measured by examining the child's ability to produce the word when an appropriate referent is presented. Intervention of this kind has resulted in significant lexical learning on the part of SLI children, as can be seen from the work of Leonard/Schwartz/Allen et al. (1989), Leonard/Schwartz/Chapman et al. (1982), Olswang/Bain/Dunn/Cooper (1983), Olswang/Bain/Rosendahl et al. (1986), Schwartz (1988), and Schwartz/Leonard/Messick/Chapman (1987). The second type of lexical treatment is designed to facilitate SLI children's 'word-finding' ability, that is, their ability to recall and produce presumably-known words when needed. This type of treatment is concerned with increasing the children's knowledge of individual words beyond simple word-referent associations (e. g. pointing out a word's superordinate category), and with providing the child with strategies for retrieving words from memory. The recent investigations of McGregor/Leonard (1989) and Wing (1990) serve as good examples.

The burgeoning literature on teaching pragmatic skills has been no less noteworthy. The communicative behaviors that have been taught to SLI children include: (1) topic initiations referring to past and future events (Bedrosian/Willis 1987); (2) requests for objects and actions (Olswang/Kriegsmann/Mastergeorge 1982); (3) requests for additional information (Dollaghan/Kaston 1986); and (4) the use of language for purposes of pretending (Skarakis-Doyle/Woodall 1988).

3.2. Understanding the Interrelationships

Although it has always been recognized that language is an intricate system of interrelationships, clinicians working with SLI children have too often had to settle for one of two extremes – either working with single features of language in isolation, or working with a wide range of features without being clear as to how these features are connected. There are some recent signs that this picture is changing. For example, Connell (1986 b) recognized that errors such as *them* for *they* in preverb position (e. g. **them like Brenda*) may be related to the omission of auxiliary verbs and verb inflections. Specifically, he hypothesized that SLI children showing such errors had not acquired the notion of subjecthood, which requires preverb pronouns of nominative case and verb markers that agree with the preverb noun phrase in number and person. Consequently, he taught pronoun case and certain verb features as a package, and found rather sweeping changes in the children's use of other verb features presumably linked to subjecthood.

Another type of study that sheds new light on the interactions within language is exemplified by the work of Johnston/Blatchley/Olness (1990). These investigators taught two miniature languages to SLI and normally-developing children. The unfamiliar nouns in the language referred to fantasy animals that played either an agent or patient role. Unfamiliar verbs were used to refer to the actions that the agent performed on the patient. In addition, a novel suffix was attached to the noun serving as the patient. One of the languages possessed the word order agent + patient + suffix + action, the other action + agent + patient + suffix. The investigators found that the SLI children had a tendency to direct most of their limited resources toward one characteristic of the language (e. g. the perceptually salient suffix that appeared at the end of the sentence in one of the languages) at the expense of another characteristic (word order). Studies of this type can provide valuable information concerning how language material might be organized to promote efficient learning by SLI children.

4. Summary

Significant progress has been made in language treatment with SLI children. Although it is unlikely that the heterogeneity of this population will ever permit the determination of a single treatment procedure and set of goals to prescribe, it is equally clear that a variety of teaching approaches are effective, for a range of language skills. Gains made during treatment are usually generalized and maintained, and often result in a narrower language ability gap between SLI children and their normally-developing peers. Unfortunately, the long-term language deficiencies seen in some of these children even with treatment make it obvious that much work remains to be done.

5. References

Bedrosian, J. & Willis, T. (1987). Effects of treatment on the topic performance of a school-age child. *Language, Speech, and Hearing Services in Schools, 18,* 158–167.

Brooks, A. & Benjamin, B. (1989). The use of structured role play therapy in the remediation of grammatical deficits in language delayed children: Three case studies. *Journal of Childhood Communication Disorders, 12,* 171–186.

Cole, K. & Dale, P. (1986). Direct language instruction and interactive language instruction with language delayed preschool children: A comparison study. *Journal of Speech and Hearing Research, 29,* 209–217.

Connell, P. (1986 a). Acquisition of semantic role by language-disordered children: Differences between production and comprehension. *Journal of Speech and Hearing Research, 29,* 366–374.

Connell, P. (1986 b). Teaching subjecthood to language-disordered children. *Journal of Speech and Hearing Research, 29,* 481–492.

Connell, P. (1987). An effect of modeling and imitation teaching procedures on children with and without specific language impairment. *Journal of Speech and Hearing Research, 30,* 105–113.

Culatta, B. & Horn, D. (1982). A program for achieving generalization rules to spontaneous discourse. *Journal of Speech and Hearing Disorders, 47,* 174–180.

Damico, J. (1988). The lack of efficacy in language therapy: A case study. *Language, Speech, and Hearing Services in Schools, 19,* 51–66.

Dollaghan, C. & Kaston, N. (1986). A comprehension monitoring program for language-impaired children. *Journal of Speech and Hearing Disorders, 51,* 264–271.

Hargrove, P., Holmberg, C., & Zeigler, M. (1986). Changes in spontaneous speech associated with therapy hiatus: A retrospective study. *Child Language Teaching and Therapy, 2,* 266–280.

Hughes, D. & Carpenter, R. (1989). Short-term syntax learning and generalization effects. *Child Language Teaching and Therapy, 5,* 202–220.

Huntley, R., Holt, K., Butterfill, A., & Latham, C. (1988). A follow-up study of a language intervention programme. *British Journal of Disorders of Communication, 23,* 127–140.

Johnston, J., Blatchley, M., & Olness, G. (1990). Miniature language system acquisition by children with different learning proficiencies. *Journal of Speech and Hearing Research, 33,* 335–342.

Leonard, L. (1981). Facilitating linguistic skills in children with specific language impairment. *Applied Psycholinguistics, 2,* 89–118.

Leonard, L., Schwartz, R., Allen, G., Swanson, L., & Loeb, D. (1989). Unusual phonological behavior and the avoidance of homonymy in children. *Journal of Speech and Hearing Research, 32,* 583–590.

Leonard, L., Schwartz, R., Chapman, K., Rowan, L., Prelock, P., Terrell, B., Weiss, A., & Messick, C. (1982). Early lexical acquisition in children with specific language impairment. *Journal of Speech and Hearing Research, 25,* 554–564.

McGregor, K. & Leonard, L. (1989). Facilitating word-finding skills of language-impaired children. *Journal of Speech and Hearing Disorders, 54,* 141–147.

Nye, C., Foster, S., & Seaman, D. (1987). Effectiveness of language intervention with the language/learning disabled. *Journal of Speech and Hearing Disorders, 52,* 348–357.

Olswang, L. & Bain, B. (in press). Language intervention research applied to clinical decision-making. In P. Tallal (Ed.), *The neural basis of developmental language disorders.* Oxford: Oxford University Press.

Olswang, L., Bain, B., Dunn, C., & Cooper, J. (1983). The effects of stimulus variation on lexical learning. *Journal of Speech and Hearing Disorders, 48,* 192–201.

Olswang, L., Bain, B., Rosendahl, P., Oblak, S., & Smith, A. (1986). Language learning: Moving performance from a context-dependent to -independent state. *Child Language Teaching and Therapy, 2,* 180–210.

Olswang, L. & Coggins, T. (1984). The effects of adult behavior on increasing language delayed children's production of early relational meanings. *British Journal of Disorders of Communication, 19,* 15–34.

Olswang, L., Kriegsmann, E., & Mastergeorge, A. (1982). Facilitating functional requesting in pragmatically impaired children. *Language, Speech, and Hearing Services in Schools, 13,* 202–222.

Rice, M., Sell, M., & Hadley, P. (1990). The social interactive coding system (SICS): An on-line, clinically relevant descriptive tool. *Language, Speech and Hearing Services in Schools, 21,* 2–14.

Ripley, K. (1986). The Moor House School remedial programme: An evaluation. *Child Language Teaching and Therapy, 2,* 281–300.

Schwartz, R. (1988). Early action word acquisition in normal and language-impaired children. *Applied Psycholinguistics, 9,* 111–122.

Schwartz, R., Chapman, K., Terrell, B., Prelock, P., & Rowan, L. (1985). Facilitating word combination in language-impaired children through discourse structure. *Journal of Speech and Hearing Disorders, 50,* 31–39.

Schwartz, R., Leonard, L., Messick, C., & Chapman, K. (1987). The acquisition of object names in children with specific language impairment: Action context and word extension. *Applied Psycholinguistics, 8,* 233–244.

Skarakis-Doyle, E. & Woodall, S. (1988). The effects of modeling upon the verbal elaboration of a language disordered child's pretend play. *Human Communication, 12,* 29–35.

Thal, D. & Goldenberg, T. (1981). Programming diversity of response: A method for teaching flexibility of language use. *Journal of Childhood Communication Disorders, 5,* 54–65.

Warren, S. & Kaiser, A. (1986). Generalization of treatment effects by young language-delayed children: A longitudinal analysis. *Journal of Speech and Hearing Disorders, 51,* 239–251.

Warren, S., McQuarter, R., & Rogers-Warren, A. (1984). The effects of mands and models on the speech of unresponsive language-delayed preschool children. *Journal of Speech and Hearing Disorders, 49,* 43–52.

Weismer, S. & Murray-Branch, J. (1989). Modeling versus modeling plus evoked production training: A comparison of two language intervention methods. *Journal of Speech and Hearing Disorders, 54,* 269–281.

Wing, C. (1990). A preliminary investigation of generalization to untrained words following two treatments of children's word-finding problems. *Language, Speech, and Hearing Services in Schools, 21,* 151–156.

Laurence B. Leonard, West Lafayette, Indiana (USA)

64. Acquired Aphasia in Children

Childhood language disorders have generally been classified into two types (Freud 1897/1968; Ludlow 1980). One type occurs prior to the emergence of language and has been termed developmental or congenital language disorder. Developmental language disorders may be labeled as being primary, when no other sensory or cognitive impairment is present to account for the dysfunction, or secondary, when it can be attributed to another dysfunction such as mental retardation or a hearing loss. Developmental language disorders presumably result from nervous system dysfunction (see Ludlow 1980; Swisher 1985), although the specific nature of the nervous system impairment may not always be known. The other type of childhood language disorder occurs after normal language acquisition has commenced, and has been termed acquired childhood aphasia, or simply childhood aphasia, and is the focus of this review.

1. Incidence of Childhood Aphasia

The first reports on childhood aphasia (Bernhardt 1885; Clarus 1874; Cotard 1868; Freud 1897/1968) appeared shortly after the classic studies of adult aphasia by Broca (1861) and Wernicke (1874). Despite the early interest in childhood aphasia, there has been much less interest in childhood aphasia over the years since these first reports. One explanation often given for the relative lack of research on childhood aphasia is that it is considered to be a 'rare' disorder. This explanation, though, needs clarification as to whether neural dysfunction that will produce an aphasia in an adult is rare in children, or, given a dysfunction that would produce an aphasia in an adult, aphasia rarely occurs. With regard to the former issue, it is certainly true that lesions frequently producing aphasia in adults such as unilateral cerebrovascular disorders are much less frequent in children. Unilateral lesions do occur, though, and the later issue is of much greater theoretical interest. Cotard (1868), a student of Charcot, was, perhaps, the first to question whether acquired childhood aphasia even existed. He claimed that children with hemiplegia, whichever the side of the lesion, never presented with aphasia, even when the entire left hemisphere was atrophied. This view was soon challenged, however, by Bernhardt (1885), who maintained that aphasia was not rare in children, and that it was a frequent symptom of infantile hemiplegia, even though he considered it to be a transient symptom.

In order to investigate the rarity of aphasia given a unilateral lesion, Satz/Bullard-Bates (1981) reviewed the childhood aphasia literature. They selected studies for inclusion in their evaluation based on the following criteria: a) speech was present before the onset of the lesion; b) hand preference was known before lesion onset; c) patients were under the age of 16 at the time of lesion; d) there was evidence that the lesion was unilateral; and e) the presence or absence of aphasia had been assessed after the injury. Of 21 studies, including 929 cases, only five studies met their criteria, including 68 cases (35 of which were right-handed and suffered left hemisphere lesions). Comparing the frequency of aphasia in right-handed children and adults following unilateral left hemisphere lesions, Satz/Bullard-Bates found that the percentage of children suffering from aphasia was actually greater than the percentage of adults suffering from aphasia. Table 64.1 shows a comparison between incidence for childhood aphasia, based on cases of childhood aphasia from Carter/Hohenegger/Satz (1982) and Hecaen (1983), and adult aphasia, from the review by Satz/Bullard-Bates (1981). It seems from these data safe to conclude, then, that children are not less susceptible to aphasia given a unilateral lesion. The rarity of aphasia in children must, therefore, refer to the less frequent nature of unilateral lesions, not less of a likelihood of aphasia following lesions that tend to produce aphasia in adults.

Children	*# of cases*	*# of Aphasics*	%
Left Hemisphere Lesion	114	85	75
Right Hemisphere Lesion	78	11	14
Adults	*# of cases*	*# of Aphasics*	%
Left Hemisphere Lesion	708	414	58
Right Hemisphere Lesion	648	20	3

Table 64.1: Incidence of Aphasia after Unilateral Lesions in Right-Handers

Adapted from Cater/Hohenegger/Satz (1982), Satz/Bullard-Bates (1981), and Hecaen (1983).

2. Ontogeny of Hemispheric Dominance

The incidence of childhood aphasia following unilateral lesions has been of great use in evaluating developmental models of speech dominance. One such prominent model has been advanced by Lenneberg (1967) and has been labeled the equipotentiality hypothesis.

> "Apparently, there is a period in infancy in which the hemispheres are still equipotential ... during the first two years of life cerebral dominance is not yet well established ... At the beginning of language development both hemispheres seem to be equally involved: the dominance phenomenon seems to come about through a pro-

> gressive decrease in involvement of the right hemisphere" (Lenneberg 1967, 151).

Lenneberg, therefore, believed that prior to the first two years of life, cerebral dominance is not well established and that both hemispheres equally participate in language. As the child gets older, according to Lenneberg, dominance is established as the right hemisphere becomes decreasingly involved in language. Much of the development of cerebral dominance was proposed to occur between the ages of two and five, but, he contends, continues to progress until puberty. The concept that the right hemisphere becomes less involved in language with age, resulting in an increase in language asymmetry, has been termed the progressive lateralization hypothesis. Although progressive lateralization is usually attributed to Lenneberg, the idea can be traced to Marie (1922):

> "The inborn centers which we know (and they are not numerous) are always bilateral and very clearly symmetrical. The motor centers of the limbs, the centers of vision, have their locations in each of the two hemispheres in symmetrical regions ... How can we admit the existence of an inborn center for speech which would be neither bilateral nor symmetrical?" (180; cited in translation by Dennis/Whitaker 1977, 93). "Far from processing a center of speech at birth, each individual must, by his own effort, create one; and it is in the left parietotemporal zone that this occurs. Why? Perhaps simply because the nerve elements of the left hemisphere develop a little before those of the right hemisphere" (181; cited in translation by Dennis/Whitaker 1977, 94).

According to Lenneberg's view, then, one would expect the frequency of aphasia to occur equally often after left and right hemisphere lesions occurring prior to age two, resulting in a greater frequency of aphasia following right hemisphere lesions in children than adults.

Since Lenneberg (1967) hypothesized that prior to age 2 the two cerebral hemispheres are equally involved in speech, we would expect that the frequency of aphasia would be equivalent after unilateral left and right hemisphere lesions that occur prior to age two. Penfield/Roberts (1959) reported on the frequency of aphasic symptoms in patients who had cortical excisions for the treatment of epilepsy before and after age two. We can see from Table 64.2 that the frequency of aphasia following left hemisphere excisions in children less than two years of age is much greater than following right hemisphere excisions. Ten of the 22 right-handers with left hemisphere excisions showed signs of aphasia whereas none of the 58 patients with right hemisphere excisions showed signs of aphasia. The Penfield and Roberts study, therefore, does not support one of the predictions following from Lenneberg's model.

	Early (< age 2)		
	# of cases	*# of Aphasics*	%
Left Hemisphere	22	10	46
Right Hemisphere	58	0	0
	Late (> age 2)		
	# of cases	*# of Aphasics*	%
Left Hemisphere	157	115	73
Right Hemisphere	196	1	0.5

Table 64.2: Aphasia Onset After Unilateral Lobectomy

Adapted from Penfield/Roberts (1959)

Since Lenneberg also hypothesized that the right hemisphere plays a decreasing role in language from ages two through puberty, we would expect that the frequency of "crossed aphasia", i. e. aphasia resulting from right hemisphere lesions in right-handers, would decrease with age. The incidence of crossed aphasia in studies typically ranges between .4% (Hecaen 1976) and 4% (Rasmussen/Milner 1977) in adults, whereas for children estimates range between 7% (Woods/Teuber 1978) and 47% (Basser 1962). The greater reported incidence of crossed aphasia in children compared to adults has been taken as evidence for maturation hypotheses of cerebral lateralization; the view that, initially, both hemispheres are involved in language but that the left hemisphere becomes more dominant for language with age. A more critical examination of the literature, however, raises serious questions with regard to the crossed aphasia data in children. For example, the Basser study, which reported the greatest percentage of crossed aphasia in the literature, has been seriously questioned because of the inclusion of subjects with evidence of bilateral lesions (see Woods/Carey 1979).

In a critical review of childhood aphasia studies, using criteria similar to those found in the Satz/Bullard-Bates report, Carter/Hohenegger/Satz (1982) did not find an increased incidence of crossed aphasia in children compared to adults. Similarly, Hecaen (1983), after adding 30 new cases of unilateral lesions in children to a previous sample (Hecaen 1976), also did not find a significantly greater frequency of crossed aphasia in children. Using the data presented in Table 64.1 we can estimate the frequency of crossed aphasia in children to be about 14%. However, this figure includes the cases in the Basser (1962) study, which was criticized for including cases with evidence of bilateral damage. When the cases from the Basser study are excluded, the frequency of crossed aphasia is only 8%, but this figure is still outside the range typically reported for adult aphasia. Carter/Hohenegger/Satz, however, argued that many cases in the childhood aphasia literature are trauma victims, which may have sustained undetected bilateral damage, and, furthermore, that some of the subjects in the literature had not had their handedness adequately tested, which may further contaminate the data with misidentified left-handers. When Carter/Hohenegger/Satz excluded cases of trauma and insufficient testing of handedness, they estimated the frequency of crossed aphasia in children to be zero (although this estimate is based on only four cases of right hemisphere lesions). The Penfield/Roberts (1959) unilateral lobectomy data (see Table 64.2) also do not show any evidence that the frequency of crossed aphasia declines with age.

The incidence data, therefore, do not provide much support for Lenneberg's equipotentiality hypothesis. It is interesting to note in this context that Lenneberg's usage of 'equipotentiality' differs in a very substantial way from the way it was originally used by Lashley (1921; see Satz/Strauss/Whitaker 1990 for a discussion of this issue). Lashley used the term to refer to the capacity of certain brain areas to mediate functions impaired by damage to other areas of the brain.

> "The term "equipotentiality" I have used to designate the apparent capacity of any intact part of a functional area to carry out, with or without reduction in efficiency, the functions which are lost by destruction of the whole. This capacity varies from one area to another and with the character of functions involved. It probably holds only for the association areas and for functions more complex than simple sensitivity or motor co-ordination" (1964, 25).

Notice, therefore, that in Lenneberg's usage, equipotentiality is used to refer to two or more area's equal contribution towards a function during normal development. In contrast, in the original usage by Lashley, the term refers to the potential for a brain area to contribute, with or without a reduction in proficiency, to a function previously involving a different brain area. Another critical distinction in the use of the term is that for Lenneberg, the activation would precede any lesion, whereas for Lashley, the activation would follow the lesion. The marked differences in the usage of equipotentiality has led to confusion in the meaning of this concept in the literature. The incidence of childhood aphasia in the literature does not support Lenneberg's usage of equipotentiality but is not inconsistent with respect to Lashley's usage. We will reconsider Lashley's use of equipotentiality when we discuss recovery from childhood aphasia later in this chapter.

Kinsbourne/Hiscock (1983) have characterized theories of ontogenetic specialization as either emphasizing change during the lifespan or remaining invariant. Since there has been relatively little support for Lenneberg's emphasis on change as outlined in his version of the equipotentiality and progressive lateralization hypotheses, the alternative viewpoint, emphasizing invariance, has gained increasing acceptance. The invariance hypothesis roughly states that the left hemisphere is dominant for speech at birth and that the right hemisphere acquires speech only after the left hemisphere is damaged. Since the childhood aphasia data raises serious questions about the symmetrical nature of language early in development, as well as an increasing asymmetry with age, the invariance hypothesis appears to be a reasonable alternative explanation. However, just as there have been different uses of the term equipotentiality, there have also been different uses of progressive lateralization. A less frequent usage of progressive lateralization has been advanced by Luria (1973, 77).

> "The third fundamental law governing the work of the second brain system ... can be expressed as the law of progressive lateralization of functions, implying their progressive transfer from the primary cortical areas to the secondary and ultimately, to

> tertiary areas ... The left hemisphere (in right-handed persons) has become dominant; it is this hemisphere which begins to be responsible for speech functions, whereas the right hemisphere, unconnected with the activity of the right hands or with speech, has remained subdominant."

Whereas Lenneberg has characterized progressive lateralization as representing increasing asymmetry resulting from a decreased participation of the right hemisphere in language, Luria describes progressive lateralization to be a progressive development of language within the left hemisphere. More specifically, Luria proposed that development within the left hemisphere proceeds from the primary to the tertiary areas within the cortex. Progressive development of the brain from primary to tertiary areas has been supported in a review of anatomical data on cortical development based on studies of myelination, cortical width, and neuronal density by Campbell/Whitaker (1986).

There has been a tendency in neuropsychology to focus on the lateral representation of cognitive functions for neurpsychological models of cognition, sometimes at the exclusion of the two other dimensions of the brain (anterior–posterior and inferior–superior). Kinsbourne/Hiscock (1983) remind us that development proceeds along all three dimensions of space; any adequate model of language development will, therefore, need to account for changes in neuropsychological relationships along all three dimensions.

Whether the childhood aphasia incidence data fit the models of equipotentiality and progressive lateralization depends on whose definition is used. We have shown that the incidence of childhood aphasia data do not provide much support of Lenneberg's usage of these terms but they are not inconsistent with either Lashley's use of equipotentiality or Luria's use of progressive lateralization. As previously noted, the invariance hypothesis was largely a response to the inability of Lenneberg's model to fit the childhood aphasia data. However, the invariance model, because it does not allow for 'change' is inconsistent with Luria's model of progressive intrahemispheric development. Furthermore, the invariance model has trouble accounting for the often reported fact that aphasia manifests itself differently in children and adults. Models hypothesizing developmental change in language have usually been used to account for the differing manifestations of childhood and adult aphasia.

The question whether adult and childhood aphasia differ and the ability of intrahemispheric developmental changes similar to those expressed in Luria's progressive lateralization hypothesis will be the next focus of attention in this chapter. This will be followed by a consideration of the literature on recovery from childhood aphasia and the ability of Lashley's equipotentiality hypothesis to account for those data.

3. Symptoms of Childhood Aphasia

One of the issues of greatest debate within the childhood aphasia literature has been to what extent childhood aphasia is similar to adult aphasia. In some trivial sense, of course, childhood aphasia must differ from adult aphasia since the premorbid language system of the child is going to differ from the premorbid language system of the adult. Dennis (1988) even suggests that asking whether children show adult aphasia is the wrong question to ask because it diverts attention from the more critical question whether brain-damaged children differ in their language from non-brain damaged children, a question that might be overlooked if they do not show adult patterns of aphasia. However, the issue of how childhood aphasia might differ from adult aphasia may have important implications for understanding language development.

3.1. Mutism

The classic picture of childhood aphasia that has emerged from the early studies and prevailed through much of the twentieth century has been that childhood aphasia is characterized by mutism, reduced initiative for speech, dysarthria, agrammatism, anomia, and an absence of fluent aphasia.

One of the distinguishing features of childhood aphasia has been a period of mutism immediately following onset (see e. g. Alajouanine/Lhermitte 1965; Branco-Lefevre 1950). Mutism is considered to be more frequent and longer in duration than with adults. For example, Hecaen (1976) observed that nine of his 15 hemiplegic cases had a duration of mutism ranging from five days to three months. The presence of mutism, though, clearly depends on the location of the lesion. Hecaen reported that 63% of the children in his sample with anterior lesions had mutism, whereas of the children with posterior lesions only 10% had a period of mutism.

3.2. Hypospontaneity of Speech

A reduction of spontaneous speech often follows a period of mutism and is usually of longer duration than mutism. In many cases there may be a very gradual transition from mutism to hypospontaneity of speech. Typically, hypospontaneity of speech has been regarded as part of the motoric, Broca-like aphasia thought to be prevalent in childhood aphasia. Hypospontaneity of speech, however, has also been observed following periods of predominantly fluent signs of aphasia in children (Van de Sandt-Koenderman/Smit/Van Dongen/Van Hesch 1984; Van Hout/Evrard/Lyon 1985). Hypospontaneity has been considered to be one of the hallmarks of childhood aphasia, and has been attributed to dysfunction of an "initiator" of speech associated with subcortical structures (Van Hout/Seron 1983).

3.3. Dysarthria

Dysarthria is also a frequent symptom of childhood aphasia (Alajouanine/Lhermitte 1965) but may be mild and transitory (Hecaen 1983). The frequency of dysarthria appears to depend on the age of the child and the location of the lesion; being more frequent in younger children and after anterior lesions of the dominant hemisphere (Hecaen 1983).

3.4. Agrammatism

A deficit in syntax has been recognized since the earliest reports of childhood aphasia (Bernhardt 1885). The nature of the syntactic deficit, however, has not been well established. Alajouanine/Lhermitte (1965) maintained that children with aphasia tend to use simplified syntax rather than make errors of syntax as do adults with agrammatism. Dennis (1980) described expressive and receptive agrammatism in a nine year old girl with a left temporoparietal infarct and noted that lower levels of syntactic structure are better preserved.

Aram and her co-workers have conducted some of the few systematic studies of syntax in children with aphasia (Aram/Ekelman/Rose/Whitaker 1985; Aram/Ekelman/Whitaker 1986). They found that syntactic impairments are one of the most reliable differences between children with early left and right hemisphere damage. Whether her results can be generalized to childhood aphasics, though, is unclear because so many of her subjects had brain damage prior to the emergence of language. The degree of syntactic dysfunction appears to be positively related to the severity of the injury (Van de Sandt-Koenderman/Smit/Van Dongen/Van Hesch 1984).

3.5. Anomia

Naming impairments in children with acquired aphasia is another frequent symptom of childhood aphasia. Hecaen (1983), for example, reported that 44% of his left-hemisphere sample (15/34) had a naming disorder and that it was persistent. Only left hemisphere lesions tend to reliably produce a naming disorder (see e. g. Aram/Ekelman/Rose/Whitaker 1985; Van Dongen/Visch-Brink 1988; Vargha-Khadem/O'Gorman/Watters 1985), but performance has also been found to be depressed in children with right hemisphere lesions. Aram/Ekelman/Whitaker (1987) suggested that whereas children with left hemisphere lesions have lexical retrieval problems causing naming impairment, in children with right hemisphere lesions naming problems may be due to impulsivity and visual-spatial problems. No association between location of lesion within the left hemisphere and naming impairment has been found (Aram/Ekelman/Whitaker 1987; Hecaen 1983).

3.6. Paraphasias

Early studies noted the striking absence of paraphasias in children with acquired aphasia. For example, Alajouanine/Lhermitte (1965) and Hecaen (1976) stated that paraphasias were rare. Studies by Van Hout/Evrard/Lyon (1985) and Visch-Brink/Van de Sandt-Koenderman (1984), however, maintained that paraphasias are not rare in childhood aphasia. Van Hout/Evrard/Lyon (1985) suggested that the discrepancy between early reports of the rarity of paraphasias and the more recent reports challenging the rarity of paraphasias may be due to several factors: a) that the paraphasias in children tend to be transient and may resolve within days; they may, therefore, have been missed by some investigators, b) since childhood aphasics are generally reluctant to speak, paraphasic errors may be noticed only on formal examination, and c) as Woods/Teuber (1978) suggested, inclusion of children only with hemiplegia in the early studies of childhood aphasia may have biased the sample towards children with anterior lesions.

3.7. Speech Comprehension

The early studies on childhood aphasia also reported the rarity of auditory comprehension deficits (e. g. Bernhardt 1885). Hecaen (1976), though, noted their occurrence but found that they were usually limited to the acute stages of the disorder. Alajouanine/Lhermitte (1965) found auditory comprehension deficits in about a third of their patients. These deficits were found to resolve by six months post-onset. Auditory comprehension deficits are most frequently found after left hemisphere lesions (Aram/Ekelman/Rose 1985; Vargha-Khadem/O'Gorman/Watters 1985); but Hecaen (1976) could not find intrahemispheric location to be a factor. Auditory comprehension deficits are most frequently found in cases of Landau-Kleffner syndrome (Cooper/Ferry 1978), suggesting that etiology may be a critical factor in their occurrence.

3.8 Repetition

Although the ability to repeat is less frequently noted than other aspects of speech, some studies have reported repetition to be impaired (Hecaen 1976), especially with regard to children showing signs of fluent aphasia (Van Dongen/Loonen/Van Dongen 1985).

3.9. Written Language

According to Hecaen (1976), written language problems are the most frequent and persistent problems found among children with acquired aphasia. Alajouanine/Lhermitte (1965) reported that written language problems are always present and are more severe than problems of oral language. Of the written language symptoms, writing problems appear to be more frequently found than reading problems (Alajouanine/Lhermitte 1965; Hecaen 1976).

3.10. Pragmatics

To date, we are not aware of any systematic studies of pragmatic aspects of language. This is an extremely important aspect of language that certainly deserves more attention.

Although it is possible to generate a general picture of the symptoms of childhood aphasia, there are innumerable unresolved issues within this field. Many of the controversies undoubtedly result from the uncontrolled variables across studies including age of the child at the time of the lesion, the age of the lesion, the age of the child at the time of testing, the location of the lesion, and the nature of the cognitive/behavioral test used. Etiology has also been shown to be a critical variable in studies of childhood aphasia. For example, as previously mentioned, auditory comprehension deficits are much more frequent in children with the Landau-Kleffner syndrome than is the case with other etiologies. Children with closed head injury tend to show 'subclinical aphasia' (Sarno 1980) and non-specific linguistic deficits (Ewing-Cobbs/Fletcher/Levin/Eisenberg 1987), whereas children with cerebrovascular accidents tend to show more specific deficits in the areas of phonology, semantics, morphology, and pragmatics (Dennis 1980). Clearly, future studies will need to take these factors into account if we are to fully understand childhood aphasia. Particular attention will need to be paid to etiology. It may no longer be defensible to group together childhood aphasics of varying etiology.

3.11. Non-fluency

Perhaps the greatest debate within the childhood aphasia literature to date has occurred over the issue of non-fluent aphasia in children. As previously noted, earlier studies emphasized the predominance of non-fluent aphasia in childhood aphasia. Some have challenged this characterization and instead argued that this pattern of non-fluent aphasia so frequently reported in the literature is an artifact of: a) some of the early studies including only childhood aphasics with hemiplegia, thereby, biasing the childhood aphasics selected towards those with anterior lesions (Woods/Teuber 1978), or, b) that some of the fluency signs may have been transient and therefore missed by investigators if not examined at a crucial stage following the lesion, or c) that since hypospontaneity of speech is so prevalent, fluent signs may have been missed if not specifically tested (Van Hout/Evrard/Lyon 1985). Since there is no doubt that fluent signs can appear in childhood aphasia, the issue cannot be whether the non-fluent aphasic pattern is invariant, but rather whether fluent aphasia in children is less frequent than in adults (and if so, why?).

To question the long-standing view that childhood aphasia is predominantly of the non-fluent type, studies using a large number of unselected childhood aphasics are needed showing that the frequencies of fluent aphasia in children are comparable to those found in adults. To date, most of the studies using a relatively large number of childhood aphasics, such as those conducted by Hecaen (1983) and Satz/Bullard-Bates (1981) have found that non-fluent aphasia is the predominant type. Many of the more recent studies, while supporting the presence of the fluent variety in childhood aphasia, have not conducted the type of study needed to question the prevailing view. Of the recent studies that have used unselected samples, Visch-Brink/Van de Sandt-Koenderman (1984) reported that eight of their 14 children demonstrated paraphasias, but did not report the number who would be classified as fluent, non-fluent, or mixed according to their criteria of rate and mean length of utterance; Van Hout/Evrard/Lyon (1985) reported positive signs of aphasia in 11 of 16 patients, but noted that the positive signs tended to recover faster, "in some cases within a few days", in children than in adults; and Paquier/Van Dongen (1990), classified only seven of their 42 children as fluent aphasics.

Several factors complicate the issue of fluency in childhood aphasia. First, as pointed out by Kerschensteiner/Poeck/Brunner (1972), definitions of fluency and non-fluency vary across studies. Agreed upon definitions are, therefore, definitely needed. Second, the clinical picture appears to vary with the age of the onset of aphasia such that the older the child at the time of injury the greater the frequency of fluent signs of aphasia. Third, the location of the lesion is a factor, with posterior lesions more frequently resulting in positive signs (as with adults). Fourth, the time of the examination following the onset of aphasia is important, with the fluent signs tending to appear earlier during the course of recovery (often disappearing days or weeks following the onset of aphasia). While there have been many recent studies demonstrating that fluent signs do appear in some childhood aphasics there have been no recent large scale studies of unselected samples of childhood aphasia that would cause us to reconsider earlier claims that the type of aphasia in children differs from adults, and is predominantly non-fluent in nature.

3.12. Explanation of Childhood Versus Adult Symptoms

From the perspective of understanding the development of language, the issue of whether non-fluent aphasia is the predominant form of aphasia in children is less crucial than whether the pattern of aphasia in children differs in some way from that found with adults. Given the description of the common symptoms of aphasia in children, there seems to be a number of aspects where the pattern of aphasia in children differs from that found in adults, in addition to the apparently predominant non-fluent nature, including: longer periods of mutism, the predominance of hypospontaneity, the infrequency of auditory comprehension deficits, and more transient paraphasias. Finding a difference between childhood and adult symptoms of aphasia suggests that continued development of language must be taking place between childhood and adulthood, and, thus, would be inconsistent with views of development emphasizing invariance. Such a finding would, though, be consistent with the progressive lateralization hypothesis advanced by Luria (1973), as discussed above. Since Luria proposed that development proceeds from primary to secondary to tertiary areas, it is presumably this aspect of 'progressive lateralization' that would ultimately explain any difference between the childhood and adult forms of aphasia.

How, then, would progressive lateralization more specifically explain differences between the childhood and adult types of aphasia? According to Campbell/Whitaker (1986), based on anatomical studies of postnatal cortex, maturation proceeds predominantly in an anterior-posterior direction, with structures maturing first in the peri-Rolandic region and later in the occipito-parieto-temporal region. Furthermore, if we assume, as suggested by Goldman and her colleagues (e. g. Goldman 1979; Goldman/Galkin 1978; Goldman/Rosvold 1972), that less mature brain regions are functionally more uncommitted, then injury to such an area would permit greater plasticity and reorganization to occur. The emerging model, therefore, suggests that the typical childhood aphasia pattern, prolonged mutism, hypospontaneity, and non-fluency, should be the result of damage to the more mature, anterior dominant hemisphere areas. The greater plasticity of the posterior areas of the dominant hemisphere, then, would account for the less frequent (and more transient) fluent signs of childhood aphasia, such as fluency, auditory comprehension deficits, and paraphasias, along with the greater recovery from the non-fluent aphasia frequently reported in childhood aphasia.

Recent studies have provided support for this model. For example, Ferro/Crespo (1988) found that the preponderance of non-fluent aphasias in young adult stroke patients occurred from lesions in the perirolandic and subcortical regions. Similarly, Hecaen/Perenin/Jeannerod (1984) reported that most of the symptoms found in childhood aphasia, including the rarer symptoms of auditory and visual comprehension deficits were more common after anterior lesions. They speculated that, "the anterior region of the left hemisphere is more engaged in diverse aspects of language in the child than in the adult, even though the specialization of this region is already fixed for verbal expression" (Hecaen/Perenin/Jeannerod 1984, 285).

Recovery, then, may be the result of intra- and interhemispheric mechanisms of reorganization. A more detailed discussion of equipotentiality and mechanisms of sparing becomes even more relevant when we consider the recovery from childhood aphasia in more detail.

4. Recovery and Sparing of Function

Since the earliest studies of childhood aphasia, it has been recognized that recovery from aphasia in children is much more dramatic than in adults (Bernhardt 1885; Clarus 1874; Freud 1897). These early observations have been supported by twentieth century reports as well (Alajouanine/Lhermitte 1965; Basser 1962; Benson 1972; Byers/McLean 1962; Geschwind 1974; Guttmann 1942; Hecaen 1976; Lenneberg 1967; Woods/Teuber 1978).

The first major twentieth-century paper was by Guttmann (1942). This study consisted of 30 unilateral cases of children 14 years and younger, only 10 of which were available for long-term study. Moderate to complete recovery in speech was observed for all but one of the cases. Basser (1962) reported repeated observation data on 30 children, ages 2 to 9 years, who sustained an acute hemiplegia (left = 15, right = 15) after the onset of speech. An initial non-fluent aphasia was observed in most of the cases. In a subsequent evaluation, (3 months to two years after onset), Basser reported significant recovery in all cases.

A similar recovery course was reported in a subsequent paper by Lenneberg (1967) for patients ranging from 3 to 18 years. All of the children were aphasic at the initial examination, but only two had a persistent aphasia, both were adolescents when the lesion occurred (ages 15 and 18 years, respectively), whereas for children under the age of 11 at the time of the injury recovery was complete.

Alajouanine/Lhermitte (1965) reported on a 1-year follow-up study of 32 children (ages 6–15 years), all of whom were aphasic at initial contact following injury to the left hemisphere. At subsequent testing, 24 of the children had regained "normal or nearly normal language" (659). In contrast, the remaining eight children, most with large cerebral lesions, showed a less favorable course. Byers/McLean (1962), in a follow-up study of ten children (ages 3–15 years) with unilateral vascular lesions, reported complete restitution of speech function.

Hecaen (1976) reported follow-up data on the language status of 17 children (ages 3–19 years) who became aphasic following unilateral left brain injury. Spontaneous recovery was noted in a majority of the cases. However, most of the patients were reported to show long-term difficulties in writing and naming, as previously noted.

Woods/Teuber (1978) reported data on 25 aphasic patients who ranged in age from 2 to 15 years at onset. At follow-up testing four years later, 21 of the cases showed spontaneous recovery of speech. In each of these cases, the lesion occurred before 8 years of age. The four cases who remained aphasic ranged in age from 8 to 13 years at the time of the lesion.

In a later study of 27 children with predominant vascular injury to the left hemisphere, Woods/Carey (1979) reported nearly complete sparing of speech in those children whose lesion onset was before the first birthday (N = 11). In approximately half of the children who became aphasic post-insult, all (N = 7) recovered speech if their lesion was before 8 years of age.

Van Dongen/Loonen (1977) reported aphasia status three years after brain injury in 14 right-handed children who ranged in age from 4 to 14 years at onset. Spontaneous recovery was observed in half of the cases. Unfortunately, it is unclear whether recovery was more associated with lesion onset (i. e. early) or type (i. e. unilateral).

Martins/Ferro (1990) examined a number of factors influencing recovery of acquired aphasia in 29 children with unilateral left brain injury after language acquisition. Twenty-two children (76%) recovered completely from the aphasia, as measured by quantitative measures of language ability.

Better recovery was found for vascular and trauma cases than with encephalitis, which, incidentally, is more likely to cause more severe and diffuse brain injury. Interestingly, recovery was closely associated with age at insult, with 100% aphasia recovery in children under age seven. In fact, all of the persistent cases of aphasias were observed in children whose lesions occurred after age 7 years.

The importance of age of insult in predicting recovery from aphasia was documented carefully in a study by Vargha-Khadem/O'Gorman/Watters (1985). The authors measured aphasia and language status in 3 groups of children: 28 patients with left hemisphere injury, 25 with right hemisphere injury, and 15 normal control subjects. Both lesioned groups were also divided by age of insult (Early = prenatal to 5 years, and Late = 5–14 years) and all children were assessed at least 2 years post-insult. With respect to aphasia course, all children in the early left hemisphere group recovered completely and only one child in the older left hemisphere group remained aphasic. With respect to language course, subtle naming difficulties were observed in the early left-lesioned group. However, the impairments were most pronounced for the older left-lesioned group, "... with the pattern being the later the age of acquisition of injury, the more obvious the deficits. This pattern is more evident with respect to naming rather than auditory comprehension deficits and is consistent with the reported finding that there is a relative preponderance of expressive to receptive disorders in acquired left hemisphere injuries" (Vargha-Khadem/O'Gorman/Watters 1985, 692).

A final recent study reported aphasia, language and intellectual recovery in 37 carefully diagnosed children with unilateral vascular accidents, 17 left [10 prenatal, 7 post-natal (mean age 5.4 years)] and 20 right [9 prenatal, 7 post-natal (mean age = 6.11); (Riva/Pantaleoni/Milani/Devoti 1990)]. The authors found complete recovery from aphasia in both of the left-damaged groups (virtually all of whom were left-handed and probably pathological left-handers).

The weight of the evidence clearly supports the characteristic pattern of faster recovery in childhood aphasia. What remains less clear is the mechanism for the greater sparing of function. Previously, it was mentioned that greater recovery of speech after left hemisphere brain damage in children might be facilitated by mechanisms of intra- and interhemispheric reorganization of uncommitted brain areas. The most direct support for an intrahemispheric mechanism of reorganization comes from the seminal report by Lamar Roberts (Penfield/Roberts 1959). This study also provides direct support for interhemispheric reorganization, as well, and the data have been tabulated so as to reflect both outcomes.

Table 64.2 presents the results of aphasia following left-sided lobectomy in nonaphasic adult epileptic patients whose lesion onset was after age two. Inspection of this table shows that 73% of right hemisphere patients became aphasic after operation on the left hemisphere. The incidence of aphasia after a left lobectomy before age two was a much lower 46%. The absence of aphasia in the majority of these early lesion onset cases likely reflects the effects of speech reorganization in the right hemisphere after injury to the critical speech zones in the left hemisphere. The mechanism of reorganization is probably facilitated by latent and equipotential structures in the right hemisphere that are activated after injury to the dominant or leading hemisphere.

In contrast, the onset of aphasia, which was much less frequent in these early left-sided lesion cases probably reflects, in part, the effects of speech reorganization structures within the injured left hemisphere. As noted above, these posterior structures are hypothesized to represent the substrate for ontogenetically later complex cognitive and linguistic operations (e. g. semantic).

The most direct support for an interhemispheric mode of reorganization is based on results using the sodium amytal procedure developed by Juhn Wada (Wada/Rasmussen 1960). The presence of speech arrest in only the right hemisphere, points to an interhemispheric reorganization. However, the presence of speech arrest in only the left hemisphere could reflect an intrahemispheric maintenance or reorganization of speech. The latest review of this literature is by Satz/Strauss/Wada/Orsini (1988) where four studies are reviewed, representing the few known sources that report parametric data on lesion focus, lesion type, age of onset of damage, handedness and hemispheric speech dominance.

The four studies are: (1) Rasmussen/Milner (1977), where the sodium amytal technique was used to assess hemispheric representation of speech, (2) Penfield/Roberts (1959), where speech was assessed following left temporal lobectomies, (3) Strauss/Satz/Wada (1990), where the sodium amytal technique was used on 53 consecutive left brain-damaged cases, and (4) Orsini (1984), where a dichotic verbal listening task was used on 40 consecutive children and adolescents with verified left focal seizures. From these studies, patients were classified as being either left hemisphere dominant for speech or atypical, representing either bilateral or right hemisphere dominance for speech. The results are presented in Table 64.3, which shows the percentage of left versus atypical speech cases by age of lesion onset (Early < 6 years; Late > 6 years).

Onset	*Left*	*Atypical*
Early	107/262 (41%)	155/262 (59%)
Late	377/473 (80%)	96/473 (20%)

Table 64.3: Percentage Speech Type by Lesion Onset across Studies

Adapted from Satz (1991)

The results show that early left focal brain injury (before age 6 years) is associated with a dramatic shift from the expected pattern of left hemisphere speech dominance observed in normal populations (approximately 96%) versus the present series (107/262 = 41%). Inspection of Table 64.3 also shows that this difference was due to a dramatic increase in the percentage of atypical speech dominance in the early left brain injury cases (Early = 59%; Later = 20%).

Onset	*Left*	*Atypical*
Early	35/107 (33%)	127/155 (82%)
Late	102/377 (27%)	43/96 (45%)

Table 64.4: Percentage MLH by Speech Type by Lesion Onset Across Studies

Adapted from Satz (1991)

A similar pattern was found for handedness (see Table 64.4). Early left brain damage was associated with a striking increase in the incidence of manifest left-handedness (MLH) [162/262 = 62%] compared to non-brain-injured populations (approximately 10%), most of which are accounted for by the atypical group (left = 33%, atypical = 82%). This suggests that the interhemispheric shift in speech was associated with a corresponding shift or alteration in hand preference. This pattern, however, is not invariant. There were cases of unimodal (speech only) and bimodal (speech and hand) transfer. Furthermore, a bimodal shift was associated with an earlier onset of damage than the unimodal shift and a lower incidence of bilateral speech organization.

When cases of interhemispheric versus intrahemispheric speech organization were compared across studies, it was found that time of onset of damage was also associated with type of hemispheric speech organization after left brain injury. In each study, there was a much higher incidence of early damage in cases of interhemispheric reorganization of speech (62% vs. 22%).

The most dramatic finding of these studies is that the earlier the left hemisphere dysfunction (i. e. before 12 months), the greater the likelihood of a bimodal interhemispheric reorganization (including a shift in both speech and handedness). Lesions occurring between the ages of 12 and 72 months are more likely to result in either a unimodal interhemispheric shift in speech, a bilateral or less complete form of hemispheric reorganization, or an intrahemispheric maintenance or reorganization of speech. In each of the latter three cases, the likelihood of a corresponding shift in handedness is lower than with lesions occurring before the first birthday, which are more likely to result in a bimodal hemispheric reorganization. It is hypothesized that this latter type of hemispheric reorganization probably accounts for instances of sparing following left hemisphere injury while the former modes of reorganization account for instances of recovery in speech. Unfortunately, it is unclear whether the rate and/or degree of recovery is related to the type of intra- or interhemispheric reorganization.

Before concluding this discussion of recovery, let us briefly return to an earlier issue — the uses of the terms equipotentiality and progressive lateralization. The results of research on recovery from childhood aphasia provide further support that Lenneberg's (1967) use of these terms is inadequate. In addition to finding little support for his notion that the two hemispheres equally contribute to language early in development, the recovery data imply that intra- and interhemispheric mechanisms contribute to the recovery picture, data not accounted for by Lenneberg's use of these terms. In contrast, the incidence and recovery data are consistent with Lashley's (1921) use of equipotentiality (implying that uncommitted brain areas may possess the ability to take on functions normally attributed to another area of the brain that has been damaged) and Luria's use of progressive lateralization (implying that there are intrahemispheric brain areas involved in speech that develop in a progression from primary to tertiary areas), and therefore, are the recommended use of these terms.

5. Conclusions

This chapter provides a brief update of the current status of childhood aphasia, focusing primarily on the incidence of aphasia, aphasia type and recovery from aphasia. The incidence data show that childhood aphasia is not rarer than adult aphasia, given a unilateral lesion to the dominant hemisphere. The less frequent nature of childhood aphasia can be attributed to only the less frequent nature of unilateral lesions to the dominant hemisphere in children. The pattern of the incidence data, especially the low frequency of crossed aphasia in children, argue against Lenneberg's (1967) equipotentiality hypothesis of speech development. However, the original use of equipotentiality as put forth by Lashley is consistent with these data.

As was noted by the earliest writers, the type of aphasia typically found in children differs from that found in adults, with the predominant type being the non-fluent variety. It has been clearly demonstrated that all types of aphasia found in adults appear in children, but from even the most recent studies of unselected cases, non-fluent aphasia still appears to be the predominant type. Finding that aphasia manifests itself differently in children than in adults suggests that language representation in the brain undergoes changes during development, and therefore is inconsistent with the invariance hypotheses of language. It has been argued that Luria's hypothesis of progressive lateralization is more consistent with the data on childhood aphasia.

Studies on recovery from childhood aphasia show that recovery of speech is greater in children than adults. Data have also been reviewed that suggest there are intra- and interhemispheric mechanisms of recovery. Although it is beyond the scope of this present chapter, it should be noted that the greater recovery of speech in children appears to occur at a cost. There are data suggesting that interhemispheric mechanisms for recovery of speech may 'crowd-out' functions normally represented in the right hemisphere (e. g. visual-spatial functions; see Strauss/Satz/Wada 1990 for a discussion of these issues in humans and LeVere/Gray-Silva/LeVere 1988 for a discussion in non-humans). One issue that needs to be addressed is why this type of reorganization takes place after early left brain injury, especially considering that there is no evidence that the left hemisphere allows for comparable reorganization after early right hemisphere lesions (Dennis 1980; Lansdell 1969). Satz/Strauss/Whitaker (1990) suggested that interhemispheric reorganization may be facilitated by the more diffuse representation of functions within the right hemisphere and its slower rate of maturation.

If interhemispheric reorganization 'crowds out' visual-spatial functions, which are normally represented within the right hemisphere, then it is reasonable to question to what extent more inferential and holistic aspects of language, thought to be represented within the right hemisphere, such as interpretation of familiar phrases (Van Lancker/Kempler 1987), may also be affected by reorganization within the right hemisphere. Similarly, future research should address whether intrahemispheric organization also occurs at a cost, namely at the expense of functions normally found to be represented within the left hemisphere.

The study of childhood aphasia has profound implications for our understanding of how language develops, the ontogeny of cerebral lateralization, and plasticity and recovery of function in the nervous system. It should be clear from the preceding review that the results from childhood aphasia studies have significantly shaped the critical questions to be addressed in future research, among them being the mechanisms involved in progressive lateralization, intra- and interhemispheric reorganization, and 'crowding out' of non-speech functions.

6. References

Alajouanine, T. H. & Lhermitte, F. (1965). Acquired aphasia in children. *Brain, 88,* 653–662.

Aram, D. M., Ekelman, B. L., Rose, D. F., & Whitaker, H. A. (1985). Verbal and cognitive sequelae following unilateral lesions acquired in early childhood. *Journal of Clinical and Experimental Neuropsychology, 7,* 55–78.

Aram, D. M., Ekelman, B. L., Whitaker, H. A. (1986). Spoken syntax in children with acquired unilateral hemisphere lesions. *Brain and Language, 27,* 75–100.

Aram, D. M., Ekelman, B. L., & Whitaker, H. A. (1987). Lexical retrieval in left and right brain lesioned children. *Brain and Language, 32,* 61–87.

Basser, L. S. (1962). Hemiplegia of early onset and the faculty of speech with special reference to the effects of hemispherectomy. *Brain, 85,* 427–460.

Benson, D. F. (1972). Language disturbances of childhood. *Clinical Proceedings Children's Hospital of Washington, 28,* 93–100.

Bernhardt, M. (1885). Über die spastische Cerebralparalyse im Kindesalter (Hemiplegia spastica infantilis), nebst einem Exkurs über: "Aphasie bei Kindern". *Archiv für Pathologische Anatomie und Physiologie und für Klinische Medizin, 102,* 26–80.

Branco-Lefevre, A. F. (1950). Contribuicao para o estudo da psicopatologia da afasia en criancas. *Archivos Neuro-Psiquiatria (Sao Paulo), 8,* 345–393.

Broca, P. (1861). Sur le siege de la faculte de language articule avec deux observations d'aphemie (Porte de Parole). Paris.

Byers, R. K. & McLean, W. T. (1962). Etiology and course of certain hemiplegias with aphasia in childhood. *Pediatrics, 29,* 376–383.

Campbell, S. & Whitaker, H. A. (1986). Cortical maturation and developmental neurolinguistics. In J. E. Obrzut & G. W. Hynd (Eds.), *Child Neuropsychology.* 55–72. New York: Academic Press.

Carter, R. L., Hohenegger, M. K., & Satz, P. (1982). Aphasia and speech organization in children. *Science, 218,* 797–799.

Clarus, A. (1874). Über Aphasie bei Kindern. *Jahresbuch der Kinderheilkunde, 7,* 369–400.

Cooper, J. A. & Ferry, P. C. (1978). Acquired auditory verbal agnosia and seizures in childhood. *Journal of Speech and Hearing Disorders, 43,* 176–184.

Cotard, J. (1868). Etude sur l'atrophie partielle du cerveau. These de Paris.

Dennis, M. (1980). Strokes in childhood I: Communicative intent, expression, and comprehension after left hemisphere arteriopathy in a right-handed nine-year-old. In R. W. Reiber (Ed.), *Language development and aphasia in children. 45–67.* New York: Academic Press.

Dennis, M. (1988). Language and the young damaged brain. In T. Boll & B. K. Bryant (Ed.), *Clinical neuropsychology and brain function: research, measurement, and practice. 85–123.* Washington D. C.: American Psychological Association.

Dennis, M. & Whitaker, H. A. (1977). Hemispheric equipotentiality and language acquisition. In S. J. Segalowitz & F. A. Gruber (Eds.), *Language development and neurological theory. 93–105.* New York: Academic Press.

Ewing-Cobbs, L., Fletcher, J. M., Levin, H. S., & Eisenberg, H. M. (1987). Language functions following closed head injury in children and adolescents. *Journal of Clinical and Experimental Neuropsychology, 5,* 575–592.

Ferro, J. M. & Crespo, M. (1988). Young adult stroke: Neuropsychological dysfunction and recovery. *Stroke, 19,* 982–986.

Freud, S. (1968). Infantile cerebral paralysis. (L. A. Russin, trans.). Coral Gables: University of Miami Press (Originally published 1897).

Geschwind, N. (1974). Late changes in the nervous system: An overview. In D. G. Stein, J. J. Rosen, & N. Butters (Eds.), *Plasticity and recovery of function in the central nervous system. 467–508.* New York: Academic Press.

Goldman, P. S. (1979). Neuronal plasticity in primate telencephalon. Anomalous projections induced by prenatal removal of frontal cortex. *Science, 202,* 768–770.

Goldman, P. S. & Galkin, T. W. (1978). Prenatal removal of frontal association cortex in the fetal rhesus monkey. Anatomical and functional consequences in post-natal life. *Brain Research, 152,* 451–485.

Goldman, P. S. & Rosvold, H. E. (1972). The effects of selective caudate lesions in infant and juvenile rhesus monkeys. *Brain Research, 43,* 53–66.

Guttmann, E. (1942). Aphasia in children. *Brain, 65,* 205–219.

Hecaen, H. (1976). Acquired aphasia in children and the autogenesis of hemispheric specialization. *Brain and Language, 3,* 114–134.

Hecaen, H. (1983). Acquired aphasia in children: revisited. *Neuropsychologia, 21,* 581–587.

Hecaen, H., Perenin, M. T., & Jeannerod, H. (1984). The effects of cortical lesions in children: Language and visual functions. In C. R. Almli & S. Finger (Eds.), *Behavioral biology of early damage (Vol. 1). 277–299.* New York: Academic Press.

Kerschensteiner, M., Poeck, K., & Brunner, E. (1972). The fluency-non-fluency dimension in the classification of aphasic speech. *Cortex, 8,* 233–247.

Kinsbourne, M. & Hiscock, M. (1983). Asymmetries of dual-task performance. In J. B. Hellige (Ed.), *Cerebral hemisphere asymmetry: Method, theory, and application. 255–334.* New York: Praeger.

Lansdell, H. (1969). Verbal and nonverbal factors in right-hemisphere speech: Relation to early neurological history. *Journal of Physiological and Comparative Psychology, 69,* 734–738.

Lashley, K. S. (1921). Studies of cerebral function in learning. The effects of long continued practice upon cerebral localization. *Journal of Comparative Psychology, 1,* 453–468.

Lashley, K. (1964). *Brain mechanisms and intelligence a quantative study of injuries to the brain.* New York: Hafner Publishing Co.

Lenneberg, E. (1967). *Biological foundations of language.* New York: Wiley.

LeVere, N. D., Gray-Silva, S., & LeVere, T. E. (1988). Infant brain injury: the benefit of relocation and the cost of crowding. In S. Finger, T. E. LeVere, C. R. Almli, & D. G. Stein (Eds.), *Brain Injury and Recovery. 133–150.* New York: Plenum.

Ludlow, C. L. (1980). Children's language disorders: recent research advances. *Annals of Neurology, 7,* 497–507.

Luria, A. R. (1973). *The working brain.* New York: Basic Books.

Marie, P. (1922). Existe-t-il dans le cerveau humain de centres innes ou preformes de langage? *La Presse Medicale, 17,* 117–181.

Martins, I. P. & Ferro, J. (1990). Recovery from acquired aphasia in children and lesion size in the temporal lobe. Paper presented at NATO Advanced Workshop on Acquired Aphasia in Children. Sintra, Portugal, September 13–15.

Orsini, D. L. (1984). Early brain injury and lateral development. Doctoral Dissertation, State University of New York, Stony Brook.

Paquier, P. & Van Dongen, H. R. (1990). Fluent aphasias in children. Paper presented at NATO Advanced Research Workshop on Acquired Aphasia in Children. Sintra, Portugal, September 13–15.

Penfield, W. & Roberts, L. (1959). *Speech and Brain mechanisms.* Princeton: Princeton University Press.

Rasmussen, T. & Milner, B. (1977). The role of early left-brain injury in determining lateralization of cerebral speech functions. *Annals of NY Academy of Sciences, 299,* 355–369.

Riva, D., Pantaleoni, C., Milani, N., & Devoti, M. (1990). Late sequelae of right versus left hemisphere lesions. Paper presented at NATO Advanced Research Workshop on Acquired Aphasia in Children. Sintra, Portugal, September 13–15.

Sarno, M. T. (1980). The nature of verbal impairment after closed head injury. *Journal of Mental and Nervous Disease, 168,* 685–692.

Satz, P. (1991). Symptom pattern and recovery outcome in childhood aphasia: a methodological and theoretical critique. In I. Martins, A. Van Hout, & H. R. Van Dongen (Eds.), *Acquired Aphasia in Children. 95–116.* The Netherlands: Kluwer Academic Publishers.

Satz, P. & Bullard-Bates, C. (1981). Acquired aphasia in children. In M. T. Sarno (Ed.), *Acquired aphasia. 399–426.* New York: Academic Press.

Satz, P., Strauss, E., Wada, J., & Orsini, D. L. (1988). Some correlates of intra- and interhemispheric speech organization after left focal brain injury. *Neuropsychologia, 26,* 345–350.

Satz, P., Strauss, E., & Whitaker, H. (1990). The ontogeny of hemispheric specialization: Some old hypotheses revisited. *Brain and Language, 38,* 596–614.

Strauss, E., Satz, P., & Wada, J. (1990). An examination of the crowding hypothesis in epileptic patients who have undergone the carotid amytal test. *Neuropsychologia, 28,* 1221–1227.

Swisher, L. (1985). Language disorders in children. In J. K. Darby (Ed.), *Speech and language evaluation in neurology: childhood disorders. 33–97.* Orlando: Grune and Stratton.

Van Dongen, H. R. & Loonen, M. C. B. (1977). Factors related to prognosis of acquired aphasia in children. *Cortex, 13,* 131–136.

Van Dongen, H. R., Loonen, M. C. B., & Van Dongen, K. J. (1985). Anatomical basis of acquired fluent aphasia in children. *Annals of Neurology, 17,* 306–309.

Van Dongen, H. R. & Visch-Brink, E. G. (1988). Naming in aphasic children: analysis of paraphasic errors. *Neuropsychologia, 26,* 629–632.

Van Hout, A., Evrard, P., & Lyon, G. (1985). On the positive semiology of aquired aphasia in children. *Developmental Medicine and Child Neurology, 27,* 231–241.

Van Hout, A. & Seron, X. (1983). L'aphasie de l'enfant. *Mardaga,* Bruxelles. 193.

Van Lancker, D. R. & Kempler, D. (1987). Comprehension of familiar phrases by left- but not by right-hemisphere damaged patients. *Brain and Language, 32,* 265–277.

Van de Sandt-Koenderman, W., Smit, I., Van Dongen, K., & Van Hesch, J. (1984). A case of acquired aphasia and convulsive disorders: some linguistic aspects of recovery and breakdown. *Brain and Language, 21,* 174–183.

Vargha-Khadem, F., O'Gorman, A. M., & Watters, G. V. (1985). Aphasia and handedness in relation to hemispheric side, age of injury and severity of cerebral lesion during childhood. *Brain, 108,* 677–696.

Visch-Brink, E. G. & Van de Sandt-Koenderman, M. (1984). The occurrence of paraphasias in the spontaneous speech of children with acquired aphasia. *Brain and Language, 23,* 256–271.

Wada, J. & Rasmussen, T. (1960). Intracarotid injection of sodium amytal for the lateralization of cerebral speech dominance. *Journal of Neurosurgery, 17,* 266–282.

Wernicke, C. (1874). *Der aphasische Symptomenkomplex.* Breslau: Max Cohen and Weigert.

Woods, B. T. & Teuber, H. L. (1978). Changing patterns of childhood aphasia. *Annals of Neurology, 3,* 273–280.

Woods, B. T. & Carey, S. (1979). Language deficits after apparent recovery from childhood aphasia. *Annals of Neurology, 5,* 405–409.

Paul Satz, Los Angeles, California (USA)/
Richard Lewis, Claremont, California (USA)

65. Language Acquisition and Development with Sensory Impairment: Hearing-Impaired Children

1. Factors Affecting Language Acquisition

Describing the pattern and nature of language acquisition in the presence of a hearing impairment is complex because there are so many variables that can affect the process. Whether the reader's concern is to understand the impact of a hearing-loss on language acquisition in any individual or to gain a more general view of the process, it is necessary to be aware of the factors involved. These factors include the type and degree of hearing impairment; age of onset and detection; the methods used to treat the impairment, to communicate and educate; the language models available in the home and community; the intellectual and remaining sensory abilities of the child.

1.1. Onset and Incidence of Hearing Loss

A hearing loss can be either present at birth or be acquired after birth. The critical factor for language acquisition is whether the loss occurs before, during or after the primary period of language acquisition. Where the loss is prelingual, the effect on language acquisition is most marked. The effects of a loss occurring during development have proved difficult to evaluate although age of onset has been a variable considered in some large-scale studies (Bamford/Mentz 1979). A hearing loss acquired after language has fully developed has little effect on linguistic competence although communication is impaired. — Carrel (1977, 3) states that although worldwide an incidence of more than 1 in 1000 births with hearing loss have been reported, these represent more severe losses. He estimates that a true incidence would be, for the U.S.A., 1 in 200, taking into account milder losses which are more difficult to detect in infancy. An increase in incidence due to hearing loss associated with middle ear effusion means that 6% of 4 year olds and 3–4% of 7 year olds are affected (Carrel 1977, 3).

1.2. Degree and Type of Hearing Loss

The degree of hearing loss tends to vary with the type and cause of impairment. More severe and profound losses are usually found in sensorineural impairments where the cochlea and auditory nerve are damaged, though mild and moderate losses can also result. Some hearing losses are so profound that the child lacks any appreciable response to sound within the range of intensities and frequencies associated with speech perception. Failure of the conductive mechanism of the middle and outer ear tends to produce losses of mild to moderate degree, especially when resulting from a condition common in childhood, otitis media with effusion, commonly called 'glue ear'. (This name is derived from the sticky glue-like secretions that form in the middle-ear and impair its function). The average loss reported is 15–30 dB. (Chalmers/Stewart/Silva/Mulvena 1989, 22). A conductive loss characteristically affects speech frequencies equally across the speech range (Klein/Rapin 1988). Sensorineural losses tend to be prelinguistic and persist throughout language development. Although some conductive losses are prelinguistic (e. g. Treacher-Collins disease and other hereditary conditions producing malformation of the conductive mechanism), the most common form of conductive loss, due to otitis media with effusion, usually starts in infancy or early childhood and is characteristically transient or fluctuating. — Sensorineural losses vary in the frequencies that are affected. One type of sensorineural hearing impairment affects the higher speech frequencies while hearing in the lower frequencies is preserved so the child may appear to have some intact hearing. Failure to hear consonants, though, means that spoken language becomes unintelligible to the child. Unless audiometry is used to assess hearing across the whole range of speech frequencies, children with high frequency losses can be misdiagnosed as suffering from developmental receptive aphasia (Bishop/Rosenbloom 1987). — The causes of hearing impairment are significant in that some aetiologies are frequently associated with additional sensory, motor or intellectual impairments which will further complicate language development (DiBartolomeo/Gerber 1977). While some causes of hearing impairment are being eliminated (e. g. rubella through the immunisation of females of child bearing age) others, especially those associated with preterm birth, are on the increase. It has been estimated that around 50% of congenital hearing losses are due to genetic causes (Carrel 1977) and several different modes of inheritance are involved (DiBartolomeo/Gerber 1977). The high incidence of inherited impairments means that 3–9% (Quigley/Kretschmer 1982, 16) of hearing-impaired children are born to hearing-impaired parents. This has social and cultural implications affecting language acquisition (cf. 1.3.). — Functional hearing ability for language acquisition depends on the level of residual hearing available to the child. In most cases of sensorineural loss the deficit is bilateral although unilateral losses occur. At one time, a hearing loss affecting one ear only was thought to be of little significance because the hearing in the second ear was sufficient for language acquisition. Research suggests, however, that a unilateral loss may affect educational achievement. (Culbertson/Gilbert 1986; Klee/Davis-Dansky 1986). — Typically, in describing subjects in studies of language acquisition, the degree of hearing loss is indicated by reference to the degree of residual hearing in the better ear. The levels of hearing loss for selected frequencies across the speech range, measured by pure-tone audiometry, are averaged. The resulting value may also be classified indicating the degree of hearing loss: i. e. profound, severe, moderate and mild. However there is considerable variability in the way these terms relate to average decibel values (Conrad 1979, 41; cf. Green 1978). As a general guide, losses of below 40 dB. are considered 'mild', 41–70 dB. 'moderate', 71–90 dB. 'severe', and greater than 90 dB. 'profound'. This is a crude method of indicating functional hearing ability since it masks differences in thresholds across frequencies which affect the way speech is perceived. Although the degree of impairment strongly relates to measures of language development it does not alone predict either the rate and success of linguistic development or educational achievement (Bamford/Mentz 1979; Conrad 1979, 247 ff). — In addition to the factors already discussed, language acquisition depends on measures taken to remedy hearing loss. Three different types of remediation can be considered but these can only be implemented after the loss has been detected. The age of detection may also affect outcome. The Commission of the European Community (1979) found that only approximately 10% of children born in European Economic Community countries in 1969, with a hearing impairment, had been diagnosed by 12 months and 45% were not diagnosed until after 3 years of age.

1.2.1. Medical Treatment

Diagnosis and detection are normally considered medical responsibilities. Once a hearing impairment has been diagnosed, treatment aims to correct or improve the functioning of the hearing mechanism. In the past treatment was limited to correcting failures in the conductive mechanism, most frequently due to otitis media with effusion. A variety of measures can be taken to restore the functioning of the middle ear but until the early part of the 1980's no treatment existed for sensorineural hearing loss. Since that time cochlear implants have been developed to treat sensorineural losses where the cochlea is damaged. This involves implanting electrodes that directly stimulate the auditory nerve. At first these were single channel devices which could only give information on the presence and duration of speech sound but more sophisticated multichannel devices can now give more information about the speech signal. Although a controversial treatment for children with prelinguistic sensorineural loss, some implants have been performed.

1.2.2. Audiological Treatment

Audiological treatment aims to provide appropriate amplification to compensate for the hearing loss as early as possible in the child's development. The amplification provided should be appropriate for the sound characteristics of the environments in which the hearing aid will be used, and the type and severity of loss. Audiological advances include methods of neonatal detection, more reliable infant screening, and assessment of hearing loss which relates more directly to the ability to perceive speech as well as the development and refinement of hearing-aids. Improvements in hearing aids aim to reproduce closely the conditions of unaided sound reception, particularly in conditions where children normally encounter spoken language. Some aids use tactile as well as auditory channels to transmit acoustic information (cf. 6.2.3.).

1.2.3. Educational Treatment

Educational treatment reflects advances in medicine and audiology. Earlier detection has led to greater provision for intervention in the prelinguistic period based on parental involvement in early language acquisition and made possible research on prelinguistic development. Improvements in hearing aids has encouraged integration of hearing-impaired children in mainstream education. — The history of research into language acquisition in the prelingually hearing-impaired has been dominated by the controversy concerning methods of communication which favor either oral language acquisition through the amplification of residual hearing and lip-reading (oral/aural method), or the acquisition of natural sign language and finger-spelling (manual method). A partial resolution of the controversy followed the introduction of methods of communication which combined oral and manual methods. 'Pure' forms of the manual and oral approaches are still used in Britain and the U.S.A., but the predominance of oral approaches has been redressed in the last decade. Newer approaches marry oral/auditory methods with manual methods in various ways. As a result there are now a variety of communication methods which employ manual means to supplement oral/aural communication: (i) approaches which use the vocabulary of natural sign languages adapted to run simultaneously with spoken language and reflecting the organization of spoken language; (ii) artificial sign languages which have been developed mainly to convey the structure of the spoken language which they accompany. — In English these tend to emphasize the inflectional morphology of the language: (iii) systems that employ hand signals to supply phonetic information not available through residual hearing and lip-reading. There are five main systems of communication in widespread use. Sign languages are composed of manual gestures and employ grammars distinct from those of spoken languages. Sign language uses spatial organization to accomplish linguistic and grammatical functions. Sign languages have functioned as a primary means of communication for deaf people for centuries. They are transmitted from one generation to another and vary in form between nations, regions and social groups. American Sign Language is also known as Ameslan or A.S.L. and British Sign Language as B.S.L. Finger-spelling uses a manual alphabet which has 26 handshapes to represent the letters of the written alphabet and allows an exact representation of written English. Different methods of finger spelling employ either one or two hands. Finger spelling usually supplements natural sign and is used for proper names and words for which no sign is available. Oral/aural methods employ speech for expression and residual hearing and lip-reading for understanding other speakers. Educators who use this method emphasize the early and consistent use of high quality, appropriate amplification and auditory training to optimize residual hearing. Early versions of this method favored specific language and speech training. Modern versions prefer more natural communicative methods that emphasize aural training rather than training in speech, language and lip-reading. Total Communication is variously and loosely interpreted. When first introduced it suggested the use of all means and aids to communication: speech, amplification, signing, finger-spelling, natural gesture, pantomime, reading, writing, drawing pictures. However, there was no specification as to how these means should be combined. It has come to mean simultaneous use of speech with some form of sign and finger-spelling. There are numerous ways in which these combinations can function. There are a number of simultaneous methods used in the U.S.A. and Britain which employ artificially devised sign systems or systems that combine natural and devised signs simultaneously with spoken language. The aim of these systems is to represent the structure of spoken language in signed form. Where English is the spoken language there is usually a means of representing the inflectional system of the language. Paget Gorman Sign System, Signed English, Signing Exact English and Seeing Essential English are such systems. These should be distinguished from the simultaneous use of natural signs with speech where the signs follow spoken language word order. This is known as Signs Supporting English. Cued Speech is a different type of system. It uses eight handshapes in four positions close to the lips. The handshapes and lip patterns together clarify the ambiguities of the phonemes that are present in visual speech reception (cf. 6.1.). It cannot function independently as a manual communication system and assists the use and development of oral language. Although devised for use with English (Cornett 1967) it has been adapted for other languages.

1.3. Sociolinguistic Background

The languages used in primary language acquisition with the hearing-impaired are usually determined by the language use in the family home and the immediate social community. Approximately 10% of children are born into families where one or both parents are hearing-impaired. Although language use in the home is not simply determined by the hearing status of the parents, when parents have a prelingual hearing impairment they may use sign language with their children. There may also be siblings and members of the extended family who provide a signing community. Although sign language may be acquired at home, oral language may be used in school and the structure of spoken language will be needed for literacy. Sign language flourishes where the hearing-impaired associate informally. This happens in schools devoted to the education of the hearing-impaired even though oral language is the medium of instruction. Children from oral home environments may acquire a form of sign language by this means. Thus many hearing-impaired children are acquiring language in a bilingual situation. Two different forms of signing may exist in school environments: natural sign language in informal contacts between hearing-impaired children and a form of pidgin sign language used with and by hearing teachers who have learned sign language as adults for classroom use. Language usage is even more complex in the wider deaf community with a continuum between sign language and spoken language. (Lawson 1981). Little recognition of bilingual language acquisition has been made in studies of either oral or sign language acquisition.

1.4. Additional Advantages and Disadvantages

Some children with hearing impairment have additional disabilities. The cause of the hearing impairment can also cause visual and intellectual impairments. Most research concerns children with single disabilities since the complexity of multiple disability is hard to untangle and generalizations cannot easily be made. — Variability in linguistic and academic achievement has largely been attributed to degree of hearing loss and intelligence. Cognitive abilities such as the form and availability of codes for memory have been shown to be related to success (Bamford/Mentz 1979; Conrad 1979, 247 ff).

2. Conductive Hearing Loss

A conductive hearing loss results when the capacity to transmit sound to the inner ear from the air is reduced relative to the capacity to transmit sound through the bone of the skull. This occurs when there is damage or malformation of the external ear, the ear drum or middle ear. A variety of conditions lead to conductive hearing loss in childhood but the most prevalent cause in younger children (under 6 years) is middle ear effusion or 'glue ear'. There are many terms used to denote this condition. These relate to the nature of the effusion which typically changes during the course of the disease. Otitis media is inflammation of the middle-ear, the air-filled space containing the bones that connect the eardrum to the oval window of the inner ear. Normally these bones and the eardrum act as a mechanical transducer for transmitting sound from the ear canal to the auditory nerve ending in the cochlea. If the Eustachian tube is obstructed for any reason, the air in the middle ear tends to be reabsorbed, fluid collects and may then become infected. The fluid reduces the efficiency of sound conduction and this results in a hearing impairment. The condition can be acute and/or chronic. Chalmers/Stewart/Silva/Mulvena (1989, 2) suggest that there is a clear cut clinical distinction between acute otitis media accompanied by pain, with or without ear discharge, and chronic effusions that have hearing impairment as a symptom. Losses due to otitis media are mild, rarely exceeding 40 dB. The loss improves when the infection subsides or is treated and the fluid is absorbed or drained surgically. Episodes may recur frequently or the condition may persist. The hearing loss therefore is usually transient. The average duration of episodes is 29—30 days but 9—32% are chronic cases lasting up to 12 weeks. In a small percentage of cases (2—10%) the condition has been known to persist for 1—4 years (Chalmers et al. 1989, 11). Persistent or frequent episodes are most likely to produce an effect on language acquision especially when they occur during the early language learning period. The condition can often predate the onset of language, as indicated by estimates of prevalence levels as high as 49% in the first year of life and 61% in the second (Klein/Rapin 1988). Given the high incidence of 'glue ear' it is likely to coincide with other conditions affecting language acquisition, such as specific language learning difficulties. In Down's Syndrome and clefts of the hard and soft palate the causes of the otitis media are linked to these conditions. – The critical question is whether in children with no other disability the hearing loss associated with this condition produces sufficient reduction in auditory acuity and exposure to language models to affect language acquisition. A further question is whether there are persistent effects on speech discrimination as a result of this transient loss. If this were so it would lend support to the suggestion that there is a critical period for exposure to speech sounds in the development of the auditory system.

2.1. Research Findings – Early Studies

Although the hearing loss associated with 'glue ear' is normally equally distributed across speech frequencies, the most vulnerable aspects of speech perception are those associated with low energy consonants in the higher frequencies. Dobie/Berlin (1979) used computer simulation to discover what linguistic information would be lost with a 20 dB. hearing loss. They identified three types of loss: consonants, particularly those marking important morphological distinctions; unstressed words; inflections and intonation contouring. Thus language structure as well as phonology could be affected by losses resulting from 'glue ear'. These receptive difficulties could also result in delayed development of expressive language forms. Early studies tended to establish an association between early otitis media and later language delays (Holm/Kunze 1969; Needleman 1977). However, there was little consensus on the nature and extent of the effects on language in early studies.

2.2. Methodological Difficulties in Research

The shortcomings of these early studies were highlighted by a series of critical reviews. The most influential were by Ventry (1980) and Paradise (1981). These reviews underline the methodological problems that beset research. Paradise lists the methodological flaws identified in early retrospective studies that compared otitis prone and otitis free subjects. First, since onset is often insidious and the age of onset variable, a hearing loss can go unrecognized unless subjects are regularly tested. The persistence and severity of the hearing loss is also hard to establish without objective measures of middle ear function repeated at regular intervals. Early studies were retrospective rather than prospective and used unreliable reports from medical records and parents for information about diagnosis and history. Subjects were often poorly matched particularly on variables which could affect language development like sex, disadvantage and language learning experiences. Often the hearing at the time of language assessment was not tested. If the loss was present during language assessment the performance would be affected and this would not be a valid or reliable result. Subject samples were often small and unrepresentative. The testing of subjects was not done 'blind' so that experimenter effects could operate. Finally, in reporting results there was a selective emphasis on positive rather than negative findings. With some exceptions (Dalzell/Owrid 1976), a distinction between the effects of the untreated loss on concurrent language development and the long-term effects after treatment or recovery were not made. There are other problems in designing research. The effect of a mild intermittent loss will depend on success in detection and treatment which may be related to other indices of advantage and disadvantage such as variations in health care provision. Even where a link between otitis media with effusion and language delay is demonstrated it is difficult to demonstrate that this is causative.

2.3. Recent Research

Subsequent research has employed a number of strategies to overcome these difficulties: These include descriptive longitudinal studies (e. g. Brookhouser/Goldgar 1987) where repeated testing was used to identify individuals with middle ear malfunction, the frequency and duration of episodes, and the severity of the hearing deficit. These authors found an association between otitis media and later language delay. Roberts/Sanynl/Burchinal et al. (1986), in a longitudinal follow-up study investigated the relationship between the occurrence of otitis media with effusion during the first three years and subsequent verbal performance and found no evidence of an association between measures. Klein/Rapin (1988), cite a research review of over 50 studies of language achievements in children with recurrent otitis media and conclude that the cause-effect relationship between early recurrent otitis media and later cognitive and language impairment remains uncertain. A methodologically rigorous study of a large sample reported by Chalmers et al. (1989, 156) concludes "Deficits in language development, speech articulation, reading, ... first identified at 5 years were found to persist into middle childhood years and were still present at age 11." However, it should be noted that the effects on language development, even where reported, are relatively mild compared with those which result from a persistent prelingual hearing loss. – Given the variability in outcome in any group of children suffering recurrent otitis media and the high prevalence of the condition it might be a more useful research strategy to identify factors which predict good and poor outcome.

3. Prelingual Hearing Loss: Research Questions

A prelingual hearing loss is persistent and cannot normally be corrected except through amplification. Current knowledge of the process of language acquisition and the linguistic achievements of the prelingually hearing-impaired is the product of research going back over 50 years or more. Given the variety of approaches, subjects and aspects of language studied there can be no typical picture. Even if additional disabilities and differences in intelligence are ignored there are still a number of factors affecting language development: degree of hearing loss, language medium, age of diagnosis. – The description of language development concerns different aspects of language ability and can be divided into oral (see 4.) and sign language (see 7.). Competence in written language (see 5.) is a common goal for children from whatever medium of communication is employed. Lip-reading (see 6.), although emphasized in oral methods, is an ability developed to some degree by all prelingually impaired. – As well as describing different aspects of language development, studies have varied in their purpose. The research questions have changed over time. – The controversy concerning methods of communication (see 1.2.3.) meant that the purpose of numerous early studies was to evaluate the relative success of competing approaches to communication in fostering language acquisition. Studies tended to concentrate on success in lip-reading and written language because poor intelligibility made it difficult to transcribe spoken language. There were also difficulties in comparing oral language competence with sign language because methods of describing and analyzing sign language were lacking. – Until descriptions of sign language and its structure began to appear, research concentrated on children acquiring oral language. Studies on sign language acquisition did not start appearing until the early 1970's. The spread and development of new combinations of communication methods, implemented in a variety of settings and in different ways, mean that there are many different forms of language acquisition which could be investigated and described. Any attempt to draw a general or comparative picture of current linguistic achievements, in all these communication forms, would be both premature and misleading. – Some studies, carried out in the seventies, of the linguistic achievements of children in oral programmes were proactive in stimulating changes in teaching methods. However, these studies addressed the effects of hearing-impairment on achievement of stages in language acquisition rather than investigating the nature of the process. Cross-sectional studies provide no more than a snapshot; to understand the dynamic nature of language acquisition, longitudinal studies are more effective and there have been too few of these. – Most research studies have focussed on language acquisition in children with substantial, moderate to profound sensorineural losses. With the exception of Davis (1986), there have been relatively few studies of children with mild to moderate persistent losses. Nevertheless, these are of importance because they could provide important comparisons with intermittent mild hearing loss already described in section 2. The linguistic achievements of the prelinguistic hearing-impaired cannot be regarded as fixed. Results may change over time reflecting scientific advances, resources and policies which affect age of detection, type and availability of hearing aids, and causes of hearing impairment. Much research has attempted to determine if oral language acquisition is delayed or deviant in the hearing-impaired child but the value and purpose of this effort has rarely been explicitly examined. It was partly motivated by the controversy over methods of communication and language use: the oralists seeking to demonstrate that language acquisition was merely delayed and not distorted through the perceptual difficulties encountered (see 4.1.). Others, with different motives, sought to establish that the inherent difficulties in speech perception for the hearing-impaired led to a form of acquisition that is different in character from that of hearing children. This line of enquiry led to questioning whether it is possible to learn a language designed for the auditory system primarily through the visual modality. More sensitivity to the sociolinguistic pattern of language use has encouraged the recognition of the bilingual nature of language acquisition in the hearing-impaired. Studies need to consider the effect that acquiring different languages at different stages of development can have on the form of language acquired. However, not only are two different languages being acquired, but the languages are organized differently; oral language depending on temporal patterning while sign language depends on spatial organization. — Growing awareness of the effect of preverbal experience on the nature of language acquisition and the effects of a communication disability on conversational experience are some recent questions that are being studied. Investigating cognitive models in all aspects of language processing is also a current area of research. The evaluation of technical advances including cochlear implants and vibrotactile aids are of both practical and theoretical significance.

4. Oral Language

Oral language is used to distinguish spoken language from sign language and refers not only to understanding and using speech but to language used for reading and writing as well. References unless otherwise stated are to children in oral language programmes. For an extended review see Mogford (1988).

4.1. Delayed or Deviant?

The debate as to whether oral language acquisition is delayed or deviant has been protracted but the nature of this distinction has rarely been discussed in depth. There is general agreement that oral language acquisition is 'delayed' if the forms produced are normally immature or if the order in which structures are acquired is similar in the hearing-impaired to hearing children of a younger age. When researchers ask if language is delayed, they want to find out if the language acquisition process for the hearing-impaired child represents individual recreation of language. It is argued, particularly by supporters of oral approaches, that since hearing-impairment is a peripheral disorder and the cognitive abilities which support language acquisition are unimpaired, the process of acquisition should be similar in character though slower in pace to the hearing child. Critics argue that this ignores the different developmental and social context in which language is acquired when a delay occurs (cf. 4.2.2.). In addition, the effect of the perceptual difficulties experienced may lead children to develop different strategies for learning and processing language. These strategies will result in hearing-impaired children producing structures not found in hearing children and acquiring the structures of language in a different order. Others argue that the communication methods used mean that the way that oral language is experienced and the interaction in which language is learned are different, which may be reflected in differences in the way language is acquired. — The term 'deviant' has been variously defined: to refer to structures inadmissible in adult grammar and not normally found as immature forms; to an atypical order of acquisition; or to an imbalance in elements used compared with hearing children at a similar stage. There is little disagreement that with severe or profound hearing losses acquisition is slow compared to hearing children of the same chronological age. Controversy surrounds additional deviation. The argument has concerned all aspects of language: phonology, syntax, semantics and pragmatics. Whatever the answer to the delayed/deviant debate, descriptions of the nature of oral language development are significant when comparisons are made with the acquisition of natural sign language (see section 7.).

4.2. Prelinguistic Development

Early diagnosis facilitates the study of prelinguistic development which can be divided into two areas; (i) prelinguistic vocalization and babbling and (ii) preverbal communication.

4.2.1. Prelinguistic Vocalization and Babbling

A study by Lenneberg/Rebelsky/Nichols (1965) established that early vocalization (cooing) emerges even though auditory-vocal models and auditory feedback are unavailable but that hearing plays a role in maintaining and developing early vocalization. Subsequent research suggested that there are qualitative and quantitative differences in the babbling of hearing-impaired infants compared with hearing infants. Although babbling emerges at a comparable age it decreases in frequency in the subsequent period (Stoel-Gammon/Otomo 1986). Smith (1982) also found similarities with hearing infants up to 15 months when labial consonants predominated in samples of hearing-impaired babbling. This suggests that visual cues were beginning to influence vocalizations. The lack of a satisfactory common framework to describe stages in preverbal development has made it difficult to compare studies. Oller's (1986) recent framework uses acoustic and perceptual parameters to distinguish early (marginal) and later (canonical) babbling. The latter exhibits most acoustic parameters characteristic of adult speech. Oller recorded marginal babbling in severely/profoundly deaf infants but canonical babbling failed to develop in the first year. He concludes that there are similarities and differences between the vocalizations of hearing-impaired and hearing infants and an auditory handicap delays the development of some properties of syllables that make pre-speech vocalizations appear speech-like to adults. The non-speech like characteristics and infrequency of pre-speech vocalizations may be linked to findings that mothers of hearing-impaired children tend to ignore, or talk through, their infant's vocalizations rather than incorporating them in preverbal exchanges as occurs with hearing infants (Cheskin 1982; Gregory/Mogford/Bishop 1979).

4.2.2. Preverbal Communication and Early Language

Bruner (1975) argued that some aspects of preverbal communication are linked to the emergence of early language. These include vocal imitation of the adult by the child, joint visual attention and turn-taking. Lack of hearing and reliance on the visual channel has been found to delay or interfere with these preverbal abilities. This alters the nature of early language acquisition in that verbal labelling by the infant, which arises out of shared visual attention to objects, is delayed and first words are more likely to concern interpersonal events (Gregory/Mogford 1981). Curtis/Prutting/Lowell (1979) found that some stages of semantic development were passed through before spoken language appeared so that these were not repeated in the early verbal period. Gregory/Mogford (1981) also found greater cognitive maturity was reflected in early semantic development in that hearing-impaired children encoded meanings for abstract qualities of size and color earlier than language-matched hearing children. The extended preverbal period has an effect on the language addressed to the hearing-impaired child. Nienhuys/Horsborough/Cross (1985) found that although hearing mothers were able to adapt their language levels to those of the early language of hearing-impaired children they also reduced the complexity of the cognitive content of their language.

4.3. Phonology

The development of phonology in hearing children is evident in the development of stable and rule-governed speech forms that gradually approximate to adult speech forms by 4–5 years of age when the child's speech is intelligible to adult speaker/listeners. Speech intelligibility is impaired by a hearing impairment (Conrad 1979, 204 ff; Markides 1970). However, it is important to separate phonology from phonetic aspects of speech development. A phoneme is not an acoustic entity but a linguistic abstraction and a way of categorizing the distinctions employed in spoken language. There are two aspects of phonology; the segmental and suprasegmental. The segmental aspect refers to the contrastive system of speech sounds (vowels and consonants); the suprasegmental includes intonation and stress. Phonetic aspects of speech, vocal quality and phonetic accuracy, are affected by the lack of auditory feedback control and auditory access to speech models. The development of phonology, the linguistic element in speech development, concerns the control of segmental and suprasegmental features to make meaningful distinctions. The auditory sense is primarily involved in the acquisition of phonology in the hearing child, although visual cues from articulatory movements also play a part (Dodd 1987). It is possible to develop a mature phonology when visual cues are absent as demonstrated in severe congenital visual impairment, although early development is slower and different due to the absence of lip-read information (Mills 1987). The hearing-impaired child relies more on visual information of articulatory movements to extract the phonological structure of language as the hearing impairment increases (Erber 1974 b). Is it possible to acquire the segmental aspects of phonology from the visual channel via lip-reading alone, or is such an ability dependent on the auditory modality? Although lip-reading does not allow the same acuity of speech perception as hearing (see. 6.1.), there is evidence that children with severe and profound prelingual hearing losses can develop knowledge of the phonological structure of their language which can be used in a variety of tasks requiring use of a phonological code. Case studies by West/Weber (1973) and Oller/Kelly (1974) found the use of phonemic contrasts and consistent phonological processes which were similar to patterns of phonological development in younger hearing children. Dodd (1976), in a group study of profoundly impaired children 9–12 years, found consistent forms in 85% or more items although all subjects had phonemes missing from their repertoires. These phonemes were those acquired later in hearing children although normally before six years of age. Dodd also found that the rules governing consonant use were similar to those of young hearing children. Other reports indicate considerable delays in phonological development in speech that persist into early adolescence (Abberton/Fourcin/Hazan 1986, 3 ff). Despite the considerable delay in development, there is evidence that where a hearing impairment is so severe as to restrict speech perception almost entirely to the visual modality it is possible to extract rules and regularities of the phonology of the language. Dodd (1987) argues that a stable and abstract system of phonology can be acquired primarily through lip-reading. – Can this abstract knowledge of phonology be employed in a variety of tasks? In hearing children the phonology of a language may also be employed in silent reading, spelling and working memory. Certain metalinguistic tasks employing rhymes and homophones also depend on a knowledge of phonology. Dodd/Hermelin (1977) concluded from a series of studies that hearing-impaired children are able to do tasks requiring phonological coding in ways resembling the hearing, even children who rely entirely on lip-reading for speech perception. This ability was also found in children in a total communication programme (see 1.2.3.) (Dodd 1987). This surprised the researchers who had expected that this group might use a code derived from print or sign rather than lip-reading. It is unclear whether this result was due to the superior language ability of the group in the total communication programme. Not all hearing-impaired children, however, have access to a phonological code. Where this ability is present, there is evidence of greater competence in reading, lip-reading and speech intelligibility (Conrad 1979, 244). Although a relationship with intelligence can be demonstrated, this ability to use a phonological code is not predicted entirely by either intelligence or hearing loss as it is presently measured. Given the relative lack of sophistication in measuring residual hearing in studies of this kind, it is not surprising that the relationship between the degree and type of hearing has not yet been related to the development of phonology. And although it is possible in an experimental task to demonstrate access to a phonological code through unaided lip-reading, this does not exclude the possibility that some degree of auditory input together with lip-read cues play a part in the acquisition of phonology.

4.4. Syntax

The acquisition of the syntax of oral language is the most severely affected aspect of language in the prelingually hearing-impaired. The nature of this impairment has emerged as research methods have grown in sophistication. – Until the mid-1960's research was largely confined to written language and described structural development which was delayed, simple, stereotyped and inflexible. This approach failed to demonstrate the hearing-impaired child's developing mastery of the syntactic rules of language or the strategies employed in either comprehension or production of oral language forms in writing and speaking. For a fuller account of this early research see reviews by Cooper/Rosenstein (1966); Swisher (1976). – During the 1970's, investigators of the development of comprehension and production of spoken language were preoccupied with the delay/deviance dichotomy. Using standardized language tests, it was possible to determine the order of acquisition of the syntactic structures of English in comparison with hearing children. Studies by Presnell (1973), Geers/Moog (1978) and Davis (1977) came to the conclusion that acquisition was not only delayed but also deviant. The children in these studies had hearing losses ranging from moderate to profound. Two other studies (Brown 1984; Wilcox/Tobin 1974) used small samples of children with less severe losses and reported results suggesting a language delay. In a larger scale study in Britain, Bamford (1979, 73 ff) analyzed samples of spoken language for 263 children, aged 8–15 years with hearing-impairments ranging from mild to profound and intelligence levels from I.Q. 64–150 on the W.I.S.C. performance scale. Samples were analysed using L.A.R.S.P. (Crystal/Fletcher/Garman 1976, 1 ff), which profiles the structures of English at clause, phrase and word level over seven stages corresponding to normal grammatical development. This study found that development was both delayed and deviant (Bamford/Mentz 1979). For the purposes of the study, 'deviant' was defined as uneven distribution of the frequency of structures at word, phrase and clause level. Development was considered delayed because samples were lacking in the recursive features, complex sentences and sentence connectivity expected in hearing children of comparable age. Hearing loss, intelligence and age were positively associated with development while age of onset, age of diagnosis and social class were only weakly associated with outcome. Another large scale investigation (Quigley/Power/Steinkamp 1977) in the U.S.A., using a specially devised Test of Syntactic Abilities, studied 450 children, 10–18 years, from various programmes. A considerable delay in the acquisition of English sentence structures was found: 18 year olds with hearing-impairment were unable to perform as well as 10 year old hearing children. Since the order of acquisition also differed, development was considered to be deviant. In written language, structures were identified that were not used by hearing students. In contrast, the Bamford study of spoken language found few such examples. Bamford/Mentz (1979) suggest that the processes involved in writing may lead to deviant structures or that the bias towards subjects with milder hearing losses in their study accounts for this finding. An important observation made by Quigley/Power/Steinkamp (1977) was that hearing-impaired children tended to process recursive structures in terms of word order and to treat all sentences as Subject-Verb-Object. Bishop (1983) investigated 79 severely and profoundly impaired children, 8–15 years, and their ability to comprehend structures in spoken, written and signed (artificial) form. Although there was greater difficulty and delay in understanding spoken forms, there was also evidence in the written and signed forms of systematic errors suggesting particular strategies were used for decoding. These strategies involved using the order of mention of items and imposing a subject-verb-object interpretation on recursive or embedded structures. Explanations for this linear processing are: (i) that they result from learning temporally ordered material through the visual channel that is primarily adapted for learning spatially organized material; (ii) that it is the product of teaching methods that emphasize particular simple structures at the expense of others; (iii) that there is interference from sign language structure which uses spatial rather than temporal ordering principles in grammar. There have been no investigations of these explanations although similar strategies have been noted in other groups with language disability (Bishop 1982, Quigley/King 1981).

4.5. Semantics

Little systematic attention has been given to the study of semantics. What is known comes from three different approaches. Firstly, investigations of lexical semantics began with normative comparisons with the hearing child and established that a delay was evident. It was suggested that some areas of experience might receive greater/lesser lexical representation because of differential sensory experience resulting from the hearing-impaired child's visual orientation to the world. Further, concepts predicated on auditory experience, those of time and the ordering of events, were considered to give greater difficulty. A second suggestion was that abstract words were fewer than concrete words in the lexicons of the hearing-impaired. Tweney/Hoeman/Andrews (1975) found, contrary to prediction, that the degree of abstraction in the lexicon was comparable for hearing and hearing-impaired adolescents. Some semantic fields were less well represented, particularly the field connected with words related to sounds. The third approach concerns the development of semantic relations. Comparisons between young hearing-impaired and hearing children matched for stage of language development in structural terms established that hearing-impaired infants exhibited the same semantic functions and communicative intentions but development was delayed (Skarakis/Prutting 1977). – It is sometimes suggested that the hearing-impaired experience difficulty with metaphorical aspects of language. Iran-Nejad/Ortony/Rittenhouse (1981) first established that providing reading material is within the syntactic competence of hearing-impaired children, these children are able to select metaphoric titles for simple stories as well as language-matched hearing children, if they are given some practice. This has been interpreted as indicating a difficulty in knowing when to interpret language in a metaphorical way because the ability is only demonstrated in such exercises.

4.6. Pragmatics

Since non-verbal elements can supplement oral linguistic forms there appears no reason why uses of language and intentions expressed by hearing-impaired children should be restricted. On the other hand, pragmatic skills are highly dependent on other areas of language development, particularly syntax. Curtis/Prutting/Lowell 1979) found in preschool children, across communicative contexts, that the range of intentions expressed was age-appropriate though the amount of communication and verbal ability to express these intentions was less than in hearing children of a similar age. Schirmer (1985) in contrast found that hearing-impaired children were delayed in using communicative functions. — Conversation is the main vehicle for assessment of pragmatic skills but, unlike other areas of competence, conversational abilities are the product of at least two speakers. The difficulties which oral hearing-impaired children experience in understanding and being understood can alter the character of their conversations as well as the contributions of their conversational partners. Wood/Wood/Griffiths et al. (1982) and Wood/Wood (1984) in observing classroom conversations between teachers and pupils communicating orally, noted that teachers exhibited high levels of control which were related to low levels of initiative and shorter conversational turns from the children. Teachers found difficulty in understanding the children and spent turns establishing understanding before a topic could develop. In these investigations and in a subsequent study of dinnertime conversations at home (Bodner-Johnson 1991), it was found that children with severe to profound hearing loss were able to interpret conversational moves and their meaning with few mistakes and to appreciate the obligations placed on them for reply. However, they were less successful in developing conversation and initiating themselves. — Wilbur (1977) investigating another aspect of pragmatics, cohesive devices used in narratives, found that hearing-impaired children had difficulties with the selection of indefinite and definite articles to indicate new or previously mentioned referents across sentence boundaries. Correct usage depends on the knowledge of the listener and the linguistic context. Wilbur maintains that these devices were used correctly at sentence level, which suggests that the problem was not syntactic but pragmatic; that is knowing when to use these devices. This could be explained by teaching methods which he maintained concentrated on teaching sentence structures and not on connected discourse.

5. Written Language

An understanding of the hearing-impaired child's mastery of written forms of language emerged from studies of educational achievement. At first these were attempts to evaluate competing educational programmes so that understanding the pattern of acquisition and the cognitive processes employed was relatively neglected. The difficulties experienced by the hearing-impaired are at first puzzling because access to written language is unaffected by a hearing loss. However, a well developed language system, usually internalized from spoken language use, seems the necessary foundation for reading. The study of the development of reading in the hearing-impaired helps to unravel the complex relationship between mastery of spoken and written forms of language. — Oral language acquisition was first studied through samples of written language because this avoided problems of poor speech intelligibility. Early studies provided descriptions of language produced using sentence length, type-token ratio, the frequency of different parts of speech, and number and types of errors made. Samples from written language were often quoted as well, since these measures failed to characterize the language sufficiently. The terms repeatedly used to describe the language were 'rigid', 'stereo-typed' and 'telegrammatic', the latter term referring to the predominance of 'content' as opposed to 'function words'. As with spoken language, opinions differed as to whether the language described was delayed or deviant. Later studies approached language using linguistically based approaches which give a better description and understanding of the nature of written language of the hearing-impaired (Quigley/Kretschmer 1982, 81 ff for review; Quigley/Montanelli/Wilbur 1976). At the age of 16–18 years, hearing-impaired adolescents had mastered the simpler structures of English in their written language but in some respects their writing differed from Standard English. Difficulties were noted with noun inflections, determiners, and with verb forms, particularly the auxiliary. Few attempts were made to employ complex structures and a preference for subject-verb-object simple sentences was demonstrated. These features probably account for previous findings which described written language as simple, rigid and stereo-typed.

5.1. Spelling

Studies of spelling ability (e. g. Hoeman/Andrews/Florian et al. 1976) suggest that this is one linguistic function in which hearing-impaired children are equal to or more advanced than hearing children. Dodd (1979) has suggested that this is the result of access to two routes to spelling: one which uses a visual route and a graphemic code; and the other, phoneme to grapheme correspondence rules which require a speech-based code. However, both Hoeman et al. (1976) and Dodd (1979) found that hearing-impaired children showed fewer errors of a phonetic character compared with hearing children. Dodd argues that some ability to use phoneme to grapheme rules can be demonstrated in children who are orally educated and that lip-reading skills play a part in the ability to use the phonemic route to spelling. Questions concerning spelling are linked with lip-reading and the acquisition of underlying phonological forms of spoken language (see sections 6.2.3. and 4.3.).

5.2. Reading

Research, which has used a variety of reading tests, studying children from different educational programmes, has repeatedly demonstrated the difficulty that hearing-impaired children experience in mastering reading. The achievements of school-leavers are disappointing (see Quigley/Kretschmer 1982 for a review). Mastery of written language is highly dependent on the mastery of spoken (oral) language which typically predates the acquisition of literacy. Hearing children map what they read onto what they know about the language: the knowledge of the structure and content of the language and possible messages to be conveyed helping the children to construct understanding from what they are able to recognize in print. The hearing-impaired child, however, is faced with learning both how to recognize what is represented by print and the structure of the language. The difficulties experienced by the hearing-impaired in understanding oral language in print are similar to those found in understanding spoken language even though the perceptual problems in reading are of course greatly reduced. The nature of the difficulties the hearing-impaired child experiences in understanding written text indicates that the problems of language comprehension experienced in spoken language are not simply or directly the result of difficulty in lip-reading, but are due to the inability to use the structures of oral language as a means of decoding language meaning. Here the debate about different methods of instruction taps some potentially interesting questions. Is it successful communication or the knowledge of the structure of oral language which is most important in learning to read? The mastery of written forms are difficult for children who have not yet mastered oral language structure. However, are children who communicate through sign language more or less proficient at mastering written language? If the problem lies in communication, then children who successfully develop sign language should have fewer problems with the written form and should be faced with a task similar to children acquiring a second language on entering school. Unfortunately, the answer to these questions is not clear cut because reading is not a simple unitary process. Disentangling the effects of language delay on communication, which results in a reduction in cultural understanding and world knowledge from difficulties in the teaching of reading, is one problem. Different abilities are involved at different stages of the learning process. Beginning readers depend on some abilities more than others, for example a linguistically-based code for recognition of novel words (Hanson/Liberman/Shankweiler 1984). Later, with increased experience of print, comprehension will then depend more on ability to use syntactic structures to decode meaning. As has been already discussed, both these abilities are affected by a hearing impairment. In addition, success in learning to read may be affected by teaching methods, the timing of instruction and the suitability of the materials used in the teaching process.

6. Lip-Reading

The understanding of lip-reading (speech-reading) has developed over the last two decades. However, a developmental account of its role in oral language acquisition in the hearing-impaired is lacking. (For a detailed review see Mogford 1987).

6.1. The Role of Lip-Reading in Language Acquisition

Lip-reading was once regarded as a compensatory visual-perceptual skill developed by the hearing-impaired for speech perception. For the prelingually hearing-impaired child with severe or profound hearing loss, who was acquiring oral language, lip-reading represented the primary means for acquisition even though information about the speech signal from observation of articulatory movements is considerably less than that available from an auditory signal. Lip-read information is limited by distance and poor illumination of the speaker's face (Erber 1971, 1974 a). Erber (1974 b) concluded that 40 English consonant and vowel phonemes produce only 16 discriminable units. In experiments with hearing subjects, Binnie/Montgomery/Jackson (1974) and Dodd (1977) showed that, for consonants, place of articulation is best conveyed through vision. However, voicing and manner are largely conveyed through hearing. This implies these features are difficult to detect visually. Erber (1974 b) concluded that the same would be true for hearing-impaired subjects. When a sign language or finger-spelling is used with speech, lip-reading is only one of several forms in which linguistic information is carried. The degree of reliance on lip-reading varies with severity of hearing impairment. While children with mild hearing-impairment make use of lip-read information intermittently, for example, when learning new lexical items, those with more severe hearing losses rely on lip-reading at all times. This places constraints on the management of interpersonal interaction, for the lip-reader needs to visually monitor the face of the speaker. Perception of conversational exchanges can be incomplete because monitoring speakers, in turn, is very difficult. — While lip-reading was regarded as a compensatory skill, the linguistic and cognitive components of the skill were not understood. This was reflected in the variety of methods used to assess lip-reading which often failed to control for the level of general linguistic development of those assessed. Research has now established that auditory experience of speech enhances visual speech recognition and that visual speech cues are used with greater skill by the hearing (Dodd 1980). For the hearing, the development of lip-reading is the product of a bi-modal process: distinctions available through audition can serve as a basis for determining the visual distinctions that correlate with acoustic features. For the hearing-impaired, as the hearing loss increases, the degree of reliance on visual speech information through lip-reading can be assumed to increase despite technical improvements in hearing aids and the emphasis in oral programmes on auditory training. As lip-reading improves with the degree of residual hearing (Conrad 1979, 186), it seems that for the hearing-impaired also, lip-reading is enhanced through input from two sensory modalities even though the quantity and quality of information from the auditory channel is relatively reduced.

6.2. Lip-Reading Research

Lip-reading is defined in different ways by different researchers and hence the abilities measured also vary. For example, lip-reading can be equated either with comprehension of spoken sentences with aided hearing or the ability to recognize phonemes in permissible nonsense words without the use of hearing aids. Often in measuring lip-reading there has been no attempt to control for receptive language ability and so it is not possible to separate difficulties due to lack of linguistic knowledge from the visual-perceptual task of speech perception. Lip-reading has been investigated for a number of different reasons. Firstly, lip-reading has frequently been investigated when assessing the relative merits of methods of education for the prelinguistically deaf. Different methods place different degrees of emphasis on lip-reading and its training. — Secondly, individual differences in lip-reading skill in children from similar educational programmes have been the focus of research. Thirdly, the nature of the linguistic and cognitive processes involved in lip-reading with the prelingually deaf child has been investigated: a relationship between lip-reading and other linguistic abilities including spelling, reading and speech is indicated. — In research, lip-reading is studied under ideal conditions which removes the task from the normal demands of interaction. Under normal language learning circumstances, conditions are rarely optimal. A comprehensive account of the development of lip-reading and its role in language acquisition should include the development of appropriate gaze patterns that allow lip-reading to be integrated with interpersonal interaction and tasks that demand visual attention.

6.2.1. Lip-Reading and Educational Methods

Some evaluations of different communication methods used in language acquisition introduced confounding socio-cultural and aetiological factors. For example, comparisons of deaf children reared by deaf (signing) parents and those reared by hearing (oral) parents ignored factors that varied systematically with parental hearing status. There appears to be no evidence that any manual form of communication interferes with lip-reading skills or that additional training in lip-reading confers any advantage. However, research which reflects the bilingual nature of language development suggests that the timing of exposure to manual communication may affect the development of lip-reading skills in the longer term (Parasnis 1983).

6.2.2. Predicting Success in Lip-Reading

Individual differences in lip-reading have frequently been reported even when the degree of hearing loss and methods of communication are controlled. One variable frequently examined is intelligence, although tests of lip-reading and intelligence used have varied between studies. A review of studies by Farwell (1976) stressed variability in the correlations reported for lip-reading and intelligence. Conrad (1979, 192) highlighted some studies omitted from this review which reported significant correlations between lip-reading and intelligence. Some investigators found a positive correlation between intelligence and lip-reading skill which was stronger for better lip-readers but weaker at the lower ranges of ability. Other variables have been investigated and the most reliable finding is that lip-reading measures show a close relationship with other measures of language ability. This is not surprising when lip-reading is the primary means of language reception. However, significant correlations have also been found with finger-spelling and sign usage (Meadow 1968) where the medium of communication is not primarily spoken language. – Conrad (1979, 186) broke new ground by measuring lip-reading relative to the language competence of each individual. Language competence was assessed through the written medium. He found weak significant correlations with intelligence for subjects already grouped by severity of hearing loss. – Attempts to explain poor lip-reading in terms of specific learning difficulties have failed. A different approach examined competence in a range of visual-perceptual skills with varying degrees of relevance to lip-reading, including visual memory. This research shed little light on the specific cognitive processes involved in visual speech recognition because it lacked an adequate model of the processes.

6.2.3. Lip Reading and Memory Codes

Auditory speech perception entails a coding mechanism for immediate storage of material until completion of higher level processing. Visual speech perception also requires a compatible memory storage system. In auditory perception this has been shown to be based on a phonological code. This code is also implicated in other linguistic skills, such as learning to read (Hanson/Liberman/Shankweiler 1984), spelling and speech production (Dodd 1979). Are the hearing-impaired able to develop a phonological code which can be used for working memory in visual speech recognition? Dodd/Hermelin (1977) concluded that the ability to store and use phonological information in an experimental task was not dependent on the auditory modality. However, it is possible that residual hearing was involved in the development of this ability. Conrad (1979, 114) showed that in prelingually hearing-impaired school-leavers there were individual differences in the use of a phonological code in an immediate memory task, which varied with hearing loss and intelligence. This suggests two sources of information about the speech signal help to develop a speech-based code although a profound hearing loss did not entirely preclude the use of an internal speech code. Conrad (1979, 193 ff) also demonstrated a relationship between the use of a speech-based code and lip-reading when hearing loss and intelligence were controlled. This relationship broke down at profound levels of hearing impairment. – The development of vibrotactile aids allows the hypothesis that two independent channels of information promote the development of lip-reading skill and a phonological code to be tested. These hearing aids convert acoustic speech signals to a tactile form to supplement lip-reading. Trials with early devices used artificially deafened subjects but there is some evidence that they can enhance success in lip-reading for prelingually hearing-impaired subjects also (De Filippo 1984).

6.2.4. The Development of Lip-Reading

Scientific and educational opinion has been profoundly pessimistic about the ability of severely and profoundly hearing-impaired to acquire oral language through the medium of lip-reading. (Conrad 1979, 203; Brasel/Quigley 1977) Lip-reading appeared to be an inefficient way of communicating information to the hearing-impaired compared with communication that involved combinations of methods or the printed word (Gates 1971). These views lead to the introduction of communication methods that use a variety of visual forms to enhance language learning. However, despite the central role given to lip-reading in oral language development, there have been few attempts to study lip-reading developmentally other than recording correlations of skill with chronological age and plotting the rate of progress by age. This implies the nature of the skill is the same throughout the course of development which is unlikely. There is limited evidence that the process changes with development, as is the case with oral language comprehension (Green/Green/Holmes 1980, 1981; De Filippo 1982). A complete developmental account would also include interactional gaze patterns permitting the development of visual speech processing.

7. Sign Language Acquisition

For many years the sign languages used in deaf communities were stigmatized by the hearing and not accorded the status of a language. This was the case although as many as three-quarters of the deaf adults in the United States were estimated to use American Sign Language in 1969. Linguistic description of sign languages began in 1960 with William Stokoe who worked on Ameslan, American Sign Language. This was followed by the work of Klima/Bellugi (1979, 1 ff). Similar work in Britain on British Sign Language (Brennan 1981) and in France led to similarities between sign languages and between spoken and signed languages being recognized. This work established properties of formal structuring and organizational principles, e. g. constrained systems of features, rules based on underlying forms, recursive grammatical processes. The research also described those characteristics peculiar to sign languages which demonstrated that at all structural levels sign languages are influenced by the modality. It was found that sign languages had levels analogous to phonology, morphology and syntax but adapted to the visuo-spatial modality. — Some features of Ameslan acquisition were reported by Schlesinger/Meadow. This study (Schlesinger/Meadow 1972, 45 ff) reported on two children of deaf parents, growing up in homes using Ameslan. This and other studies began to establish that, in spite of the difference in modality, the milestones and the nature of language acquisition were similar to that of hearing children acquiring oral language. Also the nature, rate and language acquired contrasted markedly with comparative data for hearing-impaired children acquiring oral language (Gregory/Mogford 1981). Schlesinger/Meadow (1972, 87 ff) also stressed that the quality of interaction and experience of language and communication was more relaxed and natural than for deaf children who were learning oral language. One reason for the more advanced and rapid acquisition of sign as a first language in the hearing-impaired when parents are sign language users is that the child's exposure to language models is not delayed or dependent on diagnosis as with hearing-impaired children in hearing families learning oral language. Such comparisons of language acquisition might suggest that one medium of language acquisition is better than another. Such conclusions cannot be drawn from these studies because they do not provide a controlled evaluation of different communication methods. In addition to differences in age of exposure to language models, the situations are not comparable in many ways. — Sign language acquisition in families where sign language is acquired from competent signing adults is different from instances where a form of signing is learned from hearing parents whose first language is oral and who have no experience of communicating with the hearing-impaired. These parents acquire a second language, in a different modality, at the same time modelling this for their hearing-impaired child. In addition, it is rare for hearing parents to choose to sign exclusively to their child, preferring what Meadow (1980, 23) has termed bi-modal communication, using a combination of signed and spoken English simultaneously, with signs following the pattern of spoken language (see section 1.2.3.). Native signers may be employed to provide language models for hearing-impaired children of hearing parents (Fletcher 1987, 153) but the situation is still not comparable with children who learn sign language from parents who are competent signers. Schlesinger/Meadow (1972, 45 ff) also studied the language of two children whose hearing parents were using both signed and spoken English. The children, both diagnosed towards the end of their first year, began bimodal acquisition at different ages, 15 and 37 months (Schlesinger/Meadow 1972, 82 ff). Early acquisition showed similarities with the acquisition of spoken English by hearing children, but later differences in grammatical development were found. These were explained in terms of the perceptual salience of morphemes in the visual and auditory modes. – The nature of the language acquisition task for deaf children learning sign languages has been further elucidated by Bellugi and her associates (Bellugi/van Hoek/Lillo-Martin/O'Grady 1988). Bellugi argues that the iconic nature of much sign could make the mapping of meaning onto form easier. Longitudinal and cross-sectional studies of American Sign Language acquisition from onset to 10 years of age have found precisely the same order of acquisition for parallel stages at similar ages as hearing children learning spoken languages. They have also found important discontinuities between preverbal gesture and the early linguistic system though superficially signs/gestures may look identical. In these studies there are examples of errors that demonstrate that the child acquiring sign language does not simply imitate the models that he observes. As with hearing children learning spoken language, the mistakes are evidence of the child's acquisition of a rule based system. These studies seem to indicate that language acquisition can be unimpaired if the deaf child is exposed to a language which is easily perceived. This is the case with sign language even though it uses organizational principles suited to the visual system. – A further aspect of sign language acquisition concerns the reported creation of sign language by children who are unable to profit from the oral models presented by hearing parents. Goldin-Meadow/Feldman (1975) reported that prelingual hearing-impaired children were able to create a sign language to communicate, employing invented signs which they began to combine in ways similar to the first two word combinations in hearing children. However, there have been few other studies that have reported this phenomenon. Indeed, in a similar study Gregory/Mogford (1981) found no evidence of this. The reason for this difference has not been satisfactorily explained.

8. Summary and Conclusions

The character of language development in the prelingually hearing-impaired seems to depend primarily on the form of language which the child acquires and the availability of interaction with competent users of the language. Studies of sign language acquisition in children whose families communicate using sign language show considerable agreement. The pattern, rate and characteristics of the process are similar and parallel to those of hearing children acquiring spoken language. This contrasts strongly with the process of spoken language acquisition in children with hearing parents and accomplishments of prelingually impaired children in learning to read and write, whatever the form of their first language. Even though there are some able individuals who successfully develop oral language, the average pattern of development shows considerable delay in developing linguistic competence. Opinions seem to differ about the developmental, social and educational significance of this delay. There is evidence that the delay and difficulty experienced in understanding and using spoken language affects the learning process itself, altering patterns of interaction between the children and parents, siblings and teachers. When language delay leads to attempts to teach language, this may further affect the character of the language acquired. The difficulties experienced by children with more severe prelingual hearing loss, particularly in lip-reading, and the fact that only a minority of children are born into families who use sign, has encouraged a greater use of simultaneous methods of communication at home and school. Most of these methods, it should be noted, still aim to enable the child to acquire the structure of spoken language. The additional manual forms function to make the structure of spoken language easily accessible through vision. Although there have been studies to evaluate the effect of these approaches on different aspects and stages of language acquisition, a comprehensive review of language acquisition through simultaneous presentation has not been undertaken. There are many versions of simultaneous communication methods and even those methods that go under the same name may vary in many subtle ways: in the way they are used; and when and how they are introduced. Preliminary reports describe simultaneous methods in use. They suggest that there is often a gap between what is intended and the language input that occurs. This is sometimes because speakers of oral language have difficulty acquiring more than a simple vocabulary of signs: the grammar of sign language being based on different organizational principles from spoken language. Another problem is coordinating sign and speech. Sign makes use of spatial devices and is more economical in time than speech. Trying to sign and speak simultaneously can result in reduced verbal forms. — Studies of language acquisition in the hearing-impaired have mainly concentrated on children with severe and profound hearing loss. Less attention has been given to those with mild, moderate and unilateral hearing losses. Evidence so far tends to indicate a pattern of language delay which though not severe can still provide educational and social difficulties. — The effect of a hearing deficit acquired during language acquisition is harder to assess. Considerable resources have been invested in studies of the effect of the most common, mild form of childhood hearing impairment that results from middle ear effusion. Improved research methods make the results of studies more reliable but still there is no consensus about the effects. Those delays that have been described are not severe. Differences between children with recurrent episodes and those not effected may persist into later childhood but it is difficult to establish how significant these differences are for individual achievement and why the difficulties persist. If otitis media with effusion has lasting effects on speech discrimination, even after spontaneous recovery or treatment, this is of considerable practical and theoretical concern. There are several possible alternative explanations for the persisting effects of transient hearing loss and these need to be elaborated and then investigated. — The study of language acquisition in the prelingually impaired is not only of practical significance but can also contribute to the understanding of language acquisition in children without impairment. The nature and success of sign language acquisition suggests that any species-specific predisposition to acquire language must be relatively independent of the modality through which it is acquired.

9. References

Abberton, E., Fourcin, J., & Hazan, V. (1986). Phonological competence with profound hearing loss. *Speech, Hearing and Language. Work in Progress.* 3—14. University College, London.

Bamford, J. (1979). The design of the study. In J. Bench & J. Bamford (Eds.), *Speech-hearing tests and the spoken language of hearing-impaired children. 73—110.* London: Academic Press.

Bamford, J. & Mentz, L. (1979). Spoken language: grammar. In J. Bench & J. Bramford (Eds.), *Speech-hearing tests and the spoken language of hearing-impaired children. 381—471.* London: Academic Press.

Bellugi, U., van Hoek, K., Lillo-Martin, D., & O'Grady, L. (1988). The acquisition of syntax and space in young deaf signers. In D. Bishop & K. Mogford (Eds.), *Language development in exceptional circumstances. 132—149.* Edinburgh: Churchill Livingstone.

Binnie, C. A., Montgomery, A. A., & Jackson, P. L. (1974). Auditory and visual contributions to the perception of consonants. *Journal of Speech and Hearing Research, 17,* 619—630.

Bishop, D. V. M. (1982). Comprehension of spoken, written and signed sentences in childhood language disorders. *Journal of Child Psychiatry and Psychology, 23,* 1—20.

Bishop, D. V. M. (1983). Comprehension of English syntax by profoundly deaf children. *Journal of Child Psychology and Psychiatry, 24,* 415—434.

Bishop, D. & Rosenbloom, L. (1987). Classification of childhood language disorders. In W. Yule & M. Rutter (Eds.), *Language development and disorders, 16—41.* Oxford: Mackeith Press with Blackwell Scientific.

Bodner-Johnson, B. (1991). Family conversation style: Its effect on the deaf child's participation. *Exceptional Children, 57,* 502—509.

Brasel, K. & Quigley, S. P. (1977). The influence of certain language and communication environments in early childhood on the development of language in deaf individuals. *Journal of Speech and Hearing Research, 20,* 95—107.

Brennan, M. (1981). Grammatical processes in British Sign Language. In B. Woll, J. Kyle, & M. Deuchar (Eds.), *Perspectives on British Sign Language and deafness. 120—135.* London: Croom Helm.

Brookhouser, P. E. & Goldgar, D. E. (1987). Medical profile of the language-delayed child: otitis prone versus otitis free. *International Journal of Paediatric Otorhinolaryngology, 12,* 237—271.

Brown, J. (1984). Examination of grammatical morphemes in the language of hard of hearing children. *Volta Review, 86,* 229—238.

Bruner, J. (1975). From communication to language: A psychological perspective. *Cognition, 3,* 255–287.

Carrel, R. E. (1977). Epidemiology of hearing loss. In S. E. Gerber (Ed.), *Audiometry in infancy. 3–17.* New York: Grune and Stratton.

Chalmers, D., Stewart, I., Silva, P., & Mulvena, A. (1989). *Otitis media with effusion in children – The Dunedin Study.* Oxford: MacKeith Press with Blackwell Scientific.

Cheskin, A. (1982). The use of language by hearing mothers of deaf children. *Journal of Communication Disorders, 15,* 145–153.

Commission of the European Community. (1979). *Childhood deafness in the European Community.* Contract No. 359-77-9. Ec. 1. UK. Luxembourg: C.E.C. Committee on Medical and Public Health Research.

Conrad, R. (1979). *The deaf schoolchild: language and cognitive function.* London: Harper and Row.

Cooper, R. L. & Rosenstein, J. (1966). Language acquisition in deaf children. *Volta Review, 68,* 58–67.

Cornett, O. (1967). Cued speech. *American Annals of the Deaf, 112,* 3–13.

Crystal, D., Fletcher, P., & Garman, M. (1976). *The grammatical analysis of language disability: A procedure for assessment and remediation.* London: Edward Arnold.

Culbertson, J. L. & Gilbert, L. E. (1986). Children with unilateral sensorineural hearing loss: cognitive, academic and social development. *Ear and Hearing, 7,* 38–42.

Curtis, S., Prutting, C. A., & Lowell, E. L. (1979). Pragmatic and semantic development in young children with impaired hearing. *Journal of Speech and Hearing Research, 22,* 534–552.

Dalzell, J. & Owrid, H. L. (1976). Children with conductive deafness: A follow-up study. *British Journal of Audiology, 10,* 87–90.

Davis, J. M. (1977). Reliability of hearing-impaired children's responses to oral and total presentations of The Test of Auditory Comprehension of Language. *Journal of Speech and Hearing Disorders, 42,* 520–527.

Davis, J. M. (1986). Effects of mild and moderate hearing impairments on language, educational and psychosocial behaviour in children. *Journal of Speech and Hearing Disorders, 51,* 53–62.

De Filippo, C. L. (1982). Memory for articulated sequences and lipreading performance of hearing-impaired observers. *Volta Review, 31,* 134–146.

De Filippo, C. L. (1984). Laboratory projects in tactile aids to lipreading. *Ear and Hearing, 5,* 211–227.

DiBartolomeo, J. R. & Gerber, S. E. (1977). Pathology of hearing loss. In S. E. Gerber (Ed.), *Audiometry in infancy. 17–44.* New York: Grune and Stratton.

Dobie, R. A. & Berlin, C. I. (1979). Influence of otitis media on hearing and development. *Annals of Otology, Rhinology and Laryngology, 88, (Suppl. 60),* 48–53.

Dodd, B. (1976). The phonological systems of deaf children. *Journal of Speech and Hearing Disorders, 41,* 185–198.

Dodd, B. (1977). The role of vision in the perception of speech. *Perception, 76,* 31–40.

Dodd, B. (1979). The spelling abilities of profoundly pre-lingually deaf children. In U. Frith (Ed.), *Cognitive processes in spelling. 423–440.* London: Academic Press.

Dodd, B. (1980). The interaction of auditory and visual information in speech perception. *British Journal of Psychology, 71,* 541–549.

Dodd, B. (1987). Lip-reading, phonological coding and deafness. In B. Dodd & R. Campbell (Eds.), *Hearing by eye: The psychology of lip-reading. 177–190.* New Jersey: Lawrence Erlbaum.

Dodd, B. & Hermelin, B. (1977). Phonological coding by the prelinguistically deaf. *Perception and Psychophysics, 21,* 413–417.

Erber, N. P. (1971). Effects of distance on the visual reception of speech. *Journal of Speech and Hearing Research, 14,* 848–857.

Erber, N. P. (1974a). Angle, distance and illumination on normal reception of speech. *Journal of Speech and Hearing Research, 17,* 99–112.

Erber, N. P. (1974b). Visual perception of speech by deaf children. Recent developments and continuing needs. *Journal of Speech and Hearing Disorders, 39,* 178–185.

Farwell, R. M. (1976). Speech reading: a research review. *American Annals of the Deaf, 121,* 19–30.

Fletcher, L. (1987). *Language for Ben. A deaf child's right to sign.* London: Souvenir Press.

Gates, R. R. (1971). The reception of verbal information by deaf students through a television medium. A comparison of speech reading, manual communication and reading. *Proceedings of the Convention of the American Instructors of the Deaf. 513–522.* Washington: U.S. Government Printing Office.

Geers, A. & Moog, J. (1978). Syntactic maturity of spontaneous speech and elicited imitations of hearing-impaired children. *Journal of Speech and Hearing Disorders, 43,* 380–391.

Goldin-Meadow, S. & Feldman, H. (1975). The creation of a communication system: A study of deaf children of hearing parents. *Sign Language Studies, 8,* 225–236.

Green, D. S. (1978). Pure tone air-conduction testing. In J. Katz (Ed.), *Handbook of clinical audiology. 98–109.* Baltimore: Williams and Wilkins.

Green, K.W., Green, W. B., & Holmes, D.W. (1980). Speech reading abilities of young deaf children. *American Annals of the Deaf, 125,* 906–908.

Green, K.W., Green, W. B., & Holmes, D.W. (1981). Speech reading skills of young normal and deaf children. *American Annals of the Deaf, 126,* 505–509.

Gregory, S. & Mogford, K. (1981). Early language development in deaf children. In B. Woll, J. Kyle, & M. Deuchar (Eds.), *Perspectives on British Sign Language and deafness. 218–237.* London: Croom Helm.

Gregory, S., Mogford, K., & Bishop, J. (1979). Mothers' speech to young hearing impaired children. *Teacher of the Deaf, 3,* 42–43.

Hanson, V. L., Liberman, I. Y., & Shankweiler, D. (1984). Linguistic coding by deaf children in relation to beginning reading success. *Journal of Experimental Child Psychology, 37,* 378–393.

Hoeman, H.W., Andrews, C. E., Florian, V. A., Hoeman, S. A., & Jensema, C. J. (1976). The spelling proficiency of deaf children. *American Annals of the Deaf, 121,* 489–493.

Holm, V. A. & Kunze, L. H. (1969). Effect of chronic otits media on language and speech development. *Paediatrics, 43,* 833–839.

Iran-Nejad, A., Ortony, A., & Rittenhouse, R. (1981). The comprehension of metaphorical uses of English by deaf children. *Journal of Speech and Hearing Research, 24,* 551–556.

Klee, T. M. & Davis-Dansky, E. (1986). A comparison of unilaterally hearing-impaired children and normal-hearing children on a battery of standardised language tests. *Ear and Hearing, 7,* 27–37.

Klein, S. K. & Rapin, I. (1988). Intermittent conductive hearing loss and language development. In D. Bishop & K. Mogford (Eds.), *Language development in exceptional circumstances. 96–109.* Edinburgh: Churchill Livingstone.

Klima, E. S. & Bellugi, U. (1979). *The signs of language.* Cambridge, Mass: Harvard University Press.

Lawson, L. (1981). The role of sign in the structure of the deaf community. In B. Woll, J. Kyle, & M. Deuchar (Eds.), *Perspectives on British Sign Language and deafness. 166–177.* London: Croom Helm.

Lenneberg, E. H., Rebelsky, G. F., & Nichols, I. A. (1965). The vocalisations of infants born to deaf and to hearing parents. *Human Development, 8,* 23–37.

Markides, A. (1970). The speech of deaf and partially-hearing children with special reference to factors affecting intelligibility. *British Journal of Disorders of Communication, 5,* 126–140.

Meadow, K. P. (1968). Early manual communication in relation to the child's intellectual, social and communicative functioning. *American Annals of the Deaf, 113,* 29–41.

Meadow, K. P. (1980). *Deafness and child development.* London: Arnold.

Mills, A. E. (1987). The development of phonology in the blind child. In B. Dodd & R. Campbell (Eds.), *Hearing by eye: The psychology of lip-reading. 145–161.* New Jersey: Lawrence Erlbaum.

Mogford, K. (1987). Lip-reading in the prelingually deaf. In B. Dodd & R. Campbell (Eds.), *Hearing by eye: The psychology of lip-reading. 191–212.* New Jersey: Lawrence Erlbaum.

Mogford, K. (1988). Oral language acquisition in the prelinguistically deaf. In D. Bishop & K. Mogford (Eds.), *Language development in exceptional circumstances. 110–113.* Edinburgh: Churchill Livingstone.

Needleman, H. (1977). Effects of hearing loss from early recurrent otitis media on speech and language development. In B. F. Jaffe (Ed.), *Hearing loss in children. 640–649.* Baltimore: University Park Press.

Nienhuys, T. G., Horsborough, K. M., & Cross, T. G. (1985). A dialogic analysis of interaction between mothers and their deaf or hearing preschoolers. *Applied Psycholinguistics, 6,* 121–140.

Oller, D. K. (1986). Metaphonology and infant vocalisation. In B. Lindblom & R. Zetterstrom (Eds.), *Precursors of early speech. 21–36.* Basingstoke: Macmillan.

Oller, D. K. & Kelly, C. A. (1974). Phonological substitution processes of a hard-of-hearing child. *Journal of Speech and Hearing Disorders, 39,* 65–74.

Paradise, J. L. (1981). Otitis media during early life; how hazardous to development? A critical review of the literature. *Paediatrics, 68,* 869–873.

Parasnis, I. (1983). Effects of parental deafness and early exposure to manual communication on cognitive skills and field independence of young deaf adults. *Journal of Speech and Hearing Research, 26,* 588–594.

Presnell, L. (1973). Hearing-impaired children's comprehension and production in oral language. *Journal of Speech and Hearing Research, 16,* 12–21.

Quigley, S. P. & King, C. M. (1981). An invited article: Syntactic performance of hearing-impaired and normal individuals. *Applied Psycholinguistics, 1,* 329–356.

Quigley, S. P. & Kretschmer, R. E. (1982). *The education of deaf children. Issues, theory and practice.* London: Arnold.

Quigley, S. P., Montanelli, D., & Wilbur, R. (1976). Some aspects of the verb system in the language of deaf students. *Journal of Speech and Hearing Research, 19,* 536–550.

Quigley, S. P., Power, D. J., & Steinkamp, M. W. (1977). The language structure of deaf children. *Volta Review, 79,* 73–84.

Roberts, J. E., Sanynl, M. A., Burchinal, M. R., Collier, A. M., Ranney, C. T., & Henderson, F. W. (1986). Otitis media in early childhood and its relationship to later verbal and academic performance. *Paediatrics, 78,* 428–430.

Schlesinger, H. S. & Meadow, K. (1972). *Sound and sign. Childhood deafness and mental health.* Berkeley: University of California Press.

Schirmer, B. R. (1985). An analysis of the language of young hearing-impaired children in terms of syntax, semantics and use. *American Annals of the Deaf, 130,* 15–19.

Skarakis, E. A. & Prutting, C. A. (1977). Early communication: semantic functions and communicative intentions in the communication of the preschool child with impaired hearing. *American Annals of the Deaf, 122,* 382–391.

Smith, N. (1982). Some observations concerning pre-meaningful vocalisations of hearing impaired infants. *Journal of Speech and Hearing Disorders, 47,* 439–442.

Stoel-Gammon, C. & Otomo, K. (1986). Babbling development of hearing-impaired and normally hearing subjects. *Journal of Speech and Hearing Disorders, 51,* 33–40.

Swisher, L. (1976). The language performance of the oral deaf. In H. Whitaker & H. A. Whitaker (Eds.), *Studies in neurolinguistics, Vol. II. 59–93.* London: Academic Press.

Tweney, R. D., Hoeman, H. W., & Andrews, C. E. (1975). Semantic organisation in deaf and hearing subjects. *Journal of Psycholinguistic Research, 4,* 61–73.

Ventry, I. M. (1980). Effects of conductive hearing loss. Fact or fiction? *Journal of Speech and Hearing Disorders, 45,* 143–156.

West, J. & Weber, J. A. (1973). A phonological analysis of the spontaneous language of a 4-year old hard-of-hearing child. *Journal of Speech and Hearing Disorders, 38,* 25–35.

Wilbur, R. (1977). An explanation of deaf children's difficulty with certain syntactic structures in English. *Volta Review, 79,* 85–92.

Wilcox, J. & Tobin, H. (1974). Linguistic performance of hard-of-hearing and normal hearing children. *Journal of Speech and Hearing Research, 17,* 286–293.

Wood, D. & Wood, H. A. (1984). An experimental evaluation of the effects of five styles of teacher conversation on the language of hearing-impaired children. *Journal of Child Psychology and Psychiatry, 25,* 45–62.

Wood, D. J., Wood, H. A., Griffiths, A. J., Howarth, S. P., & Howarth, C. I. (1982). The structure of conversations with 6- to 10-year-old deaf children. *Journal of Child Psychology and Psychiatry, 23,* 295–308.

Kay Mogford-Bevan, Newcastle (U.K.)

66. Language Acquisition and Development with Sensory Impairment: Blind Children

1. Theoretical and Methodological Issues

1.1. Models of Language Acquisition

In those models of language development which have their basis within linguistic theory, in particular those models which assume an innate, specifically linguistic, component, sensory impairment involving lack of vision should not result in any problems with the acquisition of the formal properties of language (see Chomsky's claim in his debate with Piaget (Piattelli-Palmarini 1980, 171)). Data from blind children provide therefore a testing ground for such predictions.

If language acquisition is viewed as dependent on cognitive development, if only in part, then clearly problems in cognitive development might predict problems in language for blind children. This possibility of prediction is dependent on the assumption of close links between specific areas of cognition and specific areas of language. The cognitive development of blind children certainly appears to be different in some areas (Warren 1977) but it is not clear that these areas are always relevant to language. The data from blind children are of interest in this complex issue particularly in relation to aspects of their semantic development.

Within a social-interactive framework the way adults interact in communication with blind children and the kind of language that serves as input will directly affect the process of language acquisition. Much recent work on language-disordered populations has been done within this framework, although little direct causal relationship between input and acquisition has been indicated.

Research on blind children's language has been done within a variety of frameworks, although a large number of studies have been observational. Two larger studies (Burlingham 1972; Fraiberg 1977) were within a psycho-analytic perspective.

1.2. Methodological Issues

1.2.1. Definition of Blindness

In order to research the relationship between the lack of vision and language acquisition, it is important that the subjects in a particular study form a homogeneous group. This is difficult to control for. Visual handicap varies from no perception of light through to extreme short-sightedness. Blindness is a legal definition which varies between countries. Blindness can also be a functional concept related to a particular task; thus a person may be able to identify features on objects when held close but be functionally blind in terms of orientation at a distance. It is also very difficult to assess visual acuity accurately in very young children.

1.2.2. Age of Onset

Comparable to hearing-impaired children, the onset of blindness is important as a variable in a research population. Visual experience during the period of language acquisition should not be underestimated, particularly in relation to the use of nonverbal communicative behaviors.

1.2.3. Frequency of Visual Handicap

Figures on the occurrence of blindness in different countries are difficult to come by. In Western industrial societies approximately 2 children in 10,000 are born blind; 18 become blind in the course of later life. This figure is far higher in other societies, where blindness frequently results for example from eye infection. In Western societies blindness as a result of difficult post-natal care in premature babies (retro-lental fibroplasia) is declining. So too is blindness which is the result of a genetic condition, through the preventive effects of genetic counselling.

Apparently increasing is the occurrence of blindness with another handicap. Conservative figures average around 50%; some studies indicate a figure as high as 90% (Jan/Freeman/Scott 1977). Research on the effects of lack of vision need a population in which blindness is the only problem. This population is difficult to find. At the young age at which most language acquisition research needs to take place it is also difficult to be sure of the diagnosis, that is to be sure that blindness is the only handicap. Many studies have taken the form of case studies for these reasons. Through the lack of homogeneity in the populations studied, the comparison and interpretation of results become also problematic.

2. Phonology

2.1. Babbling

Almost all studies which begin in the prelingual period record a normal onset of babbling (e.g. Junefelt 1987; Mills 1987; Warren 1977). Fraiberg (1977) judged the amount of babbling in the ten blind infants she observed to be less than in sighted infants but it was not quantified in this study. Rowland (1984) found the frequency of vocalization in the five infants she observed to be within normal ranges but that the vocalizations occurred at different points in the interaction from sighted children. This point will be resumed later (5.1.). In summary, babbling seen as a precursor to the acquisition of speech sounds does not seem to differ greatly from babbling in sighted children.

2.2. Perception of Speech Sounds

Few studies have been done in this area and seemingly none with young blind children. Semzova (1961), in an audiometric study of 38 blind children (7–16 years), found no difference. Lucas (1984) found better identification of mispronounced words in a story context in children aged between five and seven years, but no detailed phonological analysis was carried out of the material. There is a great deal of work still to be done here, particularly in relation to differences which have been found in speech sound production.

2.3. Production of Speech Sounds

2.3.1. Early Production

A longitudinal study of three young blind children (1–2 years, German-speaking) indicated a clear influence of blindness on the acquisition of speech sound production (Mills 1983; Mills 1987). An analysis was made of the production of consonants categorized according to the visibility of the articulation of the consonant. Thus sounds with highly visible articulation (labials, labio-dentals) were compared with sounds with a less visible articulation (alveolars, velars etc.). The blind children made more errors than the sighted children on the consonants with a highly visible articulation (41% vs. 21%). On the production of consonants with a less visible articulation the sighted and blind children did not differ. Thus the sighted children have an advantage in their acquisition of the visible consonants.

The pattern of substitution errors made is also slightly different for blind children. Whereas sighted children rarely substitute a sound from a different visual category for a target sound, blind children do this more frequently (34% such errors vs. 10%). This finding has been substantiated by later work (Dodd 1983; Mulford 1989).

2.3.2. Effect on Early Vocabulary

As has been found for sighted children, the pattern of phonological acquisition also affects the vocabulary produced at this age. Since this pattern is different in blind children, it is also reflected in their attempted words: they produce far fewer words containing a highly visible consonant compared to sighted children. The predominance of labials in the early lexicon has been explained by distributional factors and/or physiological factors but clearly the role of visual information must be included here (Vihman/Macken/Miller et al. 1985). It must also be included in a model of phonological acquisition since its absence produces a different pattern of acquisition in blind children.

2.3.3. Adult Phonology

Detailed studies of later phonological acquisition are not available. One study of sound production in blind teenagers (Göllecz 1972) indicated differences in lip movements for the articulation of vowels, but minimal differences in acoustic properties. This appears to be due to a compensatory restriction of the oral resonance chamber. This constitutes a different endpoint of acquisition for blind children in articulatory terms but not in phonological terms.

2.3.4. Phonological Disorder?

The different pattern of acquisition found in younger children does not lead necessarily to a disorder, but means a temporary delay in a specific area of phonology. Some studies do report a higher incidence of articulation problems in older blind children (Elstner 1983; Miner 1963) but it is not clear which particular areas are problematic. Since the populations investigated in these studies are large and multiply-handicapped children are not explicitly excluded, the question arises if blindness is the cause of these problems.

3. Morphology and Syntax

3.1. Language Onset

Several studies report a delay in the onset of language, that is the occurrence of the first word (e. g. Fraiberg 1977; Reynell 1978). Others report a delay in the acquisition of combining two words. These studies are often difficult to interpret since full information on other aspects of development are missing: it is not clear if another handicap is involved. Secondly in the studies cited above, many of the blind children's language measures fell within the normal range, although the mean for the group indicated a delay. It is clear then that blindness does not mean a necessary general delay in morphology and syntax.

Mulford (1989) summarizes results from 14 more recent case studies and finds no major delay in early development. She suggests that the discrepancy between earlier and later studies can possibly be explained by the shift in the cause of blindness in Western industrial societies. As mentioned above, retro-lental fibroplasia (RLF) has declined rapidly over the last twenty years but was a main cause of blindness before then. This condition is caused by the administration of too much oxygen to premature babies. Subsequent research has indicated that too much oxygen can also result in Minimal Brain Damage (MBD), so that earlier populations of blind children may well have included several MBD children.

3.2. Delay in the Verbal Auxiliary

There are no indications of major problems in syntax or morphology. However, in a study of three blind children, Landau/Gleitmann

(1985) recorded a significant delay in the acquisition of the verbal auxiliary in English. This delay in the acquisition of a highly specific aspect of syntax is related to a feature of maternal input. The mothers of blind infants use more imperatives and for longer than mothers of sighted children do on average, and they ask fewer questions. This results in a lower frequency of the verbal auxiliary in English maternal speech. The same relation between input and acquisition of the verbal auxiliary had already been found for sighted children and is one of the few areas in which a clear causal relation can be traced between the form of input and the child's acquisition of language. The delay in this specific area does not seem to have any major consequences for the further acquisition of English. The question can be asked whether the implications might not be more (or less) severe in languages which use different structures in imperatives and questions.

3.3. Syntax/Pragmatics Interface

Most work indicates no problems in older blind children (Maxfield 1936). However, one study with Dutch-speaking children has shown problems in morphology and syntax in both blind and severely visually-impaired children aged between five and ten years (Wegener-Sleeswijk 1986). Two of these children were RLF children with low IQ's, but of the remaining 17 children 11 made significantly more grammatical errors in a spontaneous speech sample than sighted peers. These children were not significantly different however on measures of complexity of morphology and syntax, that is in use of past tense forms, subordination etc. The errors that they produce frequently involve the omission of constituents and appear to be related to the children's attempts to produce longer utterances and to apply the complex rules of ellipsis. The problems of these older blind children appear to be more related to the correct pragmatic application of the syntactic rules, rather than to the control of the formal aspects of the syntactic rules themselves, that is the syntax and pragmatics interface (Mills/Wegener-Sleeswijk 1991). These children also had separate problems in pragmatics which will be discussed below (see 5.6.).

3.4. Summary

From the evidence discussed above it seems that blind children do not have serious problems with the acquisition of syntax and morphology. Only a small delay can be seen in the area of the verbal auxiliary in English. Otherwise more serious delays appear to be related to blindness occurring with other disabilities. This suggests that vision is not crucial for acquisition of these formal aspects of language, which would be in accordance with formal theories of language acquisition (see 1.1.).

4. Semantics

4.1. Early Lexicon

Several researchers have examined the acquisition of the early lexicon in blind children (Andersen/Dunlea/Kekelis 1984; Bigelow 1987; Dunlea 1989; Landau/Gleitman 1985). The descriptive findings are similar but their conclusions vary (Mulford 1989).

Most studies indicate a normal acquisition of the first 50 words. The spread of the words across different semantic categories is comparable with that of sighted children. A few differences are observed: for example that blind children have more words associated with parent/child routines. They also have more terms for sounds but fewer deictic terms. They also have fewer terms for animals, and more terms related to household items compared with sighted children. Such minor differences are related to the differing experience of the blind children, thus they have more experience of household items and less of animals which sighted children usually gain through book-reading etc. Differences in interpretation occur mainly in relationship to the apparent conceptual development (see 4.2.).

4.2. Semantic and Conceptual Development

Blind children do appear to have restricted experience in comparison with' sighted children. Related to this is the frequent observation that blind children rarely generalize new words to other objects of the same category: for example *dog* will be used for the one known dog and not for other dogs. This under-generalization, and related lack of over-generalization (otherwise common in this early period of development), has been interpreted as evidence for a delay in the ability of blind children to sort and categorize (Anderson/Dunlea/Kekelis 1984; Dunlea 1984). In the spontaneous behavior of the two children studied (up to 3;4), no sorting was observed and the children would not categorize objects on request. This interpretation has been challenged by work with 22 older children (4–6 years) in which no lack of ability to categorize was evident as compared with the sighted controls (Dobslav 1991). These blind children were also able to formulate the distinguishing properties of objects. There were only some minor differences in the type of properties named: functional properties were named by blind children but particularly those which were related to the activity of the object itself or those which the child itself carried out. This difference is again related to the type of information a blind child has access to but does not indicate a general cognitive or linguistic deficit.

Overextensions, where they do occur in blind children, are on the basis of mainly tactile properties, necessarily not visual properties as in most sighted children. This indicates again that their language development may be different in some respects but that the processes of acquisition do not fundamentally differ.

4.3. Verbalism

This term was introduced by Cutsforth (1932) to describe the use of language which does not have a conceptual basis. Since blind children have a sensory deficit, it was assumed that they could not have a conceptual basis for many terms and that their speech was full of verbalisms, indicative of 'loose thinking'. This label has been disputed by many researchers, although it has been used even recently by Rogow (1986) to describe the speech of both blind children and adults.

Landau/Gleitman (1985) showed in their longitudinal study of one child (up to 5) that words with even a high visual content such as the verbs *to see* and *to look* are not meaningless for the child but have a gradually developing meaning which approximates the adult form. At the age of three years the child interpreted the two verbs as 'haptically be aware of' and 'haptically explore' respectively. But by the age of five years she knew that sighted adults could not see an object which was behind a barrier, although they could have felt it. Landau and Gleitman's general conclusion is that blind children will use the information that they have to build up the meaning of items with a visual component, starting with the information which is most accessible for them, that is in the haptic modality.

4.4. Terms Related to Space

Blind children are still making errors at age six years with spatial deictic terms such as *this* and *here* (Mulford 1981). Mulford relates this finding to a delay in the acquisition of the cognitive concept of space, due to the lack of visual information.

The use of personal pronouns can also involve deixis and their acquisition may therefore be related to the acquisition of the concept of space (Loveland 1984). The use of first and second person pronouns involves a shift of perspective and this shift in perspective appears to be difficult for blind children. They continue to make errors with *I* and *you* longer than sighted children. This problem may however also be related to the frequency of pronouns in the input. (Errors in gender in pronouns also take longer to disappear in blind children than in sighted (Mulford 1981)).

Blind children have been shown to acquire spatial prepositions in terms of comprehension and production with some delay but with variation in the order of acquisition. Bigelow/Bryan (1982) showed that blind children can understand the prepositions *in*, *on* and *under* more readily in relationship to themselves than for the relationship between two objects. In understanding spatial relations between objects, blind children acquire prepositions referring to the vertical dimension first as do sighted children (Mills 1988). However they take longer to acquire prepositions referring to the horizontal dimension, particularly the horizontal frontal dimension. Blind children take longer to learn that fronting is relevant to the use of these prepositions, and also to learn to apply that knowledge.

4.5. Summary

From the results in the area of semantic acquisition there appear to be some clear differences in the order of acquisition, some of which may be related to a delay in the acquisition of some cognitive concepts. There is little evidence, however, to suggest that blind children have general problems in their conceptual development. Their acquisition of some semantic areas is different but not obviously deficient.

5. Pragmatics, Input, and Interaction

5.1. Pre-verbal Communication

Pre-verbal communication is considered important for the onset and further development of language in the child particularly by those researchers who adopt a social-interactive model of language acquisition. A few studies exist on this period of development in blind children and in general offer some support for this model.

Gaze and gestures are not available as signals to indicate communicative intentions in general and selection of topic for interaction in particular. Adults interacting with blind children have to learn to pick up other signals which indicate direction of attention and communicative intent. Fraiberg (1977) in a general developmental study of ten blind children observed frequent failure in this area. Als/Tronick/Brazelton (1980) report on successful preverbal interaction and a good development in one blind child; four children studied by Preisler (1990) also show more successful interaction and good communicative development. Studies by Dunlea (1989), Rowland (1983) and Urwin (1983) indicate the problems that appear to arise in this early interaction and relate them to problems in language development. The pre-verbal blind infants were best able to communicate affective states. They also were able to express more general desires such as for the repetition of a play routine by crying, vocalization and some hand movements. All the children did have problems in directing attention to an object. Two of the mothers observed by Rowland clearly failed to repond as frequently to the vocalizations of their children and these children were considerably more delayed in their language development.

All three children observed by Rowland (1983, 1984), however, showed a different pattern of vocalization compared with sighted children. They produced fewer vocalizations during and after the vocalizations of the adult: they vocalized rather more when alone. Rowland interprets this different pattern as a result of blindness and of the increased importance of the auditory environment, which blind children try to avoid 'cluttering' with their own vocalizations.

5.2. Functions of Early Language

Several studies have examined the functions for which blind children use their language in the early stages and some of these have related the development to input. Just as for sighted children, requests form a category which emerges early, but in blind children the first requests are those related to self with requests for objects emerging around 20 months (Urwin 1983). Dunlea (1989) found this category of requests to be dominant around two years. Perez-Pereira/Castro (1990 a), in a study of a blind and sighted twin pair, found that requests decreased similarly in both children (up to the age of 4 years) in favor of questions. However, the blind twin did have in total more functions related to self than the sighted child, e. g. action related to self, reports of internal states.

Kekelis/Andersen (1984) report more labelling in the early language (up to 22 months) but Perez-Pereira/Castro (1990 a) do not have such a clear finding in the older twins: the sighted child between 2;6 and 3;6 had in fact more labels than the blind child. Kekelis and Andersen relate their finding to a higher incidence of labels in the input speech to the younger children, which they interpret as an impediment to the development of other functions in the language of the child. This would not appear to be a generalizable result however.

Kekelis and Andersen also found fewer attributions and descriptions in the language input to the younger children, a surprising finding since it would seem obvious that blind children need more verbal information about the environment in order to organize experience. The children's language also reflected less use of these functions. The blind twin of Perez-Pereira and Castro also used these functions less than her sighted sister but they do not relate this to input. One can interpret this observation as being a result of greater self-orientation rather than necessarily a product of input.

Adults talking to young blind children tend to initiate topics more than adults talking to sighted children of the same age (Kekelis/Andersen 1984; Urwin 1983). Kekelis and Andersen also observed that almost half the topics introduced by the adults were related to contexts and referents which the child could not perceive and that the adults have difficulty in establishing what the child is interested in. They interpret this as an impediment to blind children in the development of language oriented to the environment. Both studies found that the topics introduced by the children were mainly self-oriented.

As discussed above (3.2.), input from the adult does appear to have an effect on the acquisition of the verbal auxiliary in English. The characteristic of the input was that adults were being more directive and therefore using fewer questions involving the auxiliary. A highly directive interactive style is associated with children at an early stage of language development and Kekelis/Andersen (1984) interpret this as an indication that input and interaction progress at a lower rate for blind children, thus producing a slower rate of development in the children. This causal effect is not proven, however.

5.3. Imitation

It has been noted by many researchers that blind children in the early stages of acquisition produce many more imitations of adults' utterances than sighted children. Most of these imitations are inappropriate conversationally, whether from sighted or blind children, but the fact that blind children produce more of such utterances and for longer has led to a clinical classification of their speech as 'echolalic'. Since this is a clinical symptom of autistic children, an association has been made between blind and autistic children by some researchers.

Prizant (1984) reviews the literature on this and suggests that imitation may occur more often in blind children for various reasons such as acquisition style, better developed rote memory, problems in segmentation due to lack of contextual information. He argues that it is not necessarily to be interpreted as a clinical symptom. Perez-Pereira/Castro (1990 b) present data from the blind twin which confirms a greater use of imitation, but repetition with modification and formulaic speech are also used more. They interpret this as a route into language acquisition, a method of practising structures, much as Speidel (1989) argues for sighted children.

5.4. Verbal Interaction: Older Children

It has been reported for some younger blind children that they do not verbalize as much as their sighted peers. Studies of older children (4 to 9 years) indicate however a greater amount of verbalization (Olson 1983; Schwartz 1983). This appears to be related to the function of maintaining interaction in the absence of the availability of visual cues such as eye gaze, smiles and other non-verbal behavior, although social and cultural differences in turn-taking routines may have an influence on the amount of verbalization (see 5.4.).

Workman (1986) reports that in children under five years adults could influence the amount of peer-peer interaction, including verbal interaction, when the adult gives the blind child information about the social environment, that is who is present, what the activities are, etc. Difficulties in obtaining this information, which is a prerequisite to initiating a conversation, seem to impede younger blind children (see 5.5.). Blind children also are reported to use more questions in their interactions (Erin 1986; Maxfield 1936), which Erin suggests is a reflection of the need to gain access to precisely this information.

McGinnis (1981) observed that slightly younger blind children (3 to 5 years) frequently used questions to change topic and did this more often than sighted peers. This too may be a reflection of turn-taking mechanisms (see 5.5.).

5.5. Turntaking

Blind people have limited access to the non-verbal cues in regulating turns either as speaker or listener. Early turntaking is supposed to be established in the pre-verbal stage and the lack of eye-contact and smiling in blind infants are a problem for the sighted parents in establishing this proto-conversational organization. Fraiberg (1977) relates this lack of reaction signals to problems in establishing a parent-child bond.

In beginning a conversation it is necessary to obtain the attention of the addressee and to direct attention to the topic of discourse if appropriate. This is frequently done non-verbally. Younger blind children use non-visual alternative means such as touching the addressee, pinching, calling the addressee's name (Mulford 1983) but they are more frequently unsuccessful and can become discouraged in initiating discourse.

Facial expression is muted in blind children (and adults), smiling is less frequent as are head nods (Parke/Shalcross/Anderson 1980; Warren 1977)). All these behaviors can function as feedback signals in conversation but since they are used less by blind children (and adults), other feedback signals must be acquired. No detailed research has been done on this so far.

It is known from work on blind adults (Junefelt/Mills 1990) that the turntaking patterns are different from sighted adults and are an adaption of the sighted patterns in their own culture. This adaptation varies in effect according to whether the culture can be described as floor-yielding or floor-seizing. Blind children must learn these patterns and adaptations but how this acquisition proceeds is not yet clear.

5.6. Assessment of Listener

In order to make the content and formulation of conversation efficient, it is necessary to assess the information to which the listener has access either directly or indirectly. Children take considerable time in acquiring this ability but blind children seem to take even longer. Their language is more frequently pragmatically deviant because of a failure to take the listener correctly into account (Wegener-Sleeswijk 1986). This is also comparable with autistic children and may be related to a slower development of a theory of mind as has been suggested for that group (cf. art. 78).

6. Conclusions

In summary it can be said that blind children with no other handicap will develop language without major delay or deficiency. In some aspects they are clearly different. These differences provide evidence for the role of vision in models of language acquisition and indicate the variety of routes of acquisition which such models must account for.

7. References

Als, J., Tronick, E., & Brazelton, T. (1980). Affective reciprocity and the development of autonomy: the study of a blind infant. *Journal of the American Academy of Child Psychiatry*, *19*, 22–40.

Andersen, E. S., Dunlea, A., & Kekelis L. S. (1984). Blind children's language: resolving some differences. *Journal of Child Language*, *11/3*, 645–664.

Bigelow, A. (1987). Early words of blind children. *Journal of Child Language*, *14*, 47–58.

Bigelow, A. & Bryan, A. (1982). The understanding of spatial prepositions 'in', 'on' and 'under' in blind and sighted pre-school children. Paper to the Canadian Psychological Association Conference, Montreal.

Burlingham, D. (1972). *Psychoanalytic studies of the sighted and the blind.* New York: International Universities Press.

Cutsforth, T. D. (1932). The unreality of words to the blind. *The Teachers' Forum*, *4*, 86–89.

Dobslav, G. (1991). *Da kann ich nur das Wort sagen. Eine vergleichende Analyse der Kategorisierungsleistungen und der Inhalte von Wortbedeutungen über Objekte bei blinden und sehenden Vorschulkindern.* Doctoral dissertation, University of Bielefeld, Germany.

Dodd, B. (1983). The visual and auditory modalities in phonological acquisition. In A. E. Mills (Ed.), *Language acquisition in the blind child: normal and deficient. 57–61.* London: Croom Helm.

Dunlea, A. (1984). The relationship between concept formation and semantic roles: some evidence from the blind. In L. Feagans, C. Garvey, & R. Golinkoff (Eds.), *The origins and growth of communication. 224–243.* Norwood: Ablex.

Dunlea, A. (1989: *Vision and the emergence of meaning in blind and sighted children's language.* Cambridge: C.U.P.

Elstner, W. (1983). Abnormalities in the verbal communication of visually-impaired children. In A. E. Mills (Ed.), *Language acquisition in the blind child: normal and deficient. 18–41.* London: Croom Helm.

Erin, J. N. (1986). Frequencies and types of questions in the language of visually-impaired children. *Journal of Visual Impairment and Blindness*, *80*, 670–674.

Fraiberg, S. (1977). *Insights from the blind.* New York: Basic Books.

Göllecz, V. (1972). Über die Lippenartikulation der von Geburt an Blinden. In S. Hirschberg, G. Szépe, & E. Vass-Kovoics (Eds.), *Papers in interdisciplinary speech research. 85–91.* Budapest: Akadémiai Kiadó.

Jan, J. E., Freeman, R. D., & Scott, E. P. (1977). *Visual impairment in children and adolescents.* New York: Grune & Stratton.

Junefelt, K. (1987). *Blindness and child-adjusted communication.* Doctoral dissertation, University of Stockholm, Sweden.

Junefelt, K. & Mills, A. E. (1990). Turntaking in blind and sighted multiparty conversations: Swedish and Dutch compared. Paper to the International Pragmatics Conference, Barcelona, Spain.

Kekelis, L. S. & Andersen, E. (1984). Family communication styles and language development. *Journal of Visual Impairment and Blindness*, *78*, 54–64.

Landau, B. & Gleitman, L. R. (1985). *Language and experience: evidence from the blind child.* Harvard: Harvard University Press.

Loveland, K. A. (1984). Learning about points of view: spatial perspective and the acquisition of 'I/you'. *Journal of Child Language*, *11*, 535–556.

Lucas, S. A. (1984). Auditory discrimination and speech production in the blind child. *International Journal of Rehabilitation Research*, *7/1*, 74–76.

Maxfield, K. E. (1936). *The spoken language of the blind pre-school child.* New York: Archives of Psychology, No. 201.

McGinnis, A. R. (1981). Functional linguistic strategies of blind children. *Journal of Visual Impairment and Blindness*, *75*, 210–214.

Mills, A. E. (1983). Acquisition of speech sounds in the visually-handicapped child. In A. E. Mills (Ed.), *Language acquisition in the blind child: normal and deficient. 46–56.* London: Croom Helm.

Mills, A. E. (1987). The acquisition of phonology in the blind child. In B. Dodd & R. Campbell (Eds.), *Hearing by eye: experimental studies in the psychology of lipreading. 145–161.* Hillsdale, NJ: Erlbaum.

Mills, A. E. (1988). Visual handicap. In D. Bishop & K. Mogford (Eds.), *Language development in exceptional circumstances. 150–164.* Edinburgh: Churchill Livingstone.

Mills, A. E. & Wegener-Sleeswijk, B. (1991). The syntactic-pragmatic interface: some blind children's problems. Paper to the Groningen workshop on language disorders.

Miner, L. E. (1963). A study of the incidence of speech deviations among visually-handicapped children. *New Outlook for the blind, 57*, 10–14.

Mulford, R. C. (1981). *Talking without seeing: some problems of semantic development in blind children.* Doctoral dissertation, Stanford University, USA.

Mulford, R. C. (1983). Referential development in blind children. In A. E. Mills (Ed.), *Language acquisition in the blind child: normal and deficient. 89–107.* London: Croom Helm.

Mulford, R. C. (1989). First words of the blind child. In M. D. Smith & J. L. Locke (Eds.), *The emergent lexicon: the child's development of a linguistic vocabulary. 136–160.* New York: Academic Press.

Olson, M. R. (1983). A study of the exploratory behaviour of legally blind and sighted preschoolers. *Exceptional Children, 49*, 130–138.

Parke, K. L., Shalcross, R., & Anderson, R. J. (1980). Differences in coverbal behavior between blind and sighted persons during dyadic communication. *Journal of Visual Impairment and Blindness, 74*, 142–146.

Perez-Pereira, M. & Castro, J. (1990 a). A pragmatic analysis of the language of a blind child compared to that of her sighted twin. Paper to International Pragmatics Conference, Barcelona, Spain.

Perez-Pereira, M. & Castro, J. (1990 b). Some strategies used by a blind child in the acquisition of language. Paper to the 4th European Developmental Psychology Conference, Stirling, Great Britain.

Piattelli-Palmarini, M. (1980). *Language and learning.* Cambridge: Harvard University Press.

Preisler, G. (1990). Communicative development in young blind children. In G. Conti-Ramsden & C. Snow (Eds.), *Communicative development.* 130–152. Cambridge: CUP.

Prizant, B. M. (1984). Toward an understanding of language symptology of visually-impaired children. In A. M. Sykanda, J. E. Jan, & S. J. Blockberger (Eds.), *Insight in sight. 70–87.* Vancouver: CNIB.

Reynell, J. (1978). Developmental patterns of visually-handicapped children. *Child Care, Health and Development,* 4/5, 291–303.

Rogow, S. M. (1986). Semantics and the blind child. *Semiotica, 62*, 297–312.

Rowland, C. (1983). Patterns of interaction between three blind infants and their mothers. In A. E. Mills (Ed.), *Language acquisition in the blind child: normal and deficient. 114–132.* London: Croom Helm.

Rowland, C. (1984). Pre-verbal communication of blind infants and their mothers. *Journal of Visual Impairment and Blindness, 78*, 297–302.

Schwartz, T. J. (1983). Social cognition in visually-impairment and sighted children. *Journal of Visual Impairment and Blindness, 77*, 377–381.

Semzova, M. I. (1961). Besonderheiten der Erkenntnistätigkeit blinder Kinder im jüngeren Schulalter. *Die Sonderschule, 6/6*, 336–340.

Speidel, G. E. (1989). Imitation: a bootstrap for learning to speak. In G. E. Speidel & K. E. Nelson (Eds.), *The many faces of imitation in children. 15–39.* Berlin: Springer.

Urwin, C. (1983). Dialogue and cognitive functioning in the early language of blind children. In A. E. Mills (Ed.), *Language acquisition in the blind child: normal and deficient. 142–161.* London: Croom Helm.

Vihman, M. M., Macken, M. A., Miller, R., Simmons, H., & Miller, J. (1985). From babbling to speech: a reassesment of the continuity issue. *Language, 61/1*, 397–445.

Warren, D. H. (1977). *Blindness and early childhood development.* New York: American Foundation for the Blind.

Wegener-Sleeswijk, B. (1986). *Ik voel wat geks, wat roods.* M. A. thesis, University of Amsterdam, Netherlands.

Workman, S. H. (1986). Teachers' verbalizations and the social interaction of blind preschoolers. *Journal of Visual Impairment and Blindness, 80*, 532–534.

Anne E. Mills, Amsterdam (Netherlands)

67. Language Acquisition and Development in Persons with Mental Retardation

1. Introduction

The American Association on Mental Retardation defines mental retardation in terms of measured intelligence and adaptive behavior. Mentally retarded persons exhibit significantly subaverage performance on standardized general intelligence tests, two or more standard deviations from the mean, associated with significant deficiencies in the ability to meet "the standards of maturation, learning, personal independence, and/or social responsibilities that are expected for his or her age level and cultural group" (Grossman 1983, 11). Language is related to both aspects of this definition. It is common to think of measured intelligence in terms of a small number of information processing activities such as stimulus encoding, memory storage, memory retrieval, metacognitive activities, and reasoning (see Carroll 1976; Sternberg 1984). Persons with mental retardation exhibit deficiencies in virtually all domains of cognitive functioning (see Brooks/Sperber/McCauley 1984; Ellis 1979). To the extent that these abilities are necessary for language acquisition, then we would expect the development of language by mentally retarded persons to be delayed. Language is also important to the adaptive functioning of retarded persons. It is an important tool for taking in knowledge, conceptualizing the world, and thinking. It also gives children a useful method for controlling their environment (Jones/Robson 1979). Therefore, language acquisition and development has been one focus of research conducted with mentally retarded persons (see e. g. Rosenberg 1982; Schiefelbusch/Copeland 1968; Schiefelbusch/Lloyd 1974). This review will highlight this research. I will first review studies that examine the relationship between several components of linguistic performance and mental retardation, then focus on language functioning as it relates to several specific syndromes in mental retardation.

2. Elements of Language Acquisition

2.1. Phonology

Articulation problems are common in mentally retarded persons (see Fawcus/Fawcus 1974; Ingram 1976). In one study, the incidence of articulation disorders ranged from 65 to 95 percent across etiologies (Schlanger/Gottsleben 1957), with the highest incidence reported for Down syndrome individuals.

Dodd (1976) examined consonant errors in 10 mentally retarded children with Down syndrome, 10 retarded children without Down syndrome, and 10 nonretarded children. Groups were approximately matched on mental age (MA) (36 and 48 months) and social background. Mean chronological ages (CAs) were approximately 43 months in the nonretarded sample and 128 months in the retarded samples. Subjects took part in a picture naming task and a lexical imitation task. Despite extensive criticism levied against many of Dodd's procedures (see Rosenberg 1982), some conclusions seem reasonable. In the main articulatory error categories investigated – cluster reduction, production of consonant harmony, and simplification of the phonological system (see Smith 1973) – the Down syndrome subjects made more errors than the other two groups, who did not differ on any of the measures. Also, the Down syndrome subjects' errors did not conform to expectation based on the performance of the other mentally retarded subjects. However, it did not appear that this difference was a qualitative difference in language performance (cf. Rosenberg 1982).

Stoel-Gammon (1980) studied four retarded children with Down syndrome. Mean length of utterances (MLUs) ranged from 1.22 to 2.06 and CAs from 46 to 75 months. Approximately three hours of spontaneous speech were recorded for each child. Her analyses of consonant errors led her to conclude the following. First, the majority of errors made by her subjects were not due to an inability to produce the sounds. Her subjects could produce most of the English phonemes. Second, the errors were regular and predictable from adult forms. Third, the errors were similar to those reported in the speech of nonretarded children of similar MLUs.

To the extent that the findings of these studies generalize to other ability levels and etiologies, it appears that the development of the phonological system of retarded individuals is slower than that of nonretarded individuals. But, there does not appear to be a qualitative difference in phonetic processing.

2.2. Syntax

The development of syntax seems to be particularly difficult for persons with mental retardation. Mentally retarded individuals exhibit deficits in the understanding and production of grammatical structures (Bridges/Smith 1984; Kernan 1990), understanding various transformations (Cromer 1975), and mastering morphological structures (Dever 1972). Several examples are described in this section.

Bridges/Smith (1984) compared the ability of 24 Down syndrome children (mean CA = 11.1 years; verbal comprehension age range 2.5 to 5.2 years) with that of 24 nonretarded children (mean CA = 3.0 years; verbal comprehension age range 2.5 to 5.2 years). Children were required to act out events in eight active and eight passive sentences. Analysis of the relationship between the ability to act out sentences and verbal comprehension age revealed that the Down syndrome and nonretarded children exhibited similar performance curves. However, the performance of the Down syndrome children lagged behind their verbal comprehension age by about one year for active sentences and one-half year for passive sentences.

Kernan (1990) compared the comprehension of syntactically ordered sequence in 14 mentally retarded adults with Down syndrome (mean IQ = 56.0) and 14 without Down syndrome (mean IQ = 56.9). Subjects took part in three tasks. On Task 1, subjects manipulated objects in a sequence visually demonstrated by the experimenter. In Task 2, the visual demonstration was paired with a verbal description of the sequence and subjects were asked to verbally indicate what happened first. In Task 3, only the verbal description was provided. The sequences were either naturally or arbitrarily ordered. Both groups of subjects performed best on Task 1 and worst on Task 3. Although delayed, the retarded subjects' pattern of performance matched that of nonretarded children and adolescents. However, the non-Down syndrome subjects out-performed the Down syndrome subjects on every task and on 36 of the 40 sentences. So, while they performed in similar fashion, the Down syndrome subjects performed at a level below that of the non-Down syndrome subjects.

Abbeduto/Furman/Davies (1989) used the *Test for Reception of Grammar* (Bishop 1982) to examine the relationship between receptive language and cognitive development in individuals with mental retardation. Sixty school age mentally retarded subjects (IQ range 40 to 79) and 60 nonretarded subjects took part, with twenty subjects per group functioning at MA levels of 5, 7, and 9 years. In general, their results indicate that the receptive language of school age retarded children is below expectations based on MA. However, this deficiency did not hold up at every level of MA tested. The retarded subjects who had MAs in the 5 year range were performing at appropriate levels of receptive language, although the authors suggest that this finding may be specific to the test used.

The combined results of these studies are consistent with the general literature. Syntax development follows a similar pattern for retarded and nonretarded persons. However, the development of syntax is seriously delayed, even beyond expectations based on cognitive development. In addition, it appears that this delay may be greater for retarded persons with Down syndrome relative to those of other etiologies (e. g. Evans 1977; Kernan 1990).

2.3. Semantic Processing

Semantic processing is important for many aspects of linguistic competence. In this section I review studies that investigate three of these areas: (1) the understanding of semantic relations associated with the expression of simple sentences, (2) the acquisition of information about word meanings when novel words are presented in context, and (3) the content and organization of lexical memory.

The relative abilities of 12 mentally retarded and 12 nonretarded individuals to understand semantic relationships expressed in various verbal context was studied by Duchan/Erickson (1976). (Twelve language-disordered children also included will not be discussed.) The mentally retarded subjects had CAs of 48 to 93 months, IQs of 50 to 80, and a mean MLU of 1.67. The nonretarded subjects had CAs of 18 to 31 months, and a mean MLU of 1.56. The verbal contexts were telegraphic two-word speech (grammatical morphemes absent), expanded speech (grammatical morphemes present), and partially nonsensical speech. The semantic relations included agent-action, action-object, possessive, and locative. There were main effects associated with type of relation and type of utterance, but the mentally retarded and nonretarded subjects did not differ on either dimension. When matched on MLU, retarded and nonretarded children understood the semantic relations expressed in simple sentences in a similar manner. In addition, research has shown that this similarity extends to the analysis of spontaneous speech for subjects matched on MLU (Coggins 1979; Layton/Sharifi 1979).

A recent study examined the 'fast mapping' ability of mentally retarded children and MA-matched nonretarded children (Chapman/Kay-Raining Bird/Schwartz 1990). Fast mapping refers to the ability to acquire information about novel word meanings after limited exposure (usually once or twice) to the word in linguistic and event contexts. Subjects were 48 retarded individuals with Down syndrome (mean CA = 12.54 years; mean MA = 4.58 years) and 48 nonretarded children (mean CA = 4.16 years; mean MA = 4.71 years). They were approximately equal on vocabulatory comprehension, syntax comprehension, and expressive vocabulary. The subjects with Down syndrome exhibited an expressive language deficiency as evidenced by a fewer number of words, fewer different words, lower percent of complete and intelligible utterances, and a smaller MLU observed in a 12 minute narrative. In the exposure task, children were asked to hide objects that included an object with a novel referent ('koob'). Various tests of comprehension and production followed. There were no significant differences in the ability of Down syndrome and nonretarded children to: (1) infer that the object and novel referent were connected (i. e., they were willing to hide the object being referred to with the novel word), (2) comprehend the novel referent after one exposure, (3) recall where the novel object was hidden, and (4) produce the novel referent correctly when asked. Thus, the Down syndrome subjects exhibit fast mapping skills that were similar to expectations based on MA and exceeded expectations based on expressive language abilities.

The nature and organization of semantic memory has been the focus of a number of studies (e. g. Davies/Sperber/McCauley 1981; Merrill 1985; Sperber/Davies/Merrill/McCauley 1982; Sperber/Ragain/McCauley 1976). Sperber et al. (1976; Experiment 1) examined the availability of category information to retarded adolescents (mean IQ = 60; mean CA = 16.3 years; mean MA = 7.25 years) using a semantic priming procedure. In their version of the task, subjects labeled pictures of objects. Pictures were presented in successive pairs in which the objects were either categorically related to each other (e. g. dog-cow) or not related to each other (e. g. table-cow). When a picture is preceded by a picture of a categorically related object, the time to name the second picture of the pair is reduced. This 'priming effect' is assumed to reflect knowledge of the categorical relationship expressed in the two pictures (that of 'animalness' in the above example). In several studies, the magnitude of semantic priming exhibited by mentally retarded individuals has been found to be similar to that of nonretarded individuals (Davies et al. 1981; Sperber et al. 1976; 1982). The most detailed analysis of semantic priming indicates that the magnitude of the priming effect, and by inference knowledge of category relationships, is more related to MA than to CA (Sperber et al. 1982). But, even though mentally retarded individuals exhibit a knowledge of these category relationships, they often fail to access and use that information when it is prudent to do so (Sperber et al. 1976; Experiment 2), and when they do, they retrieve it less efficiently than do nonretarded persons (Sperber et al. 1982). It has been suggested that this latter result may be due to some general deficit in attentional processing (see Merrill 1985; Sperber/McCauley 1984).

The research findings across these three aspects of semantic processing are consistent with those reported for phonetic and syntactic differences of retarded and nonretarded individuals. Semantic development follows the same general pattern, albeit delayed, for mentally retarded and normally developing individuals.

2.4. Communication Skills

It is known that mothers of nonretarded children adjust their speech to the level of their children (cf. Snow 1977). Several studies have been conducted to determine whether mothers of mentally retarded children also adjust their level of speech in this fashion (e. g. Cunningham/Reuler/Blackwell/Deck 1981; Peterson/Sherrod 1982; Rondal 1978). One intent of these studies was to determine if lower quality verbal interactions between mothers and retarded children may inhibit their children's language development. However, when subjects are matched on MLU, mothers of retarded and nonretarded children are similar on most syntactic, semantic, and pragmatic features of language (see e. g. Rondal 1978). The few longitudinal investigations that have been conducted also suggest that the adjustments in speech that mothers do make to their retarded children are systematically related to changes in the children's language and general level of cognitive functioning (e. g. Mauer/Sherrod 1987; McConkey/Martin 1984).

In spite of the similarities in the communication styles exhibited by mothers of retarded and nonretarded children, some important differences exist. Mothers of retarded children are more dominant and directive in their communicative style and generally less responsive to the communicative behavior of their children (Cunningham et al. 1981; Mahoney/Robenalt 1986). But, this difference in style may be related to the communicative responsiveness of the retarded children (Jones 1977; Mahoney/Robenalt 1986; Mauer/Sherrod 1987). Mentally retarded children are generally less active communicators, do not initiate communication as frequently, and exhibit poor timing in turn-taking interactions with their mothers than developmentally matched nonretarded children (Fischer 1987; Jones 1977). However, with mentally retarded children who are more active and responsive in their own communication styles, mothers are much more responsive and less dominant and directive (Mahoney 1988; Mahoney/Robenalt 1986). Whether such differences in communication style impact upon the language development of their children is a current topic of investigation (Hoff-Ginsberg 1986; Yoder 1989; Yoder/Kaiser 1989).

Researchers have also investigated general communication skills of mentally retarded children and adults. The results of most studies suggest that functional communication skills of mentally retarded persons are at least on par with and may exceed expectations based on measured verbal abilities (e. g. Abbeduto/Rosenberg 1980; Bedrosian/Prutting 1978; Coggins/Stoel-Gammon 1982; Leifer/Lewis 1984; Price-Williams/Sabsay 1979).

Leifer/Lewis (1984) compared the conversational response skills of one group of nonretarded subjects (mean CA = 20.8 months; mean MLU = 1.25) with a group of retarded subjects matched on CA (mean CA = 20.5 months) but not on linguistic ability (MLU = 0), and with a group of retarded subjects matched on MLU (mean MLU = 1.12) but not on CA (mean CA = 4.0). Children were taped in free play interactions with mothers. Children's responses (verbal and nonverbal) were coded as appropriate if the response matched the pragmatic intent of mothers' questions, inappropriate if they did not, and indeterminate if they were unclear. The CA-matched retarded subjects were seriously deficient in their ability to appropriately respond to mothers' questions, whereas the MA-matched retarded subjects exhibited greater conversational response skills than the nonretarded subjects.

Bedrosian/Prutting (1978) examined the communicative competence of mentally retarded adults in four conversational settings: conversations with a speech-language pathologist, with peers, with parent/guardian, and with a six-year-old nonretarded boy. The subjects were three males and one female (CAs 23–28 years; IQs 29–39). The researchers recorded conversations in each setting over a three month period. They were primarily interested in the conversational relationships of the mentally retarded in terms of the dimensions of dominance-submission and control across the various settings. Only one of the subjects ever assumed the dominant position in the conversations and was only able to do so in conversations with peers and the child. With respect to control, the authors found that the retarded individuals generally used similar types of control to those used by nonretarded adults. However, it was also noted that there were individual differences in the types and frequencies of control used by the retarded adults. Finally, all of the subjects were able to use requests for restatement to signal when a communication breakdown had occurred.

Price-Williams/Sabsay (1979) recorded conversational interactions of nine institutionalized Down syndrome men (CA = 29 to 49 years; IQ = 17 to 26). Their communicative activities were reported to be very effective. In summarizing 15 hours of recorded conversations between the subjects and each other and the subjects and members of the hospital staff, the authors reported a wide range of communicative skills exhibited by their subject including, for example, greeting exchanges, appropriate turn-taking behaviors, and effective linguistic and nonlinguistic strategies for securing the attention of their intended listener. Their subjects were also able to modify conversational styles to prevent and correct failures in communication.

These selected studies reveal a general asymmetry between communicative competence and linguistic competence for mentally retarded persons. Communicative competence appears to be greater than expected based on linguistic competence. However, recent data suggests that this advantage may not extend to all aspects of communication. Mundy/Sigman/Kasari/Yirmiya (1988) found that young children with Down syndrome exhibited nonverbal social interaction skills that exceeded their measured MAs, but were deficient relative to MAs in making nonverbal requests for objects or assistance with objects. It may be important to try to evaluate patterns of strengths and weakness in the communicative competence of mentally retarded persons.

3. Specific Syndromes

Persons with mental retardation are not a homogeneous group. Mental retardation is the result of a variety of etiologies. All of these conditions do not lead to identical patterns of cognitive performance. Therefore, some discussion of how language differences manifest themselves in specific syndromes resulting in mental retardation is important. In this section I consider three syndromes: Down syndrome, fragile-X syndrome, and Williams syndrome.

3.1. Down Syndrome

Down syndrome is a chromosomal abnormality resulting from the presence of extra chromosomic material in the body (from chromosome 21). The maximum level of cognitive functioning expected for most is an MA of approximately 4–5 years. Down syndrome individuals also exhibit physical symptoms that may be associated with defective speech. Abnormalities include a larynx located too high in the neck, an edematous tongue that groves improperly for several speech sounds and is impaired in motility, and undersized mouth cavity, a protruding tongue, and hypotonia of the speech muscles (Benda 1949; Buddenhagen 1971). They also exhibit a high incidence of auditory problems, the major cause of which is otitis media (Balkany 1980).

Language development, although delayed, is quite similar for Down syndrome and normally developing children. Menn (1985) has reported that phonological development is seriously delayed in individuals with Down syndrome. However, the sequence of development parallels that of normal children. Share (1975) observed a one-year delay in the onset of meaningful one-word utterances, but the number of words that could be understood and used was comparable to MA matched nonretarded children (Mein/O'Connor 1960). When they begin to combine two and three words in an utterance, they understand the same relational meanings as normally developing children matched on MLU (Layton/Sharifi 1979). A conclusion of many reviews is that there is no compelling evidence of qualitative differences in language development between Down syndrome and normally developing children (Bloom/Lahey 1978; Kiernen 1985; Rosenberg 1982).

Despite similarities in the acquisition of language by children with and without Down syndrome, there is a growing belief that the conclusion of language delay without deviance is not entirely correct and may be misleading (see Fowler 1990; Rondal 1988). Fowler (1990) argues for a specific syntactic deficit associated with Down syndrome, and points to a literature that indicates deficits in syntax that far exceed expectations based on general cognitive functioning (e. g. Thompson 1963; Wisniewski/Miezejeski/Hill 1988). Even in the domain of communication there appear to be asynchronies with respect to different aspects of the communication system. Lexical difficulties are less severe than syntactic difficulties (Evans 1977; Hartley 1982) and functional communication skills are often much greater than verbal ability (e. g. Coggins/Carpenter/Owings 1983; Scherer/Owings 1984).

Fowler suggests that while general descriptions of language may be similar for retarded persons with and without Down syndrome, the reasons for their language delays may not be. Non-Down syndrome individuals may be limited by general intellectual ability. Down syndrome individuals may be limited by a specific language deficit (cf. Fowler 1990).

3.2. Williams Syndrome

Williams syndrome is a rare metabolic disorder associated with moderate to severe mental retardation (Williams/Barrett-Boyes/Lowe 1961). Features of the syndrome include a narrowing of the aorta, and an unusual facial structure consisting of a stellate or 'starlike' pattern in the iris, medial eyebrow flare, an upturned nose, and thick lips with an open mouth posture (Jones/Smith 1975). However, despite impairments in intellectual functioning, delays in attaining motor milestones, and early delays in language development (Thal/Bates/Bellugi 1988), older individuals with Williams syndrome exhibit a surprising facility with linguistic processing (Bellugi/Marks/Bihrle/Sabo 1988) and verbal IQ scores significantly greater than performance IQ scores (Udwin/Yule/Martin 1986).

Bellugi et al. (1988) report on three Williams syndrome children. Their CAs were 11, 15, and 16 years, and full scale IQ scores were approximataly 50. They could not perform tasks that would have placed them in Piaget's stage of concrete operations. They appeared particularly deviant on tests of spatial cognition. Their scores were low on tasks of spatial orientation, spatial arrangement, and drawing. However, they were able to quickly and accurately recognize and discriminate unfamiliar faces. So, even within the visual/spatial domain some aspects of cognition were less deviant than expected.

The most striking aspect of the cognitive performance of these children was their facility with language. Bellugi et al. report vocabularies that far exceed MA expectations (age-equivalent scores of 9.0 to 11.7 years) and MLUs ranging from 8.6 to 13.1. Down syndrome individuals of similar MAs exhibited MLUs of 3.0 to 3.5. Bellugi et al. describe the expressive language of older Williams syndrome children as "complex in terms of morphological and syntactic structures including full passives, embedded relative clauses, a range of conditionals and multiple endings" (Bellugi/Marks/Bihrle/Sabo 1988, 183). On tests of grammatical comprehension, the children consistently performed at levels that exceeded MA expectations, and exhibited a high degree of metalinguistic ability in making judgements of grammaticality.

Research on individuals with Williams syndrome is relatively new. A longitudinal profile of the acquisition and development of language in these individuals should prove interesting.

3.3. Fragile-X Syndrome

Fragile X syndrome is a recently identified chromosome abnormality that primarily affects males. Most males affected with fragile X syndrome exhibit a large head circumference in infancy, long ears, a large lower jaw, and testicular enlargement in postpubertal males (Sutherland/Ashforth 1979; Turner/Frost 1980). The majority function in the moderately retarded range, although retardation can be severe. Females may be affected, but the degree of their retardation is often less severe.

Paul/Cohen/Breg et al. (1984) reported on three adolescents with fragile X syndrome. They had CAs of 13.75, 10.5, and 10 years and nonverbal IQs of 40, 50, and 70. MAs were 5.5, 5.25, and 7 years. Subjects were given a battery of speech and language evaluations, including an analysis of spontaneous speech. All children exhibited poorer performance on tests of productive syntax than on tests of receptive language, difficulties in articulation when using connected speech despite performing well on single words in tests of articulation, and poor vocal imitation performance.

Sudhalter/Cohen/Silverman/Wolf-Schein (1990) compared the linguistic performance of 9 retarded males with Down syndrome (mean CA = 13.9), 12 with fragile X syndrome (mean CA = 15.65), and 12 with autism unrelated to fragile X (mean CA = 11.75). Mean scores on the Vineland Adaptive Behavior scale ranged from 50.75 to 56.33 across groups. Communication domain age equivalent scores ranged from 5.33 to 5.88. Socialization age equivalent scores were 8.34 for the Down syndrome, 6.15 for the fragile X, and 3.80 for the autistic subjects. Subjects were videotaped in a 30 minute session that consisted of 10 minutes of free play, 10 minutes of interaction with a familar adult, and 10 minutes of interaction with an unfamiliar adult. The males affected by fragile X exhibited language that was different from both the Down syndrome and the autistic individuals. The fragile X subjects engaged in more deviant language than the Down syndrome subjects, and the deviant language of the fragile X subjects was distinctly different from the language of the autistic subjects.

Wolf-Schein/Sudhalter/Cohen et al. (1987) also reported that subjects with fragile X exhibited more jargon, echolalia, and perseveration in their speech than did subjects with Down syndrome. However, it is not clear from these data whether this is a pattern of deviance that is specific to fragile X syndrome or simply a pattern that distinguishes it from Down syndrome. A comparison with other etiologies will be required before this issue can be resolved.

4. Summary

The research discussed here indicates that mentally retarded individuals exhibit serious deficiencies in the development of language in general, with the most severe difficulties associated with the development of syntax. However, it is clear that many persons with mental retardation exhibit very effective general communication skills. There is currently some debate as to whether or not individuals whose retardation is the result of different etiologies also exhibit diverse patterns of language development. It may be informative to examine specific patterns of language deficits as they relate to specific syndromes that result in mental retardation. But it is important to recognize that searching for language characteristics that are specific to every syndrome that results in mental retardation may not be fruitful given the variability of language skills observed both within and across etiologies (Rondal 1988).

5. References

Abbeduto, L., Furman, L., & Davies, B. (1989). Relation between the receptive language and mental age of persons with mental retardation. *American Journal on Mental Retardation, 93*, 535–543.

Abbeduto, L. & Rosenberg, S. (1980). The communicative competence of mildly retarded adults. *Applied Psycholinguistics, 1*, 405–426.

Balkany, T. (1980). Otologic aspects of Down's syndrome. *Seminars in Speech, Language, and Hearing, 1*, 39–57.

Bedrosian, J. L. & Prutting, C. A. (1978). Communicative performance of mentally retarded adults in four conversational settings. *Journal of Speech and Hearing Research, 21*, 79–95.

Bellugi, U., Marks, S., Bihrle, A., & Sabo, H. (1988). Dissociation between language and cognitive functions in Williams syndrome. In D. Bishop & K. Mogford (Eds.), *Language development in exceptional circumstances. 177–189.* New York: Churchill Livingstone.

Benda, C. E. (1949). *Mongolism and cretinism.* New York: Grune and Stratton.

Bishop, D. (1982). *Test for Reception of Grammar.* Department of Psychology, University of Manchester.

Bloom, L. & Lahey, M. (1978). *Language development and language disorders.* New York: Wiley.

Bridges, A. & Smith, J. (1984). Syntactic comprehension in Down's syndrome children. *British Journal of Psychology, 75*, 187–196.

Brooks, P., Sperber, R., & McCauley, C. (Eds.) (1984). *Learning and cognition in the mentally retarded.* Hillsdale, NJ: Erlbaum.

Buddenhagen, R. G. (1971). *Establishing vocal verbalization in mute mongoloid children.* Champaign, III: Research Press.

Carroll, J. B. (1976). Psychometric tests as cognitive tasks: A new look at the structure of the intellect. In L. B. Resnick (Ed.), *The nature of intelligence. 27–56.* Hillsdale, NJ: Erlbaum.

Chapman, R. S., Kay-Raining Bird, E., & Schwartz, S. E. (1990). Fast mapping of words in event contexts by children with Down syndrome. *Journal of Speech and Hearing Disorders, 55*, 761–770.

Coggins, T. E. (1979). Relational meaning encoded in the two word utterances of Stage 1 Down syndrome children. *Journal of Speech and Hearing Research, 22*, 166–178.

Coggins, T. E., Chapter, R. L., & Owings, N. O. (1983). Examining early intentional communication in Down's syndrome and nonretarded children. *British Journal of Disorders of Communication, 18*, 98–106.

Coggins, T. E. & Stoel-Gammon, C. (1982). Clarification strategies used by four Down's syndrome children for maintaining normal conversational interaction. *Education and Training of the Mentally Retarded, 17*, 65–67.

Cromer, R. F. (1975). Are subnormals linguistic adults. In N. O. O'Connor (Ed.), *Language, cognitive deficits, and retardation. 169–187.* London: Butterworths.

Cunningham, C. E., Reuler, E., Blackwell, J., & Deck, J. (1981). Behavioral and linguistic development in the interactions of normal and retarded children and their mothers. *Child Development, 52*, 62–70.

Davies, D., Sperber, R. D., & McCauley, C. (1981). Intelligence-related differences in semantic processing speed. *Journal of Experimental Child Psychology, 31*, 387–402.

Dever, R. (1972). A comparison of the results of a revised version of Berko's test of morphology with the free speech of mentally retarded children. *Journal of Speech and Hearing Research, 15*, 169–178.

Dodd, B. (1976). A comparison of the phonological systems of mental age matched normal, severely subnormal and Down's syndrome children. *British Journal of Communication Disorders, 11*, 27–42.

Duchan, J. F. & Erickson, J. G. (1976). Normal and retarded children's understanding of speech relations in different verbal contexts. *Journal of Speech and Hearing Research, 19*, 767–776.

Ellis, N. R. (Ed.) (1979). *Handbook of mental deficiency, psychological theory and research.* Hillsdale, NJ: Erlbaum.

Evans, D. (1977). The development of language abilities in mongols: A correlational study. *Journal of Mental Deficiency Research, 21*, 103–117.

Fawcus, M. & Fawcus, R. (1974). Disorders of communication. In A. M. Clarke & A. D. B. Clarke (Eds.), *Mental deficiency: The changing outlook. 3rd Edition. 592–627.* London: Methuen.

Fischer, M. A. (1987). Mother-child interaction in preverbal children with Down syndrome. *Journal of Speech and Hearing Disorders, 52*, 179–190.

Fowler, A. E. (1990). Language abilities in children with Down syndrome: Evidence for a specific syntactic delay. In D. Cicchetti & M. Beeghly (Eds.), *Children with Down syndrome: A developmental perspective. 302–328.* New York: Cambridge University Press.

Grossman, H. J. (1983). *Classification in mental retardation.* Washington, DC: American Association on Mental Deficiency.

Hartley, X. Y. (1982). Receptive language processing of Down's syndrome children. *Journal of Mental Deficiency Research, 26*, 263–269.

Hoff-Ginsberg, E. (1986). Function and structure in maternal speech: Their relation to the child's development of syntax. *Developmental Psychology, 22*, 155–163.

Ingram, D. (1976). *Phonological disability in children.* New York: Elsevier.

Jones, O. H. M. (1977). Mother-child communication with prelinguistic Down's syndrome and normal infants. In H. R. Schaffer & J. Dunn (Eds.), *The first year of life: Psychological and medical implications of early experience. 175–195.* New York: Wiley.

Jones, A. & Robson, C. (1979). Language training in the severely mentally handicapped. In N. R. Ellis (Ed.), *Handbook of mental retardation, psychological theory and research. 367–400.* Hillsdale, NJ: Erlbaum.

Jones, K. L. & Smith, D. W. (1975). The Williams elfin facies syndrome: A new perspective. *Journal of Pediatrics, 86*, 718–723.

Kernan, K. T. (1990). Comprehension of syntactically indicated sequence by Down's syndrome and other mentally retarded adults. *Journal of Mental Deficiency Research, 34*, 169–178.

Kiernan, C. (1985). Communication. In A. M. Clarke, A. D. B. Clarke, & J. Berg (Eds.), *Mental Deficiency: The changing outlook. 4th Edition. 584–638.* London: Methuen.

Layton, T. L. & Sharifi, H. (1979). Meaning and structure of Down's syndrome and nonretarded children's spontaneous speech. *American Journal of Mental Deficiency, 83*, 439–445.

Leifer, J. & Lewis, M. (1984). Acquisition of conversational skills by young Down syndrome and nonretarded children. *American Journal of Mental Deficiency, 84*, 610–618.

Mahoney, G. (1988). Maternal communication style with mentally retarded children. *American Journal on Mental Retardation, 92*, 352–359.

Mahoney, G. & Robenalt, K. (1986). A comparison of conversational patterns between mothers and their Down syndrome and normal infants. *Journal of the Division of Early Childhood, 10*, 172–180.

Mauer, H. & Sherrod, K. (1987). Context of directives given to young children with Down syndrome and nonretarded children: Development over two years. *American Journal of Mental Deficiency, 91*, 579–590.

McConkey, R. & Martin, H. (1984). A longitudinal study of mothers' speech to preverbal Down syndrome infants. *First Language, 5*, 41–55.

Mein, R. & O'Connor, N. (1960). A study of oral vocabularies of severely subnormal patients. *Journal of Mental Deficiency Research, 4*, 130–143.

Menn, L. (1985). Phonological development: Learning sounds and sound patterns. In J. Berko-Gleason (Ed.), *The development of language. 77–113.* Columbus, Ohio: Merrill.

Merrill, E. C. (1985). Differences in semantic processing speed of mentally retarded and nonretarded persons: Comparison of short- and longterm memory processing. *American Journal of Mental Deficiency, 90*, 71–80.

Mundy, P., Sigman, M., Kasari, C., & Yirmiya, N. (1988). Nonverbal communication skills in Down syndrome children. *Child Development, 59*, 235–249.

Paul, R., Cohen, D. J., Breg, W. R., Waxton, M., & Herman, S. (1984). Fragile X syndrome: Its relationship to speech and hearing disorders. *Journal of Speech and Hearing Disorders, 49*, 328–332.

Peterson, G. & Sherrod, K. (1982). Relationship of maternal language to language development and language delay of children. *American Journal of Mental Deficiency, 86*, 391–398.

Price-Williams, D. & Sabsay, S. (1979). Communicative competence among severely retarded persons. *Semiotica, 26*, 35–63.

Rondal, J. (1978). Maternal speech to normal and Down's syndrome children matched for mean length of utterance. *Monograph of the American Association on Mental Deficiency.* Washington, D. C.: American Association on Mental Deficiency.

Rondal, J. (1988). Down's syndrome. In D. Bishop & K. Mogford (Eds.), *Language development in exceptional circumstances. 165–176.* New York: Churchill Livingstone.

Rosenberg, S. (1982). The language of the mentally retarded: Development, processes and intervention. In S. Rosenberg (Ed.), *Handbook of applied psycholinguistics: Major thrusts of research and theory. 329–392.* Hillsdale, NJ: Erlbaum.

Scherer, N. J. & Owings, N. O. (1984). Learning to be contingent: Retarded children's responses to their mothers' requests. *Language and Speech, 27,* 255–267.

Schiefelbusch, R. & Copeland, R. (Eds.) (1968). *Language and mental retardation: Empirical and conceptual considerations.* New York: Holt, Rinehart and Winston.

Schiefelbusch, R. L. & Lloyd, L. L. (Eds.) (1974). *Language perspectives – Acquisition, retardation, and intervention.* Baltimore, Md: University Park Press.

Schlanger, B. B. & Gottsleben, R. H. (1957). Analysis of speech defects among the institutionalized mentally retarded. *Journal of Speech and Hearing Disorders, 22,* 98–103.

Share, J. B. (1975). Developmental progress in Down's syndrome. In R. Koch & F. F. de la Cruz (Eds.), *Down's syndrome (mongolism): Research, prevention, and management. 78–86.* New York: Bruner/Mazel.

Smith, N. V. (1973). *The acquisition of phonology.* Cambridge: Cambridge University Press.

Snow, C. (1977). Mother's speech research: From input to interaction. In C. E. Snow & C. A. Furguson (Eds.), *Talking to children: Language input and acquisition. 1–37.* Cambridge: Cambridge University Press.

Sperber, R. D., Davies, D., Merrill, E. C., McCauley, C. (1982). Cross-category differences in the processing of subordinate-superordinate relationships. *Child Development, 53,* 1249–1253.

Sperber, R. D. & McCauley, C. (1984). Semantic processing efficiency in the mentally retarded. In P. Brooks, R. Sperber, & C. McCauley (Eds.), *Learning and cognition in the mentally retarded. 141–163.* Hillsdale, NJ: Erlbaum.

Sperber, R. D., Ragain, R. D., & McCauley, C. (1976). Reassessment of category knowledge in retarded individuals. *American Journal of Mental Deficiency, 81,* 227–234.

Sternberg, R. J. (1984). Toward a triarchical theory of human intelligence. *Brain and Behavioral Sciences, 7,* 269–315.

Stoel-Gammon, C. (1980). Phonological analysis of four Down's syndrome children, *Applied Psycholinguistics, 1,* 31–48.

Sudhalter, V., Cohen, I. L., Silverman, W., & Wolf-Schein, E. G. (1990). Conversational analyses of males with fragile X, Down syndrome, and autism: Comparison of the emergence of deviant language. *American Journal on Mental Retardation, 94,* 431–441.

Sutherland, G. R. & Ashforth, P. L. (1979). X-linked mental retardation with macroorchidism and the fragile X site Xq27 or 28. *Human Genetics, 48,* 117–120.

Thal, D., Bates, E., & Bellugi, U. (1988). Language and cognition in two children with Williams syndrome. *Journal of Speech and Hearing Research, 32,* 489–500.

Thompson, M. M. (1963). Psychological characteristics relevant to the education of the pre-school mongoloid child. *Mental Retardation, 1,* 148–151.

Turner, G. & Frost, D. (1980). X-linked mental retardation, macroorchidism, and the Xq27 fragile site. *Journal of Pediatrics, 96,* 837–841.

Udwin, O., Yule, W., & Martin, N. D. T. (1986). Age at diagnosis and abilities in idiopathic hypercalcaemia. *Archives of Disease in Childhood, 61,* 1164–1167.

Williams, J. C. P., Barrett-Boyes, B. G., & Lowe, J. B. (1961). Supravalvular aortic stenosis. *Circulation , 24,* 1311–1318.

Wisniewski, K. E., Miezejeski, C. M., & Hill, A. L. (1988). Neurological and psychological status of individuals with Down syndrome. In L. Nadel (Ed.), *The psychobiology of Down syndrome. 315–343.* Cambridge, MA: MIT Press.

Wolf-Schein, E. G., Sudhalter, V., Cohen, I. L., Fisch, G. S., Hanson, D., Pfadt, A. G., Hagerman, R., Jenkins, E. C., & Brown, W. T. (1987). Speech-language and the fragile-X syndrome: Initial findings. *Journal of the American Speech and Hearing Association, 29,* 35–38.

Yoder, P. J. (1989). Maternal question use predicts later language development in specific language disordered children. *Journal of Speech and Hearing Disorders, 54,* 347–355.

Yoder, P. C., & Kaiser, A. P. (1989). Alternative explanations for the relationship between maternal verbal interaction style and child development. *Journal of Child Language, 16,* 141–161.

Edward C. Merrill, Tuscaloosa, Alabama (USA)

68. Patterns of Interaction and Communication in Language Development Disorders

1. Introduction

Many developmental psychologists espouse the meta-theory or 'philosophy' that caregiver-child interactions are an important source of the child's development. That the child does not acquire his/her abilities in a social vacuum is especially true in the case of language development. The child needs a language environment and a caregiver for communicative and interactive exchanges. He/she would not be able to acquire language just by listening to the radio or television (e. g. Sachs/Bard/Johnson 1981).

The so-called Motherese research has furnished the very important result that mothers talk in a different way to their language-acquiring children than to older children and adults. They use a special speech style which can be characterized by various features on molecular and molar level. Although many empirical findings take conflicting sides in the question whether certain types of features are conducive to language growth or not, the correlational research to date suggests that at least the following six structures and interactive features of the mothers' input exert an influence on the child's rate of language acquisition (Cross 1978, Hoff-Ginsberg 1985, 1986, Nelson/Carskaddon/Bonvillian 1973, Newport/Gleitman/Gleitman 1977, Olsen-Fulero 1982, Smolak/Weinraub 1983, for summary see Grimm 1990, Hoff-Ginsberg/Shatz 1982, Menyuk 1988): Frequency of

- inverted yes/no questions
- wh-questions
- partial repetitions of child's utterances
- partial self-repetitions with or without modifications
- expansions
- conversation-eliciting questions or, more generally speaking, a conversation eliciting maternal interaction style.

The theoretically significant question is how to conceptualize the underlying functional relationships that lead to the empirically established correlations. In the literature these data patterns are mainly interpreted within a 'maternal influence model' (Yoder/Kaiser 1989). Specifically it is asked how these structural or interactive features of maternal language can directly or indirectly influence language acquisition. It would certainly be shortsighted to assume very simple effects. There is no direct transfer from the maternal mouth into the child's mind. It is the child who must make the language input offered to him usable for himself. Since we cannot look into children's heads, we can only offer theoretically plausible interpretations as to how a facilitation effect may come about (Grimm 1990, Hoff-Ginsberg 1986). Obviously, a specific structural or interactional feature or cluster of features may have many "properties at different levels that make them both communicatively salient and linguistically informative" (Hoff-Ginsberg/Shatz 1982, 9) and thus may help the child directly or indirectly in solving the language learning problem (a) by highlighting and exemplifying structural characteristics and (b) by eliciting conversation and thus increasing the opportunity for language learning. In the following we will mention a few exemplary interpretations to illustrate the reasoning within this research tradition (for a more detailed discussion see e. g. Hoff-Ginsberg/Shatz 1982). The most robust finding is that mothers' use of auxiliaries in inverted yes/no questions influences the rate at which their children develop the auxiliary system. Since the auxiliaries appear in first position in such sentences ("Have you seen this?", "Will you pick up the doll?") they are perceptively salient and are particularly taken note of by children. It is also true for wh-questions ("Where do you want to go?", "What is this?") that the elements of verb phrases are made prominent by the transformation of the canonical sentence structure. Partial repetitions of the mother's own or of the child's utterances might help in segmentation and in specifying constituent boundaries. For example, when the mother says "Du kannst die Tassen hierher stellen. Die Tassen. Hierher." ["You can put the cups here. The cups. Here."] she illustrates the particular structural segments of the sequence, thereby facilitating the identification of these segments for the child. The positive influence of expansions could result from the fact that the child can compare two consecutive utterances with each other (Grimm 1985). When the child says "Ich bin des, ich Fuß brocht" ["That's me, I broken foot"] and the mother responds "Das bist du, als du den Fuß gebrochen hast" ["That's you when you broke your foot"] then it appears as if the mother were teaching language with intent. She offers the child something like a good verbal form or 'gestalt' for the intended content. Thus the child has the opportunity to compare his/her own utterance with this model and can recognize where words have been corrected or added.

As Hoff-Ginsberg (1986) has shown, conversation-eliciting speech (in contrast to simple directive speech, see Olsen-Fulero 1982) may also facilitate language acquisition because it encourages the child to produce and practice language. Pure quiz questions such as "What does the cow say?" display no or even a negative empirical relationship to language acquisition. These questions are simple to answer and do not challenge the child's language production abilities. Real information-demanding questions and reflexive questions, however, are suited to get the child working on language. For example, if the child's previous utterance was not understood, he/she must try to reformulate it in order to express more clearly what he/she wants to say.

Obviously the assumption that some specific structural and/or interactional features might aid language acquisition throughout the course of development is theoretically and empirically unwarranted. In fact, it has been proposed that fine-tuning in the sense of the continual adjustment of child-directed speech to a child-appropriate level is an important candidate for facilitating language acquisition (e. g. Cross 1977). However, the empirical findings are somewhat at odds so that at best there is mixed evidence for the language facilitating influence of fine-tuning (for a review see Snow/Perlmann/Nathan 1987). It is nevertheless important to raise this issue here, since the question whether and in which ways mothers of language disordered children adjust themselves semantically and syntactically to the language level of their children plays an important role in determining the communicative environment of these children, as will be shown later in this chapter.

The research on language input to language disordered children addresses four main questions:

(a) Are the grammatical features and interactional patterns similar to those provided to normally developing children?
(b) Are there differences in the directiveness and the initiative behavior between mothers of language disordered children and those of normal language children? Should one interpret these differences in the sense of a child-driven maternal adjustment or rather as an instructional intent?
(c) What are the consequences of the language environment provided to disordered children on the language development of these children?
(d) What are the consequences of the language input on the cognitive development of the child?

Of course we will not be able to give any final answers to these questions; the number of comparative studies is too limited. There is especially a lack of longitudinal and follow-up studies so that reflections on the consequences of mother's language input must remain highly speculative.

As we will see, with a few exceptions all studies involved English-speaking children. Consequently, the validity of the inferences drawn must be quite limited. During the last few years research with normally developing children which has taken a 'cultural context' view has questioned the supposition that there is a best way to speak to children in order to facilitate language development (see for example Shatz/Grimm/Wilcox/Niemeier-Wind in press). However, research on language disordered children is still determined by the assumption that there must be a generally valid way of 'teaching' language. This, however, can only be demonstrated on the basis of intercultural studies.

This review focuses on the four main questions already outlined. In particular dyads with specifically language impaired (SLI) or (to use another term) dysphasic children, with autistic children, and with mentally retarded children are included. Whereas at least in previous studies the question was discussed whether the language input to SLI children and to autistic children is deficient and causally responsible for these children's developmental disorder, the speech style in the case of mental retardation has always been interpreted as being reactive.

Dealing with these three different developmental disorders together only makes sense if we can expect to find similar input structures and interactional patterns. However, this does not exclude the possibility that there may also be communication patterns which are specific to one of the forms of language disorder.

The material cited is selective. This is partly to keep this review within bounds but primarily because we wish to report results that are based on a fairly sound methodology. The following restrictions in the coverage should thus be noted. We will neither take into consideration studies with poorly defined or very small samples, nor studies with inadequate statistical data analysis or where it is unclear according to which criteria the material was analyzed. Further, we will not consider comparisons between mothers and fathers or other adults nor will we report on peer interactions. There are simply too few empirical studies in these areas, and those existing are theoretically not very convincing. Thus, for example, it remains completely open to which theoretical conclusions differences in speech style between mothers and fathers can lead.

2. Input: Mothers' Speech to Language Disordered Children

2.1. General Interaction Variables

The quality of the dialogue between mother and child can be evaluated according to whether they have a 'common ground' and whether their communicative exchange displays reciprocity. It is certainly true that the child's willingness to actively use language for communication depends on the quality of the dialogue. And the engagement in communication again has to do with language acquisition. These relationships have induced researchers of language development disorders to investigate the hypothesis that the quality of communicative exchanges between mothers and their disordered children is poorer than the quality of exchanges with normal children.

A very robust result is the finding that mothers of SLI children as well as mothers of mentally retarded children show far more directiveness than mothers of normal children. This result remains valid independent of whether the control children were matched according to language level, mental age, or chronological age. Nearly all studies showed the concurrent result that the mothers of the SLI children use significantly more initiatives and imperatives than mothers of normal children (Bondurant/Romeo/Kretschmer 1983, Conti-Ramsden 1990, Conti-Ramsden/Friel-Patti 1983, Grimm 1983, Moseley 1990).

On the basis of a rating with the Caldwell Inventory of Home Stimulation Wulbert/Inglis/Kriegsmann/Mills (1975) found additional evidence that the mothers of SLI children displayed less emotional and verbal responsiveness and less involvement than mothers of age-matched normal controls and of Down syndrome children. Since comparatively low Caldwell scores were found through the socioeconomic strata, it appears justified to conclude that language impairment had a stronger influence on the mother-child relationship than socioeconomic factors.

That the higher proportion of directive utterances in mothers of SLI children also holds across differing situations has been clearly demonstrated by Bondurant/Romeo/Kretschmer (1983). They compared the language behavior of 14 mothers with 2;5–5;0-year-old SLI children to 14 mothers with age-matched normally developing children in a structured and in an unstructured situation. In the unstructured (15-minute) free play situation "each mother and her child were seated on the floor facing each other with (preselected) toys on the floor between them. ... The mother was then instructed to encourage her child to play with the toys." (Bondurant/Romeo/Kretschmer 1983, 235). In the structured situation mother and child were again seated on the floor facing each other. But only the mother, not the child, "was able to see a constructed model farm built from a commercially produced set. A comparable set was scattered on the floor" (235) and the mother was instructed to help her child build the farm. In both situations the mothers of the SLI children showed significantly less acceptance utterances; in the structured situation they asked significantly less questions and – most interestingly – in the free play situation they provided over twice as many directions and produced numerically more rejection utterances in comparison to the mothers of the normal children. The authors therefore ascertain quite correctly that "the mothers of the language delayed were extremely more directive than the mothers of normal children" (240).

It is quite impressive that alone 8 of 13 analyzed studies with mentally retarded children likewise produced evidence that the mothers display pronounced directive behavior (Cardoso-Martins/Mervis 1985, Cunningham/Reuler/Blackwell/Deck 1981, Davis/Stroud/Green 1988, Eheart 1982, Hanzlik/Stevenson 1986, Mahoney/Fors/Wood 1990, Maurer/Sherrod 1987, Tannock 1988). Cunningham et al. (1981) examined the verbal and behavioral interactions of 18 mothers with their mentally retarded and 18 mothers with their normal children matched for socio-economic status and for mental age as indicated by the Peabody Picture Vocabulary Test Score. The dyads were observed in 15-minute free play and 15-minute structured task situations. During free play the mothers were instructed to interact with their child as they might do at home; in the structured task they had to have their child tidy up the toys and complete three puzzles. Compared to the controls the mothers of the mentally retarded were much more directive during both settings, i. e., they exerted more control over their children's play and gave more commands and command-questions (cf. however, Davis/Stroud/Green 1988). On the other hand, their children proved less interactive. Thus the results of Cunningham/Reuler/Blackwell/Deck (1981) as well as the studies of Eheart (1982) and Tannock (1988) have been interpreted to suggest that the mothers' directive behavior is dependent on the passivity of their mentally retarded children. In Tannock's study the mothers of 11 mentally retarded and 11 normal children individually matched for communicative ability, mental age and demographic variables were observed while interacting with their children during 15-minute free play situations. The mothers of the retarded children not only exhibited a higher level of interactional activity than the control mothers; in addition, an inverse relationship between mother's and child's interactional activity was observed. The partial correlations controlling for variations in children's level of communication were highly significant, the partial correlation being $r_p = -.80$ for retarded and $r_p = -.74$ for non-retarded dyads (Tannock 1988, 161).

The reason why the frequent initiatives and imperative utterances of the mothers of language disordered children are likewise to be regarded as reactive behavior and not in the sense of a trait is because the language disordered children behave very passively in dialogue. We will return to this aspect later.

At this point it is important to recognize that the high directiveness of mothers of language disordered and of mentally retarded children does not necessarily imply a low sensitivity and responsiveness (see e. g. Crawley/Spiker 1983), as some authors seem to claim. In fact the mothers do display responsiveness in the sense that they react to their children's language behavior. Thus only very occasionally has empirical evidence been brought (e. g. Cunningham/Reuler/Blackwell/Deck 1981, Eheart 1982, Wulbert/Inglis/Kriegsmann/Mills 1975) that these mothers show lower responsiveness than the mothers of normal children. There are, however, far more indications that the way in which the mothers of the developmentally disordered respond to their children's behavior differs from that of normal children's mothers. Thus Cross (1981) ascertained that mothers of SLI children produce significantly more non-informative responses than mothers of normal, language age-matched children. In addition, Moseley (1990) found that the mothers of SLI children produced 40 % nonsustaining utterances whereas the mothers of the MLU-matched normal controls produced only 21 %. Further, the mothers of SLI children significantly more often used recasts as 'meaning illocutions' (requests, assertives, directives) than as 'cohesion illocutions' (responsives, regulatives) in comparison to mothers of MLU-matched control children. The higher frequency of the 'meaning illocutions' is interpreted by Conti-Ramsden (1990, 269) as "effort to actively engage the child in dialogue and maintain the interaction, or a consequence of interacting with a passive partner in conversation". However, this interpretation does not help in understanding why the mothers' utterances are so often semantically unrelated to their children's utterances. For example Mahoney/Fors/Wood (1990) found that mothers of mentally retarded children used more 'mands' that were not systematically linked to their children's behavior than control mothers. Very important is also the additional observation that they directed their 'attention requests' onto things that were not within their children's attentional focus. The conclusion that the mothers of retarded children make only restricted attempts to provide a shared focus of attention and to elaborate on a semantic topic with their children is also supported by the finding that they introduce more 'topic switches' (Tannock 1988) than control mothers and that they more frequently use semantically unrelated utterances (Peterson/Sherrod 1982). An interesting aspect is that in the same study the mothers of the SLI children produced even more semantically unrelated utterances than the mothers of the mentally retarded children.

Whereas the findings with regard to mothers of language disordered and mentally retarded children are very similar, the results from studies involving mothers of autistic children take another track. Earlier studies have postulated that deficient parent-child-interactions play a causal role with regard to the language deficits of autistic children, the mothers in particular being blamed for being poorer at communicating meaning and mood, being less responsive to the children's requests and giving poorer instructions and more ambiguous information than mothers of normal children (Goldfarb/Goldfarb/Scholl 1966, Goldfarb/Yudkovitch/Goldfarb 1973). That the low frequency of language in autistic children may be caused and maintained by a lack of reinforcement for verbalization, a lack of encouragement to speak, and a lack of correction of language has been suggested by Howlin/Cantwell/Marchant et al. (1973). Basing on psychoanalytical theory the social environment on the whole was made responsible for the genesis of autism. It was claimed that the mothers were not warm, supportive, and accepting, but cold, rigid, and rejecting (e. g. Bettelheim 1967; see also art. 78).

However, all these assumptions have proved to be untenable. In a study by Rutter/Bartak/Newman (1971), the behavior of mothers and fathers of 14 intelligent autistic children ("purest kind of autism") and 11 children suffering from developmental receptive aphasia was evaluated. There were no differences in the ratings for the categories 'emotional warmth', 'empathy', and 'enthusiasm'. In accordance with this, comparisons between parents of autistic children and MLU-matched normal children have not furnished any differences with regard to reinforcement of vocalizations, encouragement to speak, or correcting of errors (Wolchik 1983, Wolchik/Harris 1982). Wolchik compared 10 mothers and fathers of autistic children at the age of 29–74 months and with average intelligence (again "purest kind of autism") with 10 mothers and fathers of MLU-matched control children between the age of 6 and 25 months. Since, as already pointed out, no differences in reinforcement, encouragement, and correction behavior could be found, the conclusion appears justified that deviant parent-child verbal interactions do not play an etiological part in the language disabilities of autistic children (Wolchik 1983, 177). However, this conclusion, although certainly correct, does not necessarily imply that the language environment is optimal for the language development of the autistic child. It could perhaps be the case that the autistic child might need a special and enriched language model. Whereas Wolchik's study only involved parents of higher functioning autistic children, a recent study by Konstantareas/Zajdeman/Homatidis/McCabe (1988) compared the maternal speech styles of 10 verbal and higher functioning with 10 nonverbal and lower functioning autistic children as the "two main subgroups of the heterogeneous population of autistic children" (649). The higher functioning children (2f, 8m) were between 28 and 112 months old and had a nonverbal IQ between 68 to 117; their language level lay between 2 and 7 years. The lower functioning children (2f, 8m) were between 29 and 117 months old; they had no speech and an IQ-measurement could not be made.

Of 10 investigated assumptions 7 could be confirmed: (a) the mothers of the lower functioning autistic children control their children's actions more, reinforce more motoric behavior and use shorter MLUs. (b) The mothers of the higher functioning autistic children answer questions more often and also offer more prompts for spoken language, they expand correct spoken language more often, reinforce more language related behavior, and have longer MLUs.

As with the mothers of the mentally retarded and the SLI children, directiveness is interpreted as reaction to difficulties on the part of the child.

In summary: In order to evaluate the affective and communicative quality of the mother-child dialogue it was investigated on the molar level whether mothers of developmentally impaired children differ – among other characteristics – in their responsiveness, directiveness and emotional warmth from mothers whose children do not display any developmental disorders. The main result is that the dialogues with the disordered children are more unbalanced in that these mothers direct and maintain the dialogue by means of their initiatives far more than the mothers of normal children. This directive behavior is mainly interpreted as being adaptive in the cases of language impaired, mentally retarded, and autistic children. The mothers are guided to their own behavior style by their children's passivity. That this reaction can be connected with semantically unrelated utterances and with unmotivated topic changes, i. e. with communication styles which do not fulfill the functions of encouraging language usage in the child, will be treated in more detail later in this chapter.

2.2. Structural Properties of Mother's Speech

It is plausible to assume that children will develop problems in acquiring language when their language input is poor and restricted. On the molecular level the data-providing function (see Hoff-Ginsberg 1986) of mothers' speech can be studied in at least two respects. On the one hand we can analyze the maternal language input according to its structural features and investigate – among other things – how long and complex the utterances are, whether certain word orders predominate or whether certain word classes such as prepositions are used. On the other hand we can investigate the so-called 'language teaching strategies' the mothers use. In order to do this we need to accomplish a formal on-line analysis of dialogue. The aim is to find out whether and how often mothers directly tack on to their children's utterances by repeating, correcting, or expanding them. It is rather surprising that up to now studies have shown only few or even no differences at all in the structural and strategic characteristics of the mothers of dysphasic, mentally retarded, or autistic children as compared to the mothers of normal children matched according to the level of their cognitive and/or language development.

2.2.1. Grammatical Features

Studies for example by O'Kelly-Collard (1978), Rondal (1978), Cunningham/Reuler/Blackwell/Deck (1981), and Davis/Stroud/Green (1988), have revealed that the utterances of mothers of mentally retarded children do not differ significantly from utterances of mothers of normal children in terms of MLU, number of propositions per utterance, sentence complexity, and in the number of ungrammatical sentences. The assumption that the mothers of developmentally disordered children formally adapt to their child's language ability is also supported for autistic children: Findings reported by Konstantareas/Zajdeman/Homatidis/McCabe (1988) show that the mothers of lower functioning autistic children produced utterances with shorter MLU than mothers of higher functioning autistic children.

One of the main hypotheses in searching for the causes of specific language impairment was that the maternal language input is deficient and therefore not suitable to serve as a model for language learning. This hypothesis was self-evident since SLI children do not display any obvious neurological, sensory, or cognitive disorders which could account directly for their language deficits. Interestingly, it was the failure to prove that mothers of dysphasic children offer their children a clearly deficient language model (see Leonard 1987 for a review) which stimulated highly sophisticated studies focusing on causal factors in the SLI children themselves.

Even though there is a strong tendency to believe that the language of mothers of dysphasic children does not differ in its structural characteristics from that of mothers of language-matched normal children (see e. g. Cunningham/Siegel/van der Spuy et al. 1985, Grimm 1987, Grimm/Weinert 1990, Lasky/Klopp 1982, Peterson/Sherrod 1982), contradicting empirical evidence must also be considered in order to modify the over-simplified hypothesis that the mothers of the dysphasic children are completely adapted to their children's developmental level. For example Cross (1981), who compared the utterances of 10 mothers of SLI children between the ages of 3;10 and 5;1 years with the utterances of 10 mothers of normal language-matched children between the ages of 1;8 and 2;6 years, drew attention to evidence that the mothers of the SLI children produced significantly more unintelligible, disfluent, totally degraded, and run-on sentences; in addition they produced significantly less utterances per turn (but see Peterson/Sherrod 1982). In a comparative study with 10 mothers of SLI children (2;11 – 5;5 years) and 10 mothers of younger children (1;7 – 3;1 years) Schodorf/Edwards (1983) found that the first group of mothers, in addition to more sentence fragments and fewer words also produced sentences with a lower MLU. Accordingly, the authors state that the SLI child is exposed to a different type of linguistic environment; the child received a shorter, simpler input during a teaching situation, and overall reduced input, in terms of total utterances spoken by the parents, during free play (Schodorf/Edwards 1983, 79).

2.2.2. Specific Discourse Features

In their study Schodorf/Edwards (1983) also made out distinct differences in the so-called 'language teaching strategies': the mothers of the SLI children (SLI mothers) responded to their children's utterances significantly less often with expansions and ready-mades but more often with corrections. Moseley (1990) found supportive data that the SLI mothers also imitate their children's utterances significantly less often. In clear contradiction to this, however, Cross (1981) discovered significantly more imitations of their children's utterances in the SLI mothers. However, with respect to expansions, her data again do correspond to those presented by Schodorf/Edwards (1983).

In contrast to the findings cited above, Lasky/Klopp (1982) could not find any differences in the language teaching strategies at all. This overall similarity between groups of mothers parallels the results of studies comparing mother-child dyads with language-matched control children to dyads with mentally retarded (Gutman/Rondal 1979, O'Kelly-Collard 1978, Peterson/Sherrod 1982, Rondal 1978) and autistic children (Wolchik 1983, Wolchik/Harris 1982). It is also supported by Grimm (1984, 1986, 1987) in a study involving German-speaking SLI children. The utterances of the mothers of 8 dysphasic children (ages: 3;9–4;8 years) and 8 MLU-matched normally developing children (ages: 2;1–2;11 years) were compared in a longitudinal design. At the first investigation timepoint the mothers of the dysphasic and control children were remarkably similar in their tendency to imitate, to correct, and to transform their children's preceding utterances or parts thereof. One year later the mothers still did not differ significantly in their imitations and corrections. However, they now did differ significantly in the frequency of transforming their child's immediate preceding utterance. These transformations consist in systematic variations of the sentence pattern underlying the child's utterance, for example, in formulating the child's question as an answer and vice versa (e. g.: Child: "Wo is mein Buch?" ["Where is my book?"] – Mother: "Da ist dein Buch." ["There is your book"]. Child: "Der kann das nicht" ["He can't do it."] – Mother: "Kann der das nicht?" ["Can't he do it?"]). As argued by Grimm (1987, 19), the mothers of the dysphasic children employ this constructive teaching strategy significantly less often than the mothers of the normal children at the timepoint "at which the children have learned to articulate correctly and form simple sentences with correct word order". This form of reacting to the child's language progress is difficult to understand given the fact that the mothers of the normal children responded to the language progress of their children significantly more often with these teaching strategies. Could it be that the mothers of the dysphasic children were already satisfied with their children's progress and that they believed their children were not capable of learning much more? If this were actually the case, their language behavior could be interpreted as an adaptation to a consistently low level of competence. Or do the mothers consider their children to have made such good progress that they no longer need so much support as they used to? This could then probably be interpreted as an overestimation of the child's independent learning ability. Of course, we do not really know the reasons and can only speculate. The fact remains, however, that in contrast to the mothers of normally developing children the mothers of developmentally disordered children at some point in development seem to make comparatively less effort to demonstrate syntactic rules to their children by using systematic variation of their child's sentence patterns. It is an open question why this is so and why they do not on the contrary continue to support their children in their laborious language progress by offering them an enriched language input. In any case it might be presumed that the mothers of the dysphasic children were less finely-tuned to their children's language progress than the mothers of normally developing children.

In summary, some investigations clearly indicate that mothers of developmentally disordered children as well as mothers of language-matched or mental age (MA) matched normal children formally adapt their speech to their child's level of language development; in addition they both use various language teaching strategies. However, there might be differences in the processes and results of calibration (see also Cunningham/Reuler/Blackwell/Deck 1981 for dyads with retarded children).

In his review, Leonard (1987) stressed the finding that mothers of SLI children react quite as sensitively to their children's language abilities as mothers of normal language children. From this he inferred that speech input characteristics cannot be the stuff from which theories of specific language impairment or developmental dysphasia should be made. We feel that the last word has not yet been spoken. The findings of Cross (1981), Cunningham/Reuler/Blackwell/Deck (1981), Grimm (1987), Lasky/Klopp (1982), and Schodorf/Edwards (1983) should stimulate further longitudinal studies over a longer period of time on the reciprocal relationship between the maternal language model and the language progress made by developmentally disordered children.

3. Discourse Features in Language Disordered Children

3.1. Participating Behavior

We have already seen that mothers of disordered children usually show more initiatives than mothers of MA- or language-matched controls. This could be interpreted on the one hand as a 'dynamic adaptation' in the sense that the mothers try "to increase the participation of a developmentally immature child" (Tannock 1988, 155) and thus "may facilitate the child's development of conversational skills". On the other hand it is also reasonable to suspect that the mothers' pronounced initiative behavior is not child-driven but is controlled by an instructional intent on the mother's part to teach her developmentally disordered child something. The mothers so to say take up the reins in order to promote their child's learning process. We will discuss these two propositions later in detail. The point to be made here is that based on either of these theoretical accounts the prediction can be derived that disordered children are less active in dialogue than normally developing children are. A pronounced passivity is predicted either as a response to maternal control behavior, i. e. the high directive and initiative behavior of their mothers, or as stimulating this maternal behavior.

First of all, there is convincing empirical evidence that disordered children produce comparatively less initiatives in dialogue. This has been shown for mentally retarded children (Cunningham/Reuler/Blackwell/Deck 1981, Eheart 1982; but see Mahoney/Fors/Wood 1990, Tannock 1988 for less clear empirical evidence) compared to younger MA- or language-matched controls as well as for SLI children compared to language or age-matched controls (Conti-Ramsden 1990, Conti-Ramsden/Friel-Patti 1983, 1984, Cunningham/Siegel/van der Spuy et al. 1985, Moseley 1990).

In addition there are some studies indicating that disordered children may be less responsive in dialogue (Cunningham/Reuler/Blackwell/Deck 1981, Eheart 1982, Mahoney/Fors/Wood 1990), but the results are by no means clear cut. For example, Eheart (1982) compared the responsiveness of 8 mentally retarded children (age: 3;3–4;9) and 8 younger normally developing children (age: 2;0–2;7) matched for play behavior. Although the mentally retarded children responded to their mother's initiations significantly more often in terms of absolute frequencies, the differences in the percentages of responding pointed in the opposite direction, since their mothers initiated twice as many interactions as the mothers of the controls did. In the study of Tannock (1988) the retarded children again did not differ in their conditional probability to respond given the mother had taken a turn. And finally, in the study by Cunningham/Reuler/Blackwell/Deck (1981) the tendency to show lower responsiveness was more pronounced for the retarded children with low compared to high MA. Thus, although developmentally disabled children seem to be less initiative and more passive in dialogue, the empirical evidence suggests that they do not ignore their mother's questions and initiations, but – like normal children – share their mother's focus of attention (e. g. Leonard 1986, Moseley 1990 for SLI children; Eheart 1982, Mahoney/Fors/Wood 1990, Tannock 1988 for mentally retarded children).

Obviously this cannot hold for autistic children, since a "pervasive lack of responsiveness to other people" (American Psychiatric Association) is one of the diagnostic characteristics of these children. Thus, the 18 autistic children studied by Sigman/Mundy/Sherman/Ungerer (1986) displayed a much lower frequency of attention sharing behavior with their caregivers than either of two MA-matched control groups of mentally retarded and normally developing children. Interestingly enough, this study also suggests that even autistic children may be responsive to some maternal directions. Actually, the autistic children under study appropriately responded to positive maternal commands that were predominantly "aimed at behavior regulation rather than social interaction or joint attention" as often as the control groups did (Sigman/Mundy/Sherman/Ungerer 1986, 653).

3.2. Children's Processing of Their Mother's Speech

The interaction research reviewed is clearly biased towards the analysis of maternal speech. Up to the present almost all studies have neglected to investigate whether disordered children differ from normal children with respect to how often and in which way they openly process their mother's language input. This is an important question since differences in language processing may allow inferences to be drawn regarding the operation of different acquisition mechanisms.

The only existing longitudinal study of SLI children's processing of maternal speech is that mentioned above by Grimm (1984, 1986, 1987, 1993). This study is therefore to be reviewed in more detail. Eight dysphasic children (mean age: 4;2 years) and 8 younger MLU-matched normal language children (mean age: 2;6 years) were observed in semi-structured interaction situations with their mothers, and an analysis was made of the way in which the children openly processed their mother's speech. All the children's utterances that were formally related to the directly preceding maternal utterances were registered. In a second step, these formally related children's utterances were coded according to two main strategies of language processing (see for instance Grimm 1984, 43–44, Grimm 1987, 16):

(1) Elementaristic strategy, in the sense of picking out one single word or phrase from the immediately preceding maternal utterance. E. g. Mother: "Es hat ein Rad verloren" ["It has lost a wheel"]; Child: "Rad" ["Wheel"].
(2) Gestalt-like/holistic strategy comprising two substrategies:
    (a) The child imitates the whole sentence or picks out more than one phrase. E. g. Mother: "Da können wir ja noch eins bauen" ["Here we can build one again"]; Child imitates with omission: "Da können eins bauen" ["Here can build one"]. Mother: "Wir bauen ein Schloß" ["We are building a castle"]; Child modifies: "Wir Schloß bauen" ["We castle build"].
    (b) The child transforms his/her mother's preceding sentence. E. g. Mother: "Und das da, das ist die größte" ["And this here, this is the biggest"]; Child: "Und das da? Größte?" ["And this here? Biggest?"]. Mother: "Wo ist der Teufel?" ["Where is the devil?"]; Child: "Da ist der Teufel" ["There is the devil"].

During the one-hour interaction situation on average 14 % of the younger normal language children's utterances related formally in the defined sense to the maternal utterances. This was true for only 7 % of the SLI children's utterances. This significant quantitative difference is interesting since, as already mentioned above (cf. 2.2.), the mothers of the normal and of the dysphasic children did not differ in how often their utterances were formally related to their child's immediately preceding utterances; the average for both groups was 24 %. Grimm interpreted these data as evidence that on the one hand almost every fourth utterance the mothers directed towards their children was teaching-oriented. On the other hand, the younger normal language children were more learning-oriented than the dysphasic children. Or in other words: In the dyads with the dysphasic children one could observe much teaching but little learning.

Even more important than this quantitative difference is the qualitative finding that the normal language children significantly more often made use of the gestalt-like strategy of processing than the dysphasic children, who restricted themselves mainly to the elementaristic processing of their mother's input. One year later this difference still existed.

The evidence concerning mentally retarded children is less clear. Although Gutman/Rondal (1979) obtained a significant difference in the number of both 'modified' and 'total echoics' of maternal utterances when comparing 21 Down syndrome and 21 MLU-matched control children, this result is not readily interpretable as showing a deficit in the retarded children's use of a valuable language learning strategy. This is especially the case since the Down syndrome children were much older (age: 3;2–12;0 compared to 2;0–2;7 for the controls), had higher mental ages (Gutman/Rondal 1979, 452) and produced more 'intraverbals' than the nonretarded control children.

In summary we may conclude that the SLI children under study processed incoming language in a different way, at least during the earlier stages of language learning. If it is correct that different acquisition mechanisms underly and are responsible for different processing strategies (e. g. Bates/Bretherton/Snyder 1988) then the most important task is to find out the mechanisms leading to the deficient use of the gestalt-like strategy in SLI children. As one line of research it seems promising to look for memory restrictions.

Because of its limited capacity short-term memory may be regarded as the bottleneck of information processing. Therefore, structural and/or procedural deficits in short-term memory may cause problems in the registration, processing and storing of language input, thus leading to a deficient individual data base for language learning. A second, though not necessarily independent hypothesis is that the dysphasic children – who have been shown to be very poor in dealing with rhythm (e. g. Kracke 1975, Lea 1980) – have problems in exploiting the rhythmic-prosodic structure of speech in language processing and in acquiring the underlying rule system (for empirical evidence see Weinert 1991, 1992).

4. The Concept of Maternal Adjustment Revisited

4.1. Maternal Adjustment Versus Socialization Style

In any naturalistic dyadic interaction we have to deal with bidirectional effects. Thus one of the main topics has been whether the more passive language disordered child is created by a directive and initiative mother or whether the mother's directiveness is just a reactive adaptation to the child's passivity. Even if, as shown above, the empirical findings seem to speak in favor of the latter effect, this cannot imply that the reactive adaptation to the child's passivity must always be evaluated positively: the mothers' reactive directiveness might dampen the children's initiatives, thereby contributing to a firm establishment of the children's passivity. This is an important issue for intervention.

Particularly in the literature on retarded children the question has been discussed whether the adaptation of mothers to their child's passivity is dynamic in the sense that the mothers are finely tuned to their child's level of participation in dialogue or whether this maternal adaptation is not child-driven but is rather the result of an instructional intent. The mothers are convinced that they must teach their child something and therefore they employ a rather rigid socialization strategy.

Above all, two types of empirical results have been interpreted in support of the dynamic adaptation hypothesis: First, the correlational evidence already reviewed (see 2.1.) suggests an inverse relationship between the mother's and the child's interactional activity (Tannock 1988; see also Cunningham/Reuler/Blackwell/Deck 1981, Eheart 1982). This suggests that either one or both interaction partners react to the conversational behavior of the other; obviously, however, correlational data preclude causal interpretations and experimental data are thus urgently needed. A second hint to a dynamic maternal adaptation is given by Tannock's (1988) results. Although the mothers of the 11 Down syndrome children (age: 1;3–4;9) under study exerted significantly greater control in terms of turn-taking, topic and response control than the mothers of the younger normal children matched for developmental age and level of communication, there were no group differences in the proportion and in the conditional probabilities of maternal response control. Thus, given the child's antecedent behavior, the mothers showed comparable responses.

However, there is accumulating evidence that the dynamic adaptation hypothesis does not account for all group differences in general interaction variables. First, in the study by Tannock (1988) the differences in maternal topic control remained significant even when proportions and conditional probabilities were computed. Second, basing on their results, Mahoney/Fors/Wood (1990) argue that the differences in the quality and quantity of the children's interactive behavior were not as pronounced as the child-driven hypothesis presupposes. Third, an 'instructional intent' interpretation of maternal behavior is suggested by the fact that the mothers of the mentally retarded children not only produced more but also more demanding 'action requests' than the control mothers. In addition, the maternal requests were less directly linked to their children's current activity (Mahoney/Fors/Wood 1990). And finally, at least in some studies (Davies/Stroud/Green 1988) differences in interaction style between mothers of mentally retarded and normally developing children were only found in free play situations and disappeared in instruction situations, where the mothers of the control children proved as directive as the mothers of the retarded children.

In summary, each of the two hypotheses seems to partly account for the observed group differences in maternal interaction style. The question, however, which effects – positive or negative – the directive and initiative communication behavior of the mothers of developmentally disordered children exerts on the child's developmental progress needs to be examined by experimental procedures.

4.2. To Which Child Abilities and Features Do Mothers Adjust?

What similarities and differences in maternal language input exactly mean is rather unclear. One of the main reasons for this is that, as already mentioned, we only have limited knowledge of which specific abilities the children bring into the dialogue and in which way they react to their mothers. When the mothers of language disordered children adapt to the language production abilities of their children, this might be interpreted as a favorable adjustment if the comprehension abilities of the children are very similar to the production abilities. However, if the children's comprehension abilities are clearly better than their production abilities, then it is questionable whether a maternal speech style adapted only to the production abilities can support the child's further language development. Only very few studies deal with this problem. Cunningham/Siegel/van der Spuy et al. (1985) for example inferred from their result that the maternal MLU is greater than the SLI children's MLU that the mothers show fine-tuning with regard to their children's comprehension. This data base is, however, rather meager. Additional investigations are urgently needed to explore whether the mothers of children with better comprehension than production abilities differ in the complexity of interactive variables such as expansions and recasts from those mothers whose children have comparable production and comprehension abilities.

A second argument is that maternal adjustment to the language level of the language disordered children might then be dysfunctional for cognitive development if the children's cognitive abilities are better developed than the language abilities. We find this developmental discrepancy in SLI children since – per definition – these children have an average nonverbal IQ despite their language deficits.

There are indications in the literature that the speech style of mothers of dysphasic children is indeed primarily guided by the language level of their children (e. g. Grimm 1983, 1986, Moseley 1990, Peterson/Sherrod 1982, Schodorf/Edwards 1983).

As outlined in 2.2.1., SLI mothers were found to produce, for instance, a shorter and simpler input than mothers of normal children. In addition, Grimm (1986, 181) showed that the questions asked by the eight mothers of the dysphasic children she investigated differed significantly from the questions of the eight mothers of the normal MLU-matched children. Thus, questions of the type *Say it more exactly* were put significantly more often by the SLI mothers. E. g.: Mother: "Was siehst du alles?" ["What can you see there?"]. Child: "Das ist ein Mann" ["That is a man"]. Mother: "Was für ein Mann?" ["What kind of man?"].

In contrast, the mothers of the normal language children significantly more often asked questions of the type *Say it by yourself*. E. g. Child: "Was ist das?" ["What is that?"]. Mother: "Ja, was kann das denn sein?" ["Well, what could it be?"].

Grimm's interpretation of these differences was that the SLI mothers question their children in a rigid way whereas the control mothers encourage their children to think about things by themselves. Interestingly, a positive correlation ($r = .47$) was found between questions of the type *Say it by yourself* and the child's MLU one year later.

On the whole, the dialogues with dysphasic children give the impression of reduced mutuality and connected herewith of reduced semantic meaning or content. In order to prove the assumption that SLI mothers adapt primarily to their children's reduced speech production ability, thereby neglecting their more advanced language comprehension and cognitive abilities, Grimm (1991) chose the following three groups-design in order to isolate the otherwise inseparably confounded factors of language and cognition: (a) dyads with SLI children, (b) dyads with normal language-matched and therefore much younger children, and (c) dyads with normal age-matched children. Thus, the SLI children share their limited productive speech ability with the younger children, and with the age-matched children they share their experience and knowledge of the world. The cognitive quality of the mother's and children's utterances was analyzed according to the coding system developed by Blank/Franklin (1980). In this system, four levels of conceptual complexity are differentiated, ranging from simple naming utterances or naming questions up to the verbalization of causal relationships or theoretical conclusions. As hypothesized, the SLI mothers' utterances were far more similar in their conceptual complexity to the utterances of the mothers of the language-matched younger children than to the utterances of the mothers of the age-matched children. It was even the case that the utterances of the SLI mothers were in part significantly less conceptually complex than the utterances of the mothers of the younger children. And most interestingly of all, even the SLI children produced higher level initiatives more often than their mothers.

Without going into more detail here, it could be clearly demonstrated that the dysphasic children are primarily offered initiatives with low 1-level quality, which are even below the standard of what is considered appropriate for cognitively less advanced younger children. In contrast, the mothers of the younger children exceeded the level shown by their children, in that they produced distinctly fewer level 1 initiatives and distinctly more initiatives at the next, conceptually more complex level. This development-promoting aspect in the sense of fine-tuning was completely lacking in the SLI mothers. Since the additional analyses of answering behavior also showed very clearly that the SLI mothers produced significantly more answers at the conceptually simplest level in comparison to all other mothers, even though the previous initiatives of the SLIchildren and the younger children were very similar, Grimm concluded that the SLI mothers' information is adapted primarily to the perceived limited language production ability and not to the children's age-appropriate knowledge of the world. Her interpretation is that from the deficient language performance in the easily perceptible production area the mothers infer an overall immaturity and therefore apply an unspecific 'toddler teaching strategy'. Or put otherwise: The reductive adaptation to the children's language production level has as a negative side-effect a non-adaptive restriction of the cognitive quality of the verbal utterances produced.

That the 'toddler teaching strategy' is not restricted to developmental dysphasia but is also adopted by mothers of deaf children was demonstrated by Nienhuys/Horsborough/Cross (1985) who also used the Blank/Franklin scheme for analyzing the conceptual complexity of the utterances of mothers of two- and five-year-old deaf and hearing children. In addition, the results presented by Matey/Kretschmer (1985) show that mothers of normally intelligent hearing-impaired children do not differ in their communication style from mothers of mentally retarded Down syndrome children.

These accumulated findings certainly need to be taken into account in intervention. The mothers should be informed that they may not confound their children's speech production with their mental ability. They should refrain from using a generalized language instruction style and recognize that conceptually more complex topics can well be expressed in simple words.

5. References

Bates, E., Bretherton, J., & Snyder, L. (1988). *From first words to grammar. Individual differences and dissociable mechanisms.* Cambridge: Cambridge University Press.

Bettelheim, B. (1967). *The empty fortress: Infantile autism and the birth of the self.* New York: Free Press.

Blank, M. & Franklin, E. (1980). Dialogue with preschoolers: A cognitively-based system of assessment. *Applied Psycholinguistics, 1,* 127–150.

Bondurant, J. L., Romeo, D. J., & Kretschmer, R. (1983). Language behaviors of mothers of children with normal and delayed language. *Language, Speech and Hearing Services in Schools, 14,* 233–242.

Cardoso-Martins, C. & Mervis, C. B. (1985). Maternal speech to prelinguistic children with Down syndrome. *American Journal of Mental Deficiency, 89,* 451–458.

Conti-Ramsden, G. C. (1990). Maternal recasts and other contingent replies to language-impaired children. *Journal of Speech and Hearing Disorders, 55,* 262–274.

Conti-Ramsden, G. C. & Friel-Patti, S. C. (1983). Mothers' discourse adjustments to language-impaired and non-language-impaired children. *Journal of Speech and Hearing Disorders, 48,* 360–367.

Conti-Ramsden, G. C. & Friel-Patti, S. C. (1984). Mother-child dialogues: A comparison of normal and language impaired children. *Journal of Communication Disorders, 17*, 19–25.

Crawley, S. B. & Spiker, D. (1983). Mother-child interactions involving two-year-olds with Down syndrome: A look at individual differences. *Child Development, 54*, 1312–1323.

Cross, T. (1977). Mothers' speech adjustments: The contribution of selected child-listener variables. In: C. Snow & C. Ferguson (Eds.), *Talking to children: Language input and acquisition. 151–188.* Cambridge, England: Cambridge Univ. Press.

Cross, T. (1978). Mothers' speech and its association with linguistic development in young children. In N. Waterson & C. Snow (Eds.), *The development of communication. 199–216.* Chichester: Wiley.

Cross, T. G. (1981). The linguistic experience of slow language learners. In A. R. Nesdale, C. Pratt, R. Grieve, J. Field, D. Illingworth, & J. Hogben (Eds.), *Advances in child development: Theory and research. 110–121.* Nedlands, Western Australia: NCCD.

Cunningham, C. E., Reuler, E., Blackwell, J., & Deck, J. (1981). Behavioral and linguistic developments in the interactions of normal and retarded children with their mothers. *Child Development, 52*, 62–70.

Cunningham, C. E., Siegel, L. S., van der Spuy, H. I. J., Clark, M. L., & Bow, S. J. (1985). The behavioral and linguistic interactions of specifically language-delayed and normal boys with their mothers. *Child Development, 56*, 1389–1403.

Davis, H., Stroud, A., & Green, L. (1988). Maternal language environment of children with mental retardation. *American Journal on Mental Retardation, 93*, 144–153.

Eheart, B. (1982). Mother-child interactions with nonretarded and mentally retarded preschoolers. *American Journal of Mental Deficiency, 87*, 20–25.

Goldfarb, W., Goldfarb, N., & Scholl, M. H. (1966). The speech of mothers of schizophrenic children. *American Journal of Psychiatry, 122*, 1220–1227.

Goldfarb, W., Yudkovitch, E., & Goldfarb, N. (1973). Verbal symbols to designate objects: An experimental study of communication in mothers of schizophrenic children. *Journal of Autism and Childhood Schizophrenia, 3*, 281–298.

Grimm, H. (1983). Vergleichende kategoriale Analyse sprachlicher Handlungsmuster in Mutter-Kind-Dyaden. In D. Boueke & W. Klein (Eds.), *Untersuchungen zur Dialogfähigkeit von Kindern. 249–268.* Tübingen: Narr.

Grimm, H. (1984). Zur Frage der sprachlichen Wissenskonstruktion. Oder: Erwerben dysphasische Kinder die Sprache anders? In E. Oksaar (Ed.), *Spracherwerb, Sprachkontakt, Sprachkonflikt. 30–53.* Berlin: de Gruyter.

Grimm, H. (1985). Der Spracherwerb als Lehr-Lern-Prozess. *Unterrichtswissenschaft, 1*, 6–16.

Grimm, H. (1986). Ontogenese der Sprache als Fortsetzung nicht-sprachlichen Handelns. In H. G. Bosshardt (Ed.), *Perspektiven auf Sprache. Interdisziplinäre Beiträge zum Gedenken an Hans Hörmann. 166–184.* Berlin: de Gruyter.

Grimm, H. (1987). Developmental dysphasia: New theoretical perspectives and empirical results. *The German Journal of Psychology, 11*, 8–22.

Grimm, H. (1990). Über den Einfluß der Umweltsprache auf die kindliche Sprachentwicklung. In K. Neumann & M. Charlton (Eds.), *Spracherwerb und Mediengebrauch. 99–110.* Tübingen: Narr.

Grimm, H. (1991). Entwicklungskritische Dialogmerkmale in Mutter-Kind-Dyaden mit dysphasisch sprachgestörten und sprachunauffälligen Kindern. Paper presented at the 10th Meeting of Developmental Psychology, Cologne, Germany, 25.–27. 9. 1991.

Grimm, H. (1993). Syntax and morphological difficulties in children with specific language impairment (developmental dysphasia): Implications for diagnosis and intervention. In H. Grimm & H. Skowronek (Eds.), *Language acquisition problems and reading disorders: Aspects of diagnosis and intervention.* 25–63. New York: de Gruyter.

Grimm, H. & Weinert, S. (1990). Is the syntax development of dysphasic children deviant and why? New findings to an old question. *Journal of Speech and Hearing Research, 33*, 220–228.

Gutman, A. J. & Rondal, J. A. (1979). Verbal operants in mothers' speech to nonretarded and Down's syndrome children matched for linguistic level. *American Journal of Mental Deficiency, 83*, 446–452.

Hanzlik, J. R. & Stevenson, M. B. (1986). Interaction of mothers with their infants who are mentally retarded, retarded with cerebral palsy, or nonretarded. *American Journal of Mental Deficiency, 90*, 513–520.

Hoff-Ginsberg, E. (1985). Some contributions of mothers' speech to their children's syntactic growth. *Journal of Child Language, 12*, 367–385.

Hoff-Ginsberg, E. (1986). Function and structure in maternal speech: Their relation to the child's development of syntax. *Developmental Psychology, 22*, 155–163.

Hoff-Ginsberg, E. & Shatz, M. (1982). Linguistic input and the child's acquisition of language. *Psychological Bulletin, 92*, 3–26.

Howlin, P., Cantwell, D., Marchant, R., Berger, M., & Rutter, M. (1973). Analyzing mothers' speech to young autistic children: A methodological study. *Journal of Abnormal Child Psychology, 1*, 317–339.

Konstantareas, M. M., Zajdeman, H., Homatidis, S., & McCabe, A. (1988). Maternal speech to verbal and higher functioning versus nonverbal and lower functioning autistic children. *Journal of Autism and Developmental Disorders, 18*, 647–655.

Kracke, I. (1975). Perception of rhythmic sequences by receptive aphasic and deaf children. *British Journal of Disorders of Communication, 10*, 43–51.

Lasky, E. Z. & Klopp, K. (1982). Parent-child interactions in normal and language-disordered children. *Journal of Speech and Hearing Disorders, 47*, 7–18.

Lea, J. (1980). The association between rhythmic ability and language ability. In F. M. Jones (Ed.), *Language disability in children. 217–230*. Lancaster: MTP Press.

Leonard, L. B. (1986). Conversational replies of children with specific language impairment. *Journal of Speech and Hearing Research, 29*, 114–119.

Leonard, L. B. (1987). Is specific language impairment a useful construct? In S. Rosenberg (Ed.), *Advances in applied psycholinguistics (1): Disorders of first-language development. 1–39*. Cambridge: Cambridge University Press.

Mahoney, G., Fors, S., & Wood, S. (1990). Maternal directive behavior revisited. *American Journal on Mental Retardation, 94*, 398–406.

Matey, C. & Kretschmer, R. (1985). A comparison of mothers' speech to Down's syndrome, hearing-impaired, and normal-hearing children. *Volta Review, 87*, 205–213.

Maurer, H. & Sherrod, K. B. (1987). Context of directives given to young Down syndrome and nonretarded children: Development of two years. *American Journal of Mental Deficiency, 91*, 579–590.

Menyuk, P. (1988). *Language development. Knowledge and use*. Boston: Scott, Foresman & Comp.

Moseley, M. J. (1990). Mother-child interaction with preschool language-delayed children: structuring conversations. *Journal of Communicative Disorders, 23*, 187–203.

Nelson, K. E., Carskaddon, G., & Bonvillian, J. D. (1973). Syntax acquisition: impact of experimental variation in adult verbal interaction with the child. *Child Development, 44*, 497–504.

Newport, E. L., Gleitman, H., & Gleitman, L. R. (1977). "Mother, I'd rather do it myself": some effects and non-effects of maternal speech style. In C. Snow & C. A. Ferguson (Eds.), *Talking to children: Language input and acquisition. 109–150*. Cambridge: Cambridge University Press.

Nienhuys, T. G., Horsborough, K. M., & Cross, T. G. (1985). A dialogic analysis of interaction between mothers and their deaf or hearing preschoolers. *Applied Psycholinguistics, 6*, 121–140.

O'Kelly-Collard, M. (1978). Maternal linguistic environment of Down's syndrome children. *The Australian Journal of Mental Retardation, 5*, 121–126.

Olsen-Fulero, L. (1982). Style and stability in mother conversational behavior. *Journal of Child Language, 9*, 543–564.

Peterson, G. A. & Sherrod, K. B. (1982). Relationship of maternal language to language development and language delay in children. *American Journal of Mental Deficiency, 86*, 391–398.

Rondal, J. A. (1978). Maternal speech to normal and Down's syndrome children matched for mean length of utterance. In C. E. Meyers (Ed.), *Quality of life in severely and profoundly mentally retarded people: Research foundations for improvement. 193–265*. Washington D. C.: American Association of Mental Deficiency.

Rutter, M., Bartak, L., & Newman, S. (1971). Autism – a central disorder of cognition and language? In M. Rutter (Ed.), *Infantile autism: Concepts, characteristics and treatment. 148–171*. Edinburgh: Churchill.

Sachs, J., Bard, B., & Johnson, M. L. (1981). Language learning with restricted input: Case studies of two hearing children of deaf parents. *Applied Psycholinguistics, 2*, 33–54.

Schodorf, J. K. & Edwards, H. T. (1983). Comparative analysis of parent-child interactions with language-disordered and linguistically normal children. *Journal of Communication Disorders, 16*, 71–83.

Shatz, M., Grimm, H., Wilcox, S., & Niemeier-Wind, K. (in press). Culture-specific speech styles in Germany and the United States: Mothers' modal verbal expressions and two-year-olds' modal development. *Child Development*.

Sigman, M., Mundy, P., Sherman, T., & Ungerer J. (1986). Social interactions of autistic, mentally retarded and normal children and their caregivers. *Journal of Child Psychiatry and Psychology, 27*, 647–656.

Smolak, L. & Weinraub, M. (1983). Maternal speech: strategy or response? *Journal of Child Language, 10*, 369–380.

Snow, C. E., Perlman, R., & Nathan, D. (1987). Why routines are different: toward a multiple-factors model of the relation between input and language acquisition. In K. E. Nelson & A. van Kleeck (Eds.), *Children's language, Vol. 6. 65–97*. Hillsdale, N. J.: Lawrence Erlbaum Associates.

Tannock, R. (1988). Mothers' directiveness in their interactions with their children with and without Down syndrome. *American Journal of Mental Retardation, 93*, 154–165.

Weinert, S. (1991). *Spracherwerb und implizites Lernen. Studien zum Erwerb sprachanaloger Regeln bei Erwachsenen, sprachunauffälligen und dysphasisch-sprachgestörten Kindern*. Bern: Huber.

Weinert, S. (1992). Deficits in acquiring language structure: The importance of using prosodic cues. *Applied Cognitive Psychology (Special Edition)*.

Wolchik, S. A. (1983). Language patterns of young autistic and normal children. *Journal of Autism and Developmental Disorders, 13*, 167–180.

Wolchik, S. A. & Harris, S. L. (1982). Language environments of autistic and normal children matched for language age: A preliminary investigation. *Journal of Autistic and Developmental Disorders, 12*, 43–55.

Wulbert, M., Inglis, S., Kriegsmann, E., & Mills, B. (1975). Language delay and associated mother-child interactions. *Developmental Psychology, 1*, 61–70.

Yoder, P. J. & Kaiser, A. P. (1989). Alternative explanations for the relationship between maternal verbal interaction style and child language development. *Journal of Child Language, 16*, 141–160.

Hannelore Grimm, Bielefeld (Germany)
Sabine Weinert, Bielefeld (Germany)

69. Disorders of Written Language Development: Definitions and Overview

This article will focus mainly on developmental disorders of reading and will deal only occasionally with spelling.

1. Learning to Read: The Alphabetic Principle and Stage Models of Reading Development

The process of learning to read is dependent on the writing system. The alphabetic writing system used in so many literate languages involves correspondence of letters (graphemes) and speech sound units (phonemes). This 'alphabetic principle' defines a 'productive writing system' (Perfetti 1985) because from a small, definite number of graphic signs an indefinite number of words may be constructed. Such economy in writing production seems to be paralleled by a similar advantage in learning alphabetic systems. In contrast to the Chinese system, for instance, the alphabetic system does not require an enormous number of specific paired-associates of sign and meaning to be stored in memory. Instead, when the learner has acquired the relatively few grapheme-phoneme-correspondences and has also learned about the context dependency of the various sound representations of a single letter he can apply this knowledge directly, grapheme by grapheme, or, in the case of grapheme clusters, by analogy (cf. Goswami 1986, 1988) to reading or 'decoding' any word or non-word. This task might be easier in languages like Finnish or Polish, with very transparent and regular relations between spelling and pronunciation.

'True' alphabetic writing, i. e. writing arbitrary signs that represent words and not objects or concepts, pays for economy by loss of 'ideographic' or pictorial concreteness. To acquire the alphabetic principle, the learner must first focus on the formal aspect of speech, i. e. speech sounds and phonology, and understand the abstract nature of the 'phoneme' (Valtin 1984). Such abstraction occurs because the phoneme does not represent one fixed sound but instead refers to a set of slightly different pronunciations of, say, 'p' depending on the patterns of the surrounding vowels and consonants in a word. To add to the difficulties, neither in listening nor in speaking can the flow of speech be separated into phonemes as natural or physical units (cf. Liberman/Cooper/Shankweiler/Studdert-Kennedy 1967). Second, the reader needs to exert cognitive control over his eye movements. Before starting to read, no saccadic eye movements in a specified direction are required. A further major problem is the focussing of attention on the relevant parts of words or texts in order to draw information. Third, the human species is not only endowed by nature to learn and use oral language for communication but is also socialized smoothly into it. Considered on a world scale, with billions of illiterates, this does not apply to written language (Kamhi/Catts 1989). Thus it seems plausible that learning to read (and to spell) takes a lot of conscious resources and effort and may easily be doomed to failure whenever the subtle balance of interacting biological, cognitive, psychosocial and environmental factors is disturbed by slight but cumulative deprivations in one or more of these areas.

Up to now, development in reading has been described by means of catalogues of skills to be acquired or by developmental stages.

Learning to read requires a set of prerequisite skills (e. g. Gibson/Levin 1976) which cannot be separated easily from the actual skills of decoding. The question as to which prerequisites are necessary and/or sufficient and in what order they develop is yet to be answered (Morais/Alegria/Content 1987). Many researchers in reading development (e. g. Clay 1970, Ehri 1979, Perfetti 1985, Rozin/Gleitman 1977) have listed the following language processes:
- phonemic analysis
- segmenting and discriminating sounds
- associating sound and phonetic codes and retrieving them from memory
- blending of sounds
- becoming aware that words are units in speech, even if not marked either auditorily or semantically
- developing phonological awareness.

The latter skill is regarded as the most important and the most difficult to acquire. Without developing an understanding or at least having access to the phonological organization of language as prerequisite for discovering the alphabetic principle, even decoding of two-phonemic units will prove extremely difficult (Valtin 1984).

As visual processes are listed (e. g. Gibson 1971, Venezky 1976):
- recognizing letters (discriminating distinctive features)
- recognizing clusters of letters
- recognizing the serial order of letters from left to right
- cognitive control of eye movements.

Finally, to guarantee steady improvement of reading, the isolated skills have to be coordinated and integrated by proficiency processes (cf. Perfetti 1985, Samuels 1976):
- integrating graphic and linguistic information
- combining and coordinating linguistic and visual processes.

In stage theories of reading development it is assumed that all children pass through an ordered sequence in learning word recognition. Authors of stage theories (Frith 1985, Høien/Lundberg 1988, Marsh/Friedman/Welsh 1981, Mason 1980, Seymour/MacGregor 1984) have proposed from 3 to 4 stages, differently labeled. The frequently cited, original model by Frith (1985) may be sketched as follows: In their first unguided attempts at reading children will use the same perception and memory skills for decoding printed material as for other visual objects and events. A linkage of spoken and printed words, defined by minimal cues, is established by a process of paired-associate learning. This is the stage of 'logographic' reading. Of course, this strategy of pre-alphabetic reading will break down when the 'sight vocabulary' exceeds fifty to eighty printed words in a very short time. Because of inaccuracies and increasing difficulties in recognizing unfamiliar words, it is necessary to use the strategy of sequential decoding or the 'alphabetic' stage, using knowledge of letter-sound relations. This stage has been recognized by many authors (e. g. Weigl 1976) as the most important 'qualitative jump'. In spontaneous writing children give many examples of 'phonetic' spelling, which is orthographically incorrect but is based on inventive letter-sound correspondences. The third, 'orthographic' stage or hierarchical decoding is reached when the learner masters the deviation from 'normal sound' and uses conditional spelling rules, e. g. those governing the stretching of vowels. – To represent the specific interplay of reading and spelling in stimulating development Frith (1985, 1986) differentiated the three stages of her original model into two substages each, so that either reading or writing functions "as the pacemaker of the strategy" (Frith 1985, 310) characteristic of the stage in question – logographic, alphabetic or orthographic. For German-speaking countries it was slightly modified by Günther (1986) to the effect of further subdivisions in each stage. More detail to stage-specific variation dependent on individual development and method of instruction came from Ellis/Cataldo (1990), Scheerer-Neumann (1989) and Seymour/Elder (1986). The general model was questioned on theoretical grounds by Eichler (1986) and on theoretical as well as empirical grounds by Stuart/Coltheart (1988) and Wimmer/Hartl/Moser (1990). Especially for German-speaking children the existence of a logographic stage is questionable.
– Compared to models of the reading process stage theories do not describe the component processes in detail. Instead the focus is on qualitative changes in reading strategies, i. e. on how children approach the word recognition task. The evidence cited in support of

stage concepts demonstrates in general that phonological processing and integration of component processes (proficiency) improve in the course of reading development. Errors in reading and spelling allow ex post conclusions with regard to the developmental stage of word processing. As is the problem with all outcome measures reading errors and other reading results do not address the details of reading processes. Particularly on higher levels of reading skills (sequential or hierarchical decoding) the interpretation of mere outcomes is questionable. Since the eye-voice-span is considerable, supposed reading errors could prove to be errors of recall. To some degree, stage theories also appear to be influenced by the specific type of reading instruction and by the regularity of sound-spelling relations in a language.

– More recent models of written language acquisition, based on a connectionist framework, postulate a set of functionally different modules and routes of transmission. Models of this type are proposed by Seidenberg/McClelland (1989) and Van Orden/Pennington/Stone (1990).

2. Reading Disorders: Definitions, Methods and Some History

As a rule, current definitions of reading disorders do not refer to existing definitions of reading. Rather they refer to deviation from or discrepancy to a norm such as general achievement or intelligence. This type of definition goes back to a medical model of reading disorders. In reviewing the history of ideas and concepts in research of reading disorders up to the present, three general routes can be detected:

- from the idea of a unitary syndrome via the search for a few categorical subtypes to the description of reading disorders in a multi-dimensional space;
- from exclusionary definitions to a more comprehensive and positive delimitation of reading disorders;
- from a medical model of reading disorders searching for organismic causes and associated symptoms to a psychological and educational model focusing on reading difficulties per se and on processes of learning and instruction.

– Despite gradual convergence and restriction to phonological processing skills as the key variable in first reading disorders, research in this field for the last two decades is still burdened by an enormous diversity of methods, definitions and concepts. This diversity makes evaluation of empirical findings extremely difficult since many unaccounted interactions of designs, sampling, measurement and concepts produce a barely manageable host of results (Stanovich 1988b, 1989, 1990a, b).

2.1. Defining by Discrepancy from Potential: Dyslexia

Fortunately, in societies where formal schooling is obligatory, most children master the complex skill of reading to a functional degree. Against this background, cases of children with otherwise normal achievement but 'unexpected' failure in learning to read were highly salient and attracted early attention in the medical profession. The notion that there are children with specific reading difficulties of supposedly constitutional origin ('congenital word blindness') is credited to Morgan (1896) at the turn of the century and was made popular by the writings of Hinshelwood (1917), besides others (cf. Ellis 1985, Warnke 1990). Hinshelwood also seems to have been the first to link reading difficulties to disorders of the left brain hemisphere. This idea was taken up and expanded by Orton (1937) who is thought to be responsible for the theory that specific reading difficulties (dyslexia) go back to deviations in the distribution of visual information processing between the two cerebral hemispheres. Orton was the first to speak of developmental alexia (i. e. absolute inability to read) so that dyslexia came to stand for the wider range of 'incomplete alexias' (Harris/Hodges 1981). He is also known for adding letter reversals and word confusions to the diagnosis of 'dyslexia'. So it gradually became quite common to think of dyslexia as a unitary syndrome with associated neurological and behavioral manifestations. In German-speaking countries the equivalent term, with a similar history, is 'legasthenia' (Ranschburg 1916).

Amongst the many and various definitions of dyslexia or legasthenia, that formulated by the World Federation of Neurology from 1968 is perhaps the most widely quoted:
"(Dyslexia is) a disorder manifested by difficulty in learning to read despite conventional instruction, adequate intelligence and sociocultural opportunity. It is dependent upon fundamental cognitive disabilities which are

frequently of constitutional origin" (Critchley 1970, 11).

The host of definitions may be classified (Marx 1985) as follows:
(1) Etiological definitions, e. g. "Reading weakness or legasthenia I call ... that inferiority of mental equipment in consequence of which children of school age can't acquire verbal reading during the first grades, despite normal sensory abilities" (Ranschburg 1916, 111).
(2) Descriptive definitions, like the one by the World Federation of Neurology quoted above or the one by Linder, which has become a classic in German-speaking countries: "Unter Legasthenie verstehen wir eine spezielle und aus dem Rahmen der übrigen Leistungen fallende Schwäche im Erlernen des Lesens (und indirekt auch des selbständigen orthographischen Schreibens) bei sonst intakter (oder im Verhältnis zur Lesefähigkeit) relativ guter Intelligenz." ["Legasthenia is conceived of as a specific weakness in learning to read (and indirectly also in learning to spell correctly), in the context of generally better school achievement and of intact or relatively good intelligence, compared to reading skill"] (Linder 1951, 100).
(3) Operational definitions, e. g. "Als Legastheniker gelten Kinder mit mindestens durchschnittlicher Begabung (IQ $\geq$ 90), deren Leistungen im Lesen und Rechtschreiben jeweils einem Prozentrang von $\leq$ 15 (T $\leq$ 40) entsprechen." ["Children are ranked as legasthenics when they score at or below percentile 15 (T $\leq$ 40) in reading and spelling, and when their intelligence is at least average (IQ $\geq$ 90)"] (Niemeyer 1974, 28). Or: "A dyslexic is a child who is normal or above at least in non-verbal IQ, two years behind in reading achievement, and with a reading disability that is not explainable primarily by social, economic, motivation or emotional factors" (Perfetti 1985, 180).

As is evident from these examples, most authors start out in their definitions from deviations from norms but not from a common base in concepts and methods. They agree that the term dyslexia (or legasthenia) should be reserved for the subgroup of 'unexpected' reading disabled and not applied to poor reading in general.

2.2. Problems with Definition by Exclusion

Definitions may be more or less comprehensive or explicit, but most if not all are exclusionary in character. Thus, some poor readers are excluded from the group of dyslexics by factors that might contribute to reading disorders in general: low intelligence, poor schooling, sensory deficits, brain damage etc. In addition, the definition of dyslexia by exclusion raises some other serious problems (Kamhi/Catts 1989). First, the definitions depend solely on the discrepancy between reading achievement and general achievement, or intelligence, or chronological age or grade level. However, measurements of reading achievement and intelligence overlap to some degree. By different reading measures different children are assigned accordingly to the group of the disabled (Rudel 1985, Schlee 1976). Second, the exclusion of children with IQs below 90 from the group of dyslexics implies that these children display other disorders. This view is contradicted by those authors who point out that there is continuity of dyslexic disorder across all ranges of intelligence (Ellis 1985, Thomson 1984) and that performance profiles of dyslexics cannot be distinguished reliably from those of poor readers (Taylor/Satz/Friel 1979). Third, since environmental causes are excluded, the search for deprivations in educational experience tends to be neglected (Vellutino 1979). Last and most regrettably, definition by exclusion has often facilitated neglect of the low-intelligent poor reader (Schlee 1976).

In conclusion, according to Rutter (1978, 12), this type of definition looks like "a counsel of despair": "A negative definition of this kind not only fails to aid conceptual clarity but also it implies that dyslexia cannot be diagnosed in a child from a poor or unconventional background. In short it suggests that if all the known causes of reading disability can be ruled out, the unknown (in the form of dyslexia) should be invoked".

2.3. Methods and Paradigms in Search for Causes and Consequences

In the search for causes of reading disorders five designs to cope with different methodological problems can be distinguished:
– (1) Extreme-groups design: Up to the seventies, the host of comparisons done with this design finally demonstrated that performance or achievement differences between the comparison groups will occur on the condition that the skills measured are directly or indirectly linked to literacy skills. Unequivocal evidence with regard to causal direction cannot be expected from this design (Valtin 1975, 1978/79) since reading difficulties might be

cause as well as effect of the observed deficits in the dependent variables measured; both lower performance might also be the effect of a third, unknown determinant. The value of research in this design lies mainly in confirming supposed correlations on which base more incisive hypotheses for research on causal relations may be generated.

— (2) Reading-level match design: In this design, which was introduced by Guthrie (1973) into research on reading difficulties, an older group of reading disordered children is matched on reading level with a younger group of 'normal' readers. Reading level is measured by reading age. Whether reading age is measured by word recognition and decoding or by tests of reading comprehension, or by both makes an important difference. When equating reading level, performance differences in correlated variables cannot be reduced to differences in reading achievement. On the other hand, as in the extreme-groups comparison, the observed differences in cognitive and other characteristics should not be interpreted as causes of reading disorder — as is sometimes erroneously done (Bradley/Bryant 1978, Treiman/Hirsh-Pasek 1985). Recently, different authors (Goswami/Bryant 1989, Jackson/Butterfield 1989, Stanovich/Nathan/Zolman 1988, Vellutino/Scanlon 1989) have critically dealt with scope and limits of this design.

— (3) Garden-variety control design: In this design, two groups of reading disabled children are compared — 'dyslexic' children with at least average intelligence but low reading achievement, and generally backward children of the same reading level but also low in intelligence. Differences (e. g. Jorm/Share/Maclean/Matthews 1986) or similarities (e. g. Taylor/Satz/Friel 1979) in associated variables between these groups are seen as evidence for or against the formation of subgroups in the reading disordered population.

— (4) Longitudinal design: Supposed prerequisite skills and abilities (e. g. phonological awareness) are measured before school entrance to predict criterial literacy achievement at successive stages (e. g. Skowronek/Marx 1989). If first measures are really taken before formal reading instruction starts, confounding of predictor and criterion achievement is avoided. Close examination of times of predictor measurements and considering the extent to which reading is already offered in kindergarten (in the Anglo-American educational system) raises doubts whether in some studies (e. g. Butler/Marsh/Sheppard/Sheppard 1985, Lundberg/Olofsson/Wall 1980, Share/Jorm/Maclean/Matthews 1984, Vellutino/Scanlon 1987) confounding really has been avoided (Marx 1989).

— (5) Intervention-design: Inadequately developed prerequisite or predictor skills relevant to acquisition of literacy are trained for a fixed period of time up to a predetermined level of competence. Ideally, the deficits should be not only diagnosed but also remedied before entering school. If post-training comparisons with control children matched in prerequisite skills show that trained children perform better in reading and spelling, the positive causal influence of these skills on literacy achievement is demonstrated. The well-controlled study by Lundberg/Frost/Petersen (1988) clearly shows that the trained skills (phonological awareness) are necessary but not sufficient for the acquisition of literacy. Training in school or in close cooperation with schools (e. g. Bradley/Bryant 1985, Mannhaupt 1990) incurs the risk that specific effects of intervention in relevant skills cannot be separated clearly since intervention interacts in unknown ways with ongoing reading instruction. Again, confounding of predictor and criterion measurements seems possible (cf. Ehri 1989).

2.4. Approaches in Subtyping of Reading Disorders

As is the case in learning disabilities in general and as already mentioned above the field of reading disorders is plagued by heterogeneity. Evidence shows that poor readers differ from normals in a broad range of dimensions — cognitive, attentional, perceptual-motor, social-emotional, basic skills and strategies — and the individual patterns of deficits may vary enormously (Kavale/Nye 1986, Miles 1983, Stanovich 1986a, Zielinski 1980).

To reduce complexity and make this diversity more intelligible — for reasons of theory development, of better diagnosis and more specific treatment — researchers and clinicians made early efforts at classification of distinct patterns of disorders. Indeed, it seems still a major concern to professionals to identify more homogeneous subgroups and bring order to an otherwise amorphous field (Adelman/Taylor 1985).

— To this end, a comprehensive and standardized description of relevant phenomena is required. However, there are doubts whether this requirements is fulfilled to an acceptable degree (Kavale/Forness 1987). How reading order is defined, whether by exclusion or by inclusion, will also exert a major influence on the results of subtyping. Including all poor readers will probably lead to many and not clearly separable groups whereas selective sampling of 'dyslexics' only, according to strict psychometric criteria will render homogeneous groupings differing along few causal lines.

There are two approaches to subgrouping: classification by clinical inference, i. e. by applying various theoretical distinctions and organizing data patterns intuitively, and the more recent approach of classification by multivariate descriptive statistics such as Q-factor analysis and cluster analysis. In the following each approach will be characterized by a few representative studies. Detailed critical reviews treating both conceptual and methodological issues are given by Fletcher/Satz (1985), Kamhi/Catts (1989), Kavale/Forness (1987), Malatesha/Dougan (1982) and Satz/Morris (1981).

– (1) Clinical inference: The most obvious distinction, grounded in very basic though largely unexamined assumptions about categorical differences in cognitive and neuropsychological characteristics, is between dyslexics and 'garden-variety' poor readers (Gough/Tunmer 1986). Rutter/Yule (1975), for instance, addressed this distinction and found that 'generally backward readers' could indeed be distinguished from 'specific reading retarded' (or dyslexics for our purposes). The authors based the distinction on two lines of evidence: First, they got a 'hump' at the lower end of the reading achievement residuals distribution, i. e. significantly more under achievers than could be predicted from normal distribution. Second, they found the two groups to differ on various neurological and behavioral characteristics, whereas deficiencies in oral and written language performance were equally prevalent in both groups. These and other differential results appeared very cogent so that the old distinction seemed confirmed. Since then, various authors have questioned its validity (Rodgers 1983, Share/McGee/McKenzie et al. 1987, Taylor/Satz/Friel 1979, Van der Wissel/Zegers 1985) because of flaws in method or because the findings could not be replicated in well-controlled samples. To quote one of the concluding statements, the comparisons on a wide array of measures showed "that the dyslexic subgroup could not be distinguished from the nondyslexic poor readers along any of several dimensions, including the initial severity and progression of reading disturbance, frequency of reversal errors, familial reading and spelling competencies, math skills, neuro-behavioral performance, or personality functioning." (Satz/Morris 1981, 113).

– Another influential and frequently cited study of the clinical type is that of Boder (1973). Her classification of developmental dyslexia is based on direct quantitative and qualitative measures of reading and spelling. Boder found three subtypes of dyslexic children: the dysphonetic (comprising 67 %) with deficiencies in analyzing and blending sounds, the dyseidetic (10 %) with rather intact phonological skills but impaired storing of visual patterns of letter strings, and a mixed, practically alexic group (23 %). Lacking statistical verification and replication, the merit of this study lies primarily in a rich clinical description and heuristic quality. Error types used by Boder may also occur in younger normal children beginning to read so that their specific diagnostic value for dyslexics is seriously doubted. Perfetti (1985) has also noted that the difference between the dysphonetic and the dyseidetic might rest only upon spelling ability.

– Summarizing their critical comments on clinical-inference studies reviewed, Satz/Morris (1981, 120) state that "subject selection, sample size, tests and observer rules are quite different." Also, the terms used for description are highly abstract and carry surplus meaning that may mask finer distinctions or even be misleading. Furthermore, most studies did not include independent comparison groups of normal and non-dyslexic poor readers in order to control for the uniqueness of achievement profiles in dyslexic subtypes.

– (2) Statistical classification: Quantitative analysis of multivariate data sets entered the study of subtypes in reading disability about ten years ago. Among the first authors to use this method were Petrauskas/Rourke (1979). Factor analysis (Q-technique) applied to a broad range of neuro-psychological measures from a (preselected) group of dyslexic readers and a small group of normal readers resulted in three reliable subgroups which classified just 50 % of the subjects. It should be noted that two (of 27) normal readers were classified into subtype 3, together with 11 dyslexic readers. The authors' main conclusion was that language deficiencies were dominant in variables associated with specific reading retardation, whereas other deficiencies, e. g. of a visuo-perceptual kind, were involved to a much lesser degree.

– Supplementing the often-used cross-sectional design in a more recent study (Morris/Blashfield/Satz 1986), which is part of the Florida Longitudinal Project, longitudinal data from normal and reading disabled children were analyzed. This study combined factor analysis with cluster analysis. Clustering resulted in three groups of poor readers: Type A children showed deficient verbal skills throughout the seven-year-interval whereas early deficits in perceptual-motor skills disappeared. Type B children, from average family background, started with average performance at kindergarten age but showed increasing weaknesses in the verbal-conceptual dimension at school age. Type C children rated below average on all measures. This group is rarely found in other classification studies which most often focus on the dyslexic and therefore miss the less intelligent (IQ below 90) and educationally deprived characteristic of Type C.

– The two studies mentioned above exemplify only few of the problems inherent in quantitative classification. To sum up the major caveats from various sources (cf. particularly Kavale/Forness 1987, Satz/Morris 1981) one has to keep in mind that

- the Q-factor technique is controversial, especially the use of correlations as a measure of similarity between subjects, and on data in which the assumption of linearity is dubious;
- clustering methods are of more heuristic value since they are not well-tested statistically; – by clustering methods any data set ("garbage in, clusters out") can be organized; thus the data set must first be tested for real clustering tendencies;
- what subtypes and labels emerge from clustering depends on what samples of subjects and tests have been used; e. g. standardized tests of reading/spelling achievements may probe a much too restricted range of relevant skills;
- only part of the sample may be grouped into clusters, and clusters may overlap so that reading retarded are grouped with normal subjects;
- external validation of subtypes is often neglected.

Aside from these criticisms and even though the many studies diverging in theoretical assumptions and methods do not combine to consistent patterns, subtyping research in the clinical-inferential mode as well as in quantitative classification has added to our knowledge of reading/spelling disorders. Generally, it confirmed hypotheses about components of literacy skills, clarified the context of associated abilities and language development and stressed the need for more comprehensive and formalized description of the field.

3. Reading Disorders: Alternative Conceptions

For about two decades the 'medical model' of dyslexia as a unitary, neuro-psychological 'syndrome' has been challenged by an alternative, 'educational-psychological' approach (Scheerer-Neumann 1979, Snowling 1987). It is argued that children with difficulties in reading acquisition should be identified directly on the basis of (deficient) learning processes and not on the basis of indirect signs or remote symptoms. Today, many signs formerly held as highly diagnostic of 'dyslexia' are no longer valid: they have been uncovered as normal developmental features, the most prominent examples being reversal and sequencing errors (e. g. b/d, was/saw) which have, among other things, turned out as an instance of base-rate fallacy (Stanovich 1986a). In many years of clinical work with dyslexic children Miles (1983) developed a 'dyslexia test' examining diverse performances which are commonly thought to be characteristic of dyslexia like right-left discrimination, repeating polysyllabic words etc. His results speak for an enormous heterogeneity: no single symptom occurred in all of over 200 cases whereas some children failed in only one or two of the items.

Generally, disorders of basic visual processes, of intersensory integration and of serial order recall have been discredited as causes of reading disorder by a host of evidence from well-controlled studies and from evaluations of visually oriented remedial instruction (Kavale/Mattson 1983, Vellutino 1979). The more experiments succeeded in isolating perceptual factors, the less poor and good readers differed in these factors (Stanovich 1986a). Yet this general conclusion does not preclude that a minor group of poor readers may be characterized by some sort of visual deficit – although this is probably more specific to the task of reading than to 'basic visual processes'. It might be rooted in insufficient encoding, storing and/or accessing of visual-orthographic memory patterns (Stanovich 1988b).

3.1. The Role of Phonological Processing

Under the converging influence of developmental psychology, psycholinguistics and models of information processing in cognitive psychology, the search for causal factors in developmental disorders of written language has focussed on skills of auditory analysis of speech sounds and of processing phonological information. These skills are directly involved in cracking the alphabetic code (Gough/Hillinger 1980, LaBerge/Samuels 1974). There is ample evidence now that deficits in processing of speech sound information in its various aspects characterize the majority of poor readers – from implicit sensitivity to sound structure of speech to explicit segmenting of phonemes (Ellis/Cataldo 1990, Valtin 1984), and from phonological encoding to retrieving phonological memory codes (Wagner/Torgesen 1987). Which specific causal relations exist between reading achievement and phonological processing skills (cf. Ehri 1989, Morais/Alegria/Content 1987) is still controversial. It is discussed whether these skills are prerequisite to or a consequence of reading instruction or whether – most probably – the relation is a reciprocal one, phonological processing and reading interacting by mutual stepwise support (cf. Wagner/Torgesen 1987). Nevertheless, summarizing the evidence these conclusions seem warranted:

– Children who already in preschool appear sensitive for units of speech below the syllable and/or for rhyming and alliteration have a reliable prognosis for not becoming reading disabled (Bryant/Bradley/Maclean/Crossland 1989, Ellis/Large 1987, 1988, Maclean/Bryant/Bradley 1987, Tunmer/Nesdale 1985).

– Children with language disorders in preschool age are predicted as reading disordered if language disorders persist up to school entrance (Bishop/Adams 1990). On the other hand, language disorders do not prevent children from developing phonological skills, even though with some lag, to about the same level reached by children without language problems (Bishop/Edmundson 1987a, b).

– Children who in preschool age undergo an extended training in phonological skills show, as a group, better achievement in reading than an untrained comparison group (Lundberg/Frost/Petersen 1988).

– Children who in first grade undergo a phonological skill training combined with acquiring the letters of the alphabet as a rule show better achievement in reading/spelling than children who were trained separately or who were offered only one of these training modes (Bradley 1988, Bradley/Bryant 1985, Wise/Olson/Anstett et al. 1989).

– Children who achieve in reading/writing below their age or – depending on definition of sample – general intellectual ability frequently show difficulties in segmenting speech (Frith/Snowling 1983, Liberman/Shankweiler 1979).

– To adult illiterates, it is very difficult to master tasks of phonological awareness, if they succed at all (Mann 1986, Morais/Cary/Alegria/Bertelson 1979).

– Children who have learned a non-alphabetic writing system or who have not been explicitly taught how to segment speech sounds, are able to learn alphabetic reading (Read/Zhang/Nie/Ding 1986, Seymour/Elder 1986).

– At least for decoding processes only rudimentary intellectual abilities are required (Cossu/Marshall 1990).

Focussing on the role of phonological processing reinforces a wider view of language development in general. As pointed out above, there is growing evidence that poor readers have more pervasive language problems. Relevant reviews (e. g. Catts 1989b) demonstrate that in many cases reading disorder reflects a language problem persisting from early years to adulthood. Late utterance of first words and morphologic or syntactic deficiencies may precede difficulties in learning to read and to spell, and problems in learning from print are to follow (Johnson/Blalock 1987).

Returning to the problems of defining developmental dyslexia (or legasthenia), the way is now paved for a more satisfying inclusionary definition that resorts to this wider context of complex language development: "Dyslexia is a developmental language disorder that involves a specific deficit(s) in the processing of phonological information. The disorder is generally present at birth and persists into adulthood. A prominent characteristic of the disorder is a specific reading disability. Preceding, accompanying, and following this reading disability, the disorder manifests itself in various difficulties in phonological coding, including problems in encoding, retrieving, and using phonological codes in memory. In addition, difficulties may be observed in speech production and in the metalinguistic awareness of speech sound segments" (Catts 1989a, 58).

3.2. Dimensional Continuity of Reading Disorders: the Phonological-Core Variable-Difference Model

Search for homogeneous subtypes is not the only way to deal with well-known heterogeneity of reading disorders. Discussing general principles of classification Morris/Satz (1984) distinguish three models. The first is hierarchical, as known from classifications into families, genera and species in biology, placing subjects into distinct, non-overlapping, systematically related subsets. The field of reading disorders might be apt, as we have seen, for the second, categorical mode of subtyping. However, when the search for 'homogeneous' subtypes provides unclear results a third mode of classification may recommend itself: the dimensional model that orders subjects along axes in a multi-dimensional space. Categorical classification assumes heterogeneity with clustering. In contrast, the dimensional models admits heterogeneity without clustering – which might be the more realistic frame for ordering reading problems. It seems a well-founded opinion of many authors (e. g. Ellis 1985, Olson/Kliegl/Davidson/Foltz 1985, Seidenberg/Bruck/Fornarolo/Backman 1985, Share/McGee/McKenzie et al. 1987) that we are not dealing with discrete entities of dyslexia like 'expected' or 'garden-variety' poor reading but with graded continuity. As Andrew Ellis (1985) remarked, the proper analogy for dyslexia might not be a disease like measles, but instead a condition like obesity, with people forming a continuum from the extreme lean to the overly fat.

What dimensions are proper candidates for spreading the above mentioned multidimensional space? Defining dyslexia with reference to (at least) normal intelligence or causally attributing it to deficits of intersensory integration or visual perception or any other general mono-cause means relying on what Fodor (1983) calls 'horizontal' abilities, i. e. global abilities independent of the material (e. g. alphabetic script) on which they are to operate. This impresses as somewhat paradoxical since from the beginnings of theorizing about reading disorders the assumption of specificity was clearly implied (Hall/Humphreys 1982). Consequently, Stanovich (1988a) judges any view invoking global processes, also of the more recent type such as general linguistic awareness or generalized metacognitive functioning (Torgesen 1977), to be "on the wrong track". Instead, one should look for in Fodor's sense 'vertical' and domain-specific processing mechanisms that are closely tied to the reading task and lead to fast automatic functioning on the basic level of word recognition (Gough/Tunmer 1986, Perfetti 1985, Vellutino 1979). Adults reading texts within their ability level show fairly autonomous word recognition, without support from context (Seidenberg/Bruck/Fornarolo/Backman 1985, Stanovich/West 1983). This line of argument meets with much of the above cited evidence concerning the linkage of phonological processing to proficiency in reading/spelling. In sum, phonological processing has been demonstrated as uniquely contributing to variance in reading skill after intelligence and other cognitive measures have been partialled out (Bradley/Bryant 1985, Lundberg/Olofsson/Wall 1980, Tunmer/Nesdale 1985). So it appears as sufficiently independent of other more global cognitive abilities to qualify for the postulated modular, domain-specific key ability.

In the model of 'phonological-core variable-difference' proposed by Stanovich (1988b) to account for 'heterogeneity without clustering', phonological processing stands for the core of deficient performance in reading disorders common to both dyslexics and 'garden-variety' poor readers whereas 'variable-differences' is to take care of the contrasts between the two groups. These contrasts originate from the dyslexic readers' general cognitive abilities being average or even superior. Compared to generally backward readers, their better 'horizontal' abilities enable dyslexics to compensate for inferior word recognition by richer vocabulary, memory and world knowledge when reading comprehension is the criterion of achievement. On the basis of findings from experiments of context use by dyslexic children Snowling (1987, 137) comes to similar conclusions: "Hence, in the face of phonological difficulties, the reading development of dyslexic children may be fostered by the use of stored lexical and semantic information as well as by use of more general knowledge resources". On the other hand, the garden-variety poor readers with phonological deficits – which might not be as severe

as those of dyslexics – and inferior general cognitive abilities would show a broad-based developmental lag in reading achievement; Stanovich (1988b) provides evidence for this lag from longitudinal comparisons.
– Admittedly, this model neglects a group of dyslexics which, though relatively small, is marked by different authors: so-called morphemic dyslexics (Seymour/MacGregor 1984) with difficulties in using the direct, visual-orthographic route of accessing the lexicon. However, the model would predict all other processing characteristics in reading performance of the visual-orthographic group similar to the phonological-deficit group. Another complication not covered by the model is the existence of 'Matthew-effects' (Stanovich 1986b), i. e. progressive falling back in reading achievement and, as a consequence, in more global cognitive performance of the reading disordered compared to normal achievers.

The above ideas fit well with the dimensional model inaugurated by Ellis. Passing through his "complete and unbroken gradation of intermediate dyslexics" (Ellis 1985, 192), linking the 'pure' psychometrically defined dyslexic to the 'pure' generally backward reader, "we will move from a processing deficit localized in the phonological core to the global deficits of the developmentally lagging garden-variety poor reader" (Stanovich 1988b, 602).

4. References

Adelman, H. S. & Taylor, L. (1985). The future of the LD field: a survey of fundamental concerns. *Journal of Learning Disabilities, 18*, 423–427.

Bishop, D. V. M. & Adams, C. (1990). A prospective study of the relationship between specific language impairment, phonological disorders and reading retardation. *Journal of Child Psychology and Psychiatry, 31*, 1027–1050.

Bishop, D. V. M. & Edmundson, A. (1987a). Language-impaired 4-year-olds: distinguishing transient from persistent impairment. *Journal of Speech and Hearing Disorders, 52*, 156–173.

Bishop, D. V. M. & Edmundson, A. (1987b). Specific language impairment as a maturational lag: evidence from longitudinal data on language and motor development. *Developmental Medicine and Child Neurology, 29*, 442–459.

Boder, E. (1973). Developmental dyslexia: a diagnostic approach based on three atypical reading-spelling patterns. *Developmental Medicine and Child Neurology, 15*, 663–687.

Bradley, L. (1988). Making connections in learning to read and to spell. *Applied Cognitive Psychology, 2*, 3–18.

Bradley, L. & Bryant, P. E. (1978). Difficulties in auditory organisation as a possible cause of reading backwardness. *Nature, 271*, 746–747.

Bradley, L. & Bryant, P. E. (1985). *Rhyme and reason in reading and spelling*. Ann Arbor: The University of Michigan Press.

Bryant, P. E., Bradley, L., Maclean, M., & Crossland, J. (1989). Nursery rhymes, phonological skills and reading. *Journal of Child Language, 16*, 407–428.

Butler, S. R., Marsh, H. W., Sheppard, M. J., & Sheppard, J. L. (1985). Seven-year longitudinal study of the early prediction of reading achievement. *Journal of Educational Psychology, 79*, 349–361.

Catts, H. W. (1989a). Defining dyslexia as a developmental language disorder. *Annals of Dyslexia, 39*, 50–64.

Catts, H. W. (1989b). Phonological processing deficits and reading disabilities. In A. G. Kamhi & H. W. Catts (Eds.), *Reading disabilities: a developmental language perspective, 101–132.* Boston: College-Hill.

Clay, M. M. (1970). An increasing effect of disorientation on the discrimination of print: a developmental study. *Journal of Experimental Child Psychology, 9*, 297–306.

Cossu, G. & Marshall, J. C. (1990). Are cognitive skills a prerequisite for learning to read and write? *Cognitive Neuropsychology, 7*, 21–40.

Critchley, M. (1970). *The dyslexic child.* Springfield, Ill.: Thomas.

Ehri, L. C. (1979). Linguistic insight: threshold of reading acquisition. In T. G. Waller & G. E. MacKinnon (Eds.), *Reading research: advances in theory and practice. Vol. 1. 63–114.* New York: Academic Press.

Ehri, L. C. (1989). The development of spelling knowledge and its role in reading acquisition and reading disability. *Journal of Learning Disabilities, 22*, 356–365.

Eichler, W. (1986). Zu Uta Frith' Dreiphasenmodell des Lesen (und Schreiben) Lernens. Oder: Lassen sich verschiedene Modelle des Schrifterwerbs aufeinander beziehen und weiterentwickeln. In G. Augst (Ed.), *New trends in graphemics and orthography. 234–247.* Berlin: De Gruyter.

Ellis, A. W. (1985). The cognitive neuropsychology of developmental (and acquired) dyslexia: a critical survey. *Cognitive Neuropsychology, 2*, 169–205.

Ellis, N. & Cataldo, S. (1990). The role of spelling in learning to read. *Language and Education, 4*, 1–28.

Ellis, N. & Large, B. (1987). The development of reading: as you seek so shall you find. *British Journal of Psychology, 78*, 1–28.

Ellis, N. & Large, B. (1988). The early stages of reading: a longitudinal study. *Applied Cognitive Psychology, 2*, 47–76.

Fletcher, J. M. & Satz, P. (1985). External validation of learning disability subtypes. In B. P. Rourke (Ed.), *Neuropsychology of learning disabilities: essentials of subtype analysis. 40–64.* New York: Guilford Press.

Fodor, J. (1983). *Modularity of mind.* Cambridge, Ma.: MIT Press.

Frith, U. (1985). Beneath the surface of developmental dyslexia. In K. E. Patterson, J. C. Marshall, & M. Coltheart (Eds.), *Surface dyslexia: neuropsychological and cognitive studies of phonological reading. 301–330.* London: Erlbaum.

Frith, U. (1986). Psychologische Aspekte des orthographischen Wissens: Entwicklung und Entwicklungsstörung. In G. Augst (Ed.), *New trends in graphemics and orthography. 218–233.* Berlin: De Gruyter.

Frith, U. & Snowling, M. (1983). Reading for meaning and reading for sound in autistic and dyslexic children. *British Journal of Developmental Psychology, 1*, 329–342.

Gibson, E. J. (1971). Learning to read. In H. Singer & R. B. Ruddell (Eds.), *Theoretical models and processes of reading. (2. Ed.). 315–334.* Newark D. E.: International Reading Association.

Gibson, E. J. & Levin, H. (1976). *The psychology of reading (2. Ed.).* Cambridge, Ma: MIT Press.

Goswami, U. (1986). Children's use of analogy in learning to read: a developmental study. *Journal of Experimental Child Psychology, 42*, 73–83.

Goswami, U. (1988). Children's use of analogy in learning to spell. *British Journal of Developmental Psychology, 6*, 21–33.

Goswami, U. & Bryant, P. (1989). The interpretation of studies using the reading level design. *Journal of Reading Behavior, 21*, 413–424.

Gough, P. B. & Hillinger, M. (1980). Learning to read: an unnatural act. *Bulletin of the Orton Society, 30*, 171–196.

Gough, P. B. & Tunmer, W. E. (1986). Decoding, reading, and reading disability. *Remedial and Special Education, 7*, 6–10.

Günther, K. B. (1986). Ein Stufenmodell der Entwicklung kindlicher Lese- und Schreibstrategien. In H. Brügelmann (Ed.), *ABC und Schriftsprache: Rätsel für Kinder, Lehrer und Forscher. 32–54.* Konstanz: Faude.

Guthrie, J. T. (1973). Models of reading and reading disabilities. *Journal of Educational Psychology, 65*, 9–18.

Hall, J. & Humphreys, M. (1982). Research on specific learning disabilities: deficits and remediation. *Topics in Learning and Learning Disabilities, 2*, 68–78.

Harris, T. L. & Hodges, R. E. (1981). *A dictionary of reading.* Newark, D. E.: International Reading Association.

Hinshelwood, J. (1917). *Congenital word blindness.* London: Lewis.

Høien, T. & Lundberg, I. (1988). Stages of word recognition in early reading acquisition. *Scandinavian Journal of Educational Research, 32*, 163–182.

Jackson, N. E. & Butterfield, E. C. (1989). Reading-level-match design: myths and realities. *Journal of Reading Behavior, 21*, 387–412.

Johnson, D. & Blalock, J. (1987). *Adults with learning disabilities. Clinical studies.* New York: Grune & Stratton.

Jorm, A. F., Share, D. L., Maclean, R., & Matthews, R. (1986). Cognitive factors at school entry predictive of specific reading retardation and general reading backwardness: a research note. *Journal of Child Psychology and Psychiatry, 27*, 45–54.

Kamhi, A. G. & Catts, H. W. (1989). Reading disabilities: terminology, definitions and subtyping issues. In A. G. Kamhi & H. W. Catts (Eds.), *Reading disabilities: a developmental language perspective. 35–66.* Boston: College-Hill.

Kavale, K. & Forness, S. (1987). The far side of heterogeneity: a critical analysis of empirical subtyping research in learning disabilities. *Journal of Learning Disabilities, 20*, 374–383.

Kavale, K. & Mattson, P. (1983). "One jumped off the balance beam": meta-analysis of perceptual motor training. *Journal of Learning Disabilities, 16*, 165–173.

Kavale, K. & Nye, C. (1986). Parameters of learning disabilities in achievement, linguistic, neuropsychological and social behavioral domains. *Journal of Special Education, 19*, 443–458.

LaBerge, D. & Samuels, S. J. (1974). Toward a theory of automatic information processing in reading. *Cognitive Psychology, 6*, 293–323.

Liberman, A. M., Cooper, F. S., Shankweiler, D., & Studdert-Kennedy, M. (1967). Perception of the speech code. *Psychological Review, 74*, 431–461.

Liberman, A. M. & Shankweiler, D. (1979). Speech, the alphabet, and teaching to read. In L. B. Resnick & P. A. Weaver (Eds.), *Theory and practice of early reading, Vol 2. 109–132.* Hillsdale, N. J.: Erlbaum.

Linder, M. (1951). Über Legasthenie (Spezielle Leseschwäche), 50 Fälle, ihr Erscheinungsbild und Möglichkeiten der Behandlung. *Zeitschrift für Kinderpsychiatrie, 18*, 97–143.

Lundberg, I., Frost, J., & Petersen, O. (1988). Effects of an extensive program for stimulating phonological awareness in preschool children. *Reading Research Quarterly, 23*, 263–284.

Lundberg, J., Olofsson, A., & Wall, S. (1980). Reading and spelling skills in the first school years predicted from phonemic awareness skills. *Scandinavian Journal of Psychology, 21*, 263–284.

Maclean, M., Bryant, P. E., & Bradley, L. (1987). Rhymes, nursery rhymes and reading in early childhood. *Merrill-Palmer Quarterly, 33*, 255–282.

Malatesha, R. N. & Dougan, D. R. (1982). Clinical subtypes of developmental dyslexia: resolution of an irresolute problem. In R. N. Malatesha & P. G. Aaron (Eds.), *Reading disorders: varieties and treatments. 69–92.* New York: Academic Press.

Mann, V. A. (1986). Phonological awareness: the role of reading experience. *Cognition, 24*, 65–92.

Mannhaupt, G. (1990). Strategieausbildung zur Lautstrukturanalyse mit Hilfe von abstrakten und konkreten Symbolen während des frühen Schriftspracherwerbs. Universität Bielefeld: Unpublished Doctor's Thesis.

Marsh, G., Friedman, M., & Welsh, V., (1981). A cognitive-developmental approach in reading acquisition. In T. G. Waller & G. E. MacKinnon (Eds.), *Reading research: advances in theory and practice, Vol. 3. 199–221.* New York: Academic Press.

Marx, H. (1985). *Aufmerksamkeitsverhalten und Leseschwierigkeiten.* Göttingen: Hogrefe.

Marx, H. (1989). Zeitliche Ausgangspunkte und ihre Auswirkungen auf Anlage und Aussage von Längsschnittstudien zur frühen Identifikation und Prädiktion von Lese-Rechtschreibschwierigkeiten. Universität Bielefeld: SFB 227, Preprint Nr. 23.

Mason, J. M. (1980). When do children begin to read: an exploration of four year old children's letter and word reading competencies. *Reading Research Quarterly, 15*, 203–227.

Miles, T. R. (1983). *Dyslexia: the pattern of difficulties.* London: Granada.

Morais, J., Alegria, J., & Content, A. (1987). The relationships between segmental analysis and alphabetic literacy: an interactive view. *Cahiers de Psychologie Cognitive, 7*, 1–24.

Morais, J., Cary, L., Alegria, J., & Bertelson, P. (1979). Does awareness of speech as a sequence of phones arise spontaneously? *Cognition, 7*, 323–331.

Morgan, P. (1896). A case of congenital word blindness. *British Medicine Journal, 2*, 1378.

Morris, R., Blashfield, R., & Satz, P. (1986). Developmental classification of reading disabled children. *Journal of Clinical & Experimental Neuropsychology, 8*, 371–392.

Morris, R. & Satz, P. (1984). Classification issues in subtype research: an application of some methods and concepts. In R. N. Malatesha & H. A. Whitaker (Eds.), *Dyslexia: a global issue. 52–62.* Dordrecht/The Hague: Martinus Nijhoff Publishers.

Niemeyer, W. (1974). *Legasthenie und Milieu.* Hannover: Schroedel.

Olson, R., Kliegl, R., Davidson, B., & Foltz, G. (1985). Individual and developmental differences in reading disabilities. In G. E. McKinnon & T. Waller (Ed.), *Reading research: advances in theory and practice, Vol. 4. 57–64.* London: Academic Press.

Orton, S. T. (1937). *Reading, writing and speech problems in children.* New York: Norton.

Perfetti, C. A. (1985). *Reading ability.* New York: Oxford University Press.

Petrauskas, R. & Rourke, B. (1979). Identification of subtypes of retarded readers: a neuropsychological multivariate approach. *Journal of Clinical Neuropsychology, 1*, 17–37.

Ranschburg, P. (1916). *Die Leseschwäche (Legasthenie) und Rechenschwäche (Arithmasthenie) der Schulkinder im Lichte des Experiments.* Berlin: Springer.

Read, C., Zhang, Y.-F., Nie, H.-Y., Ding, B.-Q. (1986). The ability to manipulate speech sounds depends on knowing alphabetic writing. *Cognition, 24*, 31–45.

Rodgers, B. (1983). The identification and prevalence of specific reading retardation. *British Journal of Educational Psychology, 53*, 369–373.

Rozin, P. & Gleitman L. R. (1977). The structure and acquisition of reading II: the reading process and the acquisition of the alphabetic principle. In A. S. Reber & D. L. Scarborough (Eds.), *Toward a psychology of reading. 55–141.* Hillsdale, N. J.: Erlbaum.

Rudel, R. (1985). The definition of dyslexia: language and motor deficits. In F. Duffy & N. Geschwind (Eds.), *Dyslexia: a neuroscientific approach to clinical evaluation. 33–54.* Boston: Little, Brown.

Rutter, M. (1978). Prevalence and types of dyslexia. In A. L. Benton & D. Pearl (Eds.), *Dyslexia. 3–28.* New York: Oxford University Press.

Rutter, M. & Yule, W. (1975). The concept of specific reading retardation. *Journal of Child Psychology and Psychiatry, 16*, 181–197.

Samuels, S. J. (1976). Hierarchical subskills in the reading acquisition process. In J. T. Guthrie (Ed.), *Aspects of reading acquisition. 162–179.* Baltimore: The Johns Hopkins University Press.

Satz, P. & Morris, R. (1981). Learning disability subtypes: a review. In F. J. Pirozzolo & M. C. Wittrock (Eds.), *Neuropsychological and cognitive processes in reading. 109–141.* New York: Academic Press.

Scheerer-Neumann, G. (1979). *Intervention bei Lese-Rechtschreibschwäche.* Bochum: Kamp.

Scheerer-Neumann, G. (1989). Entwicklungsprozesse beim Lesenlernen: Eine Fallstudie. In M. Beck (Ed.), *Schriftspracherwerb – Lese-Rechtschreibschwäche. 15–38.* Tübingen: DGVT-Tübinger Reihe.

Schlee, J. (1976). *Legasthenieforschung am Ende?* München: Urban & Schwarzenberg.

Seidenberg, M. S., Bruck, M., Fornarolo, G. & Backman, J. (1985). Word recognition processes of poor and disabled readers? Do they necessarily differ? *Applied Psycholinguistics, 6*, 161 – 180.

Seidenberg, M. S. & McClelland, J. L. (1989). A distributed developmental model of word recognition and naming. *Psychological Review, 96*, 523 – 568.

Seymour, P. H. K. & Elder, L. (1986). Beginning reading without phonology. *Cognitive Neuropsychology, 3*, 1 – 36.

Seymour P. H. K. & McGregor, C. J. (1984). Developmental dyslexia: a cognitive experimental analysis of phonological, morphemic and visual impairments. *Cognitive Neuropsychology, 1*, 43 – 82.

Share, D. L., Jorm, A. F., Maclean, R., & Matthews, R. (1984). Sources of individual differences in reading acquisition. *Journal of Educational Psychology, 76*, 1309 – 1324.

Share, D. L., McGee, R., McKenzie, D., Williams, S., & Silva, P. A. (1987). Further evidence relating to the distinction between specific reading retardation and general reading backwardness. *British Journal of Developmental Psychology, 5*, 35 – 44.

Skowronek, H. & Marx, H. (1989). The Bielefeld longitudinal study on early identification of risks in learning read and write. In M. Brambring, F. Lösel & H. Skowronek (Eds.), *Children at risk: assessment, longitudinal research and intervention. 268 – 294.* Berlin/New York: de Gruyter.

Snowling, M. (1987). *Dyslexia. A cognitive developmental perspective.* London: Basil Blackwell.

Stanovich, K. E. (1986a). Cognitive processes and the reading problems of learning-disabled children: evaluating the assumption of specificity. In J. K. Torgesen & B. Y. L. Wong (Eds.), *Psychological and educational perspectives on learning disabilities. 85 – 159.* New York: Academic Press.

Stanovich, K. E. (1986b). Matthew effects in reading: some consequences of individual differences in the acquisition of literacy. *Reading Research Quarterly, 21*, 360 – 406.

Stanovich, K. E. (1988a). The right and wrong places to look for the cognitive locus of reading disability. *Annals of Dyslexia, 38*, 154 – 177.

Stanovich, K. E. (1988b). Explaining the differences between the dyslexic and the garden-variety poor reader: the phonological-core variable-difference model. *Journal of Learning Disabilities, 21*, 590 – 604.

Stanovich, K. E. (1989). Various varying views on variation. *Journal of Learning Disabilities, 22*, 366 – 369.

Stanovich, K. E. (1990a). Concepts in developmental theories of reading skills: cognitive resources, automaticity, and modularity. *Developmental Review, 10*, 72 – 100.

Stanovich, K. E. (1990b). A call for an end to the paradigm wars in reading research. *Journal of Reading Behavior, 22*, 221 – 231.

Stanovich, K. E., Nathan, R. G., & Zolman, J. E. (1988). The developmental lag hypothesis in reading: longitudinal and matched reading-level comparisons. *Child Development, 59*, 71 – 86.

Stanovich, K. E. & West, R. F. (1983). On priming by a sentence context. *Journal of Experimental Psychology: General, 112*, 1 – 36.

Stuart, M. & Coltheart, M. (1988). Does reading develop in a sequence of stages? *Cognition, 30*, 139 – 181.

Taylor, H. J., Satz, P., & Friel, J. (1979). Developmental dyslexia in relation to other childhood reading disorders: significance and clinical utility. *Reading Research Quarterly, 15*, 84 – 101.

Thomson, M. (1984). *Developmental dyslexia: its nature, assessment, and remediation.* London: Edward Arnold.

Torgesen, J. K. (1977). Memorization processes in reading-disabled children. *Journal of Educational Psychology, 72*, 141 – 160.

Treiman, R. & Hirsh-Pasek, K. (1985). Are there qualitative differences in reading behavior between dyslexics and normal readers? *Memory and Cognition, 13*, 357 – 364.

Tunmer, W. E. & Nesdale, A. R. (1985). Phonemic segmentation skill and beginning reading. *Journal of Educational Psychology, 77*, 417 – 427.

Valtin, R. (1975). Ursachen oder Artefakte? Kritische Bemerkungen zum methodischen und theoretischen Konzept der Legasthenieforschung. *Zeitschrift für Pädagogik, 21*, 407 – 418.

Valtin, R. (1978/79). Dyslexia: deficit in reading or deficit in research? Critical comments on the methodological and theoretical aspects of research on Legasthenie. *Reading Research Quarterly, 14*, 201 – 221.

Valtin, R. (1984). Awareness of features and functions of language. In J. Downing & R. Valtin (Eds.), *Language awareness and learning to read. 227 – 260.* Berlin: Springer.

Van der Wissel, A. & Zegers, F. E. (1985). Reading retardation revisited. *British Journal of Developmental Psychology, 3*, 3 – 19.

Van Orden, G. C., Pennington, B. F., & Stone, G. O. (1990). Word identification in reading and the promise of subsymbolic psycholinguistics. *Psychological Review, 97*, 488 – 522.

Vellutino, F. R. (1979). *Dyslexia: theory and Research.* Cambridge: Lawrence Erlbaum.

Vellutino, F. R. & Scanlon, D. M. (1987). Phonological coding, phonological awareness, and reading ability: evidence from a longitudinal and experimental study. *Merrill-Palmer Quarterly, 33*, 321 – 363.

Vellutino, F. R. & Scanlon, D. M. (1989). Some prerequisites for interpreting results from reading level matched designs. *Journal of Reading Behavior, 21*, 361–385.

Venezky, R. L. (1976). Prerequisites for learning to read. In J. R. Levin & V. L. Allen (Eds.), *Cognitive learning in children. Theories and strategies. 163–185*. New York: Academic Press.

Wagner, R. K. & Torgesen J. K. (1987). The nature of phonological processing and its causal role in the acquisition of reading skills. *Psychological Bulletin, 101*, 192–212.

Warnke, A. (1990). *Legasthenie und Hirnfunktion. Neuropsychologische Befunde zur visuellen Informationsverarbeitung*. Bern/Stuttgart/Toronto: Huber.

Weigl, E. (1976). Schriftsprache als besondere Form des Sprachverhaltens. In A. Hofer (Ed.), *Lesenlernen: Theorie und Unterricht. 82–98*. Düsseldorf: Schwann.

Wimmer, H., Hartl, M., & Moser, E. (1990). Passen "englische" Modelle des Schriftspracherwerbs auf "deutsche" Kinder? Zweifel an der Bedeutsamkeit der logographischen Stufe. *Zeitschrift für Entwicklungspsychologie und Pädagogische Psychologie, 22*, 136–154.

Wise, B., Olson, R., Anstett, M., Andrews,. L., Terjak, M., Schneider, V., Kostuch, J., & Kriho, L. (1989). Implementing a long-term computerized remedial reading program with synthetic speech feedback: hardware, software, and real-world issues. *Behavior Research Methods, Instruments & Computers, 21*, 173–180.

Zielinski, W. (1980). *Lernschwierigkeiten*. Stuttgart: Kohlhammer.

Helmut Skowronek/Harald Marx, Bielefeld (Germany)

70. Developmental Dyslexia and Language Disorders

1. Introduction

Impairments in language skills are common in dyslexic children. Parental reports show that they often learn to talk later than normal and, in interviews, they may show evidence of less complex language than normal children of the same age; it is also common for dyslexic children to show higher performance, than verbal, IQ scores. Language, however, is a complex system that can break down in different ways. Linguists stress the different levels of analysis necessary for adequately describing language processing. In particular, we need to distinguish between semantic processes concerned with meaning; syntactic processes concerned with grammar; phonological processes concerned with the sound structure of language; and pragmatics concerned with language use. These different levels of language clearly interact during processing. In dyslexic children, there is considerable evidence for the primary deficit being in phonological processing.

2. Spoken Language Deficits in Dyslexic Children

2.1. Phonological Awareness

Phonological awareness refers to the ability to reflect explicitly on the sound structure of spoken words. Most research on phonological awareness has been concerned with its predictive relationship to reading in unselected samples of children. There is considerable evidence showing that phonological awareness tasks are among the best predictors of reading skill and, typically, these relationships can be shown to account for significant amounts of variance in reading skill, even after the effects of intelligence have been partialled out (see Goswami/Bryant 1990, 4 and Wagner/Torgesen 1987 for recent reviews).

The strongest evidence for a link between phonological awareness and learning to read has been produced by Bradley and Bryant. In their first study, they compared a large group of dyslexic children with normal children of the same reading age and IQ on a sound categorization task (Bradley/Bryant 1978). Dyslexic children were much worse on this auditory task than normal children who were some 3½ years younger, but read at the same level. This established that dyslexic children have difficulty in categorizing words on the basis of their sound and that this difficulty is not simply a consequence of their poor reading skills.

Bradley/Bryant (1983) set out to test whether difficulties with sound categorization were a cause of reading difficulties. This was a longitudinal study. At the beginning, the sound categorization ability of over 400 4- and 5-year-old children was assessed before they started to learn to read. Over three years later, their reading and spelling ability and verbal intelligence were assessed. Performance on the sound categorization task was predictive of later reading scores, even when measures of intelligence and memory were taken into account.

To try to check that this correlation between early sound categorization skills and reading reflected a causal influence, Bradley and Bryant included a training study. Sixty-five children who initially were poor at sound categorization were split into four groups. One group was trained in sound categorization, and a second in addition to this was taught letter-sound correspondences. There were also two control groups: one group was taught to group words according to semantic categories and the other received no training. After training, spread over two years, the group that had been taught sound categorization and letter sound correspondences was some 8 to 10 months ahead of the untaught control group in reading scores. The group that had only been taught to categorize sounds was about 4 months ahead of the control group in reading, but this difference was not statistically significant.

These results fail to clinch the argument for the causal role of sound categorization in learning to read. To prove this would require evidence that the group taught only to categorize words on the basis of their sound was significally ahead of the group taught to categorize on the basis of meaning. There was a tendency for this to happen, but not to a statistically reliable degree.

Nonetheless, the association between phonological awareness and reading ability is highly robust, having been obtained in a number of studies. Lundberg/Olofsson/Wall (1981) gave a large group of Swedish children a battery of measures of phonological awareness. They found that these tests were predictive of reading scores 1½ years later. A similar result to this has also been obtained by Stanovich/Cunningham/Cramer (1984), who found that a battery of measures of phonological awareness administered before starting to learn to read, predicted success in reading a year later. The different tests of phonological awareness were highly intercorrelated, suggesting that they were measuring some common underlying skill.

More recently, attention has been drawn to the fact that different types of phonological awareness may develop at different rates and bear different relationships to the process of learning to read. This argument has been developed most fully by Goswami/Bryant (1990, 97). Their argument depends upon recognizing that there are different levels of analysis for spoken words and awareness of these develops at different rates.

They stress the importance of the syllable, and two sub-syllabic units; namely, the onset and the rime. Within each syllable of English, the rime comprises the vowel and succeeding consonants, if any; the onset refers to the consonant or cluster which precedes the vowel. So, for example, the monosyllabic word *string* consists of an onset, /str/, and a rime, /ing/. One task that taps young children's sensitivity to rimes is rhyme detection; for example, asking children to pick the odd (nonrhyming) word out from a group of four spoken words (Bradley/Bryant 1978). As we have seen, this task can be performed quite adequately by four- and five-year-olds, before they have learned to read, and is highly predictive of their later success in reading and spelling. The ability to segment words by phonemes appears later, possibly as a consequence of learning to read. It is a very difficult task for young children and shows serious impairment in dyslexic children. Goswami/Bryant (1990, 97) argue, following a review of a very large number of studies, that it is awareness of onset and rime that is crucial to learning to read, whereas awareness of smaller speech segments (phonemes) arises at least partly as a consequence of learning to read.

2.2 Verbal Repetition Deficits

Clinical reports often comment upon the tendency for dyslexic children to mispronounce words or produce Spoonerisms; for example, saying *par cark* for *car park*. Snowling (1981) asked dyslexic children to repeat a series of words of 2, 3 and 4 syllables and also a series of analogous nonwords derived from the words by changing one or two phonemes to others that were made either in the same place in the mouth or in the same manner. She compared their performance with that of a group of younger normal readers, who were matched with the dyslexics in terms of reading ability. Interestingly, while the dyslexics were as good as the control group when repeating the words, they made significantly more errors when repeating the nonwords. This difficulty was interpreted in terms of problems with the segmentation operations required for compiling new motor articulation programs that were needed for the repetition of nonwords.

Snowling / Goulandris / Bowlby / Howell (1986) extended these findings to confirm that dyslexic children have specific difficulty with nonword repetition. In this experiment, subjects were required to repeat high-frequency words, such as *dog* and *trick*, low-frequency words, such as *glades* and *chef*, and nonwords made up by changing the first phoneme of the high-frequency words, such as *tog* and *drick*. All of the stimuli were of one-syllable, and they were presented either in a clear background, or with noise masking that was designed to reduce the signal to noise ratio. The dyslexic children were 10-year-olds, reading on average at the 8-year level.

The first clear finding of the study was that although noise masking increased the error rate in the repetition task, it did so to the same extent for dyslexics as for normal readers. Therefore, it could be concluded that the dyslexics did not have any differential difficulty with the auditory perception of the word and nonword stimuli they had to repeat. However, there were interesting group differences with respect to the repetition of different stimulus types. None of the children had any difficulty in repeating high-frequency words but, interestingly, the dyslexics could repeat low-frequency words only as well as younger reading-age matched controls. In repeating nonwords, however, dyslexic children made even more errors than younger children reading at the same level. This was a striking finding that confirmed earlier reports of nonword repetition deficits in dyslexic children. The problems could not be attributed to perceptual difficulties because the dyslexics were affected no more by noise masking than the control group, and it could not be attributed to peripheral articulation difficulties, because in that case their pronunciation of all words should have been affected. The conclusion that they had specific difficulties with the segmentation processes required in order to assemble a new motor program, therefore, seemed the most likely explanation.

It could be argued that a direct consequence of this difficulty in processing nonwords for pronunciation would be a delay in the acquisition of new lexical entries in the spoken language system. Initially, all unfamiliar words are 'nonwords' to a young child until, through learning, lexical entries are created for them. Dyslexics' difficulty in repeating low-frequency items, relative to age-matched controls fits in with this hypothesis, suggesting that they might be slower to expand their spoken vocabulary of words than expected, given their I.Q. Also consonant with this view is the finding of naming difficulties in dyslexics.

2.3. Auditory Perceptual Problems

The language deficits with which we have been concerned arguably could be related to difficulties first in establishing, and later in accessing, adequate phonological representations. A number of studies have suggested that these problems may themselves be perceptual in origin. That is, developmental difficulties with speech perception could interfere with phonological processing. Brandt/Rosen (1980) investigated the perception of stop consonants (e. g. d) by dyslexic and normal readers. They found that the dyslexics performed like children at an earlier developmental stage, a finding similar to that of Godfrey/Syrdal-Lasky/Millay/Knox (1981), who found that dyslexics were inconsistent in their phonetic classification of auditory cues in both discrimination and identification tasks. More recently, Reed (1989) carried out several experiments that pointed to the existence of a perceptual deficit in some dyslexic children.

In Reed's study, dyslexics had more difficulty in determining the order in which two stop consonants or two brief tones were presented than normal readers of the same age (7 to 10 years). In contrast, temporal order judgments that involved steady state vowels caused no difficulty. Similarly, the dyslexic children had more difficulty with a word identification task in which an auditorily presented word had to be matched with one of two pictures, differing by a single phoneme; e. g., *goal* paired with a pictorial representation of GOAL and BOWL. They were also less consistent in their phonemic categorization of stimuli, as evidenced by poorer identification of syllables in synthetic speech that were near a phoneme category boundary, as well as by poorer discrimination of syllable pairs that crossed the category boundary.

Taken together, these findings seemed to suggest that the dyslexic children had difficulty with the perception of brief auditory cues, a difficulty that could plausibly account for their impaired performance on a range of phonological processing tasks.

So far, the evidence we have reviewed paints a fairly clear picture as to the language deficits that are characteristic of dyslexic children. Foremost among these are difficulties with the processing of speech sounds, which, undoubtedly, would interfere with the child's developing awareness of the phonological structure of words and also with the establishment of adequate phonological representations of spoken words. These deficits may also be directly implicated in reading failure.

3. Written Language Deficits in Dyslexic Children

There is ample evidence that children make use of a sight vocabulary when reading, and they also can resort to the use of phonological strategies when presented with unfamiliar words. Furthermore, it seems clear that awareness of the phonological structures of words will be central to the development of decoding competence since this relies upon knowledge of correspondences between letters and letter sequences and sounds. It can be predicted, therefore, that dyslexics will have more difficulty with the acquisition of phonological reading strategies than normally developing children.

3.1. Phonological Deficits in Reading

3.1.1. Evidence from Single Word-Reading Tasks

Words in English orthography vary in the directness of mapping sound onto spelling. Experimental studies often contrast regular words with irregular (or exception) words. The logic here is that irregular words should be read less well by children and adults according to the extent to which they utilize rules about spelling patterns in order to decode them. If dyslexics are poor at using such rules, they might be expected to show little difference in their ability to read regular and irregular words, as compared to normal children reading at the same level. Frith/Snowling (1983) found that dyslexic children were not susceptible to a regularity effect in their reading. While normal readers read a greater number of regular than matched irregular words, dyslexic children did not. Along similar lines, Szeszulski/Manis (1987) asked dyslexic readers to read regular and irregular words and nonwords comparing their performance with that of normal readers who were reading at the same grade level. Among children reading at the second-grade level, there were some interesting group differences; there was a larger regularity effect for normal readers, although the effect was apparent in both groups, and the dyslexics made fewer rule-based pronunciations of nonwords than the control group. These results from group comparisons suggest that dyslexics are less skilled in the use of decoding strategies.

3.1.2. Evidence from Nonword Reading

One advantage of focusing on nonword reading in comparisons of dyslexic and normal readers is that nonwords are unfamiliar items. Reading them, therefore, taps into the processes that are used in learning to read which, by implication, are deficient in dyslexic readers. Snowling (1981) asked subjects to read monosyllabic and disyllabic nonwords of varying complexity. Overall, the dyslexics were slower and more error prone than reading-age matched controls when reading the nonwords aloud and they found the longer and more complex nonwords particularly difficult.

Since this early study, many others have examined nonword reading skill in dyslexics. There is not space here to review these numerous studies (for a full review see Snowling/Rack 1991). Suffice it to say that although a number of studies have challenged the view, there is considerable empirical support for the position that dyslexic children have specific difficulties with the acquisition of phonological reading strategies as indicated by specific difficulties in reading nonwords. This is particularly true when a stringent criterion of normal IQ is applied in the selection of dyslexic readers and when they are compared with normal readers matched for reading comprehension (Aaron 1989). This does not rule out the possibility, however, that some dyslexics may develop their use of grapheme-phoneme correspondence rules, following an initial setback and use them in a number of reading tasks; for example, in lexical decision.

4. Individual Differences Amongst Dyslexic Children

Dyslexic children have difficulties with many tasks that require explicit phonological processing. Studies of their reading have suggested that their problems are mainly with the development and use of phonological strategies. It is tempting to argue that these weaknesses in the use of phonological reading strategies are caused by their weak underlying phonological skills. However, a major problem for this argument is that the findings are based entirely on group studies. By their very nature, group studies average across subjects and, therefore, overlook individual differences. These individual differences are of potential importance in theorizing about the specific impact of cognitive deficits on the acquisition of reading skills.

While good evidence in favor of distinct subtypes is certainly lacking (Seymour 1986, 250; Treiman/Hirsh-Pasek 1985), most systematic studies of individual differences among dyslexics have revealed important variations in their reading and spelling skills. Researchers utilizing a cognitive-neuropsychological approach have provided unequivocal evidence that individual dyslexic children, studied at one point in time, can vary qualitatively with respect to their patterns of reading (and spelling) performance. First, developmental dyslexics who have a specific problem with phonological reading strategies, as revealed by their superior word reading ability compared to their nonword reading skill, have been likened to neurological patients with acquired phonological dyslexia following brain damage (Campbell/Butterworth 1985; Seymour/MacGregor 1984; Temple/Marshall 1983). In contrast, dyslexics who have relatively less difficulty with phonological reading strategies but have problems with direct lexical strategies, as evidenced by problems with the reading of irregular words, have been labelled developmental surface dyslexics (Coltheart/Masterson/Byng et al. 1983) or developmental morphemic dyslexics (Seymour 1986).

The findings of cognitive-neuropsychological studies have enhanced our understanding of the different ways in which reading can break down following brain damage and, to some extent, as the consequence of developmental difficulties, but attempts to link these impairments with underlying processing deficits have been limited. Campbell/Butterworth (1985) speculated that the problems encountered by their subject, R.E., a developmental phonological dyslexic, stemmed from this individual's inability to carry out phonemic parsing because of her extremely limited short-term memory capacity. However, since R.E. was already an adult by the time that she was studied, much of their argument remains conjecture, as does that of Funnell/Davidson (1989), who have recently described a similar case.

Moreover, even within one so-called 'subtype', there is variation: Snowling/Stackhouse/Rack (1986) described seven developmental phonological dyslexics all of whom read nonwords significantly less well than expected, given their word recognition levels. Closer examination of the phonological skills of the individuals case by case suggested that the precise locus of their deficit affected the nature of the 'dyslexia' that they exhibited. Among dyslexics of lower reading age, this could be seen very clearly by an examination of their spelling errors. Perhaps most importantly, it might be deduced that phonological skills are a good predictor of future prognosis. In order to explore this possibility, longitudinal studies are needed for the purpose of mapping the cognitive profiles of individual dyslexic children and conducting ongoing follow-up of these children for an extended period of time to discern their eventual outcome in terms of reading and spelling processes.

To this end, one of the children originally studied by Snowling/Stackhouse/Rack (1986), J.M., has been followed for now some six years. When first assessed, J.M. had problems primarily with output phonology (segmentation, memory, and repetition difficulties), and these difficulties persist to date, although he is now 14 years old (Hulme/Snowling 1991). Interestingly, J.M. still cannot read nonwords effectively, and his spelling is markedly dysphonetic, despite several years of remediation that included phonics training (Snowling/Hulme 1989). One aspect of J.M.'s performance that may be of importance is that his visual skills are excellent. We have, therefore, speculated that he has learned to read by relying on his visual strengths.

Potentially, then, individual case studies provide powerful tools for exploring the relationships between cognitive deficits and reading failure. The case of J.M. provides excellent confirmation for the picture emerging from group studies: there is a highly specific association between phonological deficits in the processing of both spoken and printed words.

5. Higher-Level Language Difficulties in Dyslexic Children?

A possible objection to the argument we have put forward, both with respect to single case and group studies, is that we have focused solely upon the processing of single words in spoken language and in reading tasks. Our argument has been that most dyslexic children's primary deficit is with the phonological aspects of language. However, a number of recent studies have suggested difficulties with syntactic processing. Bowey (1986), for example, showed that there was a strong correlation between a measure of syntactic awareness and decoding skill, and that good readers performed at a higher level on tasks designed to tap the ability to judge grammatical wellformedness than poor readers. A problem with these studies, and others of similar ilk, is that it is possible that certain syntactic structures (for example, relative clauses) are only encountered with any degree of frequency in written language. It follows that poor readers will have had less exposure to such structures than good readers and so will have difficulty in dealing with them. In the absence of data from reading-age matched controls, it is not possible to judge the validity of these findings.

Similarly, there have been a number of reports concerning the language comprehension abilities of dyslexic readers (Byrne 1981; Stein/Cairns/Zurif 1984). Together, these studies have contributed to the formulation of the "structural lag hypothesis," which asserts that dyslexics are delayed in their acquisition of certain syntactic structures (Shankweiler/Crain 1986). However, recent work has suggested that, rather than lacking knowledge of certain syntactic structures that emerge late in language acquisition, poor readers are subject to processing limitations that cause comprehension failure in particular contexts. In this regard, Macaruso/Bar-Shalom/Crain/Shankweiler (1989) presented groups of good and poor seven-year-old readers with spoken sentences containing temporal terms; for example, *Before you push the car, push the horse* and *After you pick up the truck, pick up the horse*. The children were asked to move toys in line with the instructions in the test sentences.

One experiment explored their performance when processing load was varied. One manipulation of processing load was brought about by adding pronominal modifers to half of the test sentences; for example, *Push the second smallest horse before you push the car*. A second manipulation was of context, so that subjects were first asked to choose one of the toys and then this item was included in the subordinate clause, thereby making the context helpful. Poor readers were found to make more errors with the interpretation of the complex noun phrases than with the simple versions, and also to have fewer problems in the context conditions. Overall, the results went against the structural lag hypothesis and suggested, instead, that poor readers are subject to processing limitations. It can be argued that these processing limitations arise because of their phonological deficits and, more specifically, their memory coding problems.

Turning to written language processing, there is virtually no evidence that dyslexic children have difficulties with syntactic or comprehension processes which cannot be explained by the basic difficulty that they have with decoding skills (Perfetti/Goldman/Hogaboam 1979; Stanovich 1986). In fact, Stanovich (1980) argued that poor readers are likely to use context more during reading than good readers, to compensate for their slow decoding speed. In line with this position, Frith/Snowling (1983) found that dyslexic readers were as good as reading-age matched controls at selecting the missing words in a written text, using a modified cloze procedure. In short, we would argue that experiments exploring language processing beyond the single word level have failed to find deficits in dyslexia which cannot be explained in terms of relatively low-level phonological difficulties such as word-finding and short-term memory problems. These data underscore the specificity of the problem facing dyslexic readers, a problem that resides in the processing of speech-based material and one that has an impact on the development of phonological coding capacities for both written and spoken language.

6. Treatment Implications

Despite the enormous number of published studies on developmental dyslexia, there has been scarcely any research directed at the question of how best to treat these difficulties. A number of studies carried out in dyslexia clinics in U.K., using variants of multi-sensory teaching techniques have reported gains in reading performance but these studies have lacked appropriate experimental controls, limiting their validity (Andrews/Shaw 1986; Hornsby/Miles 1980). In Canada, Lovett/Ransby/Barron (1988) compared the effectiveness of three teaching regimes, one providing training in word recognition and decoding skills, one in both oral and written skills and one in 'classroom survival skills', an alternative treatment control. There was a post-training advantage for readers defined as accuracy disabled and rate disabled, for those who received the training in word recognition and decoding. Once again, however, it is difficult to evaluate the specific aspects of treatment which led to gains, given the realistic but, therefore, uncontrolled teaching regimes.

The predominant approach to teaching dyslexic children recognizes their difficulty with sounds. The most popular teaching schemes embody highly structured phonic teaching with explicit emphasis on learning to relate spelling patterns to sound (Hornsby 1985). There is, however, a dearth of empirical evidence to substantiate claims for the effectiveness of these approaches. Moreover, there is reason to suppose that these methods, which involve teaching children to decode words phoneme by phoneme, will place a burden on skills of phonemic awareness, short-term memory, and sound blending, all of which tend to be deficient in dyslexic children. It may be the case that some dyslexic children fail to respond to these programmes for reasons related to the extent and severity of their (phonological) impairment, and learn to read using an alternative whole-word approach. Certainly, J.M., whom we discussed earlier, has been taught by these methods, yet he has evidently learned to read slowly and without developing phonological reading strategies (Snowling/Hulme 1989).

A possible reason for the failure of phonic methods to help J.M. and some other dyslexics is that the traditional phonic approach to teaching these children is based on a very crude theoretical position: dyslexic children are deficient in phonic skills and they need to be taught them explicitly. In fact these techniques may simply place excessive demands upon many dyslexic children's ability to deal with speech sounds. The work described earlier concerned with phonological awareness and the distinction between the sub-syllabic units, onset and rime, is relevant here.

The predictive relationship between the ability to detect rhymes and learning to read most likely arises because children use their knowledge of the shared sound similarities between words to categorize the written versions of these words. Hence, knowing that TRAIN, BRAIN and MAIN rhyme may allow a child to read *brain* and *main* by analogy with *train* (Goswami 1988) and to spell them alike. This work leads naturally, therefore, to a tentative suggestion for a method for teaching dyslexic children to read and spell. Since we know that sensitivity to rhyme normally develops prior to sensitivity to phonemic units, teaching methods should capitalize on the relative ease of segmenting words into onset and rime units. Analysis of words into onset and rime units should increase sensitivity to mappings between groups of letters and sound segments (e. g. /ight/ is pronounced /ite/), and thereby facilitate the learning of spelling patterns to sound relationships. In essence, teaching through onset-rime divisions may represent a fruitful new approach because it will encourage the development of analytic reading strategies without overburdening the dyslexic's weak phonological skills.

There is some preliminary evidence from experimental studies to support this approach to teaching. Bradley/Bryant (1983) found that training children to categorize words according to their sounds (onsets and rimes) in combination with training in representing the sounds of words with letters led to significant improvements in these children's reading and spelling skills. More recently, Wise/Olson/Treiman (1990) have looked directly at teaching normal children to read words divided into onset and rime units, using a computer. The word to be learnt was presented on a monitor screen and groups of letters within the word could be separately highlighted. At the same time a text-to-speech system would produce the sound of the part of the word which was highlighted. Sometimes the division of the word coincided with the onset/rime division, sometimes it did not. They found that words taught by separating them into onset and rime were learned better than those that were not. However, this was far from a realistic teaching study. The children were only seen once, and we do not know whether such learning would be durable or show generalization. Nevertheless, this study provides an excellent starting point for more realistic teaching studies. It seems possible that methods based on the onset rime distinction may prove particularly useful for dyslexic children.

7. Conclusions and Future Directions

There can be little doubt, to our minds, that research in this field has made massive strides forward in recent years. The research reviewed here indicates with some precision the range of phonological deficits that affect many dyslexic children. Furthermore, there are good grounds for believing that these phonological deficits play a role in causing these children's reading difficulties. What then should research in the near future be trying to achieve?

There are three issues which, to us, stand out as being important and worthy of more scrutiny. The first is to continue to forge explicit links between underlying phonological deficits and problems in learning to read and to spell. There is by now no doubt that many dyslexic children experience difficulties with a wide variety of phonological skills such as phonological awareness and nonword repetition. A major issue is to relate these deficits more explicitly to the patterns of reading and spelling difficulties in these children.

The second issue follows directly from the first and concerns the problem of individual differences. The charge that experimental psychologists too often ignore individual differences amongst their subjects is far from novel. In the field of dyslexia it is potentially very important, however. It is a truism that dyslexic children, like normal children, differ. We badly need more precise information about these differences and the origin (in terms of underlying cognitive processes) of different patterns of reading and spelling problems. Such knowledge is of great theoretical interest in terms of understanding the cognitive processes involved in learned to read. In practical terms such knowledge undoubtedly will have an important bearing upon the development of teaching techniques.

This brings us to our final issue which concerns remediation. We have spent relatively little time in this chapter talking about remediation. This, we would argue, is an unfortunate reflection upon our current state of knowledge. The balance of research in this area has been very much to focus on the difficulties that characterize dyslexic children rather than how these difficulties can be treated. To some extent this is defensible, before trying to tackle a problem it is undoubtedly useful to have an accurate description of its nature. Having read this far, we hope people will agree with our view that we now know a considerable amount about the nature of dyslexia; the time is now ripe to turn to studies which directly confront treatment. We have made some fairly specific suggestions about the implications of current knowledge about the cognitive deficits in dyslexic children for teaching. It is to be hoped that in the near future these important practical issues are given more attention in research studies. Studies of treatment and its effectiveness in the long term are very powerful ways of assessing the adequacy of our current theories about the underlying causes of dyslexia.

Authors' note: This chapter was written while the first author was in receipt of MRC Grant No. G 8801538 N and while the second author was in receipt of a Nuffield Foundation Social Science Research Fellowship.

8. References

Aaron, P. G. (1989). Qualitative and quantitative differences among dyslexic, normal and non dyslexic poor readers. *Reading & Writing*, *1*, 291–309.

Andrews, N. & Shaw, J. (1986). The efficacy of teaching dyslexics. *Child: care health and development*, *12*, 53–62.

Bowey, J. A. (1986). Syntactic awareness in relation to reading skill and ongoing reading comprehension. *Journal of Experimental Child Psychology 41*, 282–299.

Bradley, L. & Bryant, P. E. (1978). Difficulties in auditory organisation as a possible cause of reading backwardness. *Nature*, *271*, 746–747.

Bradley, L. & Bryant, P. E. (1983). Categorising sounds and learning to read: a causal connexion. *Nature*, *301*, 419–421.

Brandt, J. & Rosen, J. (1980). Auditory-phonemic perception in dyslexia: categorised identification and discrimination of stop consonants. *Brain & Language*, *9*, 324–327.

Byrne, B. (1981). Deficient syntactic control in poor readers: is a weak phonetic memory code responsible? *Applied Psycholinguistics*, *2*, 201–212.

Campbell, R. & Butterworth, B. (1985). Phonological dyslexia and dysgraphia in a highly literate subject; a developmental case with associated deficits of phonemic awareness and processing. *Quarterly Journal of Experimental Psychology*, *37 A*, 435–475.

Coltheart, M., Masterson, J., Byng, S., Prior, M., & Riddoch, J. (1983). Surface dyslexia. *Quarterly Journal of Experimental Psychology*, *35 A*, 469–496.

Frith, U. & Snowling, M. (1983). Reading for meaning and reading for sound in autistic and dyslexic children. *British Journal of Development Psychology*, *1*, 329–342.

Funnell, E. & Davidson, M. (1989). Lexical capture: a developmental disorder of reading and spelling. *Quarterly Journal of Experimental Psychology, 41 A*, 471–487.

Godfrey, J., Syrdal-Lasky, A., Millay, K., & Knox, C. (1981). Performance of dyslexic children on a speech perception test. *Journal of Experimental Child Psychology, 32*, 401–424.

Goswami, U. (1988). Orthographic analogies and reading development. *Quarterly Journal of Experimental Psychology, 40 A*, 329–268.

Goswami, U. & Bryant, P. (1990). *Phonological skills and learning to read.* London: Erlbaum.

Hornsby, B. (1985). A structured phonetic-linguistic method for teaching dyslexics. In M. Snowling, M. (Ed.), Children's written language difficulties. *119–133.* Windsor: NFER-Nelson.

Hornsby, B. & Miles, T. (1980). The effects of a dyslexia centered teaching programme. *British Journal of Educational Psychology, 50*, 236–242.

Hulme, C. & Snowling, M. (1991). Deficits in output phonology cause developmental phonological dyslexia. *Mind and Language, 6,* 130–134.

Lovett, M., Ransby, M., & Barron, R. (1988). Treatment, subtype and word type in dyslexic children's response to remediation. *Brain & Language, 34*, 328–349.

Lundberg, I., Olofsson, A., & Wall, S. (1981). Reading and spelling skills in the first school years predicted from phonemic awareness skills in kindergarten. *Scandinavian Journal of Psychology, 21*, 159–173.

Macaruso, P., Bar-Shalom, E., Crain, S., & Shankweiler, D. (1989). Comprehension of temporal terms by good and poor readers. *Language and Speech, 32*, 45–67.

Perfetti, C., Goldman, S., & Hogaboam, T. (1979). Reading skill and the identification of words in discourse context. *Memory and Cognition, 7*, 273–282.

Reed, M. (1989). Speech perception and the discrimination of brief auditory cues in reading disabled children. *Journal of Experimental Child Psychology, 48*, 270–292.

Seymour, P. H. K. (1986). *Cognitive analysis of Dyslexia.* London: Routledge and Kegan Paul.

Seymour, P. H. K. & MacGregor, C. (1984). Developmental dyslexia: a cognitive experimental analysis of phonological, morphemic and visual impairments. *Cognitive Neuropsychology, 1*, 43–82.

Shankweiler, D. & Crain, S. (1986). Language mechanisms and reading disorder: a modular approach. *Cognition, 24*, 139–164.

Snowling, M. (1981). Phonemic deficits in developmental dyslexia. *Psychological Research, 43*, 219–234.

Snowling, M. & Hulme, C. (1989). A longitudinal case study of developmental phonological dyslexia. *Cognitive Neuropsychology, 6*, 379–401.

Snowling, M., Goulandris, N., Bowlby, M., & Howell, P. (1986). Segmentation and speech perception in relation to reading skill. *Journal of Experimental Child Psychology, 41*, 489–507.

Snowling, M. J. & Rack, J. P. (1991). Dyslexia: deficits in grapheme-phoneme correspondence? In J. Stein (Ed.), *Vision and Visual Dyslexia. 189–195.* London: MacMillan.

Snowling, M. J., Stackhouse, J., & Rack, J. P. (1986). Phonological dyslexia and dysgraphia: a developmental analysis. *Cognitive Neuropsychology, 3*, 309–339.

Stanovich, K. E. (1980). Toward an interactive-compensatory model of individual differences in the development of reading fluency. *Reading Research Quarterly, 16*, 32–71.

Stanovich, K. E. (1986). Cognitive processes and the reading problems of learning-disabled children: Evaluating the assumption of specificity. In J. Torgeson & B. Wong (Eds.), *Psychological and educational perspectives on learning disabilities. 58–84.* New York: Academic Press.

Stanovich, K. E., Cunningham, A. E., & Cramer, B. B. (1984). Assessing phonological skills in kindergarten children: Issues of task comparability. *Journal of Experimental Child Psychology, 38*, 175–190.

Stein, C., Cairns, H., & Zurif, E. (1984). Sentence comprehension limitations related to syntactic deficits in reading-disabled children. *Applied Psycholinguistics, 5*, 305–322.

Szeszulski, P. & Manis, F. (1987). A comparison of word recognition processes in dyslexic and normal readers at two different reading age levels. *Journal of Experimental Child Psychology, 44*, 364–376.

Temple, C. & Marshall, J. (1983). A case study of developmental phonological dyslexia. *British Journal of Psychology, 74*, 517–533.

Treiman, R. & Hirsh-Pasek, K. (1985). Are there qualitative differences in reading behavior between dyslexics and normal readers? *Memory and Cognition, 13*, 357–364.

Wagner, R. & Torgeson, J. (1987). The nature of phonological processing and its causal role in the acquisition of reading skill. *Psychological Bulletin, 101*, 192–212.

Wise, B., Olson, R., & Treiman, R. (1990). Subsyllabic units as aids in beginning readers word learning: Onset-rime versus post-vowel segmentation. *Journal of Experimental Child Psychology, 49*, 1–19.

Margaret Snowling, Newcastle upon Tyne (United Kingdom)/
Charles Hulme, York (United Kingdom)

71. Developmental Dyslexia and Cognitive Processes

1. Methodological Issues: Trying to Establish Causes

In the present chapter we will consider some of the many studies concerned with cognitive deficits in dyslexic children. One important aim will be to evaluate the likelihood that the deficits described are causes of these children's reading difficulties.

It may be comparatively straightforward to measure the extent of dyslexic children's reading problems and describe some associated difficulties. It is much more difficult, however, to try to show the underlying causes of their reading problems.

Most of the evidence we have about dyslexia comes from studies which compare dyslexic with normal readers of the same age. Studies of this sort reveal a number of differences between normal and dyslexic children in, for example, language and memory tasks. These studies provide important clues as to the possible causes of the reading problem, but they are in themselves logically incapable of demonstrating causes. Effectively, what they show is a correlation between performance on a given task and reading ability.

Logically there are three possible explanations for correlations of this sort. It may be, as commonly suggested, that a task that is performed badly by dyslexic children taps a cause of their reading difficulty. Alternatively, the causal connection could be of the opposite form; their poor performance on a task could be a consequence of not having learned to read. A third possibility is that some deficits may be irrelevant to the reading difficulty. If dyslexic children show neurological immaturity, it seems likely that their performance on many psychological tasks will deviate from that of normal children; but many of these deviations may be quite irrelevant to the cause of their reading problems.

There are three ways of reducing the ambiguities of such correlational findings. First, one may add a further control group matched for reading achievement and IQ but whose reading is appropriate for their age, i.e. a younger control group (e.g. Bradley/Bryant 1978). If the dyslexic children are inferior on a given measure in comparison to such a group, this difference cannot be attributed to their lack of reading experience or ability. The probability of it being related to the cause of the reading problem is therefore increased.

The logic behind this type of comparison is in fact exactly the same as in longitudinal studies. In these studies measurements of certain abilities are made in children before they have started to learn to read. Their progress in reading is then followed and related to these early measurements. If these measures are predictive of later reading failure at least one can be sure that this does not depend upon the effects of such failure.

The results of longitudinal studies, or those in which subjects are matched for reading age, still have a major problem of interpretation because any deficits found which relate to dyslexia may be irrelevant to its cause. Interpretations here will be guided by the logical relationship between the task and the process of learning to read. A causal interpretation in such a case can be strengthened by forging explicit links between the observed deficit and the dyslexics' difficulties. For example, if it could be shown that some dyslexic children have poor visual memories, the causal status of this finding might be supported by showing that their spelling errors tended to be visually dissimilar to the correct form of the word, but similar phonetically (c.f. Boder 1973).

The third and most direct (and also the most difficult) way out of this correlational problem is to perform training studies aimed at correcting the inferred deficit and observe the effects of this on reading. Although difficult to conduct, studies of this type probably provide the most direct route for demonstrating the causes of dyslexia. A problem for studies of this type, however, is that some deficits that we find in dyslexic children, which seem likely candidates as causes of their reading problem, may not be amenable to improvement by training.

It will be clear from all this, that the problems facing us in trying to establish the causes of dyslexia are formidable. Once we accept the idea that different causes may operate in different cases (see below) and that there may be multiple causes that interact in complex ways, the task becomes even more daunting. We will try, nevertheless, in what follows to assess the likelihood that various findings do tap a cause of the reading problem.

2. Visual Problems

If dyslexic children had some generalized weakness in perceiving and remembering visual patterns, such as words, this would provide a good explanation for difficulties in learning to read. There has been a large amount of research addressed to testing this idea. Most of this research provides a clear answer: for most dyslexic children problems of visual perception and memory are not the cause of their problems. Much of this research has been reviewed in detail before (see, for example, Hulme 1981, 33; Jorm 1983); it will be sufficient here to summarize some of the more prominent findings of the older studies in this area.

Vellutino and his colleagues have demonstrated normal visual memory abilities in dyslexic children in several studies. Vellutino/Pruzek/Steger/Meshoulham (1973) showed Hebrew words to normal and dyslexic children and asked them to draw them from memory. Both groups did this equally well though children who were learning to read Hebrew, not surprisingly, did better than either group. This experiment looked at short-term memory. In a further study, long-term memory for Hebrew letters was assessed by recognition either immediately, or after 24 hour or six-month delays. Once again there were no differences between normal and dyslexic children (Vellutino/Steger/DeSetto/Phillips 1975). Dyslexic children have also been found to perform normally on visual paired-associate tasks (Goyen/Lyle 1971; Vellutino/Steger/Pruzek 1973). The tasks in these studies are demonstrably similar in their visual requirements to learning to read, and yet dyslexic children perform normally on them. Taken together therefore they argue persuasively against the idea that dyslexic children typically have visual problems that cause their reading problems. More recently there have been attempts to revive the idea of a visual deficit as a cause of dyslexia using different tasks. We will consider three such attempts in some detail now.

2.1. Eye Movements

Skilled reading involves the control of complex sequences of eye movements. Eye movements were one of the first aspects of reading to attract interest in the studies of experimental psychologists. It was soon noticed that people who read poorly showed abnormal eye movements (Tinker 1958). As Tinker pointed out, however, the peculiar eye movements of poor readers were a consequence and not a cause of their poor reading.

Recently this old idea about the cause of reading difficulties has resurfaced. Pavlidis (1981) reported that a group of dyslexic children showed erratic eye movements when asked to track a series of sequentially illuminated lights. He argued that these disordered eye movements might be a direct cause of the reading problem, or alternatively both the reading and eye movement problems might reflect some underlying 'general sequencing disability'.

It is now clear that this alleged problem with the control of eye movements is not a reliable correlate of dyslexia. Three separate studies have failed to replicate Pavlidis's findings. Brown/Haegerstrom/Portnoy/Adams et al. (1983) and Stanley/Smith/Howell (1983) found absolutely no difference in the eye movements of normal and dyslexic children when tracking sequences of lights. Most convincingly Olson/Kliegl/Davidson (1983) set out to conduct an exact replication of Pavlidis's study, and as in the other two attempted replications, found no difference between dyslexic and control children's eye movements. It seems an inescapable conclusion that, contrary to the original claims of Pavlidis, dyslexic children do not have difficulty with such tasks. There may be very rare cases of individuals with neurological damage who show grossly abnormal eye movements which interfere with their ability to read (e. g. Pirozzolo/Rayner 1978). There is no evidence, however, that a significant number of dyslexic children suffer from some basic deficit in the control of eye movements that prevents them from learning to read.

2.2. Eye Dominance

The old idea that dyslexia might relate to the lateralization of visual function was advanced by Dunlop/Dunlop/Fenelon (1973) using a test to determine the 'dominant' or 'reference' eye. In this test the child looks down two tubes so that each eye has a view of one of two similar slides. In both slides there is a picture of a house with a central front door and the subject is asked to fixate the centre of this door. In one slide there is a small tree to the left of the front door and in the other there is a larger tree to the door's right. To begin with the tubes converge and the subject has the impression of a fused image of a single house with a tree on either side of the door. When the tubes are made to diverge, before fusion breaks down, most subjects apparently get a strong impression that one of the trees moves towards the door. The eye whose image remains static is said to be the 'dominant' or 'reference' eye. The neurological basis of this effect is little understood.

Dunlop/Dunlop/Fenelon (1973) reported that crossed reference i. e. a reference eye on the opposite side to the preferred hand, was associated with dyslexia. They proposed a causal theory on the basis of these findings suggesting that the failure to develop an appropriate reference eye leads to perceptual problems which interfere with learning to read. Just why crossed reference should be so crucial in this respect is not clear.

This idea was pursued by Stein/Fowler (1982). They studied a large group of dyslexic children and a matched group of normal children who were classified as showing 'fixed' or 'unfixed' dominance. Contrary to Dunlop/Dunlop/Fenelon many of the dyslexic children showed unfixed dominance whilst crossed dominance was less common in the dyslexic children than the normals. Stein/Fowler (1985) then reported an intervention study designed, by occluding one eye, to produce fixed ocular dominance in dyslexic children. They claimed that occluding one eye had beneficial effects both on ocular dominance and reading progress, and concluded a causal factor (at least for some children) had been identified. Unfortunately there are a number of problems with this study which make such conclusions far from secure.

These problems include the fact that allocation to treatment and control groups was not random, and that the characteristics of the children in the different groups in terms of their ages, reading ages and IQs are not given. In a detailed critique of this study Bishop (1989) conducted a reanalysis of the data and found no evidence for the importance of ocular dominance as a cause of dyslexia.

One final problem concerning this research is the failure of other studies to confirm the association between ocular dominance and reading problems. Both Bishop/Jancey/Steel (1979) and Newman/Karle/Wadsworth et al. (1985) in large unselected groups of children did not find any evidence of an association between reading problems and the Dunlop test of ocular dominance.

2.3. Brief Visual Displays

Many studies show that dyslexic children have difficulty in dealing with rapid visual displays. An early example of this is in the work of Lyle/Goyen (1975). They looked at the recognition of abstract shapes presented in a tachistoscope to normal and dyslexic children. Dyslexic children were less accurate in recognizing the forms but only at very brief exposures. There was no difference between the groups at longer exposure durations, and both groups were similarly affected by making the discriminations required more difficult. More recently the idea of an association between deficits on tasks involving rapid visual displays and dyslexia has been pursued further by Lovegrove/Martin/Slaghuis (1986) who argued that a low-level visual deficit in a large proportion of dyslexic children may be a cause of their reading problems. They summarize a large body of carefully conducted studies of visual processing in dyslexic children and provide three major types of evidence concerning their visual abilities. (1) The function relating visible persistence to spatial frequency differs in dyslexic compared to control children. (2) On measures of pattern contrast sensitivity there are small but consistent differences between dyslexics and controls. Dyslexics are less sensitive than controls to low spatial frequency gratings but are equally, or more sensitive to high spatial frequencies. (3) With flickering gratings, dyslexics are less sensitive at all flicker rates but particularly so at high rates. These results are taken as evidence that retarded readers have a deficit in the visual transient subsystem (Kulikowski/Tolhurst 1973). In a fourth series of experiments, designed to measure the sustained subsystem, no differences between retarded readers and normal children were found. The idea of a deficit in the transient system of retarded readers appears to offer a useful link between a varied set of findings.

The idea that such a deficit is responsible for these children's reading difficulties seems highly implausible, however. Hulme (1988) argued that the visual requirements of the tasks used to assess the functioning of the transient system in these experiments are remote from the conditions experienced by children learning to read, and that the hypothesis predicts that dyslexic children should have most difficulty when reading prose rather than when reading isolated words. In fact the opposite pattern seems to characterize the majority of dyslexic children. Hulme argued that the deficit demonstrated in these experiments is most likely an irrelevant correlate of these children's reading difficulties, possibly related to their neurological immaturity.

2.4. Individual Differences Amongst Dyslexic Children and the Role of Visual Problems

It seems an inescapable conclusion that visual perceptual and memory problems are not a cause of the reading difficulties of most dyslexic children. A persistent idea, however, is that there may be a minority of dyslexic children whose reading difficulties do stem from visual difficulties (Hulme/Snowling 1988). Recently evidence for this view has come from a case study of a development dyslexic, J.A.S., studied when an adult by Goulandris/Snowling (1991). J.A.S. had good phonic decoding skills but in her reading she confused homophones (e. g. pair-pare; pair-pear) which require the use of visual information to discriminate their meaning when presented in isolation. Her spelling was highly error prone but extremely phonetic, suggesting a poor memory for the visual appearance of words. In line with this hypothesis J.A.S. had severe visual memory deficits, these deficits we believe are a plausible cause of her reading failure. We badly need more studies of cases such as J.A.S. whose reading and spelling difficulties seem related to visual deficits. The best evidence we have so far indicates that such cases are probably quite rare.

3. Verbal Memory Problems

This is one area that has been investigated a great deal in dyslexic children. Learning to read draws heavily upon verbal memory and it is clear that problems in this area are likely causes of reading problems.

3.1. Short-term memory

A common measure of short-term memory is digit span: the number of digits a child can repeat in correct serial order immediately after hearing them. As is usual in short-term memory tasks, here the person has to remember a small amount of information for a relatively short time and the order of recall is important. There is ample evidence that dyslexic children typically do poorly on digit-span tests and other measures of short-term memory (Jorm 1983, Siegel/Linder 1984). Moreover, the claim has often been made that their memory problems are attributable to difficulties with the use of phonological codes (Shankweiler/Liberman/Mark et al. 1979). This claim was based on findings that they did not exhibit the classic phonemic confusability effect in short-term memory (memory for lists of rhyming items being shorter than memory for lists of nonrhyming items.).

The validity of this claim was first questioned by Hall/Wilson/Humphreys et al. (1983) who showed that, provided the level of task difficulty was equated for good and poor readers, they were equally susceptible to phonemic confusability effects in memory. A series of studies by Johnston and colleagues provide corroborative evidence (Holligan/Johnston 1988; Johnston 1982, Johnston/Rugg/Scott 1987). For example, Johnston/Rugg/Scott (1987) compared groups of poor readers (of average or below average intelligence) with age-matched and Reading Age-matched controls on memory span tests, having first adjusted task-difficulty for each child by pre-testing performance on memory for lists of dissimilar items. Performance of the four groups at two age levels (eight and eleven years) was then assessed when recalling strings of phonemically similar letters (e. g. b, c, d, g, p). All groups here showed a phonemic similarity effect. It can be concluded that dyslexic children are, on average, subject to impairments of verbal short-term memory though it does not seem to be the case that they use different coding processes. Thus, dyslexic and normal readers show evidence of speech-based coding of information, as assessed by the occurrence of the phonemic similarity effect (see Hulme/Tordoff 1989, for discussion of the mechanisms responsible for this effect and its development).

An important question is how short-term memory problems in dyslexics might hinder learning to read. Short-term memory is often held to serve as a working memory system when reading (Baddeley/Hitch 1974), the idea being that this system is used to keep track of the order of words in phrases and sentences (e. g. Kleiman 1975). Impairments of short-term memory might, therefore, be expected to lead to problems in the comprehension of prose, particularly when word order is crucial to the meaning. However, there is no evidence that dyslexic children have any particular difficulties with reading prose, over and above those attributable to their difficulties in identifying words.

It is less obvious how short-term memory problems could create difficulties in learning to identify individual words which is where, we would argue, the dyslexic's problems lie (cf. Aaron 1989). One possibility, however, is that these problems lead to difficulties with phonic blending. When decoding a word that is not known the child must produce a set of possible pronunciations for the letters in the word. These separate sounds must then be blended to produce a possible pronunciation for the word as a whole. Beginning readers can often be heard to go through this process overtly. Torgeson/Wagner/Balthazar et al. (1989) showed that beginning readers find blending tasks easier if the individual sound segments are presented at a fast rate, thereby reducing memory load. Thus, it is indeed possible that short-term memory problems could make the blending procedure difficult for dyslexic children.

Torgeson/Rashotte/Greenstein et al. (1988) tested this possibility. They compared a group of dyslexic children selected for low digit-span scores with normal readers, and a group of dyslexic children with normal digit spans, on a sound blending test from the Illinois Test of Psycholinguistic Abilities. In this test a series of words and nonwords is spoken to the child, one at a time, in segmented form (e. g. *b-a-g*) and the child is asked to say the word (bag). The dyslexic children with low spans were very much worse on this task than the normal readers, or the dyslexic children with normal spans, who did not differ. It seems likely that some dyslexic children's short-term memory problems contribute to the difficulties they have with phonics.

An alternative explanation for the short-term memory problems of dyslexic children is that they are a consequence, and not a cause, of their reading problems. Perhaps learning to read brings improvements in short-term memory. One approach to this is to compare dyslexic children with normals of the same reading age. When this is done the groups do not differ on short-term memory tasks but it is always possible that this is because of the age-advantage which then accrues to the dyslexics.

A better approach is to conduct longitudinal studies, where memory is assessed before children start to learn to read. The evidence from this sort of study on the whole suggests that memory difficulties precede reading difficulties. Jorm/Share/MacLean/Mathews (1984) gave a large group of 5-year-olds a sentence memory task on entry to school. They tested all the children again on the memory test when they were almost 7, and also gave them an IQ and a reading test. Memory scores at first testing correlated with later reading scores when the effects of age and IQ were partialled out. This indicates that good memory scores before learning to read are predictive of later success in reading and is consistent with the possibility of a causal influence of memory ability on reading ability. It is worth noting that the memory test used here, involving sentences, differs from conventional short-term memory tasks which involve meaningless strings of items. However, Mann/Liberman (1984) assessed memory for unrelated strings of words in kindergarten children before they started reading and found that this did correlate with reading scores one year later.

In conclusion, it seems quite possible that the short-term memory problems commonly found in dyslexic children do contribute to their difficulties in learning to read. The most obvious way in which this might come about is because of difficulties with phonic blending. In addition short-term memory problems may lead to difficulties in holding partially decoded words in mind whilst they are compared with the pronunciations of words retrieved from long-term memory. The idea that short-term memory problems are causally related to reading problems is far from firmly established however. It is clear that there is an association between short-term memory problems and reading problems. The slight inconsistencies in the evidence on this probably reflect the fact, very nicely demonstrated by Torgeson/Rashotte/Greenstein et al. (1988), that these problems are not characteristic of all dyslexic children. The time would now seem ripe for studies designed to show that this association reflects a causal link between memory problems and reading problems. The natural way to do this would be to conduct training studies which attempt to improve the short-term memory abilities of dyslexic children. If such training was effective and led to improvements in reading this would be good evidence for a causal connection.

3.2. Long-term Memory

Even if short-term memory problems were of no consequence as causes of reading difficulties, it might still be the case that problems with more durable forms of memory were important. Rather surprisingly, studies of long-term memory in dyslexic children are less common than those of short-term memory.

One long-term memory task that has been studied a good deal is paired-associate learning. Here the child has to make an arbitrary association between a stimulus and a response. The most relevant task to learning to read is visual-verbal paired-associate learning. Here the child has to learn a name to go with some visual stimulus (often an abstract shape). The evidence from paired-associate tasks is very clear: when these tasks involve a verbal component, dyslexic children almost invariably perform more poorly than normal children of the same age (Hulme 1981, 42).

It is plausible that difficulties of this sort could lead to problems in learning to read. In the early stages of learning to read, children may develop a considerable sight vocabulary by simply learning arbitrary associations between certain patterns of letters and their spoken counterparts. A child who has difficulty with paired-associate learning will have difficulty at this most elementary stage in learning to read. The other major way of learning to read is by phonics. Here the child learns rules relating the letters used to spell words to their constituent sounds. A necessary step for this to happen is that the child learns the sounds of the letters. This again is an example of paired-associate learning and many dyslexic children have profound difficulty in mastering the names and sounds of letters.

Another way of exploring the long-term memory system of normal and dyslexic readers is by the use of recognition memory or cued recall tasks. Here the evidence is relatively consistent in pointing to the tendency for normal readers to make use of phonological memory codes, and for this tendency to be reduced in dyslexics (Byrne/Shea 1979; Mark/Shankweiler/Liberman/Fowler 1977). However, Olson/Davidson/Kliegl/Davies (1984) found this phonetic confusability effect decreased with age for normal readers but increased for dyslexics. This shows the dyslexics were delayed in the acquisition of these codes but they were by no means completely deficient. These findings, together with analyses of error data in this experiment are compatible with the hypothesis that the absence of phonological coding strategies at a specific developmental stage, might induce the use of compensatory (visual) memory strategies.

In line with this 'compensation' hypothesis, Rack (1985) found differences between 12- to 13-year old dyslexics and younger Reading Age-matched controls, suggesting that dyslexics used orthographic codes in cued recall whereas normal readers used phonological codes. In the first part of this experiment, subjects carried out a rhyme judgement task on pairs of words and, in the second part, they were shown one item from each pair and they had to recall the item which had appeared with it previously. Dyslexic and normal readers performed as well as each other in the rhyme judgements and their overall levels of recall were the same (note that the normal children were younger). However, while normal readers recalled a greater number of the rhyming stimuli, regardless of orthographic similarity, the dyslexics recalled more of the orthographically similar items, irrespective of rhyming similarity. These results suggested that the dyslexics were relying less upon the use of phonological memory codes than their younger Reading Age-matched controls. A similar result was reported by Holligan/Johnston (1988) comparing eight-year-old poor readers with age- and Reading Age-matched controls. In a recognition memory task, following written rhyme judgements, the poor readers tended to choose orthographically similar pairs whereas the normal controls chose phonologically similar pairs.

Thus, it is quite plausible that dyslexic readers have difficulty with the use of phonological codes in long-term memory. These difficulties could create significant problems during reading which requires the ongoing retrieval of phonological information in response to the visual input of printed words.

3.2.1. Naming Deficits

Another task that requires the retrieval of phonological information from long-term memory is naming. Word finding difficulties are often reported in dyslexic children and experimental studies using rapid automatized naming tasks (RAN) usually report deficiencies in dyslexics. The classic study of this was by Denckla/Rudel (1976) who gave normal children and dyslexic children random lists of objects, colours, letters and numbers to name as fast as possible. The dyslexic children were very much slower here and, although appropriate analysis is not reported, it looks as though the older dyslexic children were actually slower than younger normal children of the same reading age. The dyslexic children's difficulty here is probably not simply a consequence of their poor reading skill.

Extending these findings, Katz (1986) used the Boston Naming Test, to compare the performance of dyslexic eight-year-old readers with average and good readers of the same age. The Boston test requires the naming of pictured objects presented without contextual cues. The dyslexic children were less able to label the objects and had particular difficulty with low-frequency names and polysyllabic words. In fact, naming performance correlated with reading skill even when the children's receptive understanding of the names was controlled. In an extension of this study, Rubin/Zimerman/Katz (1989) found that poor readers did not differ from good readers in their ability to select the initial phonemes or rhymes of object names they had not produced spontaneously and they were equally able to use initial phoneme prompts to retrieve the names. Overall these findings from studies of naming deficits are consistent with the view that dyslexic children experience relatively specific problems in retrieving phonological information from long-term memory.

One difficulty with these studies is that they did not include a Reading Age comparison group. In the absence of this control group, the possibility that the naming problems are a consequence of the reading difficulty cannot be ruled out. To address this question, Snowling/van Wagtendonk/Stafford (1988) asked dyslexic children to name objects either following picture presentation or following a spoken definition, and they compared their performance with that of children of the same age as well as with children of a similar level of reading ability. All subjects found it more difficult to name the items following spoken definition but the group differences in performance were similar on both tasks. Essentially, dyslexics made more naming errors than children of the same age and a similar number to children of the same reading level.

To confirm this finding, a second experiment carefully matched dyslexic children with normal readers of the same age and who scored at the same level on the British Abilities Scales test of Word Definitions, a vocabulary test. The two groups were then presented with a receptive vocabulary test in which one of four pictures had to be selected to match a spoken word, and subsequently with a naming task. The results were clear cut; dyslexics did as well as controls on the receptive vocabulary test but made more errors on the naming task.

In summary, dyslexic children have naming difficulties which are unexpected given their age and I.Q., and are out of line with their receptive vocabulary. This suggests that they have difficulty in retrieving the phonological representations of words that they know. However, since they do not seem to be any worse at this than younger children of the same reading age, this might be a consequence of their reading difficulty. Logically however, such a possibility does not seem particularly appealing. There seems no compelling theoretical reason to expect reading to produce such changes in retrieval from long-term memory. An alternative view is that these naming deficits are one manifestation of an underlying weakness in information processing systems dealing with phonological information which are causally related to these children's reading difficulties.

4. Conclusions and Future Directions

In the present chapter we have focussed on some of the prominent cognitive deficits associated with developmental dyslexia. In discussing these deficits we have paid particular attention to the difficulties inherent in trying to demonstrate the causes of these children's difficulties in learning to read.

The evidence concerning visual perceptual and visual memory difficulties shows that these are not areas of difficulty for most dyslexic children. Some of the best documented difficulties of this type, such as those in tasks that tap the functioning of the visual transient sub-system, seem highly implausible as causes of the reading problems in dyslexia. Nevertheless, we argued that it is important not to lose sight of the fact that different children may experience difficulties in learning to read for different reasons. It appears that there may be a minority of children whose reading difficulties stem from an underlying deficit in visual processing. We understand relatively little about the nature of the visual deficits in these cases however and we badly need further studies of this issue.

In contrast to the picture that emerges from studies of visual perceptual tasks, evidence from memory tasks indicates that dyslexic children commonly experience difficulties with verbal, but not with visual, memory tasks. These difficulties occur with both short- and long-term verbal memory tasks and may plausibly be related to their reading difficulties; though definite evidence for such a causal relationship is lacking. These deficits on verbal memory tasks, may relate to the difficulties with other language tasks, particularly those involving phonological information, that we discussed in the last chapter (cf. art. 70). An important task for future studies is to clarify the relationship between these different verbal difficulties in dyslexic children and relate them more explicitly to the patterns of reading and spelling difficulties they experience. Such studies ideally might lead to suitable training studies to evaluate the feasibility of ameliorating these deficits. If such studies were successful they would provide powerful evidence bearing on the causes of these children's difficulties, and also have the important practical benefit of leading directly to better forms of treatment.

Authors' Note: This chapter was written while the first author was in receipt of a Nuffield Foundation Social Science Research Fellowship and while the second author was in receipt of MRC Grant No. G 8801538 N.

5. References

Aaron, P. G. (1989). Qualitative and quantitative differences among dyslexic, normal and non dyslexic poor readers. *Reading & Writing*, *1*, 291–309.

Baddeley, A. D. & Hitch, G. (1974). Working memory. In G. H. Bower (Ed.), *The psychology of learning and motivation (Vol. 8). 47–90.* New York: Academic Press.

Bishop, D. (1989). Unfixed reference, monocular oclusion, and developmental dyslexia – a critique. *British Journal of Opthalmology*, *73*, 209–215.

Bishop, D. V. M., Jancey, C., & Steel, A. McP. (1979). Orthoptic status and reading disability. *Cortex*, *15*, 659–666.

Boder, E. M. (1973). Developmental dyslexia: a diagnostic approach based on three atypical reading-spelling patterns. *Developmental Medicine and Child Neurology*, *15*, 663–687.

Bradley, L. & Bryant, P. E. (1978). Difficulties in auditory organisation as a possible cause of reading backwardness. *Nature*, *271*, 746–747.

Brown, B., Haegerstrom-Portnoy, G., Adams, A. J., Yingling, C., Galin, D., Herron, J., & Marcus, M. (1983). Predictive eye movements do not discriminate between dyslexic and control children. *Neuropsychology*, *21*, 121–128.

Byrne, B. & Shea, P. (1979). Semantic and phonetic memory codes in beginning readers. *Memory and Cognition*, *7*, 333–338.

Denkla, M. B. & Rudel, R. G. (1976). Rapid automatised naming: Dyslexia differentiated from other learning disabilities. *Neuropsychologia*, *14*, 471–479.

Dunlop, D. B., Dunlop, P., & Fenelon, B. (1973). Vision-laterality analysis in children with reading disability: The results of new techniques of examination. *Cortex*, *9*, 227–236.

Goulandris, N. & Snowling, M. (1991). Visual memory deficits: a possible cause of developmental dyslexia? *Cognitive Neuropsychology*, *8*, 127–154.

Goyen, J. D. & Lyle, J. G. (1971). Effect of incentives on retarded and normal readers on a visual associate learning task. *Journal of Experimental Child Psychology*, *11*, 274–280.

Hall, J., Wilson, K., Humphreys, M., Tinzman, M., & Bowyer, P. (1983). Phonemic similarity effects in good vs. poor readers. *Memory and Cognition*, *11*, 520–527.

Holligan, C. & Johnston, R. S. (1988). The use of phonological information by good and poor readers in memory and reading tasks. *Memory and Cognition*, *16*, 522–542.

Hulme, C. (1981). *Reading retardation and multisensory teaching*. London: Routledge & Kegan Paul.

Hulme, C. (1988). The implausibility of low-level visual deficits as a cause of children's reading difficulties. *Cognitive Neuropsychology*, *5*, 369–374.

Hulme, C. & Snowling, M. (1988). The classification of children's reading difficulties. *Developmental Medicine and Child Neurology*, *37*, 167–169.

Hulme, C. & Tordoff, V. (1989). Working memory development: The effects of speech rate, word length and acoustic similarity on serial recall. *Journal of Experimental Child Psychology*, *48*, 1–19.

Johnston, R. S. (1982). Phonological coding in dyslexic readers. *British Journal of Psychology*, *73*, 455–460.

Johnston, R. S., Rugg, M., & Scott, S. (1987). Phonological similarity effects, memory span and developmental reading disorders: The nature of the relationship. *British Journal of Psychology*, *78*, 205–211.

Jorm, A. F. (1983). Specific reading retardation and working memory: A review. *British Journal of Psychology*, *74*, 311–342.

Jorm, A. F., Share, D. L., MacLean, R., & Mathews, R. (1984). Phonological confusability in short-term memory for sentences as a predictor of reading ability. *British Journal of Psychology*, *75*, 393–400.

Katz, R. (1986). Phonological deficiencies in children with reading disability: Evidence from an object naming task. *Cognition*, *22*, 225–257.

Kleiman, G. M. (1975). Speech recoding in reading. *Journal of Verbal Learning and Verbal Behaviour, 14*, 323–339.

Kulikowski, J. J. & Tolhurst, D. J. (1973). Psychophysical evidence for sustained and transient detectors in human vision. *Journal of Psychology, 232*, 149–162.

Lovegrove, W., Martin, F., & Slaghuis, W. (1986). A theoretical and experimental case for a visual deficit in specific reading disability. *Cognitive Neuropsychology, 2*, 225–267.

Lyle, J. G. & Goyen, J. G. (1975). Effect of speed of exposure and difficulty of discrimination on visual recognition of retarded readers. *Journal of Abnormal Psychology, 84*, 673–676.

Mann, V. & Liberman, I. Y. (1984). Phonological awareness and verbal short-term memory: Can they presage early reading success? *Journal of Learning Disabilities, 17*, 592–599.

Mark, L. S., Shankweiler, D., Liberman, I., & Fowler, C. (1977). Phonetic recoding in the beginning reader. *Memory and Cognition, 5*, 623–629.

Newman, S. P., Karle, H., Wadsworth, J. F., Archer, R., Hockly, R., & Rogers, P. (1985). Ocular dominance, reading and spelling: a reassessment of a measure associated with specific reading difficulties. *Journal of Research in Reading, 8*, 127–138.

Olson, R. K., Kliegl, R., & Davidson, B. J. (1983). Dyslexic and normal readers' eye movements. *Journal of Experimental Psychology: Human Perception and Performance, 9*, 816–825.

Olson, R. K., Davidson, B. J., Kliegl, R., & Davies, S. E. (1984). Development of phonetic memory in normal and disabled readers. *Journal of Experimental Child Psychology, 37*, 187–206.

Pavlidis, G. Th. (1981). Do eye movements hold the key to dyslexia? *Neuropsychologia, 19*, 57–64.

Pirozzolo, F. J. & Rayner, K. (1978). The neural control of eye movements in acquired and developmental reading disorders. In H. Avakian-Whitaker & H. A. Whitaker (Eds.), *Advances in neurolinguistics and psycholinguistics*. New York: Academic Press.

Rack, J. (1985). Orthographic and phonetic coding in normal and dyslexic readers. *British Journal of Psychology, 76*, 325–340.

Rubin, H., Zimerman, S., & Katz, R. (1989). Phonological knowledge and naming ability in children with reading disability. *Reading & Writing, 1*, 393–404.

Shankweiler, D., Liberman, I., Mark, L., Fowler, C., & Fischer, F. (1979). The speech code and learning to read. *Journal of Experimental Psychology: Human Learning and Memory, 5*, 531–545.

Siegel, L. & Linder, B. (1984). Short-term memory processes in children with reading and arithmetic disabilities. *Developmental Psychology, 20*, 200–207.

Snowling, M., van Wagtendonk, B., & Stafford, C. (1988). Object naming deficits in developmental dyslexia. *Journal of Research in Reading, 11*, 67–85.

Stanley, G., Smith, G. A. & Howell, E. A. (1983). Eye movements and sequential tracking in dyslexic and control children. *British Journal of Psychology, 74*, 181–187.

Stein, J. F. & Fowler, S. (1982). Diagnosis of dyslexia by means of a new indicator of eye dominance. *British Journal of Ophthalmology, 66*, 332–336.

Stein, J. F. & Fowler, S. (1985). Effect of monocular occlusion on visuo motor perception and reading in dyslexic children. *Lancet, July 13*, 69–73.

Tinker, M. (1958). Recent studies of eye movements in reading. *Psychological Bulletin, 55*, 215–231.

Torgeson, J., Rashotte, C., Greenstein, J., Houck, G., & Portes, P. (1988). Academic difficulties of learning disabled children who perform poorly on memory span tasks. In H. L. Swanson (Ed.), *Memory and learning disabilities: Advances in learning and behavioral disabilities*. Greenwich, Conn: JAI Press.

Torgeson, J. K., Wagner, R. K., Balthazar, M., Davis, C., Morgan, S., Simmons, K., Stage, S., & Zirps, F. (1989). Developmental and individual differences in performance on phonological synthesis tasks. *Journal of Experimental Child Psychology, 47*, 491–505.

Vellutino, F. R., Pruzek, R. M., Steger, J. A., & Meshoulham, U. (1973). Immediate visual recall in poor and normal readers as a function of orthographic-linguistic familiarity. *Cortex, 9*, 368–384.

Vellutino, F. R., Steger, J. A., DeSetto, L., & Phillips, F. (1975). Immediate and delayed recognition of visual stimuli in poor and normal readers. *Journal of Experimental Child Psychology, 19*, 223–232.

Vellutino, F. R., Steger, J. A., & Pruzek, J. M. (1973). Inter- versus intra-sensory deficit in paired-associate learning in poor and normal readers. *Canadian Journal of Behavioral Science, 5*, 111–123.

Charles Hulme, York (United Kingdom)/ Margaret Snowling, Newcastle upon Tyne (United Kingdom)

72. Single and Multiple Component Developmental Dyslexias

1. History and Background

It is nearly a century since the term "congenital word-blindness" was introduced (Morgan, 1896) to refer to cases of reading disability which occur developmentally as a selective impairment and without recognisable etiology. The name was taken from the term "word-blindness" which had been coined in 1877 by Kussmaul to refer to acquired disorders of reading resulting from brain damage. Kussmaul noticed that "a complete text-blindness may exist, although the powers of sight, the intellect and the powers of speech are intact."

From the first suggestion of congenital word-blindness as a clinical entity, similarities were conjectured between it and acquired word-blindness which resulted from neurological injury or disease. In both conditions word without letter-blindness was discovered (Dejerine 1892; Kerr 1897) and Fisher (1910) speculated that a congenital aplasia of the angular gyrus, a structure known to be damaged in many cases of acquired word-blindness, might underly problems in learning to read. Hinshelwood (1917) was particularly concerned with the similarities between the two groups of disorders. He made the connection explicit and stated the following:

"The complex processes involved in vision proceed smoothly and harmoniously during health in the region of the unconscious cerebration, but when disease disturbs the delicate mechanism of the brain, there are revealed to us glimpses of its intimate working, a knowledge of which we would not acquire otherwise. It is for this reason that we have studied at such length the symptoms of acquired word-blindness, the knowledge of which will enable us to interpret and explain the phenomena of the congenital form. An adequate knowledge of former condition is an essential preliminary to the proper understanding of the latter. It is the absence of this necessary and fundamental knowledge which has given rise to much of the ambiguity and vagueness which characterise many recent accounts of this condition." Despite Hinshelwood's recommendations, most subsequent researchers were not concerned with such comparisons between congenital and acquired word-blindness. Systematic investigations of the *developmental reading disorders* in the light of acquired disorders of reading did not re-surface until the 1970's.

During the 20 th Century many different terms have been applied to refer to the condition which Morgan (1896) and Hinshelwood (1900; 1917) called "Congenital Word-Blindness". Among these were Strephosymbolia (Orton 1928), Specific Dyslexia (Hallgren 1950), Constitutional Dyslexia (Skysgaard 1942), Developmental Alexia (Orton 1937), Analfabetia Partialis and Congenital Dyslexia (Hinshelwood 1917). Currently, the term *developmental dyslexia* is widespread in use among neuropsychologists and neurologists, though educational psychologists, teachers and others often prefer the term Specific Reading Retardation or Specific Reading Disability. The term Developmental Dyslexia will be employed here and is used to refer to children in whom there is a significant discrepancy between the reading level which would be expected on the basis of their general intelligence and other skills and the reading level which they attained. These reading disorders exist despite the absence of any conspicious reason why education has not progressed normally. The term Developmental Dyslexia is not generally used to encompass those children who are learning disabled in a more general way and have difficulty in the acquisition of many different skills and abilities. However, there is no reason why the types of analysis which will be discussed below cannot also be applied to other children independent of their level of intellectual development.

Previous chapters in this volume have documented the cognitive neuropsychological analyses which have been prevalent throughout the 1980s and early 1990s. One of the justifications for the case study methodology employed in these investigations is the heterogeneity of patients. Investigations in which patient performance was averaged across the group would mask the individual performance profile of each subject. The objective is not to categorise neurological patients into boxes but to utilise a method of analysis of the patient's performance which is interpretable in relation to a single model of the cognitive process of interest. One objective is to gain a better understanding of the nature of the patient's difficulty with a view to subsequent remediation. Another objective is to use the dissociations in the patient's performance to expand the model of normal cognitive systems.

Up until the advent of cognitive neuropsychology, it was popular to investigate reading disorders in children using a group study methodology. However, such group studies assumed a degree of homogeneity which now appears unwarranted. There is a limitation to the amount of information which may be obtained with group studies if the group involved is not homogeneous with respect to the factor under investigation. Since the early 1960s a number of researchers have pointed out that developmental dyslexics do not all display similar patterns of disability. The multiple-syndrome nature of developmental dyslexia has increasingly been stressed.

Some of the early attempts to categorise the developmental dyslexias into subgroups describe symptom complexes or constellations of features which were believed to co-occur in particular dyslexic populations. Some of the features involved in these constellations did not relate to the reading process itself. However, with increasing investigation of these disorders it has been difficult to substantiate these different syndrome groups. While certain symptoms will sometimes occur together, in other children there is fractionation and they occur apart.

The cognitive neuropsychology methodology has therefore been applied to the developmental dyslexias in a similar way to its application to the acquired dyslexias. Detailed psycho-linguistic analyses have been carried out on individual cases of developmental dyslexia in order to see whether the patterns of reading performance may be interpreted in relation to a single model of reading development. The patterns of performance described have been compared with the patterns of performance which have emerged from comparable analysis with the acquired dyslexias. For certain syndromes directly analogous conditions have been described, but for others a pure developmental analogue has been more elusive.

In 1980 Shallice/Warrington divided the acquired dyslexias into those that they refer to as single-component dyslexias and those which they refer to as multiple-component dyslexias. The single-component dyslexias including phonological dyslexia could be interpreted in relation to a model of normal reading by postulating a single abnormality in the system. The syndrome of deep dyslexia was perceived as being more complex with the necessity of multiple impairments to the underlying system and was referred to as a multiple component dyslexia. The extent to which the developmental dyslexias may be considered as single or multiple-component developmental dyslexias will now be discussed.

2. Surface Dyslexia

The term *surface dyslexia* was introduced by Marshall/Newcombe (1973). They describe the case of a 45 year old man, J. C., who had sustained at the age of 20, a severe penetrating missile wound to the left temporo-parietal region. J. C. had only very mild residual aphasic symptoms but had a persistent reading disorder. He was particularly sensitive to the regularity of spelling of the words he was trying to read. Words with regular spelling to sound patterns were read more easily than those with irregular spelling to sound patterns. This means that *captain* is an easy word to read and *yacht* is a difficult word to read for a surface dyslexic. The pattern of errors was of a characteristic nature. Mis-readings suggested the application of a rule-based system for working out pronunciations. Marshall/Newcombe (1973) described these errors as "partial failures of grapheme-phoneme conversion". The phonetic value of some letters are affected by the letters which surround them. J. C. had difficulty using this context of a letter within a word to achieve its pronunciation. Thus, errors were made on ambiguous letters. Voiced consonants were sometimes produced in unvoiced form e. g. *disease* "deceased". Silent letters were assigned phonetic values e. g. *island* "izland". The "rule of e" was rarely applied e. g. *bike* 'bik". Vowel digraphs which represent one sound were generally read as only one of the component letters. In addition consonant clusters provoked difficulty and there were stress errors. J. C. also had greater difficulty in reading long words than in reading short words. Word imageability and frequency did not affect reading performance and there was no particular difficulty in pronouncing aloud unfamiliar non-words or unfamiliar regular words. Nor was there any particular difficulty in reading aloud short grammatical functional word such as *in*, *on* and *but*. So, J. C. like all surface dyslexics found it easier to read regular than irregular words and made regularisation errors. In 1981 Coltheart predicted that this pattern of reading performance would lead to particular difficulty with homophonic stimulae. He predicted that even when these words were read aloud correctly there would be confusion as to their meaning. Thus, if asked to read the words *blue* and *blew* a surface dyslexic would read them aloud correctly but would not know which item was being read when they were being asked what the word meant. This homophone confusion has been found to be a consistent characteristic of surface dyslexia.

The suggestion that this pattern of reading performance might also be found within the developmental dyslexias was first discussed by Holmes (1973). In her doctoral thesis, she described cases of children with developmental reading disorder whose pattern of reading performacne appeared to mimic that of acquired surface dyslexia. This hypothesis received substantiation by Coltheart/Masterson/Byng et al. (1983) who described in detail a case of *developmental surface dyslexia* which was compared to a case of acquired surface dyslexia. C. D. an 18 year old girl of average intelligence but with a reading age of 10 years, displayed a significant regularity effect on reading aloud. Her errors showed the application of a rule-based system e. g., *bear* → "beer"; *subtle* → "subtill'. She also displayed homophone confusion. For example, she defined *pane* as something which hurts.

Thus, in many features the case description of Coltheart/Masterson/Byng et al. (1983) directly parallels the earlier case descriptions of acquired surface dyslexia.

The cases of acquired surface dyslexia have received several theoretical interpretations. Dual route models of reading suggest that reading may be accomplished by a phonological reading route which parses a word, assigns a phonological representation to each of the parsed segments and then blends these together to produce the pronunciation. Alternatively, a semantic or lexical reading route allows a word to trigger a representation in the input-logogen system, a word-store postulated by Morton (1969) to include entries which have variable thresholds. The output of the logogen system activates a semantic representation. This semantic representation contains the meaning associated with the word. This meaning-based code then activates an output logogen which stores the words ultimate pronunciation. The semantic reading route is dependent upon the meaning of the word but does not attend to the structural pronunciation of the word. In triple-route models a third route, the direct reading route, passes directly from input to output logogens bypassing the semantic system.

Acquired surface dyslexia can be explained in relation to a dual or triple route model in terms of the impairment of both the semantic and direct reading route but the relative preservation of the phonological reading route, leading to an over-emphasis on phonological reading. This means that regular words are read accurately and there is no difficulty with non-words or function words, but words with irregular letter to sound patterns produced difficulty leading, to both regularity effect and regularisation errors. Since meaning is only assigned subsequent to the activation of pronunciation from the rule based system there is homophone confusion.

A comparable theoretical interpretation can be postulated for developmental surface dyslexia. In this case it is argued that the development of the direct reading route and of the semantic reading route are impaired in some way. Nevertheless, the phonological reading route has developed effectively and the child is able to read aloud many regular words. The error pattern is dominated by regularisation errors and there is particular difficulty with irregular words. Homophones are confused because meaning is assigned after pronunciation has been attained.

One of the difficulties with the original case description described by Coltheart/Masterson/Byng et al. (1983) is that their surface dyslexic C. D. also had difficulty with phonological route reading. The phonological reading route in this case has not developed well. This laid the case open to subsequent criticism. However, it would be a mistake to conclude that surface dyslexia is always associated with impaired development of the phonological reading route, in addition to the defective development of the other reading systems. Other surface dyslexics have been described who show much better development of the phonological reading route. In these cases the dissociation between the development of the routes is clearer and crisper. A clear example of this sort has been described by Temple (1984a). Temple describes a case of surface dyslexia in a child with epilepsy. This child, N. G., was able to read regular words whether familiar or unfamiliar with perfect accuracy. Irregular words frequently provoked regularisation errors. All of N. G.'s reading performance could be accounted for by the strict application of a rule based system. His phonological route performed excellently. Control children of a similar reading age to N. G. were compared to him on their reading performance with regular and irregular words. Although all the children showed small trends in favour of regularity effects, none showed the degree of regularisation effect that N. G. displayed. His performance lay outside the control range. N. G. was also significantly poorer than the control children at reading irregular words. Finally N. G. displayed homophone confusion. Eleven out of 22 words read correctly were defined as their respective homophones.

Whilst N. G. is a pure case of developmental surface dyslexia and in many ways he resembles the acquired case described by Bub/Cancelliere/Kertesz (1985), several other cases of developmental surface dyslexia have also been described in which there is a clear dissociation between the development of their phonologically based reading skills and their impaired development of other reading skills.

There are several other theoretical explanations which may be produced to account for the patterns of reading disorder in surface dyslexia. Shallice and Warrington have produced a theoretical explanation for acquired surface dyslexia which varies a little from the traditional two and three route models (Shallice/Warrington 1980; Shallice/Warrington/McCarthy 1983). They assume that within the phonological reading route the stored orthographic to sound correspondences are not restricted to graphemes. They suggest that there are correspondences for various sizes of orthographic unit. These include graphemes, consonant clusters, subsyllabic units, syllables and morphemes. They postulate a 'visual word form' system which can detect letter groups of different sizes and then send information about them to corresponding units in the phonological system. Shallice and Warrington assume that as a result of neurological pathology, when the route is impaired larger units are affected more severely than the smaller units. Increasing impairment leads to increased reliance on smaller and smaller units. In surface dyslexia therefore reliance is on orthographic units which are too small to cope effectively with the notorious irregularity of English orthography. Shallice and Warrington's model also differs from that of Marshall and Newcombe in that they abandon the direct route and incorporate it into their expanded phonological route.

In Shallice and Warrington's terms the developmental surface dyslexic is using small orthographic units as a basis for processing in the phonological route and has failed to develop the ability to process larger segments.

Analogy theorists have argued that there is no need for multiple routes to reading aloud, and that all words are read by a single route. Unfamiliar words are read by analogy with previously known words. Although analogy theory has had some success in accounting for developmental surface dyslexia it cannot account successfully for some of the other forms of dyslexia which will be discussed below. Some of the ideas of analogy theory have resurfaced in modified form within the parallel distributed processing models which have been a contemporary interest. These models and systems can successfully mimic aspects of learning to read and the performance pattern of surface dyslexia but again the other dyslexic disorders are problematic. Temple (1985a) has discussed some variation within the pattern of performance of developmental surface dyslexics and has suggested that both they and acquired surface dyslexics could be interpreted more fully if her expanded model is utilised which includes a broader version of the phonological reading route.

If the dual route model of reading is postulated then developmental surface dyslexia may be interpreted as a single component developmental dyslexia in which there is impaired development of the lexical-semantic reading route but relatively normal development of the phonological reading route. If a triple route model of reading development is invoked then there must be impaired development of both the lexical-semantic reading route and also of the direct reading route but with relative preservation of the phonological reading route. In this sense the deficit is no longer single component since two different reading routes are postulated to be impaired.

Nevertheless a unified description can be expressed of developmental surface dyslexia by saying that phonological reading skills have developed normally but non-phonological processes have not become properly established.

It is generally assumed that reading has been introduced into our civilisation after the end of the evolutionary processes which produced homo-sapiens and his apparently superior cortical development. In this case the reading mechanisms which are being discussed must be parasitic upon mechanisms which previously evolved within the brain to carry out some alternative process. If there is selective impairment in the development of some non-phonological processes, a question arises as to the underlying cognitive basis of these deficits. What is the system whose impairment has led to difficulty with these non-phonological processes? What was it used for before man developed reading within his cognitive repertoire. Marshall (1984; 1987) gets around this type of discussion by suggesting that reading may have entered our cognitive repertoire far earlier than we have previously realised. He suggests that we have been biased by the preserved written records but that we have no evidence that reading was not in existence prior to this time. He suggests that the reading system is 'preformed' in structure and that experience and education fills out the system's content.

Other, such as Ellis (1985; 1987) have suggested that the system which normally builds up the reading skills required for lexical-semantic reading processes are dependent upon systems which are adapted for analysing visually similar complex patterns. He suggests that the processes involved in face recognition could be relevant in this regard. He postulates that cases of surface dyslexia may be associated with difficulty with some forms of face recognition. However, there is little evidence to substantiate this idea. Preliminary investigations do not indicate a high degree of correlation between face recognition skills and word recognition skills. Indeed, the evidence suggests that these processes are dependent upon different systems within the brain and may be fractionated as a result of neurological insult and developmentally.

It remains possible that some other form of selective visual memory for complex configurational items is impaired in children with surface dyslexia but there is, as yet, no substantiation of this view.

Marcel (1980) pointed out that the reading patterns of normal children often resemble those of surface dyslexia. Current models of reading development are often in a post-Piagetian stage style. In these models, processes involved in the acquisition of phonological reading skills precede those involved in the processes of lexical-semantic reading. Thus, for example, in Frith's (1985) model of reading development there are three reading stages. The first stage concerns *logographic reading*. In this stage words are recognised as complete entities. This form of reading functions on a variation of an abstracted template matching. The words are not decomposed into their constituent sounds nor into their constituent orthographic components. The child identifies the whole word and selects as a vocal response a word within his or her vocabulary. This preliminary reading system is able to learn to recognise the first few words in a child's reading vocabulary. Subsequently the child progresses to an alphabetic stage of reading development. Within the *alphabetic stage* the child learns to master the associations between letters and sounds so that they are able to 'sound out' words to attain their pronunciations. It is at this stage that their pattern of performance resembles that of some developmental surface dyslexics and acquired surface dyslexics. However, for the normal child according to Frith (1985) reading development continues into the orthographic stage. Within the *orthographic stage* major sub-components of words are identified rapidly. Orthographic reading is normal adult reading. Words are not systematically sounded out prior to recognition. Morphemic units are easily and rapidly recognised and blended together. In relation to Frith's model (1985) of normal reading development, surface dyslexia may be interpreted as arrestment at the alphabetic stage. Follow-up studies of surface dyslexics indicate that they do not go on to develop an orthographic reading process (Temple 1987) rather their alphabetic system continues to expand but they are increasingly handicapped as time passes since in English the proportion of irregular words which have to be acquired increases with the increase in complexity of the language as the child goes through the educational process. Developmental surface dyslexia therefore makes greater impact in the later educational years.

The reaction time studies of Seymour (1986) indicate that surface dyslexics whom he refers to as morphemic dyslexics have response times which lie outside those of normal children. Thus, although the overall pattern of surface dyslexics resemble the pattern of some normal children they are distinguishable from them.

The case descriptions of surface dyslexia have been rather sparse in number, although the syndrome has now been described in relation to a variety of different European languages. It would appear that developmental surface dyslexia is less common than developmental phonological dyslexia.

3. Phonological Dyslexia

The term 'phonological alexia' was first used by Beauvois/Derouesné (1979), to describe a French patient with an acquired reading disorder. Subsequently, phonological alexia or acquired *phonological dyslexia* has been described in many other languages. The dominant characteristic of acquired phonological dyslexia is that the patients have difficulty with reading non-words or unfamiliar words. Misreading of non-words results either from failed attempts to decode analytically or attempts to produce a word which resembles the non-word. So, for example, the French patient described by Beauvois and Derouesné presented with the word *vina* said "c'est presque vinaigre". In comparison word reading is good. Individual words are read aloud with high levels of accuracy. Misreadings consist of morphological errors, in which the base of the word is read correctly but an affix is dropped, added or substituted; visual errors in which the response shares 50 % of the letters of the stimulus; and omissions. There can also be function word substitutions, where one short grammatical word is substituted for another. There is much variation in the characteristics of the reported cases of acquired phonological dyslexia but the salient feature is that non-word reading is impaired in relation to word reading. Some acquired phonological dyslexics are reported to be more successful at reading non-words that are homophonic with real words than pronouncable but non-homophonic non-words. Thus, *floo* is easier than *ploo* (Beauvois/Derouesné 1979; Patterson 1982). The validity of this claim has been questioned: in reported cases, visual similarity to real words has often been a confounding factor (Martin 1982; Patterson 1982). Acquired phonological dyslexia has been given the opposite theoretical interpretation to that of acquired surface dyslexia. It is suggested that the phonological reading route has become selectively impaired as a result of neurological injury whereas lexical and semantic reading routes and direct reading routes are intact. Shallice/Warrington (1980) consider that whereas surface dyslexia is a multiple component dyslexic syndrome, requiring more than one functional lesion for explanation, phonological dyslexics have a highly selective deficit involving grapheme phoneme translations. Phonological dyslexia is therefore a single component dyslexic syndrome.

The first description of *developmental phonological dyslexia* was provided by Temple/Marshall (1983). They described the case, H. M., of a 17 year old girl. Speech appeared early with no apparent abnormality and milestones were reported to be normal. There was no clear-cut history of specific reading difficulty although there was comment that the mother's brother did not learn to read well. There was no history of serious family illness and H. M. had no known neurological abnormality. H. M. came to the attention of the education authorities prior to her formal examinations at school when attempts were made to obtain extended time limits for her.

H. M. was found to be of good intelligence with a verbal I.Q. of 114 and a performance I.Q. of 115. She had a single word reading age of 10 years 11 months on the Schonell test and a reading age for accuracy of 9 years 7 months on the Neale test. H. M. was significantly poorer at reading aloud non-words than at reading words. Errors consisted of either neologisms such as *fex* → "feg"; *klower* → "kanowla" or were lexicalisations in which the non-word was read as a word with some visual similarity to the stimulus. Examples of lexicalisations are as follows: *chait* → "chit": *inlect* → "inlet": *fince* → "finish". Reading of whole words proceeded with relatively good accuracy. Errors in whole word reading were of a specific nature. A number were morphological errors in which the base of the word was read correctly but an affix was dropped, added or substituted. Examples of these errors were *beautiful* → "beauty"; *removal* → "remove"; *weigh* → "weight". In total for H. M., 16 % of all errors were morphological paralexias. She made only a small number of neologistic responses. Her other errors were either visual paralexias or visuo-semantic paralexias e. g. *thinness* → "thickness"; *arrange-*

ment → "agreement"; *politics* → "policies"; *liquor* → "liqueur".

Whilst H. M. did not have difficulty with function word reading when the function words were presented in isolation, she did have significant difficulty in dealing with function words and the grammatical endings of words in text reading. She was presented with the following passage: "Among animals the fox has no rival for cunning. Suspicious of man, who is its only natural enemy, it will, when pursued, perform extraordinary feats, even alighting on the backs of sheep to divert its scent trail." She read it as follows: "Among*st* animals the fox has no rival*s* for cunning. *Surprisingly*, of man, who is its only natural enemy *at* will, *with* pursued perform*ance* extraordinary feat, even alighting on the backs of sheep to divert its scent *trial*." This pattern of reading is paragrammatic (Kleist 1934). H. M. did not display any significant level of homophone confusion nor did she make regularisation errors or display any form of regularity effect. Her pattern of reading performance is explicable in relation to a model of normal reading by saying that she has had difficulty in developing the phonological reading route.

Many further cases of phonological dyslexia in children have been described (e. g. Temple 1984 b; c; Snowling/Stackhouse/Rack 1986; Campbell/Butterworth 1985; Seymour 1986). There have also been descriptions in a variety of European languages. This pattern of reading impairment in children appears to be relatively pervasive amongst the developmental dyslexias.

Long term follow up by Temple (1990) of a developmental phonological dyslexic A. H., indicates that the pattern of reading performance persists in character over time. Six years after initial investigation A. H. continued to show a pattern of phonological dyslexia. The overall qualitative characteristics of his reading had not altered or resolved with time. His overall level of performance had however improved and he had developed strategies to deal with a number of his difficulties. In the long term there is some evidence that phonological dyslexia is less handicapping than surface dyslexia since it is possible to build up a very large repertoire of words which can be instantly recognised. Difficulties only emerge if reading aloud is required particularly of long unfamiliar items and difficult names. For a surface dyslexic the problem is more extreme because of the degree of irregularity in the language. Surface dyslexia in languages such as Spanish and Italian in which the orthographic script is regular in relation to its spelling sound pattern is much less problematic and may only appear on occasional dialect words.

In the traditional group studies of developmental dyslexia, it is observed that children with developmental dyslexia on average have greater difficulty than normal on sound related tasks and phonological processing tasks. Pennington/Van Orden/Smith et al. (1990) narrow this difficulty to phonemic awareness rather than phonemic perception, (retrieval of phonology), or articulatory speed. However, not every dyslexic child has difficulty with phonological tasks. Temple (1987) has argued that whilst phonological dyslexics have difficulty with phonological tasks surface dyslexics are unimpaired. Phonological dyslexia is associated with difficulty on rhyming tasks and sound segmentation tasks even when these are presented in purely oral format. It is therefore possible that underlying the poor development of the phonological reading route there is a fundamental deficit in the sound based aspects of language processing. Evidence of a direct association however, is not yet substantiated and both of these deficits may merely be correlational symptoms of some other underlying impairment.

A study of *callosal agenesis* (Temple/Jeeves/Vilarroya 1989) has indicated that these children have impairment on phonological processing tasks. They have difficulty with sound segmentation tasks and they have difficulty with rhyming tasks. If such impairments are causal in developmental dyslexia one would also expect these children to display developmental dyslexia. However, the investigation by Temple/Jeeves/Vilarroya (1990) indicates that the previously studied children with callosal agenesis do not have developmental dyslexia in the sense that their word recognition skills are at a normal level for age. Given that the definition of developmental dyslexia requires that a child is not attaining the level expected for age and intelligence these children do not conform to such a description. However, a detailed investigation of the pattern of their reading performance indicated that their reading style was not normal. Whereas their reading of whole words and irregular words was accurate, their reading of non-words was impaired. Thus, whilst their overall word-recognition levels were good the pattern of their reading performance indicated an impairment in the development of the phonological reading route. There was no impairment in their ability to develop the lexical-semantic reading route and their level of competence with this reading system was sufficiently great that they did not display overt dyslexic symptoms on formal word recognition reading tests. This pattern of performance would be consistent with the notion that underlying phonological difficulties could be causal in creating difficulty with the development of the phonological reading route but cannot in and of themselves be causal in producing an overall pattern of developmental dyslexia.

Phonological dyslexia is not easily explicable in relation to models of normal reading development. Frith's model of reading development (1985), as described earlier, refers to three different stages of reading development: logographic, alphabetic and orthographic. Whereas surface dyslexia could be described as arrestment of reading development at the alphabetic stage, phonological dyslexia cannot be explained in relation to arrestment at a particular stage. The phonological dyslexics appears to have acquired orthographic reading skills without going through the alphabetic stage. The only alternative explanation is to suggest that they have a significantly expanded logographic reading system which is able to incorporate thousands of words. No such logographic reading system has ever been described in normal children.

If phonological dyslexics have attained an orthographic reading stage without going through an alphabetic reading stage then Frith's model for reading development does not refer to a series of stages which are invariant in order. In traditional models the series of stages in developmental schemes are invariant in order and each must be passed through before one can progress to the subsequent stage. The existence of phonological dyslexia may suggest that there are alternative models to reading acquisition and that not all children proceed through the same detailed set of stages. The question then arises whether phonological dyslexia reflects a peculiar variant which is never manifest in the normal population or whether amongst the children who develop reading normally there are also children who proceed to an orthographic stage without fully mastering the alphabetic stage or proceed to master the alphabetic stage later in time. If this were true then it would indicate individual differences in the acquisition of reading. These differences might emerge in later reading styles and Baron/Strawson (1976) have pointed out that adult reading styles vary. They describe both Phonecian and Chinese readers. The Phonecian readers show enhanced abilities in phonological reading whereas the Chinese readers show enhanced abilities in non-phonological reading. Such variations in the development of reading and reading styles could easily be accommodated by suggesting that the multiple routes in a reading model may develop relatively independently of each other. The patterns of performance in data gathered from the developmental dyslexics is consistent with the notion that these systems can be fractionated in this way and may develop in relative isolation. Such patterns of performance cannot be accounted for in relation to any single stage model of reading development.

Morton (1989) has attempted to break down one way in which an information processing model of reading incorporating multiple reading routes could be developed. However, he incorporates into his model a fixed order in the acquisition of components so that the model ties in with the single multiple stage reading acquisition system. This may be unnecessarily restrictive.

Phonological dyslexia is a common form of developmental dyslexia in which there is severe difficulty in the development of the phonological reading route. The early case description by Coltheart/Masterson/Byng et al. (1983) of surface dyslexia also had a mild impairment of the phonological reading route but it was above argued that this case was unrepresentative of surface dyslexia as a whole and that in other cases of developmental surface dyslexia the phonological reading route is intact. However, some argue that phonological reading deficits are always present in developmental dyslexia but in surface dyslexia their presence is rather mild and can be overlooked whereas in phonological dyslexia their effect is more profound. Such theorists could argue that developmental dyslexics may be placed along a scale in relation to their degree of phonological impairment. For the opposing view in which surface dyslexics have a phonological reading route which is normal and appropriate to their age and intelligence, there is a qualitative as well as a quantitative distinction between phonological and surface dyslexia.

4. Deep Dyslexia

The first of the acquired dyslexias to be described using a cognitive neuropsychological framework was *deep dyslexia* which was described in 1966 by Marshall/Newcombe. They described a patient G. R. who made a characteristic type of error which has subsequently been named a semantic error. When presented with single words out of context to read aloud, G. R. would substitute words which were related in meaning though not in visual appearance or in pronunciation. Thus for example when presented with the word *parrot*, he read it as "canary". These semantic errors attracted a great deal of interest and investigation. Although the next case of deep dyslexia was not described until the early 1970's there have now been many descriptions in a range of languages. The syndrome has been difficult to interpret in any simple way in relation to contemporary reading models.

The patients have no phonological reading skills at all and are completely unable to read any non-words or pronounce aloud any individual letters. They have complete impairment of the phonological reading route. However, there is further disruption of the semantic-lexical reading route since semantic errors are prevalent and they also make morphological errors. Moreover, their overall level of reading performance is much poorer than in phonological dyslexia, with greatest ease of reading for high frequency and concrete words with well elaborated meaning. More unusual words or more abstract words are difficult to read. Deep dyslexia according to the classification of Shallice/Warrington (1980) is certainly a multiple component dyslexic disorder and in relation to contemporary reading models as many as four or five deficits have been required to be postulated to account for the full range of features.

Coltheart (1980) proposed that the reading performance in deep dyslexia could be accounted for by suggesting that it reflected reading emanating from the right hemisphere of the brain. He noted the similarity between many of the characteristics of deep dyslexic reading and the characteristic of reading described in the isolated right hemisphere of the commissurotomy patients. The commissurotomy patients provided evidence that the right hemisphere of the brain does not have phonological reading skills and when required to read aloud concrete words has a tendency to substitute words with similar meanings though no obvious relationship in phonological pattern or visual appearance (Zaidel 1981). This pattern of reading performance has also been described in the isolated right hemisphere of left hemispherectomy patients. There has been much subsequent debate and argument about this theoretical interpretation, since others argue that the pattern of reading performance in deep dyslexia emanates from an impaired left hemisphere and does not result from right hemisphere reading. However, recent imaging studies support the Coltheart hypothesis (Coltheart/Weekes/Savage et al. 1991).

Developmental deep dyslexia has been an elusive disorder. If the reading disorder which represent the developmental dyslexias are interpretable in relation to a comparable reading model to that used to explain the acquired dyslexias, then in principle developmental deep dyslexia should exist. One possible explanation for its rare appearance is that the numerous deficits required to produce deep dyslexia in the neurological patient seldom co-occur in the developing child or if they do they may be sufficiently severe to prohibit the development of reading at all. There have been a small number of descriptions of children who do produce some semantic errors in reading aloud and some of whose characteristics resemble those of deep dyslexia. Such descriptions have been provided by Johnston (1983) and Siegel (1985). Temple (1988) showed that her subject K. S., a nine year old boy, made semantic errors at a level significantly above that that would be expected on the basis of chance. He also had severe difficulty with phonological processing. However, all the case descriptions to date have either related to children of rather limited intellectual ability, or children of very limited overall reading ability. Even the case K. S. described by Temple (1988) referred to a child where there was a question relating to the degree of his hearing ability. A partial hearing ability could be sufficient to significantly impair the development of the phonological reading route. In K. S. this was combined with an impairment of visual memory. In combination the deficits may have produced something which resembled deep dyslexia.

Amongst normal children learning to read, Seymour/Elder (1986) have described occasional semantic errors. Their study addressed a group of Scottish children whose reading instruction did not include explicit phonological instruction. In the early logographic phase of reading development some of these children made occasional semantic errors. In relation to the models of reading development postulated by Frith and others it could be argued that developmental deep dyslexia, when it does occur, reflects arrestment at the logographic stage of reading development. However, Temple (1988) compared the incidence of errors of the semantic component in her subject K. S. with the errors of a semantic component described by Seymour/Elder (1986) in their studies of normal reading development in Scottish children. The incidence of these errors types for K. S. was significantly above those for the control children. It therefore, appears that the reading pattern described for K. S. is not a simple arrestment of the logographic stage of development.

Wimmer/Hummer (1990) argue a logographic strategy for normal or poor readers is very limited and does not arise naturally when the writing system is phonologically transparent as in German and grapheme-phoneme correspondences are part of the instruction. So if developmental deep dyslexia is ever described in German it may be more significantly different from the normal pattern than is evident in English.

5. References

Baron, J. & Strawson, C. (1976). Use of orthographic and word-specific knowledge in reading words aloud. *Journal of Experimental Psychology: Human Perception and Performance, 2*, 386–393.

Beauvois, M. F. & Derouesné, J. (1979). Phonological alexia: Three dissociations. *Journal of Neurology, Neurosurgery and Psychiatry, 42*, 1114–1124.

Bub, D. N., Cancelliere, A., & Kertesz, A. (1985). Whole-word and analytic translation of spelling to sound in a non-semantic reader. In K. E. Patterson, J. C. Marshall & M. Coltheart (Eds.). *Surface Dyslexia. 15–34*. Hillsdale, N. J.: Erlbaum.

Campbell, E. & Butterworth, B. (1985). Phonological dyslexia and dysgraphia and a highly literate subject: A developmental case with associated deficits of phonemic processing. *Quarterly Journal of Experimental Psychology, 37A*, 435–477.

Caramazza, A., Miceli, G., & Villa, G. (1986). The role of the (output) phonological buffer in reading, writing and repetition. *Cognitive Neuropsychology, 3*, 37–76.

Coltheart, M. (1980). Deep dyslexia: A right hemisphere hypothesis. In M. Coltheart, K. E. Patterson, & J. C. Marshall (Eds.). *Deep Dyslexia. 326–380*. London: Routledge and Kegan Paul.

Coltheart, M., Masterson, J., Byng, S., Prior, M., & Riddoch, J. (1983). Surface dyslexia. *Quarterly Journal of Experimental Psychology, 35A*, 469–495.

Coltheart, M., Weekes, B., Savage, K., Simpson, L., Zurinsky, Y., & Gordon, E. (1991). Deep dyslexia and right hemisphere reading — a regional cerebral blood flow study. Paper presented at the meeting *Deep Dyslexia*. Birbeck College, October.

Dejerine, J. (1892). Contribution a l'etude anatomopathologique et clinique des differentes varieties de decite verbale. *Compte Rendues des Seances de la Society de Biologie, 4*, 61–90.

Derouesné, J. & Beauvois, M. F. (1979). Phonological processes in reading: data from alexia. *Journal of Neurology, Neurosurgery and Psychiatry, 42*, 1125–1132.

Ellis, A. W. (1985). The cognitive neuropsychology of developmental (and acquired) dyslexia: A critical survey. *Cognitive Neuropsychology, 2*, 169–206.

Ellis, A. W. (1987). On problems in developing culturally transmitted cognitive modules. *Mind and Language, 2*, 242–251.

Fisher, J. H. (1910). A case of congenital word blindness (inability to learn to read). *Transactions of the Ophthalmological Society, 30*, 216–225.

Frith, U. (1985). Beneath the surface of developmental dyslexia. In K. E. Patterson, J. C. Marshall, & M. Coltheart (Eds.). *Surface Dyslexia. 301–330*. Hillsdale, New Jersey: Erlbaum.

Hallgren, B. (1950). Specific Dyslexia ("congenital word blindness"): a clinical and genetic study. *Acta Psychiatrica et Neurologica Scandinavica Supplement, 65*.

Hinshelwood, J. (1900). Congenital word-blindness. *Lancet, 1*, 1506–1508.

Hinshelwood, J. (1917). *Congenital Word Blindness*. Glasgow: H. K. Lewis.

Holmes, J. (1973). Dyslexia: A neurolinguistic study of traumatic and developmental disorders of reading. Unpublished PhD thesis, University of Edinburgh.

Johnston, R. S. (1983). Developmental deep dyslexia? *Cortex, 19*, 133–140.

Kerr, J. (1897). School Hygiene, its mental, moral and physical aspects. *Journal of the Royal Statistical Society, 10*, 613–680.

Kleist, K. (1934). *Gehirnpathologie*. Leipzig: Barth.

Kussmaul, A. (1877). Disturbances of Speech. *Ziemssen's Cyclopaedia, 14*.

Marcel, T. (1980). Surface dyslexia and beginning reading: a revised hypothesis of the pronunciation of print and its impairments. In M. Coltheart, K. E. Patterson, & J. C. Marshall (Eds.) *Deep Dyslexia. 227–258*. London: Routledge & Kegan Paul.

Marshall, J. C. (1984). Toward a rational taxomy of the developmental dyslexias. In R. N. Malatesha and H. A. Whitaker (Eds.). *Dyslexia: A Global Issue. 45–58.* The Hague: Nijhoff.

Marshall, J. C. (1987). The cultural and biological context of written languages: Their acquisition, deployment, and breakdown. In J. R. Beech and A. M. Colley (Eds.) *Cognitive Approaches to Reading. 15–30.* Chichester: John Wiley.

Marshall, J. C. & Newcombe, F. (1966). Syntactic and semantic errors in paralexia. *Neuropsychologia, 4*, 169–176.

Marshall, J. C. & Newcombe, F. (1973). Patterns of paralexia: A psycholinguistic approach. *Journal of Psycholinguistic Research, 2*, 175–199.

Martin, R. C. (1982). The pseudohomophone effect: the role of visual similarity in non-word decisions. *Quarterly Journal of Experimental Psychology, 34A*, 395–409.

Morgan, W. P. (1896). A case of congenital word-blindness. *British Medical Journal, 2*, 1378.

Morton, J. (1969). Interaction of information in word recognition. *Psychological Review, 76*, 165–178.

Morton, J. (1979). Word recognition. In J. Morton and J. C. Marshall (Eds.) *Psycholinguistic Series, 2, 107–155.* Cambridge, Mass: MIT Press.

Morton, J. (1989). An information-processing account of reading acquisition. In A. Galaburda (Ed.), *From Reading to Neurons. 43–66.* Cambridge, MA: MIT Press.

Newcombe, F. & Marshall, J. C. (1980). Transcoding and lexical stabilization in deep dyslexia. In M. Coltheart, K. E. Patterson, & J. C. Marshall (Eds.). *Deep Dyslexia.* 176–188. London: Routledge & Kegan Paul.

Newcombe, F. & Marshall, J. C. (1981). On psycholinguistic classification of the acquired dyslexias. *Bulletin of the Orton Society, 31*, 29–44.

Newcombe, F. & Marshall, J. C. (1985). Reading and writing by letter sounds. In K. E. Patterson, J. C. Marshall, & M. Coltheart (Eds.). *Surface Dyslexia. 35–51.* Hillsdale, N. J.: Erlbaum.

Orton, S. T. (1928). Specific reading disability strephosymbolia. *Journal of the American Medical Association, 90*, 1095–1099.

Orton, S. T. (1937). *Reading, Writing and Speech Problems in Children.* New York: Norton.

Patterson, K. E. (1982). The relation between reading and phonological coding: Further neuropsychological observations. In A. Ellis (Ed.). *Normality and Pathology in Cognitive Functions. 77–111.* London: Academic Press.

Pennington, B. F., Van Orden, G. C., Smith, S. D., Green, P. A., & Haith, M. M. (1990). Phonological processing skills and deficits in adult dyslexics. *Child Development, 61*, 1753–1778.

Seymour, P. H. K. (1986). *Cognitive Analysis of Dyslexia.* London: Routledge & Kegan Paul.

Seymour, P. & Elder, L. (1986). Beginning reading without phonology. *Cognitive Neuropsychology, 3*, 1–36.

Seymour, P. & MacGregor, C. J. (1984). Developpment dyslexia: A cognitive analysis of phonological, morphemic and visual impairments. *Cognitive Neuropsychology, 1*, 43–82.

Shallice, T. & Warrington, E. K. (1980). Single and multiple component central dyslexic syndromes. In M. Coltheart, K. S. Patterson, & J. C. Marshall (Eds.). *Deep Dyslexia. 119–145.* London: Routledge & Kegan Paul.

Shallice, T., Warrington, E. K., & McCarthy, R. (1983). Reading without semantics. *Quarterly Journal of Experimental Psychology, 35A*, 111–138.

Siegel, R. (1985). Deep dyslexia in childhood? *Brain and Language, 216*, 16–17.

Skydsgaard, H. B. (1942). *Den konstitutionelle dyslexi.* Kobenhavn.

Snowling, M., Stackhouse, J., & Rack, J. (1986). Phonological dyslexia and dysgraphia: A developmental analysis. *Cognitive Neuropsychology, 3*, 309–339.

Temple, C. M. (1984a). Surface dyslexia in a child with epilepsy. *Neuropsychologia, 22*, 569–576.

Temple, C. M. (1984b). New approaches to the developmental dyslexias. In Rose, C. (Ed.). *Progress in Aphasiology. 223–232.* London: Plenum Press.

Temple, C. M. (1984c). Developmental analogues to acquired phonological dyslexia. In R. N. Malatesha & H. A. Whitaker (Eds.). *Dyslexia: A Global Issue. 143–158.* The Hague: Nijhoff.

Temple, C. M. (1985a). Surface dyslexia: Variation within a syndrome. In K. Patterson, J. C. Marshall, & M. Coltheart (Eds.). *Surface Dyslexia.* 269–288. Hillsdale, N. J.: Erlbaum.

Temple, C. M. (1985b). Reading with partial phonology. *Journal of Psycholinguistic Research, 14*, 523–541.

Temple, C. M. (1987). The nature of normality, the deviance of dyslexia and the recognition of rhyme. *Cognition, 27*, 103–108.

Temple, C. M. (1988). Red is read but eye is blue: A case study of developmental dyslexia and follow-up report. *Brain and Language, 34*, 13–37.

Temple, C. M. (1990). Foop is still Floop: A six year follow-up of phonological dyslexia and dysgraphia. *Reading and Writing: An Interdisciplinary Journal, 2*, 209–221.

Temple, C. M., Jeeves, M. A., & Villaroya, O. (1989). Ten, pen, men: Rhyming skills in two children with callosal agenesis. *Brain and Language, 37*, 548–564.

Temple, C. M., Jeeves, M. A., & Villaroya, O. (1990). Reading in callosal agenesis. *Brain and Language, 39*, 235–253.

Temple, C. M. & Marshall, J. C. (1983). A case study of developmental phonological dyslexia. *British Journal of Psychology, 74*, 517–533.

Wimmer, H. & Hummer, P. (1990). How German-speaking first readers read and spell: Doubts on the importance of the logographic stage. *Applied Psycholinguistics, 11*, 349–368.

Zaidel, E. (1981). Reading by the disconnected right hemisphere aphasiological perspective. In Y. Zotterman (Ed.). *Wenner-Gren Symposium on Dyslexia. 67–91.* London: Plenum Press.

Christine M. Temple, Essex (United Kingdom)

73. Treatment of Developmental Reading and Spelling Disorders

1. The Scope of Remedial Approaches

The scope of remedial approaches to reading and spelling disability is very impressive. It ranges from medication to psychotherapy and from motor training to direct instruction of reading and spelling. This heterogeneity is partially due to the fact that the different scientific disciplines contributing to the analysis of reading disability (education, psychology, linguistics, medicine) are also involved in conceptualizing intervention. Furthermore, some remedial methods have been developed in an applied context and their theoretical foundations are rather coarse.

Table 73.1 gives a survey of different therapeutic approaches. Whereas all aim to improve the disabled child's reading and spelling, there is a distinction in terms of the level at which therapy is directed: Intervention is either directed at the child's cognitive abilities, the reading and spelling processes themselves, the emotional behavior, the sensory organs or the brain. The present chapter will give a survey of all treatments, concentrating, however, on the different branches of the 'Direct Instruction' approach. The theoretical background of each approach and method will be elaborated as it is presented.

Although remedial teaching is required to be adaptive to the child's particular problems, so far no treatment has been found to be differentially effective for specifically reading disabled children as compared to generally backward readers. Consequently, studies using samples from either population will not be reported separately. Further, there is no other classificatory scheme for disabled readers and spellers from which appropriate treatment programs could be convincingly deduced.

Psychological and educational intervention
- Training of perceptual and cognitive abilities ('Prescriptive teaching')
- Training reading and spelling ('Direct instruction')
  - Promoting the alphabetic strategy (training phoneme analysis and synthesis)
  - Improving orthographic skills
    - Structural approaches
    - Lexical approaches
      - Behavior modification
      - Training memory stategies
- The language experience approach
- Psychotherapy

Medical and neurological approaches
- Ophtalmological intervention
- Pharmacotherapy
- Methods related to laterality

Table 73.1: Survey of different therapeutic approaches in intervention with reading and spelling disabled children

2. Methodological Issues in Evaluating Intervention

Considering the high quality research on the analysis of reading disabled children's cognitive abilites and processes (Hulme/Snowling cf. art. 71, Snowling/Hulme cf. art. 70 for review), one would expect to find comparable efforts also in the realm of intervention. However, this is not the case. Only few intervention studies reach the methodological standards required for empirical research. There are several reasons for this. On the one hand, there is the urgent need to help reading and spelling disabled children; on the other hand, methodological difficulties in evaluative studies are almost unsurmountable:

- Consensus exists that reading disabled children need to be taught in an adaptive, individual manner. Yet in empirical designs all children should be preferably treated by the same method.
- Consensus again exists that reading and spelling disabled children need to be treated for an extended period of time in order to show substantial improvement; however, it is very difficult to control long-term treatment.
- In all intervention studies, control groups present immense problems: For ethical reasons it is not possible to treat control children with any type of placebo over a longer period of time or simply leave them untreated. Yet, if no control group is involved it is difficult to estimate the size of regression, the Hawthorne effect and 'normal' development and learning.
- There are also many variables which are difficult to control, although they basically can be controlled or at least documented. These include on the child's side the particular type of the reading and spelling problem and other cognitive variables, motivation, and social background, and on the therapist's side enthusiasm, optimism, and a positive relationship to the child. Particularly the latter variables are rarely controlled.

The present chapter will focus mainly on intervention studies which were basically well-designed, although they could not circumvent all the methodological shortcomings mentioned above. However, for the benefit of completeness, some remedial approaches will be presented, even when no appropriate data are available.

3. Psychological and Educational Approaches

The majority of therapeutic approaches for reading and writing disabled children are rooted in the psychological and educational domain. While many educational programs developed in the sixties and early seventies intended to strengthen underlying psychological abilities (cf. 3.1.) there is now a tendency to directly train reading and spelling skills (cf. 3.2.1.). Within the skill oriented approach, different theoretical systems like behaviorism and cognitive psychology have influenced the development of training programs.

3.1. The Training of Perceptual and Cognitive Abilities ('Prescriptive Teaching')

The training of perceptual and cognitive abilities, which is known as 'Prescriptive Teaching', is still part of everyday remedial teaching (Lewis 1983). The basic idea is the following: Reading disabled children usually show deficits in a number of perceptual and cognitive abilities (as compared to high achievers) and these should be compensated as a prerequisite for reading and spelling. Training programs have been developed in the area of visual perception (e. g. Frostig/Horne 1964), of auditory perception, in the motor or visual-motor domain (e. g. Delacato 1963, Kephart 1960) and in various linguistic areas. None of the areas is directly related to the partial processes of reading and spelling. The materials used in these programs (e. g. Frostig/Horne 1964) are often nonverbal and are thus motivating for children who have failed in reading and spelling tasks.

However, the approach has not been found to be effective. At best progress is observed in the ability trained; yet there is no transfer to reading and spelling. This is particularly true for the visual domain which is often favored by teachers. Larsen/Hammill (1975) and Arter/Jenkins (1979) in reviewing a large number of studies found that the majority of methodologically acceptable studies do not support the effectiveness of 'Prescriptive Teaching'.

The training of 'basic' cognitive abilities also does not necessarily increase the effect of subsequent direct teaching. Edler/Ostrau/Schulze (1978) trained third grade disabled spellers to use more efficient problem solving strategies in visual tasks. Appropriate strategies were modeled and taught by a method of verbal self-control (see Meichenbaum/Goodman 1969). After 12 training sessions the trained children showed better performance in most of the tasks used in training; however, there was no transfer to spelling (not even a Hawthorne effect). The children then participated in a spelling program; they profited from this training, but no more than a previously untrained control group. Training in visual attention had not improved the children's cognitive prerequisites for direct spelling instruction.

Several reasons why the 'prescriptive teaching' approach has failed can be given. Concepts such as 'visual perception' or 'auditory perception' do not seem to be valid entities in the sense that they can be trained as such and manifest themselves in a variety of different tasks. It is known from the information processing literature that the processes involved in visual tasks depend on the stimulus material and the specific task requirements (Neisser 1967). Hence transfer of training between nonverbal and verbal stimuli can hardly be expected. The child who confuses ⟨d⟩ and ⟨b⟩ has to learn with which visual stimulus to associate the phoneme /d/; training visual discrimination with pictorial stimuli is irrelevant to the problem.

The conclusion that training needs to be specific to reading and writing is supported by studies from the auditory domain. Whereas a general auditory discrimination training does not affect reading (see Sabatino 1973 for review), improving phoneme analysis skills in kindergarten leads to better reading scores in first grade (e. g. Lundberg/Frost/Peterson 1988). Programs training phonological skills will be discussed in more detail in a subsequent section (3.2.2.) as a branch of the 'Direct Instruction' approach.

3.2. Direct Instruction

There is no doubt that direct instruction is the most effective approach to improve literacy in reading and spelling disabled children (Branwhite 1983, Lewis 1983). 'Direct Instruction' refers to programs which basically implement reading and writing instruction, starting if necessary at a first grade level. Although there are differences in detail, common elements are found in almost all remedial approaches using direct teaching: Consensus exists that, whatever the method, teaching should be adaptive, i. e. be tailored to the child's present knowledge and progress (Hornsby/Miles 1980, Thomson 1988). Many studies show improvement in reading disabled children's reading and writing with different types of direct instruction (Scheerer-Neumann 1979). Indeed, it appears somewhat difficult for a treated group not to display at least a short-term effect as compared to a control group. The reason for this is rather obvious: Reading disabled children usually experience a 'teaching deficit' because the instruction offered to them at school outstrips their actual needs. So any type of adaptive help is almost predestined to have some positive effect. However, if a program is really effective, it should not just show statistically significant improvement as compared to a control group, but also substantial effects with regard to the child's chronological age. Yet substantial effects can only be found in long-term studies and these present the methodological problems pointed out above. However, in spite of methodological shortcomings, good evidence can be found in large-scale and long-term studies indicating that within comprehensive and intensive programs direct instruction really can boost childrens' achievements in reading and spelling (Balow/Fuchs/Kasbohm 1978, Hornsby/Miles 1980, Thomson 1988). The severely reading and spelling retarded children in Thomson's (1988) study increased their reading and spelling ability by almost four years within a treatment period of two and a half years. Previous pessimism (e. g. Silberberg/Silberberg 1969) is not justified.

3.2.1. Direct Instruction within a Developmental Perspective

The theoretical foundations of the different methods within direct instruction approach are quite heterogeneous. While some programs are based on recent experimental evidence on poor readers' deficiencies in the phonological and structural components of reading (e. g. Bradley/Bryant 1983, Scheerer-Neumann 1981), others are rooted in more general therapeutic theories (e. g. the behavior modification approach) and still others are rather eclectic in origin (e. g. Thomson 1988). It is surprising that the literature on efficient spelling instruction for poor spellers (e. g. Hulme 1981) does not seem to be integrated in more general issues of memory development. At times, different theoretical assumptions lead to similar methods: Orton (1937) believed dyslexics' problems to be mainly visual (he coined the term 'strephosymbolia'), but this assumption was not confirmed empirically. His coworkers Gillingham/Stillman (1969) developed a training program based mainly on phonics. Their idea was to teach children according to their strengths and not according to their weaknesses. Today similar methods are uses under the presumption that reading and spelling disabled children have problems in the phonological domain.

Whereas the theoretical backgrounds of different therapeutic programs are heterogeneous, their goals seem to fit well into a model of reading and spelling development which has recently been published by Frith (1985) (see also Marsh/Friedman/Welch/Desberg 1981). Frith proposes that children's predominant reading and spelling strategies change during the acquisition of literacy; the stages she postulates are the logographic, the alphabetic and finally the orthographic stage. The logographic strategy in reading refers to the instant recognition of familiar words; there is no process of phonological assembly. Logographic writing is writing by rote. The alphabetical strategy is basically a phonological strategy. In reading it translates graphemes into phonemes in a systematic, sequential way. Alphabetic spelling implies the segmentation of words into their constituent phonemes and the translation of phonemes into graphemes. The orthographic strategy is again more 'direct', since it uses abstract orthographic patterns for word recognition and spelling. While reading and spelling disabled children seem to be quite proficient in logographic processing (Rozin/Gleitman 1977), they primarily have problems with the alphabetic strategy: There is abundant literature demonstrating poor readers' and spellers' deficits in phonological skills like phoneme analysis and phoneme synthesis which are basic components of alphabetic processing (see Kamhi/Catts 1989, Snowling/Hulme cf. art. 70, and Wagner/Torgeson 1987 for review). However, difficulties often persist up to the orthographic stage (Seymour/McGregor 1984). Although the question is still open whether orthographic problems are mainly due to a delayed alphabetic stage or rather are an issue in themselves, it is obvious that they need to be treated. There seem to be less problems with reading comprehension once basic decoding skills are acquired. Therefore only training programs are reported which are directed at promoting either the alphabetic or the orthographic strategy.

3.2.2. Promoting the Alphabetic Stategy

Taking a look at the actual methods used in direct remedial instruction, it is apparent that exercises directed at alphabetic processing are most often preferred in the initial stages of teaching. Indeed, phoneme-grapheme-correspondences, phoneme analysis and phoneme blending are at the core of effective remedial programs (Gillingham/Stillman 1969, Hornsby/Miles 1980, Kossow 1972). However, the programs and in particular the evaluative studies differ with respect to the actual methods used to promote alphabetic processing.

a) Comprehensive 'Phonics' Approaches

The phonics approach usually includes the teaching of letter and sound correspondences, phoneme analysis tasks, phoneme blending tasks, and a thorough control of reading material which increases slowly in difficulty on several dimensions. One of these dimensions is consonant-vowel-structure, another the number of syllables per word. Some programs which start with phonics include two additional features: The programs developed by Kossow (1972) and by Dummer/Hackethal (1984) teach the child to become conscious of the movements of his/her speech organs when pronouncing sounds (see also Skjelfjord 1976). Although there are no data on the effectiveness of this particular feature of the programs, it fits very well with observations on the actual processes involved in children's phonemic analysis: Children tend to analyze their own articulation (Schreuder/van Bon 1989, Skelfjord 1976).

An additional feature of the programs developed by Kossow (1972) and Dummer/Hackethal (1984) is the introduction of hand signs corresponding to single phonemes. This method is believed to be particularly helpful for children with severe reading problems. Again, we do not have any good data on the effectiveness of this method, but many remedial teachers like to use it. It is not quite clear, though, why hand signs should be effective. Some of Kossow's signs are related to the visual form of the letter and some to articulatory movements (e. g. /e/, /i/ refer to the opening of the mouth when pronouncing the vowels) so the sign could serve as an additional memory code. It is also possible that the child might be helped by the clear sequential order of signing which models the spoken word much better than the parallel visual input of the written word.

Williams (1979) tested a comprehensive phonics program (The ABD of reading = Analysis, Blending, Decoding) with generally learning disabled children in a field study. The children (7–10 years of age) were trained daily for a period of two years. The author reports that in comparison to an untrained control group the trained children made outstanding progress on phonemic tasks as well as in reading and spelling. A similarly impressive effect was found in a field study by Wallach/Wallach (1979). First grade low-income children were given daily additional training in phoneme analysis, letter-sound correspondences, decoding of simple regular words, and in reading regular classroom reading material. The differences in reading and writing achievement between the trained children and an untrained control group were not only statistically significant, but also "sufficiently large in their magnitude to be important in practical terms" (Wallach/Wallach 1979, 212).

Working with older children (M = 11 years) Lovett/Ransby/Barron (1988) studied the effect of training word recognition and decoding skills as compared to a more general language program which included comprehension of oral language, reading, and written composition. Although both groups scored higher on a word recognition task and in a reading test than a control group after 40 treatment sessions, it was the 'decoding' group which gained most.

In long-term studies with school-children a variety of phonological tasks is used and these are complemented rather early by a word training; it is thus difficult to isolate the effects of the different phonological tasks.

b) Training Phoneme Analysis and Synthesis

Several studies have looked at the effects of a phoneme analysis and/or blending training in a more controlled setting (Ball/Blachman 1988,1991, Bradly/Bryant 1983, Content/Morais/Alegria/Bertelson 1982, Fox/Routh 1984, Hohn/Ehri 1983, Kerstholt/van Bon/Schreuder 1991, Lie 1991, Mannhaupt 1990, Rosner 1971, Tornéus 1984, Treiman/Baron 1983, Vellutino/Scanlon 1984). Unfortunately, most of these used unselected preschoolers as subjects; hence the results may not be directly transferable to reading disabled children. Still, some issues are probably of general relevance.

The main result of the cited studies is the finding that, while phonemic analysis does not seem to develop spontaneously in preschool children (in contrast e. g. to sensitivity to rhymes), it can be trained quite successfully (e. g. Ball/Blachman 1991, Bradley/Bryant 1983, Lundberg/Frost/Peterson 1988). Effects are visible even after a very short training period (e. g. Content/Kolinsky/Morais/Bertelson 1986). Secondly, the training of phonemic analysis and blending in kindergarten has been shown to directly improve reading and spelling skills (Ball/Blachman 1991, Fox/Routh 1984) or to accelerate the acquisition of reading and writing in the early school years (Bradley/Bryant 1983, Lundberg/Frost/Peterson 1988).

In a long-term setting training is also effective for children with low scores on pretest. In Bradley/Bryant's (1983) study the children trained on phoneme categorization tasks during preschool and first grade attained better scores in reading and writing as compared to an untrained control group even several years after training ended. Tornéus (1984) showed that training in phoneme segmentation and blending in first grade had a particularly strong effect on children with low pretest scores in phonological tasks. Lie (1991), who also trained first graders, found that children of lower intelligence profited most from phonological training in posttest reading and spelling.

What method of teaching phonological skills is most effective and shows optimal transfer for later reading and writing? In her review of training studies, Lewkowicz (1980) concluded that the most effective phonological tasks are those which are most closely related to reading and spelling, i. e. sequential phonemic analysis (as compared e. g. to a positional analysis of single phonemes) and blending. This conclusion has been confirmed empirically by Lie (1991), who studied the influence of a 'positional phoneme analysis' training (which sound do you hear in the beginning of a word? in the middle? at the end?) compared to a complete 'sequential analysis' training during kindergarten on later reading and writing. Whereas there was no differential effect on reading ability at the end of first grade, the children trained in complete sequential analysis reached better scores in spelling. However, the differential effect was reduced by the end of second grade.

Another important issue is the question whether phonemic analysis should be complemented by some kind of visual structure or even by letters. Lewkowicz/Low (1979) found a positive effect of visual squares representing the number of phonemes early in training (see also Elkonin 1973). Hohn/Ehri (1983) showed that phoneme analysis can be promoted even more by introducing the corresponding letters. The authors argue that letters provide the children with a mental symbol system for representing the phonemes.

The superiority of a letter condition in phoneme analysis tasks has not been supported unequivocally in studies using reading disabled children. Confirmative evidence comes from Bradley/Bryant (1983) who introduced plastic letters in their second year of training for one group of children. On the other hand, Mannhaupt (1990), who trained phonemic segmentation in low achievers in the second half of first grade, did not obtain differential effects between a letter and a blank tile condition. Working with older reading disabled children (7–10 years of age) Kerstholt/van Bon/Schreuder (1991) could not confirm the advantage of a training condition with letters and/or squares as visual support. Thus it seems that the introduction of letters within a phoneme training program is mainly effective for preschoolers who might not be aware of the structure of an alphabetic writing system prior to training. This interpretation can be supported by data from Cunningham (1990), who found better transfer from a phoneme segmentation training to reading when the children (1st grade) were explicitly introduced to the value and utility of phoneme awareness for the activity of reading. Older reading disabled children who have already learned the basics of the correspondence between the spoken and the written language apparently do not profit as much from letters as support for phonemic analysis.

In future research, efforts definitely need to be directed at training phonological skills in reading disabled children; mere extrapolation from preschool studies is certainly not justified. What is also needed is an analysis of the microstructure of phoneme segmentation. First attempts have found onset and rime (e. g. c-at) as possible functional units (Schreuder/van Bon 1989, Wise/Olsen/Treiman 1990). Schreuder/van Bon (1989) also looked at the influence of word structure on phonemic analysis and found that different parts of a word influence each other so that a strictly serial model for phoneme segmentation cannot be adequate.

In conclusion of this section it should be mentioned that although phoneme analysis and blending certainly are important partial processes of reading and spelling, they need not necessarily be trained in isolation. Ehri (1987) and Morais/Alegria/Content (1987) argue that phonological skills are acquired while learning to read and to spell. Particularly in 'creative spelling' (Read 1986) children are constantly required to analyze words into their constituent phonemes (cf. 4.).

3.2.3. Improving Orthographic Skills

While segmentation and blending single phonemes seem to be necessary skills for attaining literacy in an alphabetic script like English, they are not sufficient for advanced reading and writing. The competent reader and speller has to deal with many words which do not conform to simple phoneme-grapheme correspondences; these words either display higher order phonographic, graphotactic, or morphemic structure or are orthographically irregular. There are basically two different educational approaches to teach children how to cope with regular but complex and irregular words: The 'structural' approach introduces the child to higher order regularities of the written language; the 'lexical' or 'word-specific' approach teaches strategies for directly learning the orthographic code of regular and/or irregular words. In long-term programs these approaches are usually combined.

a) Structural Approaches

Although not all programs using a structural approach are theory oriented, basic research has provided overwhelming evidence that orthographic structure is used in mature reading and writing (Gibson/Shurcliff/Yonas 1970, Glushko 1979, Seidenberg 1987, Taft 1979, 1987 and others). The higher order regularities can be phonographic, graphotactic or morphemic in origin. Although more evidence is emerging constantly (see Coltheart 1987 for review), the exact nature of the utilization and – particularly – the acquisition of orthographic structure is still open for further research. Gibson/Shurcliff/Yonas (1970) believe that invariant spelling patterns are being learnt; Goswami (1986) suggests that children may use analogies to extract rules. Connectionist models of reading acquisition (Seidenberg/McClelland 1989) may be opening new research avenues.

There is evidence that reading and writing disabled children do not make as much use of orthographic structure as better readers and spellers (Guthrie/Seifert 1977, Manis/Morrison 1985, Morrison/Manis 1982, Scheerer-Neumann 1981). While Guthrie/Seifert (1977) regard this deficit as a consequence of delayed reading acquisition rather than as a basic cause of reading retardation, Manis/Morrison (1985) feel that reading disabled children have general difficulties in learning complex and inconsistent rules.

In any case, the utilization of orthographic structure is basically teachable. Graphophonic regularities in reading can be taught by rules like "'i' before 'e'". Insight into the morphemic structure of words allows children to take avantage of building blocks like the ⟨ed⟩-ending of the past tense in English or the suffix ⟨ig⟩ in German (Siemens 1985). The syllable structure of long words in particular can also be used to facilitate decoding. Scheerer-Neumann (Scheerer-Neumann 1981, Scheerer-Neumann/Ahola/König/Reckermann 1978) trained reading disabled third graders how to segment written words into syllables using the vocalic center group as reference. The children were quite proficient at phoneme blending, but had problems in decoding long words. After only 12 training sessions there was a considerable decrease in oral reading errors particularly for words with three or more syllables. Syllables are very helpful as segments because they are the units of spoken language and as such are easily accessible to the children (Liberman/Shankweiler/Liberman et al. 1977).

Within syllables onset and rime might be useful structural segments. Wise/Olson/Treiman (1990) trained first graders to read a set of four letter words: The scores on post-test were better for those words which had been presented during training in onset-rime segmentation than those in a post-vowel segmentation condition. However, using Dutch third graders as subjects, van Bosch (1991) failed to replicate this facilitatory effect. Whether the discrepancy is due to differences in subjects' age or to structural differences between written English and Dutch is questionable. It is conceivable that in English the rime more often has a decisive effect on the preceding vowel than in Dutch.

The structural approach is frequently used in remedial spelling. The programs developed by Hornsby/Miles (1980) and Thomson (1988) make intensive use of orthographic regularities. In Germany this approach has been proposed by Kossow (1972) and Scheerer-Neumann (1988). Scheerer-Neumann taught spelling rules to poor fifth-grade spellers of average intelligence who were basically proficient in the alphabetic strategy. The rules selected included capitalization of nouns and morphemic constancy, i. e. graphemic constancy of morphemes even in words with a deviant pronunciation. The pupils learned the orthographic rules and how to apply them; additionally some of the relevant words were also taught lexically by the 'look-cover-write-check' method. The posttest included a subset of the trained words as well as untrained words in order to investigate a possible transfer effect. After 30 – 35 training sessions distributed over 4 months errors related to the trained orthographic regularities decreased by 45% with trained words and by 38% with transfer words. This result shows both a very good transfer effect, suggesting that orthographic regularities really had been learnt and could be applied, as well as an effect of word-specific training. On the other hand there was almost no transfer effect to words whose structural difficulties had not been trained. Thus, although there was evidence for transfer to new words when they had the same structure as the trained words, there was almost no transfer to new orthographic structures.

b) Lexical (Word-Specific) Approaches

Lexical or word-specific approaches in remedial reading and spelling instruction rely solely on the direct teaching of the orthographic properties of words. The basic idea is that children systematically build up a reading or spelling vocabulary with single words as units. Word training procedures have been developed within diverse theoretical traditions: For behavior modification approaches single words are manageable units of reading and writing behavior. Cognitive models of reading and spelling assume that phonological and orthographical processes are complemented by direct access of the stored orthographic representations of words (the 'orthographic lexicon', Coltheart 1989), and/or their constituent morphemes. Finally, single word training is also an issue in human memory research (e. g. Hulme 1981).

– Behavior Modification

Within the behavior modification approach learning to read is considered as operant discrimination learning. Consequently, the correct reading or writing of a word is positively reinforced (Machemer 1972) or, alternatively, errors are punished in a response-cost system (Reuter 1977). Since no assumptions are made about the nature of the cognitive processes involved in reading and writing, the children receive no hints as to the linguistic or psychological structure of the words trained. Instead great care is given to the number and spacing of the trials: The words to be learned are repeated several times during a training period according to a scheme which is derived from learning theory; distributed practice with shorter intervals for newly introduced words has been shown to be more effective than massed practice (see Kerr/Lambert 1982, for review). This technique can easily be implemented and has been shown to be very effective even with parents as trainers (Machemer 1972). Some programs also control the rehearsal behavior during each trial: Murphy/Hern/Williams/McLaughlin (1990) observed that the copy-cover-write-check procedure combined with systematic repetitions lead to better results in spelling than more traditional training methods. Lenz/Singh/Hewett (1991) suggest that it is the component of directed rehearsal which makes "overcorrection" a powerful procedure in academic remediation.

Some training studies conducted within the cognitive reading research tradition have also used repeated presentations of words to improve word recognition. It seems rather easy to increase a child's reading accuracy and speed in word recognition by systematically practising a set of words. That it is in fact word-specific knowledge which is acquired by this type of procedure is demonstrated by the absence of a transfer effect to untrained words (Fiedorowicz 1986, Reitsma/Dongelmans 1988).

– Training Memory Stategies

Whereas behavior modification methods mainly control the number and spacing of trials and rehearsals, memory strategies can also be modified more directly. The vast literature on memory development has convincingly shown that younger children do not use as effective memory strategies as older children (e. g. Ornstein/Naus 1978; for a review see Hagen/Jongeward/Kail 1975, Ornstein 1978). Reading disabled and generally learning disabled children resemble chronologically younger children (Bauer 1979, Bauer/Newman 1991, Dallago/Moely 1980). When learning the spelling of new words spelling disabled children often display an impulsive, non-strategic behavior; they do not take enough time and commit more errors than their peers (Kossow 1972). There is also a vast literature showing that the use of more efficient memory strategies can be trained (Hagen/Hargrave/Ross 1973; for review, see Bauer 1987, Hagen/Jongeward/Kail 1975). The task therefore is to determine which strategies are most effective to retain the orthographic code of words. There are some short-term experimental studies on this question which are also relevant for comprehensive remedial programs. The main issue refers to the modality of the code used: This is the classic question whether learning is most efficient using the visual, the auditory or the kinesthetic modality, or a combination of any two or three. Gillingham/Stillmann (1956) proposed a strategy they called 'simultaneous oral spelling'; while copying (later in training writing by rote) a word the child names each letter. Since this procedure involves a visual, an auditory, and a motor component it is often referred to as 'multisensory teaching'. The importance of the motor component has also been stressed by Fernald (1943) and by Montessori (1913). Hulme (1981) tested the efficiency of different spelling codes experimentally and some other studies have followed. In a very convincing study Hulme/Bradley (1984) found that retarded spellers (M = 11 years) profited most from simultaneous oral spelling compared to a condition without letter naming and a condition which used letter cards instead of writing. Performance under the 'simultaneous oral spelling' condition improved even 4 weeks after training. The results were dissimilar for normal readers who were chronologically younger (M = 6 years, 8 months) but of the same spelling age: They did not show any differential effects under the various conditions. In a study using an intraindividual design Bradley (1981) found that merely pronouncing the word while writing was not as helpful as simultaneous spelling. That simply pronouncing the word is not as efficient as simultaneous spelling is not surprising, since the spoken word does not contain the complete orthographic information.

Taken together, these results show that multiple coding improves the memory performance of retarded readers. This is in agreement with basic memory research. Paivio (1971) has demonstrated that items which can be coded both visually and verbally are better retained in memory. The question then remains, why the additional auditory code does not improve spelling in normal readers. Although Hulme/Bradley (1984) do not report relevant data it is probable that normal spellers use some type of verbal code spontaneously. For languages with more regular phoneme-grapheme correspondences like German, this verbal code seems to be the 'overpronunciation' of the word with respect to its spelling rather than the letter names (Scheerer-Neumann 1986a). When 'multisensory' training is regarded as an instance of multiple code learning, it should also be helpful to include structural properties of the word as an additional code (e. g. the morphemic structure of a word like "child/ish").

Most importantly, Hulme/Bradley's (1984) data fit the picture of inefficient memory strategies in poor spellers, which can be improved by training. This conclusion is supported by research showing that in spelling instruction particularly poor spellers need a memorization set in order for successful learning to come about. Bosman/de Groot (1991) found that copying a stimulus word while it was still in view was totally ineffective for poor spellers (grade 1), while it had a small effect in good spellers. The low level performance of poor spellers probably has to do with their inability to spontaneously generate additional codes while copying. The finding that a memorization set is necessary for appreciable retention to come about conforms with the idea of the child as an active learner whose task it is to select and code information. This is very different from the conception of the orthographic lexicon as a store of 'photographic word-pictures' which has been prominent among teachers for many years (Scheerer-Neumann 1986b). There are some additional data which demonstrate active processes in spelling acquisition: Kauffman/Hallahan/Haas et al. (1978) and Hasselbring (1982) found greater improvement in spelling when the children were shown their errors together with correct spellings instead of the correct spellings alone. This finding demonstrates that children do not just store correct spellings but rather pay attention to the letters they missed before.

Word training programs can be implemented very well by a microcomputer. A computer program has the advantage of being easily adapted to a child's basic level and daily performance, a feature which is essential for spelling disabled children. Adaptive spelling programs for disabled spellers have been reported among others by Hasselbring (1982) and Breuninger/Betz (1989).

3.3 The Language Experience Approach

The 'Language experience approach' or 'whole language approach' stresses the child's own language as a bridge from oral to written language (e. g. Hildreth 1965). The child's attention is focussed on the functional aspects rather than on the structural properties of written language. Instead of basal readers, children's literature is used as reading material as early as possible. Children are encouraged to communicate by writing even at a stage where they cannot be expected to avoid spelling errors. Errors are not only tolerated but considered as signs of certain developmental stages (Read 1986).

Stahl/Miller (1989) have recently completed a meta-analysis of a large number of studies comparing the effectiveness of the language experience approach with a basal reader approach. They found that, overall, the approaches were similar in their effectiveness, although there were also differential results. The language experience approach was more effective in teaching children concepts about print and reading at the kindergarten level. Unfortunately, the authors did not look specifically at slow learners; yet data are reported on disadvantaged children and a large overlap between the learning disabled and the disadvantaged population can be assumed. The disadvantaged children also profited from the language experience approach at the kindergarten level; however, at the first grade level the basal reader approach proved more effective. The authors conclude that – in Downing's (1979) terms – the language experience approach is more efficient in the 'cognitive phase', when children become aware of print and reading, but that the basal reader approach is more helpful during the 'mastering phase'.

The advantage of the basal reader approach on the skill acquisition phase complies with a presupposition underlying most remedial approaches particularly within the direct instruction tradition: Most of them explicitly demand a step-by-step procedure where nothing is left to chance and no transfer is expected from the child (Dummer/Hackethal 1984, Hornsby/Miles 1980, Thomson 1988). On the other hand, the language experience approach does rely upon learning which is not explicitly taught. In practice, both approaches can be combined to a certain extent. It is possible to use the highly motivating elements from the language experience approach, have children read and write on their own very early and still introduce elements of the written language in a rather systematic form. In a study which included kindergarten and first grade Sawyer (1988) found best results for children who were poor phoneme segmenters when a combination of a phonics and a language experience approach was used. Spontaneous, creative writing, one important element of the language experience approach, implies extensive practice in phoneme analysis since the children often want to write words whose spelling they are not familiar with. They have to construct these words out of known elements, usually phoneme-grapheme correspondences. Although words constructed by children in creative spelling are frequently not yet correct orthographically, early spelling errors do not seem to have a negative effect on later orthographic skills: Clarke (1988) found that creative writing even leads to better spelling achievements at the end of first grade than more traditional teaching methods. Creative writing can be facilitated by a text processor (e. g. Levin/Boruta/Vasconcellos 1983) which can also be used for checking the spelling. Computers offer new possibilities to help reading disabled children; the scope has not yet been fully explored.

3.4. Psychotherapy

Psychotherapy has been suggested by Axline (1947) and others as a treatment of reading disability. There may indeed be cases where reading disability should be viewed as neurotic behavior and treated accordingly. However, in the majority of cases, emotional and behavioral problems in reading disabled children are secondary to their failure at school. Constant problems in important school subjects affect most children's self concept severely. Most school systems are not flexible enough to allow children to progress at their own pace. Thus for some children psychotherapy is needed as a precondition for more direct instruction. Child guidance institutions usually offer integrated remedial programs including counseling, help in emotional problems and remedial instruction (e. g. Betz/Breuninger 1987). Unfortunately, there are no appropriate data to document the influence of each line. It would be of particular interest to find out whether successful remedial instruction has in itself a positive effect on the child's emotions and behavior.

4. Medical and Neurological Approaches

4.1. Ophthalmological Intervention

Although reading disability is defined as a condition without sensory dysfunction, some subtle visual perceptual problems may occur in reading disabled children. Binocular instability has been suggested as one possible disorder; unstable fixation degrades the visual stimulus and might thus interfere with reading (Stein/Fowler 1982). The argument that many good readers also show the same condition (Newman/Karle/Wadsworth et al. 1985) does not necessarily disprove the point, since unstable fixation might be compensated by superior linguistic skills. Occlusion of one eye has been proposed as a remedy for children with ocular instability. A positive effect has been claimed by Stein/Fowler (1985); however, the data are not entirely conclusive. Another alleged remedy in the visual domain is the use of a tinted overlay or tinted lenses. Reports of improved reading with this method are mainly anecdotal. However, there are two recent case studies which show a tremendous qualitative improvement in the children's reproduction of visual patterns with tinted overlays (Hannell/Gole/Dibden et al. 1991): Whereas the reproductions appear to be fairly normal under the condition of tinted overlays, the contours appear to be 'fuzzy' under normal viewing conditions. One of the children introspectively reported a 'furriness' in the perception of normal black and white print. The mechanism why tinted lenses should be helpful for some children is not yet clear; it is, however, known that tinted lenses slow the transmission of impulses along the primary visual pathway.

Eye-movements are another topic in the field of poor reader's visual perception. Extensive research in eye-movements has basically shown that deviant behavior in this domain is a by-product rather than a cause of reading disability (Pirozzolo 1983). Pavlidis' (1981) contradicting results have not been replicated (e. g. Olson/Kliegl/Davidson 1983). However, this chapter is not yet closed. Bassou/Pugh/Granie/Morucci (1991) have recently reported on divergent eye-movements during reading in some children, i. e. their eyes moved in different directions while reading. However, the authors are very cautious in interpreting their results. It is also open for questions what remedies could be developed if divergent eye-movements really would turn out to be a major stumbling block for reading disabled children. In any case, it seems that only a minority of reading disabled children are afflicted with visual-perceptual problems. Individual diagnoses are certainly indicated.

4.2. Pharmacotherapy

In the past decades the drug Ritalin had the reputation of improving reading disabled children's achievements. However, Gittelman/Klein/Feingold (1983) have shown convincingly that reading disabled children receiving both Ritalin and specific reading instruction perform no better on reading measures than a control group receiving specific reading instruction and a placebo. More recent studies investigated the effects of the drug Piracetam which is supposed to be a 'nootropic' drug, influencing specifically the 'higher' functions of the brain, particularly those which normally reside in the left cerebral hemisphere. It has also been hypothesized that it influences transcallosal transfer, but apparently there is no sound evidence for this assumption (Wilsher 1986). Some experimental studies show that Piracetam improves verbal short-term memory in normal adults (i. e. college students) (e. g. Dimond/Brouwers 1976). Thus it is not very surprising that in several well designed double blind studies the drug has also been shown to improve reading in reading disabled children (e. g. Conners/Reader 1987). However, although significant improvement on some reading measures was found in the experimental groups as compared to placebo control groups, the extent of the effects seems to be rather small and thus of questionable practical relevance. It is also not clear which cognitive processes are affected by the drug. It could be that children just performed better on a posttest; alternatively the effect could be attributable to more efficient learning at school. These questions might be answered by appropriate experimental designs.

4.3. Methods Related to Laterality

Delacato (1963) has been the main proponent of the idea that motor training — like throwing a ball — can promote a consistent lateral dominance and thereby improve reading and spelling in disabled children. This approach turned out to be a blind alley: Although the relationship between laterality in the sense of the functional differentiation of the two hemispheres and reading disability is still under discussion, there has been no sound evidence that motor training has any influence on reading and spelling (Arter/Jenkins 1979).

However, there has been a recent attempt to influence directly the two hemispheres' involvement in the reading task. Bakker/van Leeuwen/Spyer (1987) claim that they can accelerate slow readers' performance by flashing words to the left hemisphere and improve inaccurate but fast reading by flashing words to the right hemisphere. While the basic idea that the hemispheres contribute differentially to literacy is well taken, Bakker's et al. (1987) empirical evidence is not entirely conclusive due to the lack of convincing control groups.

5. Future Research

This chapter has reviewed a wide scope of remedial approaches. Empirical evaluation of the different methods has not been sufficient so far. Even in studies with adequate research designs the dependent variables are mostly too coarse; simple pre- and posttests using scores from reading or spelling tests as criterion give a clue as to the general efficiency of a program but do not convey any insight into the processes which were actually altered by the training. However, this insight is needed if programs are to be implemented successfully under conditions which do not exactly reproduce every single variable of the original research study. As a first step in understanding the actual learning processes, the children's reading and spelling problems should be analyzed in detail before training. Secondly, the programs should specify exactly what skill or partial process they intend to improve and hence predict which differential effects are expected. Differential prediction is not only important for the evaluation of a program but can also serve as support — or rejection — of the underlying theory.

6. References

Arter, J. A. & Jenkins, J. R. (1979). Differential diagnosis-prescriptive teaching: A critical appraisal. *Review of Educational Research, 49,* 517—555.

Axline, V. (1947). Nondirective therapy for poor readers. *Journal of Consulting Psychology, 11,* 61—69.

Bakker, D., van Leeuwen, H. M. P., & Spyer, G. (1987). Neuropsychological aspects of dyslexia. In D. Bakker, C. Wilsher, N. Debruyne, & N. Bertin (Eds.), *Developmental dyslexia and learning disorders. 30—39.* Basel: Karger.

Ball, E. W. & Blachman, B. A. (1988). Phoneme segmentation training: Effect on reading readiness. *Annals of Dyslexia, 38,* 208—225.

Ball, E. W. & Blachman, B. A. (1991). Does phoneme awareness training in kindergarten make a difference in early word recognition and developmental spelling? *Reading Research Quarterly, 26*, 50–66.

Balow, B., Fuchs, D., & Kasbohm, M. (1978). Teaching nonreaders to read: An evaluation of the Basic Skill Centers in Minneapolis. *Journal of Learning Disabilities, 11*, 351–354.

Bassou, L., Pugh, A. K., Granie, M., & Morucci, J. P. (1991). Binocular vision in reading: A study of the eye movements of ten year old children. Paper presented at the 7th European Conference on Reading. Edinburgh, Scotland, August 1991.

Bauer, R. H. (1979). Memory, acquisition, and category clustering in learning disabled children. *Journal of Experimental Child Psychology, 27*, 365–383.

Bauer, R. H. (1987). Control processes as a way of understanding, diagnosing, and remediating learning disabilities. In H. L. Swanson (Ed.), *Memory and learning disabilities: suppl. 2. Advances in learning and behavioral disabilities. 41–81.* Greenwich, CT: JAI Press.

Bauer, R. H. & Newman, D. R. (1991). Allocation of study time and recall by learning disabled children at different ages. *Journal of Experimental Child Psychology, 52*, 11–21.

Betz, D. & Breuninger, H. (1987). *Teufelskreis Lernstörungen.* Weinheim: Beltz.

Bosman, A. & de Groot, M. B. (1991). Differential effectiveness of reading and non-reading tasks in learning to spell. Paper presented at the 7th European Conference on Reading, Edinburgh, Scotland, August 1991.

van Bosch, K. (1991). *Poor reader's decoding skills. Effects of training, task and word characteristics.* Unpublished Ph.D. dissertation, Nijmegen, Netherlands.

Bradley, L. (1981). The organisation of motor patterns for spelling: An effective remedial strategy for backward readers. *Developmental Medicine & Child Neurology, 23*, 83–91.

Bradley, L. & Bryant, P. E. (1983). Categorizing sounds and learning to read: A causal connection. *Nature, 301*, 419–421.

Branwhite, A. B. (1983). Boosting reading skills by direct instruction. *British Journal of Educational Psychology, 53*, 291–298.

Breuninger, H. & Betz, D. (1989). Der Einsatz des Computers in der außerschulischen Lerntherapie. In I. M. Naegele & R. Valtin (Eds.), *LRS in den Klassen 1–10, 113–118.* Weinheim: Beltz.

Clarke, L. K. (1988). Invented vs. traditional spelling in first grader's writings. *Research in the Teaching of English, 22*, 281–309.

Coltheart, M. (Ed.) (1987). *The psychology of reading. Attention & Performance XII.* London: Lawrence Erlbaum.

Coltheart, M. (1989). Functional architecture of the language-processing system. In M. Coltheart, G. Sartori, & R. Job (Eds.), *The cognitive neuropsychology of language. 1–25.* London: Lawrence Erlbaum.

Conners, C. K. & Reader, M. (1987). The effects of piracetam on reading achievement and visual event-related potentials in dyslexic children. In D. J. Bakker, C. Wilsher, H. Debruyne, & N. Bertin (Eds.), *Developmental dyslexia and learning disorders: Diagnosis and treatment. 75–90.* Basel: Karger.

Content, A., Kolinsky, R., Morais, J. & Bertelson, P. (1986). Phonetic segmentation in prereaders: Effects of corrective information. *Journal of Experimental Child Psychology, 42*, 49–72.

Content, A., Morais, J., Alegria, J., & Bertelson, P. (1982). *Cahiers de Psychologie Cognitive, 2*, 259–269.

Cunningham, A. E. (1990). Explicit versus implicit instruction in phonemic awareness. *Journal of Experimental Child Psychology, 50*, 429-444.

Dallago, M. & Moely, B. E. (1980). Free recall in boys of normal and poor reading levels as a function of task manipulations. *Journal of Experimental Child Psychology, 30*, 62-78.

Delacato, C. (1963). *The diagnosis and treatment of speech and reading problems.* Springfield, Ill.: Thomas.

Dimond, S. J. & Brouwers, E. Y. M. (1976). Improvement of human memory through the use of drugs. *Psychopharmacology, 49*, 307–309.

Downing, J. (1979). *Reading and reasoning.* Edinburgh: Chambers/ NewYork: Springer Verlag.

Dummer, L. & Hackethal, R. (1984). *Handbuch zum Kieler Leseaufbau.* Kiel: Veris Verlag.

Edler, M., Ostrau, R., & Schulze, K. (1978). *Rechtschreibtraining mit Legasthenikern.* Unpublished Diplom-Thesis, Ruhr-Universität Bochum, Germany.

Ehri, L. (1987). Learning to read and spell words. *Journal of Reading Behavior, 19*, 5–31.

Elkonin, D. B. (1973). The psychology of mastering the elements of reading. In B. Simon & J. Simon (Eds.), *Educational psychology in the U.S.S.R. 165–179.* London: Routledge & Kegan Paul.

Fernald, G. (1943). *Remedial techniques in basic school subjects.* New York: McGraw Hill.

Fiedorowicz, C. A. M. (1986). Training of component reading skills. *Annals of Dyslexia, 36*, 318–334.

Fox, B. & Routh, D. K. (1984). Phonemic analysis and synthesis as word attack skills: Revisited. *Journal of Educational Psychology, 76*, 1059–1061.

Frith, U. (1985). Beneath the surface of developmental dyslexia. In K. E. Patterson, J. C. Marshall, & M. Coltheart (Eds.), *Surface dyslexia. 301–330.* Hillsdale, N. J.: Lawrence Erlbaum.

Frostig, M. & Horne, D. (1964). *The Frostig program for the development of visual perception: Teacher's guide*. Chicago: Follett.

Gibson, E., Shurcliff, A., & Yonas, A. (1970). Utilization of spelling patterns by deaf and hearing subjects. In H. Levin & J. Williams (Eds.), *Basic studies on reading. 57–73*. New York: Basic Books.

Gillingham, A. & Stillman, B.W. (1956). *Remedial training for children with specific disability in reading, spelling, and penmanship*. Cambridge, Mass.: Educators Publishing Service.

Gittelmann, R., Klein, D. F., & Feingold, I. (1983). Children with reading disorders – II. Effects of methylpheniate in combination with reading remediation. *Journal of Child Psychology and Psychiatry, 24*, 193–212.

Glushko, R. J. (1979). The organization and activation of orthographic knowledge in reading aloud. *Journal of Experimental Psychology: Human Perception and Performance, 5*, 674–691.

Goswami, U. (1986). Children's use of analogy in learning to read: A developmental study. *Journal of Experimental Child Psychology, 42*, 73–83.

Guthrie, J.T. & Seifert, M. (1977). Letter-sound complexity in learning to identify words. *Journal of Educational Psychology, 69*, 686–696.

Hagen, J.W., Hargrave, S., & Ross, W. (1973). Prompting and rehearsal in short-term memory. *Child Development, 44*, 201–204.

Hagen, J.W., Jongeward, R.H., & Kail, R.V. (1975). Cognitive perspectives on the development of memory. In H.W. Reese (Ed.), *Advances in Child Development and Behavior, 10*, 57–101.

Hannell, G., Gole, G. A., Dibden, S. N., Rooney, K. F., & Pidgeon, K.J. (1991). Reading improvement with tinted lenses: a report of two cases. *Journal of Research in Reading, 14*, 56–71.

Hasselbring, T. S. (1982). Remediating spelling problems of learning-handicapped students through the use of microcomputers. *Educational technology, 22(4)*, 31–32.

Hildreth, G. H. (1965). Experience related reading for school beginners. *Elementary English, 42*, 280–297.

Hohn, W. & Ehri, L. (1983). Do alphabet letters help prereaders acquire phonemic segmentation skills? *Journal of Educational Psychology, 75*, 751–762.

Hornsby, B. & Miles, T. R. (1980). The effects of a dyslexia-centered teaching programme. *British Journal of Educational Psychology, 50*, 236–242.

Hulme, C. (1981). *Reading retardation and multisensory teaching*. London: Routledge & Kegan Paul.

Hulme, C. & Bradley, L. (1984). An experimental study of multi-sensory teaching with normal and retarded readers. In R. N. Malatesha & H. A. Whitaker (Eds.), *Dyslexia: A global issue. 431–443*. The Hague: Martinus Nijhoff.

Kamhi, A. G. & Catts, H.W. (Eds.) (1989). *Reading disabilities: A developmental language perspective*. Boston: College-Hill.

Kauffman, J. M., Hallahan, P., Haas, K. Brame, T., & Boren, R. (1978). Imitating children's errors to improve their spelling performance. *Journal of Learning Disabilities, 11*, 217–222.

Kephart, N. C. (1960). *The slow learner in the classroom*. Columbus: Merrill Publishing Company.

Kerr, M. M. & Lambert, D. L. (1982). Behavior modification of children's written language. *Progress in Behavior Modification, 13*, 79–108.

Kerstholt, M., van Bon, W., & Schreuder, R. (1991). Training in phonemic segmentation: The effect of alphabet letters as visual support. Paper presented at the 7th European Conference on Reading, August 1991, Edinburgh, Scotland.

Kossow, H.-J. (1972). *Zur Therapie der Lese- und Rechtschreibschwäche*. Berlin: Deutscher Verlag der Wissenschaften.

Larsen, S. C. & Hammill, D. D. (1975). The relationship of selected visual-perceptual abilities to school learning. *Journal of Special Education, 9*, 281–291.

Lenz, M., Singh, N. N., & Hewett, A. E. (1991). Overcorrection as an academic remediation procedure. *Behavior Modification, 15*, 64–73.

Levin, A., Boruta, M. J., & Vasconcellos, M.T. (1983). Microcomputer-based environments for writing: A writer's assistant. In A. C. Wilkinson (Ed.), *Classroom computers and cognitive science, 219–223*. New York: Academic Press.

Lewis, R. B. (1983). Learning disabilities and reading: Instructional recommendations from current research. *Exceptional Children, 50*, 230–240.

Lewkowicz, N. K. (1980). Phonemic awareness training: What to teach and how to teach it. *Journal of Educational Psychology, 72*, 686–700.

Lewkowicz, N. K. & Low L.Y. (1979). Effect of visual aids and word structure on phonemic segmentation. *Contemporary Educational Psychology, 4*, 238–252.

Liberman, I. Y., Shankweiler, D., Liberman, A. M., Fowler, C., & Fischer, F. W. (1977). Phonetic segmentation and recoding in the beginning reader. In A. S. Reber & D. L. Scarborough (Eds.), *Towards a psychology of reading. 207–225*. New York: Wiley.

Lie, A. (1991). Effects of a training program for stimulating skills in words analysis in first-grade children. *Reading Research Quarterly, 26*, 234–250.

Lovett, M.W., Ransby, M. J., & Barron, R.W. (1988). Treatment, subtype, and word type effect in dyslexic children's response to remediation. *Brain & Language, 34*, 328–349.

Lundberg, I., Frost, J., & Petersen, O. (1988). Effects of an extensive program for stimulation phonological awareness in preschool children. *Reading Research Quarterly*, *23*, 263–284.

Machemer, P. (1972). Entwicklung eines Übungsprogramms für Eltern zur Behandlung von Legasthenikern nach verhaltenstherapeutischem Modell. *Schule und Psychologie*, *19*, 336–346.

Manis, F. R. & Morrison, F. J. (1985). Reading disability: A deficit in rule learning. In L. S. Siegel & F. J. Morrison (Eds.), *Cognitive development in atypical children*. *1–26*. New York: Springer.

Mannhaupt, G. (1990). *Strategieausbildung zur Lautstrukturanalyse mit Hilfe von abstrakten oder konkreten Symbolen während des frühen Schriftspracherwerbs*. Ph. D. Dissertation. Universität Bielefeld, Germany.

Marsh, G., Friedman, M., Welch, V., & Desberg, P. (1981). A cognitive-developmental theory of reading acquisition. In G. E. Mackinnon & T. G. Waller (Eds.), *Reading research: Advances in theory and practice*, *55–141*. New York: Academic Press.

Meichenbaum, D. H. & Goodman, J. (1969). Training impulsive children to talk to themselves: A means of developing self-control. *Journal of Abnormal Psychology*, *77*, 115–126.

Montessori, M. (1913). *Selbstätige Erziehung im frühen Kindesalter*. Stuttgart: Julius Hoffmann.

Morais, J., Alegria, J., & Content, A. (1987). The relationships between segmental analysis and alphabetic literacy: An interactive view. *Cahiers de Psychologie Cognitive*, *7*, 415–438.

Morrison, F. J. & Manis, F. R. (1982). Cognitive processes and reading disability: A critique and proposal. In C. J. Brainerd & M. Pressley (Eds.), *Verbal processes in children*, *59–93*. New York: Springer-Verlag.

Murphy, J. F., Hern, C. L., Williams, R. L., & McLaughlin, T. F. (1990). The effects of the copy, cover, compare approach in increasing spelling accuracy with learning disabled students. *Contemporary Educational Psychology*, *15*, 378–386.

Neisser, U. (1967). *Cognitive psychology*, New York: Appleton-Century-Crofts.

Newman, S. P., Karle, H., Wadsworth, J. F., Archer, R. Hockly, R., & Rogers, P. (1985). Ocular dominance, reading and spelling: A reassessment of a measure associated with specific reading difficulties. *Journal of Research in Reading*, *8*, 127–138.

Olson, R. K., Kliegl, R., & Davidson, B.J. (1983). Eye movements in reading disability. In K. Rayner (Ed.), *Eye movements in reading*, *457–479*. New York: Academic Press.

Ornstein, P. A. (Ed.), *Memory development in children*. Hillsdale, N. J.: Erlbaum 1978.

Ornstein, R. A. & Naus, M. J. (1978). Rehearsal processes in children's memory. In P. A. Ornstein (Ed.), *Memory development in children*, *69–99*. Hillsdale, N. J.: Erlbaum 1978.

Orton, S. T. (1937). *Reading, writing and speech problems in children*. New York: Norton.

Paivio, A. (1971). *Imagery and verbal processes*. New York: Holt, Rinehart and Winston.

Pavlidis, G. T. (1981). Do eye-movements hold the key to dyslexia? *Neuropsychologia*, *19*, 57–64.

Pirozzolo, F. J. (1983). Eye movements and reading disability. In K. Rayner (Ed.). *Eye movements in reading*, *499–521*. New York: Academic Press.

Read, C. (1986). *Children's creative spelling*. London, Boston & Henley: Routledge & Kegan Paul.

Reitsma, P. & Dongelmans, J. (1988). Het effect van oefeningen met wisselrijen voor leeszwakke kinderen. *Tijdschrift voor Orthopedagogiek*, *27*, 248–265.

Reuter, P. E. (1977). Legasthenie– eine Verhaltensstörung? *Praxis der Kinderpsychologie und Kinderpsychiatrie*, *26*, 254–265.

Rosner, J. (1971). *Phonic analysis training and beginning reading skills*. Pittsburgh Learning Research and Development Center Publication Series, No. 9.

Rozin, P. & Gleitman, L. R. (1977). The structure and acquisition of reading II: The reading process and the acquisition of the alphabetic principle. In A. S. Reber & D. L. Scarborough (Eds.), *Towards a psychology of reading*, *55–141*. Hillsdale, N. J.: Lawrence Erlbaum.

Sabatino, D. A. (1973). Auditory perception: Development, assessment and intervention. In L. Mann & D. A. Sabatino (Eds.), *The first review of special education*. Philadelphia. Buttonwood Farms.

Sawyer, D. J. (1988). Studies of the effects of teaching auditory segmenting skills within the reading program. In R. L. Masland & M.W. Masland (Eds.), *Preschool prevention of reading failure*, *121–142*. Parkton, Md: York Press.

Scheerer-Neumann, G. (1979). *Intervention bei Lese-Rechtschreibschwäche*. Bochum: Kamp.

Scheerer-Neumann, G. (1981). The utilization of intraword structure in poor readers: Experimental evidence and a training programme. *Psychological Research*, *43*, 155–178.

Scheerer-Neumann, G. (1986a). Sprechen, Denken und Rechtschreiben. *Grundschule*, *18/6*, 20–24.

Scheerer-Neumann, G. (1986b). Wortspezifisch JA – Wortbild NEIN. Ein letztes Lebewohl an die Wortbildtheorie. Teil 1.: Rechtschreiben. In H. Brügelmann (Ed.), *ABC und Schriftsprache – Rätsel für Kinder, Lehrer und Forscher*, *171–185*. Konstanz: Faude Verlag.

Scheerer-Neumann, G. (1988). *Rechtschreibtraining mit rechtschreibschwachen Hauptschülern auf kognitionspsychologischer Grundlage: Eine empirische Untersuchung*. Opladen: Westdeutscher Verlag.

Scheerer-Neumann, G., Ahola, H., König, U., & Reckermann, U. (1978). Die Ausnutzung der sprachlichen Redundanz bei leseschwachen Kindern: I. Nachweis des spezifischen Defizits. *Zeitschrift für Entwicklungspsychologie und Pädagogische Psychologie 10*, 35–48.

Schreuder, R. & van Bon, W. H. J. (1989). Phonemic analysis: effect of word properties. *Journal of Research in Reading, 12*, 59–78.

Seidenberg, M. S. (1987). Sublexical structures in visual word recognition: Access units or orthographic redundancy? In M. Coltheart (Ed.). *Attention and Performance 12, 245–263*. Hillsdale, N. J.: Lawrence Erlbaum.

Seidenberg, M. S. & McClelland, J. L. (1989). A distributed, development model of word recognition and naming. *Psychological Review, 96*, 523–568.

Seymour, P. H. K. & McGregor, C. J. (1984). Developmental dyslexia: A cognitive developmental analysis of phonological, morphemic, and visual impairments. *Cognitive Neuropsychology, 1*, 43–82.

Siemens, H. (1985). Die Morphem-Methode – ein Überblick. In M. Bergk & K. Meiers (Eds.), *Schulanfang ohne Fibeltrott, 166–178*. Bad Heilbrunn: Klinkhardt.

Silberberg, N. & Silberberg, M. (1969). Myths in remedial education. *Journal of Learning Disabilities, 2*, 209–217.

Skjelford, V. (1976). Teaching children to segment spoken words as an aid in learning to read. *Journal of Learning Disabilities, 9*, 297–306.

Stahl, S. A. & Miller, P. D. (1988). Whole language experience approaches for beginning reading: A quantitative research synthesis. *Review of Educational Research, 59*, 87–116.

Stein, J. F. & Fowler, S. (1982). Ocular motor dyslexia. *Dyslexia Review, 5*, 25–28.

Stein, J. F. & Fowler, S. (1985). Effect of monocular occlusion on visuomotor perception and reading in dyslexic children. *Lancet, July 13*, 69–73.

Taft, M. (1979). Lexical access via an orthographic code: The basic orthographic syllable structure (BOSS). *Journal of Verbal Learning and Verbal Behavior, 18*, 21–39.

Taft, M. (1987). Morphographic processing: The BOSS re-emerges. In M. Coltheart (Ed.), *Attention and Performance 12, 265–279*. Hillsdale, N.J.: Lawrence Erlbaum.

Thomson, M. (1988). Preliminary findings concerning the effects of specialized teaching on dyslexic children. *Applied Cognitive Psychology, 2*, 19–31.

Tornéus, M. (1984) Phonological awareness and reading: A chicken and egg problem? *Journal of Educational Psychology, 76*, 1346–1358.

Treiman, R. & Baron, J. (1983). Phonemic-analysis training helps children benefit from spelling-sound rules. *Memory & Cognition, 11*, 382–389.

Vellutino, F. R. & Scanlon, D. M. (1984). Phonological coding, phonological awareness, and reading ability: Evidence from a longitudinal and experimental study. *Merrill-Palmer Quarterly, 33*, 321–363.

Wagner, R. & Torgeson, J. (1987). The nature of phonological processing and its causal role in the acquisition of reading skills. *Psychological Bulletin, 101*, 192–212.

Wallach, M. A. & Wallach, L. (1979). Helping disadvantaged children learn to read by teaching them phoneme identification skills. In L. B. Resnick & P. A. Weaver (Eds.), *Theory and practice of early reading. Vol. 3. 197–215*. Hillsdale, N. J.: Lawrence Erlbaum.

Williams, J. (1979). The ABD's of reading: A program for the learning disabled. In L. B. Resnick & P. A. Weaver (Eds.), *Theory and practice of early reading, vol. 3. 179–195*. Hillsdale, N. J.; Lawrence Erlbaum.

Wilsher, C. R. (1986). Developmental dyslexia and the nootropic concept. *Early Child Development and Care, 26*, 207–228.

Wise, B., Olson, R., & Treiman, R. (1990). Subsyllabic units as aids in beginning reader's word learning: Onsetrime versus post-vowel segmentation. *Journal of Experimental Child Psychology, 49*, 1–19.

Gerheid Scheerer-Neumann, Bielefeld (Germany)

74. Hyperlexia and Precocious Reading

1. Definitions and Issues

Since the introduction of the term 'hyperlexia' to the psychological literature over two decades ago, the consensus definition of this condition has been: precocious and uninstructed reading recognition ability, emerging in the preschool years and appearing in the context of delayed or disordered cognitive and language functioning (e. g., Welsh/Pennington/Rogers 1987). Ironically, the original term coined by Silberberg/Silberberg (1967) did not include the criterion of cognitive or behavioral disorder, although more than half of their original subject sample did manifest some condition suggesting cerebral dysfunction (Silberberg/Silberberg 1967). The authors proposed that exceptional word decoding skills may be an example of a physiological variant (Hallgren 1950) that distributes normally across the population and varies independently from other normal variants, such as intelligence. However, the majority of studies on hyperlexia have not adequately tested the Silbergs' proposal by examining this isolated precocity in a range of both typical and atypical populations of children.

The vast majority of research and clinical case reports exploring the phenomenon of hyperlexia have involved children whose reading proficiency is concomitant with some form of behavioral pathology. This approach dove-tailed with an early and influential literature on savant and 'splinter' skills in the severely retarded (Bergman/Escalona 1948; Eisenberg/Kanner 1956; Kanner 1943; Mahler/Elkisch 1953; Parker 1919; Philipps 1930). There is, after all, a strong motivation to understand the remarkable achievement of a mentally-retarded, noncommunicative, autistic child who exhibits an 'island of ability' with regarded to word decoding skills. The phenomenon in which reading recognition far outstrips comprehension and general intelligence is obviously more salient in the context of cognitive impairment, and thus, the burgeoning research literature became dominated with studies of children with a variety of diagnoses, such as autism or 'autistic features', hyperactivity, language and speech disorders or childhood schizophrenia (Aram/Rose/Horwitz 1984; Cobrinick 1974; 1982; Elliot/Needleman 1976; Fontenelle/Alarcon 1982; Frith/Snowling 1983; Goldberg/Rothermel 1984; Graziani/Brodsky/Mason/Zager 1983; Healy/Aram/Horwitz/Kessler 1982; Huttenlocher/Huttenlocher 1973; Mehegan/Dreifuss 1972; Richman/Kitchell 1981; Siegel 1984; Silberberg/Silberberg, 1967; 1971; Snowling/Frith 1986; Welsh/Pennington/Rogers 1987; Whitehouse/Harris 1984).

Irrespective of the substantial overlap between autism and hyperlexia (Whitehouse/Harris 1984), precocious reading is clearly not a pathognomonic sign of autism (Cobrinick 1982), nor is the behavior restricted to this diagnosis. Snowling/Frith (1986) recently concluded that hyperlexia was not a syndrome-specific phenomenon after finding that both autistic and nonautistic mentally retarded children exhibited a similar decoding precocity and comprehension deficit. Whereas all of the studies cited above, excepting one (Richman/Kitchell 1981), included at least some low-IQ children in their samples, it is also the case that the range of IQ scores represented in many subject samples is quite broad. For example, in the Whitehouse/Harris (1984) sample of 20 autistic children who exhibited precocious reading, the IQ scores ranged from 20 to 144! The wide range of psychological disorders and IQ levels represented in the hyperlexia literature may support a plasticity view of the condition (Bender 1966), in which accelerated word recognition skill is dissociated from the other cognitive and language impairments resulting from various forms of brain dysfunction.

Thus, we have a situation in which most of the research regarding hyperlexia involves behaviorally and/or intellectually impaired children. However, the phenomenon is observed in a variety of clinical syndromes and across a broad band of intellectual function. There has been much theoretical debate as to the connection between hyperlexia and developmental dyslexia (e. g., DeHirsch 1971; McClure/Hynd 1983), as well as evidence suggesting similarities in the reading processes utilized by hyperlexic readers and individuals with the acquired syndrome of surface dyslexia (Aram/Rose/Horwitz 1984; Welsh/Pennington/Rogers 1987). However, there has been a general lack of integration of the respective literatures involving hyperlexia and normal precocious reading. This chapter will explore possible parallels between the reading behaviors exhibited by 'classic' hyperlexics and by developmentally normal precocious readers. By building a bridge between the two separate literatures, one can begin to address whether the word decoding facility observed in hyperlexic children is also exhibited by behaviorally normal children, suggesting that this precocity is not a symptom of pathology. Documenting the existence of accelerated word decoding skills in a wide range of children will have implications for the normal physiological variant position of Silberberg/Silberberg (1971).

2. Mechanisms Underlying Hyperlexic Reading

The recent empirical literature examining hyperlexia can be characterized as falling into two 'camps' with regard to the mechanisms hypothesized to underlie the condition. One position emphasizes the cognitive impairments characterizing hyperlexia, such as the absence of an internal organizing framework to guide text comprehension. A second position suggests that hyperlexia represents accelerated cognitive skills in the areas of visual and/or auditory memory or phonological processing. Neither framework alone has generated a complete description of the full range of cognitive strengths and weaknesses characteristic of hyperlexic.

The comprehension deficit has been attributed to deficiencies in the ability to structure, categorize and associate the semantic and syntactic information necessary for meaningful processing (Fontenelle/Alarcon 1982; Healy/Aram/Horwitz/Kessler 1982; Huttenlocher/Huttenlocher 1973; Richman/Kitchell 1981; Snowling/Frith 1986). For example, Healy/Aram/Horwitz/Kessler (1982) interpreted the data as reflecting a lack of interaction between the 'bottom-up' perceptual decoding skills and 'top-down' conceptual processing to give text meaning. Similarly, Snowling/Frith (1986) found that retarded hyperlexic children exhibited comprehension deficits that reflected ineffective use of sentence context and generally poor metacognitive skill. Overall, the studies focusing on cognitive weaknesses view hyperlexia as a deficit condition rather than as a precocity and, with few exceptions (e.g., Healy/Aram/Horwitz/Kessler 1982) in-depth investigations of 'bottom-up' decoding skills have been lacking.

Research examining the strengths of the hyperlexic reader originally evaluated the proposal that superior single-word reading resulted from advanced memory abilities for unrelated auditory and visual stimuli (Cain 1969; Goodman 1972) that have been observed in some hyperlexic children. In this research, word recognition was generally interpreted as rote memory for the visual gestalt or total configuration of the word (Cobrinick 1974; 1982; DeHirsch 1971; Elliot/Needleman 1976; Fontenelle/Alarcon 1982), rather than the result of decoding individual graphemic units.

However, this exclusive visual memory interpretation has been compromised by recent evidence demonstrating that reading is guided to a large extent by grapheme-phoneme correspondence (GPC) rules. Evidence of GPC rule use derives from studies demonstrating adequate, and even advanced, nonword reading in hyperlexic children (Frith/Snowling 1983; Goldberg/Rothermel 1984; Healy/Aram/Horwitz/Kessler 1982; Siegel 1984; Welsh/Pennington/Rogers 1987). Moreover, hyperlexic children often are more accurate reading 'regular' words that correspond to GPC rules than 'irregular' words that violate these rules (Aram/Rose/Horwitz 1984; Welsh/Pennington/Rogers 1987), suggesting a greater reliance on phonological decoding of words than on direct access to the lexicon (Welsh/Pennington/Rogers 1987). An empirical question requiring further examination is the degree to which superior visual and auditory memory abilities contribute to the development of an effective GPC rule system in these children.

Clarification regarding the areas of reading-related strength and weakness in hyperlexic children can be achieved by using general intelligence as a baseline for expected reading achievement. Given this approach, it appears that reading recognition, as defined by single word reading, is a relative strength as compared to general intelligence. This exceptional word decoding performance appears to be facilitated by precious and advanced phonological processing according to GPC rules. In contrast, single-word reading comprehension is generally commensurate with IQ and, therefore, is not a specific deficit per se. When reading comprehension of hyperlexic children has been found to be a specific area of weakness, comprehension has been evaluated with connected discourse requiring the effective use of an intact knowledge base, metacognitive control processes and other topdown strategies (e. g., Snowling/Frith 1986). It is certainly possible that reading comprehension of single words is limited by the child's general intellectual level; whereas, the additional demands of integrating prose stresses the fragile system and limits comprehension skills to an even greater degree.

It must be noted that there is still a lack of agreement as to the reading profile that best defines the phenomenon of hyperlexia. Both McClure/Hynd (1983) and Snowling/Frith (1986) have suggested that 'true' hyperlexia' be reserved for those children exhibiting advanced word decoding and impaired comprehension in relation to IQ. Irrespective of the currently unresolved nosological issues, a consistent theme emerging from the study of hyperlexia is the apparent functional dissociation between the phonological and semantic processing systems underlying reading (Snowling/Frith 1986; Welsh/Pennington/Rogers 1987). The independence of cognitive mechanisms underlying reading is consistent with current models of reading (Perfetti 1985) and this theoretical proposal has been supported by the descriptions of reading behavior in acquired brain lesion cases (Patterson/Marshall/Coltheart 1986).

3. Parallels with Normal Precocious Reading

For years there have been anecdotal reports by parents and educators of early reading observed in normal children (Torrey 1973), as well as curriculum-based studies of preschool readers in the education literature (Durkin 1970). In an unselected group of four-year-olds attending a university-operated preschool, Mason (1980) found that the largest percentages of children read words through the use of nonlinguistic context or through visual recognition of very frequent words. By far, the smallest category of children employed what Mason called letter-sound analysis in which multisyllabic words were read through accurate phonological decoding. Interestingly, it is just this skill that appears to be accelerated in hyperlexic readers in spite of concomitant behavioral and/or intellectual impairments.

To date, the most systematic program of research on normal children who read precociously has been conducted by Jackson and her colleagues (Jackson/Biemiller 1985; Jackson/Donaldson/Cleland 1988; Mills/Jackson 1989). This research has evaluated the specific reading-related skills and more general cognitive patterns exhibited by a group of kindergarten children identified by their teachers as advanced readers. Essentially, teachers were asked to nominate children that they thought were reading at or above the third-grade level. It is important to note that the term 'reading' referred to reading comprehension, as well as reading recognition. Thus, there is a subjective difference between most research on hyperlexia and these studies of precocious reading; the former usually defines advanced reading in terms of word recognition alone, while the latter focuses on reading with comprehension.

Nonetheless, the findings of this set of studies provide interesting points of comparison with the data base on hyperlexic reading, and together the two research domains have important implications for theories of normal reading acquisition and development. Jackson (Jackson/Biemiller 1985; Jackson/Donaldson/Cleland 1988) found that efficiency in lower-order skills, such as letter identification speed and phonological decoding, were facilitative of early reading, but not necessarily a prerequisite. In fact, the authors concluded that no single lower-order skill was responsible for reading precocity, and instead, overall verbal ability, a superior knowledge base, and metacognitive strategies may contribute to reading success. Many of their findings converged on the notion that the strengths of these precocious readers were top-down executive abilities that effectively utilized the bottom-up perceptual information in the text. In a follow-up study of these children at 10 to 12 years, Mills/Jackson (1989) found that it was general verbal ability that was as good a predictor of current reading comprehension as early reading-related skills. Although as a group the precocious readers were advanced in both lower-level perceptual skills and higher-level conceptual strategies, within-group analyses found these reading processes to be uncorrelated.

How do these findings regarding normal precocious reading compare and contrast with the characterization of hyperlexic readers in the clinical literature? One important similarity is that both literature provide empirical support for the independence of different systems underlying reading. Specifically, phonological skills and semantic skills appear to function relatively independently of each other in both developmentally normal readers and clinically diagnosed hyperlexics. In addition, both samples of readers exhibit a dissociation of GPC decoding ability from overall intelligence and/or verbal ability (Jackson/Butterfield 1986). Therefore, both literatures support the notion first advanced by Silberberg/Silberberg (1967): word decoding may represent a normal physiological variant that distributes independently of other normal variants such as IQ. Given that a superiority in word decoding has been found in such diverse clinical populations as the mentally retarded, autistic, language disabled, as well as in behaviorally normal children, this precocity is clearly not a pathognomonic marker of any one clinical condition, nor does it appear to be symptomatic of general neurological dysfunction.

A key difference between the literatures that limits direct comparison lies in the definition of precocious reading. Normal early readers were advanced in both reading comprehension and word decoding, and these precocities were in relation to age and not to intelligence. The sample of children studied by Jackson and colleagues had an average IQ of 128 and, thus, comprehension and decoding skills at the third grade level did not represent a striking deviation from intelligence. For example, the estimates of mental age for verbal intelligence and for reading comprehension were nearly equivalent in this kindergarten group. In contrast, hyperlexic readers have frequently been found to exhibit decoding skills that far exceed their general or verbal IQ levels. However, like precocious readers, their reading comprehension scores are generally commensurate with intelligence.

A second point of divergence between the two reading groups involves the degree to which top-down processes deriving from an intact knowledge base and metacognitive strategies aid the development of advanced reading skills. In the case of precocious readers, it appears that a 'good balance' between top-down integrative processes and bottom-up perceptual processes is most responsible for their advanced reading levels (Jackson/Biemiller 1985). In fact, it may general verbal ability that contributes most to continued success in reading in the later school years (Mills/Jackson 1989). This stands in striking contrast to the typical characterization of the hyperlexic child in which bottom-up and top-down reading skills may fail to interact at all to give text meaning (Healy/Aram/Horwitz/Kessler 1982). Clearly, the strong suit for hyperlexic readers is word decoding according to GPC rules, and not strategic use of text context and knowledge base, as has been found for normal precocious readers. However, recall that the criterion for advanced reading is often different for these two groups of advanced readers. Given that superior reading recognition with comprehension is typical of the normal precocious reader, it is not surprising that top-down processes would play a more prominent role.

4. Conclusions

Thus, two themes have emerged from this review of the hyperlexia and precocious reading literatures. First, it appears that underlying reading mechanisms can function relatively independently from one another and from general intelligence, and that word decoding in particular may be a modular skill that represents a physiological variant (Silberberg/Silberberg 1967). Second, as traditionally studied, hyperlexic children with concomitant clinical conditions and developmentally normal precocious readers differ with regard to the relative contributions to superior reading of bottom-up perceptual processes and top-down semantic processes.

This chapter will close with a brief description of one study conducted in our laboratory that provides an interesting bridge between the hyperlexia and precocious reading literatures. Pennington/Johnson/Welsh (1987) conducted a case study of a child with superior intelligence and no signs of autism or neurological dysfunction who, nevertheless, exhibited precocious, uninstructed reading prior to age 3. The child's reading strengths and weakness in relation to IQ were examined with many of the same measures used by Welsh/Pennington/Rogers (1987) to study autistic hyperlexic readers, facilitating a direct comparison of performance profiles. Like the precocious readers studied by Jackson and others, this subject had above-average intellectual endowment and reading comprehension commensurate with this ability level. However, unlike the precocious readers, this child did not exhibit a particular strength in conceptual, integrative, or metacognitive skills. Instead, this subject demonstrated an outstanding ability to decode words according to GPC rules that far exceeded general intelligence, similar to the autistic hyperlexic readers studied by Welsh/Pennington/Rogers (1987). Thus, again there is evidence for a dissociation between word decoding mechanisms and general ability in a behaviorally normal child. This precocity far outstripped other above-average intellectual and reading-related skills, but was not in itself a sign of behavioral pathology, neurological dysfunction, or language disorder as some have suggested (e. g., DeHirsch 1971; McClure/Hynd 1983; Richman/Kitchell 1981; Snowling/Frith 1986).

In conclusion, the continued exploration of hyperlexic reading in a variety of clinical and nonclinical samples should provide important insights regarding the typical and atypical course of reading acquisition and development. A promising avenue for future research would be the application of similar criteria and methodologies for the study of advanced reading in both clinical and nonclinical samples of precocious readers. At present, there is a lack of convergence and integration between the research programs exploring hyperlexia and normal precocious reading, although the apparent parallels in the underlying processes and mechanisms would seem to warrant such a collaboration in the future.

5. References

Aram, D. M., Rose, D. F., & Horwitz, S. J. (1984). Developmental reading without meaning. In R. M. Malatesha & H. A. Whitaker (Eds.), *Dyslexia: A global issue. 517–531.* Nato ASI Series.

Bender, L. (1966). The concept of plasticity in childhood schizophrenia. In P. H. Hoch & J. Zubin (Eds.), *Psychopathology of schizophrenia. 354–365.* New York: Grune & Stratton.

Bergman, P. & Escalona, S. (1948). Unusual sensitivities in very young children. *Psychoanalytic study of the child.* New York: International University Press, V. 3 and 4.

Cain, A. C. (1969). Special "isolated" abilities in severely psychotic young children. *Psychiatry, 32,* 137–149.

Cobrinick, L. (1974). Unusual reading ability in severely disturbed children: Clinical observations and a retrospective inquiry. *Journal of Autism and Childhood Schizophrenia, 4,* 163–175.

Cobrinick, L. (1982). The performance of hyperlexic children on an "incomplete words" task. *Neuropsychologia, 20,* 569–577.

DeHirsch, K. (1971). Are hyperlexics dyslexics? *The Journal of Special Education, 5,* 243–245.

Durkin, D. (1970). A language arts program of pre-first grade children: two-year achievement report. *Reading Research Quarterly, 4,* 543–565.

Eisenberg, L. & Kanner, L. (1956). Early infantile autism, 1943–1955. *American Journal of Orthopsychiatry, 26,* 556–566.

Elliot, D. E. & Needleman, R. M. (1976). The syndrome of hyperlexia. *Brain and Language, 3,* 339–349.

Fontenelle, S. & Alarcon, M. (1982). Hyperlexia: Precocious word recognition in developmentally delayed children. *Perceptual and Motor Skills, 55,* 247–252.

Frith, U. & Snowling, M. (1983). Reading for meaning and reading for sound in autistic and dyslexic children. *British Journal of Developmental Psychology, 1,* 329–342.

Goldberg, T. E. & Rothermel, R. D. (1984). Hyperlexic children reading. *Brain, 107,* 759–785.

Goodman, J. (1972). A case of an "autistic savant": Mental function in the psychotic child with markedly disrepant abilities. *Journal of Child Psychology, Psychiatry, 13,* 267–273.

Graziani, L. J., Brodsky, K., Mason, J. C., & Zager, R. P. (1983). Variability in IQ scores and prognosis of children with hyperlexia. *American Academy of Child Psychiatry, 22,* 441–443.

Hallgren, B. (1950). Specific dyslexia: A clinical and genetic study. *Acta Psychiatrica et Neurologica,* Supplement 65.

Healy, J. M., Aram, D. M., Horwitz, S. J., & Kessler, J. W. (1982). A study of hyperlexia. *Brain and Language, 17,* 1–23.

Huttenlocher, P. R. & Huttenlocher, J. (1973). A study of children with hyperlexia. *Neurology, 23,* 1107–1116.

Jackson, N. E. & Biemiller, A. J. (1985). Letter, word, and text reading times of precocious and average readers. *Child Development, 56,* 196–206.

Jackson, N. E. & Butterfield, E. C. (1986). A conception of giftedness designed to promote research. In R. J. Sternberg & J. E. Davidson (Eds.), *Conceptions of giftedness. 151–181.* New York: Cambridge University Press.

Jackson, N. E., Donaldsen, G. W., & Cleland, L. N. (1988). The structure of precocious reading ability. *Journal of Educational Psychology, 80,* 234–243.

Kanner, L. (1943). Autistic disturbances of affective contact. *Nervous Child, 21,* 217–250.

Mahler, M. S. & Elkisch, P. (1953). Some observations on disturbances of the ego in a case of infantile psychosis. *Psychoanalytic study of the child.* New York: International University Press, V. 8.

Mason, J. M. (1980). When do children begin to read: An exploration of four year old children's letter and word reading competencies. *Reading Research Quarterly, 2,* 203–227.

McClure, P. H. & Hynd, G. W. (1983). Is hyperlexia a severe reading disorder or a symptom of psychiatric disturbance? Nosological considerations. *Clinical Neuropsychology, 5,* 145–149.

Mehegan, C. C. & Dreifuss, F. E. (1972). Exceptional reading ability in brain damaged children. *Neurology, 22,* 1105–1111.

Mills, J. R. & Jackson, N. E. (April, 1989). *Predictive significance of early giftedness: The case of precocious reading.* Paper presented at the biennal meeting of the Society for Research in Child Development, Kansas City, MO.

Parker, S. W. (1919). Pseudo-talent for words. *Psychology Clinics, 11,* 1–7.

Patterson, K. E., Marshall, J., & Coltheart, M. (Eds.) (1986). *Surface dyslexia.* Hillsdale, NJ: Erlbaum.

Pennington, B. F., Johnson, C., & Welsh, M. C. (1987). Unexpected reading precocity in a normal preschooler: Implications for hyperlexia. *Brain and Language, 30,* 165–180.

Perfetti, C. A. (1985). *Reading ability.* New York: Oxford University Press.

Philipps, A. (1930). Talented imbeciles. *Psychology Clinics, 18,* 246–265.

Richman, L. C. & Kitchell, M. M. (1981). Hyperlexia as a variant of developmental language disorder. *Brain and Language, 12,* 203–212.

Siegel, L. (1984). A longitudinal study of a hyperlexic child: Hyperlexia as a language disorder. *Neuropsychologia, 22,* 577–585.

Silberberg, N. E. & Silberberg, M. C. (1967). Hyperlexia: Specific word recognition skills in young children. *Exceptional Children, 34,* 41–42.

Silberberg, N. E. & Silberberg, M. C. (1971). Hyperlexia: The other end of the continuum. *Journal of Special Education, 5,* 233–267.

Snowling, M. & Frith, U. 81986). Comprehension in "hyperlexic" readers. *Journal of Experimental Child Psychology, 42,* 392–415.

Torrey, J. (1973). Learning to read without a teacher. In F. Smith (Ed.), *Psycholinguistics and reading.* 147–157. New York: Holt, Rinehart, & Winston.

Welsh, M. C., Pennington, B. F., & Rogers, S. (1987). Word recognition and comprehension skills in hyperlexic children. *Brain and Language, 32,* 76–96.

Whitehouse, D. & Harris, J. C. (1984). Hyperlexia in infantile autism. *Journal of Autism and Developmental Disorders, 14,* 281–289.

Marilyn C. Welsh, Greeley, Colorado (USA)

75. Aspects of Metalinguistic Abilities in Specific Language Impairment (Developmental Dysphasia) and Dyslexia

1. Metalinguistic Abilities: Theoretical Framework

Theoretical discussions of the nature and development of metalinguistic abilities abound in the literature (Bialystok 1986; Bialystok/Ryan 1985a,b,c; Cazden 1972, 1975; Clark 1978; Hakes 1980, 1982; Karmiloff-Smith 1986; Mattingly 1972; Menyuk 1985, 1991; Tunmer/Bowey 1984; Tunmer/Herriman 1984; van Kleek 1982, 1984a,b; Vygotsky 1962). The relation between metalanguage and metacognition has been debated (cf. Bialystok/Ryan 1985c; van Kleeck 1982, 1984a), and various cognitive frameworks underlying metalinguistic skills have been proposed (Bialystok/Ryan 1985a,c; Karmiloff-Smith 1986; van Kleeck 1982). Theorists have recognized varying levels of meta-abilities from intuitive to conscious knowledge. However, definitions of metalinguistic abilities have generally focused on the endpoint involving conscious awareness of language units and rules. For example, van Kleeck (1982, 237) defines metalinguistic skill as "the ability to reflect consciously upon the nature and properties of language." The distinction between linguistic and metalinguistic abilities has been depicted in a number of ways in the literature. It has been suggested that metalinguistic tasks require that language be treated as 'opaque', in contrast to typical listening and speaking situations in which language is 'transparent' (Cazden 1972, 1975). Similarly, metalinguistic awareness has been characterized as entailing the ability to treat language as an object of thought (Ehri 1975; Tunmer/Bowey 1984), and a contrast has been made between primary linguistic activities involved in speaking and listening and secondary linguistic activities involved in conscious language knowledge (Mattingly 1972). It is typically assumed that metalinguistic awareness requires some degree of primary linguistic competence for the child to reflect on (van Kleeck 1982), and that metalinguistic activities are more difficult in that they demand higher degrees of cognitive control (Bialystok/Ryan 1985a,c; Hakes 1982).

There is considerable disagreement regarding the hypothesized role of metalinguistic skills in language acquisition. Clark (1978) has espoused the view that the motivating force for language development is children's realization of the inadequacy of their own version of language, which prompts a move to the next stage of development. This claim is based on a variety of types of evidence for language awareness in young children, including spontaneous self-repairs, corrections of utterances of other speakers, and language play. Likewise, Menyuk (1991) has advanced the notion that children achieve awareness of linguistic categories and relations as language is acquired and that these meta-abilities may be the catalyst for developmental change. Specifically, she contends that awareness evolves as children compare what is known about language to the linguistic input they receive. As these comparisons are made, children may observe discrepancies which lead them to make modifications in the representations of their linguistic knowledge. Within this framework, Menyuk has proposed a three-stage progression in the development of metalinguistic skills ranging from intuitive use of linguistic knowledge to conscious language knowledge to automatic processing of this knowledge. In contrast to the views of Clark (1978) and Menyuk (1991), Karmiloff-Smith (1986) has argued that metalinguistic awareness has little or no role to play in language acquisition macrodevelopmentally. Other researchers have adopted the stance that explicit metalinguistic judgments serve a minimal function in first language acquisition, but have pointed to the importance of these abilities in the development of literacy skills (Hakes 1982; Kamhi/Catts 1989a; Kamhi/Koenig 1985). These conflicting viewpoints likely stem, at least in part, from differing definitions of metalinguistic abilities (cf. Bialystok/Ryan 1985c) and different ideas about what constitutes evidence of language awareness.

Since the 1970's theorists have emphasized the linguistic bases of reading (Mattingly 1972; Perfetti 1985; Stanovich 1986; Vellutino 1977, 1979). This has led to an increasing interest in the role of metalinguistic skills in the development of literacy (Bialystok/Ryan 1985a,c; Hakes 1982; Tunmer/Bowey 1984; Tunmer/Herriman 1984). Varying views have been expressed concerning the relationship between metalinguistic awareness and reading. Some researchers have stressed the notion that certain metalinguistic skills are a prerequisite for learning to read (Mattingly 1972, 1984). Others have suggested that conscious awareness of language is an outgrowth of reading experience and instruction (Vygotsky 1962). More recent evidence has prompted a number of researchers to hypothesize a bidirectional interaction between metalinguistic and reading abilities (Catts 1989; Downing 1984; Ehri 1979). Tunmer/Bowey (1984) contend that the following four categories of metalinguistic abilities are implicated in beginning to skilled reading: word awareness (recognizing that sentences are composed of and can be divided into individual words), phonological awareness (knowledge that words consist of sounds), grammatical awareness (an understanding that sentences follow certain syntactic and semantic rules), and pragmatic awareness (knowledge of rules governing connected discourse). Tunmer and Bowey hypothesize that word and phonological awareness are related to reading performance during the early stages of reading when the focus is on decoding. Grammatical and pragmatic awareness are thought to play a greater role at later stages of skilled reading as children develop text comprehension skills.

2. Populations Exhibiting Deficits in Metalinguistic Awareness

Deficits in metalinguistic abilities have been documented in two groups of children who are the focus of this chapter. The first group consists of children who have been identified in the literature as having specific language impairment (SLI) (cf. Lahey 1988). These children display substantial problems in oral language functioning that cannot be attributed to emotional disturbance, deficits in hearing, oral motor function, or general intelligence (Johnston 1988; Tallal 1988). Historically, the term 'developmental dysphasia' has also been used to refer to these children (Lahey 1988). The second population of children who exhibit difficulties in language awareness are children who have marked reading impairment in the absence of intellectual, sensory, emotional, or environmental deficiencies (Harris/Hodges 1981; Perfetti 1985). These children are alternately referred to in the literature as dyslexic or reading disabled (RD) (Kamhi/Catts 1989b). These terms will be used interchangeably throughout this chapter. Research has demonstrated the heterogeneous nature of reading disabilities and the existence of various distinct subgroups of dyslexic children (see review by Kamhi/Catts 1989b). The concern here is with the large proportion of RD children who clearly exhibit language-related difficulties (Perfetti 1985; Vellutino 1977); though it can be argued that language problems are implicated at some level in all reading disabilities (cf. Kamhi 1989).

3. Relation Between Developmental Language Disorders and Reading Disabilities

There is evidence that a substantial number of children with early histories of oral language deficits experience academic difficulties when they enter school and that these children are particularly at risk for reading and written language problems (Aram/Ekelman/Nation 1984; Aram/Nation 1980; Hall/Tomblin 1978; Stark/Bernstein/Condino et al. 1984). The issue of a language-learning disorder 'connection' and the possibility of changes in the symptoms of language disability over time have been discussed by Maxwell/Wallach (1984), among others. Nevertheless, as Kamhi/Catts/Mauer et al. (1988) have pointed out, researchers have identified a group of school-age SLI children who are apparently distinct from the more general population of learning disabled and RD children (Johnston/Ellis Weismer 1983; Liles 1987; Savich 1984). Although dyslexic children have been found to perform within normal range on standardized language tests (Hessler/Kitchen 1980), many children with reading disabilities exhibit subtle linguistic deficits that are not revealed by these measures of oral language functioning. A comprehensive review of this research is provided by Roth/Spekman (1989). Compared to normally developing children, studies have demonstrated that RD children evidence various deficiencies in language abilities including word finding problems (Denckla/Rudel 1976; German 1982), syntactic and morphological deficits (Stein/Cairns/Zurif 1984; Vogel 1977), deficits in figurative language skills (Lee/Kamhi 1990) and in narrative discourse (Feagans/Short 1984). Yet, direct comparisons of oral language abilities in SLI and RD children indicate that the children with reading problems outperform the SLI children (Lee/Kamhi 1990; Masterson/Kamhi 1985).

Various researchers have speculated about the link between oral language deficits and reading impairment (Donahue 1986; Kamhi 1989; Kamhi/Catts 1986; Kamhi/Catts/Mauer et al. 1988). Donahue (1986) has proposed that within the reading disabled population at least three subgroups of language disorders exist. The first subgroup consists of children with more severe language problems who are identified during the preschool period as language impaired. The second group of students are those who are not identified as having problems before entering school. These children may have phonological processing deficits that interfere with decoding skills in beginning reading; or they may have subtle higher-order linguistic deficits that impact upon text comprehension and 'reading to learn' at about the fourth grade (Chall 1983). The third subgroup suggested by Donahue are children who fail to develop adequate reading abilities for a variety of reasons such as problems in motivation or attention. Although these children began school with age-appropriate language abilities, their reading difficulties result in less experience with the more complex, literate vocabulary and syntactic structures that characterize written language (cf. Nippold 1988) and lead to a complex interplay between limitations in oral language proficiency and restricted reading abilities. Clearly, the relation between oral language disorders and reading problems is not straightforward, but we can conclude that children who exhibit problems in one of these areas are at risk in the other area as well.

4. Experimental Studies of Metalinguistic Skills Evidenced by SLI Children

Recently there has been increasing interest in the development of language awareness in SLI children. Anecdotal reports of metalinguistic deficiency in SLI children were provided by Wiig/Semel (1976). The majority of experimental investigations since that time have involved studies focusing on grammatical judgment tasks (Buday/Newhoff/Perry 1983; Fujiki/Brinton/Dunton 1987; Kamhi/Koenig 1985; Liles/Shulman 1981; Liles/Shulman/Bartlett 1977; Perry/Newhoff/Buday 1983) or tasks tapping lexical or phonological awareness (Kamhi/Catts 1986; Kamhi/Koenig 1985; Kamhi/Lee/Nelson 1985). In addition, there have been a few investigations of communicative awareness exhibited by children with language disorders (Lee/Kamhi/Nelson 1983; Meline/Brackin 1987). To date, the only longitudinal study of SLI children's metalinguistic abilities is one conducted by Liebergott/Menyuk/Chesnick/Korngold (1988, as cited by Menyuk 1991). Liles/Schulman/Bartlett (1977) examined metalinguistic skills in 5 to 8-year-old normally developing and SLI children who were matched for age and receptive vocabulary level. They compared the groups' proficiency in judging and correcting sentences containing errors of syntactic agreement, lexical restriction, and word-order in an attempt to determine what factors children apply to their definition of grammaticality. Normal language controls identified significantly more agrammatical sentences involving syntactic agreement and word-order violations than the SLI subjects. SLI subjects not only recognized fewer errors than the controls, they also displayed a disparity between their identification accuracy level and correction level in that they recognized errors they could not correct. This was particularly the case for the syntactic errors. In a follow-up study, Liles/Shulman (1981) compared the performance of SLI and normal language children (5;4 – 6;7) on a grammatical judgment task and a comprehension task to assess whether the ability to make grammatical judgments about a form is related to comprehension of the form. Although both groups performed similarly on the comprehension task, the SLI children scored significantly worse on the judgment task than the normal language subjects.

Several other studies have also demonstrated deficits in SLI children's grammatical awareness. Fujiki/Brinton/Dunton (1987) compared SLI and normally developing first, second, and third graders' performance on a judgment and correction task involving three types of errors: syntactic omission, word order, and syntactic number agreement. They found a significant difference between the normal language and SLI first and second grade groups on this task. Studies by Newhoff and colleagues (Buday/Newhoff/Perry 1983; Perry/Newhoff/Buday 1983) have indicated that older SLI children (9 to 14-year-olds) evidence greater difficulty than language age-matched controls in identifying and explaining why sentences were 'wrong' that contained errors on -s morphemes (plural, possessive, third-person singular, contractible auxiliary is) and tense-marking morphemes (past -ed, progressive -ing, past irregular).

Kamhi/Koenig (1985) examined metalinguistic abilities in SLI and normal language controls (4 to 7 years of age) who were matched on receptive language level and mental age. SLI subjects scored significantly lower than controls on sentences containing syntactic errors; however, the two groups were comparable in terms of identification and correction of semantic and phonological errors. Like the Liles/Shulman (1981) study, these results do not support the notion that comprehension deficits can account for the language impaired children's limitations in grammatical awareness given that subjects in both groups were matched on receptive language skills. Further, the SLI children's scores on the language measures were not correlated with their performance on the syntactic judgment task. It is likely that the nature of the phonologically anomalous sentences (e.g. *John has two tig [big] cars*) in the Kamhi/Koenig study contributed to the lack of differences between groups. Other studies have found correction of phonological errors to be at least as difficult as correction of syntactic errors (Smith/Tager-Flusberg 1981). Kamhi/Koenig note that children may have been attending primarily to semantic and syntactic features of the sentence rather than focusing on phonological judgments. Similar findings have been reported by Kamhi/Catts (1986). They found that SLI children scored significantly poorer than normal language controls on a morpheme judgment task, but the groups displayed comparable performance on tasks tapping lexical and phonological awareness. Task variables again appeared to impact on these demonstrated findings. The control subjects demonstrated a ceiling effect on the word division tasks, whereas the phoneme segmentation task was too difficult for all subjects. Using a syllable segmentation task to assess phonological awareness, Kamhi/Catts/Mauer et al. (1988) also failed to find a significant difference between the performance of SLI and normal language controls.

On the other hand, evidence that SLI children's metalinguistic deficits extend beyond problems in making grammatical judgments has been provided by an investigation by Kamhi/Lee/Nelson (1985). The performance of SLI children (3 to 6 years of age) was compared to a group of mental age-matched (MA) controls and a language age-matched (LA) group. Subjects were presented sentence and word division tasks based on tasks used by Fox/Routh (1975) with normal 3 and 4-year-olds. These tasks included dividing sentences into words, dividing bisyllabic words into syllables, and dividing monosyllabic words into sounds. A second experimental procedure involved a series of questions designed to tap word awareness (e. g. *Say a short word. What makes that a short word*?). Responses were assigned developmental stage scores based on Papandropoulou/Sinclair's (1974) findings with normally developing children. The results indicated that SLI children performed significantly worse than both control groups in dividing sentences and words. Less than half of the SLI subjects could divide any of the sentences or bisyllabic words into smaller units, compared to all of the MA group and over 70 % of the LA group. Dividing monosyllabic words into their component sound units was especially difficult for the SLI children. Only 2 SLI subjects (15 %) could perform the task in contrast to 80 % of the MA group and over half of the LA group. Significant differences were found in the distribution of stage scores for the word awareness task, with the MA group's performance being superior to the SLI and LA groups. Kamhi/Lee/Nelson (1985) contend that these findings suggest that SLI children do not just have difficulty in accessing extant language knowledge, but are also restricted in their ability to acquire knowledge about linguistic elements that compose sentences and words such that they are at risk for reading problems.

Investigations of SLI children's communicative awareness have also revealed deficits. Lee/Kamhi/Nelson (1983) presented ten unintelligible sentences to children in a 30-minute play session. SLI children rarely made requests for clarification whereas the normal language children asked for clarification in the majority of instances. Lee et al. have suggested that SLI are less sensitive to their own communicative needs than normally developing children; therefore, language impaired children assume it is their fault when they fail to understand. These findings concur with the results of studies by Meline and colleagues (Meline 1986; Meline/Meline 1983) regarding the reticence of SLI children when confronted with a communicative obstacle. Meline/Brackin (1987) further investigated SLI children's awareness of inadequate messages employing a paradigm used by Robinson/Robinson (1977) with normally developing 5 and 6-year-olds. Stories were presented which included a speaker and listener. In the story, the speaker makes a vague request and his intention is not understood. Subjects were asked to determine whose fault it was that the speaker did not get what he wanted. SLI and younger controls matched on receptive language abilities were predominately listener-blamers in contrast to age-matched controls who were speaker-blamers. Meline and Brackin discuss their findings in terms of Bialystok/Ryan's (1985 a, c) model of cognitive requisites underlying metalinguistic abilities. They consider various explanations for the poor performance by the SLI children, including a lack of specialized knowledge, inexperience with analytical problem solving, lack of cognitive control, and insensitivity to their own communicative needs. Similarly, learning disabled children have been characterized as exhibiting 'passivity' in conversational situations. They have also been found to be less likely to request clarification of inadequate messages than controls, though they detected comprehension problems as well as the normal language subjects so the problem was not one of lack of awareness (Donahue/Pearl/Bryan 1980).

Liebergott et al. (1988, as cited by Menyuk 1991) have conducted a longitudinal investigation of metalinguistic development over a three-year period in three groups of children (N = 135): SLI children; 'iffy' children who had displayed early language delays, but had outgrown the difficulties to a large extent; and very-low-birth-weight premature children. At the start of the study, children ranged in age from 4;6 to 5;6. On a battery of standard language measures, the SLI group scored lowest, the iffy group's performance fell in the middle, and the premature children obtained the highest scores. Performance on the language measures was compared to scores on a battery of metalinguistic tasks which were designed to tap awareness of categories and relations at various levels of language including phonological, lexical, 'semantactic', and discourse. Menyuk reports that the three groups differed from each other on the metalinguistic battery in the same way they did on the battery of standard language measures. A cluster analysis indicated that some of the children in the other two groups scored as poorly as the SLI children on the metalinguistic tasks. The SLI group was reconstituted to include these low-performing iffy and premature subjects. Significant differences were found between this lowest achieving group and the other subjects at each of the three time periods tested. Different developmental patterns were observed across the groups. In contrast to the other children, those in the lowest performing group (which primarily consisted of SLI children) did not demonstrate steady improvement in metalinguistic abilities. With the exception of the area of discourse (a story recall task), this group's abilities on the metalinguistic battery improved slowly and plateaued at the midpoint of the study. It should be noted that the tasks in this study designated as requiring metalinguistic processing included measures such as comprehension of complex sentences and story recall that many researchers would consider to tap primary linguistic abilities rather than metalinguistic awareness (though the tasks are just listed, not described). Therefore, these findings reflect a somewhat different view of metalinguistics than that adopted in the studies described previously.

In summary, there is increasing evidence that children with specific language impairment exhibit deficits in metalinguistic abilities relative to normal language children matched on chronological age, mental age, or receptive language level. Results from experimental studies have consistently demonstrated that SLI subjects perform significantly more poorly than controls on tasks measuring grammatical awareness. A limited number of investigations of SLI children's communicative awareness have also pointed to deficiencies in that area. Mixed results have been reported regarding SLI children's lexical and phonological awareness, which may underlie beginning reading skills. There is also evidence that SLI children display different patterns of metalinguistic development than normally developing children, though more investigations are needed that clearly distinguish acquisition of primary language abilities from language awareness.

5. Experimental Investigations of the Relation Between Metalinguistic Skills and Reading Development/Disabilities

The aspect of metalinguistic abilities that has received the greatest attention in terms of its relation to reading is phonological awareness. Research employing a variety of experimental paradigms, across different languages and varying ages of subjects, has consistently found a strong positive relation between children's phonological awareness and their reading abilities (Blachman 1984; Blachman/James 1985; 1986 as cited by James 1988; Cossu/Shankweiler/Liberman et al. 1988; Fox/Routh 1975; Liberman/Shankweiler/Fischer/Carter 1974; Lundberg/Olofsson/Wall 1980; Mann/Liberman 1984; Rosner/Simon 1971; Share/Jorm/Maclean/Matthews 1984; Stanovich/Cunningham/Cramer 1984; Zifcak 1981). There appears to be a reciprocal relation between phonological awareness and reading skills such that awareness of phonological aspects of the language may be both a precursor of reading development and a result of reading experience (Ehri 1979, Perfetti/Beck/Bell/Hughes 1987; Stanovich 1986). Studies examining children's metalinguistic abilities prior to the initiation of formal reading instruction, have demonstrated that early sound awareness is a good predictor of later literacy (Bradley/Bryant 1983; Lundberg/Olofsson/Wall 1980; Maclean/Bryant/Bradley 1987; Mann/Liberman 1984;

Stanovich et al. 1984). Maclean et al. (1987) conducted a 15-month longitudinal study of preschoolers' performance on rhyming and alliteration tasks. They found that 3-year-olds exhibited rudimentary phonological awareness skills and that performance on these phonological tasks predicted the ability to read words at 4 years of age. Most studies have compared kindergartners' awareness of phonemes, rhyme, and syllable structure to their reading skills in first grade. However, the impact of informal literacy instruction has not been controlled. In an attempt to take this factor into account, Bradley/Bryant (1983) included as subjects only 4 to 5-year-olds who evidenced no reading abilities on a standardized reading test. Their findings indicated that awareness of rhyme and alliteration was significantly correlated to reading skills three years later. On the other hand, some phonological awareness skills are apparently not requisite for reading but emerge with reading instruction (Ehri 1989; Perfetti/Beck/Bell/Hughes 1987). For example, the findings of Perfetti et al. indicated that children's phoneme deletion skills develop only after some reading experience. Further insight into the impact of reading instruction on phonological awareness has been gained from cross-cultural investigations and studies of illiterate adults (Morais/Bertelson/Cary/Alegria 1986; Read/Ruyter 1985; Read/Zhang/Nie/Ding 1986). Results of these studies have indicated that more advanced phonological analysis skills involving explicit awareness of phonemic segments seem to be dependent upon instruction in an alphabetic orthography. For more comprehensive discussions of the relationship between phonological awareness and reading abilities refer to Bailet (1991), Blachman (1984), Catts (1989), and Wagner/Torgesen (1987).

A limited number of investigations have examined children's word awareness and grammatical awareness in relation to reading skills. Studies have shown that it is difficult for young children to separate words from their referents (Ianco-Worral 1972) and to segment utterances into words (Ehri 1975). Notable improvement in word awareness is observed once children begin to learn to read (Francis 1973; Papandropoulou/Sinclair 1974). Furthermore, awareness of aurally presented word boundaries has been found to be a significant predictor of reading achievement in beginning first graders (Evans/Taylor/Blum 1979; McNinch 1974). With respect to grammatical awareness, research has demonstrated that the ability of elementary school-aged children, adolescents, and adults to identify and revise agrammatical sentences is significantly correlated with reading performance (Blachman/James 1985, 1986 as cited by James 1988; Flood/Menyuk 1983; Forrest-Pressley 1983; Menyuk/Flood 1981). Blachman/James (1985; 1986 as cited by James 1988) conducted a longitudinal study of metalinguistic and reading abilities in first, second, and third grades. Subjects were presented a set of oral language tasks and a battery of reading achievement measures. The metalinguistic tasks included a grammatical judgment and correction task involving word order and morphological errors, a word referent task, a riddle task that involved lexical or structural ambiguity, and a phoneme segmentation task. The results indicated that grammatical awareness and phonological awareness were significantly correlated to reading achievement in beginning readers (grades 1 and 2) and were significant predictors of reading performance. Word awareness was not strongly related to reading achievement. The ability to explain ambiguity in riddles, which reflects both grammatical and word awareness, was most strongly correlated to more skilled reading that involved text comprehension. Blachman and James contend that these findings are consistent with Tunmer/Bowey's (1984) hypotheses about the role of various aspects of metalinguistic skills in reading development.

Metalinguistic investigations of children with deficient reading skills have primarily focused on phonological awareness. Poor readers have been shown to have more difficulty than good readers in detecting rhymes, segmenting speech into phonemic and syllabic units, and deleting, substituting and manipulating phonemes (Bradley/Bryant 1978; Bryant/Bradley 1981; Fox/Routh 1975, 1980; Katz 1986; Lenchner/Gerber/Routh 1990; Liberman/Shankweiler/Fischer/Carter 1974; Morais/Cluytens/Alegria 1984; Snyder/Downey 1991). An investigation by Bradley/Bryant (1978) examined rhyming and alliterative skills in dyslexic children and controls matched on reading level who were 3½ years younger than the dyslexic subjects. Subjects were instructed to select the odd item that did not belong with the others in a series of spoken words. Dyslexic subjects scored significantly lower on this task than the younger normal readers. Fox/Routh (1980) employed a task in which they asked first grade children to *say just a little bit* of spoken syllables. Subjects consisted of children identified as having average, mildly depressed or severely depressed reading skills. Those with severely depressed reading abilities were unable to divide syllables into phonemes in contrast to the two other groups who performed quite well on the task. The ability of third grade RD children to identify the number of syllables in words was examined by Katz (1986). The task involved asking subjects to decide whether or not the names of pictured objects had the same number of syllables (object names were usually one or three syllable in length). Even when the RD subjects demonstrated that they knew the names of the objects, they performed worse than the normal readers in making length judgments. Snyder/Downey (1991) investigated phonological awareness in normally achieving and RD students (ages 8 – 14 years) using a pig latin task designed to assess the ability to manipulate phonological elements. The normally achieving subjects performed significantly better than the RD subjects on this task even when differences between the groups' short-term auditory memory skills were statistically removed. Lenchner et al. (1990) compared the performance of third and fourth graders identified as poor vs. good readers on six different measures of phonological awareness that evaluated the ability to segment, blend, and manipulate phonemes. Results indicated that for the poor readers, scores on the phoneme deletion and substitution tasks were significantly correlated with decoding and word attack skills. The deletion task was deemed to be the most valid of the tasks used, in that it correlated most highly with the other phonological awareness tasks and with the decoding measures.

A few investigations have compared metalinguistic abilities exhibited by dyslexic children to that of children with other types of deficits. In a large-scale study of first grade children, Felton/Wood (1989) found that children with impaired reading skills performed significantly more poorly than children with attention deficit disorder on phonological awareness tasks, as well as on confrontation and rapid automatized naming tasks. Two studies by Kamhi and his colleagues (Kamhi/Catts 1986; Kamhi/Catts/Mauer et al. 1988) have compared phonological processing abilities and metalinguistic skills of RD and SLI children. In the Kamhi/Catts (1986) study, three groups of children (6 to 9 years of age) served as subjects: RD children with no history of speech-language impairment, SLI children, and normally developing controls. The three groups were matched for mental age on a nonverbal measure of intelligence. Six tasks were administered that assessed phonological, lexical, and morphological awareness. Phonological processing abilities were additionally assessed via word and sentence repetition tasks. The metalinguistic measures consisted of sentence division, bisyllabic and monosyllabic word division, elision (phoneme deletion), phoneme segmentation, and a morpheme judgment and correction task. The elision task (used by Rosner/Simon 1971) required the child to determine what would be left if a particular sound (first or last) were deleted from a word, e. g. (t)all. The segmentation task involved a tapping procedure used by Liberman/Shankweiler/Fischer/Carter (1974) in which children indicated the number of phonemes in spoken syllables. The findings rather surprisingly revealed that the performance of RD and SLI children was equivalent on measures of phonological lexical, and morphological awareness. The SLI children scored significantly lower than the RD subjects only on measures of word and sentence repetition (i. e. production tasks). Both the RD and SLI subjects performed significantly worse than normal language controls on the morpheme judgment task. The performance of the RD subjects was significantly poorer than that of the controls on the sentence division task and the elision task. Regression analyses indicated that elision task scores were the best predictor of reading performance, accounting for roughly 50 % of the variance for each of three reading measures. Performance on the word repetition task, on the other hand, was the best predictor of language abilities. Further investigation of phonological processing abilities of RD and SLI children by Kamhi/Catts/Mauer et al. (1988) revealed similar findings. That is, dyslexic children performed significantly better than SLI subjects only on a multisyllabic word repetition task. The scores of the two experimental groups were not significantly different on a syllable segmentation task, though the dyslexic subjects' performance was significantly worse than that of the normally developing controls. These investigations support the findings from studies reviewed previously which indicate that RD and SLI children display deficits in various aspects of metalinguistic abilities compared to children who are developing oral and written language skills normally. They do not, however, provide any evidence that children with reading impairment can be distinguished from those with oral language disorders on the basis of language awareness skills.

Based on the existing literature, we can conclude that metalinguistic abilities play an important role in reading and reading disabilities. Numerous studies have demonstrated a strong relationship between phonological awareness and reading performance. Grammatical awareness and word awareness have also been shown to be linked to literacy skills. The bulk of the evidence might seem to suggest that dyslexic children are primarily deficient in phonological awareness skills in contrast to SLI children who are mainly lacking in grammatical awareness abilities; however, the little information that is available concerning direct comparisons of these two groups performing the same tasks does not support this interpretation.

6. Claims Regarding the Role of Metalinguistics in Language Disorders and Reading Disabilities

Factors that have motivated the investigation of metalinguistic abilities in SLI children include the following: 1) a desire to characterize the interaction between the development of language performance and linguistic awareness (Liles/Shulman/Bartlett 1977); 2) consideration of the metalinguistic demands of language assessment and remediation procedures (Kamhi/Koenig 1985; van Kleeck 1984b); 3) concern that metalinguistic deficits may place SLI children at risk for reading problems (James 1988; Kamhi/Lee/Nelson 1985); and 4) a search for underlying causes of developmental language impairment (Menyuk 1991). The strongest claim regarding the role of metalinguistic deficits in oral language disorders has been made by Menyuk (1991). Based on findings of metalinguistic studies of normally developing and SLI children, she puts forth the argument (which she concedes is highly speculative) that "these children are delayed in language because of metalinguizing difficulties" (Menyuk 1991, 319). Menyuk postulates that SLI children intuitively acquire knowledge of language but have problems achieving conscious awareness of that knowledge. She proposes that such awareness is needed to firmly establish linguistic representations and to retrieve them automatically. Deficits in SLI children's meta-abilities are therefore thought to disrupt the development and automatic retrieval of linguistic representations, delaying the development of language skills. Menyuk contends that alternate explanations of language delay that appeal to reduced processing rates or memorial problems might be subsumed by a metalinguistic deficit explanation which incorporates the construct of automaticity limitations. Although there has been some interest in the impact of other aspects of metalinguistic abilities on reading skills (James 1988), the vast majority of claims focus on the extensive literature dealing with the role of phonological awareness in beginning reading. A number of researchers have proposed that reading disability is linked to deficits in phonological awareness (see reviews by Stanovich 1986; Wagner 1986, 1988; Wagner/Torgesen 1987). Stanovich (1986, 393) has suggested that, "If there is a specific cause of reading disability at all, it resides in the area of phonological awareness. Slow development in this area delays early code-breaking progress and initiates the cascade of interacting achievement failures and motivational problems." Other researchers have attributed reading disability to inadequate bootstrapping of phonological awareness on orthographic awareness (Foorman/Liberman 1989). A dissenting viewpoint is represented by investigators who claim that phonological awareness is a product rather than a prerequisite of learning to read (Ehri 1989; Morais/Bertelson/Cary/Alegria 1986). Ehri (1989) adopts the position that the type of phonological deficits demonstrated by dyslexic children are primarily due to inadequate reading and spelling instruction.

It is certainly the case that there is evidence that SLI and RD children display significantly poorer performance on metalinguistic tasks than normally developing children and that reading proficiency has been shown to be correlated with aspects of linguistic awareness. However, the exact nature of the relationship between metalinguistic deficits and impairments in oral language or reading skills is unresolved. Relatively little information pertaining to SLI children is available at this point and claims regarding the role of metalinguistic deficits in oral language disorders are speculative at best. Researchers have attempted to gain insight into the causal connection between phonological awareness and reading abilities through training studies (reviewed in 7.) or advanced statistical techniques such as path analysis (Torneus 1984; Wagner 1988). Yet, a number of questions remain as to how these findings should be interpreted. Although facility in metalinguistic awareness appears to be linked to language and reading disorders, it would be imprudent to ignore the evidence concerning various other potential factors underlying specific language impairment (cf. Johnston 1988; Tallal 1988) and reading disabilities (cf. Kamhi 1989; Perfetti 1985; Stanovich 1986).

7. Clinical Implications: Assessment and Remediation

In light of the relationship between metalinguistic abilities and reading proficiency and the fact that SLI children demonstrate deficits in language awareness, it has been suggested that these skills should be assessed in all children suspected of having language or reading disabilities (James 1988, 1989). James (1989) recommends that language evaluations should incorporate measures designed to tap phonological, word, grammatical, and pragmatic awareness by means of tasks such as: segmentation of words and sentences, separation of words from their referents, judgment of grammatical acceptability of sentences, detection of ambiguity, and judgment of message adequacy and appropriateness of communicative interactions. A description of tasks that might be used for this type of informal assessment of metalinguistic awareness has been provided by James (1988). A grammatical judgment screening test for elementary school-aged children has recently been developed by Fujiki/Brinton/Dunton (1987). Based on screening test scores on this measure, approximately 82 % of SLI and normal language subjects were correctly categorized. This percentage would have been considerably higher if the scores for the third graders had not been included. Blachman (1989) has argued that despite the role that phonological awareness, in particular, seems to play in beginning reading, traditional reading readiness tests and reading assessment batteries do not place an emphasis on this ability. She notes that kindergartners' performance on measures of phonological awareness have been shown to predict reading proficiency in first grade as well as or better than reading readiness tests or intelligence measures (Stanovich/Cunningham/Cramer 1984). Blachman suggests that measures of phonological awareness such as word segmentation, sound categorization of words, or sound deletion tasks should be included in assessments of beginning readers.

The impact of metalinguistic training on reading development has been investigated in terms of phonological awareness skills. Studies with beginning readers and prereaders have demonstrated that training in phonological awareness has a positive effect on reading achievement, particularly when links are established between the sound segments of the word and the letters which represent those segments (Bradley/Bryant 1983, 1985; Fox/Routh 1984; Lundberg 1987; Treiman/Baron 1983). For an indepth review of this research refer to Blachman (1989). There is also evidence that reading instruction which incorporated a focus on phonological awareness was beneficial for learning disabled children (Williams 1979, 1980). Vellutino/Scanlon (1987) have demonstrated the effectiveness of phonemic segmentation training in improving word recognition in normal and poor readers in the second and sixth grade. It should be noted, however, that not all researchers endorse the view that metalinguistic training is an important aspect of reading instruction programs (Singer 1984). Relatively little consideration has been given to the influence of metalinguistic training on children's oral language abilities; though some investigators have suggested that clinical objectives targeting metalinguistic skills might profitably be included in remediation programs for SLI children (Kamhi/Lee/Nelson 1985; van Kleeck 1984b). Training efforts to this point have focused more on abilities that are generally subsumed under the rubric of metacognitive skills rather than metalinguistic awareness per se. In one of the few investigations in this area, Dollaghan/Kaston (1986) reported success in improving awareness of message adequacy in SLI children. A study by Olsen/Wong/Marx (1983) indicated that training cognitive control strategies had a positive influence on pragmatic awareness and language use by learning disabled children, but the trained skills failed to generalize. Westby (1989) has described means of assessing and facilitating comprehension monitoring skills for children with language and reading problems.

8. Directions for Future Research

Compared to the research examining the role of metalinguistic abilities in reading and reading disorders, there has been relatively little empirical investigation of the relationship between metalinguistic skills and oral language deficits. Future research efforts might profitably be focused in a number of directions. Additional longitudinal investigations of SLI children (extending into the school-age years) would be useful to chart the course of development in metalinguistic awareness. By comparing the development of specific linguistic relations and categories with awareness of those particular aspects of language and observing plateaus and growth spurts in both of these areas, insights might be gained about the nature of the interaction between linguistic and metalinguistic skills. There is also a need for studies that further investigate phonological and word awareness in SLI children to determine the extent which deficits in these abilities might predict difficulties in beginning reading skills for certain children with oral language deficiencies. The role of grammatical and pragmatic awareness deficits in later stages of reading deserves greater consideration. Similarly, investigation of the link between these aspects of metalinguistic awareness and other cognitive and metacognitive processes involved in comprehending both spoken and written discourse would be informative. For example, studies might assess the extent to which poor language awareness interacts with SLI and RD children's deficits in constructive cognitive processes (i. e. semantic integration and inference construction) involved in the comprehension and retention of connected discourse (Ellis Weismer 1985; Klein-Konigsberg 1984). There is also a need for training studies that explore the impact of instruction aimed at improving various aspects of metalinguistic awareness (in addition to phonological awareness) on language and reading skills in SLI and RD children. Finally, additional investigations involving direct comparisons of children with developmental language disorders and those with reading disabilities may lead to an enhanced conceptualization of the complex nature of the relationship between linguistic abilities and metalinguistic skills.

9. References

Aram, D., Ekelman, B., & Nation, J. (1984). Preschoolers with language disorders: 10 years later. *Journal of Speech and Hearing Research, 27*, 232–244.

Aram, D. & Nation, J. (1980). Preschool language disorders and subsequent language and academic difficulties. *Journal of Communication Disorders, 13*, 159–170.

Bailet, L. (1991). Development of disorders of spelling in the beginning school years. In A. Bain, L. L. Bailet, & L. C. Moats (Eds.), *Written language disorders: Theory into practice. 1–21.* Austin, TX: Pro-Ed.

Bialystok, E. (1986). Factors in the growth of linguistic awareness. *Child Development, 57*, 498–510.

Bialystok, E. & Ryan, E. (1985a). Toward a definition of metalinguistic skill. *Merrill-Palmer Quarterly, 31*, 229–251.

Bialystok, E. & Ryan, E. (1985b). On precision and the virtue of simplicity in metalinguistics: A reply to Menyuk. *Merrill-Palmer Quarterly, 31*, 261–264.

Bialystok, E. & Ryan, E. (1985c). A metacognitive framework for the development of first and second language skills. In D. Forrest-Pressley, G. MacKinnon, & T. Waller (Eds.), *Meta-cognition, cognition, and human performance, 1.* 207–252. New York: Academic Press.

Blachman, B. (1984). Language analysis skills and early reading acquisition. In G. Wallach & K. Butler (Eds.), *Language learning disabilities in school-age children. 271–287.* Baltimore, MD: Williams & Wilkens.

Blachman, B. (1989). Phonological awareness and word recognition: Assessment and intervention. In A. Kamhi & H. Catts (Eds.), *Reading disabilities: A developmental language perspective. 133–158.* Boston: College-Hill Press.

Blachman, B. & James, S. (1985). Metalinguistic abilities and reading achievement in first-grade children. In J. Niles & R. Lalik (Eds.), *Issues in literacy: A research perspective.* Thirty-fourth Yearbook of the National Reading Conference.

Bradley, L. & Bryant, P. (1978). Difficulties in auditory organization as a possible cause of reading backwards. *Nature, 271*, 746–747.

Bradley, L. & Bryant, P. (1983). Categorizing sounds and learning to read – A causal connection. *Nature, 301*, 419–421.

Bryant, P. & Bradley, L. (1981). Visual memory and phonological skills in reading and spelling backwards. *Psychological Research, 43*, 193–199.

Buday, E., Newhoff, M., & Perry, B. (1983). Metalinguistic ability in normal and language-disordered children. Paper presented at the American Speech-Language-Hearing Association Convention, Cincinnati.

Catts, H. (1989). Phonological processing deficits and reading disabilities. In A. Kamhi & H. Catts

(Eds.), *Reading disabilities: A developmental language perspective. 101–132.* Boston: College-Hill Press.

Cazden, C. (1972). *Child language and education.* New York: Rinehart & Winston.

Cazden, C. (1975). Play with language and metalinguistic awareness: One dimension of language experience. In C. Winsor (Ed.), *Dimensions of language experience. 3–19.* New York: Agathon.

Chall, J. (1983). *Stages of reading development.* New York: McGraw-Hill.

Clark, E. (1978). Awareness of language: Some evidence from what children say and do. In W. Levelt, A. Sinclair, & R. Jarvella (Eds.), *The child's conception of language. 17–44.* New York: Springer-Verlag.

Cossu, G., Shankweiler, D., Liberman, I., Katz, L., & Tola, G. (1988). Awareness of phonological segments and reading ability in Italian children. *Applied Psycholinguistics, 9,* 1–16.

Denckla, M. & Rudel, R. (1976). Naming of pictured objects by dyslexic and other learning disabled children. *Brain and Language, 3,* 1–15.

Dollaghan, C. & Kaston, N. (1986). A comprehension monitoring program for language-impaired children. *Journal of Speech and Hearing Disorders, 51,* 264–271.

Donahue, M. (1986). Linguistic and communicative development in learning disabled children. In S. Ceci (Ed.), *Handbook of cognitive, social, and neuropsychological aspects of learning disabilities. 263–289.* Hillsdale, NJ: Erlbaum.

Donahue, M., Pearl, R., & Bryan, T. (1980). Learning disabled children's conversational competence: Responses to inadequate messages. *Applied Psycholinguistics, 1,* 387–403.

Downing, J. (1984). Task awareness in the development of reading skill. In J. Downing & R. Valtin (Eds.), *Language awareness and learning to read. 27–55.* New York: Springer-Verlag.

Ehri, L. (1975). Word consciousness in readers and prereaders. *Journal of Educational Psychology, 67,* 204–212.

Ehri, L. (1979). Linguistic insight: Threshold of reading acquisition. In T. Waller & G. MacKinnon (Eds.), *Reading research: Advances in theory and practice. 63–116.* New York: Academic Press.

Ehri, L. (1989). The development of spelling knowledge and its role in reading acquisition and reading disability. *Journal of Learning Disabilities, 22,* 356–365.

Ellis Weismer, S. (1985). Constructive comprehension abilities exhibited by language-disordered children. *Journal of Speech and Hearing Research, 28,* 175–184.

Evans, M., Taylor, N., & Blum, I. (1979). Children's writing language awareness and its relation to reading acquisition. *Journal of Reading Behavior, 11,* 7–19.

Feagans, L. & Short, E. (1984). Developmental differences in the comprehension and production of narratives by reading disabled and normally achieving children. *Child Development, 55,* 1727–1736.

Felton, R. & Wood, F. (1989). Cognitive deficits in reading disability and attention deficit disorder. *Journal of Learning Disabilities, 22,* 3–13.

Flood, J. & Menyuk, P. (1983). The development of metalinguistic awareness and its relation to reading achievement. *Journal of Applied Developmental Psychology, 4,* 65–80.

Foorman, B. & Liberman, D. (1989). Visual and phonological processing of words: A comparison of good and poor readers. *Journal of Learning Disabilities, 22,* 349–355.

Forrest-Pressley, D. (1983). *Cognitive and metacognitive aspects of reading.* New York: Springer-Verlag.

Fox, B. & Routh, D. (1975). Analyzing spoken language into words, syllables, and sounds. *Journal of Psycholinguistic Research, 4,* 331–342.

Fox, B. & Routh, D. (1980). Phonemic analysis and severe reading disability. *Journal of Psycholinguistic Research, 9,* 115–119.

Fox, B. & Routh, D. (1984). Phonemic analysis and synthesis as word attack skills: Revisited. *Journal of Educational Psychology, 76,* 1059–1064.

Francis, H. (1973). Children's experience of reading and notions of units of language. *British Journal of Educational Psychology, 43,* 17–23.

Fujiki, M., Brinton, B. & Dunton, S. (1987). A grammatical judgment screening test for young elementary school-aged children. *Language, Speech, and Hearing Services in Schools, 18,* 131–143.

German, D. (1982). Word-finding substitutions in children with learning disabilities. *Language, Speech, and Hearing Services in Schools, 13,* 223–230.

Hakes, D. (1980). *The emergence of metalinguistic abilities in children.* New York: Springer-Verlag.

Hakes, D. (1982). The development of metalinguistic abilities: What develops? In S. Kuczaj (Ed.), *Language, cognition, and culture. 163–210.* Hillsdale, NJ: Erlbaum.

Hall, P. & Tomblin, J. (1978). A follow-up study of children with articulation and language disorders. *Journal of Speech and Hearing Disorders, 43,* 227–241.

Harris, T. & Hodges, R. (1981). *A dictionary of reading and related terms.* Newark, NJ: International Reading Association.

Hessler, G. & Kitchen, D. (1980). Language characteristics of a purposive sample of early elementary learning disabled students. *Learning Disability Quarterly, 3,* 36–41.

Ianco-Worral, A. (1972). Bilingualism and cognitive development. *Child Development, 43,* 1390–1400.

James, S. (1988). The development of oral language and reading. In C. Hedley & J. Hicks (Eds.), *Reading and the special learner. 91–107.* Norwood, NJ: Ablex.

James, S. (1989). Assessing children with language disorders. In D. Bernstein & E. Tiegerman (Eds.), *Language and communication disorders in children. 157–207.* Columbus: Merrill Publishing.

Johnston, J. (1988). Specific language disorders in the child. In N. Lass, L. McReynolds, J. Northern, & D. Yoder (Eds.), *Handbook of speech-language pathology and audiology. 685–715.* Philadelphia: B. C. Decker.

Johnston, J. & Ellis Weismer, S. (1983). Mental rotation abilities in language-disordered children. *Journal of Speech and Hearing Research, 26,* 397–404.

Kamhi, A. (1989). Causes and consequences of reading disabilities. In A. Kamhi & H. Catts (Eds.), *Reading disabilities: A developmental language perspective. 67–99.* Boston: College-Hill Press.

Kamhi, A. & Catts, H. (1986). Toward an understanding of developmental language and reading disorders. *Journal of Speech and Hearing Disorders, 51,* 337–347.

Kamhi, A. & Catts, H. (1989a). Language and reading: Convergences, divergences, and development. In A. Kamhi & H. Catts (Eds.), *Reading disabilities: A developmental language perspective. 1–34.* Boston: College-Hill Press.

Kamhi, A. & Catts, H. (1989b). Reading disabilities: Terminology, definitions and subtyping issues. In A. Kamhi & H. Catts (Eds.), *Reading disabilities: A developmental language perspective. 35–66.* Boston: College-Hill Press.

Kamhi, A., Catts, H., Mauer, D., Apel, K., & Gentry, B. (1988). Phonological and spatial processing abilities in language- and reading-impaired children. *Journal of Speech and Hearing Disorders, 53,* 316–327.

Kamhi, A. & Koenig, L. (1985). Metalinguistic awareness in normal and language-disordered children. *Language, Speech, and Hearing Services in Schools, 16,* 199–210.

Kamhi, A., Lee, R., & Nelson, L. (1985). Word, syllable, and sound awareness in language-disordered children. *Journal of Speech and Hearing Disorders, 50,* 207–212.

Karmiloff-Smith, A. (1986). From meta-processes to conscious access: Evidence from children's metalinguistic and repair data. *Cognition, 23,* 95–147.

Katz, R. (1986). Phonological deficiencies in children with reading disability: Evidence from an object-naming task. *Cognition, 22,* 225–257.

Klein-Konigsberg, E. (1984). Semantic integration and language learning disabilities: From research to assessment and intervention. In G. Wallach & K. Butler (Eds.), *Language learning disabilities in school-age children. 251–270.* Baltimore: Williams & Wilkins.

Lahey, M. (1988). *Language development and disorders.* New York: Macmillan.

Lee, R. & Kamhi, A. (1990). Metaphoric competence in children with learning disabilities. *Journal of Learning Disabilities, 23,* 476–482.

Lee, R., Kamhi, A., & Nelson, L. (1983). Communicative sensitivity in language-impaired children. Paper presented at the Annual American Speech-Language-Hearing Assoc. Convention, Cincinnati.

Lenchner, O., Gerber, M., & Routh, D. (1990). Phonological awareness tasks as predictors of decoding ability: Beyond segmentation. *Journal of Learning Disabilities, 23,* 240–247.

Liberman, I., Shankweiler, D., Fischer, F., & Carter, B. (1974). Reading and the awareness of linguistic segments. *Journal of Experimental Child Psychology, 18,* 201–212.

Liles, B. (1987). Episode organization and cohesive conjunctives in narratives in children with and without language disorder. *Journal of Speech and Hearing Research, 30,* 185–196.

Liles, B. & Shulman, M. (1981). Linguistic intuitions and comprehension of meaning as demonstrated by linguistically normal and linguistically deviant children. *AVISO: A Journal of Special Education,* 1–19.

Liles, B., Shulman, M., & Bartlett, S. (1977). Judgments of grammaticality by normal and language-disordered children. *Journal of Speech and Hearing Disorders, 42,* 199–209.

Lundberg, I. (1987). Phonological awareness facilitates reading and spelling acquisition. In R. Bowler (Ed.), *Intimacy with language: A forgotten basic in teacher education. 56–63.* Baltimore: The Orton Dyslexia Society.

Lundberg, I., Olofsson, A., & Wall, S. (1980). Reading and spelling skills in the first school years, predicted from phonemic awareness skills in kindergarten. *Scandinavian Journal of Psychology, 21,* 59–173.

Maclean, M., Bryant, P., & Bradley, L. (1987). Rhymes, nursery rhymes, and reading in early childhood. *Merrill-Palmer Quarterly, 33,* 255–281.

Mann, V. & Liberman, I. (1984). Phonological awareness and verbal short-term memory. *Journal of Learning Disabilities, 17,* 592–599.

Masterson, J. & Kamhi, A. (1985). Linguistic and extralinguistic influences upon children's sentence productions. Paper presented at the Annual Convention of the American Speech-Language-Hearing Association, Washington, DC.

Mattingly, I. (1972). Reading, the linguistic process, and linguistic awareness. In J. Kavanagh & I. Mattingly (Eds.), *Language by ear and eye. 133–147.* Cambridge, MA: MIT Press.

Mattingly, I. (1984). Reading, linguistic awareness, and language acquisition. In J. Downing & R. Valtin (Eds.), *Language awareness and learning to read. 9–25.* New York: Springer-Verlag.

Maxwell, S. & Wallach, G. (1984). The language-learning disabilities connection: Symptoms of early language disability change over time. In G. Wallach & K. Butler (Eds.), *Language learning disabilities in school-age children. 15–34.* Baltimore: Williams & Wilkins.

McNinch, G. (1974). Awareness of aural and visual word boundary within a sample of first graders. *Perceptual and Motor Skills, 38*, 1127–1134.

Meline, T. (1986). Referential communication skills of learning disabled/language impaired children. *Applied Psycholinguistics, 7*, 129–140.

Meline, T. & Brackin, S. (1987). Language-impaired children's awareness of inadequate messages. *Journal of Speech and Hearing Disorders, 52*, 263–270.

Meline, T. & Meline, N. (1983). Facing a communicative obstacle: Pragmatics of language-impaired children. *Perceptual and Motor Skills, 56*, 469–470.

Menyuk, P. (1985). Wherefore metalinguistic skills? A commentary on Bialystok and Ryan. *Merrill-Palmer Quarterly, 31*, 253–259.

Menyuk, P. (1991). Metalinguistic abilities and language disorder. In J. Miller (Ed.), *Research on child language disorders: A decade of progress. 387–397.* Austin, TX: Pro-Ed.

Menyuk, P. & Flood, J. (1981). Linguistic competence, reading, writing problems, and remediation. *Bulletin of the Orton Society, 31*, 13–28.

Morais, J., Bertelson, P., Cary, L., & Alegria, J. (1986). Literacy training and speech segmentation. *Cognition, 24*, 45–64.

Morais, J., Cluytens, M., & Alegria, J. (1984). Segmentation abilities of dyslexics and normal readers. *Perceptual and Motor Skills, 58*, 221–222.

Nippold, M. (Ed.). (1988). *Later language development: Ages nine through nineteen.* Boston: College-Hill Press.

Olsen, J., Wong, B., & Marx, R. (1983). Linguistic and metacognitive aspects of normally achieving and learning disabled children's communication processes. *Learning Disabilities Quarterly, 6*, 289–304.

Papandropoulou, I. & Sinclair, H. (1974). What is a word? Experimental study of children's ideas on grammar. *Human Development, 17*, 241–258.

Perfetti, C. (1985). *Reading ability.* New York: Oxford University Press.

Perfetti, C., Beck, I., Bell, L., & Hughes, C. (1987). Phonemic knowledge and learning to read are reciprocal: A longitudinal study of first grade children. *Merrill-Palmer Quarterly, 33*, 283–319.

Perry, B., Newhoff, M. & Buday, E. (1983). Normal and language-disordered children's metalinguistic awareness of the -s morpheme. Paper presented at the American Speech-Language-Hearing Association Convention, Cincinnati.

Read, C. & Ruyter, L. (1985). Reading and spelling skills in adults of low literacy. *Remedial and Special Education, 6*, 43–52.

Read, C., Zhang, Y., Nie, H., & Ding, B. (1986). The ability to manipulate speech sounds depends on knowing alphabetic writing. *Cognition, 24*, 31–44.

Robinson, E. & Robinson, W. (1977). The child's understanding of life-like communication failures. *Australian Journal of Psychology, 29*, 137–142.

Rosner, J. & Simon, D. (1971). The auditory analysis test: An initial report. *Journal of Learning Disabilities, 4*, 40–48.

Roth, F. & Spekman, N. (1989). Higher-order language processes and reading disabilities. In A. Kamhi & H. Catts (Eds.), *Reading disabilities: A developmental language perspective. 159–197.* Boston: College-Hill Press.

Savich, P. (1984). Anticipatory imagery ability in normal and language-disabled children. *Journal of Speech and Hearing Research, 27*, 494–501.

Share, D., Jorm, A., MacLean, R., & Matthews, R. (1984). Sources of individual differences in reading acquisition. *Journal of Educational Psychology, 76*, 1309–1324.

Singer, H. (1984). Learning to read and skilled reading: Multiple systems interacting within and between the reader and the text. In J. Downing & R. Valtin (Eds.), *Language awareness and learning to read. 193–206.* New York: Springer-Verlag.

Smith, C. & Tager-Flusberg, H. (1982). Metalinguistic awareness and language development. *Journal of Experimental Child Psychology, 34*, 449–468.

Snyder, L. & Downey, D. (1991). The language-reading relationship in normal and reading-disabled children. *Journal of Speech and Hearing Research, 34*, 129–140.

Stark, R., Bernstein, L., Condino, R., Bender, M., Tallal, P., & Catts, H. (1984). Four-year follow-up study of language impaired children. *Annals of Dyslexia, 34*, 49–68.

Stanovich, K. (1986). Matthew effects in reading: Some consequences of individual differences in the acquisition of literacy. *Reading Research Quarterly, 21*, 360–407.

Stanovich, K., Cunningham, A., & Cramer, B. (1984). Assessing phonological awareness in kindergarten children: Issues of task comparability. *Journal of Experimental Child Psychology, 38*, 175–190.

Stein, C., Cairns, H., & Zurif, E. (1984). Sentence comprehension limitations related to syntactic deficits in reading disabled children. *Applied Psycholinguistics, 5*, 305—322.

Tallal, P. (1988). Developmental language disorders. In J. Kavanagh & T. Truss (Eds.), *Learning disabilities: Proceedings of the national conference. 181—272.* Parkton, MD: York Press.

Torneus, M. (1984). Phonological awareness and reading: A chicken and egg problem? *Journal of Educational Psychology, 76*, 1346—1358.

Treiman, R. & Baron, J. (1983). Phonemic-analysis training helps children benefit from spelling-sound rules. *Memory and Cognition, 11*, 382—389.

Tunmer, W. & Bowey, J. (1984). Metalinguistic awareness and reading acquisition. In W. Tunmer, C. Pratt, & M. Herriman (Eds.), *Metalinguistic awareness in children: Theory, research, and implications. 144—168.* New York: Springer-Verlag.

Tunmer, W. & Herriman, M. (1984). The development of metalinguistic awareness: A conceptual overview. In W. Tunmer, C. Pratt, & M. Herriman (Eds.), *Metalinguistic awareness in children: Theory, research, and implications. 12—35.* New York: Springer-Verlag.

van Kleeck, A. (1982). The emergence of linguistic awareness: A cognitive framework. *Merrill-Palmer Quarterly, 28*, 237—265.

van Kleeck, A. (1984a). Metalinguistic skills: Cutting across spoken and written language and problem-solving. In G. Wallach & K. Butler (Eds.), *Language learning disabilities in school-age children. 128—153.* Baltimore: Williams & Wilkins.

van Kleeck, A. (1984b). Assessment and intervention: Does "meta" matter? In G. Wallach & K. Butler (Eds.), *Language learning disabilities in school-age children. 179—198.* Baltimore: Williams & Wilkins.

Vellutino, F. (1977). Alternative conceptualizations of dyslexia: Evidence in support of a verbal-deficit hypothesis. *Harvard Educational Review, 47*, 334—354.

Vellutino, F. (1979). *Dyslexia: Theory and research.* Cambridge, MA: MIT Press.

Vellutino, F. & Scanlon, D. (1987). Phonological coding, phonological awareness, and reading ability: Evidence from a longitudinal and experimental study. *Merrill-Palmer Quarterly, 33*, 321—363.

Vogel, S. (1977). Morphological ability in normal and dyslexic children. *Journal of Learning Disabilities, 10*, 292—299.

Vygotsky, L. (1962). *Thought and language.* Cambrige, MA: MIT Press.

Wagner, R. (1986). Phonological processing abilities and reading: Implications for disabled readers. *Journal of Learning Disabilities, 19*, 623—630.

Wagner, R. (1988). Causal relations between the development of phonological processing abilities and the acquisition of reading skills: A meta-analysis. *Merrill-Palmer Quarterly, 34*, 261—279.

Wagner, R. & Torgesen, J. (1987). The nature of phonological processing and its causal role in the acquisition of reading skills. *Psychological Bulletin, 101*, 192—212.

Westby, C. (1989). Assessing and remediating text comprehension problems. In A. Kamhi & H. Catts (Eds.), *Reading disabilities: A developmental language perspective. 199—260.* Boston: College-Hill Press.

Wiig, E. & Semel, E. (1976). *Language disabilities in children and adolescents.* Columbus, OH: Merrill.

Williams, J. (1979). The ABD's of reading: A program for the learning disabled. In L. Resnick & P. Weaver (Eds.), *Theory and practice of early reading. 179—195.* Hillsdale, NJ: Erlbaum.

Williams, J. (1980). Teaching decoding with an emphasis on phoneme analysis and phoneme blending. *Journal of Educational Psychology, 72*, 1—15.

Zifcak, M. (1981). Phonological awareness and reading acquisition. *Contemporary Educational Psychology, 6*, 117—126.

Susan Ellis Weismer, Madison, Wisconsin (USA)

76. Communicative Behavior with Neurotic Developmental Disorders: Elective Mutism

1. Introduction

There are two forms of psychological mutism – traumatic and elective; both are dramatic and both are rare. The main theme of this paper is an account of elective mutism.

The rarity of mutism may be the reason for the lack of a substantial literature on the subject of elective mutism. Following the original classic article by Tramer (1934), over the next half century there were only about half a dozen major contributions to the literature on this subject, culminating in the article by Kolvin/Fundudis (1981). And in the recent years there has been only one further research report of a controlled study with more than 20 electively mute children (Wilkins 1985).

2. Traumatic Mutism

This has an acute onset following a psychological or physical shock or injury. Some consider it to be an hysterical phenomenon as it is not associated with any disorder of the structures subserving speech functioning (lips, tongue, palate or vocal cords) and, furthermore, the patient is able to cough normally. The literature suggests that it is common, but a wide clinical survey has attested to its considerable rarity (Kolvin/Fundudis 1981).

3. Elective Mutism

This is the term coined by Tramer (1934) to describe a fascinating group of children, whose talking is confined to familiar situations, usually the home, and to a small group of intimates. It needs to be distinguished from the inordinate shyness that occurs relatively frequently in reception classes in school (Brown/Loyd 1975; Wright 1968), by its severity and persistence.

The literature suggests that the earliest manifestations are in the pre-school years, with the parents being unaware of significant abnormality because there has been a period of relatively normal speech development (Elson/Pearson/Jones et al. 1965; Reed 1963; Salfield 1950). Kolvin/Fundudis (1981) report that commonly an inordinate degree of shyness was present from the early years of life in the majority of cases and only in a small percentage were there indications that it had emerged for the first time at a later stage in development.

3.1. Epidemiology

From their epidemiological study, Fundudis/Kolvin/Garside (1979, 15) report a rate of 0.4 per thousand children in a total city cohort of 3,300 seven-year-olds. To put this in perspective, this is less common than broadly defined autism by a factor of two. Subsequently, the same team (Kolvin/Fundudis 1981) identified 24 electively mute children, over a period of six years, gathered from a wide survey of clinical departments of speech pathology and child psychiatry serving a large population in the North East of England. However, other workers have reported on larger samples of clinically or epidemiologically identified elective mute children. For instance, Brown/Lloyd (1975) report a prevalence of 7.2 per thousand of children who do not speak at school at the age of 5. Thus, some eight weeks after starting school, 42 out of 6072 children were not speaking, but after 12 months the rate had fallen to 0.33–0.66 per thousand. Thus, their rate of 'persistent elective mutism' is closely comparable to that reported in the Kolvin and Fundudis epidemiological survey. Brown and Lloyd's survey is complicated by ethnic factors and they used a rather broad definition of elective mutism. Nevertheless, it confirmed that persistent elective mutism is rare. Hayden (1980) reports on the results of a clinical study of 68 cases of elective mutism, based on a five-centre study in the U.S.A. However, the diagnostic criteria employed are questionable: they are rather broad and the duration of mutism was often very brief; there was inadequate specification of the settings in which the child refuses to speak, and there was diverse co-morbidity.

3.2. Diagnosis and Differential Diagnosis

A number of important themes merit consideration. First, previously there was both a tendency to emphasize the importance of motivation in the diagnosis of elective mutism and acceptance of the notion that the presence of abnormalities of speech and language precluded such a diagnosis. However, such earlier views were based on anecdotal material or small case studies without controls. As indicated above, studies of more representative series of cases indicate that such previous accounts were often misleading.

Second, in a pilot observational study of pre-school children, Kolvin/Nolan (1979) observed that unusual shyness occurred frequently, especially in girls, but this tended to be transient. The behavior consisted of a tendency to speak in a soft voice or an unwillingness to speak to their mothers or to play in the presence of strangers, combined with a tendency to cling and hide behind their mother's skirts. This reluctance to talk proved to be a transient phenomenon which is likely to reflect normal separation anxiety compounded by transient adaptation reactions to the usual stresses and unfamiliarity of the new school situations. Thus with familiarity, this anxiety diminishes and the child may begin to talk (Cantwell/Baker 1985). The latter authors suggest that many of the children in the Brown/Lloyd (1975) sample may have demonstrated this behavior.

Hence, it is not unexpected that confusion may arise with those excessively shy infant school children who do not speak when first attending school. However, shyness is not specific to elective mutism (Wilkins 1985). Hence Kolvin/Fundudis (1981) go on to suggest that a distinction needs to be made between such transient states of inordinate shyness and those behaviors which are pathological, in both severity and persistence. They therefore apply more rigorous criteria when defining elective mutism as persistent, severe and pathological shyness beyond the home situation, which is usually associated with abnormalities of temperament and of relationships of the child with his/her mother. If the mutism had been evident at the start of school life, then it had to show no signs of abating in the following year. If the mutism appeared to have a later onset, there had to be no evidence of diminution, again over a period of at least a year.

Third, there is little diagnostic difficulty with the early-onset (Kolvin/Ounsted/Humphrey et al. 1971) and the late-onset psychoses of childhood (Kolvin/Berney 1990; Kolvin et al. 1971), about which there is now considerable agreement.

Fourth, another crucial issue concerns the distinction between elective mutism and Asperger's syndrome (Asperger 1944). Although both groups of children have initial problems of social adjustment, which mainly declare themselves outside the home, there are many important differences. In both there is evidence of a lifelong personality deviation rather than an illness with a definite onset (Kolvin/Fundudis 1981; Wolff/Barlow 1979). Whereas the children with Asperger's syndrome are often described by their mothers as solitary, remote and strange, in the case of electively mute children the parents are often not aware of anything unusual until the children first attend school (Kolvin/Fundudis 1981). The children with Asperger's syndrome are described as showing obstinacy and aggressive outbursts, especially when attempts are made to persuade them to conform. However, the obstinacy of elective mutism is more usually combined with degrees of withdrawal or retreat. Next, while obsessionality is almost universal in Asperger's syndrome, it occurs only occasionally in elective mutism. By definition, none of the elective mutes speak outside the home or at school, whereas in the case of Asperger's syndrome only a few refuse to speak at school. Finally, whereas electively mute children use gestures and other forms of non-verbal communication, children with Asperger's syndrome tend not to communicate well by such means.

A further issue is the classification of children who speak rather little. We endorse, first, the view that those children who speak very little in all circumstances should not be assigned the diagnosis of elective mutism (Blake/Moss 1967), and second, the view that those children who display 'reluctant speech', i. e. they will not speak spontaneously but will answer questions which have been asked, should also be excluded from the specific diagnosis (Williamson/Sewell/Sanders/Haney 1977).

3.3 Developmental and Biological Factors

In most major studies of elective mutism there is a consistent pattern of an excess of girls to boys, which is unusual for childhood disorders (Kolvin/Fundudis 1981; Wilkins 1985; Wright 1968). In the investigation by Kolvin and Fundudis, the control group was drawn from a general population sample, whereas in Wilkins' research the elective mute sample was compared with a matched sample of clinic children who had been diagnosed as having an emotional disorder. In both studies there was an excess of birth complications but this was significant only in the former study. However, Kolvin/Fundudis (1981) report evidence of slow or uneven development compared with the controls and this included delay in onset of speech, excessive developmental mispronunciation with associated problems of speech and bowel and bladder function, and also EEG immaturity. The case-note study by Wilkins provides an account of one in three of the electively mute children having delayed speech, whereas none of the children with emotional disorders had such problems. Although he does not report any other developmental anomalies, it should be remembered that in a case-note study there has not necessarily been a specific focus on particular deficits, and therefore a lack of listing does not necessarily imply absence of deficit. To recapitulate, Wright (1968) found that about one in five of his study children had an underlying speech or language delay or problem; Kolvin/Fundudis (1981) report as many as 50 percent and Wilkins (1985) reports 33 percent.

Kolvin/Fundudis (1981) report that electively mute children are born significantly early in the sibship but Wilkins (1985) did not replicate this finding. However, electively mute children in both studies come from families of similar size as those of the controls.

3.4. Personality and Temperament

In addition to inordinate shyness and social and communication problems, a diversity of other personality and temperamental anomalies have been described in these children (Kolvin/Fundudis 1981).

Evidence of an insidious development of shyness has been reported in over 80% of cases and even in those where it appeared acute, it may well be that the essential abnormality became dramatically obvious only when the child entered the school setting (Kolvin/Fundudis 1981; Wright 1968). In addition, a wide variety of complex personality patterns often occur, such as oppositional behavior and poor malleability both at school and at home. The commonest personality pattern was of sulkiness combined with aggressiveness, with a child presenting as sulky to strangers and aggressive within the home. Many of these children are described as having powerful personalities, with 'wills of steel'. About a quarter showed a combination of shyness in social situations with submissiveness at home. Another quarter seemed to be rather sensitive children. In addition, there was an important trend for such children to be more withdrawn in relation to peers than to adults.

In addition to the above personality patterns, there were a varied group of patterns of problem behaviors in over two-thirds of the children. These included excessive and unusual motor activity. Wilkins (1985) was not able to study personality and behavior systematically, and therefore merely listed those features which occurred more frequently in the elective mutes than in children with emotional disorders. His analysis appears to play down shyness and emphasize anxiety and depression as symptoms in the elective mute group, but he does report manipulative behavior. However, it must again be stressed that a retrospective case-note study from a psychiatric clinic may not be sufficiently focused on features under scrutiny and inevitably there may be distortions in the data.

3.5 Cognitive Aspects

Again, literature review reveals few studies quoting psychometric findings with even modest-sized samples of electively mute children (Kolvin/Fundudis 1981; Wright 1968). The evidence available shows that although electively mute children as a group cover most ranges of intellectual ability as measured on non-verbal IQ, there is a distinct shift to the left. Thus, while the majority fall within the normal range of intelligence, a substantial concentration of elective mutes is found within the dull – normal and lower categories of non-verbal intelligence (Kolvin/Fundudis 1981; Wright 1968). The reason for the poorer performance on nonverbal IQ remains obscure. Nevertheless, there are a number of other features among elective mute children which may have important associations with their poorer performance: first, as indicated above, electively mute children display a wide variety of complex temperamental, personality and behavioral patterns (Kolvin/Fundudis 1981) which may vary according to the circumstances in which the child is assessed; further, underpinning these various patterns of temperamental expression is a 'will of iron' and a determination to get his/her own way.

In general terms, when electively mute children do speak – which they do within the confines of their own homes – their vocabulary, verbal conceptualisation of ideas and grammatical structure of sentences are usually normal.

3.6. Assessment

Enlisting co-operation of the electively mute child for the purpose of psychological/psychiatric assessment usually constitutes a challenge, the bases of which are the complex emotional and attitudinal expressions which accompany the refusal to talk. Thus, co-operation is best facilitated by the clinician adopting a style of communication which avoids expectation of the child to talk. In contrast, pressure by the clinican is likely to intensify the child's resistance, which is compounded by the excessive reserve/shyness and/or passive hostility which accompanies the child's refusal to talk. For younger children, drawing and play materials as a medium for preliminary interaction is often helpful. Subsequently, standardized non-verbal measures are the main source of assessment, particularly among the older children. The use of play materials and other purposeful tasks or activities can prove a helpful and meaningful way of not only engaging the child but also of obtaining a productive cognitive assessment. In those children with more highly resistant attitudes, the assessment may have to be carried out over a number of sessions with the tasks and measures being administered in a piecemeal fashion.

Skill, flexibility and patience are the guiding principles for achieving a useful and valid psychological/psychiatric assessment. They are also important for understanding the child's cognitive potential, personality, strengths and vulnerabilities and for establishing the basis of an individually tailored, multimodal, therapeutic programme.

3.7. Family and Social Factors

There is a tendency to assume that more of the families of electively mute children come from the lower end of the social class spectrum, but the evidence is that the families of these children are represented at all levels of socio-economic strata (Brown/Lloyd 1975; Kolvin/Fundudis 1981; Wright 1968). Of greater importance is the nature of the psychological dynamics within these families. The literature abounds with examples of parents with unusual personalities and psychiatric problems which are often offered as explanations for the elective mutism of their children (Elson/Pearson/Jones/Schumacher 1965; Parker/Olsen/Throckmorton 1960; Wergeland 1979). The confidence placed in these findings must be limited by the lack of controls and small sample size of the studies upon which the theories are based. Some of the factors which have been viewed as causative include the following: maternal rejection and paternal disinterest (Elson et al. 1965), maternal anxiety, fearfulness and overprotectiveness (Parker et al. 1960; Wergeland 1979), the influence of 'family secrets' and the child's fear of parental retaliation (Pustrom/Speers 1964), abusive behavior by alcoholic fathers (Adams/Glasner 1954), and the effects of a symbiotic relationship between parent and child (Browne/Wilson/Leybourne 1963). However, most of these notions derive from older publications.

Evidence from a controlled and larger study of 24 cases (Kolvin/Fundudis 1981) does not suggest the presence of a common set of family dynamics, but rather the origins appear multifactorial. In that study, one-third of the parents of electively mute children were found to have personalities that were characterized by serious or marked reserve and shyness. Taking into account all of the personality problems of the parents, irrespective of type, in two in five of the families one or other of the parents had a personality which could best be described as odd or unusual. As to psychiatric problems, severe neurotic disorder was found in one of the parents in about one-sixth of the families and depression in one of the parents, again in one-sixth, with a combination of these two disorders occurring in a number of the families. When serious psychiatric disturbance or major personality problems were considered in combination with serious marital disharmony it was found that six of ten of the families were affected. Thus, however, the disturbance in families is defined, the available evidence points to an excess of psychological morbidity in families of elective mute children compared with families of normal control children (Kolvin/Fundudis 1981). For instance, these authors noted that 20% of mothers and 16% of fathers of elective mute children had received specialist psychiatric help, compared with only 8% of mothers and 3% of fathers of normal control children.

In a study of 24 families, Wright (1968) reported a 75% rate of parental psychological disturbance. This higher rate was probably due to the inclusion of the use of a much broader definition of disturbance, for instance including the trait of parental shyness as one of the criteria. Further, as shyness in parents of electively mute children appears to be fairly common (Brown/Lloyd 1975; Kolvin/Fundudis 1981; Wright 1968), it raises the interesting possibility of a familial or even a genetic link between shyness of the parents and elective mutism of the child. The latter possibility is enhanced by the finding of a number of affected siblings (Wright 1968) or twins (Halpern/Hammond/Cohen 1971; Mora/DeVault/Schopler 1962) in different series of electively mute children. On the other hand, the influence of learning/modelling cannot be discounted.

3.8. The Aetiology of Elective Mutism

As evident above, numerous workers have postulated a diversity of psychogenic bases for elective mutism; others imply that it is a learnt pattern of behavior, and yet others implicate temperamental or personality factors which have a familial basis. Another suggestion is that it may be a secondary psychological reaction to some biologically based symptoms; for instance, some children may avoid speaking because they are teased when they mis-pronounce words (Rutter 1977); other work suggests an important maturational component. This diversity of aetiological factors suggests that the origins are multiple and the condition heterogeneous.

3.9. Intervention and Outcome

Elective mutism has been, and continues to be, a challenge to psychodynamically and behaviorally oriented psychotherapists. The reported success rates of the different methods of intervention have been variable; however, it is difficult to draw any conclusions from such studies because of the differences in diagnostic criteria used, the severity of the mutism and the criteria of improvement. For example, Wright (1968) reported that at follow-up of 19 of 24 cases, 79% had achieved 'excellent' or 'good' adjustment, whereas Kolvin/Fundudis (1981) report an adjustment rate of 46%. Further, the confidence in success rates reported in other studies is limited by small samples and poor specification of improvement criteria (e. g. Elson/Pearson/Jones/Schumacher 1965; Kupietz/Schwartz 1982; Pustrom/Speers 1964). For example Elson et al. (1965) noted that most of the children "tended to have made a fairly good adjustment" following their discharge from hospital, but that there was a "tendency to be somewhat reserved" (Elson et al. 1965, 185). The problem of defining treatment success or improvement has been further highlighted by Pustrom/Speers (1964) who report that, in three cases, after intervention some improvement was achieved in terms of readiness to talk to others, but they resisted talking to the therapist. The authors concluded that "failure to speak to his therapist represents a last-ditch stand against giving up his omnipotent control over others" (Pustrom/Speers 1964, 296). Such statements emphasize the intractability of elective mutism to psychotherapy, in that although degrees of improvement are usually reported, the spontaneity of interpersonal communication of the electively mute child is seldom fully shifted.

The emphasis of earlier treatment approaches on intrapsychic dynamics (e. g. motives, drives, personality traits) of the electively mute child and/or the parents (e. g. Browne/Wilson/Legbourne 1963; Chetnik 1973; Elson et al. 1965); have tended to give way to the more recently developed behavioral strategies (e. g. Kupietz/Schwartz 1982; Nolan/Pence 1970; Norman/Broman 1970). Such a shift is not surprising because the resistance of elective mutism to treatment has continued to pose a challenge to therapists of all persuasions. However, some reviewers conclude that behavioral therapies have been found to have greater effectiveness than the psychodynamic therapies (Kratochwill/Brody/Piersel 1979). In keeping with the more pragmatic stance of the behaviorists it has been argued that intervention should be directed not only at 'mutism' but more broadly at 'social skills' (Kratochwill/Brody/Piersel 1979). Consistent with the above is the proposal of a multidimensional management approach (Friedman/Karagan 1973) consisting of the following: a) avoidance of strategies that are likely to put pressure on the child to talk; b) inclusion of the child in small peer group activities; c) use of reading, story-telling and other verbal activities which do not make the child feel especially uncomfortable (e. g. within the family context); d) encouragement by parents for relatives and peers to visit within the electively mute child's home to create a natural social context of conversation but without putting pressure on the child to talk; e) encouragement within the classroom situation for the electively mute child to engage in non-verbal, non-threatening interpersonal relationship through the use of such activities as puzzles and workbook exercises; f) a gradual process of encouragement involving the electively mute child in a one-to-one situation where appropriate stimuli (e. g. pictures which require to be identified and labelled, e. g. *what is this*?) are used as a means of creating a spontaneous form of verbal communication on the part of the electively mute child, and then including one or two other children in the activity; g) the electively mute child and any others in whose presence the child is prepared to talk are encouraged to engage in activities outside the home. This broadbased behavioral approach seems attractive but it merits more careful evaluation.

4. References

Adams, H. M. & Glasner, P. J. (1954). Emotional involvement in some forms of mutism. *Journal of Speech and Hearing Disorders, 19*, 59–69.

Asperger, S. (1944). Die autistischen Psychopathen im Kindesalter. *Archiv für Psychiatrie und Nervenkrankheiten, 1*, 76–137.

Blake, P. & Moss, T. (1967). The development of socialization skills in an electively mute child. *Behavioral Research and Therapy, 5*, 349–356.

Brown, J. B. & Lloyd, H. (1975). A controlled study of children not speaking at school. *Journal of the Association of Workers of Maladjusted Children, 3*, 49–63.

Browne, E., Wilson, V., & Leybourne, P. C. (1963). Diagnosis and treatment of elective mutism in children. *Journal of the American Academy of Child Psychiatry, 2*, 605–617.

Cantwell, D. P. & Baker, L. (1985). Speech and language: Development and disorders. In M. Rutter & L. Hersov (Eds.), *Child and adolescent psychiatry: Modern approaches. 526–544.* London: Blackwell Publications.

Chetnik, M. (1973). The intensive treatment of an elective mute. *Journal of the American Academy of Child Psychiatry, 12*, 482–498.

Elson, A., Pearson, C., Jones, C. D. & Schumacher, E. (1965). Follow-up study of childhood elective mutism. *Archives of General Psychiatry, 13*, 182–187.

Friedman, R. & Karagan, N. (1973). Characteristics and management of elective mutism in children. *Psychology in the Schools, 10*, 249–252.

Fundudis, T., Kolvin, I., & Garside, R. (1979). *Speech retarded and deaf children: Their psychological development.* London: Academic Press.

Halpern, W. I., Hammond, J., & Cohen, R. A. (1971). A therapeutic approach to speech phobia: Elective mutism re-examined. *Journal of the American Academy of Child Psychiatry, 10*, 94–107.

Hayden, T. L. (1980). Classification of elective mutism. *Journal of the American Academy of Child Psychiatry, 19*, 118–133.

Kolvin, I. & Berney, T. (1990). Childhood schizophrenia. In B. J. Tonge, G. D. Burrows, & J. S. Werry (Eds.), *Handbook of studies on child psychiatry.* Amsterdam: Elsevier.

Kolvin, I. & Fundudis, T. (1981). Elective mute children; psychological development and background factors. *Journal of Child Psychology and Psychiatry, 22*, 219–232.

Kolvin, I. & Nolan, J. (1979). Personal observation.

Kolvin, I., Ounsted, C., Humphrey, M., & McNay, A. (1971). The phenomenology of childhood psychoses. *British Journal of Psychiatry, 118*, 385–395.

Kratochwill, T. R., Brody, G. H., & Piersel, W. C. (1979). Elective mutism in children. In G. B. Lahey & A. E. Kazdin (Eds.), *Advances in clinical child psychology. 193–239.* New York: Plenum Press.

Kupietz, S. S. & Schwartz, I. L. (1982). Elective mutism: Evaluation and behavioural treatment of three cases. *New York State Journal of Medicine, 82*, 1073–1076.

Mora, G., DeVault, S., & Schopler, E. (1962). Dynamics and psychotherapy of identical twins with elective mutism. *Journal of Child Psychology and Psychiatry, 3*, 41–52.

Nolan, J. & Pence, C. (1970). Operant conditioning principles in the treatment of an electively mute child. *Journal of Consulting and Clinical Psychology, 35*, 265–268.

Norman, A. & Broman, H. J. (1970). Volume feedback and generalization techniques in shaping speech of an electively mute boy: A case study. *Perceptual and Motor Skills, 31*, 463–470.

Parker, E. B., Olsen, J. F., & Throckmorton, M. (1960). Social casework with elementary schoolchildren who do not talk in school. *Social Work, 5*, 64–70.

Pustrom, E. & Speers, R. W. (1964). Elective mutism in children. *Journal of the American Academy of Child Psychiatry, 3*, 287–297.

Reed, G. F. (1963). Elective mutism in children: a re-appraisal. *Journal of Child Psychology and Psychiatry, 4*, 99–107.

Rutter, M. (1977). Delayed speech. In M. Rutter & L. Hersov (Eds.), *Child psychiatry: Modern approaches. 698–716.* Oxford: Blackwell Scientific Publications.

Salfield, D. M. (1950). Observations of elective mutism in children. *Journal of Mental Science, 96*, 1024–1032.

Tramer, M. (1934). Electiver Mutismus bei Kindern. *Zeitschrift für Kinderpsychiatrie, 1*, 30–35.

Wergeland, H. (1979). Elective mutism. *Acta Psychiatrica Scandinavica, 59*, 218–223.

Wilkins, R. (1985). A comparison of elective mutism and emotional disorders in children. *British Journal of Psychiatry*, *146*, 198–203.

Williamson, D. A., Sewell, W., Sanders, S., & Haney, J. (1977). The treatment of reluctant speech using contingency management procedures. *Journal of Behavior Therapy and Experimental Psychiatry*, *8*, 155–156.

Wolff, S. & Barlow, A. (1979). Schizoid personality in childhood. *Journal of Child Psychology and Psychiatry*, *20*, 29–46.

Wright, H. L. (1968). A clinical study of children who refuse to talk. *Journal of the American Academy of Child Psychiatry*, *7*, 603–617.

Israel Kolvin, London (United Kingdom)
Trian Fundudis, Newcastle upon Tyne (United Kingdom)

77. Language and Communicative Behavior in Childhood Psychosis

1. Definition

From the beginning, the definition of what is called 'schizophrenia' has always been a great problem which could not even be satisfactorily solved by the setting up of various classification systems. Meanwhile one can find countless publications dealing with the definitional and nosological problems of this term. This has resulted in considerable heterogeneity of opinion with regard to the terminological meaning and nosological differentiation of 'schizophrenia'. The same is true for childhood schizophrenia, and, as Stutte (1975) ascertained, no other term in the history of child psychiatry up to the present has undergone such changes in meaning as that of the childhood psychoses.

Even today, especially in the Anglo-American literature, the term 'childhood schizophrenia' stands for a collection of heterogeneous syndromes, which again are referred to by various labels such as 'childhood psychosis', 'infantile autism', 'atypical child'. 'symbiotic psychosis', 'dementia praecocissima', 'dementia infantilis', 'schizophrenic syndrome of childhood', 'pseudo-psychopathic schizophrenia', and 'latent schizophrenia'. Accordingly, under these terms a broad range of psychomotoric and/or neurologically impaired or retarded children are subsumed. Of course, one or two children classified under these syndromes might indeed be inflicted by a real schizophrenic psychosis and also as adults display the typical schizophrenic condition, but these remain exceptions.

The younger the child suffering from a psychotic-like condition, the greater the probability that this is due to an organic brain disturbance. This is the reason why, at diagnosis, neurological symptoms are relatively frequent (psychomotoric and speech retardation, spasticity, epileptic seizures, ataxia, disturbances in motor coordination, sensory disturbances). Even though the etiology is varied, clinicians nevertheless diagnose a childhood psychosis, since the clinical phenomenology is relatively uniform (autistic retreat, negativism, emotional unresponsiveness, motoric states of excitement, emotional frigidity, refusal to speak, disorders in language development, language deterioration, condition of dementia yet intelligent facial expression ('Prinzengesicht')). The psychopathological expressions based on heterogeneous causes are apparently relatively uniform in the age-group below 5–6 years.

It is therefore difficult to diagnose childhood schizophrenia with sufficient certainty before age 5. Because of this it should be stated quite clearly what is meant by childhood schizophrenia and how it can be distinguished from other forms of childhood psychosis, especially from early autistic disorder. The term childhood schizophrenia should be used only in such cases in which the symptoms, even when modified by age-related specificities, are similar to those shown in adulthood and in which the continuity of the early psychosis into the adult form can be confirmed by longitudinal studies up to early adulthood. The childhood psychoses, including the infantile autism according to Kanner may share some symptoms, especially negative ones, with adult schizophrenia on a phenomenological level. However, they hardly ever develop into the schizophrenic psychosis found in adults. Also, one does not find in children with so-called childhood psychoses an increased hereditary streak of schizophrenic psychoses, as is the case in childhood schizophrenia (Eggers 1973, 1978 a). Consequently, a separate chapter in this handbook will deal with childhood autism (cf. art. 78).

Various forms of infantile psychoses can be described according to the degree of maturation of individual ego functions and defense mechanisms. Taking into consideration the aspects of psychological development, French authors named these illnesses quite pertinently as 'psychoses de développement' (Duché 1971, Heuyer 1960, Michaux/Duché 1965). Such conditions would include psychoses of early onset such as the early infantile autism (Kanner 1943), the psychodefective (Bender 1953) or the no-onset-type (Despert 1938) of childhood psychosis, the pseudoneurotic psychosis (Bender 1953), the acute onset type (Despert 1938), the symbiotic psychosis (Mahler 1954) or dementia infantilis (Heller), the dementia praecocissima (de Sanctis 1908), and the syndrome of Kramer-Pollnow (1932).

The actual schizophrenic psychoses in childhood, however, require a higher degree of ego-structuring and appear later, after completion of the 5th year of age. They belong to the so-called late-onset psychoses (Kolvin 1971).

The reason for the differentiation between various forms of infantile psychosis and childhood schizophrenia is that an already differentiated level of psychological development and a higher degree of ego maturity are prerequisites for the ability to produce psychotic symptoms similar or even identical to those in adults. The ego-structuring achieved allows the genesis of guilt or inferiority feelings and the experience of ego alienation, for instance, which in their turn presuppose the sense of ego identity. Such a level of psychological integration allows only for depressive or schizophrenic psychoses known as late-onset psychoses or 'psychoses de la phase de latence' (onset rarely before the age of five) in contrast to the autistic, symbiotic or organic psychoses of early childhood (Eggers 1982).

2. Symptomatology

The frequency of childhood schizophrenia lies for under 10-year-olds between 0.5% and 1% and for 10 to 14-year-olds by 3 to 4% of total cases of schizophrenic psychoses in the general population. The detection and precise study in early childhood of psychopathological phenomena usually occurring in adults reveal that undoubtedly manic, depressive or schizophrenic symptoms may already appear before the age of 10, and that these correspond positively to adult symptoms although modified by factors related to the phase of development. Thus it is possible to evaluate age-related characteristic features of childhood schizophrenia. It is generally accepted that the younger the child, the poorer the psychopathological symptoms.

This view is correct in so far as that at early school age negative, non-productive symptoms predominate, such as poor drive, loss of interests typical for this age, autistic withdrawal from the world of child relations, inability to maintain links with relatives and friends, anxious-paranoid basic mood with a tendency to eruptions of feelings of rage, increased affective blunting and loss of age-related intentional volitional strivings as well as regressive-atavistic tendencies (encopresis, coprophagy, faecal smearing, eating of waste, fear of toilets, destructive impulses). The personality change is displayed mainly in the emotional, intentional, and social behavior. Previously animal-loving children are unmotivatedly cruel to animals. Children who used to be gentle, sensitive, and affectionate suddenly become unloving, unnaturally cold, hard, wilful, impudent and show no emotional links to previously beloved caregivers.

The disturbance in social contact is less marked in childhood schizophrenia than in other childhood psychoses. In their comparative study, Kolvin/Ounsted/Humphrey/McNay (1971) found that the poor relationships in the late-onset psychoses were "less global and more patchily present" than in the infantile psychoses. The poor relational ability with other people could be confirmed as a central feature of infantile psychosis, and as "an important but not a central feature of late-onset psychosis, with only half of these children mixing poorly or avoiding contact with adults or children" (Kolvin et al. 1971, 387).

The social contact disorder in schizophrenic children is closely related to their impoverished drive and impaired ability to react emotionally. In productive forms of childhood schizophrenia the social contact disorder is primarily a result of the child's preoccupation with often threatening delusions and hallucinatory bodily sensations. Visual and acoustic hallucinations, although seldom in childhood schizophrenia, certainly do occur before the age of 10.

For instance among other things a 7-year-old girl heard human voices in her head: "They are always saying something *you crab*, *you dirty slut*, they tell me nothing but ugly and indecent things". The child felt a snake inside her abdomen, believed she was poisoned, felt "persecuted by evil forces" and thought the food was poisoned (Eggers 1982, 84).

In contrast, in early childhood psychoses with onset before the age of 5 or in early infantile autism the communication disorder is more elementary and as a rule is not caused by productive-psychotic phenomena such as hallucinations or delusionary symptoms. At most one could suspect such productive symptoms in some of the children with an infantile psychosis on account of their behavior (e. g. a child looks as if he/she is hearing voices), but this cannot be verified. And also at a later stage, children with an infantile psychosis only seldom display true schizophrenic symptoms.

The communicative behavior of schizophrenic children is to a great extent the result of age-related delusional and hallucinatory types of experience, including so-called transitivistic depersonalisation phenomena (Eggers 1973, 1982). Children identify themselves with people, animals or even objects in their environment. Other symptoms typical of this age are seemingly delusional-hallucinatory bodily sensations and fears such as those narrated by a 10-year-old boy: "The navel bursts; the heart stops: lightning shoots through me: the sex is broken into two". Statements like *I am not myself anymore* or *I am divided into two small persons* (Ssucharewa 1967) also indicate that schizophrenic children already have splitting experiences. Moreover, delusional symptoms in children whose illness was manifested before the age of 10 frequently take the form of diffuse and unattached anxiety or cosmic threats: *The sun falls from the sky, the rain will never stop and everybody will drown*. Later symptoms include paranoid ideas of reference and of being poisoned, and also hypochondriac, religious and depressive delusional symptoms. Whereas delusional ideas are relatively transient and variable before the age of 10, they become more or less systematized in cases over the age of 12. As a rule these children have an above-average intelligence and are highly sensitive, with early manifested tendencies to brood over metaphysical or religious problems. Thus a boy who became ill at the age of 11 and showing a marked delusional system, already said the following when aged 5: "I consider this life as only a transition period". Similar expressions were used by a schizophrenic girl at the beginning of her psychosis: "One has to think of the autumn of life".

Hallucinations in psychotic children often take the form of abnormal bodily sensations. The children perceive talking or singing persons within their head or abdomen, feel animals inside their body, have the impression that smoke passes through their body, that their head becomes larger or 'crooked', that their navel bursts, their sex is broken into two, lightning shoots through their body, and cornered stones lie in their abdomen. Characteristically, schizophrenic children are more likely to have visual hallucinations than schizophrenic adults (Eggers 1973).

3. Speech and Language Behavior in Schizophrenic Children

3.1. Clinical Observations

The communication disorder is also expressed in language behavior. Although there are no systematic linguistic studies on the language behavior in childhood schizophrenia, we do have, mainly in the older literature, descriptions of language use in these children. However, schizophrenic children's speech has by no means found the same scientific interest as the speech of children with a childhood psychosis, especially of those with infantile autism. (cf. art. 78).

The language disorders in schizophrenic children (between 6–12 years of age) are not uniform, so that at times we find mutism and verbiage even in one and the same child. Some children display an unmotivated change of vocal volume, speaking to themselves loudly or softly. Their utterances appear unmotivated and unrelated, at times with fantastic and incomprehensible content or meaning. We find verbal modifications, word creations (neologisms), stringing together of seemingly meaningless words, senseless repetition of syllables, words, or phrases (verbigerations). Very typical are eccentricities in expression (e. g. a 12-year-old schizophrenic boy: "Ich bin innerlich so ausgegloist" ["I am so 'burned-out' internally"].

Atschkova (1966) reports that sometimes language use stops for no apparent reason, that some children speak to themselves in a whisper but will not answer questions and do not speak to their relatives. Kudrjawzewa (1967) observed in the children she studied neologisms, rhyming, speaking out-of-context, and meaningless talking about technical topics. She describes the monotony and poverty of language in these children. They seldom use language as a tool for communication. Thus, some authors speak of compulsive talking and verbiage in the sense of "fruchtloser Klügelei, in Vorbeireden oder Wiederholungen von Fragen" ["fruitless riddles, missing the point, or repetition of questions"] (Kudrjawzewa 1967, Stutte 1963, v. Stockert 1956). One of the oldest descriptions of language in childhood schizophrenia can be found in L. Voigt (1919, 183). He describes the process of a psychotic language disorder in a 10-year-old girl. When asked to say the Lord's Prayer, the girl first says: "Das darf man nicht" ["That isn't allowed"], but then she does begin: "Vater, Vater, Vater, unser, unser, unser, unser, im, im, im, im, Himmel, Himmel, Himmel, Himmel ..." ["Father, Father, Father, our, our, our, our, in, in, in, in, heaven, heaven, heaven, heaven"]. Also in reading she repeats each word several times, her reading being otherwise correct. Three years later, at 13 years, the girl's speech sounds very clipped, it is over-articulated, monotonous, and slow, as if memorized, the consonants are pronounced very distinctly, each word separated markedly from the following. In between, some utterances are spoken fluently, with normal, natural pronunciation and prosody. The speech content is impoverished, limited to a few short sentences, such as "will brav sein, Verzeihung, will folgen" ["want to be good, excuse me, want to be obedient"], "kann schreiben" ["can write"], "kann lesen" ["can read"], "schön lesen" ["read well"]. At 14 years of age the girl reads fluently with natural prosody and comprehension of the sentence meaning. At 15 years of age we again find verbigeration and the girl repeats stereotypically: "Ich will brav sein, ich will folgen, ich will es noch einmal versuchen" ["I want to be good, I want to be obedient, I want to try once again"].

3.2. Characteristics of Language Behavior in Schizophrenic Children

Schizophrenic children's language is often characterized by the classic authors as 'disintegrative speech'. This term covers a whole series of linguistic phenomena such as:

1. Changes in rhythm and rate of speech. Over-articulation, clipped speech, abnormal stressing of consonants in comparison to vowels, unusual stressing of phrases, rapid gabbling, or — on the other hand — abnormal stretching of words and phrases can be found.
2. Changes in speech melody (dysprosody). The children tend to use a singing intonation, which is more or less melodic, but usually at an abnormal pitch. They often fall into a singsong droning, a monotonous mumbling to themselves or they repeat some tune or other in a stereotype litany-like way. Thus a 10-year-old boy played 'orchestra', thereby referring to "Hermann" (meaning the Hermann-Hagestedt Radio Orchestra (Eggers 1973, 66)). We can also find meaningless rhyming, as in the case of a 14-year-old schizophrenic boy: "Karl May is vorbei, ach armes, deutsches Mägdelein, es kann ja nimmer sein, Ströme inhaliert, doch nicht imponiert, es ist vorbei, ich bin wie Brei, Gelenke gehören dein, das rechte ist nicht mein, es ist mir einerlei, der Tod eilt herbei" (Voigt 1919, 193).
3. Paragrammatism. This term refers to a series of deviations from normal language, which schizophrenic children have in common with schizophrenic adults, that is, in principle we do not find any differences here between 'schizophrasia' in adult and childhood schizophrenias. The language is characterized by abnormal sentence constructions, by unusual word and phoneme relations, by alterations of lexical morphemes or morphemic paraphrasing, by word-finding disorders, by incorrect word ordering, or by verbigerations. These disorders can eventually result in a proper 'word-salad'.
4. Language disintegration, paraphrasing, distraction of thought, speaking out-of-context. Here words and sentences are no longer ordered in meaningful sequences. The sentence segments are incomprehensible to the listener, at least at first hearing or sight. Thereby it must remain open whether these typical schizophrasic phe-

nomena are the result of a disturbed language production ability or rather of a thought disturbance. – This type of disorder can be demonstrated in the utterances of a 13-year-old acutely afflicted girl with optical and acoustic hallucinations, who developed very impressive delusions: "Sie sind alle mitgefahren, um die Familie zu heilen, schon die ganze Zeit, wie sie den Durchbruch gemacht haben, um mich zu führen, die Freche, die Judenstirne, steckt im Kopf, daß sie mich retten" ["They all came with, in order to heal the family, the whole time already, as they have made the break-through, in order to lead me, the impudent one, the Jewish foreheads, it's stuck in the head, that they will save me"] (Eggers 1973, 34).

Another 13-year-old girl produced typical verbigerations: "Das Feuer, das Feuer, es brennt, es brennt, es brennt ..." ["The fire, the fire, it's burning, it's burning, it's burning ..."]. She displayed a pronounced distraction in speech production. Thus, for example, her answer to the question if she wasn't feeling well was: "Bei Schlächtern nicht, der himmlische Vater sieht mehr vor Augen als ich. Ich bin schon im Haus zusammengebrochen und gehe ich so, dann sagt die eine so, dann schimpft die Elli so, durch Gottes Weisheit und Gnade ..." ["Not by butchers, the heavenly Father sees more before his eyes than I. I already broke down in the house and if I go like that, then the one will say thus, then Elli will scold so, by God's wisdom and mercy ..."] (Eggers 1973, 39).

The girl's speech was in part also characterized by derived or composed morphemic paraphrasing (Lecours/Vanier-Clement 1976). She spoke of "Erhaltungsunannehmlichkeit" ["conservation-trouble"], "Ernstlichkeit" ["earnestness"], "Apothekigkeit" ["apothecary-ness"]. Such word-creations (neologisms) can be scattered here and there in the speech productions: "Ich bin verfolgt von den Menschen. Ich will sterben, ich war schon in Vergasung, aber mein Herz wollte nicht sterben. Sie schlachten die Mädels ab. Ich habe gehört von den Leuten. Erhaltungsunannehmlichkeit. Und mir fällt alles auf die Augen" ["I am persecuted by the people. I want to die, was already in the gasification, but my heart didn't want to die. They kill off the girls. I have heard of the people. Conservation-trouble. And everything falls onto my eyes."] (Eggers 1973, 39).

Like schizophrenic adults, schizophrenic children tend to speak out-of-context. This means that a sensible conversation between clinician and patient cannot take place. The children give no context-related answers but rather appear to follow internal ideas and inspirations, that is, they are governed completely internally. Thus their answers appear strangely a-logical, senseless, eccentric, and bizarre as in the following case of a 14-year-old girl. To the question why she was lying in bed she answered: "Weil ich an die Englein glauben soll. Ich bin ein Backfisch und darum muß ich für die Kinder an die Englein glauben" ["Because I should believe in angels. I am a teenager and so I must believe in angels for the children"]. To the further question if that was a reason not to get up she answered: "Nein, aber weil der Stuhl da so dicht am Tisch steht" ["No, but because the chair is standing so near to the table"]. Asked if she was ill, she answered: "Die sagten, wenn sie von der Kirche kamen, mit dem Handschuh, mit dem Schlüssel" ["They said, when they came from Church, with the glove, with the key"]. The question where she was ailing most elicited the curiously eccentric answer: "An der Zunge" ["My tongue"] (Eggers 1973, 49 f.). The combinations in thought and language appear illogical to the listener; they are completely out of context and therefore baffling. However, the girl's last answer could refer to her thought and language disorder. For, as H. Grimm (1991) indicated, for young children the concepts tongue and language can be identical. Thus, when they are questioned about their language they may refer to their tongue.

The three cases of schizophrenic children between 12 and 14 years cited above demonstrate the schizophasic language disorders as manifested at the onset of the psychosis. This contradicts the view of Hoffman/Sledge (1984) and Kirov (1985) that "schizophasia occurs primarily in the more advanced stages of schizophrenic illness, and generally is associated with prolonged periods of social isolation and functional deterioration" (cf. art. 54). Insofar, although Hoffman's (cf. art. 54, 535 f) hypothesis appears plausible that "chronic social isolation, sustained alienation from other human beings, coupled with bizarre ideation, may, over time, cause the schizophrenic to volitionally disregard the constraints of ordinary language" this hypothesis should certainly not be generalized.

3.3 Language Characteristics in the Further Course of Childhood Schizophrenia

As shown by our longitudinal studies with 57 patients suffering from a childhood or prepuberal schizophrenia (onset of illness: 11 children at or before 11 years; 46 children between 12 and 13 years), schizophasic language disorders can still be observed after several decades in the course of the illness (mean length of follow-up: 16 years) (Eggers 1973, 1987 b). Thus, during the post-examination of a 30 year old female patient, who had fallen ill at the age of twelve, a curious disorder in the comprehension of meaning was observed, which one could perhaps best refer to as 'semantic dissociation' as an expression of a 'cognitive slipping'. The patient defined the difference between a pond and a river as follows: "Der Teich ist mit Sand besät, der Fluß ist im Wasser und wenn man das Wasser mit dem Feuer zusammentut, ist es dasselbe – beides ist gefährlich, ich weiß was gemeint ist, aber wie das zusammenhängt, weiß ich auch nicht" ["A pond is sown with sand, a river is in water and when one puts the water together with fire it is the same – both are dangerous, I know what is meant, but what the connection is, I don't know either."] She was also not able to produce correct and meaningful definitions with the essential characteristics for other terms or to formulate the essential characteristics. When asked to explain the idiom "Morgenstund hat Gold im Mund" ["The early bird catches the worm"] she answered: "Morgens darf man nicht singen oder pfeifen, sonst gibt's was Schlechtes zu hören." ["In the morning you may not sing or whistle, otherwise you will get to hear something bad."] (Why?) "Vom Meister eine verpaßt." ["Get a clout from the master"]. The word "Gold" meant "Von morgens 5 Uhr bis 7 Uhr bedeute das" ["It means from 5 o'clock to 7 o'clock in the morning"] (Eggers 1973, 29). In the answers of this patient we can find a tendency to concretism as well as a tendency to disregard the meaning of the sentence. She 'hangs on to' a specific word, and disregards the other words and phrases essential for grasping the overall meaning. In general, what the patients offer are more coincidental, associative ideas and answers which give rise to the impression of irrelevance.

3.4. Language Comprehension Disorder

The examples given demonstrate that it is not only expressive language which is disturbed in schizophrenic children and adults, but also receptive language or comprehension. This could be attributed to an impairment in the ability to generate hierarchies of individual words and phrases. The comprehension of a sentence does not come about by adding together the words, but by a logical evaluation of words according to their meaning. It seems that the individual words and phrases are seen as being equal in importance and that they are not hierarchically classifiable. This could account for the typically paralogic, strangely confused language of schizophrenic patients. It also accounts for what Beringer (1926) refers to as "der Charakter des Einfallmäßigen, Unverpflichtenden" ["the idea-like, non-committal character"] of schizophrenic utterances as well as the "Bedeutungsverschiebungen" ["shifts in meaning"] which he frequently observed in his patients.

The interpretation offered by Grinker/Holzman (1973) with regard to schizophrenic adolescents and young adults points in the same direction: "The patient may omit ideas essential for the listener to grasp the continuity (ellipsis), as if the patient assumed that the listener must know the full thoughts" (Grinker/Holzman 1973, 171).

The tendency of schizophrenic children and adolescents to treat individual words and phrases as equal in importance and to refrain from ordering them hierarchically is in agreement with recent findings by Caplan/Perdue/Tanguay/Fish (1990) and Caplan/Foy/Asarnow/Sherman (1990). These authors found a significant correlation between the extent of illogical thinking and increased distraction or decreased attentional span. The attentional deficit and the tendency for illogical thinking were evaluated on the basis of a free recall of a previously told story and a free interview. These were based on the Kiddie Formal Thought Disorder Scale (K-FTDS) (Caplan/Guthrie/Fish 1989). The associative slackening is displayed in unpredictable changes of the topic of conversation towards an unrelated topic, which makes it difficult for the listener to follow the conversation.

I have dealt elsewhere (e. g. Eggers 1991) with the difficulties experienced by schizophrenic adolescents as well as by children at high risk for schizophrenia in evaluating on the receptive level the meaning of relevant and irrelevant stimuli and in developing on the expressive level task-related solution strategies (cf. also Bunk 1991). If, like Käsermann (1983), one regards speech as a behavior "das zielgerichtet/funktional zur Lösung der Kommunikationsaufgabe (Realisierung der Intentionen) eingesetzt wird" ("which is applied purposefully/functionally to solve the communicative task (realization of intention)", then the schizophrenic's language disorder can be understood as an impairment in the generation and implementation of adequate solution strategies in coping with this communicative task. This view implies the annulment of the contrasts 'language disorder versus thought disorder', so that the controversy as to whether the language disorders of schizophrenics are the result of a cognitive disorder or of an independent verbal disorder can be considered closed.

3.5. Linguistic Results

Linguistic findings exeeding mere descriptions of the language behavior in schizophrenic children are rare and of recent publication. This is partly due to low incidence rates of childhood and prepuberal schizophrenia (Bunk/Eggers 1990, Eggers 1982).

Leaper/Emmorey (1985) performed a comparative case study with 2 schizophrenic and 2 normal children at the ages of 6 and 9 years. They analyzed speech samples from three different situations: an interview, a free picture description and the re-telling of a story. Among others, two psycholinguistic aspects were examined: First, the extent of cohesion with regard to the logical semantic relation between two sentences or sentence segments, and second, the assumed or prerequisite information on which a statement is based. Often the topics of conversation refer to something said earlier (the verbal context) or to something in the immediate environment of the speaker (the nonverbal context). In these instances, the speaker uses a presuming nominal group. With respect to the cohesion in sentence structure over all contexts, no difference was found between the normal and schizophrenic children under study, whereas there are differences between normally healthy and thought disordered schizophrenic adults. Both thought disordered children and thought disordered adults, however, refer during their descriptions and reproductions to irrelevant information and give little explicit reference to what was said previously. The discourse appears fragmentary and logically instable.

In a study of a group of schizophrenics ranging in age from 15 to 41 years, Morice/Ingram (1983) found a relationship between the syntactic complexity in spontaneous speech in the sense of the depth of logically linked clauses and age at onset of illness. The lesser the linguistic complexity, the earlier the onset of illness had been manifested. This relationship was independent of illness duration. The results indicate that there is a common factor responsible for the language disorders as well as for the general phenomenology of schizophrenic symptoms. By those authors concerned with the neuropsychological aspects of information processing in psychotic disturbances, this factor is interpreted as a central regulation factor of attentional processing (Caplan/Foy/Asarnow/Sherman 1990, Cornblatt/Erlenmeyer-Kimling 1985, Nuechterlein/Edell/Norris/Dawson 1986).

4. Differential Diagnosis

4.1. Differentiation between Language Disorders in Childhood Schizophrenia and in Infantile Autism

The fundamental difference is as follows: In autism, language cannot develop, or can only develop partially, probably on account of a serious disorder in social relationships existing from birth. In cases of childhood schizophrenia, language is as a rule at a normal developmental stage since the age levels at illness onset are higher. Language developmental disorders are typical for autistic children, as observed by Kolvin (1971) in 88% of his patients. They are far less often found in childhood schizophrenia. Only when the schizophrenic psychosis has been manifested do changes in language behavior occur. However, in a few cases and at especially early onset (prior to 5–6 years of age) the differentiation from language use in autistic children may prove difficult (Bosch 1972). Changes in language flow, a tendency for echolalia, phonographism, and neologisms can still be observed in schizophrenic children in early school years. A specific language peculiarity characteristic in autistic children is the so-called 'pronominal reversal', which is only seldom found in childhood schizophrenia (Kolvin 1971). Sentence fillers, meaningless phrases, and nonsensical words can be found far more frequently in the early childhood psychoses than in childhood and prepuberal schizophrenia. Here, the language deviation most frequently observed by Kolvin/Ounsted/Roth (1971) was a tendency to answer questions incompletely or only partially.

Typical are disorders in thought and association (vacuity and withdrawal of thought, incoherence, distraction of thought etc.) whereas they are only rarely found or completely lacking in the early childhood psychoses. One common characteristic of both childhood autism and childhood schizophrenia is the occurrence of echolalia, which, however, occurs more frequently in autistic children.

4.2. Differentiation from the Language Disorders found in Manic Psychoses

Manias or manic psychoses are extremely rare in childhood. When they do occur, one usually finds short phases with rapid shifting of phases, often within one or several days. When manic phases occur, they frequently turn into schizophrenic psychoses and then may either merge completely with the schizophrenic process or otherwise the manic-type episodes can remain and be combined with depressive, schizophrenic or schizo-affective episodes. Changes are possible and can alternate before or intermittently during the total course of the psychosis (Bunk/Eggers 1990, Eggers 1986). There are no linguistic studies on manic psychoses and purely manic episodes in the course of a schizo-affective psychosis in children and adolescents. Clinically speaking, however, it appears that the disconnectedness between the verbal utterances is not as marked as in the purely schizophrenic psychoses. This impression is supported by Hoffman/Stopek/Andreasen (1986), who found that manic speech difficulties were due to shifts from one discourse structure to another, while the schizophrenic speech disorder reflects a basic deficiency in elaborating any discourse structure.

4.3. Differentiation from Aphasic and Mutistic Language Disorders

The irregularity of language disorders in the schizophrenic child indicates that they cannot be due to an organic defect, i. e., the disorders are distinguishable from sensory or motoric aphasia. However, a small subgroup of schizophrenic adults who were afflicted in childhood can display very serious language disorders in the sense of paraphrasing or paragrammatical speech, as is typical in the aphasic speech disorder. Moreover, the question must remain open whether in the serious dysphasic language disorders in schizophrenics we are dealing with an 'intentional dysfunction' in the sense that schizophrenic patients are not able to express what they wish to say in a grammatically correct way, or whether we are dealing with a neural deficit corresponding to that of aphasics. Significant correlations between especially seriously disordered schizophrenics and complications due to birth trauma or minor neurological deficits have, however, not been found (cf. art. 54). In conclusion, the language disorders of schizophrenic patients are not as marked as in the case of aphasic patients. Also, it is possible with effort and empathy to establish a context of meaning in spite of the scattiness in speech and written language.

Among the language disorders of schizophrenic children mutism has been mentioned. This schizophrenic aphrasia is part of a complex psychotic phenomenology in contrast to psychogenic (traumatic or elective) mutism, which is not connected to any psychotic phenomenon.

5. Relationship between Language Disorders and Communicative Behavior

In human beings, it is the nature of language to serve communication. Language is not an exclusive but an essential part of our communicative behavior: "Wir kommunizieren nicht, weil wir grammatische Regeln und Wortbedeutungen gelernt haben, sondern wir lernen diese, weil wir kommunizieren" ["We do not communicate because we have learned grammatical rules and the meanings of words, but we learn these because we communicate"] (Grimm 1987, 582).

Lutz (1938/1939) pointed out the disturbance in the relational characteristic of schizophrenic children's speech. In fact, he understood schizophrenic language disorders as a specific relational disorder, whereby apart from cognitive and specifically linguistic factors, a motoric disorder (an increase or decrease in motoric activity) certainly is also partly responsible.

Even prior to onset of illness, deviations in language and thought can be found as well as in contact behavior, which differentiates subjects with a later manifestation of a schizophrenic psychosis from healthy subjects. In a follow-up study of at-risk children with schizophrenic mothers (Parnas/Schulsinger/Schulsinger et al. (1982) found that the following items differentiated the schizophrenics from the non-psychotic group: 'incoherence', 'pathology of associations', 'incongruent facial expression', 'difficulties in making friends'. Thus it is also the preverbal, facial expressive behavior which differentiates between healthy subjects and subjects at high risk for schizophrenia.

Not only in families with psychotic members, but also in families with disturbed, nonpsychotic adolescents, parental communication deviance seems to be a factor of prognostic significance with regard to the later manifestation of a schizophrenic psychosis, as could be demonstrated in follow-up studies (Douane/West/Goldstein et al. 1981, Goldstein/Rodick/Jones et al. 1978, Lewis/Rodick/Goldstein 1981).

Another high-risk study revealed that children of schizophrenic parents display lower verbal productivity and a decrease in cohesive thought in their spoken utterances, i. e., the formal and the semantic links in their utterances were looser than in healthy peers (Harvey/Weintraub/Neale 1982). The language behavior of these children at risk for schizophrenia was similar to the performance of thought-disordered adult schizophrenics, who also provided fewer links between clauses and used less informative types of cohesive ties (Rochester/Martin 1979). The described language disorders in children at high risk for schizophrenia might be associated with the fact that these children's flow of speech is more often interrupted by members of the family. The results presented by Waxler/Mishler (1971) appear to indicate this possibility.

The described disordered association, illogical thinking and the cognitive slippage in schizophrenic children find their counterpart in the difficulty in maintaining a focus of attention in family transactions, as described by Singer/Wynne (1965). A disorder in adequate focusing in adult schizophrenics can also be linguistically substantiated: Rutter (1985) examined monologues and conversations of schizophrenic patients, of patients with affective disorders, and of normal orthopaedic patients using a variant of the Cloze Procedure. The sentences in the transcribed protocols were separated and presented as a card set to raters who were blind to the subject's diagnosis and who were to attempt to re-organize the sentences into a meaningful text. The schizophrenic material was more problematic to reconstruct since it was very difficult if not impossible to recognize a reference system according to which the sentences could be ordered. In the conversation situation Rutter observed that the schizophrenic subjects and, in tendency, the affectively disordered subjects would ask questions at inapt points in the conversation and would answer questions with incorrect referential content. Rutter interprets these disorders less as the cause of cognitive deficits or thought disorders but rather as the expression of an impaired ability in taking over social roles during the schizophrenic psychosis.

6. Conclusions

Language disorders in children and adolescents display a Janus-face from the clinical-phenomenological point of view as well as in linguistic studies: It is not possible to decide whether we are dealing primarily with a cognitive, possibly neurologically caused impairment or rather with a social interaction disorder. The latter would be caused by developmental and communicative impairments. Much seems to support the view that this dichotomous question has been put incorrectly. It is the old controversy 'nature versus nurture'. Language and behavior per se, as well as schizophrenic behavior, are entirely dependent on a highly complex interaction among genetic, biological, specifically neurological, and social factors. An integrative model of thought and language disorders as well as of communicative behavior in schizophrenics still needs to be developed. An integrative-dynamic model of schizophrenia is described elsewhere (Eggers 1991).

Author's Note: I wish to thank D. Bunk and P. Wiemer for their helpful assistance.

7. References

Atschkova, M. (1966). Die Pfropf-Schizophrenie im Kindes- und Jugendalter. *Psychiatrie, Neurologie und medizinische Psychologie* (Lpz.), *18*, 292–295.

Bender, L. (1953). Childhood schizophrenia. *Psychiatric Quarterly*, *27*, 663.

Beringer, K. (1926). Denkstörungen und Sprache bei Schizophrenen. *Zeitschrift für Neurologie*, *103*, 185–197.

Bosch, G. (1972). Psychosen im Kindesalter. In K. P. Kisker, J. E. Meyer, M. Müller, E. Strömgren (Eds.), *Psychiatrie der Gegenwart*, *Band II*, *Teil I*. *873–920*. Heidelberg/Berlin/New York: Springer.

Bunk, D. (1991). *Zur Psychologie des schizophrenen Problemlösens*. Bochum: Winkler.

Bunk, D. & Eggers, C. (1990). The course of juvenile schizoaffective and schizophrenic psychoses:

The use of pattern analysis classifying the development of schizophrenia-like illnesses. In A. Marneros & M. T. Tsuang (Eds.), *Affective and schizoaffective disorders. 89–101.* Berlin/Heidelberg/New York: Springer.

Caplan, R.., Foy, J. G., Asarnow, R. F., & Sherman, T. (1990). Information processing deficits of schizophrenic children with formal thought disorder. *Psychiatry Research, 31,* 169–177.

Caplan, R., Guthrie, D., Fish, B., Tanguay, P. E., & David-Lando, G. (1989). The Kiddie Formal Thought Disorder Rating-Scale: Clinical assessment, reliability and validity. *Journal of the American Academy of Child and Adolescent Psychiatry 28,* 408–416.

Caplan, R., Perdue, S., Tanguay, P. E., & Fish, B. (1990). Formal thought disorder in childhood onset schizophrenia and schizotypal personality disorder. *Journal of Child Psychology and Psychiatry and Allied Disciplines, 31,* 1103–1114.

Cornblatt, B. A. & Erlenmeyer-Kimling, L. (1985). Global attentional deviance as a marker of risk for schizophrenia: Specificity and predictive validity. *Journal of Abnormal Psychology, 94,* 470–486.

de Sanctis, S. (1908). Dementia praecocissima catatonica. *Folia Neuro-biologica, 2,* 9.

Despert, L. (1938). Schizophrenia in children. *Psychiatric Quarterly, 12,* 366.

Douane, J., West, K., Goldstein, M. J., Rodnick, E., & Jones, J. (1981). Parental communication deviance and affective style as predictors of subsequent schizophrenia spectrum disorders in vulnerable adolescents. *Archives of General Psychiatry, 38,* 679–685.

Duché, D. J., (1971). Psychoses infantiles. *Revista portuguesa para o estudo da deficiencia mental, 1,* 445.

Eggers, C. (1973). *Verlaufsweisen kindlicher und präpuberaler Schizophrenien.* Berlin/Heidelberg/New York: Springer.

Eggers, C. (1978 a). Zur nosologischen Abgrenzung zwischen frühkindlichem Autismus und kindlicher Schizophrenie. *Bibliotheca Psychiatrica, 157,* 1–21.

Eggers, C. (1978 b). Course and prognosis of childhood schizophrenia. *Journal of Autism and Childhood Schizophrenia, 8,* 21–26.

Eggers, C. (1982). Psychoses in childhood and adolescence. *Acta paedo psychiatrica, 48,* 81–98.

Eggers, C. (1986). Schizoaffective psychoses in children and juveniles. In A. Marneros & M. T. Tsuang (Eds.), *Schizo-affective psychoses.* 202–224. Berlin/Heidelberg/New York/Tokio: Springer.

Eggers, C. (1991). Stimulus protection model of schizophrenia: Convergence of neurobiological and developmental psychological factors. In C. Eggers (Ed.), *Schizophrenia in youth. 29–40.* Berlin/Heidelberg/New York/London/Paris/Tokio/Hongkong: Springer.

Goldstein, M. J., Rodnick, E., Jones, J., McPherson, S., & West, K. (1978). Familial precursors of schizophrenia spectrum disorders. In L. Wynne (Ed.), *The nature schizophrenia.* New York: Wiley.

Grimm, H. (1987). Sprachentwicklung: Voraussetzungen, Phasen und theoretische Interpretationen. In R. Oerter & L. Montada (Eds.), *Entwicklungspsychologie. 578–636.* München/Weinheim: Psychologische Verlagsunion.

Grimm, H. (1991). Personal communication.

Grinker, R. R. & Holzmann, P. S. (1973). Schizophrenic psychology in young adults. *Archives of General Psychiatry, 28,* 168–175.

Harvey, P. D., Weintraub, S., & Neale, J. M. (1982). Speech competence of children vulnerable in psychopathology. *Journal of Abnormal Child Psychology, 10,* 373–387.

Heuyer, G. (1960). Introduction à la notion de demence en psychiatrie infantile. *Revue de Neuropsychiatrie Infantile, 8,* 83.

Hoffman, R. E. & Sledge, W. (1984). A microgenetic model of paragrammatism produced by schizophrenic speaker. *Brain and Language, 21,* 147–173.

Hoffman, R. E., Stopek, S., & Andreasen, N. C. (1986). A comparative study of manic schizophrenic speech disorganization. *Archives of General Psychiatry, 43,* 831–838.

Käsermann, M. L. (1983). Form und Funktion schizophrener Sprachstörungen. *Sprache & Kognition, 3,* 132–147.

Kanner, L. (1943). Autistic disturbances of affective contact. *Nervous Child, 2,* 217–250.

Kirov, K. (1985). Long-term study of schizophasic patients. *Psychopathology, 18,* 226–229.

Kolvin, I. (1971). Studies in the childhood psychoses. Diagnostic criteria and classification. *British Journal of Psychiatry, 118,* 381–384.

Kolvin, I., Ounsted, C., Humphrey, M., & McNay, A. (1971). The phenomenology of childhood psychoses. *British Journal of Psychiatry, 118,* 385–395.

Kramer, R. & Pollnow, H. (1932). Über eine hyperkinetische Erkrankung im Kindesalter. *Monatsschrift für Psychiatrie und Neurologie, 82,* 1.

Kudrjawzewa, W. (1967). Klinik und Verlauf der Schizophrenie des frühen Kindesalters nach den Materialien sowjetischer Untersucher. *Psychiatrie, Neurologie und medizinische Psychologie, 19,* 23–31.

Leaper, C. & Emmorey, K. (1985). The discourse of thought-disordered schizophrenic children. *Brain and Language, 25,* 72–86.

Lecours, A. R. & Vanier-Clement, M. V. (1976). Schizophrenia and jargonaphasia: A comparative description with comments on Chaika's and Fromkin‘s respective looks at "schizophrenic" language. *Brain and Language, 3,* 516–565.

Lewis, J. M., Rodnick, E. H., & Goldstein, M. J. (1981). Intrafamilial interactive behavior, parental communication deviance, and risk for schizophrenia. *Journal of Abnormal Psychology, 90*, 448–457.

Lutz, J. (1938/39). Über die Schizophrenie im Kindesalter. *Schweizer Archiv für Neurologie und Psychiatrie, 24*, 335–372.

Mahler, M. S. (1954). Childhood schizophrenia. *American Journal of Orthopsychiatry, 24*, 523.

Michaux, L. & Duché, D. (1965). Schizophrénies infantiles. *Revue du Practicien, 125*, 3295.

Morice, R. & Ingram, J. (1983). Language complexity and age of onset of schizophrenia. *Psychiatry Research, 9*, 233–242.

Nuechterlein, K. H., Edell, W. S., Norris, M., & Dawson, M. E. (1986). Attentional vulnerability indicators, thought disorders, and negative symptoms. *Schizophrenia Bulletin, 12*, 408–426.

Parnas, J., Schulsinger, F., Schulsinger, H., Mednick, S. A., & Teasdale, T. W. (1982). Behavioral precursors of schizophrenia spectrum. *Archives of General Psychiatry, 39*, 658–664.

Rochester, S. & Martin, J. R. (1979). *Crazy talk.* New York/London: Plenum Press.

Rutter, D. R. (1985). Language in schizophrenia. The structure of monologues and conversations. *British Journal of Psychiatry, 146*, 399–404.

Singer, M. & Wynne, L. (1965). Thought disorder and family relations of schizophrenics. III. Methodology using projective techniques. *Archives of General Psychiatry, 12*, 187–200.

Ssucharewa, G. (1967). Die Bedeutung der vergleichenden Berücksichtigung des Lebensalters für die Untersuchung der Verlaufsgesetzmäßigkeit der Schizophrenie bei Kindern und Jugendlichen. *Acta paedopsychiatrica, 34*, 307–320.

Stutte, H. (1963). Psychosen im Kindesalter und in der Pubertät. *Medizinische Klinik, 13*, 526–529.

Voigt, L. (1919). Über Dementia praecox im Kindesalter. *Zeitschrift für die gesamte Neurologie und Psychiatrie, 48*, 167–234.

von Stockert, F. G. (1956). Psychosen im Kindesalter. *Jahrbuch der Jugendpsychiatrie, Bd. I*, 322. Bern: Huber.

Waxler, N. E. & Mishler, E. G. (1971). Parental interaction with schizophrenic children and well siblings. *Archives of General Psychiatry, 25*, 223–232.

Christian Eggers, Essen (Germany)

78. Language and Communicative Behavior in Autistic Disorder

1. Introduction

Recently renamed Autistic Disorder (AD) in recognition of its life-long duration, Early Infantile Autism (EIA) is one of the most severe and debilitating psychopathologies of childhood and later life. It was first identified as a distinct nosologic entity by Leo Kanner (1943) in North America who also named it and by Hans Asperger (1944) in Europe who called it 'Autistic Psychopathy'. Although for a long time the term 'Kanner's syndrome' was used interchangeably with the term EIA, more recently Asperger's syndrome has been differentiated from autism by some writers (Wing 1981). Others maintain that Asperger described that subgroup of autistic children who are higher functioning and that no differentiation between high functioning autism and Asperger's syndrome is warranted at the present time (Schopler 1985).

The term EIA was employed interchangeably with such other terms as 'Psychosis of Childhood'. 'Childhood Schizophrenia', 'Symbiotic Psychosis' (Mahler 1952) and 'atypical development'. A major breakthrough in the field was made when the 'psychoses' that originate in infancy and early childhood were differentiated from those comparable conditions that appear first in adult life, with very few cases having their origins in childhood. The division was substantiated through studies by Kolvin and his collaborators (Kolvin 1971; Kolvin/Ounsted/Humphrey/McNay 1971) who were able to show that the 'early onset' cases, i. e., prior to age 5, presented different epidemiology and key characteristics than those with later onset. The former are now described as Autism and

Pervasive Developmental Disorder while the latter are classified using adult criteria for schizophrenia. Although the distinction has been disputed by some writers (Fish 1977), at the present time this is the position of many workers in the field and it is also the position of the DSM III-R.

2. Epidemiology and Classification

Partly because of the idiosyncratic nomenclature employed by clinicians in different countries to label autistic children, and partly as a result of lack of consensus on etiology, up until 1980 very little agreement existed as to what constituted the key symptoms of the syndrome. This had inevitable repercussions for both assessment and treatment practices. As well, it resulted in diluting and confusing research efforts on the disorder. In fact, many of the early studies employed very different criteria for sample selection than studies do today. Earlier studies have also tended to concentrate on the relatively higher functioning subgroup of children, the ones who did not show any neurological impairment, hence omitted the large number of moderately and severely retarded autistic children. This was not fortuitous since the prevailing etiologic view of the time was psychoanalytic (Bettelheim 1967), postulating that psychogenic factors were responsible for the condition and that autistic children were biologically intact.

A rapidly accumulating body of evidence pointing to biological factors in etiology, resulted in a corresponding broadening of the classification criteria to include the lower functioning, mentally retarded subgroup of children (DeMyer/Hingtgen/Jackson 1981). Corresponding restrictions were imposed to exclude other populations of higher functioning children who might be confused with the autistic such as the severely developmentally delayed in receptive language abilities, the attentional deficient and the borderline or atypical cases. The Diagnostic and Statistical Manual III (DSM III) (American Psychiatric Association 1980) was the first effort to adopt an atheoretical, phenomenological approach relying on explicit, operational criteria for the diagnosis (Spitzer/Endicott/Robins 1978). Despite the advantages of this system, however, considerable shortcomings have been identified by a number of writers. To an extent, these problems were remediated in the revised version, the DSM III-R (American Psychiatric Association 1987). For Autistic Disorder (AD) to be diagnosed, at least 8 criteria must be met, with at least one from each of the three main symptom clusters being present. Cases meeting fewer than the eight criteria, or having no symptom representation in each of the three symptom clusters are diagnosed as Pervasive Developmental Disorder (PDD) Not Otherwise Specified (NOS). The obvious implication is that AD, a form of PDD, represents the more serious expression of the PDD syndrome. The clear advantage of the DSM III-R classification lies in its taking care of all three criticisms levelled against the DSM III just mentioned. The age of onset is no longer crucial, which reflects evidence on the life-long course of the disorder as shown in follow-up studies (Paul 1987). As well, the categories COPDD, Atypical PDD and Residual Autism present in the DSM-III are now observed under one category, PDD, and a more comprehensive and detailed representation of the syndrome has been provided.

Despite these advantages, the DSM III-R continues to present difficulties. One of the main ones is that it does not allow for rating the severity of expression of each symptom but requires that information be expressed in a binary YES-NO fashion. This results in issues of severity not being addressed, other than by means of the AD-PDD dichotomy (Konstantareas 1988). Although efforts are under way to take into account and improve the DSM III-R criteria, not only for AD but also for other disorders, researchers and clinicians have to rely on other means to quantitatively determine degree of severity. Checklists have been developed for use over the years with many disorders including autism. Thus the Childhood Autism Rating Scale (CARS) (Schopler/Reichler/DeVellis/Daly 1980), The Behaviour Rating Instrument for Autistic and Atypical Children (BRIAAC) (Ruttenberg/Dratman/Fraknoi/Wenar 1966); The Behaviour Observation Scale for Autism (BOS) (Freeman/Ritvo/Guthrie et al. 1978) have been developed, and their psychometric properties have been reviewed (Parks 1983). The checklists have the advantage of allowing degree of severity and cutoff points for meeting the diagnosis to be addressed, factors crucial for clinical research and administrative purposes.

3. Differential Diagnosis

The three main symptom clusters to be considered are: (a) Social Interaction Deficits of a qualitative and not merely quantitative nature, (b) impairment in both nonverbal and verbal communication, and (c) restricted repertoire of activities and interests, along with stereotypical body movements. Insofar as some of the behaviors subsumed under each of these three clusters may be also displayed by children who present with other disorders, there has been a continuous attempt to better define and restrict the boundaries of the syndrome (Rutter/Schopler 1987). Existing differentiation efforts are still a subject of controversy.

3.1. Autism vs Mental Retardation

A number of authors have stressed the occurrence of autism and retardation in as many as 80 percent of autistic individuals. Kanner's (1943) exclusion of the cognitively delayed and neurologically impaired was in fact partly the result of the scant attention being paid at that time to a careful psychological evaluation of the children (cf. Wing 1989). Aside from this consideration, the crucial question for differential diagnosis is whether or not retardation without autism can be easily differentiated from the far more common retardation accompanied by autism. With the DSM III-R criteria now available, and a better appreciation of the regular and the associated characteristics of autism, it seems that this separation is not difficult for an experienced clinician. (a) With respect to socio-affective ability, one of the key differentiating features is that the social interaction deficits autistic children present are more severe than the corresponding cognitive deficits. This is not true of retardation where the social age of the child is consistent with his/her cognitive ability. Furthermore, the lack of interest in people, inability to appreciate the emotional state of others and obliviousness are absent from the behavior repertoire of mentally retarded children. (b) The qualitative deficit in language and communication so characteristic of autism, along with the severe deficits in the social use of language, are also not displayed by retarded children, and (c) the stereotypical and at times bizarre behavior of the autistic children, including insistence on the maintenance of sameness and sensory and perceptual peculiarities so typical of autism, are minimally present in the retarded-only children. In sum, none of the three main symptom clusters used to identify and define the autistic syndrome are evident in the retarded or, if present, they are much less frequently displayed by them. (d) In addition to the above distinctions, autistic children display an uneven profile of cognitive abilities and deficits that is distinct from the even profiles displayed by nonautistic retarded children. Strongest performance in the autistic is for visuospatial and concrete tasks, while weakest for abstractions or sequencing tasks (DeMyer/Hingtgen/Jackson 1981).

3.2. Autism vs Childhood Onset Schizophrenia

Since Kolvin's (1971) early work on the differentiation of the infancy onset versus later onset psychosis of childhood, very little systematic work has been carried out on this particular topic. Yet many writers have agreed, using Kolvin's work, that the two conditions are distinct (e. g. Rutter/Schopler 1987). It is important to point out that the incidence of schizophrenia appearing in childhood is extremely low. In a statewide epidemiological study in North Dakota, Burd/Kerbeshian (1987) reported an incidence of .19 in 10,000, a rate much lower than that of 4 per 10,000 or even 13.9 per 10,000 for Autistic Disorder. Despite the low incidence, it is important to keep in mind the key distinguishing features between Autistic Disorder and Childhood Schizophrenia. Schizophrenia with onset in childhood does not appear in infancy but in early or middle childhood. Grossly bizarre and disturbed behavior, language and thought disturbance in the form of delusions and hallucinations characterize its appearance. The same criteria employed for diagnosing adulthood onset schizophrenia are used (DSM III-R). In addition, there is a family history of schizophrenia in the backgrounds of such children, the course of their disorder is variable, following remissions and relapses, and they respond to psychotropic medication.

3.3. Autism vs Severe Developmental Language Disorder — Dysphasia

Dysphasia shares with autism a major communication deficit which can be receptive or expressive and is most frequently mixed. However, a number of systematic studies have shown that, compared to autism, dysphasia is a less severe and qualitatively different disorder. Dysphasic children can rely on nonverbal communication for expression. Additionally, their social delays, although present, are not as central to their difficulties.

Dysphasic youngsters are quite keen on social interaction, are alert to other children's activities and display considerable frustration when unable to use speech effectively. Although socially delayed, they do not display the 'obliviousness' and 'aloneness' of the autistic child who is particularly indifferent to the peer group. Dysphasic children as well are less likely to employ pronoun reversals such as *you* for *I* and to use neologisms and metaphorical language.

Finally, more likely than not, these language impaired children are of normal nonverbal intelligence.

3.4. Autistic-like Disorders in Individuals of Normal Intelligence

Although Asperger's (1944) publication of 'autistic psychopathy' has been almost contemporaneous to Kanner's (1943), only recently has there been interest in describing the characteristics of Asperger's syndrome children. For many workers in the field Asperger's syndrome is not really different from the AD expressed in high functioning individuals or PDD (Schopler 1985; Wing 1981). Asperger attributed the characteristics of these higher functioning people to a disturbance in personality or a 'schizoid personality disorder'. He stressed their increased adaptation with the passing of time, giving an optimistic picture of outcome. As Frith (1989) also points out, Asperger believed that autistic individuals had intelligence of a distinct flavor, opposite to conventional learning and worldly wisdom. Such intelligence he thought might be best represented by the popular view of the 'mad professor'. More recently, some workers in the field have argued in favor of distinguishing Asperger's syndrome from PDD or high functioning autism on the basis of deficits in socialization and communication that are milder than those presented by high functioning autistic individuals. As restated by Gillberg (1985) and originally stated by Asperger (1944), the diagnostic features for Asperger's are: (a) inability to relate normally to others, with social isolation and peculiarities of gaze and social naiveté, (b) pedantic and perseverative speech, (c) deviant nonverbal communication, including reduced facial expression, monotonous intonation and limited or inappropriate gestures, (d) repetitive activities and strong attachments to possessions, and (e) clumsy gross motor movements and poor coordination. Of course why such individuals may not be seen as simply representing the mildest form of the high functioning autism continuum is unclear. For the present no convincing evidence exists that would show qualitative and not merely differences in degree between the two conditions (Schopler 1985).

3.5. Later Onset Autism

This issue is only partly resolved. DeLong/Beau/Brown (1981) have reported three cases of autism following viral infection which occurred well after the third year of life. In one instance the child suffered a herpes simplex infection while in the other two the cause was unknown. There were concomitant EEG and CAT scan findings. The psychophysiological and structural changes apparently dissipated a few months later along with a full psychological recovery from symptoms in two of the three cases. Insofar as these individuals presented a clinical picture of AD after the first 30 months of life, which could be either reversible or continue for a longer period, one wonders how to classify such conditions. Thus far only these few cases have been reported but more may be reported in the future, hence this issue remains unresolved, albeit tantalizing.

Deterioration after a period of apparently normal functioning is not uncommon in autism. Roughly 50% of cases assessed in our clinic have presented this clinical picture. However, it is usually between the first and second year of life that this phenomenon appears to occur. Research on this important issue is almost non-existent.

3.6. Rett Syndrome

Of greater relevance particularly recently are cases of specific degeneration with a characteristic clinical course in female children who are concurrently or initially diagnosed as autistic. Rett (1966) was the first to describe this syndrome. More recently specific criteria for diagnosis have been published by the Rett syndrome criteria work group (Gillberg 1989). To be diagnosed as Rett's a child has to mainly show: (a) a normal head circumference at birth and deceleration of head growth between 5 months and 4 years; (b) stereotypic hand movements such as hand wringing/squeezing, mouthing and washing, rubbing automatisms, after loss of purposeful hand skills; (c) appearance of gait apraxia and truncal apraxia/ataxia between 1–4 years of age; (d) an apparently normal prenatal and perinatal period and (e) a tentative diagnosis of Rett syndrome until 2–5 years of age. Supportive criteria include breathing dysfunction, EEG abnormalities, seizures, spasticity, growth retardation and scoliosis. Needless to say that as Gillberg (1989) has also shown, not all children meet these criteria. Furthermore, all four cases he reported concurrently with Rett's syndrome meet criteria for AD. In our own series all 5 children who subsequently showed some of these symptoms and were diagnosed as Rett's had previously been diagnosed as autistic. The degeneration showed by these children is not ongoing but is rather episodic. Although some writers describe Rett's as a distinct nostologic entity not to be confused with autism, it is still far from clear if in fact this is the case. Although both AD and Rett syndrome are thought to be due to neurological abnormality, it is unclear whether it is the same abnormality that causes two different variants in phenomenology or whether the two conditions have distinct, or distinct but overlapping underlying neuropathologies (see Gillberg 1989).

3.7. Fragile X Condition

Another disorder, that has shown a comparable unclear overlapping phenomenology with AD is Fragile X condition which was first identified by Brown/Jenkins/Friedman et al. (1982), and appears mainly in males. Fragile X individuals are also likely to be cognitively low functioning and male. Many meet the clinical criteria for AD. Gillberg (1983) reported a case of triplets, all showing classic autism, moderate retardation and the Fragile X abnormality. A study by Goldfine and his team (Goldfine/McPherson/Adair et al. 1985) yielded negative results. More recently Hagerman (1989) has argued that Fragile X is the single most prevalent cause of autism in children with documented organic etiology. In view of the fact that as many as 25% of cases of autism have documented organicity (Hagerman 1989) this is a high percentage indeed. With recent improvements in genetic research and DNA technology more autistic individuals who are also Fragile X positive and show retardation will be identified. Hagerman (1989), in reviewing existing evidence, argues that in addition to such physical features as prominent ears, a long face, hyperextensible finger joints, flat feet and macro-orchidism, Fragile X individuals present with a characteristic and unique clinical picture of PDD or autism. Although they meet DSM III-R criteria they tend to show a greater degree of social avoidance with strangers than IQ-matched non Fragile autistic children. As well, they show an avoidance of social gaze, become easily anxious and such anxiety may escalate into aggressive behavior and episodic violent outbursts, particularly in the adult males. In the area of language, greater jargon, perseveration, echolalia and talking to themselves is displayed by Fragile X males with or without autism.

4. Etiology of Autistic Disorder and PDD

4.1. Environmental

Historically, when Kanner (1943) first described autism, the prevalent theoretical climate in Child Psychiatry was psychoanalytic. It was therefore understandable that a search for causation would naturally lead towards prevailing assumptions on etiology. In fact, Kanner expressed considerable ambivalence as to where responsibility for autism was to be attributed. He originally felt, on the basis of his highly select sample which consisted of professional or managerial parents, that autistic children were biologically intact. However, they were born into families with fairly rigid, obsessional, dignified and serious dispositions who were not warm, supportive and accepting of their children. Particularly blameworthy for Kanner were the mothers. Coleman/Gillberg (1985) comment on his ambivalence, however, since before his publication on autism, Kanner (1941) published a book titled *In Defence of Mothers* in which he sought to absolve them of guilt in relation to their autistic children. An environmental view was also extensively argued by Bettleheim (1967) who in the *Empty Fortress* claimed that autism was the result of inappropriate mothering. This same view was espoused by a number of other writers.

An account of the reasons why the environmental view had so many adherents has been provided by Schopler (1970). He discussed evidence on the social psychology of prejudice and scapegoating which results from ignorance and helplessness and brought it to bear on this issue. It was not until Rimland (1964), a parent and professional himself, published his book on a possible Neuronal Theory of Autism that systematic attempts were made to test the environmental view of causation. A number of studies were carried out in which the cognitive, personality, social and communication patterns of parents of autistic children were compared to those of normal, dysphoric and other populations. The bulk of the results thus far has failed to support the view that there are systematic differences in the parents of autistic versus those of normal children (Lennox/Callias/Rutter 1977). The findings have not shown them to be noncaring, to lack warmth or to be deviant. Rutter (1978) in fact also remarks that it is rather interesting that the siblings of autistic children should be indistinguishable from other normal children. Had the parents been deviant, it would be difficult to explain how they would be differentially psychonoxious to one but not to the rest of the children. Furthermore, we know that severe social deviation and psychological and physical abuse frequently result in emotional problems in children but that they do not result in autism.

In summary, the environmental theories, espoused over the years by a number of writers have failed to receive support. Parents of autistic children are indiscriminable from parents of normals (DeMyer 1979). In fact, in view of the extreme levels of stress many of these parents are subjected to, particularly the parents of the hyperirritable autistic children, it is remarkable how well they function (Konstantareas/Homatidis 1989). Although many of the mothers show reactive depression (DeMyer 1979), they are certainly not otherwise psychiatrically involved. Thus any adverse effects the parents may display appear to be the result rather than the cause of their child's difficulties.

4.2. Biological

There is an extensive body of evidence which clearly supports a biologic view of causation in Infantile Autism. These studies fall into a number of distinct categories, including genetics, pre-, peri- and neonatal complications, EEG, PEG and CAT scan findings, neuropathological and biochemical findings, and the coexistence of autism with a number of other disease entities. Only a brief review of this work is possible here.

4.2.1. Genetics

A number of twin studies have been carried out in Britain (Folstein/Rutter 1977), Scandinavia (Gillberg 1983, 1984) and the U. S. (Ritvo/Spence/Freeman et al. 1985) in which at least one of the twins was autistic. All studies have been plagued by small numbers since autism is a rare disorder and sex-matched twins are difficult to find. Results of the British study (Folstein/Rutter 1977) suggested that autism may require an inheritable cognitive deficit but it could also occur as a result of brain damage by itself. In the Scandinavian study, Gillberg (1983) reported preliminary findings in which high concordance rates were found for monozygotic (MZ) twin pairs and much lower for dizygotic (DZ) twin pairs. Also he found 100% concordance rates in the MZ twins for cognitive deficits of any kind, including retardation, severe speech and language disorders, learning disabilities or autism, compared to 21% for sex-matched DZ pairs. Finally, in the U. S. samples, Ritvo et al. (1985) found 96% concordance for MZ twin pairs and 24% for DZ pairs. However, his research methodology, involving self-selection, is questionable.

Results also show an increased risk rate from 50 to 100% for siblings, suggesting that 2 – 5% of the siblings of autistic children may themselves be autistic. Finally, there are data suggesting sex differences in the familial transmission of autism. Not only are males more likely to be affected at a ratio of 3 or 4 to 1, but autistic females once affected are more likely to display a more severe general impairment (Konstantareas/Homatidis/Busch 1989).

In conclusion, there is little doubt that at least some cases of autism are genetically caused, although there is a need for more specific evidence as to the transmission pattern or patterns involved.

4.2.2. Preconception, Prenatal, and Neonatal Complications

Recently, information has become available suggesting that a greater proportion of parents of autistic, compared to parents of retarded children, have been exposed to chemicals or are professional chemists (Deykin/MacMahon 1980; Felicetti 1981). An increased incidence of hypothyroidism in the mothers or fathers of autistic children compared to parents of normal controls has also been reported (Coleman/Rimland 1976). Prenatally, viral infections feature prominently, particularly rubella during the first trimester of pregnancy (Chess 1977). But autism related to maternal toxoplasmosis, syphilis, cytomegalovirus, varicella and the mumps and chickenpox viruses has also been reported (Coleman/Gillberg 1985). Mid trimester bleeding is another prenatal complication which is more likely to be associated with the birth of an autistic child rather than his/her sibling (Torrey/Hersh/McCabe 1975). As I indicated earlier, prenatal complications in interaction with genetics has been suggested to be associated with autism (Folstein/Rutter 1977).

Perinatal complications such as emergency Caesarean section, forceps delivery, prolonged or precipitous labour, cord problems and excess of maternal weight gain are more likely to be present in the births of autistic children than those of their siblings (Deykin/MacMahon 1980).

Of neonatal factors, DeMyer (1979) has estimated that first year illness, followed by behavioral change in the child, was present in 15% of her sample of 33 autistic children, while second year illness accounted for 18% and third year illness for 6% of the cases.

4.2.3. Electrophysiological and Brain Imaging Abnormalities

In general, longer brainstem transmission times and abnormal patterns were reported for subgroups of autistic children. A higher proportion of autistic children with abnormal tracings, 50% of them, were found by Tanguay/Edwards/Buchwald et al. (1982). The findings have been interpreted as suggesting that brainstem dysfunction may lead to distortion in auditory input at higher levels, which may account for the autistic child's cognitive and language deficits. Alternatively, such abnormalities may be incidental to a disease process affecting many parts of the brain, along with the brainstem.

Structural brain damage in autism has been examined first through pneumoencephalograms (PEG). Enlargement of the left ventricular system, and especially the left temporal horns, was found by Hauser/DeLong/Rosman (1975) in 13 of 18 cases with autism. Computerized axial tomography (CAT) scans carried out by Hier/Lemay/Rosenberger (1979) in 16 autistic patients revealed that, although they did not present with localized or diffuse brain injury, they showed a reversal of the left-right brain asymmetry in the parietal occipital region. This was shown by 57% of the autistic patients and by only 25% of other neurological patients. Since some nonautistic children also showed reverse asymmetry, the investigators considered this reversal as a risk factor for autism. Other more recent studies, relying on CAT scans, have yielded negative findings (Tsai/Jacoby/Stewart 1983). Contradictory results have also been reported for enlargement of the lateral and third ventricle. Rumsey/Duara/Grady et al. (1985) also found substantially elevated utilization of glucose throughout many parts of the brain of 10 autistic adults compared to controls. Thus far, however, no dramatic insights have been gained from the brain imaging research in autism, despite early enthusiasm. Future studies may prove more enlightening.

4.2.4. Neuropathological Research Findings

Autopsy studies have been many but poorly controlled and based on incomplete clinical histories. A recent study examined the cortex of four individuals with definite clinical features of autism throughout their lives (Williams/Hauser/Purpura et al. 1980). Although the results from two of the patients did show some abnormalities, these were subtle and limited to dendritic calibre and spine density. The other two patients had essentially no abnormalities, despite many classic clinical autistic features while they were alive. As well, a very detailed autopsy of a 29-year-old man who met criteria for autism and also suffered seizures at 21 years of age, showed lesions in the forebrain and the cerebellum (Bauman/Kemper 1985).

The contradictory results where some autopsies of autistic individuals show brain abnormalities and others do not may be explained by means of the etiological heterogeneity of the syndrome. It is also possible that in some cases of autism brain structure is relatively unremarkable but brain biochemistry is abnormal (Konstantareas 1986).

4.2.5. Biochemical Findings

High serotonin levels have been reported for autistic individuals while the reverse was found for others. High serotonin is not unique to autism and has been reported for many other mental retardation syndromes. Studies of platelet monoamine oxidase have yielded essentially negative results thus far, although elevations have been reported in isolated cases (Coleman/Gillberg 1985).

A number of other studies have been carried out over the last 15 years including examination of hormones, immune reactions, trace elements, etc. Thus far, no specific biochemical markers have been found. So, although subgroups of children sharing specific biochemical abnormalities may exist, we have not as yet been able to isolate them (Coleman/Gillberg 1985).

4.2.6. Autism among Subgroups with Other Diseases

Thus far, autism has been demonstrated to occur in some genetic disorders. Some of the possible or definite linkages are with tuberous sclerosis, neurofibromatosis (Gillberg/Forsell 1984) and Fragile X or Martin Bell syndrome. In addition, an extra X chromosome is often associated with speech and language difficulties, if not with the entire syndrome of autism (Coleman/Gillberg 1985). Among infectious diseases, exposure of mother to the rubella virus, the virus of mumps, cytomegalovirus, and oral herpes virus (HSV-1) and the genital herpes virus (HSV-2) has been found to be related to autism in the offspring. It is difficult to be certain that autism was directly caused by the given virus in any individual case. Yet for rubella the relationship is more firmly established (Chess 1977). Thus infectious agents acting prematurely or after birth may be at least partly related to the development of autism.

Of metabolic diseases, PKU appears to result in a behavior syndrome comparable to autism, if treatment is not instituted in early life. With present screening cutoff levels of 4 mg %, approximately one third of PKU patients may be missed. Of other aminoacidopathies, histidinemia has been reported to coexist with autistic symptoms. Purine autism, with increased secretion of uric acid has also been reported. Autism has also been found in cases of hyperlacticemia or lactic acidosis, with increases in the rate of lactate production relative to rate of lactate utilization (Coleman/Gillberg 1985).

Of structural disease entities, hydrocephalus has been frequently associated with autism. Malignant tumours have not been reported but occasionally lesions such as porencephaly and other abnormalities are seen in the CAT scans of autistic patients (Gillberg/Svendsen 1983). As discussed earlier, Rett's syndrome can also co-exist with autism. Of other degenerative diseases, neurocutaneous disorders such as tuberous sclerosis and neorofibromatosis have also been associated with autism in a number of cases (Lotter 1974; Wing 1975).

5. Language and Communication Deficits in Autism

That language and communication deficits are central to AD is evident in Kanner's (1943) first description. Pronominal reversal, i. e., substitution of *you* for *I*, delay in speech acquisition, noncommunicative use of speech when speech is available, idiosyncratic and inappropriate or perseverative utterances were among the language characteristics attributed to most of the original 11 cases he described. With the emergence of systematic research in the mid-sixties, particularly work on speech training by Lovaas and his collaborators at UCLA (Lovaas/Berberich/Perloff/Schaeffer 1966), the centrality of language impairment was emphasized. Since then, an impressive number of research papers and reviews have appeared on this topic. Furthermore, with advances in psycholinguistics and in cognate fields, the issue broadened to encompass both theoretical positions regarding the nature and meaning of language deficits in autism and intervention strategies to remediate them.

5.1. Language Characteristics of Autistic Individuals

5.1.1. Muteness

This ranges from total silence to the emission of inarticulate, nonpatterned vocalizations used for vocal play but no recognizable speech. Muteness has also been employed for those vocalizations that are used in a self-stimulatory manner but are devoid of meaning and even for those with minimal functional characteristics. Although rate of muteness reported for autism has varied from 28% to 61% (Fay/Schuler 1980), definition of muteness as well as diagnostic criteria used for the classification of the children and referral practices have varied over the years, hence no conclusive data on it is available.

Muteness in the young autistic child has been frequently linked with the suspicion of deafness. This is a very commonly reported phenomenon by parents and one of the first considerations in making a referral to a professional. Hyposensitivity to sound may alternate in the same child with hypersensitivity, particularly under high motivation conditions. In fact, diagnostic checklists such as the Childhood Autism Rating Scale (Schopler/Reichler/DeVellis/Daly 1980) consider this as one of the symptoms of the syndrome. There is little doubt that very rarely is an autistic child concurrently deaf and that the hyposensitivity is functional rather than organic.

5.1.2. Babbling

Babbling, which is reflected in vowel-consonant sound combinations, has adult-like intonational patterns and is repetitious, is also either completely absent or it is distorted in autistic children. In our own sample, a large percentage of children have never babbled while most of those who did have displayed either a delayed or an attenuated form of babble. Very few autistic children seem to develop babbling at the same time as normal children do. Research in this area is of necessity hampered by the retrospective nature of the information collected. Thus to quote exact percentages may be misleading at the present time. Needed is systematic research on normal timing and extent of babbling to provide a basis for the deviant characteristics of the babbling of autistic children. As well, we need to examine more systematically the relationship of the characteristics of babble of those AD children who do produce it and their other presenting characteristics. This will help us determine the relationship of this feature of normal language to the communication and other deficits of autistic children.

Some beginnings have already been made in this direction. Ricks (1975) reported that parents in his sample recalled no vocalization in their autistic children during their first year of life. But, between 3 and 5 years of age, some autistic children in his sample did babble. However, the babble was monotonous. Moreover, in contrast to normal babies and Down syndrome children of 3 to 6 years, who ignored their own babbling, the autistics did not ignore it when played back to them. When they responded to the taped babble, however, it was to repeat only their own babbling in a sameness preserving fashion, but not the babbling of other children. These findings suggested to the authors that the babbling peculiarities of autistic children are in keeping with their overall processing and adaptational pattern rather than having unique features of its own.

5.1.3. Echolalia

In contrast to babbling, some of which usually occurs before a formal assessment is undertaken, echolalia lends itself to research much more readily. In fact, it is the one key feature best recalled by students because of its striking characteristics. Additionally, it has served well in the psychoanalytic explanation of AD over the years because, like Narcissus in the Greek mythology, it reflects the egocentric style and distancing autistic children were thought to choose in an effort to actively separate themselves from others.

Echolalia is defined as the meaningless repetition of a word, phrase or sentence, without regard for the communication needs of the interlocutor. It can be immediate or delayed (Kanner 1943) and mitigated (modified) or unmitigated (Fay/Schuler 1980). Kanner (1943, 222) described at length the verbal echolalic behavior of 9 of his 11 autistic patients. He appeared to believe that echolalia was not an isolated phenomenon but rather part of the obsessional, perseverative and concrete nature of the disorder. Although some echolalic utterances appear to be routine, mechanical renditions of other people's speech, most seem to be related to events that are normally affect laden and of significance to the child and/or to his social context. This is an element of echolalia not sufficiently examined in the literature.

After years of mere description and benign neglect, and with new data provided from a number of academic disciplines, echolalia started to become a subject of scientific interest and left the realm of enigma and fascination. Since the mid – 70's, its social aspects are being examined and analyzed, much as they have been studied for other forms of language production (see Prizant 1979). Thus, although behavioral approaches have defined echolalic behavior as inappropriate and have targeted it for elimination, functional approaches have analyzed it for its possible 'communication intent'. Basing their work on the methodology of pragmatic research on normal language development, Prizant/Duchan (1981) studied immediate echolalia with four autistic children. They arrived at four structural categories: (1) noninteractive echolalia with lack of comprehension, (2) interactive echolalia with no comprehension, (3) echolalia produced noninteractively with comprehension, and (4) interactive echolalia with evidence of comprehension, the most advanced category. Of greater interest were the results of the delayed echolalia study (Prizant/Rydell 1984) which yielded a variety of functional uses, ranging from relatively automatic, non-intentional utterances to fully communicative and functional. Some of the functions described from least to most communicative were: turn-taking and verbal completion, rehearsal, self-directive, non-interactive labelling, protest, request, interactive labelling, calling, providing information, directive and affirmation (Schuler/Prizant 1985).

In analyzing the characteristics of autistic language, these authors have argued that autistic children use a gestalt processing style which contrasts sharply with the more advanced analytic mode necessary for normal language acquisition.

In sum, recent developments have provided considerable information on the characteristics and possible functions of echolalia and have linked it to a more general model of disordered information processing in autism. A comparable position has been taken by other cognitive writers in the field (Frith 1989). However, we are still far from understanding why and how such a style has evolved at all and how it precisely relates to other aspects of communication, cognition and social interaction in these children.

5.1.4. Pronominal Reversal and Metaphorical Language Use

Although much as with echolalia, pronominal reversal was thought to be the result of the socioaffective impairment and identity problems in autistic children, this is no longer believed to be the case. Of course, it is quite startling to an observer to hear a child address himself as a *you* or omit the first person pronoun *I* in using a mand such as asking for juice or a cookie. In our summer camp, for example, Marlene, a 9-year-old girl, would frequently approach us saying "want juice", omitting the relevant pronoun. On other occasions she would fearfully demand, "You go home now? Come bus, come bus?" The context had allowed us to interpret what she meant to tell us: *I want juice* and *I don't want the bus to take me home*. To the uninitiated, however, the meanings might have been different. Thus, much as with simple, unprocessed S – R connections, pronoun reversal may be interpreted to mean a 'gestalt' style of processing or automatic and mechanical repetition rather than be thought as vested with more complex personal meaning. However, this is not to indicate that this style is yet clearly understood. It is only at one level of explanation that one can state that the children's gestalt processing is responsible for this phenomenon. A number of additional pieces of information need to be explained. First, it is unclear why the child can and does acquire the proper name of the individual whom he addresses as *you* but cannot say *you* (see also Frith 1989, 127). Second, it is unclear why or when some children completely omit the pronouns while others, or the same child at different times, use a pronoun reversal pattern. Third, we need to know why and under what circumstances do the children use the pronouns correctly and under which they do not. Fourth, we need to examine the interrelationship between echolalia, promonimal reversal and metaphorical language use. Finally, we need to know other important correlates of these three phenomena, such as their relationship to other aspects of the receptive and expressive language of that child. By acquiring additional information, we may be in a better position to arrive at effective remediation.

5.1.5. Phonology, Syntax, Morphology and Prosody

For the approximately 50% of autistic individuals who speak, the obvious next question is the nature of their phonologic and syntactic competence. Bartolucci/Pierce/Streiner/Eppel (1976), compared the picture-naming ability of autistic mentally retarded and normal children, appropriately matched on non-verbal M. A. Unexpectedly perhaps, they found the same distribution of error patterns and the same frequency distribution of various phonemes for all three groups. Yet the types of rules the autistic children employed in their constructions may not be as advanced (Cantwell/Baker/Rutter 1978). Tager-Flusberg (1981) also found that autistic children did follow syntactic rules in their comprehension of language.

In our own work, we have frequently found a number of autistic children to use syncopated, foreshortened phrases in an effort to terminate the communication as quickly as possible. We have also found them to omit functors (pronouns, prepositions, adverbs, etc.) and have systematically demonstrated how to remedy this through the superimposition of signs on the relevant functors. By progressively fading out the signed functor, once the word is included in the sentence, we were able to assist the children in acquiring the missing word (Konstantareas 1984).

Turning to prosodic development, there is little doubt that prosody or 'speech melody' is disturbed in the speech productions of autistic individuals. This was identified quite early (Kanner 1943). Furthermore, the prosodic deficits are apparently in evidence even after considerable improvement in speech production.

Prosody studies in autism are few, although interest in the topic began early (Goldfarb/Braunstein/Lorge 1956). In a more recent study by Paccia/Curcio (1982), prosody in echolalic speech was examined in the context of the hypothesis that, if the prosodic contours of an echo changed, that would reflect some degree of comprehension. Results were interpreted to indicate that echolalia did include prosodic restructuring. They also argued that those echolalic children who do not manipulate the prosodic features of their speech may be more impaired linguistically than those who do.

More recent work summarized by Baltaxe/Simmons (1985) suggests that those autistic children who speak may not be prosodically as globally impaired as the earlier studies suggested. Deficits may depend on which aspect of prosody is considered. They believe that most verbal autistic individuals have both delays and abnormalities in mainly their fundamental frequency range and the linguistic information they express. In some instances, they believe the fundamental range may be too narrow or too wide, yet the stress and intonation contour may be appropriate or, conversely, the fundamental frequency range may be close to normal but intonation and stress may be inaccurate. A number of dysphasic children apparently share with the autistic their prosodic abnormalities, including a narrowed frequency range. However, overall the dysphasics in their studies tended to be less extensively impaired in their prosody and to be closer to the normal children.

In summary, studies in prosodic development, particularly of autistic children, are not many. We know that normal children reach some prosodic stability by their fourth year, although prosodic maturity is not reached until puberty. The close interrelationships between prosody and other aspects of the autistic child's language have begun to be clarified. Yet, as Baltaxe/Simmons (1985) also caution, we may find that impairment or delay in prosody and delays in other areas of linguistic functioning may occur independently in the same individual, much as with the adult aphasias. If cross influences between linguistic and prosodic elements do exist, the direction of causation also remains to be specified. Baltaxe/Simmons (1985) speculate that the constructive use of echolalia in autistic children who develop more adequate language may be due to their inability to use prosody in speech reception and expression. Being unable to break down the speech flow into units, may compel the autistic individual to use larger, unprocessed chunks in an attempt to communicate with others. In that sense, they claim, echolalia may be comparable to the early prosodic 'frames', 'matrices' and 'envelopes' normal children employ to communicate, as discussed by Bruner (1975), among others.

6. Intervention Strategies for Communication

6.1. The Speech Training Approach

Early attempts to treat autistic children were predicated on the psychoanalytic model. No special emphasis was placed on speech and language remediation. It was not until the 1960s with Ferster (1961), that learning difficulties were perceived to be crucial to the autistic child's deficits. Ferster (1961) stressed the non-existence of generalized reinforcers in these children, e. g., praise, approval and warm bodily contact, despite the children's obvious responsiveness to primary reinforcers such as food, drink, etc. Thus the learning therapists emphasized the need to build social skills, and particularly language, from scratch.

The first systematic study using operant principles to build speech or to modify the echolalic speech of autistic children was published by Lovaas/Berberich/Perloff/Shaeffer (1966). The central tenet of this position, further elaborated and modified over the years, was that speech, because of its obvious social and symbolic aspects, should be given priority in treatment attempts with this population. Elsewhere (Konstantareas 1981), the behaviorist position to speech training is presented in some detail. To summarize, a two-stage sequence was followed with the mute children. In the first, speech sounds, syllables and words were shaped through imitation, discrimination, and reinforcement out of context. Thus the child could acquire, through chaining, words such as *baba*, *mama*, *data*, etc. Additional words such as *juice*, *cookie*, *give* and so on, were introduced for imitation. Once these spoken but context-free utterances could be emitted by the child, the second stage, involving speech in context, was introduced. Here words were reinforced if emitted in response to the relevant object or in the context of an activity. Progressively phrases and sentences correctly related to the context were introduced and, when correct, were reinforced.

The systematic, well-documented and orderly application of the principles has made them very appealing to educators and therapists over the years. Thus the operant paradigm has established its credibility in a field that tended to be predominated by descriptive accounts or clinical case presentations of general efforts to help the autistic child.

The quantitative and evaluative stance of the behaviorists compelled them to re-evaluate and modify their earlier expectations that, once speech was acquired, the autistic child would become 'normal'. In an elegantly reported follow-up, Lovaas/Koegel/Simmons/Long (1973) acknowledged some of the limitations of their procedures, particularly the fact that maintenance of hard-won gains required continuation of intervention. Stimulus and response generalization and maintenance were not automatic, not only for the behaviorist technology, but for any therapeutic intervention. As well, they implied, but did not outrightly state, that the child's presenting characteristics may be crucial for his ability to acquire speech. But these were not the only difficulties. Some workers in the field complained of the wooded, flat and robot-like quality of the speech acquired through operant training. Others were also concerned about the lack of spontaneity evident in the speech of this population (Bonvillian/Nelson 1978), while still others were unable to help autistic children produce speech at all, despite extensive efforts. Hingtgen/Churchill (1969), for example, reported that after 6 hours per day five weeks, three of their four autistic children had acquired 60, 25 and 16 words each, while a fourth child could not acquire anything but sounds. A mixed outcome was also obtained by Mack/Webster/Goksen (1980) in the Clarke Institute in a follow-up of 54 autistic or autistic-like children exposed to a program akin to that developed by Lovaas/Berberich/Perloff/Schaefer (1966). Although many children acquired spoken language, others could not. This might have been surprising then but, as we shall see, it is not at all surprising now if one takes into account the child's cognitive and other deficits which may preclude speech acquisition.

Speech training strategies based on the behavioral paradigm have been increasingly directed at the very young children. The rationale behind this development, as described by Lovaas (1987), is twofold: (a) That treatment gains with the older children originally employed "have been specific to the particular environment in which they were treated, substantial relapse has been observed at follow-up, and no client has been reported as recovered" (Lovaas 1987, 3). (b) With children younger than 4 years of age, treatment for most of their waking hours for many years, and including all significant persons in all significant environments, would result in extensive gain maintenance. In addition, the possibility of successful mainstreaming into the primary school would be higher for the younger children. A significant assumption made was that very young autistic children are less likely to discriminate between environments and therefore more likely to generalize and maintain their treatment gains.

Space precludes a detailed account of experimental design, assessment and treatment procedures and outcome of this intensive intervention (cf. Lovaas 1987; Lovaas/Smith 1988). In brief, three groups of children participated: (a) An experimental, intensive behavioral group exposed on average for 40 hours per week to communication and behavior training for 2 or more years. (b) Control group 1, consisting of children with comparable characteristics to the experimental but exposed to training for less than 10 hours per week for a comparable length of time. This group was used to examine spontaneous recovery. (c) Control group 2, not exposed to specific intervention but comparable in characteristics to the other two, was used to guard against the possibility that the experimental group was particularly selected to be higher functioning or different from the usual autistic population. No random assignment was employed. Results revealed that 47% of the experimental treatment group achieved normal intellectual and educational functioning, with IQs in the normal range and successful performance in first grade in public schools. Another 40% were mildly retarded and assigned to special classes and 10% were profoundly retarded and assigned to classes for autistic and retarded children. Children in control group 1, by contrast, fared much worse. Only 2% of them achieved normal functioning, 45% were mildly retarded and 53% were severely retarded and placed in classes for autistic and retarded children. Control group 2 was not significantly different from Control group 1. Lovaas (1987) interpreted these data as providing strong support in favor of early intensive behavioral intervention. Furthermore, he argued that, for all intents and purposes, teachers could not distinguish the experimental group subjects from normal children, although he conceded that on "closer psychological assessment, particularly as these children grow older, certain deficits may remain ..." (Lovaas 1987, 8). In a commentary and critique of this report and the success claims for the intensive behavioral approach, Schopler/Short/Mesibov (1989) argued that it is impossible to determine the effects of the intervention Lovaas (1987) reported because of: (a) inappropriate choice of outcome measures, (b) subject selection bias, and (c) inadequate control groups.

6.1.1. Critique of Speech Training

The behavioral approach to speech training has been quite productive and effective, and continues to enjoy considerable popularity. It has provided a technology for assistance with speech shaping and word and phrase acquisition. However, it has not been without its criticism. The following have been the main criticisms that have been levelled against it: (1) It has tended to be mechanistic and simplistic in that it has concentrated on speech only, ignoring by and large the necessity for helping the children achieve spontaneous, functional speech (Goetz/Schuler/Sailor 1979; Konstantareas 1986). (2) Perhaps because of its emphasis on repetition and drilling, it results in stilted and flat verbal output with poor pitch, intonation and stress and the other prosodic elements of normal speech production which reflect intention. (3) It is attempted, with minor exceptions such as work by Carr and his group who use sign language (Carr 1979), with all dysfunctional children rather than a select group for which it may be more relevant (Konstantareas 1981). This may be responsible for the inability of some children to profit from it despite repeated efforts (cf. Creedon 1973; Hingtgen/Churchill 1969). (4) Perhaps because of ignoring new knowledge in the fields of developmental psychology, psycholinguistics and communication theory, it has not taken into account the crucial relevance, among other factors, of cognitive growth, information processing, socio-affective development and communication acquisition in normal children. Such information would have allowed for the development of a richer and more flexible approach to language intervention.

6.2. Simultaneous Communication Training

Partly because of the limitations of speech training with particularly the mute and the lower functioning subgroup of autistic children and partly as a result of its effectiveness once attempted with those subgroups but also with the verbal and higher functioning, speech and sign language training (simultaneous communication) has become one of the main alternatives to speech only training. It was first attempted by Creedon (1973) and by Webster/McPherson/Sloman et al. (1973) but shortly thereafter its use acquired something of a momentum, which it continues to enjoy until now. Elsewhere we reported the rationale for its use (Konstantareas 1986). In brief, among the reasons that have been considered to be important for its success have been: (1) The information processing characteristics of autistic children. Autistic children have been shown to be impaired primarily in auditory sequential processing (Hermelin/O'Connor 1970). Interestingly, in one of our studies we found the lower functioning subgroup to have suffered a greater number of and more prolonged ear infections than matched for CA normal children or functioning autistic children (Konstantareas/Homatidis 1987). Autistic children are also generally better able to code visually, spatially and kinesthetically and have most of their difficulties in encoding temporal-sequential input. Processing speech, which requires decoding and recoding, may tax their capacities to such an extent that they may not deal with it at all. Further evidence for the auditory peculiarities of these children has been provided by Condon (1975) who has reported deficits in 'self-synchrony' and 'interactional synchrony' in autistic children. Self-synchrony refers to 'entrainment' between one's vocalizations or speech and his/her body movements and interactional synchrony to the precise correspondence between the listener's movements and the articulatory structure of the speaker's utterances. Upon microkinesic analysis, Condon (1975) found delays of up to a full second, i. e., twenty-four frames of moving film. Furthermore, for many children the body movement repeated itself in a reverberatory fashion two or more times, to a single auditory signal, a phenomenon Condon calls 'multiple entrainment'. Attempts to replicate the 'Condon effect' have met with only partial success. If replicated, these findings may provide important clues to the apparently disturbed auditory universe of these children as reported by themselves (Volkmar/Cohen 1985). (2) Developmental and motivational features of the children also appear relevant to the effectiveness of sign language use with them. Interventions thus far have rarely taken into account the child's cognitive ability. Speech training techniques have been employed, for example, regardless of the child's mental age. Thus an 8-year-old child with a mental age of 11 months may be asked to speak, an activity above his cognitive competence. Although gestures, shared attention, imitation and turntaking may be highly recommended in his case, systematic speech training may be premature. Information on normal child development and the relevance of action and gesture in early communication acquisition (cf. Lock 1978) are of particular relevance in guiding intervention with the very young and/or low functioning children. If spoken language evolves phylogenetically and ontogenetically from gestures, we may need to focus our attention on these forerunners of verbal communication. Following the constructivist approach of Piaget (1963) to normal language acquisition, and regardless of the primacy given to cognition, the correspondences between the two domains are compelling (Ingram 1978). One can therefore hardly afford to ignore the relevance of cognition to intervention with autistic children. Thorough assessment of it through sensorimotor intelligence testing with the younger children and nonverbal intelligence tests, such as the Leiter International Performance Scale, for those above the mental age of 2 years, has been our practice. It is only after we have carefully assessed the children's various cognitive, communication and social abilities that we can decide on the communication system best suited to any given child (Konstantareas 1990). A comparable view has been expressed by other clinicians (cf. Watson 1985).

Aside from cognition, motivational factors are very crucial. What is reinforcing for an autistic child is frequently impossible to decide upon in advance. Also how these children avail themselves of desirable objects is very important to consider. Many autistic individuals satisfy need states by goal-directed movements aimed at the coveted object rather than use conventional linguistic means to obtain it. This goal-directed reaching has, in fact, been considered by us and by others (Schaeffer 1978) to be one of the key factors underlying spontaneity in communication by means of sign language. They frequently touch others as well when unable to obtain an object and to pull or push them toward a desired location. They use their hands to 'ask' for help in achieving their goals. This tendency of autistic individuals to be motoric and active, much as younger and immature organisms tend to be, has direct relevance to their ability to employ a system based on hand and motor movement. As well, autistic individuals tend to be impatient with small visual detail, such as the printed word, hence, their reluctance to engage in desk-related behavior.

(3) Finally, certain features of sign language render it particularly well-suited to the information processing and special characteristics of this population. For Hewes (1973), protolanguage was likely gestural. Vocalization, originally a mutation present in some individuals, became progressively selected for. The socially shy autistic children may therefore feel more comfortable with the more natural and spontaneous manner sign language affords them to express intent. Signs, being an extension of body movements, may also be easier for them to use since many of them, particularly the younger and lower functioning, do not vocalize spontaneously. The signs for *come*, *go*, *give* and *want* are examples of natural extensions of reaching or approaching others. Another feature of sign language, iconicity, has been shown to be of relevance in early sign acquisition. With normal children, Brown (1977) demonstrated that perceived iconic signs are easier to learn than non-iconic. Such signs which are 'time-bound', 'age-bound', 'culture-bound' and 'experience-bound' are perceived as similar to their referents. Using 'translucency' as a test of iconicity, Bellugi/Klima (1976) found that 50% of the 90 signs shown to their subjects could be seen as having some connection to their references. Translucency refers to the degree to which a subject can discern a relationship between a sign and its referent, after having been presented with both. With autistic children, Konstantareas/Oxman/Webster (1978) were able to demonstrate that iconic signs of the Ontario sign language for the deaf were easier to acquire than were non-iconic signs. This was especially the case for verbs and adjectives which tend to have extensive sensorimotor elements associated with them. Another characteristic of sign language relevant to its ease of acquisition by lower functioning and lower speed language processors, such as the autistic children, is the rate of its presentation. Signs were shown to

be at least twice as long as speech to process by fluent users of both signs and speech (Bellugi/Fischer 1972). A third characteristic is lack of redundancy. Sign language retains content words such as nouns, adjectives and verbs but omits functors such as the copula, articles and prepositions. Because it is an economical, low redundancy language, it may be better suited to the needs of children who have difficulty in processing information. Finally, sign language training has distinct advantages over speech training in terms of it being amenable to direct manipulation. Compared to the tongue, lips, mouth and oral cavity, the inaccessible internal structures on which we rely to produce speech, one can mold the child's hands into signs. Thus, by virtue of its reliance on accessible parts of the body, sign language seems easier to employ in early training compared to speech.

6.2.1. Implementation Studies

Creedon's (1973) paper on implementation of simultaneous communication training has constituted a basic model for interventions in this area. Since 1973, with a study by Webster et al., our group has embarked upon a series of studies aiming at clarifying intervention issues. Konstantareas/Oxman/Webster (1977) reported on a demonstration project with 6 children who were able to acquire signs over a brief, five-week summer camp period. Konstantareas/Webster/Oxman (1979) provided the outcome of a systematic effort at organizing and carrying out a simultaneous communication program with five children. Intensive and detailed evaluation of changes in social interaction and communication, as well as in a variety of other behaviors, was attempted. Results were quite promising, particularly for communication acquisition, both receptively and expressively. Spontaneous social interaction, however, did not substantially increase as a result of the intervention. However, self-help skills improved and unoccupied behavior decreased.

Once the feasibility of application was established, we examined a variety of issues which appeared to require attention. One obvious question was parental concern as to possible reduction of vocalizing and speech as a result of exposure to simultaneous communication. Oxman/Konstantareas/Leibovitz (1979) provided a negative answer to this question. Although children in our experimental group began the program with fewer vocalizations than an untreated control, they vocalized more by the program's end. The issue of whether simultaneous two-modality training (signing and speaking) would be inferior to single modality (signing and mouthing) was also examined (Konstantareas/Leibovitz 1981). Results showed that, on average, the two-modality intervention was superior. Gain maintenance and generalization for simultaneous communication was shown to be quite good, particularly for the higher functioning children who continued to be exposed to simultaneous language training after they left an intensive program (Konstantareas 1987).

6.2.2. Evaluation of Simultaneous Communication Training

Since 1973, more than 30 studies have appeared in the literature on this alternative to speech training. Most are either case studies or involve small groups of children. For selective reviews, see Bonvillian/Nelson (1978), Carr (1979), Kiernan (1983) and Konstantareas (1986). The older, mute and minimally vocal autistic children have appeared to be the best candidates for this technique but we have no evidence on best predictors for its success. Some workers in the field have proposed that children with vocal imitation skills are best suited to speech training (Carr 1979). However, a more recent study by Barrera/Sulzer-Azaroff (1983) found that echolalic autistic children benefited more in acquiring expressive labels from a simultaneous than an oral only training approach. Van Wagenen/Jensen/Worsham/Petersen (1985) also recommend the use of this approach with verbal children as a result of their own work in this area. Thus, although by default the mute and older children have been traditionally and successfully exposed to simultaneous communication, perhaps as a last resort, this need not be valid. The review of evidence presented earlier as to the goodness of fit between the presenting characteristics and needs of autistic children and the characteristics of this strategy, as well as recent work, suggest that the superimposition of signs on words may be useful with a fair number of this group and indeed other language impaired groups, as we have shown (Konstantareas 1984). Furthermore, even blind autistic and mute children can benefit (Konstantareas/Hunter/Sloman 1982). Research is required to examine the relevance of at least the following child characteristics as predictors of effectiveness of the simultaneous communication approach: receptive and expressive speech, ability to imitate words and signs, ability to respond to gestures and to words, mental age and IQ and degree of interactive ability. Only by systematically engaging in this effort can we arrive at valid predictors of communication medium, i. e., words only versus words and signs. Some efforts in examining this issue have already been made by us (Konstantareas/Blackman 1978) and by others (Yoder/Layton 1988) but much more is needed.

Aside from type of medium, one may have to consider using both approaches but successively. In our clinical work we have frequently recommended graduating from simultaneous to speech only communication, once word production had increased. We, Konstantareas (1987) and Layton/Stutts (1985) have shown that, regardless of modality of training, high verbal imitators prefer to use speech while low imitators prefer to communicate by sign. Specifically on pragmatic usage, Layton/Stutts (1985) also found that the high verbal imitators outperformed the low imitators on all communicative functions while the low imitators used mostly requests as their sole communicative function.

In conclusion, simultaneous communication training appears to be an approach well suited to many autistic children and can lead either to speech or, in those children with poor vocalization ability, to the use of signs to express basic needs. Children who, in the past, would be completely unable to communicate through speech, now have a viable, alternative means of communication, the use of elementary signs. We have found that as many as 50% of children who did not speak prior to simultaneous communication training begin to speak after exposure to this technique. This result has also been reported by others (e. g., Creedon 1973). Furthermore, this approach is not uniquely suited to autistic individuals but has been successfully attempted with retarded children and even children with severe reading disabilities (Blackburn/Bonvillian/Ashby 1984).

6.3. Other Interventions

In addition to the two main approaches to training, a variety of techniques have been employed but evidence on their effectiveness is chiefly anecdotal. Pictures of real life objects have been used with very low functioning autistic children or with those unable to shape their hands into even gross approximations to signs. Picture boards have been constructed and used well with those autistic children who respond poorly to either speech or simultaneous communication training. The Bliss Symbol System, particularly relevant to the needs of individuals with neuromuscular disorders, has also been attempted with autistic children. In one of the very few studies available on this issue, Hurlbut/Inata/Green (1982) compared the use of Bliss symbols and an iconic picture-drawing system with three cerebral palsied adolescents who had severe physical and mental disabilities and were non-ambulatory. No other diagnostic information is provided in the report. Probe data were taken to assess maintenance, stimulus and response generalization, and spontaneous usage of each system. Results revealed that all students required approximately four times as many trials to acquire the Bliss symbols as the corresponding iconic drawings. As well, they retained all drawings while they required retraining in almost all Bliss symbols. This is not surprising in view of the similarities between the representational drawings and their corresponding objects, and the much less obvious similarities between the more abstract Bliss symbols and the objects. In fact, one suspects that one of the reasons for the unavailability of published studies on the use of the Bliss system with autistic individuals may be its limited usefulness with this population. In view of the well-documented difficulties autistic children show in abstracting information and in light of our previous discussion on their processing difficulties, even the higher functioning subgroup may find the system difficult. Furthermore, the higher functioning subgroup is also likely to be verbal.

More recently, considerable interest has been expressed in Facilitated Communication. Originally discovered by Crossley and her colleagues in Australia, this technique involves helping individuals with poor verbal abilities to express themselves with the aid of the touch of another person, the facilitator. An alphabet board, a hand-held typewriter or a computer are used. The children type or point to letters aided by the touch of the facilitator who gently holds or touches the individual's arm at the elbow, wrist or the hand. The facilitator mainly assists the person not by moving his/her hand to the correct letter, but by ensuring that the person does not perseverate in hitting the same key more than once. The main published account of this technique by Biklen (1990) challenges existing theoretical views on the limited literacy abilities of particularly the mute and apparently low functioning autistic children. He reports some striking conversations with such low functioning individuals using facilitated communication. Answers to even complex questions pertaining to feeling states and requiring social reasoning capacity were spelled correctly and were logically correct in individuals thought to be cognitively quite limited and nonliteral. There has already been some controversy related to whether the facilitators merely facilitate or actually manipulate and influence the process (Crossley/McDonald 1980). As well, it was difficult for students to communicate with more than one or two facilitators, especially early on in the process. Furthermore, Biklen (1990) concedes that the method is not a uniform approach to teaching or supporting communication that can be used with each person but depends on the specific attitudinal characteristics of the facilitator, such as a non-patronizing attitude, self-effaciveness, being apologetic for asking simplistic questions, etc. Some of the descriptions provided by Biklen (1990) are suggestive of a population with considerable symbolizing and representational capacities not frequently encountered even in high functioning autistic individuals. In some instances, insofar as no information on diagnosis is provided to us, we cannot judge the relevance of the work to autism. It is at present unclear who may benefit from this approach. As well, it has, of course, not been found that facilitated communication will cure autism, although Crossley apparently believes that considerable improvement after facilitated communication is possible in terms of the behavioral characteristics of children (Biklen 1990).

As to the explanation for the apparent success of this new approach, the current hypothesis offered by its proponents is that it overcomes the apraxia many of these minimally verbal or mute individuals suffer from. How this is achieved and whether one can assess in advance who is apraxic, hence will benefit, have not yet been clarified. In some respects, however, the technique resembles sign language with mute individuals since it, too, once it is provided, allows the expression of thoughts and feelings previously blocked due to the unavailability of an expressive capacity. Remarkably, even 6-year-old autistic youngsters can apparently spell out correctly words no one explicitly taught them. They seem to have incidentally acquired them from looking at television programs and commercials.

In sum, in addition to speech and simultaneous communication training, the use of real pictures of objects or drawings of objects hold promise with some autistic children. As well, facilitated communication holds considerable promise and may turn out to be one of the most useful means of interacting with minimally verbal autistic children. We require, however, much research into the neurological underpinnings of the facilitated communication process. We also need to examine who of the autistic children, and under what conditions will benefit from any augmentative communication system.

7. Prognosis of Autistic Disorder

Considerable information on prognosis has been collected, which spans the last forty to fifty years, but much more is needed before we can fully understand the life-long characteristics of the disorder. In general, autism continues well into adulthood, although developmental changes have been documented (Paul 1987). In middle childhood there is already a movement towards tentative, albeit still deviant, social interaction. Level of functioning may determine the degree of involvement. As well, some speech may appear in those previously completely mute as well as improvement in hyperactive behavior, although stereotypical ritualistic and compulsive behavior persist.

In adolescence an estimated 10 – 35% of autistic children undergo regression and some become seizuring with a peak between 11 and 14 years of age. Paul (1987) reports that once regression is present, return to normal functioning may await until the individual reaches his/her late twenties. With increasing age social skills and language may improve somewhat. In addition, there is further improvement to the point that as many as 14% of autistic individuals no longer meet social deviance criteria for the condition. No recent studies on this issue are available, however. The language characteristics of autistic adults with typical autism may resemble those seen in schizophrenia, with loose associations, preoccupation with particular topics and semantic concreteness (Paul 1987).

8. References

American Psychiatric Association (1980). *Diagnostic and statistical manual of mental disorders* (3rd ed.). Washingthon, D. C.: Author.

American Psychiatric Association (1987). *Diagnostic and statistical manual of mental disorders* (3rd revised ed.). Washington, D.C.: Author.

Asperger, H. (1944). Die autistichen Psychopathen im Kindesalter. *Archiv für Psychiatrie und Nervenkrankheiten, 117*, 76–136.

Baltaxe, C. A. & Simmons, J. Q. (1985). Prosodic development in normal and autistic children. In: E. Schopler & G. B. Mesibov (Eds.), *Communication problems in autism. 95–125.* New York: Plenum.

Barrera, R. D. & Sulzer-Azaroff, B. (1983). An alternating treatment comparison of oral and total communication training programs with echolalic autistic children. *Journal of Applied Behavior Analysis, 16* (4), 379–394.

Bartolucci, G., Pierce, S., Streiner, D., & Eppel, P.T. (1976). Phonological investigation of verbal autistic and mentally retarded subjects. *Journal of Autism and Childhood Schizophrenia, 6*, 303–316.

Bauman, M. & Kemper, T. L. (1985). Histoanatomic observations of the brain in early infantile autism. *Neurology, 35*, 866–874.

Bellugi, U. & Fischer, S. (1972). A comparison of sign language and spoken language. *Cognition, 1*, 173–199.

Bellugi, U. & Klima, E. S. (1976). Two faces of sign: Iconic and abstract. *Annals of the New York Academy of Sciences, 280*, 514–538.

Bettelheim, B. (1967). *The empty fortress: Infantile autism and the birth of the self.* New York: Free Press.

Biklen, D. (1990). Communication unbound: autism and praxis. *Harvard Educational Review, 60*, 291–314.

Blackburn, W. D., Bonvillian, J. D., & Ashby, R. P. (1984). Manual communication as an alternative mode of language instruction for children with severe reading disabilities. *Language, Speech, and Hearing Services in Schools, 15*, 22–31.

Bonvillian, J. D. & Nelson, K. E. (1978). Development of sign language in autistic children and other language-handicapped individuals. In P. Siple (Ed.), *Understanding language through sign language research. 187–212.* New York: Academic Press.

Brown, R.W. (1977, May). Why are signed languages easier to learn than spoken languages? Keynote address National Symposium on Sign Language Research and Teaching, Chicago.

Brown, W.T., Jenkins, E. C., Friedman, E., Brooks, J., Wisniewski, K., Raguthu, S., & French, J. (1982). Autism associated with fragile-X syndrome. *Journal of Autism and Developmental Disorders, 12*, 303–308.

Bruner, J. (1975). The ontogenesis of speech acts. *Journal of Child Language, 2*, 1–19.

Burd, L. & Kerbeshian, J. (1987). A North Dakota prevalence study of schizophrenia in childhood. *Journal of the American Academy of Child and Adolescent Psychiatry, 26* (3), 347–350.

Cantwell, D., Baker, L., & Rutter, M. (1978). A comparative study of infantile autism and specific developmental receptive language disorder. IV. Analysis of syntax and language function. *Journal of Child Psychology and Psychiatry, 19*, 351–362.

Carr, E. G. (1979). Teaching autistic children to use sign language: Some research issues. *Journal of Autism and Developmental Disorders, 9*, 345–359.

Chess, S. (1977). Follow-up report on autism in congenital rubella. *Journal of Autism and Childhood Schizophrenia, 7*, 69–81.

Coleman, M. & Gillberg, C. (1985). *The biology of the autistic syndromes.* New York: Praeger.

Coleman, M. & Rimland, B. (1976). Familial autism. In M. Coleman (Ed.), *The autistic syndromes. 175–182.* Amsterdam: North-Holland.

Condon, W. S. (1975). Multiple responses to sound in dysfunctional children. *Journal of Autism and Childhood Schizophrenia, 5*, 37–56.

Creedon, M. P. (1973, March). Language development in nonverbal autistic children using a simultaneous communication system. Paper presented at the Society for Research in Child Development Meeting, Philadelphia.

Crossley, R. & McDonald, A. (1980). *Annie's coming out.* New York: Penguin.

DeLong, G. R., Beau, S. C., & Brown, F. R. (1981). III. Acquired reversible autistic syndrome in acute encephalopatnic illness children. *Archives of Neurology, 38*, 191–194.

DeMyer, M. K. (1979). *Parents and children in autism.* New York: Wiley.

DeMyer, M. K., Hingtgen, J. N., & Jackson, R. K. (1981). Infantile autism reviewed: A decade of research. *Schizophrenia Bulletin, 7*, 388–451.

Deykin, E. Y. & MacMahon, B. (1980). Pregnancy, delivery and neonatal complications among autistic children. *American Journal of Diseases of Children, 134*, 860–864.

Fay, W. & Schuler, A. L. (1980). *Emerging language in autistic children.* Baltimore: University Park Press.

Felicetti, T. (1981). Parents of autistic children: Some notes on a chemical connection. *Milan Therapy, 1* (1), 13–16.

Ferster, C. B. (1961). Positive reinforcement and behavioral deficits of autistic children. *Child Development, 32*, 437–456.

Fish, B. (1977). Neurobiologic antecedents of schizophrenia in children. *Archives of General Psychiatry, 34*, 1297–1313.

Folstein, S. & Rutter, M. (1977). Infantile autism: a genetic study of 21 twin pairs. *Journal of Child Psychology and Psychiatry, 18*, 297–321.

Freeman, B. J., Ritvo, E. R., Guthrie, D., Schroth, P., & Ball, J. (1978). The behavior observation scale for autism: Initial methodology, data analysis, and preliminary findings on 89 children. *Journal of the American Academy of Child Psychiatry, 17*, 576–588.

Frith, V. (1989). A new look at language and communication in autism. *British Journal of Disorders in Communication, 24*, 123–150.

Gillberg, C. (1983). Identical triplets with infantile autism and the fragile-X syndrome. *British Journal of Psychiatry, 143*, 256–360.

Gillberg, C. (1984). Infantile autism and other childhood psychoses in a Swedish urban region. Epidemiological aspects. *Journal of Child Psychology and Psychiatry, 25*, 35–43.

Gillberg, C. (1985). Asperger's syndrome and recurrent psychosis – A case study. *Journal of Autism and Developmental Disorders, 15*, 389–397.

Gillberg, C. (1989). The borderland of autism and Rett syndrome: five case histories to highlight diagnostic difficulties. *Journal of Autism and Developmental Disorders, 19*, 545–559.

Gillberg, C. & Forsell, C. (1984). Childhood psychosis and neurofibromatosis – more than a coincidence? *Journal of Autism and Developmental Disorders, 14*, 1–8.

Gillberg, C. & Svendsen, P. (1983). Childhood psychosis and computed tomographic brain scan findings. *Journal of Autism and Developmental Disorders, 13*, 19–32.

Goetz, L., Schuler, A. L., & Sailor, W. (1979). Teaching functional speech to the severely handicapped: current issues. *Journal of Autism and Developmental Disorders, 9* (4), 325–343.

Goldfarb, W., Braunstein, P., & Lorge, I. (1956). A study of speech patterns in a group of schizophrenic children. *American Journal of Orthopsychiatry, 26*, 544–555.

Goldfine, P. E., McPherson, P. M., Adair, G., Hardesty, V. A., Beauregard, L. Y., & Gordon, B. (1985). Association of fragile-X syndrome with autism. *American Journal of Psychiatry, 142*, 108–110.

Hagerman, R. J. (1989). Chromosomes, genes and autism. In C. Gillberg (Ed.), *Diagnosis and treatment of autism. 105–131.* New York: Plenum.

Hauser, S. L., DeLong, G. R., & Rosman, N. P. (1975). Pneumographic findings in the infantile autism syndrome. *Brain, 98*, 667–688.

Hermelin, B. & O'Connor, N. (1970). *Psychological experiments with autistic children.* Oxford: Pergamon Press.

Hewes, G. H. (1973). Primate communication and the gestural origin of language. *Current Anthropology, 14*, 5–24.

Hier, D. B., Lemay, M., & Rosenberger, P. B. (1979). Autism: Association with reversed cerebral asymmetry. *Neurology, 28*, 348.

Hingtgen, J. & Churchill, D. (1969). Identification of perceptual limitations in mute autistic children. *Archives of General Psychiatry, 21*, 68–71.

Hurlbut, B. I., Inata, B. A., & Green, J. D. (1982). Nonvocal language acquisition in adolescents with severe physical disabilities: Bliss symbol versus iconic stimulus formats. *Journal of Applied Behavior Analysis, 15*, 241–258.

Ingram, D. (1978). Sensori-motor intelligence and language development. In A. Lock (Ed.), *Action, gesture and symbol: The emergence of language. 261–290.* London: Academic Press.

Kanner, L. (1941). *In defense of mothers.* Springfield, Ill.: Charles C. Thomas.

Kanner, L. (1943). Autistic disturbances of affective contact. *Nervous Child, 2*, 217–250.

Kiernan, C. (1983). The use of nonvocal communication techniques with autistic individuals. *Journal of Child Psychology and Psychiatry, 24*, 339–395.

Kolvin, I. (1971). Studies in the childhood psychoses. I. Diagnostic criteria and classification. *British Journal of Psychiatry, 118*, 381–384.

Kolvin, I., Ounsted, C., Humphrey, M., & McNay, A. (1971). II. The phenomenology of childhood psychoses. *British Journal of Psychiatry, 118*, 385–395.

Konstantareas, M. M. (1981). Developing new avenues of communication. In M. M. Konstantareas, E. G. Blackstock, & C. D. Webster (Eds.), *Autism: A primer. 95–106.* Montreal: The Quebec Society for Autistic Children.

Konstantareas, M. M. (1984). Sign language as a communication prosthesis with language-impaired children. *Journal of Autism and Developmental Disorders, 14* (1), 9–25.

Konstantareas, M. M. (1986). Manual language: its relevance to communication acquisition in autistic children. In H. T. A. Whiting & M. G. Wade (Eds.), *Themes in motor development. 159–179.* Dordrecht: Martinus Nijhoff.

Konstantareas, M. M. (1987). Autistic children exposed to simultaneous communication training: A follow-up. *Journal of Autism and Developmental Disorders, 17* (1), 115–131.

Konstantareas, M. M. (1988). Autism: Recent developments in its assessment and treatment. *Psychiatry, 2*, 19–26.

Konstantareas, M. M. (1990). A psychoeducational model for working with families of autistic children. *Journal of Marital and Family Therapy, 16*, 59–70.

Konstantareas, M. M. & Blackman, A. (1978). Assessing preferred communication training modalities in non-verbal autistic children. Paper presented at the Research Symposium of the Canadian Society for Autistic Children, Vancouver, B. C.

Konstantareas, M. M. & Homatidis, S. (1987). Brief report: Ear infections in autistic and normal children. *Journal of Autism and Developmental Disorders, 17* (4), 585–594.

Konstantareas, M. M. & Homatidis, S. (1989). Assessing child symptom severity and stress in parents of autistic children. *Journal of Child Psychology and Psychiatry, 30*, 459–470.

Konstantareas, M. M., Homatidis, S., & Busch, J. (1989). Cognitive, communication, and social differences between autistic boys and girls. *Journal of Applied Developmental Psychology, 10*, 411–424.

Konstantareas, M. M., Hunter, D., & Sloman, L. (1982). Training a blind autistic child to communicate through signs. *Journal of Autism and Developmental Disorders, 12*, 11–11.

Konstantareas, M. M. & Leibovitz, S. F. (1981). Early communication acquisition by autistic children: Signing and mouthing versus signing and speaking. *Sign Language Studies, 31*, 135–154.

Konstantareas, M. M., Oxman, J., & Webster, C. D. (1977). Simultaneous communication with autistic and other severely dysfunctional nonverbal children. *Journal of Communication Disorders, 10*, 267–282.

Konstantareas, M. M., Oxman, J., & Webster, C. D. (1978). Iconicity: Effects on the acquisition of sign language by autistic and other severely dysfunctional children. In P. Siple (Ed.), *Understanding language through sign language research. 213–237*. New York: Academic Press.

Konstantareas, M. M., Webster, C. D., & Oxman, J. (1979). Manual language acquisition and its influence on other areas of functioning in autistic and autistic-like children. *Journal of Child Psychology and Psychiatry, 20*, 337–350.

Layton, T. L. & Stutts, N. (1985). Pragmatic usage by autistic children under different treatment modes. *Australian Journal of Human Communication Disorders, 13*, 127–142.

Lennox, C., Callias, M., & Rutter, M. (1977). Cognitive characteristics of parents. *Journal of Autism and Childhood Schizophrenia, 6*, 163–173.

Lock, A. (1978). The emergence of language. In A. Lock (Ed.), *Action, gesture and symbol: The emergence of language. 3–20*. London: Academic Press.

Lotter, V. (1974). Factors related to outcome in autistic children. *Journal of Autism and Childhood Schizophrenia, 4*, 263–277.

Lovaas, O. I. (1987). Behavioral treatment and normal educational and intellectual functioning in young autistic children. *Journal of Consulting and Clinical Psychology, 55 (1)*, 3–9.

Lovaas, O. I., Berberich, J. P., Perloff, B. F., & Schaeffer, B. (1966). Acquisition of imitative speech by schizophrenic children. *Science, 151*, 705–707.

Lovaas, O. I., Koegel, R., Simmons, J., & Long, J. S. (1973). Some generalization and follow-up measures on autistic children in behaviour therapy. *Journal of Applied Behavior Analysis, 6*, 131–166.

Lovaas, O. I. & Smith, T. (1988). Intensive behavioral treatment for young autistic children. In B. B. Lahey & A. E. Kazdin (Eds.), *Advances in Clinical Psychology, Volume II. 285–324*. New York: Plenum.

Mack, J. E., Webster, C. D., & Goksen, I. (1980). Where are they now and how are they faring: Follow-up of 51 severely handicapped speech-deficient children four years after an operant-based program. In C. D. Webster, M. M. Konstantareas, J. Oxman, & J. E. Mack (Eds.), *Autism: New directions in research and education. 93–106*. New York: Pergamon.

Mahler, M. S. (1952). On child psychoses and schizophrenia: autistic and symbiotic infantile psychoses. *Psychoanalytic Study of the Child, 7*, 286–305.

Oxman, J., Konstantareas, M. M., & Leibovitz, S. F. (1979). Simultaneous communication training and vocal responding in nonverbal autistic and autistic-like children. *International Journal of Rehabilitation Research, 2*, 394–396.

Paccia, J. M. & Curcio, F. (1982). Language processing and forms of immediate echolalia in autistic children. *Journal of Speech and Hearing Research, 25* (1), 42–47.

Parks, S. L. (1983). The assessment of autistic children: A selective review of available instruments. *Journal of Autism and Developmental Disorders, 13*, 255–267.

Paul, R. (1987). Natural history. In D. J. Cohen & A. M. Donnellan (Eds.), *Handbook of autism and pervasive developmental disorders. 121–130*. New York: John Wiley & Sons.

Piaget, J. (1963). *The origins of intelligence in children*. New York: Norton.

Prizant, B. M. (1979). An analysis of the functions of immediate echolalia in autistic children. *Dissertation Abstracts International, 39* (9-B), 4592–4593.

Prizant, B. M. & Duchan, J. F. (1981). The functions of immediate echolalia in autistic children. *Journal of Speech and Hearing Disorders, 46* (3), 241–249.

Prizant, B. & Rydell, P. J. (1984). Analysis of functions of delayed echolalia in autistic children. *Journal of Speech and Hearing Research, 27*, 183–192.

Rett, A. (1966). *Über ein cerebral-atrophisches Syndrom bei Hyperammonämie*. Vienna: Brüder Hollinek.

Ricks, D. M. (1975). Vocal communication in preverbal, normal and autistic children. In: N. O'Connor (Ed.), *Language, cognitive deficits and retardation. 75–80*. London: Butterworths.

Rimland, B. (1964). *Infantile autism*. New York: Appleton-Century-Crofts.

Ritvo, E. R., Spence, M. A., Freeman, B. J., Mason-Brothers, A., & Marazita, M. L. (1985). Evidence for autosomal recessive inheritance in 46 families with multiple incidences of autism. *American Journal of Psychiatry*, *142*, 187–191.

Rumsey, J. M., Duara, R., Grady, C., Rapoport, J. L., Margolin, R. A., Rapoport, S. I., & Cutter, N. R. (1985). Brain metabolism in autism: Resting cerebral glucose utilization as measured with positron emission tomography (PET). *Archives of General Psychiatry*, *15*, 448–457.

Ruttenberg, B. A., Dratman, M. L., Fraknoi, J., & Wenar, C., (1966). An instrument for evaluating autistic children. *Journal of the American Academy of Child Psychiatry*, *5*, 453–478.

Rutter, M. (1978). Diagnosis and definition of childhood autism. *Journal of Autism and Childhood Schizophrenia*, *8*, 139–161.

Rutter, M. & Schopler, E. (1987). Autism and pervasive developmental disorders: Concepts and diagnostic issues. *Journal of Autism and Developmental Disorders*, *17*, 159–186.

Schaeffer, B. (1978). Teaching spontaneous sign language to nonverbal children: Theory and method. *Sign Language Studies*, *21*, 317–352.

Schopler, E. (1970). Parents of psychotic children as scapegoats. *Journal of Contemporary Psychotherapy*, *4*, 17–22.

Schopler, E. (1985). Editorial: Convergence of learning disability, higher level autism and Asperger's syndrome. *Journal of Autism and Developmental Disorders*, *15*, 359–360.

Schopler, E., Reichler, R. J., DeVellis, R. F., & Daly, K. (1980). Toward objective classification of childhood autism: Childhood Autism Rating Scale (CARS). *Journal of Autism and Developmental Disorders*, *10*, 91–103.

Schopler, E., Short, A., & Mesibov, G. (1989). Relation of behavioral treatment to "normal functioning": comment on Lovaas. *Journal of Consulting and Clinical Psychology*, *57*, 162–164.

Schuler, A. L. & Prizant, B. M. (1985). Echolalia. In E. Schopler and G. B. Mesibov (Eds.), *Communication problems in autism. 163–182.* New York: Plenum.

Spitzer, R. L., Endicott, J. E., and Robins, E. (1978). Research diagnostic criteria. *Archives of General Psychiatry*, *35*, 773–782.

Tager-Flusberg, H. (1981). Sentence comprehension in autistic children. *Applied Psycholinguistics*, *2*, 5–24.

Tanguay, P. E., Edwards, R. M., Buchwald, J., Schwafel, J., & Allen, V. (1982). Auditory brainstem evoked responses in autistic children. *Archives of General Psychiatry*, *39*, 174–180.

Torrey, E. F., Hersh, S. P., & McCabe, K. D. (1975). Early childhood psychosis and bleeding during pregnancy. *Journal of Autism and Childhood Schizophrenia*, *5*, 287–297.

Tsai, L., Jacoby, C. G., & Stewart, M. A. (1983). Morphological cerebral asymmetrics in autistic children. *Biological Psychiatry*, *18*, 317–327.

Van Wagenen, L., Jensen, W. R., Worsham, N., & Petersen, B. P. (1985). The use of simultaneous communication to teach difficult verbal discriminations to an autistic and developmentally disabled child. *Australian Journal of Human Communication Disorders*, *13*, 143–152.

Volkmar, G. R. & Cohen, D. J. (1985). The experience of infantile autism: A first person account of Tony W. *Journal of Autism and Developmental Disorders*, *15*, 47–54.

Watson, L. R. (1985). The TEACCH Communication Curriculum. In E. Schopler & G. Mesibov (Eds.), *Communication problems in autism. 187–206.* New York: Plenum.

Webster, C. D., McPherson, H., Sloman, L., Evam, M. A., & Kuchar, E. (1973). Communicating with an autistic boy by gestures. *Journal of Autism and Childhood Schizophrenia*, *3*, 337–346.

Williams, R. S., Hauser, S. L., Purpura, D. P., DeLong, G. R., & Swisher, C. N. (1980). Autism and mental retardation. *Archives of Neurology*, *37*, 749–753.

Wing, L. (1975). Clinical and therapeutic approach to early autistic psychosis in children: The point of view of the research worker. (French) *Revue de Neuropsychiatrie Infantile et d'Hygiene Mentale de l'Enfance*, *23* (12), 803–818.

Wing, L. (1981). Asperger's syndrome: a clinical account. *Psychological Medicine*, *11*, 115–129.

Wing, L. (1989). The diagnosis of autism. In: C. Gillberg (Ed.), *Diagnosis and treatment of autism. 5–22.* New York: Plenum.

Yoder, P. J. & Layton, T. L. (1988). Speech following sign language training in autistic children with minimal verbal language. *Journal of Autism and Developmental Disorders*, *18*, 217–229.

M. Mary Konstantareas, Toronto (Canada)

79. Speech Disordered Children

1. Introduction

Speech disordered children are not a homogenous group. However, they all share the frustration of not being able to express their needs and thoughts intelligibly, often failing academically and being socially isolated. Speech disorders can be classified into a number of subtypes. Perhaps the most important dichotomy is that between articulatory/phonetic disorders and phonological disorders. Articulation disorder refers to an impaired ability to physiologically produce speech sounds. Phonological disorder refers to an impaired ability to use speech sounds linguistically (Grundy 1989).

Every language has a set of phonemes (speech sounds) that are combined in sequences to form words. Phonemes are the minimal linguistic units that differentiate meaning e. g. /r/ and /l/ are two phonemes in English because they distinguish word pairs like *lip* and *rip*. A phoneme is a linguistic abstraction, not an acoustic or articulatory entity. While the acoustic phonetic properties of /l/ in *lip* and *ball* vary greatly, English speakers nevertheless perceive them both as the phoneme /l/. Every language also has constraints governing how phonemes may be combined. The cluster /sv/ is illegal in English, but legal in Swedish. Most phonologically disordered children can articulate all their native language's speech sounds. Their difficulty lies in selecting and combining phonemes into sequences that constitute words in their native language.

While the incidence of developmental phonological disorder is unknown, because surveys failed to differentiate types of speech disorder, estimates range from 3 to 10% of the normal school population (Enderby/Philipp 1986). To these children, who have a specific disorder, must be added those whose speech disorder is part of a more general handicap such as hearing impairment or intellectual disability. One survey of a clinical population found that up to 60% of children referred to community speech pathology clinics are phonologically disordered (Dodd 1982). However, children diagnosed as phonologically disordered vary in terms of: the type of errors made; the detectable underlying deficits in the speech processing chain from perception to production; associated linguistic disorders; the causal and maintenance factors of their disorder; and consequently, their response to different therapeutic approaches.

2. Describing Phonological Errors

The description of mispronunciations, whether those of young children acquiring language or those of speech disordered children, was initially taxonomic or phonemic. Phonetic inventories for speech sounds appropriately produced in particular positions within word structures were listed (Fletcher 1990). Such phoneme repertoires, while valuable for articularly assessment, are limited because they provide no information about how a phoneme might be produced or omitted in a given phonetic context. For example, while a child might produce /s/ correctly in sun, /s/ might be deleted in consonant clusters e. g. [tɒp] for stop. Unlike taxonomic theory, generative phonology viewed phonology as an integral part of the grammar of a language (Chomsky/Halle 1968). One of the concerns of generative phonology is to explain the relationship between abstract mental representation of words and their actual pronunciation. Adult's underlying mental representations are assumed to contain all the phonemic contrasts needed to distinguish one word from another, but the minor non-distinctive (redundant) features, such as aspiration, are specified by phonological output rules (Hyman 1975).

Generative phonological theory provided the impetus for the description of mispronunciations in terms of phonological processes and rules (e. g. Compton 1970). Stampe (1972) defined a phonological process as the mental operation that results in the substitution of a class of sounds or sound sequences presenting a specific difficulty to the speech capacity. In Stampe's view, the child's task in learning phonology is to suppress those processes that do not occur in the adult language. For example, the following productions illustrate the phonological process of cluster reduction: [tɒp] *stop*; [kɪp] *skip*; [sip] *sleep*; [sɪ] *swing*. A taxonomic analysis would conclude that /s/ is in error for 50% of occurrences. A phonological rule analysis would state: in /s/ + consonant clusters, if the consonant is a plosive, then the /s/ deletes, but if the consonant is a continuent, then the consonant deletes. The latter analysis allows prediction of how words not contained in the language sample will be pronounced.

Both taxonomic and phonological rule analyses depend crucially on the accuracy of detailed phonetic transcriptions of disordered speech and this limitation is not always acknowledged (Carney 1979). Instrumental analyses of speech errors have shown that even skilled transcribers cannot perceive all the phonological contrasts marked. For example, Hardcastle/Morgan/Clarke (1987) used electropalatography to demonstrate articulatory differences in the pronunciation of 'heard' [t] for /ʃ/ in [tip] *sheep* as opposed to [t] in *tent*. The role of instrumentation in the description of phonological errors will obviously grow. However, our current understanding of speech errors is derived from observers' transcriptions of their perceptions.

2.1. Developmental Patterns

Most children begin to use recognisable words at about 12 months of age. By 18 months they often have a vocabulary of 50 words. The phonology of the first 50 words is often inconsistent and in some instances children render better (i. e. more adult-like) pronunciations of particular words than they do when they are slightly older and have larger vocabularies (Leopold 1947). For example, one child produced *Gladys* perfectly at 12 months. This may have been an example of protolanguage (Halliday 1975) because the word was used to elicit attention whether or not Gladys was within auditory range. However, once the child had a larger vocabulary *Gladys* was pronounced as [dædɪs], conforming to current phonological processes (Dodd 1975).

In one early study of normal development Smith (1973) described the phonological acquisition of his son. He assumed that the child's underlying representation of words corresponded directly to the adult surface form and postulated realisation rules that mapped these forms to the child's own surface (output) forms. Smith later revised his model to include a perceptual filter to account for any miscoding of words. The realisation rules implemented major strategies:

(1) consonant cluster reduction e. g. /l, r, w, j/ delete postconsonantally as in [bu] *blue*; /s/ deletes preconsonantally as in [pun] *spoon*.
(2) consonant harmony or assimilation e. g. [lɛloʊ] *yellow*.
(3) systemic simplification e. g. fricatives and affricates are realised as plosives as in [tɪp] for *ship* and *chip*.

The number and type of realisation rules implementing these strategies varies according to the level of phonological development which is loosely related to chronological age, and level of cognitive development (Macken/Ferguson 1983). Individual children can abstract idiosyncratic rules that are not common in normal development e. g. the s + consonant cluster rule described earlier. However, most children share similar sets of phonological rules and apply them consistently (Aitchison 1987) and similar normal developmental speech error phenomena have been observed across languages, e. g. Magnusson (1983) observed cluster reduction in Swedish. Children usually attain a phonological system that is consistent with that of the adults in their environment between 4 and 6 years of age.

2.2. Phonological Disorder

Phonologically disordered speech has been described in terms of features, phoneme repertoires, rule statements contrastive analyses and/or phonological processes (Fletcher 1990). Reviews of such error data from children diagnosed as phonologically disordered have led to a range of conclusions about what distinguishes disorder from normal developmental errors. Some reviewers hold that disorder merely reflects varieties of delayed development. Fletcher's (1990) review concluded that disorder arises when normal phonological development becomes delayed or 'frozen' relative to other aspects of language development. Ingram (1976) asserts that phonological disorder occurs when normal developmental processes fail to be eliminated, resulting in early processes co-existing with later ones. Others argue that disorder reflects severity in terms of the number of errors made, rather than the type of errors made (Shriberg/Kwiatowski/Best et al. 1986). These three conclusions differ in detail but have as their basic tenet that the types of phonological processes used by the population diagnosed as disordered can also be observed in the normal population.

Other researchers argue that phonologically disordered children use processes that are different from those observed during normal development. Leonard (1985) described a variety of unusual and subtle phonological behaviours associated with disorder. These included:

(1) the replacement of speech sounds that occur early in development by speech sounds that are usually acquired later e. g. substitution of [s] for all word final consonants except /p, b, and m/.
(2) additions to adult surface forms e. g. addition of syllabic nasals to word final voiced plosives: [badn] *bad*, [bɪgn] *big*.
(3) use of sounds or suprasegmental features not occuring in the child's native language e. g. marking consonant clusters with a bilabial fricative [ßes] dress (Leahy/Dodd 1987); marking plurality suprasegmentally by rising tone, higher fundamental frequency, longer duration and higher intensity. Another frequently observed characteristic of phonologically disordered children's errors is strict word structure constraints (Dunn/Davis 1983). For example, most children delete some consonants word finally during normal development, but some disordered children may mark most word final consonants with a glottal stop (Leahy/Dodd, 1987).

There are also phonologically disordered children whose speech appears to be characterised by inconsistent errors. Speech pathologists often regard inconsistency as one indicator of developmental dyspraxia, a motor programming deficit rather than a linguistically based problem (Hall 1989). Alternatively, apparently inconsistent phonological behaviour may, on closer inspection of phonetic context, be consistent. Leonard (1985) reviews some interesting examples. One 4.0 year old child demonstrated a constraint that prevented nasals and plosives from occuring in the same word e. g. [pedi and meni] *penny* (Willbrand/Kleinschmidt, 1978). Grunwell (1981) reported a 6:3 year old child who used an extremely complex rule: all adult forms containing stressed syllable initial fricatives, liquids, glides, bilabial plosives or nasals that were followed by a front vowel were realised with an apical place of articulation e. g. [bu] *blue*, but [di] *bee*, [f] *four*, but [θit] *feet*.

However, there are also reports of children whose speech is fluent but characterised by inconsistent errors both within and between words and who show no associated dyspraxic groping, repetition or soft neurological signs (Spencer 1986). The speech of children with Down Syndrome is often described as inconsistent, with children producing a variety of pronunciations for many words e. g. [h t, ti, si, ʃi] *horse* in one 15 minute language sample (Dodd/Leahy 1989). As these examples show, vowel errors may co-occur with inconsistency of consonant production (Murdoch/Porter/Younger/Ozanne 1984). While little is known about the acquisition of vowels by children developing phonology normally, Reynolds (1990) concluded that most children over 24 months of age make few vowel errors. More detailed rule analysis of apparently inconsistent errors might reveal that some children use complex, bizzare/phonological rules. Alternatively, those making inconsistent errors may constitute a distinct sub-group of phonologically disordered children.

3. Associated Underlying Deficits

Textbook overviews of articulation and phonological disorders invariably have a section where they review research which has sought correlations between speech related abilities (e. g. speech sound discrimination, motor skills) and disorder. Reviewers (e. g. Sommers 1984; Winitz 1969) usually stress that conflicting findings are the rule rather than the exception. There are two major factors contributing to these contradictory findings. Researchers employ widely differing methodologies to assess the same skills. For example, when Bountress (1984) compared the results of a single group of non-communication disordered children on three different standard assessment of speech perception, he found statistically significant differences in performance between the tests. The other, perhaps more important, factor is that many studies have assumed, incorrectly, that speech disordered children are a homogenous population. Thus different populations of speech disordered children have varied in their performance on identical tasks.

Multivariate analyses of speech disordered children indicate that subgroups exist: some perform within normal limits on measures of perception, cognition or language, and some do not (McNutt/Hamayan 1982). The need to classify subgroups of phonological disorder is now generally agreed. What remains controversial is the criteria that should be used. Grundy (1989) suggests a psycho-linguistic perspective: phonological disorder may result from the impaired operation of mental processes serving "either the productive, or the perceptive, or the organizational mechanisms of speech" (Grundy 1989, 257). However, no information is given concerning the phonological behaviours indicating the site of these three deficits.

Research studies investigating classification systems based on linguistic typologies have yielded little information. Both Arndt/Shelton/Johnson/Furr (1977) and Winitz/Darley (1980) tested large groups of children seeking associations between speech error patterns and independent variables such as measures of language, motor skills, auditory discrimination and oral stereognosis. No reliable associations were found. One plausible explanation for this failure to find any relationship between types of errors and other speech related abilities is that the linguistic typologies employed focused on speech sounds rather than phonological processes, failing to distinguish between articulatory and phonological disorders. In the discussion above (2.2) three categories of error types emerged in the description of what constituted a phonological disorder: delay (Fletcher 1990); consistent but unusual (non-developmental) phonological errors (Leonard 1985); and inconsistent phonological errors (Dodd/Leahy 1989). Perhaps these three categories may reflect the nature of the deficits underlying subgroups of phonologically disordered children.

Dodd/Leahy/Hambly (1989) tested this possibility by comparing the performance of three groups of subjects, selected according to the nature of their surface phonological errors: children using normal developmental processes that were inappropriate for their chronological age – 'delayed'; children using some consistent but nondevelopmental processes – 'deviant consistent'; and children who exhibited many apparently non-rule-governed errors – 'deviant inconsistent'. In one experiment their production errors in imitation, picture naming and spontaneous speech were evaluated. In imitation there is no need to access internal lexical representations, picture naming requires accessing the internal representation as well as generating a production plan, and spontaneous speech requires planning long utterances phonologically and syntactically and involves communicative intent. The results distinguished between the three subgroups of phonologically disordered children, providing an initial validation of the classification. The delayed group made fewer errors than the other two groups but had stable performance across the three production tasks. The inconsistent group were better in imitation than in elicited or spontaneous production. The deviant consistent group's errors increased with the complexity of the production task, indicating that the domain of some phonological processes extends across words e. g. use of one consonant to mark all consonants in an utterance (Leahy/Dodd 1987).

Other experiments comparing these three subgroups of phonological disorder have revealed that the deviant consistent group performs poorly on tasks involving detection of phonological legality of spoken nonsense words, recognition of their own phonological forms (Dodd/Leahy/Hambly 1989) and awareness of alliteration and rhyme (Brierly 1987). These findings suggest that the use of consistent but unusual phonological rules might be attributed to an impaired ability to abstract knowledge from the mental lexicon about the nature of the phonological system to be acquired. Leonard (1985) views children as active learners of their phonological system, who seek to mark, in their speech output, the contrasts between words they perceive. Consistent but bizarre solutions to the problem of marking differences might result from selecting the wrong parameters of the perceived speech signal as salient in their native phonology. If this were so, these children's deficit could be labelled cognitive and lie in Grundy's (1989) organisational level of the speech chain.

Phonologically disordered children who make inconsistent errors appear to have intact knowledge of their phonological system, not differing from controls on tasks distinguishing the deviant consistent sub-group (Dodd/Leahy/Hambly 1989; Brierly 1987). However, their performance on a series of fine motor tasks suggests that their deficit may lie in motor programming (Bradford 1990). The three subgroups of phonologically disordered children plus a matched normal control group were assessed on four tasks measuring: repetitive use of a simple motor programme (pegboard task); motor accuracy involving both perceptual and motor programming abilities; kinæsthetic memory; and, learning to pronounce novel words. The kinæsthetic memory task was the only one that failed to discriminate the inconsistent subjects from the other subgroups of phonological disorder and the normally speaking controls. These findings are in agreement with those of Sommers (1984) who concluded that the severity of speech disorder was associated with poor fine motor skill – children with inconsistent errors are perceived as particularly unintelligible. A deficit at the level of speech production (Grundy 1989), specifically motor planning, might, then, account for children who produce inconsistent phonological errors.

Children whose errors are due to the use of normal developmental processes that are inappropriate for their chronological age did not appear to have any specific deficit on the tasks that discriminated the two other subgroups of phonological disorder. This is not surprising, since they are following the normal course of development, albeit slowly. The factors underlying their delay may be more general: impoverished language learning environment, slower neurological maturation, or general cognitive delay (Powers 1971). This point leads to the question of the aetiology underlying the deficits in the speech processing chain that have been identified. Localising subgroups of phonologically disordered children's deficit is useful for planning assessment and intervention. However, it is also important to consider the origin of the deficits.

4. Causal Factors

Most speech disorders are considered to be 'functional', i. e. no established cause (Sommers 1984). However, a great deal of research effort has been spent seeking correlations between speech disorders and a wide range of factors e. g. family history of communication disorder, neurological assessment, sensory deficit and socio-economic status. This reflects the assumptions that causal factors exist and are clinically relevant. For example, Robinson's (1987) survey found that disordered children frequently had a family history of communication disorder, indicating a genetic component; and, that a range of plausible medical 'causes' (e. g. neurological illness such as meningitis, low birth weight) were recorded for a quarter of the children studied. Such diagnoses can be associated with persistent neurological deficits, although this is not invariably so. Two other frequently mentioned causes of phonological disorder are fluctuating hearing loss due to otitis media (Dickson 1984), and psychopathology (Prizant/Auder/Burke et al. 1990). A number of more controversial proposed causes of phonological disorders are discussed below.

4.1. Familial Phonological Disorders

Parents of phonologically disordered children often report other communication disordered family members who have received remediation for impaired speech or literacy. Reports of the number of children who have a family member who is also communication disordered vary between 24% (Ingram 1959) and 45.9% (Neils/Aram 1986). These studies are limited by their inclusion of a wide range of types of communication disorder. However, Neils/Aram (1986) found that 'articulation disorder' was the most common type of communication disorder reported for relatives (54.9%). More recent studies have established a familial basis for some phonologically disordered children (Lewis 1990). While description of the mode of inheritance awaits further research, Lewis' (1990) analysis suggests "either an autosomal dominant or multifactorial-polygenic mode of transmission [with] a sex-specific threshold for expression" (Lewis 1990, 168).

4.2 Language Learning Environment

Phonological acquisition is obviously dependent upon adequate exposure to the language to be learned. Current theory holds that language acquisition is the result of the process of social interaction (Halliday 1975). These interactions occur around shared activities that are appropriate for the child's focus of attention and interest in a natural situation. The adult provides language models and feedback about the child's speech. Language use is thus taught alongside form (phonology, grammar and vocabulatory). There are two major ways in which this crucial language learning experience can be disrupted.

(1) Communication Disordered Caretakers
Children acquire the language in which they are immersed. If their language model is disordered, it is likely that they will learn that disorder. As examples: many children who lisp also have mothers who lisp (Blanton 1936); hearing children of hearing impaired parents are at risk of communication impairment, particularly phonological disorder

(Schiff/Ventry 1976). The long-term effects of initial exposure to disordered language depend upon other available language learning experiences and intervention.

(2) Inadequate Exposure to Language

Individual differences between children's language learning potential preclude definition of what constitutes 'adequate exposure' for language acquisition. Nevertheless some language learning environments are associated with delayed or disordered acquisition of phonology. The one that has received most research attention is that of multiple birth children (MBC). They have been reported to have delayed communication development compared to singletons in terms of age of speech onset, syntax, vocabulary, pragmatics and phonology (Savic 1980). Their unintelligibility has led some authors to conclude that twins often share an autonomous language (Luria/Yudovich 1959). An opposing view is that twin's unintelligible speech is unintentionally disordered rather than a deliberately autonomous language (Savic 1980). Rather, their disordered speech may result from their language learning environment. Three-way communicative interactions (one adult and two children) are their norm for adult-child interactions, reducing the amount of adult modelling and feedback (Savic 1980). Further, MBC spend more time interacting with another child, reducing their exposure to adult language. A similar language learning environment can exist for siblings close in age or for children in day care. Nevertheless, many children whose primary communication partners are children of a similar age evidence normal phonological development. It would, then, be premature to draw conclusions about the contribution of the language learning environment to the acquisition of disordered phonology.

4.3. Auditory Sensation and Perception

It is a common assumption that children make speech errors because they misperceive adult speech. The misperception may be attributed to hearing impairment or an impaired ability to process auditory information. In either case, a child may store incorrect or incomplete mental representations of words which in turn give rise to spoken errors. There is no doubt that permanent hearing impairment affects speech development. Even a mild bilateral hearing loss across the speech frequency range has serious implications for speech and language development; and, children with a specific high frequency hearing loss have particular difficulties with fricatives. A more controversial causal relationship is that between phonological disorder and fluctuating hearing loss.

Many phonologically disordered children have a history of otitis media which may be associated with periods of impaired hearing. There are a number of plausible explanations that may account for this relationship:

– During episodes of hearing loss, children are likely to misperceive words. Mental representations of these misperceived words may not be corrected when normal hearing is restored (Katz/Illmer 1972).
– Children who experience frequent episodes of impaired hearing may learn to rely primarily on vision for information about the world and not attend to auditory information, even when their hearing is unimpaired (Katz/Illmer 1972).
– During the first year of life infants learn to discriminate between the phonemes of their native language. Even if no further episodes of hearing loss occur after infancy, their knowledge of their native language's system of phonemic contrasts may be impaired (Kirkwood/Kirkwood 1983).

However, the evidence concerning a causal link between episodes of otitis media and phonological disorders is far from clear-cut. Most children (75%) experience at least one episode of otitis media with effusion (OME), and well over ten percent will have recurrent episodes (Teele/Klein/Rosner 1984). Not all these children become communication disordered. While retrospective studies have consistently shown a relationship between OME and communication disorder, they are flawed because they fail to document the number and length of episodes of OME. Prospective studies of infants enrolled in early infancy should be more reliable since hearing status can be monitored throughout development. However, recent prospective studies report conflicting evidence. One study (Teele/Klein/Rosner 1984) suggested that the receptive language ability of high socio-economic status children declined with increasing number of episodes of OME, but this relationship did not hold for children from low socio-economic backgrounds. In the Wright/Sell/McConnell et al. (1988) study children's receptive and expressive language scores were considered in relation to three variables: age of first OME episode; number of episodes; and presence of hearing loss at time of testing. None of these variables significantly affected speech and language performance. The results of these studies suggest that while fluctuating hearing loss may be an important contributing factor to phonological disorder, it is rarely a sole cause.

In the absence of any sensory impairment, central auditory processing impairments are often cited as a major cause of phonological disorders (Sommers 1984; Tallal 1987). Early researchers stressed the need for assessing speech discrimination ability and 'ear training' in therapy. More recently, sophisticated assessment procedures for identifying auditory processing deficits have been devised (Willeford 1985). Katz (1983) reviewed the literature concerned with the relationship between speech disorders and phonemic synthesis (the ability to 'blend' distorted speech sounds into words). He found that children who made speech errors performed more poorly than age matched controls. However, children identified as having such a central auditory processing problem are most often described as having a wide range of impairments including receptive language, attention and memory as well as speech (Katz 1983). There is, then, little evidence for central auditory processing deficits being a cause of phonological disorders in the absence of more general learning disability.

The literature reviewed in this section leads to the conclusion that in most cases it is impossible to attribute phonological disorder to a single causal factor (see also Robinson 1987). For example, one case (Leahy/Dodd 1987) had a family history of phonological disorder, but had also suffered a series of ear infections in early childhood that may have been associated with fluctuating hearing loss. This little girl also had a highly verbal older sibling who 'interpreted' for her, contributing to the maintenance of her disorder. Perhaps a predisposition to phonological disorder can be inherited, but its emergence may be dependent on co-occurence of certain medical or language learning environment conditions. A phonologically disordered child's assessment should, then, include not only a description of the characteristics of the linguistic disorder, but also case history and psychosocial information.

5. Psycholinguistic Implications of Phonological Disorder

5.1. One Lexicon or Two?

One controversial issue in the study of children's speech errors is the number and nature of their mental representations of a word. Since phonologically disordered children have been shown to perceive differences between minimally paired words that they cannot produce, a number of researchers have proposed that children have two lexicons: one serving word recognition and the other word production (e. g. Chiat 1983). Other researchers claim that only one lexicon need be posited (e. g. Hughes 1983).

Analyses of phonologically disordered children's errors led Spencer (1986) to support a modified version of Dinnsen/Elbert/Weismer's (1981) proposal that there are two main categories of disorder, distinguished according to the nature of their output representations of words. Both groups have largely intact input representations. One group have output representations that underspecify phonemes resulting in children's surface errors. For example, *sandal* might be represented as /fricative + ændəl/ allowing variable surface realisations such as [fændəl], θændəl or sændəl]. A second group's output representations are fully specified but simpler than the adult forms e. g. /tænəl/ for *candle* resulting in consistent errors.

However, the relationship between word's underlying representations and their surface realisations is difficult to determine (Hughes, 1983). For example, one child deleted or realised consonants variably according to phonetic context – [d o:] for *dog* but [d ogi] for *doggie* (Weismer/Dinnsen/Elbert 1981). These data suggest that children's surface errors do not always reflect their 'output' lexicon's specifications for words. Rather, output constraints may be imposed subsequent to lexical retrieval of words. In the case of the previous example *dog* would be fully specified in the lexicon but a phonological process deleting word-final plosives would result in [dɒ], whereas intervocalic /g/ in [dɒgi] would be realised since it would not be constrained by the process governing word-final consonants. This hypothesis is consistent with data from treatment efficacy studies focusing on phonological processes showing generalisation from taught to untaught lexical items. For example, treatment aimed at teaching a child to produce word-final /p/ and /k/ generalised to all appropriate word final consonants (Leahy/Dodd 1987). Such evidence casts doubt on the need to posit two entirely different lexicons.

5.2. Relationships Between Speaking, Spelling and Reading

Children who have a current spoken phonological disorder are also reported to have a spelling disorder (Ham 1958). However, the spoken error is not reflected by the spelling error i. e. children don't spell words the way they say them. A correctly pronounced word is just as likely to be spelled incorrectly as a mispronounced word (Robinson/Beresford/Dodd 1982). The words most frequently spelled in error by phonologically disordered children are those where a spelling rule needs to be applied e. g. /k/ is represented orthographically by *ck* after a short vowel as in *back* but by *ke* after a long vowel as in *bake*. In contrast, words that have a strict one sound-one letter correspondence (e. g. adopt) and words that have unusual spellings (e. g. ocean) are spelled equally well by phonologically disordered children and reading age matched controls (Dodd/Cockerill 1985). In this study the most common error type for the non-speech disordered group was plausible misspellings e. g. sittee for *city*, whereas the phonologically disordered children most often produced errors that contained illegal sequences of letters e. g. zroor for *zebra*. Thus, while there is no one-to-one correspondence between speech and spelling errors, the two disorders are linked in that both reflect an impaired ability to derive and use phonological and orthographic rules.

There is also a link between reading disability and impaired phonological processing. Reading disabled children perform poorly on tasks assessing phonological awareness (Lencher/Gerber/Routh 1990). Tests of preschool children's phonological awareness are predictive of their later success in acquiring literacy (Bradley/Bryant 1983) and speech disordered children are reported to perform poorly on standard reading tests (Snowling/Stackhouse/Rack 1986). Recent evidence suggests that if either speech, spelling or reading is identified as being disordered, then some impairment also exists for the other two abilities (Dodd/Sprainger/Oerlemans 1989). These results are consistent with the hypothesis that a central impairment in processing phonological information leads to problems in speaking, spelling and reading. Identification of patterns of disorder across the three skills would provide valuable information for the construction of psycholinguistic models of children's processing of verbal information as well as providing insights into the nature of phonological disorder.

Authors note: My thanks to V. Duggirala, A. Ozanne and P. McCormack for their valuable insights. The NHMRC provided financial assistance.

6. References

Aitchison, J. (1987). *Words in the Mind.* Oxford: Basil Blackwell.

Arndt, W., Shelton, R., Johnson, A., & Furr, M. (1977). Identification and description of homogenous subgroups within a sample of misarticulating children. *Journal of Speech and Hearing Research, 20*, 263–292.

Blanton, S. (1936). Helping the speech handicapped school student. *Journal of Speech Disorders, 1*, 97–100.

Bountress, N. (1984). A second look at tests of speech sound discrimination. *Journal of Communication Disorders*, 17, 349–357.

Bradford, A. (1990). *The Motor Planning Skills of Subgroups of Speech Disordered Children.* Unpublished honours thesis, University of Queensland, Brisbane.

Bradley, L. & Bryant, P. (1983). Categorizing sounds and learning to read: a causal connection. *Nature, 301*, 419–421.

Brierly, A. (1987). *Phonological Disorder in Children.* Unpublished honour thesis, Macquarie University, Sydney.

Carney, E. (1979). Inappropriate abstraction in speech assessment procedures. *British Journal of Disorders of Communication, 14*, 123–135.

Chiat, S. (1983). Why *Mikey's* right and *my key's* wrong: the significance of stress and word boundaries in a child's output system. *Cognition, 14*, 275–300.

Chomsky, N. & Halle, M. (1968). *The Sound Pattern of English.* New York: Harper & Row.

Compton, A. (1979). Generative studies of children's phonological disorders. *Journal of Speech and Hearing Disorders, 35*, 315–340.

Dickson, S. (1984). Diagnostic principles and procedures. In S. Dickson (Ed.), *Communication Disorders: Remedial Principles and Practices. 2–45.* Glenview IL, Scott Foresman.

Dinnsen, D., Elbert, M., & Weismer, G. (1981). Some typological properties of functional misarticulating systems. In W. Dressler (Ed.), *Phonologica*

1980. 83–88. Innsbruck: Innsbrucker Beiträge zur Sprachwissenschaft.

Dodd, B. (1975). *The Acquisition of Phonological Skills in Normal, Severely Subnormal and Deaf Children.* Unpublished Ph. D. Thesis, London University.

Dodd, B. (1982). Sub-groups of phonologically disordered children. *Paper to Neurolinguistics and Speech Pathology Conference*, University of Newcastle upon Tyne, U. K.

Dodd, B. & Cockerill, H. (1985). Phonologically disordered children's spelling abilities. In J. E. Clarke (Ed.), *Beiträge zur Phonetik und Linguistik, 48. 405–415.* Hamburg: Springer-Verlag.

Dodd, B. & Leahy, J. (1989). Phonological disorders and mental handicap. In M. Beveridge, G. Conti-Ramsden, & I. Leudar (Eds.), *Language and Communication in Mentally Handicapped People. 33–56.* London: Chapman & Hall.

Dodd, B., Leahy, J., & Hambly, G. (1989). Phonological disorders in children: Underlying cognitive deficits. *British Journal of Developmental Psychology, 7*, 55–71.

Dodd, B., Sprainger, N., & Oerlemans, M. (1989). The phonological skills of spelling disordered children. *Reading and Writing, 1*, 333–335.

Dunn, C. & Davis, B. (1983). Phonological process occurrence in phonologically disordered children. *Applied Psycholinguistics, 4*, 187–207.

Enderby, P. & Philipp, R. (1986). Speech and language handicap: towards knowing the size of the problem. *British Journal of Disorders of Communication, 21*, 151–165.

Fletcher, P. (1990). The breakdown of language: Language pathology and therapy. In N. Collinge (Ed.), *Encyclopædia of Language. 424–457.* London: Rutledge.

Grundy, K. (1989). Developmental speech disorders. In K. Grundy (Ed.), *Linguistics in Clinical Practice. 3–25.* London: Taylor & Francis.

Grunwell, P. (1981). *The Nature of Phonological Disability in Children.* London: Academic Press.

Hall, P. K. (1989). The occurrence of developmental apraxia of speech in a mild articulation disorder: A case study. *Journal of Communication Disorders, 22*, 265–276.

Halliday, M. (1975). *Learning How to mean: Explorations in the Development of Language.* New York: Dover.

Ham, R. (1958). Relationship between misspelling and misarticulation. *Journal of Speech and Hearing Disorders, 23*, 294–297.

Hardcastle, W., Morgan, B. R., & Clarke, C. (1987). An instrumental phonetic study of lingual activity in articulation-disordered children. *Journal of Speech and Hearing Research 30*, 171–184.

Hughes, R. (1983). The internal representation of word final phonemes in phonologically disordered children. *British Journal of Disorders of Communication, 18*, 78–88.

Hyman, L. M. (1975). *Phonology: Theory and Analysis.* New York: Holt, Rinehart & Winston.

Ingram, D. (1976). *Phonological Disability in Children.* London: Edward Arnold.

Ingram, T. S. (1959). Specific developmental disorders of speech in childhood. *Brain, 82*, 450–467.

Katz, J. (1983). Phonemic synthesis. In E. Lasky & J. Katz (Eds.), *Central Auditory Processing Disorders. 269–296.* Baltimore: University Park Press.

Katz, J. & Illmer, R. (1972). Auditory perception of children with learning disability. In J. Katz (Ed.), *Handbook of Clinical Audiology. 540–563.* Baltimore: Williams & Wilkins.

Kirkwood, C. R. & Kirkwood, M. E. (1983). Otitis media and learning disabilities: The case for a causal relationship. *The Journal of Family Practice, 17*, 219–227.

Leahy, J. & Dodd, B. (1987). The development of disordered phonology: A case study. *Language and Cognitive Processes, 2*, 115–132.

Lencher, O., Gerber, M., & Routh, D. (1990). Phonological awareness tasks as predictors of decoding ability: Beyond segmentation. *Journal of Learning Difficulties, 23*, 240–246.

Leonard, L. (1985). Unusual and subtle phonological behaviour in the speech of phonologically disordered children. *Journal of Speech and Hearing Disorders, 50*, 4–13.

Leopold, W. (1947). *Speech Development of a Bilingual Child: A Linguist's Record. Vol. 2.* Evanston IL: Northwestern University Press.

Lewis, B. (1990). Familial disorders: Four pedigrees. *Journal of Speech and Hearing Disorders, 55*, 160–170.

Luria, A. & Yudovich, F. (1959). *Speech and the Development of Mental Processes in the Child.* London: Staples.

Macken, M., & Ferguson, C. (1983). Cognitive aspects of phonological development: Model, evidence, and issues. In K. Nelson (Ed.), *Children's language: Vol. 4.* 255–282. Hillsdale NJ.: Erlbaum.

Magnusson, E. (1983). *The Phonology of Language Disordered Children: Production, Perception and Awareness.* Lund: CWK Gleerup.

McNutt, J. & Hamayan, E. (1982). Subgroups of older children with articulation disorder. In R. Daniloff (Ed.), *Position Papers in Speech, Hearing and Language. 51–70.* Baltimore: College Hill.

Murdoch, B. E., Porter, S., Younger, R. & Ozanne, A. (1984). Behaviours identified by South Australian clinicians as differentially diagnostic of developmental articulatory apraxia. *Australian Journal of Human Communication Disorders, 12*, 55–70.

Neils, J. & Aram, D. (1986). Family history of children with developmental language disorders. *Perceptual and Motor Skills, 63*, 655–658.

Powers, M. (1971). Functional disorders of articulation: Symptomatology and etiology. In L. Travis (Ed.), *Handbook of Speech Pathology and Audiology. 837–876.* Englewood Cliffs NJ: Prentice Hall.

Prizant, B., Audet, L., Burke, G., Hummel, L., Maher, S., & Theodore, G. (1990). Communication disorders and emotional stroke behavioural disorders in children and adolescents. *Journal of Speech and Hearing Disorders, 55,* 179–192.

Reynolds, J. (1990). Abnormal vowel patterns in phonological disorder. *British Journal of Disorders of Communication, 25,* 115–148.

Robinson, R. (1987). Introduction and overview. In *Proceedings of the First International Symposium on Specific Speech and Language Disorders in Children.* 1–19. London: AFASIC.

Robinson, P., Beresford, R. & Dodd, B. (1982). Spelling errors made by phonologically disordered children. *Spelling Progress Bulletin, 12,* 19–20.

Savic, S. (1980). *How Twins Learn to Talk.* London: Academic Press.

Schiff, N. & Ventry, I. (1976). Communication problems in hearing children of deaf parents. *Journal of Speech and Hearing Disorders, 41,* 348–358.

Shriberg, L., Kwiatowski, J., Best, S., Hengst, J. & Terselie-Weber, B. (1986). Characteristics of children with phonologic disorders of unknown origin. *Journal of Speech and Hearing Disorders, 51,* 140–161.

Smith, N. (1973). *The Acquisition of Phonology.* Cambridge: The University Press.

Snowling, M., Stackhouse, J., & Rack, J. (1986). Phonological dyslexia and dysgraphia: A developmental analysis. *Cognitive Neuropsychology, 3,* 309–339.

Sommers, R. (1984). Nature and remediation of functional articulation and phonological disorders. In S. Dickson (Ed.), *Communication Disorders: Remedial Principles and Practices. 118–172.* Glenview IL: Scott Foresman & Co.

Spencer, A. (1986). Towards a theory of phonological development. *Lingua, 68,* 3–38.

Stampe, D. (1972). *A Dissertation on Natural Phonology.* New York: Garland.

Tallal, P. (1987). The neuropsychology of developmental language disorders. In *Proceedings of the First Symposium on Specific Speech and Language Disorders in Children.* 36–47. London: AFASIC.

Teele, D. W., Klein, J. D., & Rosner, B. A. (1984). Otitis media with effusion during the first three years of life and development of speech and language. *Pediatrics, 74,* 282–287.

Weismer, G., Dinnsen, D. A., & Elbert, M. (1981). A study of the voicing distinction associated with omitted word-final stops. *Journal of Speech and Hearing Disorders, 46,* 320–327.

Willbrand, M. & Kleinschmidt, M. (1978). Substitution patterns and word constraints. *Language, Speech and Hearing Services in Schools, 9,* 155–161.

Willeford, J. (1985). Assessment of central auditory disorders in children. In M. Pinheiro & F. Musiek (Eds.), *Assessment of Central Auditory Dysfunction. 239–255.* Baltimore: Williams & Wilkins.

Winitz, H. (1969). *Articulatory Acquisition and Behaviour.* New York: Meredith.

Winitz, H. & Darley, F. (1980). Speech production. In F. Lassman, R. Fisch, D. Vetter, P. LaBenz, & E. LaBenz (Eds.), *Early Correlates of Speech, Language and Hearing.* 232–265. Littleton, MA: PSG Publications.

Wright, P., Sell, S., McConell, K., Sutton, A., Thompson, J., Vaughan, W., & Bess, F. (1988). Impact of recurrent otitis media on middle ear function, hearing, and language. *Journal of Pediatrics 113,* 581–586.

Barbara Dodd, St. Lucia, Queensland (Australia)

80. Developmental Dysarthria

1. Introduction

Developmental dysarthria, a disorder of speech associated with neuropathologic conditions occurring in children, is a relatively new term in the communication disorders literature, although the disorder has existed for a very long time. Historically the term 'dysarthria' has referred to acquired neuromotor speech deficits seen in adults and has only recently come into use to describe speech disorders of children associated with disturbances in muscular control of the speech mechanism, such as is seen in cerebral palsy. Because 'developmental' neurogenic speech disorders result from insult or lesion to the brain occurring prior to or during the course of speech development, developmental and acquired speech disorders are not directly comparable. Lesions to the developing brain disrupt systems as they develop, whereas, lesions to the adult brain disrupt systems that are fully developed anatomically and physiologically.

What is known today as cerebral palsy was first described by Little in the 'Lancet' in the 19th century (Little 1843) and it was labelled Little's disease. Little's description indicated that children with the disease had neuromotor involvement of the upper and/or lower extremities and that some had involvement of the speech musculature. Later writers noted variability in the type of motor problems seen. For example, hypertonic muscles were seen in some children, whereas flaccidity and/or tremors were present in others. By the late 1800s and early 1900s, there was some agreement that several types of cerebral palsy existed, and, not long after that, classification systems began to appear in the literature (Minear 1956; Phelps 1956). For example, Minear (1956) summarized the results of a survey of the American Academy of Cerebral Palsy, indicating that at least eight different types of cerebral palsy were being observed at the time. These included (1) spasticity, (2) athetosis, (3) rigidity, (4) ataxia, (5) tremor, (6) atonia, (7) mixed, and (8) unclassifiable cerebral palsy.

Recognizing the variety of neurologic problems associated with cerebral palsy, Crothers/Paine (1959) streamlined classifications into three subtypes including spasticity, involuntary motion disorders (dyskinesia, extrapyramidal cerebral palsy), and mixed. They further differentiated spastic patients based on the topographic distribution of neuromotor signs (e. g., hemiplegia, paraplegia). These classifications of cerebral palsy continue to be used at the present time (Hardy 1983), and they remain problematic because patients within each classification are heterogeneous.

Given this heterogeneity, it is not surprising that speech disorders or dysarthrias seen in children vary as they do in adults. That is, Darley/Aronson/Brown (1969 a; 1969 b) reported the existence of several types of dysarthria, in adults, correlated with underlying neuropathology. Although the types of dysarthria seen in children with neurologic disorders have not been studied extensively, clinicians can predict with some reliability whether or not the speech musculature will be involved based on information concerning the type of cerebral palsy and the motor systems involved based on information concerning the type of cerebral palsy and the motor systems involved. For example, in spastic quadriplegia involving the upper and lower extremities of the body, speech is more likely to be involved than in spastic diplegia involving only the lower extremities because of the topographic arrangement of cortical motor control. However, the pattern of speech disruption is much more difficult to predict based upon this information. Further, not all children with neuromotor problems carry a diagnosis of cerebral palsy; that is, dysarthria may be present in children with a variety of neurologic disorders. Perhaps research with children similar to that conducted by Darley/Aronson/Brown (1969 a; 1969 b) with adults presenting with a variety of neurological impairments may lead to a better understanding of the relationship between neuropathology and speech disorders in children.

2. Etiology and Behavioral Pathology

There are many conditions that interfere with neurologic development that may occur before birth (prenatal), during or immediately following birth (perinatal), or later during early childhood (postnatal). Any of these conditions may result in dysarthria depending upon which brain mechanisms are involved. Prenatal problems include genetic factors such as blood incompatibilities of mother and child (e. g., Rh incompatibility), metabolic disturbances, and others. Problems that disrupt oxygen supply to the fetus, maternal infections, exposure to roentgenograms, chemicals, and other problems occurring during early pregnancy also may cause damage to the neurologic system of the fetus. As well, perinatal head trauma may occur in difficult deliveries either from the use of forceps during delivery or from cranial pressure exerted by contact between the baby's head and the mother's pelvis. Premature and rapid deliveries also may be problematic in that they do not allow for gradual adjustment of the fetal circulatory system to extrauterine conditions. Respiratory problems that occur during and following birth may also result in brain damage.

Other problems may occur after birth. These include infections such as encephalitis and meningitis, brain abscesses, tumors, stroke, and other encephalopathies resulting in disorders such as Reye's syndrome (Holzhauer/Campbell/Hall/Halpin 1986). Head injuries among children also are common. It has been estimated that the annual brain-injury rate per 100,000 children in the USA is 185 and that major causes of pediatric brain injury are falls, recreational activities, and motor vehicle accidents (Kraus/Fife/Cox et al. 1986).

Any of the aforementioned conditions and others may result in developmental dysarthria, depending upon the site and extent of brain damage. The neurologic basis for developmental dysarthria found in children is similar to that described for acquired adult disorders. That is, dysarthria results when, during the course of development, damage to the motor cortex, direct and indirect motor pathways, basal ganglia, cerebellum and/or peripheral nerves occurs. Brain injury in any of these areas disrupts information communicated via the final common pathway to and from the muscles involved in speech production. We should point out that brain damage affecting the motor system occurring prenatally and perinatally is often labelled cerebral palsy. When damage occurs postnatally, it may or may not be labelled cerebral palsy. For example, some head-injured children evidence motor disorders similar to those seen in cerebral palsy, but may not be labelled as such.

There are two major types of dysarthria that are commonly discussed with regard to developmental neuromotor disorders. These include spastic dysarthria and dyskinetic dysarthria. Spastic dysarthria results from infarction of the upper motoneuron system (motor cortex and/or direct and indirect motor pathways), whereas dyskinetic dysarthria results from primary involvement of the basal ganglia and connections. Mixed dysarthrias among neurologically impaired children also occur when aspects of both the upper motoneuron system and the basal ganglia are involved (Pruszewiez/Obrebowski/Zgorzalewicz 1977). Other types of dysarthria (e. g., ataxic dysarthria resulting from cerebellar infarction and flaccid dysarthria resulting from lower motoneuron involvement) appear to be less common in children than in adults (Hardy 1983).

2.1. Abnormal Movement Patterns

When the neurologic system is damaged prior to completion of its development abnormal movement patterns — not seen in adults — may be present. In a normal child, some components of the motor system develop before others and therefore dominate motor behavior until other systems are completely developed. For example, excitatory motor components develop before inhibitory ones. When the normal motor system has completely developed, some of the early motor patterns disappear, some remain but are no longer dominant, and some continue as in infancy throughout life.

When the neurologic system is damaged developmentally, early patterns of behavior that normally disappear do not. Other early dominant movement patterns that normally become nondominant, remain dominant or become exaggerated. To overcome these problems, compensatory motor patterns often develop. These retained, exaggerated, and/or compensatory behaviors result largely because normal inhibitory mechanisms do not develop. Therefore, excitatory muscle activity remains unchecked as the brain matures following a lesion. For example, the Moro embrace reflex may persist, and tonic neck reflexes and other postural reactions may become overly dominant and exaggerated.

Several writers, including Ingram (1962), Sheppard (1964), Alexander (1987) and McDonald/Chance (1964) have described specific infantile oral reflexes that involve aspects of speech production including labial, lingual, velar, pharyngeal, mandibular, laryngeal, respiratory, and others. Table 80.1, taken from McDonald/Chance (1964) provides a list of some of these reflexes involving structures used in articulation of speech. Abnormal and compensatory oral motor behaviors seen in neurologically impaired children are listed in Table 80.2, which is taken from Alexander (1987). Researchers have suggested that these and other infantile reflexive behaviors may be critical to the development of speech production in neurologically impaired children. Mysak (1963), Sheppard (1964; 1987) and others have suggested that abnormal oral motor reflex patterns may interfere with speech production. However, this assertion has been questioned. For example, Hixon and Hardy indicated that nonspeech and speech movement patterns are controlled by different neurologic mechanisms and therefore are unrelated (Hixon/Hardy 1964).

Love/Hagerman/Taimi (1980) studied the relationship between infantile oral reflexes

Reflex	Stimulus	Response
Cephalic reactions	Stroking the lobe of the ear or the nostril	Turns head away from stimulus
Facial response	Sharp tapping around mouth	Rounding and protrusion of lips as in pouting
Rooting reflex	Repeated light stroking of the cheek or around the mouth	Movement of the head as if trying to get a nipple into the mouth
Mouth opening	Sight of an object such as a nipple, finger, or tongue depressor, which is usually associated with mouth opening	Lowering of the mandible and separation of lips
Lip reflex	Tapping around the angle formed at the corner of the mouth	Involuntary movements of the lips – lip closure and pouting
Biting reflex	Object placed between teeth (or gums)	Strong, sustained elevation of the mandible
Sucking reflex	Gentle pushing and pulling on a nipple or finger placed in mouth	Alternating protruding and retracting movement of the tongue, often with elevation of the tip
Chewing reflex	Tapping with teeth or gums with a tongue blade	Alternating elevations and depressions of the mandible
Laughing	Light stroking or tickling, particularly of the sides of the thorax	Involuntary twitching of the body, opening of the mouth, disruption of breathing rhythm, often accompanied by sound production on both inhalation and exhalation
Swallowing (Oral)	Presence of food or liquid in oral cavity	Waveline motion of tongue to propel food into oropharynx
Swallowing	Contact of food or fluid with mucosa of faucial pillars and pharyngeal wall	Contraction of faucial pillars and walls of pharynx, elevation and closing of larynx, and momentary suspension of respiration

After McDonald ET & Chance B. Cerebral palsy. Englewood Cliffs, NJ: Prentice-Hall, 1964, 123. In Thompson (1988). Neurogenic articulation disorders in children. In McReynolds & D. Yoder (Eds.), *Handbook of speech-language pathology and audiology*. 548–591. Philadelphia: B. C. Decker Inc.

Table 80.1: Infantile Oral Reflexes Observed in Neurologically Impaired Children

and speech performance in 60 individuals, with cerebral palsy and found that only 25 percent of the subjects presented with infantile oral reflexes. This finding contrasted with data reported by Shepard, who found that 43 of 52 dysarthric subjects (84 percent) displayed abnormal reflex patterns (Sheppard 1964). When Love/Hagerman/Taimi examined speech performance of the 15 subjects displaying abnormal oral reflexes, eight of the children demonstrated no speech, and all but one of the remaining seven evidenced some articulatory impairment. However, a clear pattern between the number of abnormal reflexes present and the level of articulatory proficiency was not found. These data indicate that the presence of abnormal reflexes and dysarthria varies greatly across neurologically impaired children.

2.2. Spastic Disorders

Children with spastic dysarthria may have a wide range of speech problems resulting from damage to the neuromotor system. In general, hyperreflexia and hypertonia of muscle groups involved in speech production is seen. Variability across children with spastic dysarthria is common, however, because of subtle variations in patterns of brain injury.

Many children with spastic dysarthria also evidence spastic involvement of the upper and lower extremities and are classified as such. These classifications include spastic hemiplegia, spastic paraplegia, spastic diplegia, and spastic quadri- plegia. All of these motor disorders result from impairment of portions of the upper motoneuron system. It is important to understand the extent of neurologic involvement found in children carrying these classifications because they pro-

Behavior	Description
Cheek-lip retraction	Abnormal pulling back of cheeks; lips appear thin and form a tight line across mouth; often seen head and neck hyperextension and tongue retraction
Exaggerated jaw closure	Abnormal jaw closure on objects such as feeding utensils
Exaggerated tongue protrusion	Forward-backward suckling movement with exaggerated forward motion; tongue appears thick
Jaw thrusting	Strong depression of lower jaw; jaw may be stuck in open position; position occurs with head-neck hyperextension
Jaw thrusting with protrusion	Compensatory strong depression of lower jaw occurring in an attempt to close jaw
Jaw thrusting with retraction	Strong depression and retraction of lower jaw seen concomitant with head and neck hyperextension and tongue retraction
Lip pursing	Lips pursed and protruded with tension extended to the cheeks; corners of lips retracted slightly
Tongue retraction	Posterior movement of tongue into oropharyngeal area occurring with head and neck hyperextension; back of tongue appears humped; the tongue is thick
Tongue retraction with anterior elevation	Tongue assumes posterior position in oral cavity with tongue tip elevated and pushing against hard palate and alveolar ridge; compensatory for tongue instability
Tongue thrusting	Strong forward pushing of the tongue; tongue appears thick
Tonic biting	Strong jaw closure in response to tactile stimulation of biting surface of teeth or gums; jaw is stuck in closed position; increased head, neck, trunk extension occurs in attempt to overcome abnormal pattern

After Alexander (1987) Oral-motor treatment for infants and young children with cerebral palsy. Sermin Speech Lang, *8*, 87–100. In Thompson (1988). Neurogenic articulation disorders in children. In L. McReynolds & D. Yoder (Eds.), *Handbook of speech-language pathology and audiology*. 548–591. Philadelphia: B. C. Decker Inc.

Table 80.2: Abnormal and Compensatory Oral Motor Behaviors of Infants and Young Children with Cerebral Palsy

vide information on the distribution of brain damage. Because of the close proximity of corticobulbar and corticospinal tracts at the cortical level and during their course to the brain stem and spinal cord, damage to one system often occurs concomitant with the other. Therefore, classifications may be helpful in predicting the extent to which muscles involved in speech production are affected.

In spastic hemiplegia, the upper and lower extremities of one side of the body are involved, resulting from unilateral lesion of the corticospinal system. The corticobulbar system may or may not be involved; but when it is involved, dysarthria may result from hemiparesis and spasticity in the lower half of the face and oral musculature. Spastic paraplegic children present with involvement of both lower extremities while the upper extremities remain unaffected. In addition, the muscles of the torso walls may be involved, resulting in respiratory involvement and possible mild dysarthria. In a large study of speech patterns in dysarthric children, Kamalashile (1975) found only two paraplegic children with dysarthria probably because respiratory impairment often does not affect speech production, unless other aspects of the speech musculature also are affected.

The extent of neuromotor involvement in spastic diplegia exceeds that of hemiplegia and paraplegia in that the muscles of both the upper and lower extremities and the torso are involved. The spastic involvement in diplegia also often extends to the neck musculature; however, involvement of the arms and neck area are less severe than that of the legs. In children with spastic diplegia, speech production may or may not be impaired. Some children may evidence rather mild speech problems such as dysprosody resulting from involvement of the respiratory system coupled with impairment of the extrinsic laryngeal musculature. But other children may evidence severe dysarthria resulting from involvement of the oral, laryngeal, and respiratory musculature. As pointed out by Hardy (1983), oral and laryngeal motor involvement may not be extensive in these cases. However, when a marked reduction in respiratory support is present, coupled with mild dysfunction of oral and laryngeal mechanisms, significant dysarthria may result.

Spastic quadriplegia is the most severe. In children with quadriplegia, both the upper and lower extremities are involved with equal severity and motor involvement often extends to the oral and laryngeal musculature. Therefore, developmental dysarthria is often seen, and often it is severe. Speech production problems were reported in 63 of the spastic quadriplegic children studied by Kamalashile (1975).

2.3. Dyskinetic Disorders

In children with dyskinetic dysarthria, as in spastic dysarthria, variability exists with regard to the various dimensions of speech production that may be disrupted. Movement of the lips, tongue, mandible, soft palate, laryngeal mechanism, and the respiratory mechanism may be impaired secondary to involvement of the thoracic wall, laryngeal, and orofacial musculature. In children with dyskinetic dysarthria, all four extremities often are involved; therefore, they may be labelled quadriplegic, with the upper extremities being more seriously involved than the lower extremities. In general, movement patterns in impaired muscle groups are lacking in coordination, and involuntary movements such as athetosis and chorea, may be seen. Atethoid movements are usually described as slow and writhing; whereas, chorea is characterized by rapid, flailing, and jerking movements of the extremities.

3. Speech Pathology

Review of the literature focused on identification of speech pathology associated with the developmental dysarthrias is limited. Although several studies have compared performance of dyskinetic and spastic children on certain speech and nonspeech tasks, many parameters of speech production have not been studied extensively. Further, research methodologies employed in many studies have been problematic. For example, some studies have not controlled for important variables such as hearing ability and intelligence, and children presenting with wide ranges of severity have been included for study in a single group. These sources of uncontrolled variability make it difficult to draw conclusions about specific speech patterns occurring in children with dysarthria. In addition, it is interesting to note that most studies focusing on speech production problems associated with developmental dysarthria were published in the mid to late 1960s. By the 1970s, a shift in focus to prespeech, oral motor behaviors, feeding, and positioning was noted, with little discussion of speech production behavior. This shift was perhaps influenced by factors such as (1) changes in legislation affecting delivery of services in the USA to younger and more severely impaired children; (2) popularity of neurodevelopmental theories and approaches to treatment (K. Bobath 1966; 1971; 1976; B. Bobath 1967; 1971 a; 1971 b); and (3) concern with early feeding programs for neurologically impaired children (Morris 1977). Hardy (1983) appears to be the first to refocus on speech production problems in these children, specifically in children with cerebral palsy.

The following discussion will focus primarily on speech production problems. Each of the subsystems involved in speech production (respiration, phonation, resonance, and articulation) will be discussed separately and, where possible literature will be cited comparing the performance of spastic and dyskinetic dysarthric children.

3.1. Respiration

Studies of respiration in children with dysarthria have shown that breathing patterns often are disrupted in children with spastic, athetoid, and ataxic cerebral palsy. However, athetoid children appear to evidence more severe involvement than others. Athetoid children with dyskinetic dysarthria present with "varying gradations of a pattern of irregular, shallow, and noisy breathing" (Berry/Eisenson 1956, 358) resulting in disruption in volume, rate, and rhythm of speech. Some abnormal breathing patterns include rapid breathing (McDonald/Chance 1964), shallow breathing (Palmer 1952), involuntary movement of the respiratory musculature (McDonald/Chance 1964) and "reversed breathing" (Davis 1982). In a study in which the breathing patterns of 58 children with athetoid cerebral palsy were studied, Palmer (1952) reported that every subject had at least one breathing abnormality. In contrast, children with spastic dysarthria presented with relatively better respiratory control, although these children evidenced reductions in chest movement and greater abdominal breathing movement than did normal children.

There are several speech problems that may result from these and other impairments of respiratory functioning in children with dysarthria, however, malfunctioning of the respiratory system alone does not often result in significant speech production problems. It is when other subsystems of speech production are impaired along with respiration that the repiratory component becomes important. Some abnormal speech patterns that have been noted include short phrasing (Hardy 1983), frequent inspiration (Hardy 1983), reduced syllabic repetitions (Schliesser 1982) decreased rate, (Clark/Hoops 1980), and uncontrolled phonation (McDonald/Chance 1964).

3.2. Phonation

A variety of phonation problems may be seen in children with dysarthria, some of which result from impairments in respiratory functioning. Phonation problems also commonly result from abnormal body postures and reactions. For example, when hyperextension of the head occurs in the symmetrical tonic neck reflex, breathy vocal quality may result. As explained by Davis (1982), head "hyperextention biomechanically facilitates vocal fold abduction" (Davis 1982, 103). Other phonation problems result from involvement of the vagus (tenth cranial) nerve. In this case, strained vocal quality may be seen because of hypertonicity and spasticity of the intrinsic laryngeal musculature. This problem is common in spastic dysarthria.

Reactions to decreased lung volume and other compensatory learned behaviors also may contribute to hypertension of the vocal folds. For example, children with low vital capacity may use increased body tension to push expiratory air for speech production. This causes an increase in general tension in the laryngeal mechanism, and the child with dysarthria sounds as if she or he is using residual air phonation (Davis 1982).

There are three general dimensions of phonation that may be disrupted in dysarthric speakers. These include (1) pitch, which is determined by the longitudinal tension of the vocal folds, (2) loudness, which is determined by the amount of medial compression of the folds, and (3) periodicity, which is determined by patterns of vocal fold vibration. In children with dysarthria, any of these dimensions may be impaired. Pitch may be high or low, and reduced pitch range may be evident. Loudness often is reduced, and breathiness and aperiodicity may occur.

Few studies are reported in the literature that have attempted to describe phonation problems in developmental dysarthria. Early studies by Rutherford (1944) and Leith/Steer (1958) indicated, based on listener judgements, that pitch, loudness, and rate are often affected in dysarthria. Examining aspects of phonation in 48 children with athetoid cerebral palsy and 74 with spastic cerebral palsy, Rutherford reported a greater degree of impairment in the children with athetoid as compared to those with spastic cerebral palsy. Specifically, Rutherford found decreased pitch range, increased loudness, breathiness, slow speech and abnormal rhythm. Laryngeal dysfunction noted in the athetoid children included dilator spasm, constrictor spasm, and phonation out of phase with articulation. Structural and functional abnormalities of the vocal folds were less often noted in the children with spastic dysarthria, however, many phonation problems were seen in the spastic children as well.

Further study is needed in this area such that phonatory problems in developmental dysarthria can be better understood. Manifestations of phonation problems that have been reported, but that have not been well studied in children are listed in Table 80.3. In addition, possible reasons for each phonatory characteristic are listed.

3.3. Resonance

Children with dysarthria also may evidence resonatory and other articulatory problems because of insufficient velopharyngeal functioning. In one study, the authors estimated that approximately 30 percent of children with dysarthria secondary to cerebral palsy have velopharyngeal closure problems (Dawes 1958). In another study, 34 of 54 children presented with nasality (rhinophonia) (Pruszewics/Obrebowski/Zgorzalewicz 1977). These problems may result from malfunction in timing, range of motion, changes in muscle tone, reduced movement (unilateral or bilateral paresis), and/or random reflexive behaviors of the soft palate and/or posterolateral pharyngeal walls. For example, Pruszewicz/Obrebowski/Zgorzalew-

Phonatory problem	Laryngeal abnormality
Decreased sustained phonation (Pruszewicz/Obrebowski/Zgoralewicz 1977)	Decreased medial compression of vocal folds
Breathy vocal quality (Hardy 1963; Rutherford 1944)	Decreased medial compression of vocal folds
"Strained" vocal quality (Davis 1982)	Hypertension, spasticity of laryngeal musculature
Decreased loudness (Hardy 1983)	Decreased medial compression of vocal folds
Bursts of loudness (Davis 1982)	Aperiodicity resulting from involuntary activity of laryngeal musculature
Increased loudness (Rutherford 1944)	Constrictor spasm; hypertension of laryngeal musculature
Monoloudness; decreased loudness range (Hardy 1964)	Decreased medial compression of vocal folds and immobility of vocal folds
Sudden changes in pitch (Davis 1982)	Changes in longitudinal tension resulting from involuntary activity of laryngeal mechanism
Monopitch; decreased pitch range (Davis 1982)	Decreased longitudinal tension and immobility of vocal folds
Slow rate (Rutherford 1944)	Out of phase phonation and articulation
Abnormal rhythm (Rutherford 1944)	Out of phase phonation and articulation
"Residual air phonation" (Davis 1982)	Hypertension of vocal folds

After C. Thompson (1988). Neurogenic articulation disorders in children. In L. McReynolds & D. Yoder (Eds.), *Handbook of speech-language pathology and audiology.* 548–591. Philadelphia: B. C. Decker Inc.

Table 80.3: Phonation Problems Seen in Children with Developmental Dysarthria and Possible Laryngeal Abnormalities

icz reported that ten of 54 children with dyskinetic dysarthria had disordered velar functioning resulting in hypernasality; four presented with distinct velar asymmetry, and six presented with reduced bilateral movement. Physiologic problems causing perceived hypernasality were undetermined in another 22 children in the study.

Netsell (1969) discovered five abnormal velopharyngeal movement patterns seen among cerebral palsy speakers by studying simultaneous recordings of intraoral air pressure, the rate of nasal air flow, and the speech signal. Patterns noted included gradual opening, gradual closing, anticipatory closing, retentive opening, and premature opening. In children with gradual opening patterns, early segments of connected speech were produced normally, with the onset of nasal airflow occurring in later segments. In gradual closing, the opposite was observed. In anticipatory opening, nasal airflow was seen as speech was initiated and subsided thereafter, and, in children with retentive opening patterns, slow closure of the velopharyngeal port occurred during the formation of individual consonants. Finally, in premature opening, the velopharyngeal seal was broken at inappropriate times during consonant production, thereby disrupting the acoustic form of the consonant. Other patterns of velopharyngeal functioning also may be observed in children with dysarthria. For example, Kent/Netsell (1978) reported instability of velar elevation in athetoid children.

Disruptions in velopharyngeal functioning result in abnormal intraoral breath pressure needed for production of all speech sounds except nasals. Therefore hypernasality and/or nasal emission may be detected during speech production. Other speech problems such as slow rate of speech also may be noted secondary to velopharyngeal incompetence, when children compensate for slow palatopharyngeal movement.

3.4. Articulation

Articulation errors occurring in children with dysarthria have been reported by several investigators including Byrne (1959), Clark/

Hoops (1980), Irwin (1968), and Rutherford (1944). These data have indicated that children with dysarthria have complex articulation problems because of weakness, decreased range of motion, alterations in timing, changes in muscle tone, abnormal oral movement patterns such as extensor jaw thrust and tongue thrust, and other neuromotor problems of the lips, jaw, and tongue.

In general, studies have shown that dyskinetic dysarthric speakers present with more severe articulation problems than do spastics (Byrne 1959; Irwin 1968; Farmer 1980; Platt/Andrews/Howie 1980; Platt/Andrews/Young/Quin 1980). That is, spastic dysarthric speech is generally more intelligible and less articulatorily impaired than athetoid dysarthric speech. This finding is perhaps due to the many aberrations in tongue, mandibular, and lip control seen in children with extrapyramidal damage. As pointed out by Palmer (1952) athetoid children evidence difficulty in elevation of the tip of the tongue, gross clumsy tongue movement, bizarre lip closing and facial grimacing.

Studies describing articulatory errors seen in children with dysarthria have pointed out a number of error patterns, some of which appear to remain consistent as these children mature (Platt/Andrews/Young/Quin 1980). Specifically, in terms of manner of articulation, children with dysarthria evidence great difficulty with production of fricatives, affricates, and liquids in both initial and final word positions, and stops, nasals, and glides are somewhat easier at least in the initial word position. As pointed out by Byrne (1959) in a study of 61 children with developmental dysarthria with cerebral palsy aged 2 to 7 years, 75 percent of the children produced /w/, /b/, /j/, /m/, and /d/ correctly, and at least 60 percent of the children produced /n/, /h/, /g/, /k/, and /t/ correctly in the initial word position. However, these sounds were produced correctly in the final position in less than 50 percent of contexts as were fricatives and affricates in both initial and final positions. In a similar study with older dysarthric speakers, Platt/Andrews/Young/Quin (1980) indicated that these individuals continue to evidence problems with fricatives and affricates, although productions in the initial position become more accurate with age.

With regard to place of articulation, most errors are noted in production of postdental fricatives (/ð/, /θ/), alveolar fricatives and affricates (/s/, /z/, and /ʤ/), palatal liquids (/r/), and labiodental fricatives (/f/, /v/) but bilabial and velar articulations are more often produced accurately. These patterns, again, are consistent in older children and adults with developmental dysarthria although final word productions of postdental fricatives remain particularly difficult.

Phonemic errors made by children with developmental dysarthria also have been studied and classified (Byrne 1959; Farmer 1980; Platt/Andrews/Howie 1980). The most comprehensive phonemic analysis reported in the literature was completed by Platt/Andrews/Howie on their data derived from 50 congenitally dysarthric adults. Findings indicated that most errors consisted of within-manner (place and voicing errors) as compared to between-manner errors. Vowel production errors also are common, particularly in attempts to produce those in extreme positions of the vowel diagram (Byrne 1959; Platt/Andrews/Young/Quin 1980; Irwin 1968; Kent/Netsell/Bauer 1975). This is not surprising given reductions in range of motion of the tongue and other oral structures found in dysarthric children, Kent/Netsell (1978).

Difficulty performing diadochokinetic tasks (both speech and nonspeech) also has been noted among children with dysarthria (Hixon/Hardy 1964; Platt/Andrews/Young 1980; Schliesser 1982). However, mixed findings have been reported with regard to the correlation between these activities and speech production. That is, alternate motion rates using speech stimuli have correlated highly with speech intelligibility in several studies; (Hixon/Hardy 1964; Platt/Andrews/Young/Quin 1980; Schliesser 1982) whereas, conflicting results have been reported with regard to correlations between nonspeech alternate motion rates and speech intelligibility. In a study of 50 children with developmental dysarthria, Hixon/Hardy (1964) reported that of five nonspeech activities including (1) opening and closing of the lips and teeth together, (2) retracting and rounding the lips, (3) raising the tongue to the alveolar ridge and lowering it, (4) lateralizing the tongue from one corner of the mouth to the other, and (5) opening and closing the jaw, only one (lateralizing the tongue) correlated with speech production ability. In a similar study of 15 adults with developmental dysarthria aged 16 to 51 years, Schliesser (1982) found three nonspeech activities to be strongly related to severity of dysarthria. These included opening and closing the jaw, retracting the tongue to the alveolar ridge, and retracting and rounding the lips. These conflicting findings may indicate differences between younger and older individuals with dysarthria and/or reflect the great heterogeneity seen in developmental dysarthria. Whatever the source(s) of variability in these studies, one can say that most children with developmental dysarthria evidence difficulty in performance of both speech and nonspeech diadochokinetic tasks and that these problems may or may not relate to the severity of dysarthria.

4. Clinical Evaluation

Clinical assessment of dysarthria in children includes evaluation of all subsystems of speech production including respiration, phonation, resonance, and articulation. As well, evaluation of intelligibility and prosody are important. The major goals of the evaluation are to (1) identify physiologic deficits of the speech production system, (2) identify the involved speech production subsystems, (3) estimate the severity of dysarthria based on a variety of factors including intelligibility scores and ratings of speech naturalness, and (4) establish the modifiability of speech through stimulability testing and identification of compensatory strategies that may improve speech.

In testing for neuromotor speech problems the evaluation may be approached from three different levels: physiologic, acoustic, and perceptual. Each level of analysis provides different information that assists the clinician in achieving the aforementioned goals. At the physiologic level, measures of muscle activity, kinematic parameters, muscle strength, muscle endurance (fatigue), muscle tone, and aerodynamic factors are considered, whereas, acoustic analyses examine the components of the speech waveform which include frequency, intensity and duration. Perceptual measures, which are most often used clinically, provide information based on auditory judgements relevant to all subsystems of production, prosody and intelligibility.

The evaluation of dysarthria typically examines muscle function during both speech and nonspeech activities. However, the importance and meaning of data derived from the nonspeech measures is controversial as was discussed earlier. Similarly, both maximal and submaximal performance measures are taken, even though the usefulness of maximal performance measures have been questioned (Kent/Kent/Rosenbek 1987). Nonetheless, certain nonspeech maximal performance measures may be useful to the clinician (Luschei 1991; Robin/Somodi/Luschei 1991). The following sections present a speech subsystem approach to the evaluation of developmental dysarthria.

4.1. Evaluation of the Respiratory System

4.1.1. Physiologic Analyses

Evaluation of respiration in children with neuromotor speech problems should include measures of subglottic air pressure and maintenance of subglottic pressure across the vital capacity. If an individual is able to maintain a subglottic pressure of 5 cm H_2O for 5 seconds, then one can rule out the contribution of the respiratory system as the primary source of the speech production problem (Netsell/Hixon 1978). A commonly used method to measure subglottic airflow is the U-tube manometer with a leak tube to simulate glottal resistance (Netsell/Hixon 1978). A simple version of this test, using a glass of water and straw is described by Hixon/Hawley/Wilson (1982).

A second area of assessment involves the examination of respiratory movements. Dysarthric speakers may exhibit altered respiratory patterns which include exaggerated use of certain muscles, or 'paradoxic' movements in which the circumference of the abdomen is decreased (Yorkston/Beukelman/Bell 1988). The most commonly used instrument to assess chest wall movements in dysarthric speakers is the magnamometer (Hixon/Mead/Goldman 1976; Putman/Hixon 1984). Other measures of respiratory function include the vital capacity, the consistency of the lung volume level and the overall lung volume level.

4.1.2. Perceptual Measures

Perceptual observations discussed by Darley/Aronson/Brown (1975) are useful indicators of respiratory involvement in dysarthric speakers (although they may be indicative of problems at other levels of the system as well). Observations including monoloudness, excess loudness variation, loudness decay, alternating loudness, forced inspiration-expiration, and short phrases alert the clinician to possible involvement of the respiratory system. The advantage of these observations is that they can be made during conversational speech. However, taken alone, perceptual observations are often unreliable and perhaps invalid (Yorkston/Beukelman/Bell 1988).

4.2. Evaluation of the Phonatory System

4.2.1. Physiologic measures

One important indicator of phonatory function is airflow. The most common method of measuring airflow is with a pnemotachographic device (Folkins/Moon 1990), a non-invasive procedure that measures the pressure drop across a resistance that is placed in the airstream. Dysarthric speakers may have inconsistent phonatory control and, therefore, an average measure of air flow may not be reflective of the integrity of their system (Netsell/Lotz/Shaughanessy 1984). However, by using a computer to digitize the data, allowing for examination of resistance over time, inconsistencies may be quantified.

Other methods to evaluate vocal function include the stroboscope, the electroglottograph (EGG), and electromyography (EMG). A strobe is a light that flashes at a specific frequency which allows for observations of the vocal folds in various positions. The EGG is a device that measures vocal fold contact by a technique that detects current flow through tissue. Measures derived from this device reflect the opening and closing of the vocal folds and their temporal pattern. The EMG signal is a measure of the electrical activity of muscles. The muscle activity can be obtained from electrodes placed on the surface or by placing needle electrodes in the muscle.

4.2.2. Acoustic measures

Acoustic measures of vocal performance are becoming commonplace in speech pathology clinics in so much as technological advances now allow for inexpensive and easy to use instruments. The measurement of fundamental frequency can be made rather easily and clinicians can obtain objective data on habitual frequency, fundamental frequency range, and frequency variability in connected speech. Measures of vocal intensity and cycle-to-cycle change in amplitude or frequency during phonation also can be made.

Spectrograms also provide information about the acoustic components of speech. For example, during vowel production tasks, noise or weakness in patients with vocal involvement can be identified by examining spectral changes compared to normal spectra. Likewise, the acoustic spectrum, a plot of the energy contained in each of the frequencies of a complex sound (i. e., a Fourier transformation), may provide useful information about the presence or absence of vocal fold neuropathology.

4.2.3. Perceptual Measures

Darley/Aronson/Brown (1975) suggest a variety of perceptually based parameters that may be observed when diagnosing phonatory deficits in adults with dysarthria. These include pitch level, pitch breaks, monopitch, voice tremor, monoloudness, excessive loudness variation, loudness decay, alternating loudness, harsh voice, hoarse voice, breathy voice, strained-strangled voice, and short phrases. Ability to sustain steady phonation, produce reflexive sounds, and alter pitch and loudness are all indicative of phonatory function and are among the most common means of assessing vocal pathology. Poor performance on these tasks may be indicative of neurological involvement affecting one or more aspect of phonatory function including the ability to produce adequate subglottic pressures, ability to control exhalatory efforts during phonation, and hyperadduction of the folds. Impairment of the respiratory system also can reduce maximal phonation time.

The s/z ratio is another common measure of phonatory and respiratory integrity. Unlike the maximal phonation time, the s/z ratio is thought to differentiate respiratory involvement from phonatory impairment (Boone 1977). The patient is asked to sustain first an /s/, and then a /z/, for as long as possible. Individuals with normal phonatory systems should be able to sustain /s/ for as long as /z/; if there is some laryngeal abnormality, the subject should be able to produce a normal length unvoiced sound (/s/), but have a reduction in the voiced cognate. If there is respiratory insufficiency, the overall times may be reduced for both sounds.

4.3. Evaluation of the Resonatory System

4.3.1. Physiologic Measures

Because the velopharyngeal system acts as a valve upon the airstream, measures of air flow and air pressure serve as indicators of its functional adequacy. These measures are considered indirect in that the clinician must extrapolate from the aerodynamic measures velar resistance or orifice size. One easy, commonly used method for detecting air flow is to place a mirror below the nose. If there is nasal air flow, the presence of humidified air should fog the mirror.

Quantitative measurement of airflow requires the placement of a tube, with known resistance, in the airstream. The pressure drop across the constant resistance is linearly related to flow. This is the same methodology noted above for testing respiratory airflow.

Aerodynamic measures also may be used to estimate orifice size. One such method, described by Warren/DeBois (1964) does so by assuming that the area of the orifice can be determined if the differential pressure across the orifice is measured. Another method (Hixon/Bless/Netsell 1976), supplies forced oscillatory airflow simultaneously to the nasal and oral cavities (with a mask) and to a rigid walled model of the nasal and oral cavity having an adjustable orifice which mimics the VP port. The two outputs are balanced and the size of the patient's VP orifice can be inferred from the size of the model's.

Radiographic techniques still are used to examine VP function. Lateral still radiography is the oldest form of assessment of the velar port. However, these are static representation of the velum, (one picture taken at a time), and therefore are limited in usefulness for understanding speech problems. In contrast, motion picture radiography and videofluoroscopy provide useful information about the functioning and integrity of the VP port. Multiview videofluoroscopy (Skolnick 1969) allows for examination of the VP mechanism from separate views (sagittal, frontal, and base). Computerized tomographic (CT) scans also may be used to examine the soft palate. For instance, Moon/Smith (1987) recorded a series of scans of the palate, of which each scan represented a single frame that could be viewed on a video monitor.

Ultrasound is a technique used to study articulation, but has recently been applied to the study of pharyngeal wall movement as many instrumental techniques are limited in their ability to view this aspect of VP functioning. By placing a transducer on the skin below the earlobe and behind the ramus of the mandible, visualization of the pharyngeal wall is possible (Parush/Ostry 1986).

A very useful and commonly used clinical technique for visualizing the palate and its movement is endoscopy. An endoscope is an optical instrument that allows one to visualize internal body structures under a light source (part of the stroboscope described above for phonatory assessment), using fiberoptic fibers to illuminate an area of interest. Nasal endoscopy is quite popular. Using a nasal endoscope (a) the presence or absence of an adenoidal pad, (b) the extent of velar movement, (c) the size and shape of the VP port, and (d) the contribution of lateral wall movement to closure may be evaluated.

4.3.2. Acoustic Measures

The spectrograph provides information about oral-nasal coupling. However, the changes related to such coupling are subtle and may not be of clinical utility in that spectographic analysis is time consuming and requires a great deal of training. The Oral Nasal Acoustic Ratio (TONAR) is a device used to measure the relative magnitudes of oral and nasal pressure. This is an instrument that has received relatively little attention, yet the procedure is simple and highly reliable.

4.3.3. Perceptual Measures

Of course the clinician's ear is an important aspect of diagnosis. Judgments of nasality are used by the majority of clinicians to assess VP structure and function. However, even here a number of approaches exist. Visual intraoral examination is another common method of VP assessment. However one can discern movement of soft palate, but still perceive hypernasality. More than 90% of clinicians use perceptual judgement to assess the adequacy of the VP port (Schneider/Shprintzen 1980). Some approach the task by having the patient prolong the vowels /a/ and /i/ with nostrils open and closed, with change in quality across the two phonemes indicating an adequately functioning mechanism. Others use the *Iowa Pressure Articulation Test* (Morris/Spriestersbach/Darley 1961) which allows for assessment of pressure consonants which may be particularly troublesome for individuals with VP incompetence. Other clinicians use multidimensional scaling techniques.

4.4. Evaluation of the Articulatory System

4.4.1. Physiologic Measures

The most common form of evaluation is the oral motor examination. The oral motor examination includes evaluation of the peripheral speech structures at rest and during nonspeech activities, as is common in an oral peripheral examination (Dworkin/Culatta 1980). Signs of lips and facial weakness include parting of the lips at rest and asymmetry of the angles of the mouth. In addition, there may be flattening of the nasolabial fold on one or both sides and mandibular weakness may be suspected when the mandible hangs lower than normal in a resting position. The size of the tongue in relation to the oral cavity also should be checked, with a shrunken appearance of one or both sides indicating unilateral or bilateral involvement, respectively. Abnormal patterns also may be noted at rest such as anterior or posterior tongue elevation. As well, observation of the palatopharyngeal mechanism should be accomplished with the child's tongue relaxed on the floor of the mouth and with the mouth open wide. With bilateral involvement, both sides of the soft palate rest near the posterior aspect of the tongue; whereas with unilateral damage, only the weak side appears lower than normal. However, keep in mind that many normal children present with asymmetry of the soft palate; therefore, neurologic impairment cannot be inferred from this observation alone.

Other observations that may be made when the oral structures are at rest include any pocketing of food in the anterior or lateral sulci, indicating abnormal oral motor functioning. In addition, the child's ability to control oral secretions should be noted. Finally, structural relationships of the lips, jaw, tongue, and palate should be checked (e. g., tongue size, palatal arch, and maxillary arch). Children with dyskinetic dysarthria often present with a high palatal arch and narrow maxillary arch that, coupled with restricted mobility of the tongue, influences articulatory precision.

In assessment of nonspeech movement of the articulators, strength, range of motion, coordination, and accuracy of movement are assessed. Symmetry of structures is also assessed, and the presence of abnormal oral reflexive or compensatory behaviors as listed in Table 80.2 are noted. Lip-pursing also may be noted during these activities.

To assess mandibular control, range of motion is tested as the child opens and closes the mouth and moves the mandible from side to side without resistance. Movement with imposed resistance is checked to determine the strength of muscles that open and close the mandible. The examiner tests the muscles involved in opening the jaw by attempting to close the child's mouth when the child is given instructions to open the mouth as widely as possible and to try to prevent the examiner from forcing it closed. Muscles involved in closing the mouth are evaluated as the child attempts to overcome resistance when closing the mouth. This time, the examiner exerts force to keep the jaw open as the child attempts to close it.

The tongue also is checked to evaluate strength and range of motion, the latter by testing tongue protrusion, elevation, and lateralization. Upon tongue protrusion, weakness may be observed on one or both sides, and, with a unilateral weakness, the tongue deviates toward the side of weakness. Exaggerated tongue protrusion and/or tongue thrust may be observed. In tongue elevation to the upper lip and alveolar ridge and in lateralization from side to side, weakness is noted when the child is unable to move the tongue in desired directions and when slowness or irregularity of movement is noted. Tongue strength is tested by exerting pressure against it upon protrusion with a tongue blade or by observing the child's ability to place the tongue in the cheek and resist the examiner's attempts to force it inward.

Diadochokinesis is often used to test oral motor coordination. Although the usefulness of this procedure has been questioned (Kent/Kent/Rosenbek 1987; Luschei 1991) most clinicians still use this measure. Activities performed in assessment of rapid alternating motion of the lips, jaw, and tongue include (a) productions of /u/ and /i/ and repetition of /p/ for observation of the lips; (b) repetition of /t/ for observation of tongue tip articulation; (c) repeated productions of /k/ for evaluation of posterior tongue activity; and (d) repetitions of /p t k/ for evaluation of sequential motion.

Syllables per second of $/p_1/$, $/t_1/$, $/k_A/$, and $/p_1\ t_1\ k_A/$ repetitions are calculated was well as duration of sustained repetitions. Slowness (decreased number of syllables per second) and short duration of syllabic repetition often indicate neuromuscular weakness of the lips, tongue, and/or mandible. However, they also may be seen secondary to respiratory insufficiency, velopharyngeal incompetence, and/or laryngeal involvement. Observable incoordination of the articulators and abnormal rhythm (e. g., pauses between syllables or words, variable rate) also indicate neuromuscular involvement. One measure of articulatory muscle function is the EMG (described above). As previously noted, EMG activity can be observed using surface electrodes placed on the skin of the lips, jaw or even tongue (Somodi/Robin/Luschei 1990).

There are a number of instruments used to measure articulatory movement, the most common being stain gauge transducers which provide information about the displacement and velocity of a given structure. This method is most applicable to the measurement of upper and lower lip and jaw during speech and nonspeech activities. Examination of the tongue typically requires the use of X-ray or ultrasound techniques.

Force transducers have been used to examine the strength of certain oral structures or the amount of force used during given activities. The forces used during speech are estimated to be below 20% of the maximal strength of a given articulator. Fine force control has been examined in both dysarthric and apraxic adults who show differences from normal speakers (McNeil/Weismer/Adams/Mulligan 1990).

Robin and Luschei recently developed a device to measure the strength and fatigue of oral structures (Robin/Somodi/Luschei 1991). By examining the amount of pressure a person can generate while pressing on a bulb, muscle strength is estimated; whereas, fatigue is examined by calculating the duration of sustained pressure equal to 50% of maximal.

4.4.2. Acoustic Measures

Acoustic measures of articulation involve the use of the sound spectrograph. Data obtained from spectrographic recordings has been used to gain an understanding of intelligibility of dysarthric speech (Ansel/Kent 1986) and to provide insight into the underlying problems giving rise to dysarthric speech (Kent/Rosenbek 1983). Acoustic measures, like many instrumental measures, require training to use and interpret. However, they can provide useful information about the speech waveform to augment data derived from perceptual tests.

4.4.3. Perceptual Measures

Articulation tests are used to assess the sound inventory. There are several commercially available articulation tests that may be used with children with dysarthria. For many children, a single-word articulation test is appropriate; however, analysis of speech in a sentence articulation task also should be undertaken for children with sentence production ability. One test that can be recommended for testing both single words and sentences is the *Screening Deep Test of Articulation* (McDonald 1964). Because it is designed to sample sound production in a variety of phonetic contexts, it is particularly useful for children with dysarthria. These children present with restrictions in motor function; therefore, production of some sound combinations may be possible, whereas others may not be.

Regardless of the test instrument chosen, consonant errors should be analyzed with regard to place of articulation (bilabial, labiodental), manner of articulation (stop, fricative) and voicing, error type (substitution, omission, distortion), and word position of errors. A place-manner-voicing analysis provides a method for identification of patterns such as substitution of linguovelar by linguoalveolar sounds (place errors), substitution of fricatives by stops (manner errors), and substitution of voiceless by voiced sounds (voicing errors). In addition, an analysis of vowel production errors should be undertaken with regard to place (front, central, back), height (high, mid, low), tension, and lip rounding. These analyses are well described in other sources focused primarily on articulation (Bernthal/Bankson 1981).

Sound productions also should be analyzed phonetically by means of narrow phonetic transcription. Because sound distortion is common in dysarthria, resulting from weakness and incoordination of the articulators, this analysis may be particularly useful for children with dysarthria. For example, children with dysarthria may produce bilabials as fricatives instead of as stops because of incomplete lip contact.

Phonologic process analysis also may be useful in assessment of dysarthria. This analysis has been discussed by several writers (Compton 1975; Ingram 1976; Weiner 1978; Hodson 1980; Shriberg/Kwiatkowki 1980). Using phonologic process analysis, one may identify modifications or simplifications of adult phonology.

4.5. Speech Intelligibility

Speech intelligibility is commonly estimated in assessments of speech production in children and is particularly important in assessment of dysarthria. Intelligibility measures are useful for estimating the severity of speech deficits (Platt/Andrews/Young/Neilson 1978); they provide a method for evaluating the extent to which neurophysiologic impairments and abnormal systems of speech production influence speech. And they provide a functional dependent variable or outcome measure for use in evaluating the effects of treatment for some children.

Intelligibility in developmental dysarthria has received little attention, as have other aspects of speech production in this population. However, methods used to estimate intelligibility in adult dysarthric speakers may be used with children. The *Assessment of Intelligibility of Dysarthria Speech* (Yorkston/Beukelman 1984) provides a set of word and sentence stimuli that when read or produced imitatively are analyzed to yield indices of speech intelligibility. Although normative data have not been gathered for children, this test could easily be adapted for assessment of developmental dysarthria.

4.6. Prosody

Individuals with dysarthric speech often have impairments in prosody and, therefore, assessment of prosody is recommended with dysarthric children (Robin/Eliason 1991). In assessing prosody, it is recommended that emotive intonation patterns such as happy, sad, and angry be tested as well as linguistic distinctions such as interrogative versus declarative forms or sentence level stress. A detailed review of stimuli used in assessing prosody can be found in Robin/Klouda/Hug (1991). It is recommended that both perceptual judgments of prosody be made as well as acoustic studies if possible to isolate which aspect of the speech waveform (frequency, duration or intensity) is creating the prosodic disruption.

4.7. Compensatory Strategies and Stimulability Testing

A final aspect of assessment is focused on evaluation of the modifiability of abnormal speech production. This activity, sometimes referred to as diagnostic therapy (Rosenbek/La Pointe 1985), provides a basis for making prognostic statements and for planning treatment. Although the direction of this portion of the evaluation is guided by the presenting behaviors of an individual child, a few guidelines can be offered.

One major adjustment that often improves speech production is posture. The best posture for efficient speech production for most people is when the spine is straight and the head is held at midline. Therefore, attempts should be made to position children in this posture.

Other compensatory techniques are directed toward specific subsystems and overall intelligibility of speech. First, alterations in breath support may be made. For example, instructions to inhale more deeply before speaking may improve overall speech production by providing a greater amount of air volume for driving the system. Forced laryngeal adduction may also compensate for respiratory (Nober 1987) weakness and facilitate loudness variation (Rosenbek/LaPointe 1985). Next, alterations in vocal intensity might be tested. For children presenting with hypertonic muscle tone and strain strangled vocal quality, instructions to speak with reduced intensity may improve vocal quality. Conversely, for children with generalized muscular weakness and breathy vocal quality, but who appear to speak with minimal effort, instructions to speak more loudly may improve vocal quality. Finally, attempts to modify articulatory precision should be made. For example, slowing the speech rate may facilitate better articulation.

Rate modification may be extremely useful for improving intelligibility. Even though dysarthric speakers typically speak at a slower rate than normal, further rate reduction may be necessary. Yorkston/Beukelman/Bell (1988) provide an in depth review of specific motor control techniques used with adult dysarthric speakers that may also be useful with children.

Attempts also should be made to modify articulatory placement for production of errored phonemes, both in isolation and in CV segments. Given simple placement instructions, some articulatory contacts may be relatively easy for a child to accomplish. However, some articulatory postures may be more difficult because of motoric constraints. Attempts to approximate these more difficult postures should be made so that an acoustically acceptable signal is produced. For example, a child who has difficulty with the tongue tip elevation necessary for production of /t/, may be able to produce an acoustically acceptable /t/ by coupling the blade of the tongue and the alveolar ridge.

4.8. Other Assessment Considerations

Children with dysarthria, like children with other types of speech disorders, often present with a variety of additional problems. These include auditory processing, intelligence, language development, and other neuropsychologic factors (Wilson/Davidovicz 1987); visual perception; and somatosensory impairments (Hardy 1983). These factors will not be discussed here; however, it is necessary that they be considered in both assessment and treatment of these children.

5. Treatment

Treatment for developmental dysarthria is based upon the age of the child being treated, presenting behavioral deficits, severity, the clinician's theoretical framework for the development of speech in neurologically impaired children and other factors. Developed largely as an outgrowth of theories of neuromotor speech development and the clinical experience of authorities in the field, three major orientations to treatment are available, including (1) neurodevelopmental treatments focused on motor development and prespeech behavior (Alexander 1987; Bobath 1967; Bobath/Bobath 1972; Morris 1987; Mysak 1980; 1987) (2) treatments for disrupted subsystems of speech production (Hardy 1983), and (3) provision of nonspeech, alternative and augmentative communication systems (Ferrier/Shane 1987). It is necessary to point out, however, that experimental data documenting the effects of these treatments are lacking. As observed by Jaffe (1984), "treatment for dysarthria is not researched in the most recent literature" (Jaffe 1984, 163). Data are unavailable to indicate the extent to which treatment improves communicative functioning; data on subject variables important for successful application of a particular treatment have not been reported; and many treatments have not been well described. Therefore, central to this discussion is the need for applied, clinical research documenting the effects of these and other treatments for developmental dysarthria.

5.1. Neurodevelopmental Approaches

Neurodevelopmental treatment approaches such as oral motor treatment (Alexander 1987) feeding treatment (Morris 1987), and neurospeech therapy (Mysak 1980), have been developed largely for intervention with infants and young, preverbal children with cerebral palsy, emphasize positioning, handling, and sensory stimulation in an attempt to inhibit development of abnormal postures and reactions. Treatments of this type have derived from neurodevelopmental theory, suggesting that special posturing and handling inhibits abnormal movement patterns and allows facilitation of more normal movement patterns prerequisite for speech development (Bobath/Bobath 1964).

Although it is beyond the scope of this chapter to provide a detailed description of these treatment approaches, they are based on common premises that are summarized in the points below:

a. The overall goal of treatment is to facilitate normal motor development as much as possible because the development of coordinated oral motor behavior is directly influenced by movement patterns of the body.
b. Abnormal movement patterns reduce opportunity for normal movement and sensory feedback and so are inhibited through special posturing and handling techniques.
c. Normal movement patterns are facilitated by means of visual, auditory, tactile, and other stimulation methods.
d. Facilitation of normal oral motor reflexive and volitional movements provides a basis for speech production.
e. Training techniques are implemented throughout the day and are emphasized during activities of daily living such as feeling.
f. Early intervention is essential.
g. Family involvement is encouraged.

Neurodevelopmental treatments are comprehensive, encompassing a wide range of activities which are described elsewhere (see Alexander 1987; Davis 1978; Morris 1977; 1982; Mysak 1980). Specialized training is, however, necessary before implementing certain aspects of it (i. e., positioning and handling) and, several components of this treatment are controversial with regard to their effect on speech production. For example, some treatments utilized reflexive activity and as printed out earlier the relationship between reflexive activity and volitional speech behavior has been questioned. Further, data are unavailable to indicate that the accomplishment of some aspects of treatment is possible, such as training selective responding to auditory stimuli or modifying abnormal respiratory patterns. Advocates of neurodevelopmental approaches to treatment have not published data to support these or any other aspects of this treatment. These data are badly needed.

5.2. A Subsystems Approach

A perhaps more traditional approach to intervention for developmental dysarthria involves modification of disrupted subsystems of speech production identified during assessment. Treatment is focused on respiration, phonation, resonance, and articulation with the overall goal of treatment being facilitation of the best possible speech given the neuromotor limitations of a particular child. This approach to treatment is most appropriate for preschool and school-age children. Younger children and infants probably do not present with the ability to participate in treatment of this nature. Like neurodevelopmental treatment, posture and positioning are emphasized. Suggestions for posturing children and adults have been described in several sources (Hardy 1983; Morris 1987; Mysak 1980).

A subsystems approach to treatment has been recommended for both acquired and developmental dysarthria (Hardy 1983; Rosenbek/LaPointe 1985). In the following discussion, suggestions taken from the adult and child literature are summarized. Many of these interventions were borrowed from those used with other speech impaired populations (e. g., methods for managing resonance are similar to those used with individuals with cleft palate and methods for managing phonation are similar to those used with children with voice disorders). Suggestions for both speech and nonspeech training will be discussed where appropriate for each subsystem. One should keep in mind that these are only suggestions and that data supporting their use are unavailable. In fact, not one treatment study evaluating the efficacy of intervention for dysarthric children has been published to our knowledge.

5.2.1. Respiration

The major goals of intervention concentrated on respiration include (1) modification of inspiration to provide sufficient air intake for speech production, (2) modification of expiratory patterns to facilitate controlled exhalation, (3) modification of inspiration and expiration relationships, and (4) production of speech within respiratory limits. Inspiration training consists of tasks designed to gradually increase air intake. The mean duration of inhalation is measured, and a target duration is set. The child is instructed to breathe deeply, and air intake is monitored using a variety of methods: tactile monitoring of torso movement; visual monitoring of the movement of a light-weight object (such as a feather) attached to a string and suspended in front of the child's mouth, visual feedback using a spirometer. When air intake has been modified in nonspeech activities, inspiration is monitored during speaking tasks with a gradual increase in the length of spoken utterances. Finally, the optimum length of phrase produced per breath is identified, and the child is trained to inhale at these intervals.

Some caution is warranted with regard to inhalation training. This training is inappropriate for children for whom increased effort results in increased dysfunction. Further, deep inspiration prior to speech production is an atypical speech-breathing pattern; for some children, it may disrupt coordination of inspiration, expiration, and phonation. For these children, concentration on controlled exhalation may be more appropriate.

Exhalation training also often begins with nonspeech tasks, with the major goal of such training being facilitation of controlled exhalation. Blowing is one such task that has been suggested. Blowing exercises are implemented to increase the pressure and/or duration of expired air in an attempt to improve the strength and coordination of respiratory muscles. A variety of devices are available for measuring air pressure and duration during blowing such as the simple device described above by Hixon/Hawley/Wilson (1982) using a water glass and a straw. Whether or not blowing exercises improve respiratory support for speech production is, however, an empirical question, and, as pointed out be Hardy (1983) there may be no relationship between these activities. As soon as possible, controlled exhalation training should involve speech production. A logical beginning point is sustained vowel phonation with the goal being to increase the duration of phonation. Consonant productions are incorporated in strings of CV productions. During these activities, pitch and loudness should be kept constant, and consonants and vowels chosen for practice should be in the sound repertoire of the child. The Visipitch may be useful for providing visual feedback regarding pitch and loudness variation during this training.

Modification of inspiratory and expiratory relationships involves a combination of inspiration training activities and expiration training activities. Maximum inspiration is facilitated followed by controlled expiration. As with other aspects of respiratory treatment, this training may begin during nonspeech tasks and then move to speech tasks (e. g., deep inhalation followed by controlled vowel prolongation and deep inhalation followed by consonant repetitions, CV repetitions, and so on). The final aspect of respiration training is focused on connected speech production and training the child to talk within the physiologic limits of her or his mechanism.

5.2.2. Phonation

Intervention focused on improved phonation is applied in accordance with the type of laryngeal pathology seen in a particular child. As discussed in the assessment section, there are three major aspects of phonation that may be disordered, which include loudness, quality, and pitch. In children with dysarthria, any of these may be impaired. The voice may be too soft (breathy) or too loud, vocal quality may be abnormal, or pitch may be too high or too low. Treatment methods used to improve laryngeal problems secondary to neurologic involvement (dysarthria) are similar to those used to improve laryngeal problems secondary to other problems. A few of the more common treatment methods will be discussed here, keeping in mind that no data exist to support their use. For other methods, a textbook on voice disorders may be consulted (Aronson 1985).

Common problems seen in children with dysarthria concern the intensity, or loudness, dimension of phonation. Specifically, laryngeal weakness and hypo-adduction result in breathy phonation, whereas hypertonicity and hyper-adduction result in overly loud phonation. Breathy phonation may be modified by means of exercises used to increase speaking effort. These include various 'pushing' exercises as originally advocated by Froeschels/Kastein/Weiss (1955). This method simply requires simultaneous pushing with the arms and phonating. This method may not be used with some children with dysarthria, however, because in addition to weakness of the larynx, they also may evidence upper extremity weakness that precludes pushing activity. Children may also be instructed to tighten the muscles of the abdomen and oral mechanism prior to and during speech production in the hope that this effort will generalize to the laryngeal mechanism. Voiced bilabial plosives and labiodental fricatives are good speech sounds for use in practicing this activity because of the visible articulatory contact inherent in their production and a Visipitch may be utilized to evaluate any changes in intensity.

Methods to decrease loudness or adduction involve maneuvers that decrease effort and muscle tension. General muscular relaxation techniques may in some cases be helpful; however, most neurologically impaired children are probably unable to undergo procedures necessary to accomplish this (e. g., progressive muscular relaxation [Jacobsen 1976], the chewing method [Froeschels 1952]). A technique that may be useful for more children is laryngeal massage done either manually or with vibration. Aronson (1985) presents instruction in manual laryngeal message. Once relaxation has been induced, vowels, CV sequences, words, and phrases are practiced. The effects of the yawn-sigh (Boone 1977) and other easy-onset techniques also may be evaluated. For some children, reduced laryngeal tension and concomitant reduced loudness may result from use of these techniques. Similar techniques may be used for altering vocal quality (e. g., strained or strangled vocal quality seen in spasticity).

When pitch is targeted for treatment, attempts to raise pitch, lower it, or increase its variability are often therapeutic goals. This may be done by means of visual feedback such as is possible with the Visipitch. Using this type of biofeedback, the targeted pitch or pitch pattern is displayed along with the child's production. In this manner, immediate feedback is provided.

Closely related to pitch and loudness training and perhaps more important with regard to intelligibility is stress and intonation. Children presenting with monopitch and/or monoloudness also evidence reduced stress patterns or flat intonation contour in speech production. Therefore, treatment focuses on improving stress patterns. This training may begin as soon as the child is able to prolong vowels. During vowel prolongation, intonation variation is introduced. The clinician simply models a down, up, down pattern while phonating /a/ and the child imitates. Visual feedback using a Visipitch, voice light, or other instrument is also helpful during this training. As soon as the child has learned to produce a few consonants, these are incorporated into training, and when production of words and short phrases in possible, contrastive stress drills may be implemented (Rosenbek/LaPointe 1985).

5.2.3. Resonance

Treatment of abnormal resonance for children with dysarthria is approached in a manner similar to that for children with cleft palate, although some unique considerations are involved in managing dysarthria. One major treatment strategy is prosthetic or surgical management. In children presenting with significant hypernasality and nasal emission, a palatal lift or pharyngeal flap surgery may be recommended. Deciding whether or not this type of management is appropriate requires some special considerations:

a. Prosthetic or surgical management is contraindicated when other subsystems of speech physiology are severely involved such that speech production remains unintelligible even with decreased hypernasality.
b. In cases of disproportionately severe hypernasality relative to other speech subsystems, prosthetic or surgical management may be recommended to improve physiologic support for development of speech.
c. Some children may be unable to tolerate a palatal lift, for example, if a hyperactive gag reflex is present.
d. Palatal lifts may be difficult to manage for some children with dysarthria because motor involvement of the upper extremities precludes independent insertion and removal.

When prosthetic or surgical intervention is recommended and when mild to moderate cases of hypernasality are present, which preclude the use of the management strategies just described, treatment procedures may be applied to improve resonatory functioning. Nonspeech procedures include the use of whistling and blowing exercise for facilitation of oral airflow (Shprintzen/McCall/Skolnick 1975), elicitation of the gag reflex with simultaneous production of /a/ (Mysak 1980) and palatal massage (Cole 1971; Lubit/Larsen 1969; Yules/Chase 1969) for improving velopharyngeal closure. Speech tasks for improving resonance in dysarthria have not been specifically described. A logical progression of activities might begin with nonnasal vowel training, followed by nonnasal CV training, CVC, word, phrase training, and so on. During these tasks, instructions to overarticulate (open mouth wider, exaggerate oral contacts) may be given to improve oral airflow.

As with treatment focused on respiration and phonation, incorporation of visual feedback techniques is recommended during resonance activities. These may range from simple devices such as a mirror or feather placed under the child's nose to sophisticated equipment such as The Oral Nasal Acoustic Ratio (TONAR).

5.2.4. Articulation

Treatment to improve articulation in developmental dysarthria may include (1) training of nonspeech behavior in an attempt to increase strength, range of motion, and/or tone of the lips, tongue, and mandibular musculature and (2) speech training to improve speech sound production. Because oral exercises involve individual muscle groups, the practice may not improve speech production which involves the integration of several muscle groups. Further, it has been suggested that many oral exercises require movements not needed in speech production (e. g., tongue lateralization) and so are probably unnecessary.

Two types of oral exercises have been discussed: isotonic and isometric (Rosenbek/LaPointe 1985). Isotonic exercises simply involve repetitive movement of the articulators without resistance, and isometric exercises involve movement of specific structures with imposed resistance. Of course, when this type of activity is included in treatment, only those structures that appear weak need to be treated, and often only one or two movements per structure may be necessary (e. g., tongue elevation, but not protrusion and retraction).

In the accomplishment of this treatment, visual (e. g., mirror work) and tactile stimulation (e. g., tactile manipulation) may be required to facilitate desired movement patterns. Once the movements have been approximated, treatment is focused on increasing the number of repetitions of a particular movement and on increasing the duration of sustained movement with imposed resistance. It may be possible to incorporate instrumentation into this training. Netsell (1975) reported a biofeedback technique using EMG feedback in which muscle potentials were converted to audible tones. With electrodes attached to a patient's upper lip, for example, muscle activity was monitored and modified with instructions to keep the tone within a specified frequency range.

Speech training proceeds much like articulation training in other populations with regard to target selection and training activities. However, some additional considerations in treatment for developmental dysarthria are necessary. These pertain largely to the presenting neurophysiologic limitations of children with dysarthria. That is, it may be impossible for certain articulations to be accomplished due to restrictions in movement and/

or abnormal movement patterns. For example, a child who cannot accomplish linguovelar coupling is likely unable to produce /g/ or /k/. Therefore, /g/ and /k/ would be inappropriate targets for treatment. This is not to say that this child should never be trained to produce these sounds. However, postponing treatment that focuses on them may be indicated, with treatment instead focused on sounds that are within the neurophysiologic limits of the child's system. Another, perhaps unique, aspect of target selection with children with dysarthria pertains to training compensatory articulations. In many cases of developmental dysarthria, when normal articulatory coupling cannot be accomplished, compensatory placements may be trained to yield an acceptable acoustic product. The example provided earlier with regard to production of /t/ with more anterior placement of the tongue than is normal is salient here. Although training of this nature should be attempted only when attempts to train normal articulations have failed, these compensatory patterns often become targets with children with developmental dysarthria.

Articulation treatment in this population utilizes a variety of stimuli such as tactile positioning of the child's articulators, visual models of articulatory placement (e. g., pictures, drawings, and/or the clinician's model), and auditory cues (e. g., spoken models, tape recorded feedback). As soon as target behaviors are produced successfully in isolation, sound production training is done in syllable and word contexts, incorporating production in utterances of increasing length as soon as possible.

During this phase of training, attention should be given to generalization to untrained sounds, word positions, and linguistic contexts. Treatment probes designed to assess such generalization may be helpful in guiding treatment and in understanding speech acquisition in children with dysarthria. The process of generalization has not been studied in this population. Data are unavailable that indicate whether or not training in the initial position, for example, facilitates transfer to the final and medial position in words. Clinicians also do not know whether generalization occurs across sounds similar in place, manner, voicing, or a particular process. As well, the extent to which generalization from phrases to sentences to conversational speech occurs is unknown as is the extent to which trained responses are used in nontraining situations or the natural environment. In children with functional articulation disorders, articulation generalization is variable (Bankson/Byrne 1972; Powell/McReynolds 1969), therefore, it is likely to be in children with dysarthria as well.

Another focus of treatment that is related to articulation is the rate of speech production. As mentioned earlier about assessment of compensatory strategies, articulation is often improved when children are given instructions to reduce their rate of speech. When such is the case, rate reduction treatment might be incorporated into articulation training using devices such as a metronome, a flashing light, or a pacing board with the goal of treatment to facilitate production of one word per beat of the metronome, flash of the light, or touch of the pacing board. It is important to point out here that rate reduction often produces changes in pitch and loudness variation. Therefore, the clinician must decide which abnormal prosodic variable is the least disruptive to speech intelligibility: rate or intonation.

5.2.5. Intelligibility

The final consideration in a subsystems approach is concerned with speech intelligibility. Speech intelligibility reflects the interworkings of all subsystems of speech production and, therefore, provides an index for evaluating the effects of training one or several aspects of speech production. Because improved speech intelligibility is the ultimate goal of treatment, it is suggested that periodic assessment of intelligibility be undertaken to evaluate treatment effectiveness and to modify treatment when appropriate.

5.3. Nonspeech Alternative or Augmentative Communication

Another major treatment approach for dysarthria pertains to provisions of an alternative or augmentative communication system or device. These devices often are used with children with dysarthria and range from simple to complex, depending upon the presenting behaviors and abilities of the child (Ferrier/Shane 1987; Cook/Coleman 1987; McDonald/Schultz 1973). For example, simple picture communication boards may be used with some children (Vanderheiden/Harris-Vanderheiden 1976), whereas, with others, computer based systems may be provided. Selection of a nonspeech communication system is based on the child's physical ability, level of cognitive functioning, visual processing ability, and other considerations such as the communicative environment in which the system will be used. Based on the data, a system is prescribed with appropriate symbols (Clark/Woodcock 1976; Carlson 1984), vocabulary size, access mechanism, and output ability. Cook/Coleman (1987), Shane/Bashir (1980), Vanderheiden/Harris-Vanderheiden (1976) and others have discussed matching nonspeech communication systems to children.

As with other treatments for dysarthria, little data have been published indicating the benefits of providing nonspeech communication systems to nonspeaking children. Although several authors have presented case studies (Buzolich 1987; Glennen/Calculator 1985), the need for controlled experimental research in this area is apparent. Culp presents a review of outcome research, indicating that there is a high percentage of communication board rejection and a low percentage of communication board use among nonspeaking individuals and suggests specific directions for research (Culp 1987). Research evaluating the usefulness of specific alternative or augmentative communication systems and treatment methods for facilitating optimum use of these systems is badly needed.

6. Summary

This chapter has reviewed developmental dysarthria and has highlighted significant needs for research. Specifically, needs for further research to identify neuropathological disorders, other than cerebral palsy, that result in dysarthria and to delineate types of dysarthria that can be reliably identified in children have been highlighted. For example, children presenting with a variety of disorders, such as Reye's syndrome, need to be studied using neuroimaging techniques to document the site and extent of brain damage, and physiological, acoustic, and perceptual techniques to assess speech production deficit patterns. With data such as these, we may begin to better understand the relationship between neuropathology and speech pathology in brain damaged children.

This chapter also has pointed out the need for better assessment tools. For dysarthria, standardized tests designed to evaluate the various subsystems of speech production are needed. In addition, data regarding dysarthric and normal children's performance on many physiologic and acoustic measures are needed.

Finally, this chapter has pointed out that a paucity of research exists which has evaluated the effects of treatment for developmental dysarthria. We strongly suggest that single-subject experimental research designs be used to demonstrate the effects of treatment strategies summarized in this chapter. The advantages of using these designs in clinical research and guidelines for using them have been discussed in several sources including Connell/Thompson (1986), Kearns (1986), McReynolds/Kearns (1983) and, McReynolds/Thompson (1986). Clinicians and researchers working with children with developmental dysarthria are encouraged to consult these sources and to begin gathering scientific data to document the effects of treatment for these disorders.

7. References

Alexander, R. (1987). Oral-motor treatment for infants and young children with cerebral palsy. *Seminars in Speech and Language*, *8*, 87–100.

Ansel, B. M. & Kent, R. D. (1986). Acoustic predictors of speech intelligibility in cerebral palsied-dysarthric adults. Paper presented to the third biennial Clinical Dysarthria Conference, Tucson, AZ.

Aronson, A. E. (1985). *Clinical voice disorders*. An interdisciplinary approach. 2nd Edition. New York: Thieme-Stratton.

Bankson, N. & Byrne, M. (1972). The effect of a timed correct sound production task on carryover. *Journal of Speech and Hearing Research*, *15*, 160–168.

Bernthal, J. E. & Bankson, N. W. (1981). *Articulation disorders*. Englewood Cliffs, NJ: Prentice-Hall.

Berry, M. F. & Eisenson, J. (1956). *Speech disorders: Principles and practices of therapy*. New York: Appleton-Century-Crofts.

Bobath, B. (1967). The very early treatment of cerebral palsy. *Development Medicine Child Neurology*, *9*, 373–391.

Bobath, B. (1971 a). *Abnormal postural reflex activity caused by brain lesions*. London: William Heinemann Medical Books.

Bobath, B. (1971 b). Motor development: its effect on general development and application to the treatment of cerebral palsy. *Physiotherapy*, *57*, 526–532.

Bobath, K. & Bobath, B. (1964). The facilitation of normal postural reactions and movements in the treatment of cerebral palsy. *Physiotherapy*, *50*, 246–262.

Bobath, K. (1966). *The motor deficit in patients with cerebral palsy.* London: William Heinemann Medical Books.

Bobath, K. (1971). The normal postural reflex mechanism and its deviation in children with cerebral palsy. *Physiotherapy, 57,* 515–525.

Bobath, K. & Bobath, B. (1972). Cerebral palsy: Part 1: diagnosis and assessment of cerebral palsy. Part 2: the neurodevelopmental approach to treatment. In P. H. Pearson, C. E. Williams (Eds.), *Physical therapy services in the developmental disabilities.* Spingfield, IL: CC Thomas.

Bobath, K. (1976). *The motor deficit in patients with cerebral palsy.* England: Spasties International Medical Publications.

Boone, D. R. (1977). *The voice and voice therapy.* 2nd Edition. Englewood Cliffs, NJ: Prentice-Hall.

Buzolich, M. J. (1987). Children in transition: implementing augmentative communication systems with severely speech-handicapped children. *Seminars in Speech and Language, 8,* 199–213.

Byrne, M. C. (1959). Speech and language development of athetoid and spastic children. *Journal of Speech and Hearing Research, 24,* 231–240.

Carlson, F. (1984). *PicSyms categorical dictionary.* Lawrence, KS: Baggeboda Press.

Clark, C. R. & Woodcock, R. W. (1976). Graphic systems of communication. In L. Lloyd (Ed.), *Communication assessment and intervention strategies 549.* Baltimore: University Park Press.

Clark, W. M. & Hoops, H. R. (1980). Predictive measures of speech proficiency in cerebral palsied speakers. *Journal of Communication Disorders, 13,* 385–394.

Cole, R. M. (1971). Direct muscle training for the improvement of velopharyngeal function. In W. C. Grabb, S. W. Rosenstein, & K. R. Bzoch (Eds.), *Cleft lip and palate.* Boston: Little, Brown.

Compton, A. (1975). Generative studies of children's phonological disorders: A strategy of therapy. In S. Singh (Ed.), *Measurements in hearing, speech, and language,* Baltimore: University Park Press.

Connell, P. J. & Thompson, C. K. (1986). Flexibility of single-subject experimental designs. Part III. Using flexibility to design or modify experiments. *Journal of Speech and Hearing Disorders, 51,* 214–225.

Cook, A. M. & Coleman, C. L. (1987). Selecting augmentative communication systems by matching client skills and needs to system characteristics. *Seminars in Speech and Language, 8,* 153–167.

Crothers, B. & Paine, R. S. (1959). *The natural history of cerebral palsy.* Cambridge, MA: Howard University Press.

Culp, P. M. (1987). Outcome measurement: the impact of communication augmentation. *Seminars in Speech and Language, 8,* 169–181.

Darley, F. L., Aronson, A. E. & Brown, J. R. (1969 a). Differential diagnostic patterns of dysarthria. *Journal of Speech and Hearing Research, 12,* 246–269.

Darley, F. L., Aronson, A. E., & Brown, J. R. (1969 b). Clusters of deviant speech dimensions in the dysarthrias. *Journal of Speech and Hearing Research, 12,* 462–478.

Darley, F. L., Aronson, A. E., & Brown, J. R. (1975). *Motor speech disorders.* Philadelphia: WB Saunders.

Davis, L. (1978). Pre-speech. In F. D. Connor, G. G. Williamson, J. M. Siepp (Eds.), *Program guide for infants and toddlers with neuromotor and other developmental disabilities.* New York: Teachers College Press.

Davis, L. F. (1982): Respiration and phonation in cerebral palsy: A developmental model. *Seminars in Speech and Language, 8,* 101–106.

Dawes, V. A. (1958). Palatal dysfunction in cerebral palsy. Unpublished paper presented at American Speech and Hearing Association Convention, New York.

Dorland's illustrated medical dictionary. 26th Edition, Philadelphia: WB Saunders.

Dworkin, J. & Culatta, T. (1980). *D-COME: Dworkin Culatta Oral Mechanism Examination.* Nicholasville, KY: Edgewood Press.

Farmer, A. (1980). Voice onset time production in cerebral palsied speakers. *Folia Phoniatrica, 32,* 267–273.

Ferrier, L. J. & Shane, H. C. (1987). Computer-based communication aids for the nonspeaking child with cerebral palsy. *Seminars in Speech and Language, 8,* 107–122.

Folkins, J. & Moon, J. (1990). Approaches to the study of speech production. In J. Bardach & H. L. Morris (Eds.), *Multidisciplinary management of cleft lip and palate.* 707–716. Philadelphia, PA: W. B. Saunders Company.

Froeschels, F. (1952). Chewing method as therapy. *Archives of Otolaryngology, 61,* 427–434.

Froeschels, F., Kastein, S., & Weiss, D. A. (1955). A method of therapy for paralytic conditions for the mechanisms of phonation, respiration, and glutination. *Journal of Speech and Hearing Disorders, 20,* 365–370.

Glennen, S. L. & Calculator, S. N. (1985). Training functional communication board use: a pragmatic approach. *Augmentative and Alternative Communication, 1,* 134–142.

Hardy, J. C. (1983). *Cerebral palsy.* Englewood Cliffs, NJ: Prentice-Hall.

Hixon, T. J. & Hardy, J. C. (1964). Restricted motility of the speech articulators in cerebral palsy. *Journal of Speech and Hearing Research, 29,* 293–306.

Hixon, T., Bless, D., & Netsell, R. (1976). A new technique for measuring velopharyngeal orifice area during sustained vowel production: an application of aerodynamic forced oscillation principles. *Journal of Speech and Hearing Research*, *19*, 601–607.

Hixon, T., Mead, J., & Goldman, M. (1976). Dynamics of chest wall during speech production: Function of the thorax, rib cage, diaphragm, and abdomen. *Journal of Speech and Hearing Research*, *19*, 297–356.

Hixon, T. J., Hawley, J. L., & Wilson, K. J. (1982). An around-the-house device for the clinical determination of respiratory driving pressure: a note on making simple even simpler. *Journal of Speech and Hearing Disorders*, *47*, 413–415.

Hodson, B. (1980). *The assessment of phonological processes*. Danville, IL: Interstate Press.

Holtzhauer, F. J., Campbell, R. J., Hall, L. J., & Halpin, T. J. (1986). Reye's syndrome: an epidemiologic analysis of mild disease. *American Journal of Disorderd Children*, *140*, 1231–1236.

Ingram, D. (1976). *Phonological disability in children*. New York: American Elsevier.

Ingram, T. T. S. (1962). Clinical significance of the infantile feeding reflexes. *Development Medicine Child Neurology*, *4*, 159–169.

Irwin, O. C. (1968). Correct status of vowels and consonants in the speech of children with cerebral palsy as measured by an integrated test. *Cerebral Palsy Journal*, *29*, 9–12.

Jacobsen, E. (1976). *You must relax*. 5th Edition. New York: McGraw-Hill.

Jaffe, M. B. (1984). Neurological impairment of speech production: Assessment and treatment. In J. Costello (Ed.), *Speech disorders in children*. 157 ff. San Diego: College Hill Press.

Kamalashile, J. (1975). Speech problems in cerebral palsy children. *Language Speech*, *18*, 158–165.

Kearns, K. P. (1986). Flexibility of single-subject experimental designs. Part II. Design selection and arrangement of experimental phases. *Journal of Speech and Hearing Disorders*, *51*, 204–213.

Kent, R. D. & Netsell, R. (1978). Articulatory abnormalities in athetoid cerebral palsy. *Journal of Speech and Hearing Research*, *43*, 353–373.

Kent, R. D., Kent, J. F., & Rosenbek, J. C. (1987). Maximal performance tests of speech production. *Journal of Speech and Hearing Disorders*, *52*, 367–387.

Kent, R. D., Netsell, R., & Bauer, L. L. (1975). Cineradiographic assessment of articulatory mobility in the dysarthrias. *Journal of Speech and Hearing Research*, 40, 467–480.

Kent, R. D. & Rosenbek, J. C. (1983). Acoustic patterns of apraxia of speech. *Journal of Speech and Hearing Research*, *26*, 231–249.

Kraus, J. F., Fife, D., Cox, P., Ramstein, K., & Conroy, C. (1986). Incidence, severity and external causes of pediatric brain injury. *American Journal of Disordered Children*, *140*, 687–693.

Leith, W. & Steer, M. (1958). Comparison of judged speech characteristics of athetoids and spastics. *Cerebral Palsy Review*, *19*, 15–19.

Little, W. J. (1843). Course of lectures on deformation of the human frame, lecture no. 8. *Lancet*, *1*, 318.

Love, R. J., Hagerman, E. L., & Taimi, E. G. (1980). Speech performance, dysphagia and oral reflexes in cerebral palsy. *Journal of Speech and Hearing Research*, *45*, 59–75.

Lubit, E. C. & Larsen, R. E. (1969). The Lubit palatal exercise: a preliminary report. *Cleft Palate Journal*, *6*, 120–133.

Luschei, E. S. (1991). Development of objective standards of nonspeech oral strength and performance. In C. A. Moore, K. Yorston, & D. Beukelman (Eds.), *Dysarthria and apraxia of speech: Perspectives on management 3–14*. Baltimore, MD: Paul H. Brookes Publishing Co.

McDonald, E. T. & Schultz, A. R. (1973). Communication boards for cerebral palsied children. *Journal of Speech and Hearing Disorders*, *38*, 73–88.

McDonald, E. T. & Chance, B. (1964). Cerebral palsy. Englewood Cliffs, NJ: Prentice-Hall.

McDonald, F. I. (1964). *Screening deep test of articulation*. Pittsburgh: Stemwix House.

McNeil, M. R., Weismer, G., Adams, S., & Mulligan, M. (1990). Oral structure nonspeech motor control in normal, dysarthric, aphasic, and apraxic speakers: Isometric force and static position control. *Journal of Speech and Hearing Research*, *33*, 255–268.

McReynolds, L. & Kearns, K. (1983). *Single-subject experimental designs in communicative disorders*. Baltimore: University Park Press.

McReynolds, L. V. & Thompson, C. K. (1986). Flexibility of single-subject experimental designs. Part I. Review of the basics of single-subject designs. *Journal of Speech and Hearing Disorders*, *51*, 194–203.

Minear, W. L. (1956). A classification of cerebral palsy. *Pediatrics*, *18*, 841–852.

Moon, J. & Smith, W. (1987). Application of cine CT technology to the assessment of velopharyngeal activity. *Cleft Palate Journal*, *24*, 226–232.

Morris, H., Spriestersbach, D. C., & Darley, F. L. (1961). An articulation test for assessing competency of velopharyngeal closure. *Journal of Speech and Hearing Research*, *4*, 48–55.

Morris, S. E. (1977). *Program guidelines for children with feeding problems*. Edison, NJ: Childcraft Education.

Morris, S. E. (1982). *The pre-speech assessment scale*. Clifton, N. J.: Preston.

Morris, S. E. (1987). Therapy for the child with cerebral palsy: interacting frameworks. *Seminars in Speech and Language*, *8*, 71–85.

Mysak, E. (1963). Dysarthria and orthopharyngeal reflexology: a review. *Journal of Speech and Hearing Disorders*, *28*, 252–260.

Mysak, E. (1980). *Neurospeech therapy for the cerebral palsied. A neuroevolutional approach*. 3rd Edition. New York: Teachers College Press.

Netsell, R. (1969). Evaluation of velopharyngeal function in dysarthria. *Journal of Speech and Hearing Research*, *34*, 113–122 (a).

Netsell, R. (1975). Instrumentation in the rehabilitation of dysarthria. Presented at the Veterans Administration Workshop on motor speech disorders, Madison, WI.

Netsell, R. & Hixon, T. J. (1978). A noninvasive method for clinically estimating subglottic air pressure. *Journal of Speech and Hearing Disorders*, *43*, 326–330.

Netsell, R., Lotz, W., & Shaughanessy, A. (1984). Laryngeal aerodynamics associated with selected voice disorders. *American Journal of Otolaryngology*, *5*, 397–403.

Nober, E. H. (1987). Assessment of auditory processing in cerebral palsy. *Seminars in Speech and Language*, *8*, 19–39.

Palmer, M. F. (1952). Speech therapy in cerebral palsy. *Journal of Pediatrics*, *40*, 514–524.

Parush, A. & Ostry, D. (1986). Superior lateral pharyngeal wall movements in speech. *Journal of the Acoustical Society of American*, *80*, 749–756.

Phelps, W. M. (1956). Classification of athetosis with special reference to the motor classification. *American Journal of Physical Medicine*, *35*, 24–31.

Platt, L. F., Andrews, G., Young, M., & Quin, P. T. (1980). Dysarthria of adult cerebral palsy. I. Intelligibility and articulatory impairment. *Journal of Speech and Hearing Research*, *23*, 28–38.

Platt, L. F., Andrews, G., Young, M., & Neilson, P. D. (1978). The measurement of speech impairment of adults with cerebral palsy. *Folia Phoniatrica*, *30*, 50–58.

Platt, L. F., Andrews, G., & Howie, P. M. (1980). Dysarthria of adult cerebral palsy. II. Phonemic analysis of articulation errors. *Journal of Speech and Hearing Research*, *23*, 41–55.

Powell, J. & McReynolds, L. (1969). A procedure for testing position generalization from articulation training. *Journal of Speech and Hearing Disorders*, *12*, 625–645.

Pruszewicz, A., Obrebowski, A., & Zgoralewicz, B. (1977). Selected problems in the hearing, voice, and speech disturbances in the extra-pyramidal form of cerebral palsy. *Folia Phoniatrica*, *29*, 302–310.

Putman, A. & Hixon, T. J. (1984). Respiratory kinematics in speakers with motor neuron disease. In M. McNeil, J. Rosenbek, & A. Aronson (Eds.), *The dysarthrias*. San Diego: College Hill.

Robin, D. A. & Eliason, M. (1991). Speech and prosodic problems in children with neurofibromatosis. In C. Moore, K. Yorkston & D. Beukelman (Eds.), Recent advances in motor speech disorders. 137–144. Baltimore: Paul H. Brooks.

Robin, D. A., Klouda, G., & Hug, L. (1991). Neurogenic disorders of prosody. In M. P. Cannito & D. Vogel (Eds.), *Treating disordered speech motor control: For clinicians by clinicians*. 241–271. Austin, TX: Pro-Ed.

Robin, D. A., Somodi, L., & Luschei, E. S. (1991). Measurement of tongue strength and endurance in normal and articulation disordered subjects. In C. Moore, K. Yorkston, & D. Beukelman (Eds.), *Dysarthria and apraxia of speech: Perspectives on management*. 173–184. Baltimore: Paul H. Brooks.

Rosenbek, J. C. & LaPointe, L. L. (1985). The dysarthrias: description, diagnosis, and treatment. In D. L. Johns (Ed.), *Clinical management of neurogenic communicative disorders*. 97–152. Boston: Little Brown.

Rutherford, B. (1944). A comprehensive study of loudness, pitch, rate, rhythm, and quality of children handicapped by cerebral palsy. *Journal of Speech and Hearing Disorders*, *9*, 263–271.

Schliesser, H. F. (1982). Alternate motion rates of the speech articulators in adults with cerebral palsy. *Folia Phoniatrica*, *34*, 258–264.

Schneider, E. & Shprintzen, R. (1980). A survey of speech pathologists: current trends in the diagnosis and management of velopharyngeal insufficiency. *Cleft Palate Journal*, *17*, 249–253.

Shane, H. C. & Bashir, A. S. (1980). Election criteria for the adoption of an augmentative communication system: preliminary consideration. *Journal of Speech and Hearing Disorders*, *45*, 408–414.

Sheppard, J. (1964). Cranio-oropharyngeal motor patterns in dysarthria associated with cerebral palsy. *Journal of Speech and Hearing Research*, *7*, 373–380.

Sheppard, J. (1987). Assessment of oral motor behaviors in cerebral palsy. *Seminars in Speech and Language*, *8*, 57–70.

Shprintzen, R. J., McCall, G. N., & Skolnick, M. D. (1975). A new therapeutic technique for the treatment of velopharyngeal incompetence. *Journal of Speech and Hearing Disorders*, *40*, 69–83.

Shriberg, L. & Kwiatkowski, J. (1980). *Natural process analysis*. New York: Jon Wiley & Sons.

Skolnick, M. L. (1969). Video velopharyngography in patients with nasal speech, with emphasis on lateral pharyngeal wall motion in velopharyngeal closure. *Radiology*, *93*, 747–755.

Somodi, L., Robin, D. A., & Luschei, E. S. (1990). An inexpensive means of assessing strength and fatigue. Paper presented at the Annual Meeting of the American Speech, Language, and Hearing Association, Seattle, Washington.

Thompson, C. K. & McReynolds, L. V. (1988). Neurogenic articulation disorders in children. In L. McReynolds & D. Yoder (Eds.), *Handbook of Speech-Language Pathology and Audiology* 548–591. Philadelphia: B. C. Decker, Inc.

Vanderheiden, G. C. & Harris-Vanderheiden, D. (1976). Communication techniques and aids for the nonvocal severly handicapped. In L. Lloyd (Ed.), *Communication assessment and intervention strategies*. 607–652. Baltimore: University Park Press.

Warren, D. & DeBois, A. (1964). A pressure-flow technique for measuring velopharyngeal orifice area during continuous speech. *Cleft Palate Journal, 1*, 52–71.

Weiner, F. (1978). *Phonological process analysis.* Baltimore: University Park Press.

Wilson, B. C. & Davidovicz, H. M. (1987). Neuropsychological assessment of the child with cerebral palsy. *Seminars in Speech and Language, 8*, 1–18.

Yorkston, K. M. & Beukelman, D. R. (1984). *Assessment of intelligibility of dysarthric speech.* Tigard, OR: CC Publications.

Yorkston, K. M., Beukelman, D. R., & Bell, K. R. (1988). *Clinical management of dysarthric speakers.* Boston: Little, Brown and Company.

Yules, R. B. & Chase, R. A. (1969). A training method for reduction of hypernasality in speech. *Plastic Reconstruction Surgery, 43*, 180–185.

Cynthia K. Thompson, Evanston, Illinois (USA)/
Donald A. Robin, Iowa City, Iowa (USA)

81. Effects of Congenital Malformations on Speech Development

1. Introduction

Congenital craniofacial malformations constitute "experiments of nature" (Pruzansky 1973) which offer as much of a challenge to the fields of linguistics and speech science as they do to surgery, speech pathology, dentistry, psychology and other clinical specialties. These experiments often include perturbations of the speech production mechanism due to aberrant supralaryngeal vocal tract structure, and are most informative to the linguistic researcher when the associated speech is organized by a normal cognitive system possessed of a mature or developing linguistic system. Such speakers permit investigation of (a) the plasticity of the speech production mechanism for the successful realization of a phonological system, and (b) the anatomical requirements for accomplishing this task. Children with congenitally aberrant supralaryngeal vocal tracts provide an opportunity to explore the adequacy of linguistic theories in accounting both for their speech production and for the role of speech production in language acquisition.

Only rarely do congenital craniofacial malformations affect single structures. Historically, even the relatively common defect of cleft palate was diagnosed and treated without recognition of either (a) alterations in the anatomy contiguous to the cleft, such as abnormalities of the cervical spine which can affect the configuration of the pharynx, or (b) the fact that over 50% of individuals born with clefts have associated malformations, many presenting with syndromes which alter both the vocal tract and the auditory system. In such conditions as Crouzon disease and Apert syndrome, the linguist is presented with multiple perturbations of the 'normal' mechanism.

2. Cleft Lip and Palate

2.1. Introduction

Comprehensive reviews of effects of cleft lip and palate on articulation, with exhaustive literature citations, are found in Bzoch (1989), McWilliams/Morris/Shelton (1990), and Peterson-Falzone (1988). Improved surgical techniques have markedly increased the number of children with clefts who demonstrate normal development of communication skills, and there has been a recent surge of studies on the optimum age of surgical closure of the palate to prevent abnormal speech development. Based on current data on motor development, speech-motor control, and sensorimotor feedback, Kemp-Fincham/Kuehn/Trost-Cardamone (1990) suggested that there seems to be a sensitive period for development of speech motor control, and consequently phonetic development, occurring between 4 and 6 months, and that it may therefore be important to close the palate prior to or during this period. Their theoretical discussion concurs with recent reports of better speech development in babies operated within the first six months of life as opposed to babies operated at later ages (e. g., Copeland 1996).

2.2. Prelinguistic Vocalizations and Early Childhood Studies

Several recent studies have investigated prelinguistic vocalizations and the early stages of phonetic and phonologic development in children with clefts. Philips/Kent (1984) discussed weakening of the second formant by nasalization in the cries of cleft infants, but reported acoustic evidence of rhythmically organized vocalizations in their reduplicated babbling, with reduced acoustic consonant-vowel contrasts. The authors hypothesized that the reduced contrast could cause delays in acquisition of the vowel system. Salas-Provance/Kuehn (1990) compared fundamental frequency, utterance duration and syllable duration in 4 cleft palate babies and and 4 non-cleft babies from 13 to 15 months. The cleft palate babies exhibited higher mean fundamental frequencies and a restricted range of F_0. Utterance durations were longer as compared to the non-cleft babies, but syllable durations were similar.

O'Gara/Logemann (1988; 1990) analyzed the vocalizations of 51 cleft palate babies periodically between 3 and 36 months of age. The babies were divided into an 'earlier closure/greater tissue group' whose clefts were closed prior to 12 months of age (average 9.3 months) and a "later closure/lesser tissue" group who were closed after 12 months (average 14.5 months). All of the babies showed a higher frequency of use of glottal and labial place features than of intraoral place features, with the earlier closure group showing greater use of intraoral place features than the later closure group and an earlier decrease in the use of glottal placements. At 6 months of age, none of the babies in either group showed the 'alveolar takeover' (predominance of alveolar productions over labials or velars) noted to occur in normal babies. The earlier closure group showed oral stop predominance at 18 to 19 months of age, while the later closure group never showed this predominance even through 36 months of age. Pharyngeal placements occurred only sporadically in both groups. Stops exceeded fricatives in both groups at all ages studied. Both groups showed a spurt in the use of nasal fricatives (discussed below) at 30 – 31 months of age, possibly related to the increased language requirements for fricative differentiation. The earlier closure group showed an early preference for front vowels, similar to normal babies, while the later closure group was slower to develop this preference. Both groups showed a consistent preference for mid-vowels rather than high or low vowels across all ages studied.

Philips (1989) reported that surgical closure of the cleft produced a spontaneous increase in what had been limited phonetic repertoires and a concomitant decrease in the use of atypical phonological processes in toddlers with clefts.

Grunwell/Russell (1987) analyzed the 'speech-like' pre- and postoperative vocalizations of 3 cleft palate infants operated between 11 and 14 months. None were using plosives other than 'glottal plosives' prior to surgery. Post-operatively, all were using some plosive articulations but only one was using apical/laminal plosives. The authors felt that the predominance of glottal contoids and velar approximants and a marked lack of bilabial and apical/laminal contoids replicated the results of O'Gara/Logemann (1988).

Lynch/Fox/Brookshire (1983) reported that two cleft palate toddlers between the ages of 2:5 and 3:1 produced a disproportionate number of words beginning with glides and nasals, despite the fact that both reportedly had adequate velopharyngeal closure. Estrem/Broen (1989) studied 5 cleft palate toddlers, only one of whom had adequate velopharyngeal closure at the time the data was collected. These children chose and produced more words beginning with velars and glottals, and also targeted and produced more words beginning with labials and targeted fewer words beginning with alveolars. In short, the children with clefts selected words that contained sounds they were capable of producing, and they selected and produced more posterior sounds and labial sounds than did normal toddlers.

Powers/Dunn/Erickson (1990) similarly found limited phonetic inventories in 4 males aged 3:2 to 3:11 with good velopharyngeal closure. Fricatives and affricates were rarely used, and stops were limited primarily to the word-initial position. Liquids and glides, other than /w/, were also infrequently used. Glottal and pharyngeal substitutions were rarely heard. The most common phonological processes were cluster reduction, liquid simplification, final consonant deletion and backing. The authors pointed out that not all of the articulatory problems could be explained solely on the basis of present or past structural deficits. Their results coincided with those of a longitudinal study by Van Demark/Morris/VandeHaar (1979), who found that their subjects were considerably behind normal children in mastering sounds that do not require velopharyngeal closure.

2.3. Analysis of Articulation

Analysis of articulation problems in children with clefts has been approached in two ways which could be broadly termed 'cause' and 'effect.' In the former, errors have been classified according to the apparent physical etiology, i. e., labial, dental, palatal, velopharyngeal. In the latter approach, errors have been categorized both according to the normal mode of production of affected phonemes, and according to the mode of production of replacement phonemes. When replacement phonemes are studied, the relationship to observations of early vocalizations becomes apparent.

Categorization of errors based on presumed structural bases becomes inexorably tied to categorization by place of production, the exception being the structural deviation viewed as the primary culprit in 'cleft palate speech,' namely the velopharyngeal mechanism. Labial defects typically have little impact (see Peterson-Falzone 1988). Dental/occlusal anomalies and reduced width of the maxillary arch may affect linguadental, linguoalveoar and linguapalatal phonemes, although these are typically recognizable even if distorted (Peterson-Falzone 1988) unless nasal air loss is predominant or the use of compensatory articulations obscures the phonemic contrasts. Abnormal tongue carriage and deviant lingual contacts in articulation were often viewed in the older literature as indicative of defective lingual structure or innervation; current investigators view these problems as secondary to abnormal structure and function of the velopharyngeal system. Inadequate velopharyngeal closure produces nasal air loss on consonants requiring the build-up of intraoral pressure, and hypernasal resonance on vowels and vocalic segments. Children in whom such inadequacy is present during acquisition of speech motor control often develop one or more maladaptive 'compensatory articulations' (discussed below) which may persist even after an adequate velopharyngeal system has been provided through surgical or prosthetic care.

Clearly the articulatory errors found in school-age children and adults with clefts are dictated in part by the adequacy of their early care and by the status of their oral and velopharyngeal systems at the time they are tested. Bearing in mind the consequent heterogeneity of subjects in studies of 'cleft palate speech,' these studies have repeatedly shown (1) more problems with fricatives and affricates than with plosives; (2) more problems on voiceless than voiced consonants, probably related to differences in aerodynamic requirements; (3) difficulty in suppressing voicing on voiceless consonants, interpreted as a result of leakage of air through the velopharyngeal port and a consequent inability to equalize air pressure above and below the vocal folds; (4) better production of single consonants than of the same consonants occurring in clusters, possibly reflecting the effect of impaired oral structures on the ability to make rapid articulatory adjustments; (5) substitution of either nasal phonemes or 'backed' productions, the latter being an apparent attempt to make use of the vocal airstream before it escapes through an open velopharyngeal port; (6) a tendency for articulation skills to continue to improve well past the age when these skills plateau in non-cleft children; and (7) a higher than normal frequency of problems with consonants not dependent upon adequate velopharyngeal closure. (For references, see McWilliams/Morris/Shelton 1990; Peterson-Falzone 1988; Philips/Kent 1984).

The literature on cleft palate is replete with descriptions of 'compensatory articulations.' Most of these seem to represent a sacrifice of the place feature for the retention of the manner feature (Trost 1981), although the child with severely disordered articulation may substitute glottal stops for continuants and even for liquids and glides, as well as for stops. Trost (1981) listed six compensatory articulations heard in English-speaking patients: glottal stops, pharyngeal stops, pharyngeal fricatives, velar fricatives, mid-dorsum palatal stops and 'posterior nasal fricatives,' the latter being Trost's term for what older literature often called 'nasal snort'. Trost also noted that some of these articulations, particularly glottal stops, can occur simultaneously with articulatory gestures in other parts of the vocal tract, an example being bilabial closure produced simultaneously with a glottal stop. Trost-Cardamone (1985) later added "pharyngeal affricates" to the list of compensatory articulations. There are references to palatal fricatives occurring as compensatory gestures (Philips/Kent 1984; McWilliams/Morris/Shelton 1990), and there is a growing body of evidence that many, if not most, of the productions classified as "pharyngeal" fricatives may actually be laryngeal fricatives (Kawano/Isshiki/Harita/Tanokushi 1985; Witzel/Brown/Laskin/Margar-Bacal 1990).

Philips/Kent (1984) pointed out that both pharyngeal and laryngeal articulations contribute to relatively low-frequency acoustic structure for consonants, with weakened or absent cues in some spectral regions and additional (abnormal) cues in other spectral regions. In severely nasalized speech, the low-frequency nasal formant may be nearly continuously present, the effect of which is to obscure segment boundaries normally marked by changes in source excitation, manner, or place of articulation. Basic acoustic feature contrasts that are weakened or eliminated by velopharyngeal inadequacy include periodic versus aperiodic energy source, nasal versus nonnasal resonance, occluded versus nonoccluded vocal tract, voiced versus voiceless excitation, and a variety of contrasts related to place of articulation.

2.4. Timing

One of the most productive areas of research in recent years has been that of timing or motor speech coordination in speakers with repaired clefts. Aerodynamic, spectrographic, radiographic and combined photodetector-nasopharygoscopic studies have shown differences not only between cleft and non-cleft speakers in timing of speech segment durations (D'Antoni 1982; Forner 1983), but also between cleft speakers with apparent velopharyngeal competency versus those with varying degrees of incompetency on various measures of timing and coordination of the action of the laryngeal and articulatory mechanisms (Karnell/Folkins/Morris 1985; Warren/Dalston/Morr et al. 1989). It has been conjectured that these differences may be attributable, in part, to an abnormally tight mechanical linkage between the tongue and velum in speakers with repaired clefts. Forner (1983) suggested that the backing of articulatory gestures may alter the aerodynamic interaction of labial, lingual, velar, and laryngeal valving. There is an obvious cause-effect question in considering compensatory articulations and the temporal differences shown in these studies: Do compensatory articulations cause the temporal disruptions, or do the demands of attempting to coordinate laryngeal, velopharyngeal, lingual and labial activity in the presence of velopharyngeal inadequacy cause the development of compensatory articulations?

3. Apert Syndrome and Crouzon Disease

Apert syndrome (acrocephalosyndactyly Type I) and Crouzon disease (craniofacial dysostosis) are two of a large family of syndromes of "premature craniofacial synostosis." In both Apert and Crouzon, premature closure of multiple sutures of the face and skull results in significant distortions of the craniofacial complex, including a malformed neurocranium and hypoplasia of the middle third of the face contributing to decreased space in the nasal, oral and pharyngeal airways. The hypoplastic maxilla is displaced posteriorly with respect to the mandible, and the oral airway is further crowded by (a) accumulations of soft tissue along the lateral palatine shelves, and (b) a long and thick soft palate (see Peterson-Falzone 1988, for a more complete description of the features of these syndromes and for references).

The supralaryngeal structures in subjects with these syndromes may be described in brief as (a) a normal-sized tongue in severely constricted oral and pharyngeal cavities, limiting the tongue's configurational possibilities within the vocal tract, and (b) malalignment of the labial and dental articulators due to the malocclusion. While the syndromes of Apert and Crouzon are rare, affected individuals have provided important information about the use of anomalous anatomy for achieving the vowel space of a language. It is not possible to obtain comparable information by perturbing a model of the vocal tract, because it is not possible to predict how the human cognitive system will respond to the perturbations.

Because speakers with Apert syndrome or Crouzon disease must learn the phonology of their language with a vocal tract potentially restricted in its ability to achieve articulatory maneuvers, a series of acoustic and perceptual studies was undertaken to explore the ability of such speakers to maintain the normal set of vowel contrasts in English. The results of these studies may be summarized as follows:

(1) A spectrographic study of the formant structure of vowels produced in a constant /hVd/ frame by six subjects with Apert syndrome and three with Crouzon disease (all adolescents with the exception of one unoperated Apert adult) showed a marked tendency for the F_1-F_2 plots to collapse into the "schwa" or neutral vowel region (Landahl/Peterson-Falzone/Lieberman 1978). However, within this compact acoustic vowel space, the vowel tokens showed spatial organization with regard to their expected phonetic categories. The intervowel formant relationships reflected the relationships seen in normal speakers (Peterson/Barney 1952): That is, /i/ /a/ and /u/ appeared to serve as point vowels for these subjects despite the constricted vowel tracts. However, divergences and convergences between mean formant values were either too great or too small. In no subject was there a normal distribution of mean formant values for any vowel. In summary, the general relational nature of the vowel space was realized, but the vowels were not as contrastive as in normal speakers.

(2) In an in-depth study of vowels produced in a wide variety of phonetic contexts by the unoperated Apert adult male speaker, Fourier analysis and Linear Predictive Coding showed the same compact vowel space when compared to the norms of Stevens/House (1963) (Landahl/Butler/Lieberman/Peterson-Falzone 1981). In all contexts, /u/ was the most deviant vowel.

(3) Two studies of the intelligibility of the words and the identifiability of the vowels produced by the unoperated Apert adult yielded similar results (Landahl/Robinson/Peterson-Falzone 1979; Varley/Landahl/Gould 1986). Linguistic students were able to identify the words used in the study described above at the 95% level and the vowels excised from those words at the 75% level. No /u/ tokens were correctly identified, corresponding to the highly aberrant formant structure. When the excised vowel tokens were submitted to a discriminant function analysis based on data produced by nine randomly selected adult male speakers from the Peterson/Barney study of 1952, the results indicated that the listeners did much better at vowel identification that did the discriminant function analysis, suggesting that the listeners used more information than F_1 and F_2 in figuring out the speaker's vowel system. The discriminant function analysis did not do significantly better when information on F_3 was added. Durations of two short/long pairs of vowels were studied in an attempt to determine whether durational cues were assisting the listeners in identifying the excised vowels, but the results were not definitive.

(4) A vocal tract modeling study (Landahl/Gould 1987) was undertaken to investigate whether it should be physically possible for the speaker used in the above studies to produce a different type of vowel space other than the one revealed in the acoustic measurements. The results were essentially negative, that is, the vowel space computed by the programmed model was even more compact than had been observed in the previous studies with the exception of the fact that the model indicated that the speaker should have been able to produce /a/ within the normal region. The authors concluded that it may have been more important for the speaker to keep his /a/ in proper relation to the rest of his vowel space than to imitate a 'normal' /a/.

(5) A developmental study of the F_1-F_2 vowel spaces of a male and a female child with Apert syndrome (Hasner/Landahl 1987) was undertaken for comparison to the vowel spaces of normal infants (Lieberman 1980). At approximately one year of age, the vowel spaces of the Apert children did not exhibit obvious abnormal qualities. The formant frequency ranges were consistent with those reported by Lieberman (1980). The authors felt that these findings were due to the fact that the physical development of the vocal tract in Apert children is not grossly different from that of normal children at this early stage. However, longitudinal data derived from the female Apert child indicated a compact vowel space by the age of two years.

In summary, this series of studies has indicated that the experiments of nature represented by Apert syndrome and Crouzon disease do not totally preclude the articulation of human language but do have deleterious effects on the production system for realizing the linguistic system in speech.

4. References

Bzoch, K. R. (1989). *Communicative Disorders Related to Cleft Lip and Palate* (3rd edition). Boston: College-Hill.

Copeland, M. (1990). The effects of very early palatal repair on speech. *British Journal of Plastic Surgery, 43*, 676–683.

D'Antonio, L. L. (1982). An investigation of speech timing in individuals with cleft palate. Unpublished doctoral dissertation, University of California, San Francisco.

Estrem, T. & Broen, P. A. (1989). Early speech production of children with cleft palate. *Journal of Speech and Hearing Research, 32*, 12–23.

Forner, L. L. (1983), Speech segment durations produced by five and six year old speakers with and without cleft palates. *Cleft Palate Journal, 20, 2*, 185–198.

Grunwell, P. & Russell, J. (1987). Vocalisations before and after cleft palate surgery: a pilot study. *British Journal of Disorders of Communication, 22*, 1–17.

Hasner, A. & Landahl, K. (1987). Development of vowel space in children with Apert syndrome. Unpublished manuscript, Department of Linguistics, The University of Chicago.

Karnell, M. P., Folkins, J., & Morris, H. L. (1985), Relationships between the perception of nasalization and speech movements in speakers with cleft palate. *Journal of Speech and Hearing Research, 28, 1*, 63–72.

Kawano, M., Isshiki, N., Harita, Y., & Tanokushi, F. (1985). Laryngeal fricative in cleft palate speech. *Acta Otolaryngologica*, Supplement *419*, 180–188.

Kemp-Fincham, S. I., Kuehn, D. P., & Trost-Cardamone, J. E. (1990). Speech development and the timing of primary palatoplasty. In J. Bardach & Hl. Morris (Eds.), *Multidisciplinary management of cleft lip and palate. 736–745*. Philadelphia: W. B. Saunders.

Landahl, K., Butler, J., Lieberman, P., & Peterson-Falzone, S. J. (1981). Fourier and linear predictive analyses of aberrant vowel formants. In B. J. Urban (Ed.), *Proceedings of the 18th Congress of the International Association of Logopedics and Phoniatrics*. 113–118.

Landahl, K. & Gould, H. (1987). Congenital malformation of the speech tract in humans and its developmental consequences. In R. J. Ruben, T. R. Van de Water, & E. W. Rubel (Eds.), *The Biology of Change in Otolaryngology. 131–149*. Amsterdam: Excerpta Medica.

Landahl, K., Peterson-Falzone, S., & Lieberman, P. (1978). Formant frequency patterns in anomalous supralaryngeal vocal tracts. Presented before the annual convention of the American Speech-Language-Hearing Association, San Francisco.

Landahl, K., Robinson, J., & Peterson-Falzone, S. (1979). Vowel durational cues in speakers exhibiting aberrant formant frequency patterns. Presented before the American Speech-Language-Hearing Association, Atlanta.

Lieberman, P. (1980). On the development of vowel production in young children. In G. Yeni-Komshian & D. Ferguson (Eds.), *Child Phonology – Volume I: Production. 113–142*. New York: Academic Press.

Lynch, J. L., Fox, D. R., & Brookshire, B. L. (1983). Phonological proficiency of two cleft palate toddlers with school-age follow-up. *Journal of Speech and Hearing Disorders, 48*, 274–285.

McWilliams, B. J., Morris, H. L., Shelton, R. L. (1990). *Cleft palate speech* (2nd edition). Toronto: B. C. Decker.

O'Gara, M. M. & Logemann, J. A. (1990). Early speech development in cleft palate babies. In J. Bardach & H. Morris (Eds.), *Multidisciplinary management of cleft lip and palate. 717–721*. Saunders, 1990.

O'Gara, M. M. & Logemann, J. A. (1988). Phonetic analyses of the speech development of babies with cleft palate. *Cleft Palate Journal, 25, 2*, 122–134.

Peterson, G. E. & Barney, H. L. (1952). Control methods used in a study of the vowels. *Journal of the Acoustical Society of America, 24*, 175–184.

Peterson-Falzone, S. J. (1988). Speech disorders related to craniofacial structural defects, Part 2. In N. J. Lass, L. V. McReynolds, J. L. Northern, & D. E. Yoder (Eds.), *Handbook of speech-language pathology and audiology. 477–547*. Toronto: B. C. Decker.

Philips, B. J. & Kent, R. D. (1984). Acoustic-phonetic descriptions of speech production in speakers with cleft palate and other velopharyngeal disorders. In NJ. Lass (Ed.), *Speech and language: Advances in basic research and practice*, Volume 11. *113–168*. New York: Academic Press, 1984.

Philips, B. J. (1989). Phonological development of children with palatal clefts (abstract). *Folia Phoniatrica, 41*, 203–204.

Powers, G. R., Dunn, C., & Erickson, C. B. (1990). Speech analyses of four children with repaired cleft palates. *Journal of Speech and Hearing Disorders, 55*, 542–549.

Pruzanksy, S. (1973). Clinical investigation of the experiments of nature. *ASHA Reports, 8*, 63–94.

Salas-Provance, M. & Kuehn, D. P. (1990). Nonsegmental characteristics in prespeech utterances of babies with cleft palate. Presented before the American Speech-Language-Hearing Association, Seattle.

Stevens, K. & House, A. (1963). Perturbation of vowel articulation by consonantal context: an acoustical study. *Journal of Speech and Hearing Research, 6*, 111–128.

Trost, J. E. (1981). Articulatory additions to to the classical description of the speech of persons with cleft palate. *Cleft Palate Journal, 18, 3*, 193–203.

Trost-Cardamone, J. E. (1985). From diagnosis to treatment: Speech remediation for persons with cleft palates and related velopharyngeal disorders. Short course presented before the California Speech-Language-Hearing Association, Anaheim.

Van Demark, D. R., Morris, H. L., & Vandehaar, C. (1979). Patterns of articulation abilities in speakers with cleft palate. *Cleft Palate Journal, 16, 3*, 230–239.

Varley, D., Landahl, K., & Gould, H. (1986). Perceptual categorization of a compressed vowel space. *Journal of the Acoustical Society of America, 79*, Suppl. No. 1, 58.

Warren, D. W., Dalston, R. M., Morr, K. E., Hairfield, W. M., & Smith, L. R. (1989). The speech regulating system: Temporal and aerodynamic responses to velopharyngeal inadequacy. *Journal of Speech and Hearing Research, 32*, 566–575.

Witzel, M. A., Brown, S., Laskin, R. L., & Margar-Bacal, F. (1990). The laryngeal fricative in cleft palate speech: Description and diagnosis. Presented before the American Speech-Language-Hearing Association, Seattle.

Sally J. Peterson-Falzone, San Francisco, California (USA)/
Karen L. Landahl, Chicago, Illinois (USA)

82. Stuttering: Physiological Correlates and Theoretical Perspectives

1. Introduction

The purpose of this chapter is to summarize the results of investigations of the physiological bases of stuttering. Many different methodologies have been employed to assess the physiological correlates of stuttering, and the different methodologies often were motivated by distinct theories of the etiology of the disorder. Thus, this review will also discuss theoretical perspectives in relation to the physiological findings.

Stuttering is a disorder of speech with a prevalence estimated to be 1% of the world's population (Bloodstein 1981; Van Riper 1982). It is a disorder in the rhythm or natural flow of speech "... in which the individual knows precisely what he wishes to say, but at the same time is unable to say it ..." (WHO 1977, 202). The disruptions of speech or disfluencies that characterize stuttering are easily recognized by the naive listener. There are sound and syllable repetitions, silent pauses, voiced pauses, and interjections that disrupt the flow of speech.

The normal flow of sound production is the acoustic consequence of movement, which in turn is the result of an organized neural input to the motoneuron pools that innervate the muscles involved in speech. Speech requires coordinated activity in many different muscles, including orofacial, laryngeal, and respiratory muscles. Thus an organized synaptic input must be distributed over a large number of muscles, so that appropriate forces are developed in the appropriate muscles at the right time. A universal symptom of stuttering is that the distributed input to muscles is disrupted, and inputs appropriate for the continuation of speech are not generated or are overtaken by other sources of neural drive.

What are the factors that produce breakdowns in speech motor processes in stuttering? Historically, theories of the etiology of stuttering emphasized a single aspect of the disorder as the major explanatory variable. For example, stuttering has been explained as arising primarily from faulty laryngeal control (Kenyon 1943), the negative evaluations of children's speech by their parents (Johnson 1942), or as a learned anticipatory struggle response (Bloodstein 1981). Theories of stuttering proliferated, and battles were waged in the stuttering literature with a major division between those who believed in a 'physiological cause' and those who believed stuttering was 'entirely learned'. The futility of this debate has been recognized in recent years (e. g., Smith/Weber 1988), and evidence has accumulated that there is a genetic component underlying the development of stuttering (e. g., Howie 1981) and that environmental factors and learning also play important roles in the development and maintenance of disfluent behavior (e. g., Bloodstein 1981).

Currently on the theoretical front, many authors argue that single factor approaches cannot provide a complete explanation of stuttering, because many factors converge to produce the conditions we associate with this disorder. Thus, several multifactorial models of stuttering (e. g., Starkweather 1987; Wall/Meyers 1984; Van Riper 1982; Zimmermann/Smith/Hanley 1981) have appeared and are receiving widespread acceptance. Central to these models are the assumptions that (1) many different types of variables play a role in the development and maintenance of stuttering, and (2) there is considerable variation between individuals who stutter on the relative importance of each factor in the development of the disorder.

The present review of physiological factors correlated with stuttering is grounded in the integrative, multifactorial approach to stuttering that we have described in earlier papers (Zimmermann 1980 c; Zimmermann/Smith/Hanley 1981; Smith 1990). A key aspect of this multifactorial framework is that it recognizes that disruption of speech motor performance is a universal symptom of the disorder. Therefore, the long list of complex factors involved in the etiology of the disorder, e. g., psychosocial, linguistic, and cognitive factors, can be viewed as ultimately either directly or indirectly interacting with speech motor processes to produce the kinds of breakdowns characteristic of stuttering. This approach recognizes that many different kinds of measurements will contribute to our attempt to understand stuttering, e. g., sociocultural, behavioral, acoustic, and physiological measures, but that all of these levels of measurement must be integrated into a comprehensive explanation of stuttering. This approach leads us to examine linkages between different levels of measurement and to determine how various factors contribute to a disruption in speech motor processes.

For example, experimental results suggest that stuttering is correlated with linguistic complexity (Bloodstein 1981). Under the proposed multifactorial model, the challenge is to determine the link between linguistic complexity and speech motor breakdown. In summary, we believe that a theory of stuttering must be a multifactorial theory with integration of these factors accomplished through an understanding of their effects on the operation of neuromotor systems.

2. Physiological Correlates of Stuttering

Cognitive, emotional, and linguistic processes influence the planning and execution of speech motor behavior. Investigations exploring the physiological bases of stuttering have employed diverse methodologies to assess central and peripheral physiological processes underlying the various stages of speech production, including preparation and execution. In addition, a number of investigations of the physiological bases of stuttering have assessed the status of sensorimotor, autonomic, and other systems in stutterers during performance of a wide range of nonverbal motor tasks. A complete review of this literature is beyond the scope of this chapter. Therefore the following sections will outline major themes that have emerged in the search for the physiological correlates of stuttering.

2.1. Measures of CNS Function

The Orton-Travis theory that stuttering develops because normal patterns of cerebral dominance are absent (Orton 1928; Travis 1931) has had a major impact on investigations of central nervous system (CNS) processes and stuttering. Thus, investigations have focused on the search for differences in hemispheric laterality between stutterers and normal speakers. Electroencephalography (EEG) has been widely used to study human brain function. Early EEG investigations, using necessarily crude methods of data analysis (for example, the percent time of alpha), reported left/right alpha ratios that seemed to support the Orton-Travis theory (e. g., Douglass 1943). In later studies, signal averaging was used to study the laterality of event-related potentials of the brain. By measuring slow changes in the EEG, specifically the contingent negative variation (CNV), investigators attempted to obtain an index of cognitive, linguistic, and motor planning processes preceding speech production in stutterers. Results of these studies (Zimmermann/Knott 1974; Pinsky/McAdam 1980) are not consistent. Zimmermann/Knott reported that a majority of stutterers showed larger shifts over the right hemisphere preceding speech production, while the stutterers tested by Pinsky/McAdam showed the normal pattern of a larger CNV over the left hemisphere preceding speech.

Other methodologies for assessing CNS function also have produced mixed results.

Andrews/Quinn/Sorby (1972) found that three adult stutterers showed normal unilateral left cerebral dominance for speech on the intracarotid sodium amytal test. Some investigations reporting tests of dichotic listening on groups of stutterers and nonstutterers have yielded significant group differences in ear advantage, while other studies report no group differences (e. g., Curry/Gregory 1969; Dorman/Porter 1975).

In summary, there may be some deficit in the central nervous system processes subserving speech production and associated functions in individuals who stutter. The proposal that such a deficit may be found does not imply that the deficit(s) must be the same in all individuals who stutter, nor does it imply that the differences between stutterers and nonstutterers are causally related to stuttering. At this point, however, we simply do not know anything about the precise nature of these deficits nor of the significance of the differences that are reported. Our lack of understanding in this area is no doubt due to the difficulty of studying brain functions in intact, behaving human subjects and the limits of current theories of brain-behavior relationships. Advances in technologies for studying human brain functions, for example, quantitative analysis of EEG and SPECT (single photon emission computed tomography), may aid in understanding stuttering if the measures can be integrated into a general theoretical account of brain-behavior relationships.

2.2. Electromyography (EMG)

In general, investigations of muscle activity and movement (reviewed in section 2.3 below) in stutterers have been undertaken with the goal of describing abnormal activity and have not been explicitly theory driven. Activity of articulatory and laryngeal muscles has been recorded with surface and indwelling electrodes during speech production in stutterers. These investigations report that stuttered speech is characterized by excessive activity in articulatory and laryngeal muscles, oscillations of muscle activity at frequencies characteristic of normal tremor, and coactivation of antagonistic orofacial and laryngeal muscles (e. g., Fibiger 1971; Freeman/Ushijima 1978; Kalotkin/Manschreck/O'Brien 1979; McClean/Goldsmith/Cerf 1984; Smith 1989). These descriptions are widely accepted, but there are many issues that remain to be resolved before the significance of these observations to a theory of stuttering can be understood.

For example, of the investigations reporting excessive muscle activity during disfluent behavior, only two include a quantitative analysis of the EMG data (Freeman/Ushijima 1978; Kalotkin/Manschreck/O'Brien 1979); and Kalotkin/Manschreck/O'Brien failed to normalize values for comparisons across subjects. In a recent study by Smith/Denny/Wood (1991), EMG amplitude was found on average to be larger during 500 ms intervals of perceptually fluent speech following the disfluencies compared to the EMG during the disfluencies. Thus, despite the widespread impression that stuttering is associated with abnormally high levels of muscle activity, the degree, distribution across muscles, time course, and consistency across subjects of excessive muscle activity related to stuttering is not well established.

It is well established that, in stutterers, abnormal oscillations of muscle activity occur. This finding has been replicated in a number of laboratories and has led to specific hypotheses concerning the neural sources producing motor instability in stuttering (e. g., Smith 1989). The third result, listed above, co-activation of antagonistic muscles has also been a consistent finding, however the interpretation of this result often has been confused by the erroneous assumption that co-activation of antagonistic muscles is always an abnormal pattern of muscle activation. In fact, depending on the task demands, co-activation can be a preferred strategy of recruitment of muscles. For example, Smith (1989) applied a cross-correlational analysis and reported coactivation of antagonistic muscles of the jaw during disfluencies of stutterers, but this was not abnormal. The normal subjects tested demonstrated coactivation of these muscles to a similar degree during speech.

The existing EMG data on stuttering provide some clues concerning the nature of aberrant inputs to motoneuron pools innervating muscles involved in speech production. The next step is to apply more detailed methods of signal analysis to test specific hypotheses about (1) the time course of muscle activity in fluent and disfluent speech, (2) the sources in the nervous system that generate the aberrant activity, and (3) the age at which these abnormal aspects of speech motor activity develop.

2.3. Kinematic Events

Measurement of kinematic events has indicated that stuttering is characterized by abnormal chest wall movements, including increased durations of expiratory and inspiratory phases, halted movements, unusual, oppositional movements of the abdomen and rib cage, speaking on inspiration, and chest wall tremor (Fossler 1930; Seth 1934); abnormal or 'nonpredicted' positioning of the vocal folds (Conture/McCall/Brewer 1977); tonic positioning, oscillatory movements of the articulators, and a disruption in inter-articulator timing (McClean/Goldsmith/Cerf 1984, Zimmermann 1980 a; b). Caruso/Abbs/Gracco (1988) reported that normal speakers showed an invariant sequence of peak velocities of upper lip, lower lip, and jaw movements measured for a single speech gesture within a single utterance, while stutterers' fluent productions of the utterance showed reversals of this pattern. From this finding they speculated about the role of the supplementary motor area in stuttering. McClean/Kroll/Loftus (1990) replicated the methods of Caruso/Abbs/Gracco, but did not find that normal speakers demonstrated invariant velocity sequencing of these structures. For stutterers, McClean et al. reported that velocity sequencing was strongly dependent on the therapeutic history of the subject.

Kinematic analysis of articulatory events in stutterers' fluent and disfluent speech produced the important observation that even the perceptually fluent speech of stutterers is characterized by abnormal sensorimotor organization (Zimmermann 1980 a; b). This observation has been confirmed in a number of subsequent studies (e. g., Peters/Boves 1988). This is a significant result, because it led to the insight that, although perceptual judgments of stutterers' speech are dichotomous (e. g., fluent or disfluent), the processes underlying stuttering are continuous.

2.4. Measures of Autonomic Activity

In our multifactorial theoretical approach to stuttering and in many other theories of stuttering (e. g., Brutten/Shoemaker 1967), a significant factor thought to contribute to speech motor breakdown is the emotional state of the speaker. Scientists have long recognized that the physiological changes underlying emotional experience, for example, changes in heart rate, blood flow, and sweating, are mediated by activity of the autonomic nervous system (ANS). Furthermore, autonomic processes are integrated with somatic sensorimotor processes at many levels of the nervous system (Pick 1970). Therefore, investigation of ANS activity may provide important clues as to how the emotional state of the individual affects speech motor processing.

A major goal of studies of ANS activity in stuttering has been to determine if stutterers have higher levels of autonomic arousal compared to normal speakers. ANS function has been assessed in stuttering by measuring heart rate, blood flow, blood pressure, electrodermal activity, and biochemical assays. In many early studies only one autonomic measure was used, while later studies have used multiple measures, making them more sensitive to group differences and better able to distinguish sympathetic and parasympathetic influences. Results of earlier investigations produced mixed results concerning the role of the ANS in stuttering (see Weber/Smith (1990) for a review).

In contrast, two recent studies employing large numbers of subjects and simultaneous measurement of a variety of autonomic indices have produced consistent findings. Peters/Hulstijn (1984) recorded heart rate, pulse volume, and tonic and phasic skin conductance while 24 stutterers and 24 nonstutterers performed tasks including writing, mirror writing, responding to intelligence test items, silent reading, and spontaneous speech. They found no between-group differences on any autonomic measure, but they reported that for both groups, speaking was associated with relatively large increases in autonomic arousal when compared to that observed in the other tasks. Weber/Smith (1990) recorded tonic and phasic skin conductance, peripheral blood flow, and heart rate in 19 stutterers and 19 normal speakers with matched group distributions of age, sex, and educational background. Autonomic measures were recorded during jaw movements, a strenuous breath-holding task, reading, and spontaneous speech. Weber/Smith reported no group differences on any of the measures recorded for any of the tasks. They, like Peters/Hulstijn, found that speaking, for both groups of subjects, was characterized by high levels of autonomic arousal. Weber/Smith further analyzed the fluent and disfluent utterances within the stuttering subjects and found that increased sympathetic arousal was correlated with the occurrence and severity of disfluent speech.

The results reported by Peters/Hulstijn and Weber/Smith are remarkably similar. They suggest the following conclusions regarding autonomic activity and stuttering: (1) stutterers, even when engaged in disfluent speech, do not experience autonomic arousal that is outside the range of that experienced during speech by nonstutterers; (2) for both stutterers and nonstutterers, speaking is characterized by large increases in sympathetic arousal, even when compared to a strenuous physical maneuver or difficult cognitive tasks; and (3) within individuals who stutter, higher levels of sympathetic arousal tend to co-occur with speech that is perceived as disfluent. In view of these conclusions, research now needs to be directed at discovering if increased sympathetic arousal in stutterers is correlated with specific characteristics of instability in speech motor processes.

2.5. General Motor Performance in Stutterers and Nonstutterers

Many different theories of stuttering have provided impetus for investigations comparing stutterers' and nonstutterers' performance, usually by measuring aspects of timing control, on various motor tasks. The Orton-Travis theory of inadequate cerebral dominance in stuttering triggered numerous investigations by researchers in the 1920's and 30's. In many of these studies rapid, repetitive movements or reproduction of a temporal pattern by subjects moving hands, oral structures, and/or the chest wall were analyzed. In many cases, stutterers were found to perform more poorly (e. g., Blackburn 1931; Hunsley 1937), while in other studies, no differences were found (e. g., Cross 1936; Seth 1934). Recent investigations suggest that stutterer/nonstutterer differences may emerge more consistently when the task requires that the subjects generate (rather than reproduce) a rhythm (e. g., Brown/Zimmermann/Linville/Hegmann 1990), or that he plan and execute movements that involve complex temporal and spatial coding (e. g., Webster 1989).

The idea that stuttering is primarily the result of a deficit in control of the larynx led investigators to test whether stutterers differed from nonstutterers in voicing control. A study by Adams/Hayden (1976), reporting that stutterers were slower than nonstutterers in phonating the vowel /a/ in response to an auditory cue, was the first in a long series of reaction time (RT) investigations of stuttering in the 1970's and 80's. These investigations have included tests of auditory-voice reaction time, visual-voice reaction time, and tests of manual reaction time. The results of the many RT studies cannot be summarized in detail, but in general, they strongly suggest that stutterers' have longer RT's than normal speakers when the response required is a speech utterance, but that group differences with manual or other nonspeech RT responses are less consistent (Peters/Hulstijn/Starkweather 1989).

Although often motivated by distinct theories of the 'cause' of stuttering, these studies address a question central to our understanding of the disorder: Is stuttering a speech disorder that arises in part from a generalized deficit in sensorimotor organization, or is it speech specific, with no relation to other motor skills? The positive findings of the studies reviewed in this section are adequate to sustain the viability of the hypothesis that stuttering is often accompanied by a generalized sensorimotor deficit. The precise nature of such a deficit remains to be discovered.

3. Conclusion

Historically, researchers and clinicians who work in the area of stuttering have been divided into a multitude of camps with almost no agreement on what the goals of theory should be or on what data should be regarded as significant. Physiological data were dismissed by those with a behavioral approach, and behavioral data were rarely incorporated into narrow, 'physiological' explanations of stuttering. In the past few years, some degree of consensus has emerged concerning both theory and data. Both researchers and clinicians are beginning to agree that a multifactorial approach to stuttering is essential and that both behavioral and physiological data must serve as the building blocks for an integrated, multifactorial theory.

From the present review of the physiological correlates of stuttering, it can be seen that our knowledge is far from complete. In particular, information on central nervous system processes in stuttering is lacking. Much more progress has been made in understanding autonomic nervous system activity in relation to stuttering. These data are congruent with the results of many investigations that, through administration of standard personality tests, failed to find a "stuttering personality" (Bloodstein 1981). Taken together, these results weigh strongly against the hypothesis that stutterers have generally high levels of emotional reactivity (e. g., Brutten/Shoemaker 1967). What emerges instead, is the view that stuttering is a disorder that arises when a variety of factors, including normal levels of emotional stress, impact on a sensorimotor system that is vulnerable to breakdown.

Acknowledgement: Preparation of this review was supported by grant DC00559 from the NIH's National Institute on Deafness and Other Communication Disorders.

4. References

Adams, M. & Hayden, P. (1976). The ability of stutterers and nonstutterers to initiate and terminate phonation during production of an isolated vowel. *Journal of Speech and Hearing Research, 19*, 290–296.

Andrews, G., Quinn, P., & Sorby, W. A. (1972). Stuttering: an investigation into cerebral dominance for speech. *Journal of Neurology, Neurosurgery, and Psychiatry, 35*, 414–418.

Blackburn, W. (1931). A study of the voluntary movements of the diaphragm, tongue, lips and jaw in stutterers and normal speakers. *Psychological Monograph, 41*, 1–13.

Bloodstein, O. (1981). *A Handbook on Stuttering*. Chicago: National Easter Seal Society.

Brown, C., Zimmermann, G., Linville, R., & Hegmann, J. (1990). Variations in self-paced behaviors in stutterers and nonstutterers. *Journal of Speech and Hearing Research, 33*, 317–323.

Brutten, E. & Shoemaker, D. (1967). *The Modification of Stuttering*. Englewood Cliffs: Prentice Hall.

Caruso, A., Abbs, J. & Gracco, V. (1988). Kinematic analysis of multiple movement coordination during speech in stutterers. *Brain, 111*, 439–455.

Conture, E., McCall, G., & Brewer, D. (1977). Laryngeal behavior during stuttering. *Journal of Speech and Hearing Research, 20*, 661–668.

Cross, H. (1936). The motor capacities of stutterers. *Archives of Speech, 1*, 112–132.

Curry, F. & Gregory, H. (1969). The performance of stutterers on dichotic listening tasks thought to reflect cerebral dominance. *Journal of Speech and Hearing Research, 12*, 73–82.

Dorman, M. & Porter, R. (1975). Hemispheric lateralization for speech perception in stutterers. *Cortex, 11*, 181–185.

Douglass, L. (1943). A study of bilaterally recorded electroencephalograms of adult stutterers. *Journal of Experimental Psychology, 32*, 247–265.

Fibiger, S. (1971). Stuttering explained as a physiological tremor. *Speech Transmission Lab-Quarterly Program & Strategy Report, 1–2*, 1–23.

Fossler, H. (1930). Disturbance in breathing during stuttering. *Psychological Monograph, 40*, 1–32.

Freeman, F. & Ushijima, T. (1978). Laryngeal muscle activity during stuttering. *Journal of Speech and Hearing Research, 21*, 538–562.

Howie, P. (1981). Concordance for stuttering in monozygotic and dizygotic twin pairs. *Journal of Speech and Hearing Disorders, 24*, 317–321.

Hunsley, Y. (1937). Disintegration in the speech musculature of stutterers during the production of nonvocal temporal pattern. *Psychological Monograph, 49*, 32–49.

Johnson, W. (1942). A study of the onset and development of stuttering. *Journal of Speech Disorders, 7*, 251–257.

Kenyon, E. (1943). The etiology of stammering: The psychophysiologic facts which concern the production of speech sounds and of stammering. *Journal of Speech Disorders, 8*, 347–348.

Kalotkin, M., Manschreck, R., & O'Brien, D. (1979). Electromyographic tension levels in stutterers and normal speakers. *Perceptual and Motor Skills, 49*, 109–110.

McClean, M., Goldsmith, H., & Cerf, A. (1984). Lower-lip EMG and displacement during bilabial disfluencies in adult stutterers. *Journal of Speech and Hearing Research, 27*, 342–349.

McClean, M., Kroll, R., & Loftus, N. (1990). Kinematic analysis of lip closure in stutterers' fluent speech. *Journal of Speech and Hearing Research, 33*, 155–160.

Orton, S. (1928). A physiological theory of reading disability and stuttering in children. *New England Journal of Medicine, 199*, 1046–1052.

Peters, H. & Boves, L. (1988). Coordination of aerodynamic and phonatory processes in fluent speech utterances of stutterers. *Journal of Speech and Hearing Research, 31*, 352–361.

Peters, H. & Hulstijn, W. (1984). Stuttering and anxiety: The difference between stutterers and nonstutterers in verbal apprehension and physiologic arousal during the anticipation of speech and nonspeech tasks. *Journal of Fluency Disorders, 9*, 67–84.

Peters, H., Hulstijn, W., & Starkweather, C. (1989). Acoustic and physiological reaction times of stutterers and nonstutterers. *Journal of Speech and Hearing Research, 32*, 668–680.

Pick, J. (1970). *The Autonomic Nervous System: Morphological, Comparative, Clinical and Surgical Aspects*. Philadelphia, Toronto: J. B. Lippincott Company.

Pinsky, S. & McAdam, D. (1980). Electroencephalographic and dichotic indices of cerebral laterality in stutterers. *Brain and Language, 11*, 374–397.

Seth, G. (1934). Psychomotor control in stammering and normal subjects: An experimental study. *British Journal of Psychology, 49*, 139–143.

Smith, A. (1989). Neural drive to muscles in stuttering. *Journal of Speech and Hearing Research, 32*, 252–264.

Smith, A. (1990). Factors in the etiology of stuttering. *ASHA REPORTS*, Research Needs in Stuttering: Roadblocks and Future Directions, *18*, 39–47.

Smith, A., Denny, M., & Wood, J. (1991). Instability in Speech Muscle Systems in Stuttering. In H. Peters, W. Hulstijn, & W. Starkweather (Eds.), *Speech Motor Dynamics*. New York: Springer-Verlag, 231–242.

Smith, A. & Weber, C. (1988). The need for an integrated perspective on stuttering. *ASHA, 30*, 30–32.

Starkweather, C. (1987). *Fluency and Stuttering*. Englewood Cliffs, NJ: Prentice-Hall.

Travis, L. (1931). *Speech Pathology*. New York: Appleton-Centruy-Crofts.

Van Riper, C. (1982) *The Nature of Stuttering*. Englewood Cliffs, NJ: Prentice Hall.

Wall, M. & Myers, F. (1984). *Clinical Management of Childhood Stuttering*. Baltimore: University Park Press.

Weber, C. & Smith, A. (1990). Autonomic correlates of stuttering and speech assessed in a range of experimental tasks. *Journal of Speech and Hearing Research, 33*, 690–706.

Webster, W. (1989). Sequence initiation performance by stutterers under conditions of response competition. *Brain and Language, 36*, 286–300.

World Health Organization (1977). Manual of the international statistical classification of diseases, injuries, and causes of death. Geneva: World Health Organization.

Zimmermann, G. (1980 a). Articulatory dynamics of fluent utterances of stutterers and nonstutterers. *Journal of Speech and Hearing Research, 23*, 95–107.

Zimmermann, G. (1980 b). Articulatory behaviors associated with stuttering: A cineradiographic analysis. *Journal of Speech and Hearing Research, 23*, 108–121.

Zimmermann, G. (1980 c). Stuttering: A disorder of movement. *Journal of Speech and Hearing Research, 23*, 122–136.

Zimmermann, G. & Knott, J. (1974). Slow potentials of the brain related to speech processing in normal speakers and stutterers. *Electroencephalography and Clinical Neurophysiology, 37*, 599–607.

Zimmermann, G., Smith, A., & Hanley, J. (1981). Stuttering: In need of a unifying conceptual framework: *Journal of Speech and Hearing Research, 24*, 25–31.

Anne Smith, West Lafayette, Indiana (USA)/ Gerald N. Zimmermann, Iowa City, Iowa (USA)

83. Linguistic Phenomenology in Stuttering

1. Introduction

Interpretations of the stuttering-language disorder interaction fall into two broad categories. Historically, the most prominent view has been that stuttering is often accompanied by language disorder. More recently, the perspective that stuttering is a language disorder has been expressed by various authors. After a consideration of the motivation for each interpretation, some current and controversial issues in psycholinguistics will be advanced as particularly germane to stuttering research development.

2. Stuttering Accompanied by Language Disorders

From approximately 1940–1965 psychodynamic and learning theory explanations for the onset and nature of stuttering were in favor.During that period there were frequent reports that many children who stutter also have language and articulation disorders, and attempts were made to explain why these separate disorders might appear in one client. The typical interpretation invoked the construct of fear of speech. The child who stutters might be less inclined to talk for this reason, thereby retarding speech development. A more popular argument was one that is still preferred by Bloodstein (1987, 355–359); the child with a language or speech problem is more likely to receive help (formal or informal) that produces fear of speech difficulty, thereby causing stuttering.

There is a substantial literature verifying the observation that several linguistic deficits often accompany stuttering – deficits in phonology, prosody, syntax, semantics, and pragmatics. Nippold (1988) has provided a comprehensive review of this research. Because evidence accumulated that stuttering could not be explained adequately as a psychodynamic or learned behavior, the interpretations for these findings have shifted toward physiology. In addition, there is a growing interest in providing therapy for stuttering and the 'additional' language deficits as early as possible (despite Bloodstein's warning).

3. Stuttering is a Language Disorder

Several authors have developed the thesis that stuttering represents a deficit in language processing, and our view is that this perspective is more coherent than the one which suggests that stuttering may be accompanied by language disorder. The most thorough treatment of this perspective has been supplied by Wingate (1988). Our discussion will also draw heavily on an excellent review of the evidence by Duckworth (1988) and Hamre's (1984) review of language models.

Wingate (1988, ch.3) dates the formal study of language factors to the work (1935–1945) of Spencer Brown under Wendell Johnson at the University of Iowa. Based on Brown's (1945) summary of these linguistic influences on stuttering loci, subsequent references are frequently made to 'Brown's four factors'. In short, these represent (a) a phonetic factor – more stuttering on consonants than vowels; (b) a grammatic factor – more stuttering on nouns, adjectives, adverbs, and verbs; (c) a length factor – more stuttering on words longer than five letters; and (d) a sentence position influence – more stuttering on the first three words than subsequent words. Brown's interpretation was compatible with the preferred view of stuttering at that time, namely, that these four features likely conspire to render such words more salient (fear-inducing). For unknown reasons – perhaps because this psychological view seemed to 'settle the matter' – interest in pursuing linguistic correlates of stuttering was meager for two decades. Renewed interest in the 1960's seems to correspond with a growing dissatisfaction with psychological theory and more general interest in the biology of language embodied in a 'new' discipline, psycholinguistics. That is, if it is clear that one cannot defend more stuttering on nouns than prepositions because nouns induce fear, then it is reasonable to ask whether nouns are more physiologically complex as they operate in conversation.

As it turns out, Brown's data have been a rich source for recent investigators. On our view, Wingate's (1988) reanalysis of this work is particularly useful for three reasons. First, he provides a rational psycholinguistic explanation for Brown's 'four factors.' Second, he presents compelling evidence that two additional factors (discovered but ignored by Brown) have a more immediate and pervasive influence on stuttering occurrences than the other four; stutters inevitably occur during the production of syllable initial phones and stressed syllables. Third, Wingate's development of phonetic and prosodic influences is heuristic beyond theoretic implications for stuttering. His discussion also provides evidence from stuttering that may clarify several linguistic phenomena in human language (syllable structure, propositionality, sonority hierarchy and its development, nature of normal hesitation patterns, entry of prosodic decisions in a speech plan hierarchy).

From reviews of the research (cited above) it is clear that certain of Brown's six factors have been investigated moreso than others. Acoustic and physiologic phonetic studies have revealed evidence of instability in stutterers' stuttered (and fluent) articulatory gestures. Research on prosodic and syntactic complexity lends credence to the view that both influence stuttering frequency and loci. Currently, of course, conceptualization of linguistic factors is considerably different from earlier views (cf. 5. & 6.). It is likely that future research on stuttering will be fruitful to the extent that current and changing linguistic theory is applied.

To advance an understanding of linguistic influences, then, students of stuttering bear a substantial cross-disciplinary burden. As evidence accumulates, explanations for the acquisition, accomplished use, and impairment of language change. On the view that stuttering is a language disorder, it is expected that developments in psycholinguistics have potential for clarifying the acquisition, nature, and treatment of stuttering. After outlining a rather accepted view of language systems (and their hypothesized interaction with stuttering) we will present two new interpretations, Cognitive Grammar theory and the Competition Model, *vis-a-vis* their implications for stuttering research.

4. Language Systems

As a general outline, linguistic phenomenology can be grouped into five systems: Phonology, prosody, syntax, semantics, and pragmatics. Figure 83.1 illustrates one view on the relationship between these systems and stuttering.

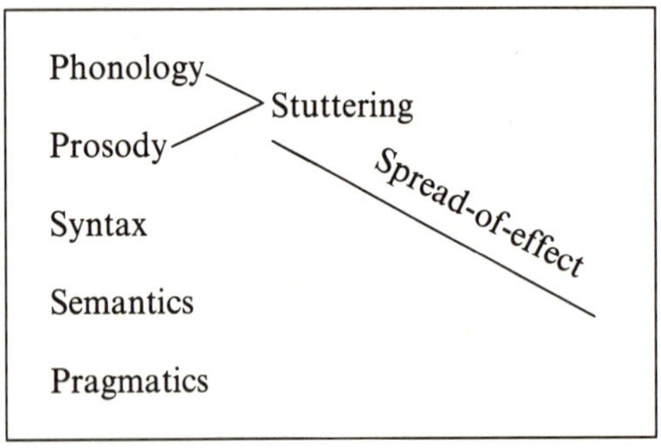

Fig. 83.1: Language Systems Model

This perspective characterizes a deficit in phonology and prosody as the *sine qua non* of stuttering. In short, each stutter verifies that. As a succinct summary of the evidence on the phonetic transition difficulty in stuttering, Wingate (1988, ch.6) presents a 'fault line' thesis that captures the regular occurrence of stutters in transition from the initial phone ('onset') to the remainder ('rime') of the stressed syllable. This approaches an observable answer to Duckworth's (1988, 67) important question: "How might deficits in language structure be related to language function?" Although Duckworth seems to suggest that 'function' relates to communicative interaction (one dimension of the 'pragmatic' system), we must also address this question in terms of (a) linguistic function for a hierarchical speech plan and (b) neurologic function for a cogent account of a stuttered event; e. g. Wingate's (1988, 239) neurolinguistic summary is that stuttering is a language production "...defect that extends beyond the level of motor execution."

4.1. Spread-of-Effect

If stuttering is a language disorder then it is reasonable to hypothesize that systems beyond the core (phonology and prosody) are also vulnerable to impairment. For each client, then, one might ask, "How pervasive is this person's language impairment?" The basic argument is that each of the systems is relatively isomorphic, contributing its unique complexity to the ultimate ease with which an utterance is rendered phonetically. This isomorphism (autonomy) of systems argument is compatible with current applications to stuttering, but it contrasts sharply with developing psycholinguistic theory (cf. 5. & 6.).

4.2. Syntax

As we have mentioned, stuttering loci and frequency appear to be positively related to syntactic complexity when MIT-Style grammar is used to construct or analyze simple vs. complex sentences. That is, the traditional grammar from which Brown (1945) extracted "parts of speech" is inadequate for parsing natural language and categorizing stutters (Wingate 1988). Cognitive grammar, a recent development, will be presented later with comment on how this might be applied to a refined clarification of the role of syntax in stuttering.

4.3. Semantics

To our knowledge, there have been no published applications of formal or generative semantic theory to investigations of stuttering. If we use the more vague construct, 'meaning,' as our referent for semantics, then there are two variables of relevance to an understanding of stuttering: Propositionality and lexical acces. Reviews of the language literature inevitably cite the classic study by Eisenson/Horowitz (1945) which revealed that significantly more stuttering occurred during the reading of meaningful (compared to meaningless) connected prose. They employed Hughlings Jackson's seminal discovery that 'propositionality' characterizes natural language commerce and is at the nexus of what aphasics cannot do with words. Eisenson and Horowitz suggested that increments in propositionality may correlate positively with increments in stuttering frequency

– and, we would add, may be associated with duration/other indices of severity.

Lexical access difficulty may contribute to those occasions when a word is only partially available and a stutter results. There is some evidence of 'word-finding' difficulty in children who stutter and this needs to be explored further. More recently, Wingate (1988) used the standard Word Fluency task – "write as many words as you can think of that begin with the letter S." Twenty adult stutterers generated significantly fewer words than the twenty nonstutterers. While he also used other tasks that suggested word access difficulty, it was the Word Fluency deficit that he found most commensurate with his "fault line" hypothesis. That is, in both stuttering and the Word Fluency task, the word-initial phone is in place but lexical access and assembly are not readily available.

With respect to investigating the semantic integrity of stutterers' language and/or determining the effects of semantic complexity on stuttered events, it may be revealing to apply lexical acquisition models for hypothesis testing. One might predict, for example, that the expression of semantic relations acquired early would be associated with less stuttering than those acquired later. It is clear that the semantic system(s) is integrated with prosodic decisions at a very early stage in utterance planning; often a word receives primary stress for purely semantic reasons.

Such rich integration among systems has been captured by the recently developed cognitive grammar theory and the Competition Model (cf. 5. & 6.) These present serious challenges to the argument that each system functions autonomously.

5. Cognitive Grammar

The theory of cognitive grammar, developed by linguist Ronald Langacker (1987), presents a radical reorientation to the characterization of linguistic structures. A number of contemporary theoretical approaches characterize grammatical structures as autonomous from other levels of language (e. g., semantics). One consequence of this imposed separation is the assumption that grammatical structures are semantically empty or arbitary. E. g., it is widely assumed that active and passive forms of a simple sentence are semantically equivalent representations of a single underlying 'deep structure.' Langacker proposes instead that grammar consist of units that are inherently symbolic. That is, syntactic structures represent conventionalized forms of meaning, as do words and inflections. Thus syntax, the lexicon, and morphology are all characterized similarly as consisting of symbolic units. A symbolic unit can be reduced to a semantic unit that stands in a symbolic relationship with a phonological unit. On this view, there is no need to posit the existence of linguistic elements that are not present in the overt expression (e. g., the well-known dummy *do*).

Cognitive grammar theory posits that active and passive sentence forms are available in a language because of the capacity of speakers to construe a situation in alternate ways. Similarly, simple past and past-progressive forms of verbs allow speakers latitude in describing actions from a particular perspective. This characterization of the interaction between speakers' cognitive capabilities and linguistic structures represents a shift away from idealized models of grammar toward models that are based upon human performance.

Speakers' employment of figurative language and so-called 'rote' expressions is of interest in a cognitive grammar framework. These elements are frequently discarded from orthodox linguistic analyses because they do not appear to be amenable to description in terms of rules. Yet they constitute much of what is produced when speakers speak. A cognitive grammar orientation accords these expressions the status of unit. As a consequence, units can vary from a single word to a phrase to an entire utterance.

Investigations of stuttering and language variables have implicitly assummed a traditional linguistic model (cf. MIT-Style grammar, 4.2.). Consequently, investigators have counted stuttered words, classified stuttered words by grammatical category, and performed transformational analyses upon samples of stuttered speech. Cognitive grammar theory has the potential to profoundly alter our view of what constitutes the unit of analysis in linguistic investigations of stuttering.

6. The Competition Model

The Competition Model (Bates/MacWhinney 1987; MacWhinney 1987) represents an attempt to ground language acquisition and language processing in biology. Its authors describe it as a model of linguistic performance rather than of linguistic competence.

As such, it seems more likely to accommodate instances of language breakdown than models that posit abstract representations of grammatical competence based upon formal logic. It represents an attempt to deal with individual differences among children acquiring language as well as with differences that exist among natural languages.

A major goal of the Competition Model is to "... delimit a set of fundamental processing mechanisms whose strength at a given point in development varies across learners in a way that can eventually be linked to fundamental differences between the learners" (Bates/MacWhinney 1987, 159). Toward this end, investigations have been carried out to determine whether various measures of linguistic performance gathered from very young children correlate with each other and with measures taken at a later age. Additional studies have been aimed at language processing skills in individuals with aphasia. These studies of children and of brain-injured adults may shed light on the cognitive abilities that underlie language use: which of these abilities develop in synchrony, and which are potentially dissociable?

The authors have explored the extent to which factors at one level of linguistic structure (e. g., phonology) influence the acquisition of forms at another level (e. g., syntax). They have observed that the distinctive patterns of language style that emerge in children can be seen in phonology, grammar, the lexicon, and even in non-linguistic social and cognitive domains. That is, there seems to be a spread-of-effect (cf. Fig. 83.1 & 4.1.) across all levels of language, brought about by the differential strength or activation of the mechanisms underlying language use.

An impressive body of evidence has accrued that suggest that some children tend to favor nominal forms in early language development while others use pronominal forms. Furthermore, the nominal users tend to be referential, expanding noun phrases, while the pronominal users have more heterogeneous vocabularies and develop more elaborate verb phrase morphology. This nominal/referential versus pronominal/expressive finding suggests a link between lexical and morphological development. Of special interest to the present work is the additional finding that the children who seem to follow a pronominal/expressive style have a greater tendency to imitate words and sentences. However, the imitation is often imprecise, leading Bates/MacWhinney to speculate that these children may be "...focussing on the suprasegmental/intonational 'packaging' of a target rather than its phonetic details" (Bates/MacWhinney, 184). Thus, a link seems to exist between phonological-prosodic development and lexical and morphological development.

7. Research Implications

In this section, reference will be made to Cognitive Grammar (**CG**) and the Competition Model (**CM**). Direction for research of four types will be presented (descriptive, developmental, comparative, and clinical).

7.1. Descriptive

What do **CG** & **CM** offer for refining our understanding of the nature of stuttering? First, they suggest caution for isolation of systems in research designs. Second, they portend novel means of approaching explanation of linguistic phenomenology in stuttering. That is, because they focus on linguistic performance rather than an idealized competence, research designed in accord with **CG** & **CM** will more likely clarify the relationship between language structure and function (cf. Duckworth's question, 4.) Consider the merits of Wingate's "fault line" hypothesis (cf. 4.3.). While his evidence supports the inference that phonetic transition difficulty is tied to a problem of lexical access and assembly, a **CG** analysis might explain the loci variability of such difficulty in discourse. Research might reveal that stutters co-occur with certain combinatorial properties of symbolic units of various sizes. On the apparent (but unexplained) deviance of stutterers' spoken stories (Wingate 1988, 217), it may be that stutterers do not possess the normal repertoire or ready availability of construal options. One might predict, then, that stutterers' stories will contain a more limited array of larger units resulting in the frequent appearance of 'rote' or conventional phrases. More generally, both **CG** & **CM** offer a direction for further research on the alleged influences of syntactic complexity, lexical access, and propositionality on stuttering.

7.2. Developmental

To our knowedge, **CG** is a linguistic theory without published application to first language acquisition. However, if partial explanation on the nature of stuttering derives from **CG** generated studies (such as those suggested in 7.1.), it will be logical to apply such findings to the stuttering acquisition issue. Of course, this issue can be addressed now; there is functionalistic correspondence between **CG** & **CM** on core constructs, and **CM** has been rigorously applied to language development questions. For example, children favoring pronominal forms (cf. 6.) use substantially more different words, and this was one characteristic of adult stutterers' spoken stories reported by Wingate (cf. 7.1.). At what age does this appear and are young stutterers more likely to be pronominal than nominal users?

CM has derived considerable support from longitudinal studies seeking correlations betwen levels of analysis (semantic, syntactic, etc.). This is probably the design of choice to investigate stuttering developmental interactions between various symbolic units or levels of analysis. E.g., Menyuk/Liebergott/Schultz (1986, 79–93) reviewed their study of 53 children over the first 3 years. They found significant positive correlations between age of achieving (a) structured CV's, (b) closed syllables, and (c) 50 different words. The longitudinal design also identifies a sound approach for comparing these correlations from normal children to correlations from children who demonstrate early dysfunction (stuttering) in phonologic-prosodic production. One logical extension of this approach would be to determine if there are earlier (than stuttering) indices of phonologic difficulty (i. e. 'protostuttering'). Considering the stages of vocal development (Vihman 1988, 72–77), there is reason to suspect a correlation between difficulty in achieving canonical babbling (6–8 months) and later stuttering – and, perhaps, later ties to lexical acquisition and access. Canonical, or reduplicated babbling (*dadada*), "constitutes the chief production milestone in the first year" (Vihman 1988, 74). It represents the first evidence of mastery of articulatory-laryngeal control to the extent that repeatable and smooth CVC phonetic transitions are available for subsequent elaboration. It may not be a coincidence that a basic failure of phonetic transition has often been described as the essence or core feature of stuttering. Are children who deviate from the typical 6–8 month achievement of canonical babbling more likely to stutter later?

The development of vocal control usually refers to modifications within a child over time ('ontogenetic'). Jason Brown (1988) has proposed a "microgenetic" (within milliseconds) account of "vocal development" that is coherent with (a) phases of childhood vocal development and (b) characteristics of different aphasias. As it turns out, his microgenetic theory can also be viewed as a neural version of **CM** and it may emerge as a useful neurolinguistic model for stuttering.

7.3. Comparative

Both **CG** & **CM** support a suspicion that errors in phonetic transition (stuttering; apraxia of speech, cf. Hamre/Harn 1979) might share with other production errors (e. g. misarticulations, slips of the tongue) a sensitivity to influences from (a) other **CM** levels and (b) **CG** construal and symbolic unit decisions. That is, evidence concerning one disorder might clarify the nature of another that is phenomenologically related. It would seem heuristic to apply descriptive research (cf. 7.1. for examples) for such a cross-disciplinary purpose. Finally, it is common for evidence from disorders to serve a comparative function to contribute to an understanding of normal language use and acquisition.

7.4. Clinical

One might view the clinical enterprise as hypothesis testing in the truest sense of that experimental construct (Hamre 1972). As knowledge develops concerning linguistic phenomenology in stuttering, determining the operation of such correlates in a single client can extend and focus diagnostic explanation, treatment planning, and measures of progress.

8. References

Bates, E. & MacWhinney, B. (1987). Competition, variation and language learning. In B. MacWhinney (Ed.), *Mechanisms of language acquisition. 157–193.* Hillsdale, NJ: Lawrence Erlbaum Associates.

Bloodstein, O. (1987). *A handbook on stuttering.* Chicago: National Easter Seal Society.

Brown, J. (1988). *The life of the mind.* Hillsdale, NJ: Lawrence Erlbaum Associates.

Brown, S. (1945). The loci of stutterings in the speech sequence. *Journal of Speech Disorders, 10,* 181–192.

Duckworth, M. (1988). Stuttering and linguistics. In M. Ball (Ed.), *Theoretical linguistics and disordered language. 51–79.* San Diego: College-Hill.

Eisenson, J. & Horowitz, E. (1945). The influence of propositionality on stuttering. *Journal of Speech Disorders, 10*, 193–197.

Hamre, C. (1972). Research and clinical practice: a unifying model. *ASHA, 14*, 542–545.

Hamre, C. (1984). Stuttering as a cognitive-linguistic disorder. In R. Curlee & W. Perkins (Eds), *Nature and treatment of stuttering: New directions. 237–259*. San Diego: College-Hill.

Hamre, C. & Harn, W. (1979). The effect of masking on apraxia: Evidence from spectrographic data. In H. Hollien & P. Hollien (Eds.), *Current issues in the phonetic sciences. 1057–1063*. Amsterdam: Benjamins.

Langacker, R. (1987). *Foundations of cognitive grammar, vol. 1: Theoretical prerequisites*. Stanford: Stanford University Press.

MacWhinney, B. (1987). The competition model. In B. MacWhinney (Ed.), *Mechanisms of language acquisition. 249–308*.Hillsdale, NJ: Lawrence Erlbaum Associates.

Menyuk, P., Liebergott, J., & Schultz, M. (1986). Predicting phonological development. In B. Lindblom & R. Zetterstrom (Eds.), *Precursors of early speech. 79–93*. Basingstoke, Hampshire (UK): MacMillan.

Nippold, M. (1988). Concomitant speech and language disorders in stuttering children: A critique of the literature. *Journal of Speech and Hearing Disorders, 55*, 51–60.

Vihman, M. (1988). Early phonological development. In J. Bernthal & N. Bankson (Eds.), *Articulation and phonological disorders, 2nd ed. 95–109*. Englewood Cliffs, NJ: Prentice Hall.

Wingate, M. (1988). *The structure of stuttering: A psycholinguistic analysis*. New York: Springer-Verlag.

Curt Hamre/William Harn, Lubbock, Texas (USA)

84. Psychological Aspects and Theories of Stuttering

1. Introduction

The controversy which carried on into the 70s as to whether stuttering should be considered either a manifestation of a psychological disorder or an organic/physiological or linguistic one, has today shifted in favour of an integrative multimodal view (Gregory 1986). The integrative models and the various accents they set, assume that stuttering in early childhood is influenced by multiple, coexisting, interacting factors of a physiological/organic, linguistic and psychological nature, which can change individually in the course of a lifetime (Friedler/Standop 1986; Peters/Starkweather 1989). Since the disorder is not assumed to be homogenous, this view of the phenomenon of stuttering can be regarded as a more restricted, idiosyncratic view with the discussion differentiated according to age groups and degrees of chronicity (Schulze/Johannsen 1986).

Since current research is concerned with delivering more and more individual, empirical proof of the importance of the different variables associates with the three bundles of factors already mentioned, it is necessary to gain a better understanding of the way the different factors interact together and with general developmental psychological processes. The extent to which the factors are etiologically important, the extent to which they influence the speech disorder qualitatively and quantitatively and the influence they have on features marking the development of the disorder and on the probability of remission must also be more fully understood.

Current trends in research and theoretical discussions show that interest now revolves around the organic/physiological and linguistic bundles of factors (Peters/Hulstijn 1987; Schulze/Johannsen 1986). In contrast, the psychological aspects, which are sometimes referred to as 'traditional' factors, are nowadays taken less systematically into consideration in terms of models and research themes (Schulze/Johannsen 1990). This development together with a paradigmatic change in favour of modular research strategies does not mean that the psychological factor has been adequately investigated or scientifically exhausted. The problems of developing models capable of showing the nature and the functioning of psychological variables of influence, would suggest that the opposite is more likely to be the case and illustrates the general scientific problems of dealing with psychological partial aspects of complex phenomena. The theoretical notions and the empirically substantiated findings relating to the importance of psychological factors of influence for childhood stuttering are reviewed synoptically below.

2. Psychological Aspects of Childhood Stuttering

With the emergence of the social and behavioral sciences (psychoanalysis, behaviourism, social psychology, communication sciences, linguistics), an increasing interest in psychosocial variables began to develop at the beginning of the 30s with a focal point in the period 1945–1970. The most widely differing models and research paradigms of these disciplines were also applied to the investigation of stuttering. The concepts which evolved during this period formed an antipole to the purely organic/physiological models and methods of treatment which had prevailed up to this time (Shames/Rubin 1986). The focal point of research has particularly influenced the practice of prevention and early treatment of stuttering or treatment concepts for childhood stuttering and it has even dominated in some countries. As already mentioned, since the beginning of the 80s we have been able to observe a renewed focusing of research and theory formation on organic/physiological (Curlee/Perkins 1985) and linguistic variables (Wingate 1988), although the amount of research into psycho-social variables must be regarded as very small in comparison to the total research effort (Schulze 1989, 55 ff).

Although, in my opinion, a definite move away from purely psychological interpretation models has become apparent in current scientific discussion, stuttering still tends to be considered a purely psychological problem by many practioners and in terms of public opinion. The patient's or the parents' anticipatory attitude is often connected with this. The aim of therapy is subsequently to change in the personality of the patient and possible organic or linguistic factors are not often taken into account.

2.1. Models: Psycho-Social Factors

The theoretical concept relating to the importance of psycho-social factors (Schulze 1989) can be subdivided into two groups:
A. The model of the psychopathological personality containing two fundamental assertions. (a) Stuttering is basically a behavioral manifestation of a neurosis. b) the child's personality disorder is closely linked to pathological features of the parents' personalities. This leads to a dialogic loss of confidence in the child and results in stuttering.
B. The model of the effectiveness of unfavourable interactional variables does not assume a fundamental psychological disorder in the child or his reference person, although the importance of individual dimensions of behavior and attitude must be regarded as central to the aetiology and course. We shall refer to more behaviorally oriented models of social interaction with a focus on immediate, open and directly observable interactional behaviors. Examples are:
(1) The diagnosogenic theory of the genesis of stuttering which was postulated as early as the 40s and which is still popular today. This attributes stuttering causally to a parental misinterpretation of normal speech disfluencies in the child (Johnson 1959).
(2) The operant conditioning concept based on learning theory which explains the onset and, in particular, the maintenance of stuttering in terms of operant conditioning processes alternating between the parents and the child (Costello 1984).
(3) Finally, the concept of the efficiency of communicative stressors which assumes powerful interaction between stutter-specific personal factors in the child and external communicative stressors (Starkweather 1987).
The systematic examination of these theoretical concepts makes it clear that we are not dealing with completely different thought models, but that most of the concepts overlap to a great degree with regard to content even though some accentuation may be different. Apart from the use of completely different terminologies and the reference to different personality theories (e. g. trait versus state model of personality; Amelang/Batussek 1990), the main difference is, in may opinion, just how fundamental the personality disorder is assumed to be in the child and the parents, and to what extent the concepts can be interpreted as etiological and to what extent they can be generalized. These theoretical

contributions are to be regarded as hypothetical attempts to examine the extremely complex interrelationship of the personal, interactional and environmental conditions in which stuttering is to be found. The following illustration shows how intricate and complex such relationship can be. It contains the variables classified as meaningful in the theoretical and clinical discussion. If we assume that childhood stuttering takes place within the framework of the infrafamilial styles of communication and interaction, it becomes clear that these can be affected by various psychosocial factors of influence. Different kinds of personal factors relating to the parents and the child are also as important as factors relating to family structure or socio-cultural parameters.

A. Personal factors relating to parents and child
(A.1) Previous socialization experiences (special socialization conditions e. g. growing up in a children's home or in a foster family, growing up when parents often move home)
(A.2) Intrapsychic structures (e. g. high level of aspiration; ambition; coping with success or failure; basic affective mood; self-control; self-assertiveness; self-confidence; strength of ego).
(A.3) Life and stress management (e. g. threshold of tolerance of everyday stress; ways of coping with critical life events such as training, re-training, illness, separation from important reference persons.
(A.4) Verbal and non-verbal communication styles of relevant reference persons (e. g. competitive communication styles: 'time pressure', 'listener loss', 'interruption', 'high speech rate', high communicative responsibilitiy; discrepancy between verbal and nonverbal behavior; multilingualism).
(A.5) Organic-physiological and psychological disorders (e. g. motoric disorder of the mouth; cognitive or linguistic retardation, stress resulting from chronic illness and rehabilitation measures, medical operations, behavior and performance disorders).

B. Family life style
(B.1) Social environment (e. g. lack or excess of external contacts, constant change of reference person, e. g. children of publicans, children of parents in migration; children whose parents often move home).
(B.2) Leisure behavior (e. g. adult-oriented leisure behavior, excessive television or video viewing; lack of separation between leisure and work spheres).
(B.3) Housing conditions (cramped, noisy living accomodation, house-building situation, frequent changes of home and locality when child is looked after while both parents are at work).
(B.4) Job satisfaction and working conditions (job/professional stress affecting family; unemployment; early retirement; irregular working hours due to shift change or duty).
(B.5) Socio-economic conditions (e. g. high level of financial stress, distraint).

C. Family structure
(C.1) Inter-generative relationship (e. g. blurring of generation boundaries; multi-generation household with conflict arising from distribution of responsibility in household and child-rearing matters).
(C.2) Intrafamilial power and role distribution (e. g. competitive or unclear role distribution in the nuclear family).
(C.3) Marital relationship (e. g. hidden or open continuous crisis; marital separation).
(C.4) Parent-child relationship (e. g. inner rejection of child or one parent; predominantly negative, punishment oriented guidance of children; frequent daily power struggles relating to everyday routine; moral overtaxing of children; coalition forming).
(C.5) Brothers-sisters relationship (hidden or open competitive relationship).

Hypothetically, these factors can influence the child's fluency directly or indirectly via such mediator variables as stress and anxiety. The high level of individual variability of relevance of such psycho-social and environmental stimuli for the development of stuttering suggests that individual vulnerability due to certain stressors is more important than the nature of the stressor (Bloodstein 1987; Van Riper 1982). — The way that children cope with such stressors on an experimental psychological level has not been well researched. In the light of recent results of stress research in adults, it must be assumed that there is a complex stress process with information processing (primary appraisals, secondary appraisals etc.) playing an important part on various levels (Jerusalem 1990). Moreover, it must be assumed that individual vulnerability and coping behavior in the child is not only determined by cognitive processes (attitudes, appraisals), but also by interrelated organic/physiological and linguistic variables which cause the stress experienced by the child to promote stuttering rather than the development of another psycho-physiological disorder. One of the problems of such descriptive models is that not much is known about the psycho-physiological processes that underlie these psychosocial variables, although their effect on fluency can be reliably determined and the individual pattern of the variables concerned can be worked out by functional analysis in individual cases (Starkweather/Gottwald/Halfond 1990).

2.2. State of Research

The enormous complexity of the factors involved in the development of stuttering makes it necessary to restrict the variables to be examined and complicates investigation. A serious problem for the interpretation of research data is that many research approaches do not clearly distinguish which of the following are to be examined: dispositional factors (e. g. heredity, pre-, peri-, postnatal influences or developmental conditions in early childhood), immediate causal factors: (factors and events immediately preceding the initial manifestation of stuttering in time or coinciding with it) or factors responsible for stabilization, chronification, generalization: (factors promoting chronification or barriers preventing remission; chronification factors reinforcing frequency and intensity or contributing to the generalization of the disorder in other areas of life). – This often results in a lack of interpretational clarity and in interpretative arbitrariness because, for example, the important process of differentiating between the cause and the psycho-social consequences of stuttering when interpreting the data can only be carried out inadequately.

The current state of research into the importance of psycho-social and interactional variables can be summarized as follows.

2.2.1. Scope of Research

The results of about 70 empirical studies have been published in the last 45 years. These aimed at specifying psycho-social variables: (parental variables, intrafamilial constellations, styles of interaction). About 3200 families have been investigated up to now. About 600 families were allocated to studies which were concerned with the issue of the typical personality features of stutterers' parents. In addition, there are several studies on mainly adult stutterers and occasional studies on children examining personal psychological variables in the stutterers themselves (Schulze 1989).

2.2.2. Research Methods

Two main methods of research are used.
a) Interviewing or testing the parents of stutterers or the stutterer him-/herself using informal and standardized test procedures (e. g. clinical depth interviews; psychometric personality tests such as MPI, MMPI, 16-PF, FPI; projective tests such as Rorschach, TAT, CAT, SCENO, Family in Animals). – In terms of life history, most studies proceed from the current situation of the stutterer and a few employ the method of retrospective questioning of adult stutterers on early childhood events or on their experience of upbringing and family climate in early childhood.
b) Direct behavioral observation of parent-child interaction in dyadic or triadic play situations (naturalistic, semi-naturalistic, experimental) recorded on video. The evaluation is carried out using methods of systematic behavioral observation (e. g. with special systems of categories or signs).

2.2.3. Study Designs

The predominant study design is the cross-sectional study with control group comparison. As a rule, a control group is formed from a non-impaired total population. The inclusion of a further control group e. g. as a control for a general factor such as 'disability' or 'language disorder' is rare. Study and control groups are normally matched according to one variable (e. g. age or sex). Other important variables such as duration of stuttering, severity of stuttering, therapy and counselling experience, developmental status, completeness of family, number of brothers or sisters etc. are seldom included as a control. As a result, the differences of variance in relevant features cannot be taken into account in such post-hoc analyses in spite of control group design. Because of the levelling of possible group differences due to the heterogenity of the disorder or the subject number which is usually low, there is an increasing demand for research to be carried out on a sub-group specific basis (Cooper 1990; Yairi 1990).

A similar research strategy contains the so-called "high density" design (Cox/Seider/Kidd 1984). Families in which stuttering occurs frequently are investigated (e. g. 5 family members must have stuttered for at least 6 consecutive months) and are compared with non-stuttering control families. This special study design makes it possible to compare stutterers and their non-stuttering relatives and stutterers and their families with non-stuttering families. The logic of this investigation approach is that the factors which are relevant to the development of stuttering should occur in a higher concentration in families containing many stutterers. These could include perinatal, medical, developmental-psychological, linguistic factors or factors associated with upbringing, social factors, personality factors and interactional factors within the family. This method is therefore very important because it enables the investigation of the multivariate conditions of stuttering in a relatively small sample and can contribute to the clarification of stutter-specific constellations of variables. The individual case study (n = 1) and the methods of comparative casuistics are being increasingly employed as a research method, particularly in the investigation of atypical conditions associates with the onset and course of stuttering (Barlow/Hersen 1984; Jüttemann 1990).

2.2.4. Variables Investigated

Early studies were primarily aimed at the empirical detection of global, static-structural personality features (e. g. neuroticism, extraversion, overprotection). However, later studies were increasingly concerned with the functional-dynamic effects of individual aspects of attitude, experience and behavior (e. g. readiness to label, level of aspiration, child-rearing and communication styles, self-confidence, perceived difference in status).

2.2.5. Results

The results of the previous empirical studies on the etiological importance of parental and interactional variables for childhood stuttering can be summarized as follows (Schulze 1989, 74 ff).

2.2.5.1. Findings Relating to Psychopathology of the Personality of the Parents

Various methods have been used to investigate hypotheses contained in some theoretical concepts and, above all, those derived from clinical descriptions. According to these hypotheses, stuttering, when considered etiologically, is the result of a personality disorder of the parents and, in particular, of the mother. There is an entire series of control group studies which use mainly standardized personality tests (MPI, MMPI, 16-PF, FPI). According to the data obtained from about 580 families, the parents of stutterers can be no more readily distinguished as a group by typical personality features or a higher occurrence of personality disorders than the nonstuttering control groups. One study without control group comparison of a group of 50 families of stutterers diagnosed 20 to 30 mothers to be neurotic, but these results could not be confirmed. The factorial analytical study of Riley and Riley (1984) suggested that in 5% of that 56 parents investigated, the parents had a psychological need for the stuttering symptoms. On the basis of this study it would appear that parental psychological disorders are involved only to a slight extent in the genesis and manifestation of childhood behavioral disorders and that the role they play is only small for stuttering.

2.2.5.2. Specific Attitudinal Characteristics of Parents

There are a series of findings suggesting that the parents of stuttering children are very demanding, over-exact, dominant and critical. Furthermore, they also show an increased tendency to diagnose 'stuttering', have a low level of tolerance of disfluency and differ according to the individual dimensions of their child-rearing styles, e. g. with respect to being consistent, their affective participation, their readiness to communicate, their conformity to norms. Although there are differences between these and the normal control groups, they cannot be considered completely certain because of the inconsistency of the findings and they should also not be interpreted as stutter specific features because of the absence of further control groups in the study designs. These differences could also be due to a general factor 'disability' since disordered behavior in children brings about a change of attitudes, feelings and behavior in the parents (e. g. concern, feelings of guilt, ambivalence of action) (Lerner/Spanier 1978). Taking into consideration the scope of the variables examined (the questionnaire in the study of Johnson (1955) contained 846 items) and the many psycho-social dimensions in which no differences were ascertained, the findings should be considered particular since they have not been confirmed in any other duplicate studies. Moreover, in some studies there were no differences in the dimensions of attitudes which were investigated in relation to the control families. In the factorial analytical study of the clinical population of Riley and

Riley (1984), the anticipatory attitudes of 5% of the parents (when measured multidimensionally) were found to be unrealistic. This also means, however, that the anticipatory attitudes of 49% of the parents of stuttering children were appropriate.

2.2.5.3. The Way Stuttering Children See Their Parents

The results of these studies show that stutterers view their parents very differently. In contrast to the control groups the following differences could be ascertained: The way the child perceives his/her parents acceptance, overprotection and control, love. Moreover, stutterers characterize their fathers retrospectively as "less cooperative and accepting stricter less fair and loving, less interested, more dictatorial". Other studies show no significant differences in the children's perception of upbringing or domestic environmental influences.

2.2.5.4. Parent-Child Interaction in Observational Studies

As a result of criticism of extremely reactive diagnostic procedures (retrospective self-reports) and measuring techniques and because of the improvement of recording and evaluation techniques (film, video, tape-recorder, computer), an increasing number of methods of direct behavioral observation have been developed for use in interactional diagnostics. Widely differing dimensions of verbal and nonverbal interactional behavior have been investigated so far with the main focus of interest on verbal interactional styles. In contrast to the results of early interactional studies which showed that parents of stutterers considerably had more negative interactional styles, there are other studies which in no way can support this. Some studies allow hypotheses which assume differences in thematic coherence, flexibility of dialogue and initiative. Other differences relate to questioning and instructional behavior, speed of mothers' speech, divergence of speech rate between mothers and fathers. However, it is necessary to point out that there has not yet been a thorough experimental investigation of these hypotheses, although some of the partial results are already considered substantiated and play an important role in prevention and early treatment (Conture 1990).

As a whole, the results of available observational studies can only be considered contradictory. Faults in study designs (lack of suitable control groups, inadequate matching) restrict the interpretation of the data considerably. However, the interactional climate must not be considered to be more negative in general terms. It is more probable to assume that interactional parameters which can generate communicative stress occur more frequently and are of a different nature in families of stutterers than in normal control families. The systematic investigation of such interactional parameters and the proof of their stutter specificity or etiological importance are still at an early stage and must be intensified before general therapeutic principles can be developed (Cooper 1990).

2.2.5.5. The Position of the Stutterer Within the Family

The findings concerned with the question of whether stutterers occupy a particular position in the family in comparison to brothers and sisters are inconsistent. – Some studies suggest that stutterers often occupy 'only child' status in the family, but other studies cannot support this. The significance of the age difference between the stutterer and his/her elder brothers and sisters could also not be confirmed.

3. Psychological Aspects of Adulthood Stuttering

Stuttering is characteristically a disorder of early childhood and is generally closely associated with motoric and linguistic developmental processes. However, in the case of stuttering in adulthood the following questions relating to psychological aspects are of importance:

A. What are the psychosocial consequences of stuttering for the sufferer and do these give rise to certain personality features or certain attitudes, feelings and behavior? A series of surveys (Baumgärtel 1984; Cox 1986; Schulze/Johannsen 1990) comparing psychological variables in the case of adult stutterers and non-stuttering control groups show that adult stutterers are slightly more anxious, more sensitive, more insecure and less self-confident in social situations. Despite considerable individual variability, group differences emerge which are interpreted as secondary psychosocial symptoms of the disorder.

Because of assumed or actual social stigmatization and because of discrimination against the stutterer in terms of his/her achievement (as exemplified by 'stutterer jokes'), increased levels of self-observation and communicative self-control can arise as a result of avoiding stuttering and concealing the disorder. Consequently, the anxiety level in the stutterer is generally slightly raised. As a result of experiencing the occasional ineffectiveness of the chosen coping strategies, the area of verbal communication, over the years and decades, becomes a constant source of failure, helplessness and injury in terms of expectation and experience and these give rise to widely varying coping mechanisms (e. g. resignation, social withdrawal, aggressiveness) (Carlisle 1986).

The psychological consequences of the disorder probably increase in proportion to their significance for the overall psychosocial situation of the patient. In addition, there are also psychological problems originating in other areas (e. g. life, marital, professional crises) or psychological disorders which are independent of stuttering. Moreover, the effectiveness of stuttering therapy (fluency shaping or stuttering modification) is dependent on the successful transfer to other life situations beyond therapy. Although this transfer often takes place spontaneously in the case of young stutterers, it can actually be considered to be the problem itself in the case of juvenile or adult stutterers who have had the disorder for many years. – Under laboratory conditions basal fluency can be established quite easily with the help of various methods (Ham 1986). – For transfer and generalization, additional psychological transfer strategies must be activated (Boberg 1983; Edelstein 1989; Webster/Poulos 1989). These are taken from various branches of clinical psychology (behavioral psychology, cognitive psychology, client-centred therapy, rational-emotive therapy). Stuttering therapy for adults should employ methods of psychological change without the therapy basically being conceived as psychotherapy. If psychological problems are predominant, psychotherapy is indicated as treatment or it should precede stuttering therapy.

B. Is there a psychogenic form of stuttering which can be interpreted etiologically and which is comparable to so-called neurogenic stuttering (Helm-Estabrooks 1986)? Dysfluency occurring unequivocally as a result of emotional trauma or within the framework of a primary psychological/psychiatric disorder is rare and is nowadays distinguished from stuttering by differential diagnostics. The etiological proof of 'psychogenic' stuttering is difficult since it is necessary to exclude a history of stuttering in the patient which existed before the sudden initial manifestation of stuttering in adulthood. A neurological disorder must also be excluded. In practice, the psycho-genesis of stuttering described by the patient and his reference persons is often questionable. Plausible explanations for certain phenomena (e. g. intra-individual variation of symptoms) are put forward out of psychological necessity and physical and emotional traumas in the family (e. g. accident, illness, separation) are considered to be the concepts causing the disorder. Although such concepts undoubtedly fulfil an important psychohygienic function (e. g. exculpation of guilt, resistance to change), they are usually not relevant as an etiological interpretation. Psychogenic stuttering is also rarely reported in the literature (Freund 1966). Individual clinical cases are documented in the context of a war neurosis and in relation to anxiety attacks, depression and other somatic complaints lacking an organic basis and in relation to schizophrenia and manic depressive psychosis.

The current main differential diagnostic criteria are: (1) a sudden initial manifestation in youth or adulthood which is closely associated with the experience of chronic stress or with the onset of an acute emotional crisis, (2) a predominantly monosymptomatic dysfluency pattern, (3) the dysfluency extends beyond the specific situations and is relatively independent of them, (4) the patient has only a slight perception of the dysfluency and (5) there is usually no stutter-specific distress (Schulze 1989; St. Louis 1986).

Using methods of differential diagnosis, it is necessary to distinguish the rare psychogenic form of stuttering and true stuttering from transitory dysfluencies which occur as a reaction to specific stress situations, in particular, situations involving communication and speech. – Interruptions to the speech flow which are closely associated with objectively and subjectively identifiable stress situations (e. g. examination situation, television interview, marriage proposal, multilingual conversation, reporting an accident e. g. from an emergency telephone) can contain the whole spectrum of severe stuttering symptoms (sentence inversions, interjections such as "ahh, ahh", word/part-word repetitions, prolongations, blockages, secondary motoric phenomena). In clinical terms, there are the following relatively consistent, typical features: The cause is known and when the stress phase is over, the fluency pattern is reestablished. There is usually no generalized speech fear or generalized speech avoidance. The distress which is often referred to as 'speech anxiety' or 'insecurity' can be very great, but it is usually limited to certain stress situations. The sufferer doesn't usually consider him-/herself to be a stutterer although he perceives his speech to be 'stuttered' or 'disjointed' in the situation.

These differential diagnostic distinctions and the development of chronic stuttering in response to psychological stress are important in terms of choosing a therapy approach. It is necessary to ascertain to what extent therapeutic work would be useful or possibly sucessful on the level of speech/speaking (speech pattern, fluency, disfluency behavior) and to what extent psychological variables (attitudes, feelings, open behavior) and the current life situation of the patient are important for treatment. It is also necessary to decide if the stutterer-therapeutic (multimodal) approach should be replaced by basic psychotherapeutic/psychiatric treatment.

4. Discussion

Although the state of research is sketchy and to some extent contradictory there exists no doubt among experts that psychosocial aspects play a certain role in the development, chronification and remission of stuttering.

According to the earlier theories and the views which are still held today by laymen and the public, the main causes of stuttering are to be found in psychological traumas or psychopathological personality features. In contrast, the dynamics of the development of stuttering and the characteristically inconsistent pattern of the disorder are explained today in terms of the effectiveness of such moderator variables as stress and emotional agitation together with organic and linguistic

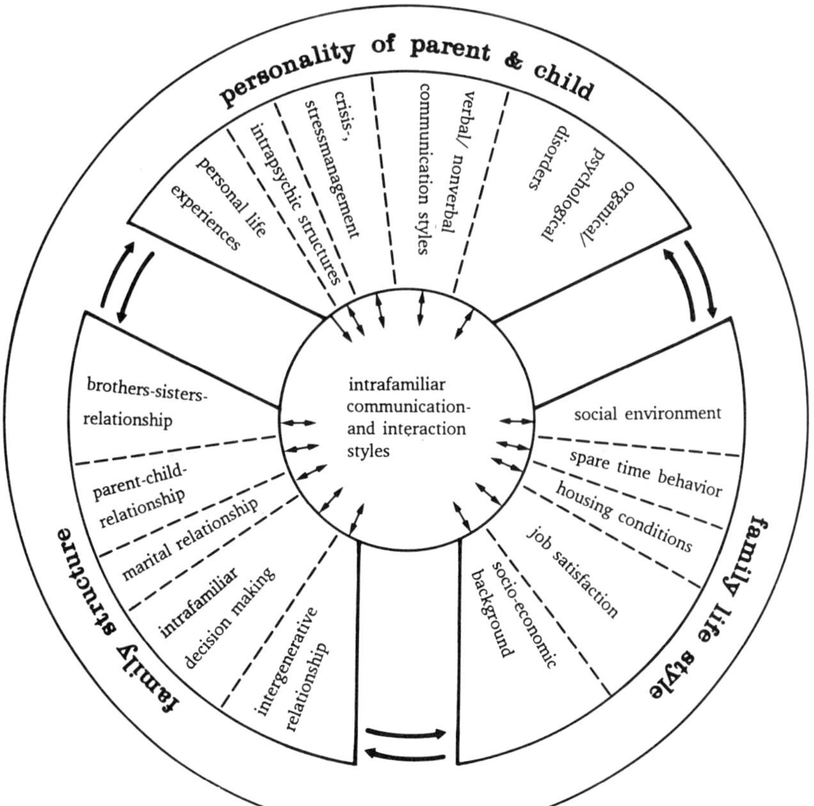

Fig. 84.1: Hypothetical variables (factors of influence) creating and changing intrafamilial styles of communication and interaction in relation to the onset and development of childhood stuttering (Schulze 1989).

factors. The heterogeneity of the findings would suggest that there are neither stutter specific factors in the child, his environment nor in the mutual relationship between the two. The breadth of the possible psychosocial factors (cf. figure 84.1) and the enormous variety of the stutter-relevant variables occurring individually in clinical practice, would seem to suggest the existence of an unspecific psychosocial context of influence. This means that each psychosocial factor can be relevant to stuttering if it contributes to the destabilization of the equilibrium of the capacities and demands which are necessary for fluent speech (Adams 1988; Starkweather 1988).

On the basis of the previous findings, it is impossible to speak in terms of typical stutterers or typical families of stutterers or typical fathers or mothers of stutterers. The extent to which psychosocial factors are involved can vary widely individually and only individual diagnostics can ascertain the importance of these in the functional analysis of behavior and in the treatment concept. It must also be decided to what extent psychological therapy elements should be integrated into the therapy approach for stuttering. On the basis of the state of research it is impossible to justify treatment for childhood stutterers that is basically oriented around family therapy, analytical child psychotherapy or client-centred play therapy. In the case of juveniles and adults the therapy design should be in accordance with the basic or predominant disorder.

A psychogenesis of stuttering which is unequivocal is extremely rare and psychotherapy is necessary. As a rule, however, stuttering therapy includes multimodal procedures and procedures based on combined methods. It combines methods of speech therapy and psychological modification methods and these should be applied and dosed carefully by the therapist in accordance with the needs of the individual case (Wendlandt 1984).

5. References

Adams, M. R. (1988). *The "Demands and capacities" model: Theoretical elaborations*. Paper presented at the Second International Oxford Dysfluency Conference. Sommerville, College Oxford, England. August 24–26, 1988.

Amelang, M. & Batussek, D. (1990). *Differentielle Psychologie und Persönlichkeitsforschung*. Stuttgart: Kohlhammer. 3rd Ed.

Barlow, D. H. & Hersen, M. (1984). *Single case experimental designs. Strategies for studying behaviour change*. New York: Pergamon Press. 2nd Ed.

Baumgärtel, F. (1984). Ein Beitrag zur Persönlichkeitsdiagnostik von Stotterern. *Bremer Beiträge zur Psychologie, 33*. Bremen: Universität Bremen.

Bloodstein, O. (1987). *A handbook on stuttering*. Chicago: National Easter Seal Society. 4th Ed.

Boberg, E. (Ed.) (1983). *Maintenance of fluency*. New York. Elsevier 1981.

Carlisle, J. A. (1986). *Tangled tongue. Living with a stutterer*. Reading: Addison-Wesley Publishing Comp.

Conture, E. (1990). *Stuttering*. Englewood Cliffs: Prentice Hall. 2nd Ed.

Cooper, J. A. (Ed.) (1990). *Research needs in stuttering: Roadblocks and future directions*. Rockville, Maryland: Asha Reports No. 18.

Costello, J. M. (1984). Operant conditioning and the treatment of stuttering. In W. H. Perkins (Ed.), *Stuttering disorders. 107–127*. New York: Thieme-Stratton Inc.

Cox, M. D. (1986). The psychological maladjusted stutterer. In K. O. St. Louis, (Ed.), *The atypical stutterer. Principles and practices of rehabilitation. 93–122*. Orlando: Academic Press.

Cox, N. J., Seider, R. A., & Kidd, K. K. (1984). Some environmental factors and hypotheses for stuttering in families with several stutterers. *Journal of Speech and Hearing Research, 27*, 543–548.

Curlee, R. F. & Perkins, W. H. (Eds.) (1985). *Nature and treatment of stuttering*. London: Taylor & Francis.

Edelstein, B. A. (1989). Generalization: Terminological, methodological and conceptual issues. *Behaviour Therapy, 20*, 311–324.

Fiedler, P. & Standop, R. (1986). *Stottern. Ätiologie, Diagnose, Behandlung*. München: Uban & Schwarzenberg. 2nd Ed.

Freund, H. (1966). *Psychopathology and the problems of stuttering. With special consideration of clinical and historical aspects*. Springfield, III.: C. C. Thomas.

Gregory, H. H. (1986). Stuttering: A contemporary perspective. *Folia Phoniatrica, 38*, 89–120.

Ham, R. (1986). *Techniques of stuttering therapy*. Englewood Cliffs: Prentice Hall.

Helm-Estabrooks, N. (1986). Diagnosis and management of neurogenic stuttering in adults. In K. O. St. Louis, (Ed.), *The atypical stutterer. Principles and practice of rehabilitation. 193–218*. Orlando: Academic Press.

Jerusalem, M. (1990). *Persönliche Ressourcen, Vulnerabilität und Streßerleben*. Göttingen: Hogrefe.

Johnson, W. (1955). A study of the onset and development of stuttering. In W. Johnson & R. R. Leutenegger (Eds.), *Stuttering in children and adults. 37–73.* Minneapolis: University of Minnesota Press.

Johnson, W. (1959). *The onset of stuttering.* Minneapolis: University of Minnesosta Press.

Jüttemann, G. (Ed.) (1990). *Komparative Kasuistik.* Heidelberg: Asanger.

Lerner, R. M. & Spanier, G. B. (Eds.) (1978). *Child influences on marital and family interaction.* New York: Academic Press.

Peters, H. F. M. & Hulstijn, W. (Eds.) (1987). *Speech motor dynamics in stuttering.* Wien: Springer.

Peters, H. F. M. & Starkweather, C. W. (1989). Development of stuttering throughout life. *Journal of Fluency Disorders, 14,* 303–321.

Riley, G. D. & Riley, J. (1984). A component model for treating stuttering in children. In M. Peins (Ed.), *Contemporary approaches in stuttering therapy. 123–172.* Boston: Little, Brown & Company.

Schulze, H. (1989). *Stottern und Interaktion. Vergleichende Untersuchung der verbalen Interaktionsstile von Eltern und ihren stotternden Kindern.* Ulm: Universität, Phoniatrische Ambulanz.

Schulze, H. (1989). Dysfluency – Syndrome. In G. Kittel (Ed.), *Kursbuch für Phoniatrie und Pädaudiologie. 103–118.* Köln: Deutscher Ärzte-Verlag.

Schulze, H. & Johannsen, H. S. (1986). *Stottern bei Kindern im Vorschulalter. Theorie, Diagnostik, Therapie.* Ulm: Universität. Phoniatrische Ambulanz.

Schulze, H. & Johannsen, H. S. (1991). Importance of parent-child interaction in the genesis of stuttering. *Folia Phoniatrica,* (43, 133–143).

Shames, G. H. & Rubin, K. (1986). *Stuttering then and now.* Columbus: C. E. Merrill Publ. Company.

St. Louis, K. O. (Ed.) (1986). *The atypical stutterer. Principles and practices of rehabilitation.* Orlando: Academic Press.

Starkweather, C. W. (1987). *Fluency and stuttering.* Englewood Cliffs: Prentice Hall.

Starkweather, C. W. (1988). *Upgrading the demands and capacities model. Paper presented at the Second International Oxford Dysfluency Conference.* Sommerville College, Oxford, England. August 24–26, 1988.

Starkweather, C. W., Gottwald, S. R. & Halfond, M. M. (1990). *Stuttering prevention: A clinical method.* Prentice Hall: Englewood Cliffs.

Van Riper, C. (1982). *The nature of stuttering.* Englewood Cliffs: Prentice Hall. 2nd Ed.

Webster, W. G. & Poulos, M. G. (1989). *Facilitating fluency. Transfer strategies for adult stuttering treatment programs.* Tucson: Communication Skill Builders.

Wendlandt, W. (1984). *Zum Beispiel Stottern. Stolperdrähte, Sackgassen und Lichtblicke im Therapiealltag.* München: Pfeiffer.

Wingate, M. E. (1988). *The structure of stuttering. A psycholinguistic analysis.* New York: Springer.

Yairi, E. (1990). Subtyping child stutterers for research purpose. In J. A. Cooper, (Ed.), *Research needs in stuttering: Roadblocks and future directions. 50–57.* Rockville, Maryland: ASHA Reports No. 18.

Hartmut Schulze, Ulm (Germany)

85. Therapy of the Stuttering Child

1. Introduction

A particularly vibrant area of stuttering treatment activity in the past two decades has been treatment of young children who stutter. Many modern clinicians have rejected Wendel Johnson's (1959) diagnosogenic theory and Bloodstein's (1987) anticipatory struggle theory so that now treatment for young children is condoned and even enthusiastically endorsed. The purpose of this chapter is, then, to review the current status of therapy for the young stuttering child (up to the age of 8 or so).

2. The Direct Treatment of Stuttering

2.1. Introduction

Direct treatments are those that attempt to change stuttered speech by methods aimed in a straightforward manner towards reducing moments of stuttering and increasing durations of nonstuttered speech. Their ultimate goal is usually the complete elimination of stuttering, resulting in normal-sounding and normal-feeling stutter-free speech. Direct treatments are essentially the only treatments that have been evaluated empirically, although there is much room for criticism of the amount and quality of that body of research. Perhaps research efforts are lacking here because researchers have believed that 'spontaneous recovery' will eliminate stuttering in many young children, although this belief has been seriously challenged (R. Ingham 1983; Martin/Lindamood 1986). Further, research aimed at discriminating which stutterers will and will not recover without formal treatment is essentially nonexistent.

2.2. The Basics of Direct Treatment with Young Stutterers

Elsewhere this writer (Costello 1983) has described the basics of direct treatment to consist of "... the most simplistic and uncomplicated kind of treatment format: ... arranging differential consequences for the occurrence of fluent utterances and moments of stuttering." The application to stuttering of these basic principles of behavior change has been thoroughly described and documented (cf. Costello 1980; 1982; Costello/Ingham 1984 a; Ingham 1984).

The first published study to test these principles with preschool-aged stutterers was the seminal study of Martin/Kuhl/Haroldson (1972). Two young children individually conversed with a puppet named Suzibelle. During these conversations a child's moments of stuttering were immediately followed by a 10-s period during which the lights illuminating Suzibelle were turned off and Suzibelle stopped talking to the child (e. g., timeout). This treatment eliminated the stuttering of both children, and a new era of stuttering treatment for children was underway.

Subsequent studies used another form of timeout, wherein the stutterer is required to stop speaking for a brief period whenever a stutter occurs. This procedure has been repeatedly shown to serve as a functional negative consequence for stuttering in older children and adults (e. g., Costello 1975; Ryan 1974) and is also quite useful for young stutterers from about the age of five. Other events that have been used with young children to consequate moments of stuttering are: saying *slow down* (Reed/Godden 1977), requiring the child to repeat the word or utterance that contains stuttering (Onslow/Costa/Rue 1990), applying response cost (removal of a token reinforcer) (Salend/Andress 1984), and clinician remarks such as *uh oh* or *there's a bumpy word* (using the child's label for stuttering). As is always the case, different stimuli will serve as functional negative stimuli for different children.

The methods described above emphasized the controlling effects of negative feedback for moments of stuttering. Other versions of the basics have concentrated on the application of positive reinforcement for nonstuttered utterances, such as stutter-free speech of a minimum duration (Peters 1977; Shaw/Shrum 1972). Myriads of stimuli are useful as positive reinforcers in such procedures: clinician praise, stickers, 'plus' marks on data sheets, etc. Token reinforcement systems are also quite powerful, as long as the exchange rate for 'back-up' reinforcers isn't too sparse. Of course, as in treatments for all other kinds of behaviors, reinforcement schedules become progressively more intermittent, and reinforcing stimuli gradually more natural, as treatment continues. As well, most clinicians design treatments that combine feedback for both nonstuttered utterances and occurrences of stuttering.

Interesting and effective applications of the basics were reported by Johnson (1984) and Onslow (1990) wherein parents were the treatment agents and the home environment was the treatment setting. Johnson taught parents to attend selectively to their children's stutter-free utterances and to ignore utterances that contained stuttering during ongoing daily activities. Onslow/Costa/Rue trained mothers of young stutterers to reinforce stutter-free utterances with praise and tangible reinforcers during formalized treatment sessions at home and during natural daily activities.

In the above examples basic contingency management was applied to the nonstuttered and stuttered speech of young children during spontaneous conversation. For some young children, however, production of a substantial amount of conversational speech may be unlikely. Stuttering severity, stutterers' reactions to their stuttering, general shyness, or even the existence of a concurrent language disorder could make stutter-free utterances of reinforceable length infrequent. Another disadvantage of conversation as a treatment medium is highlighted by research suggesting that disfluency is exacerbated by increases in sentence complexity (Gaines/Runyan/Meyers 1991; Ratner/Sih 1987) and length (Brundage/Ratner 1989; Gaines/Runyan/Meyers (1991) – variables that can fluctuate in children's spontaneous conversation. Therefore, a treatment task that is spontaneous and natural but less conversational, and that can control utterance complexity and length, would seem beneficial. This concept has become almost standard in the treatment of young children.

2.3. Extended Length of Utterance as a Treatment Strategy

The concept of designing treatment so that only very short stutter-free utterances are required in the beginning and progressively longer stutter-free utterances are gradually introduced was first described by Ryan (1974; Ryan/Ryan 1983). Ryan's program is referred to as GILCU (gradual increase in length and complexity of utterance) and adds to the basics the principles of programmed instruction and successive approximation (Costello 1977). Ryan's work with older children showed that this program was not only highly successful but was relatively simple for clinicians to learn to administer. Johnson/Coleman/Rasmussen (1978) also successfully applied the GILCU program to children in the public schools.

For use with younger children, the principles of GILCU have been operationalized in detail in a highly successful version referred to as Extended Length of Utterance (ELU) (Costello 1983). Children's stutter-free utterances are very gradually extended from 1 syllable through 2, 3, 4, 5, and 6 syllables (spontaneously generated words and phrases evoked by pictures), to connected speech utterances progressing from 3 s through 5, 10, 20 ... seconds, ultimately to 5 min of stutter-free conversation with the clinician in the clinic. Throughout the program stutter-free and stuttered responses are consequated with positive reinforcement and negative feedback, respectively.

2.4. Summary

Several characteristics of direct treatment that applies the basics with young children should be highlighted. First, the hallmarks of this kind of treatment are the use of child-appropriate response contingent differential consequences for stutter-free utterances and moments of stuttering, most often combined with requirements for the production of progressively longer stutter-free utterances (ELU). Second, this kind of treatment appears to be appropriate for all young children who stutter, irrespective of (a) the child's level of awareness or concern about stuttering; (b) the severity of stuttering; (c) who serves as treatment agent: clinician, parent, or teacher; or (d) where treatment takes place: clinic, home, or school. Third, this kind of treatment includes no instructions to the child regarding how to produce stutter-free speech. Children are left to their own devices, which may mean that they build upon their existing fluent speech or independently develop an acceptable speech pattern that meets the clinician's standards for natural-sounding, stutter-free speech at normal speaking rates.

2.5. Treatments Founded on 'Additives'

Many direct treatments described for young children add to the basics the requirement that children alter their habitual speech pattern in specific ways so as to approach speech differently and thereby reduce the occurrence of stuttering (Cooper 1987; Culp 1984; Runyan/Runyan 1986; Shine 1984). Such additives have become fundamental in the treatment of adult stutterers, which is apparently why they are suggested for use with children as well. Although additives are described by a variety of labels, certain characteristics appear to be common among them. They are: decreased speaking rate, oftentimes paired with prolongation of vowels and continuant consonants; gentle/easy onset of vocalization; control of air flow/breath management; light articulatory contacts; reduced loudness. Coppola and Yairi (1982) added rhythmic speech to this list.

Most of the reports of these procedures are based on little or no data. Among the questions in need of study are the following.

(1) Would additives be required if treatment began with only the use of the basics? In most reports, speech pattern changes are introduced into the treatment at the outset. Further, many of the treatments that use additives introduce several at the same time, and in combination with the basics. In such cases the role of the additives cannot be isolated nor can their necessity be demonstrated.

(2) Is it possible to adequately operationalize and measure the use of additives? Although speaking rate is often measured, different conventions for its measurement abound. Even more problematic: how does one measure prolongation? light contact? easy onset? airflow? And if measurement of these characteristics can be developed and agreed upon, will such measurement be able to be applied online by clinicians during treatment? This would appear to be mandatory for treatments that require children to use such additives.

(3) Are young children able reliably to manipulate their speech production so as to include alterations required by additives? Ryan (1974) mentioned that it was difficult to get young children to produce the kind of prolonged speech required by DAF treatment regimes. It is likely that this is true for other unusual manners of speaking as well, perhaps due to young children's immature motor control systems or to their lack of metalinguistic awareness (Cooper 1987). Conture (1990) attempts to deal with this problem by using elaborate analogies to "provide essential insight for the young client into what he or she *does* that interferes with speech and what is necessary to change in order to speak more fluently."

(4) What is the quality of children's speech at the end of treatment that uses additives? Reports of the outcomes of these techniques have not included assessment of the naturalness of children's posttreatment speech (cf. Martin/Haroldson/Triden 1984). If children continue to use additives to control stuttering, noticeable abnormalities in speech naturalness would be expected.

In summary, while many direct treatments with young children recommend inclusion of additives to the basic treatment paradigm, the necessity of such additions and the quality of their effect on fluency have not yet been well documented.

3. The Indirect Treatment of Stuttering

3.1. Introduction

Indirect treatments are those that attempt to change stuttered speech by methods (generally referred to as counseling) aimed at behaviors of others in the child's environment (particularly parents) and at other aspects of the child's behavior. Broadly, indirect therapies are based on the belief that certain conditions – those that provoke stress for the child (communicative or otherwise), or make the child feel generally insecure or anxious, or produce uncertainty about the ability to communicate, or that make demands beyond the child's capacities – aggravate, if not cause, the child's stuttering (e. g., Gregory 1987; Prins 1983; Starkweather/Gottwald 1990; Starkweather/Gottwald/Halfond 1990; Williams 1984). Such conditions are, then, considered to be the targets for treatment.

Most indirect therapies, although perhaps compelling in their underlying logic, are completely unsupported by empirical evidence regarding their effects (cf. Costello 1983; Ingham/Ingham 1990; Guitar 1984). This unfortunate state of affairs appears to exist for several reasons. (a) The treatments are ill-defined and suggest multitudes of potentially independent variables in need of modification. (b) Objective measurement of the amorphous independent and dependent variables dictated by these viewpoints is difficult (e. g., see Ulliana/Ingham 1984), although some efforts have been made in this direction (Cooper 1987; DeNil/Brutten 1991). (c) Outcomes of these treatments are usually confounded by accompanying direct treatments (e. g., Conture 1990; Cooper 1987; Gregory 1984; 1987; Guitar/Peters 1980; Johnson 1984; Prins 1983; Riley/Riley 1984; Rustin 1987; Rustin/Cooke 1983; Starkweather/Gottwald/Halfond 1990; Wall/Myers 1984). In the several cases where direct treatment follows a period of indirect treatment, the inference can be made that indirect treatment did not produce a completely satisfactory outcome. However, it is not possible to discern whether the preceding indirect therapy was expeditious, detrimental, or irrelevant to the eventual outcome of the direct treatment.

3.2. Indirect Therapy Directed Toward Parents

Recently, it has been suggested that rapid parental speech may aggravate a child's stuttering, perhaps by inducing fast speech in the child. This suggests that modification of parent speech rate should be a target of treatment (Johnson 1984; Gregory 1984; Prins 1983; Starkweather/Gottwald/Hanson 1990; Wall/Myers 1984). Meyers/Freeman (1985b) found that mothers of stuttering children did, indeed, speak more rapidly than mothers of nonstutterers; however, their stuttering children did not speak faster than nonstuttering children. Stephenson-Opsal/Ratner (1988) found that reductions in mother's speech rates were accompanied by decreases in their children's stuttering, but not via speech rate reductions. These researchers suggested that reduced parent speech rates may prompt changes in other aspects of the child-parent conversational interaction such as rate of turn-taking, change in demand-structure of child-directed speech, and reduced language complexity, thus allowing the child more time to 'preprogram' utterances.

Another variable suggested as a treatment target (Gregory 1984; Riley/Riley 1984; Rustin 1987; Rustin/Cooke 1983; Williams 1984) is interruptions. Meyers/Freeman (1985a) found that mothers of stuttering and nonstuttering children were more likely to interrupt a child during a disfluency than during a fluent utterance and that both children's own interruptions of mothers' speech were more likely to be disfluent than fluent. These data, however, offer no direct evidence regarding the functional relationship between stuttering and interruptions. Therefore, the recommendation that interruptions of the stuttering child's speech should be reduced appears premature as a treatment procedure.

Table 85.1 provides a partial list of other undocumented variables suggested in the literature as potential treatment targets for indirect treatments aimed at altering parent behaviors. Both hypothesized fluency interruptors and fluency facilitators are listed.

In an overview of the concept of indirect treatment for young stuttering children, Costello (1983) raised two questions that have yet to be answered satisfactorily. First, do clinicians have the right to ask families to change certain aspects of their relationship with the stuttering child, and to infer by this that the family is at least partially responsible for the child's stuttering, when little or no evidence exists that these variables do, in fact, influence the child's stuttering? Second, are clinicians effectively able to affect changes in family members' behaviors, when many of those behaviors occur in environments and under conditions not accessible to the clinician? Given the known effects of direct treatments with young children, it continues to seem reasonable to contend that "a more suitable strategy for treatment of stuttering in young children is to directly teach them to produce fluent, nonstuttered speech no matter what is going on in their natural environment" (Costello 1983).

3.3. Indirect Therapy Directed Toward the Stuttering Child

Most indirect therapies also address characteristics of the child – other than fluency and stuttering – under the assumption that modification of such characteristics produces or facilitates fluency. Suggested targets have been communication attitudes and feelings (Cooper 1987), speech avoidance and fear (Wall/Myers 1984), unduly high self-expectations (Riley/Riley 1984), and overall psychological adjustment (Wall/Myers 1984). Also suggested has been treatment of any existing concomitant communication disorder including auditory processing and oral motor discoordination (Conture 1990; Riley/Riley 1984). Changing the child's language use and pragmatics has been mentioned in terms of encouraging use of less complex vocabulary and syntax and reducing question-asking (Williams 1984), teaching the child to be a good listener and good conversationalist (Conture 1990; Gregory 1984) and to use contentional turn-taking rules – that is, not to interrupt (Conture 1990; Gregory 1984; Meyers/Freeman 1985a; Rustin/Cooke 1983; Starkweather/Gottwald/Halfond 1990; Wall/Myers 1984; Williams 1984), and helping the child develop appropriate social skills, especially in reaction to being teased (Rustin 1987; Wall/Myers 1984). Also mentioned has been instruction in relaxation skills (Rustin 1987). Yet again the major problem with this kind of indirect treatment (aside from the absence of common theoretical underpinnings, which is made obvious by the hodgepodge assortment of behaviors recommended for treatment) is that its effects are entangled with concurrent employment of the above-described parent counseling and even direct treatment of the child's stuttering. Therefore, the extent to which attention to these variables influences the eventual outcome of treatment has not been determined.

3.4. Generalization and Measurement.

Two remaining issues, either of which could fill its own chapter, remain to be briefly mentioned. First, the ultimate evaluation of the outcome of any kind of stuttering treatment rests on information regarding the generalization and maintenance of treatment effects across all aspects of the child's daily environment. Many of the reports cited herein suggest that across-settings generalization occurs spontaneously among young children, as an outgrowth of treatment; yet most of the same reports provide little more than anecdotal evidence in this regard. A review of the relevant literature by Ingham/Onslow (1987) highlights this deficit and describes the few procedures that have been used to promote generalization. They conclude that 'Train and Hope" (Stokes/Baer 1977) is the method (or nonmethod) most often relied upon.

Lastly, much has been written regarding the kind of measurement required to docu-

Fluency Interruptors
telling the child to slow down, relax, think before talking (Asha 1990)
calling attention to child's speech (Asha 1990)
correcting child's stuttered speech (Asha 1990)
quickly changing topics (Gregory 1984)
asking too many questions without waiting for reply (Gregory 1984; Rustin 1987; Rustin/Cooke 1983)
making too many verbal demands that require complex verbal responses (Prins 1983)
finishing child's statements and filling in words or guessing what child is about to say (Gregory 1984; Williams 1984)
not listening to the child (Prins 1983; Rustin 1987; Williams 1984)
smiling or frowning at inappropriate times while child is talking (Williams 1984)
hurrying the child when the child is talking (Riley/Riley 1984; Williams 1984)
making conversation unrelated to the current activity (Rustin 1987)
constantly correcting or criticizing child's verbal and nonverbal behavior (Gregory 1984; Riley/Riley 1984)
using ambiguous nonverbal communication (Rustin 1987)
allowing the child to speak in competition with others (Prins 1983; Williams 1984)
being too directive regarding child's conversation or play (Rustin 1987)
being a passive parent (Rustin 1987)
allowing child to use stuttering to manipulate parents (Riley/Riley 1984)
being inconsistent or making extreme changes in disciplinary practices (Rustin/Cooke 1983; Williams 1984)
being erratic in planning and conducting routine daily activities (Gregory 1984; Prins 1983)
arranging activity schedules that create time pressure for the child (Gregory 1984; Prins 1983)
making behavioral demands the child is unable to meet (Prins 1983)
having disagreements between parents ("verbal bickering") of any kind, in the child's presence (Williams 1984)
having disagreement between parents regarding whether or not child is a stutterer, in the child's presence (Conture 1990)
discussing how much fun parents will have when child has begun preschool or kindergarten, in the child's presence (Williams 1984)
being separated/divorced (Williams 1984)
showing negative reactions to the child's stuttering (Starkweather/Gottwald/Halfond 1990)
imposing high standards (Conture 1990; Gregory 1984; Starkweather/Gottwald/Halfond 1990; Williams 1984)
having an abnormal need for the child to stutter (Riley/Riley 1984)
bringing a sibling into the world or otherwise creating a family crisis (Gregory 1984; Williams 1984)
allowing siblings or peers to tease the child (Riley/Riley 1984; Williams 1984)
Fluency Facilitators
regularly spending more (talking) time with the child (Conture 1990; Prins 1983; Starkweather/Gottwald/Halfond 1990)
simplifying language used with child (Conture 1990; Prins 1983; Starkweather/Gottwald/Halfond 1990; Wall/Myers 1984)
reading more often to the child (Conture 1990)
directly discussing child's stuttering with the child (Starkweather/Gottwald/Halfond 1990)
enhancing child's degree of independence and self-reliance (Rustin/Cooke 1983)
enhancing child's ability to problem solve (Rustin/Cooke 1983)
increasing child's self-confidence and self-acceptance (Gregory/Hill 1984)

Table 85.1: Hypothesized fluency interruptors and fluency facilitators postulated in the literature

Selection of valid dependent variables
Reliable measurement of dependent variables
Periodic measurement of treatment effects throughout pretreatment, treatment, and posttreatment phases
Multiple measures of natural conversational speech across settings beyond the treatment environment
At least occasional use of nonreactive (covert) measures
Use of a potent treatment method for the establishment/acquisition of stutter-free speech
Inclusion of transfer activities (if necessary)
Inclusion of maintenance activities (if necessary)

Table 85.2: Features to be addressed in research on stuttering treatment effects, especially in regard to across-setting generalization (Ingham 1989)

ment stuttering treatment effects with validity and reliability (e. g., Costello/Ingham 1984 b; Ingham/Costello 1984). Table 85.2 lists eight features suggested by Ingham (1989) that should be addressed in studies purporting to demonstrate stuttering treatment effects. The conduct of such research obviously requires a major commitment of time and resources, but the last word on stuttering treatment with young children – irrespective of the approach entertained – won't be written until such research has been conducted, reported, and replicated.

4. References

ASHA (1990). Let's Talk (No. 19). *Asha, 32.*

Bloodstein, O. (1987). *A handbook on stuttering.* Chicago: National Easter Seal Society.

Brundage, S. B. & Ratner, N. B. (1989). Measurement of stuttering frequency in children's speech. *Journal of Fluency Disorders, 14,* 351–358.

Conture, E. G. (1990). *Stuttering* (2nd ed.). Englewood Cliffs, NJ: Prentice Hall.

Cooper, E. B. (1987). The Cooper Personalized Fluency Control Therapy. In L. Rustin, H. Purser, & E. Rowley (Eds.), *Progress in the treatment of fluency disorders.* 124–146. London: Taylor and Francis.

Coppola, V. A. & Yairi, E. (1982). Rhythmic speech training with preschool stuttering children: An experimental study. *Journal of Fluency Disorders, 7,* 447–457.

Costello, J. M. (1975). Time-out procedures for the modification of stuttering: Three case studies. *Journal of Speech and Hearing Disorders, 40,* 216–231.

Costello, J. M. (1977). Programmed instruction. *Journal of Speech and Hearing Disorders, 42,* 3–28.

Costello, J. M. (1980). Operant conditioning and the treatment of stuttering. In W. H. Perkins (Ed.), Strategies in stuttering therapy. *Seminars in Speech, Language, and Hearing, 1,* 311–325.

Costello, J. M. (1982). Techniques of therapy based on operant theory. In W. H. Perkins (Ed.), *Current therapy of communication disorders. General principles of therapy.* 3–11. New York: Brian C. Decker Division of Thieme-Stratton.

Costello, J. M. (1983). Current behavioral treatments for children. In D. Prins & R. J. Ingham (Eds.), *Treatment of stuttering in early childhood. Methods and issues.* 69–112. San Diego: College-Hill Press.

Costello, J. M. & Ingham, R. J. (1984 a). Stuttering as an operant disorder. In R. F. Curlee & W. H. Perkins (Eds.), *Nature and treatment of stuttering: New directions.* 187–213. San Diego: College-Hill Press.

Costello, J. M. & Ingham, R. J. (1984 b). Assent strategies for child and adult stutterers. In R. F. Curlee & W. H. Perkins (Eds.), *Nature and treatment of stuttering: New directions.* 303–333. San Diego: College-Hill Press.

Culp, D. (1984). The preschool fluency development program. In M. Peins (Ed.), *Contemporary approaches in stuttering therapy.* 39–71. Boston: Little-Brown.

De Nil, L. F. & Brutten, G. J. (1991). Speech-associated attitudes of stuttering and nonstuttering children. *Journal of Speech and Hearing Research, 34,* 60–66.

Gaines, N. D., Runyan, C. M. & Meyers, S. C. (1991). A comparison of young stutterers' fluent versus stuttered utterances on measures of length and complexity. *Journal of Speech and Hearing Research, 34,* 37–42.

Gregory, H. H. (1984). Prevention of stuttering: Management of early stages. In R. F. Curlee & W. H. Perkins (Eds.), *Nature and treatment of stuttering: New directions.* 335–356. San Diego: College-Hill Press.

Gregory, H. H. (1987). The treatment of stuttering: Recent history and contemporary issues. In L. Rustin, H. Purser, & E. Rowley (Eds.), *Progress in the treatment of fluency disorders*. 105–123. London: Taylor & Francis.

Gregory, H. H. & Hill, D. (1984). Stuttering therapy for children. In W. H. Perkins (Ed.) *Current therapy of communication disorders: Stuttering disorders*. 77–94. New York: Thieme-Stratton.

Guitar, B. (1984). The indirect treatment of stuttering. In J. M. Costello (Ed.), *Speech disorders in children: Recent advances*. 291–312. San Diego: College-Hill Press.

Guitar, B. & Peters, T. J. (1980). *Stuttering: An integration of contemporary therapies*. Memphis, TN: Speech Foundation of America.

Ingham, J. C. (1989). Generalization in the treatment of stuttering. In L. V. McReynolds & J. E. Spradlin (Eds.), *Generalization strategies in the treatment of communication disorders*. 63–81. Toronto: B. C. Decker.

Ingham, R. J. (1983). Spontaneous remission of stuttering: When will the emperor realize he has no clothes on? In D. Prins & R. J. Ingham (Eds.), *Treatment of stuttering in early childhood. Methods and issues*. 113–140. San Diego: College-Hill Press.

Ingham, R. J. (1984). *Stuttering and behavior therapy: Current status and experimental foundations*. San Diego: College-Hill Press.

Ingham, R. J. & Costello, J. M. (1984). Stutterers treatment evaluation. In J. M. Costello (Ed.), *Speech disorders in children: Recent advances*. 303–346. San Diego: College-Hill Press.

Ingham, R. J. & Ingham, J. C. (1990). Let's talk about stuttering. *Asha, 32*, (12), 42.

Ingham, R. J. & Onslow, M. (1987). Generalization and maintenance of treatment benefits for children who stutter. *Seminars in Speech and Language, 8*, 303–326.

Johnson, G. F., Coleman, D., & Rasmussen, K. (1978). Multidays: Multidimensional approach for the young stutterer. *Language, Speech, and Hearing Services in Schools, 9*, 129–132.

Johnson, L. J. (1984). Facilitating parental involvement in therapy of the preschool disfluent child. In W. H. Perkins (Ed.), *Current therapy of communication disorders: Stuttering*. 29–39. New York: Thieme-Stratton.

Johnson, W. (1959). *The onset of stuttering*. Minneapolis: University of Minnesota Press.

Martin, R., Haroldson, S., & Triden, K. A. (1984). Stuttering and speech naturalness. *Journal of Speech and Hearing Disorders, 49*, 53–58.

Martin, R., Kuhl, P., & Haroldson, S. (1972). An experimental treatment with two preschool stuttering children. *Journal of Speech and Hearing Research, 15*, 743–752.

Martin, R. & Lindamood, L. P. (1986). Stuttering and spontaneous recovery: Implications for the speech-language pathologist. *Language, Speech, and Hearing Services in Schools, 17*, 207–218.

Meyers, S. C. & Freeman, F. J. (1985a). Interruptions as a variable in stuttering and disfluency. *Journal of Speech and Hearing Research, 28*, 428–435.

Meyers, S. C. & Freeman, F. J. (1985b). Mother and child speech rates as a variable in stuttering and disfluency. *Journal of Speech and Hearing Research, 28*, 436–444.

Onslow, M., Costa, L., & Rue, S. (1990). Direct early intervention with stuttering: Some preliminary data. *Journal of Speech and Hearing Disorders, 55*, 405–416.

Peters, A. D. (1977). The effect of positive reinforcement on fluency: Two case studies. *Language, Speech, and Hearing Services in Schools, 8*, 15–22.

Prins, D. (1983). Continuity, fragmentation, and tension: Hypotheses applied to evaluation and intervention with preschool disfluent children. In D. Prins & R. J. Ingham (Eds.), *Treatment of stuttering in early childhood. Methods and issues*. 21–42. San Diego: College-Hill Press.

Ratner, N. B. & Sih, C. C. (1987). The effects of gradual increases in sentence length and complexity on children's dysfluency. *Journal of Speech and Hearing Disorders, 52*, 278–287.

Reed, C. G. & Godden, A. L. (1977). An experimental treatment using verbal punishment with two preschool stutterers. *Journal of Fluency Disorders, 2*, 225–233.

Riley, G. D. & Riley, J. (1984). A component model for treating stuttering in children. In M. Peins (Ed.), *Contemporary approaches in stuttering therapy*. 123–171. Boston: Little-Brown.

Runyan, C. M. & Runyan, S. E. (1986). A fluency rules therapy program for young children in the public schools. *Language, Speech, and Hearing Services in Schools, 17*, 276–284.

Rustin, L. (1987). The treatment of childhood dysfluency through active parental involvement. In L. Rustin, H. Purser, & E. Rowley (Eds.), *Progress in the treatment of fluency disorders*. 166–180. London: Taylor & Francis.

Rustin, L. & Cooke, F. (1983). Intervention procedures for the disfluent child. In P. Dalton (Ed.), *Approaches to the treatment of stuttering*. 47–75. London: Croom Helm.

Ryan, B. P. (1974). *Programmed therapy for stuttering in children and adults*. Springfield, IL: Charles C. Thomas.

Ryan, B. P. & Ryan, B. V. K. (1983). Programmed stuttering therapy for children: Comparison of four establishment programs. *Journal of Fluency Disorders, 8*, 291–321.

Salend, S. J. & Andress, M. J. (1984). Decreasing stuttering in an elementary-level student. *Language, Speech, and Hearing Services in Schools, 15*, 16–21.

Shaw, C. & Shrum, W. (1972). The effect of response-contingent reward on the connected speech of children who stutter. *Journal of Speech and Hearing Disorders, 37*, 75 – 88.

Shine, R. E. (1984). Direct management of the beginning stutterer. In W. H. Perkins (Ed.), *Current therapy of communication disorders: Stuttering disorders*. 57 – 76. New York: Thieme-Stratton.

Starkweather, C. W. & Gottwald, S. R. (1990). The demands and capacities model II: Clinical applications. *Journal of Fluency Disorders, 15*, 143 – 157.

Starkweather, C. W., Gottwald, S. R., & Halfond, M. M. (1990). *Stuttering prevention. A clinical method*. Englewood Cliffs, NJ: Prentice Hall.

Stokes, T. F. & Baer, D. (1977). An implicit technology of generalization. *Journal of Applied Behavior Analysis, 10*, 349 – 367.

Stephenson-Opsal, D. & Ratner, N. B. (1988). Maternal speech rate modification and childhood stuttering. *Journal of Fluency Disorders, 13*, 49 – 56.

Ulliana, L. & Ingham, R. J. (1984). Behavioral and nonbehavioral variables in the measurement of stutterers' communication attitudes. *Journal of Speech and Hearing Disorders, 49*, 83 – 93.

Wall, M. J. & Myers, F. L. (1984). *Clinical management of childhood stuttering*. Baltimore: University Park Press.

Williams, D. E. (1984). Prevention of stuttering. In W. H. Perkins (Ed.), *Current therapy of communication disorders: Stuttering disorders*. 21 – 28. New York: Thieme-Stratton.

Janis Costello Ingham, Santa Barbara, California (USA)

86. Therapy of the Stuttering Adult

Since the 1850s, the treatment of stuttering has focused on prosthetic, early pedagogic, homeopathic approaches, and, above all, practice (see Fiedler/Standop 1986; Rieber/Wollock 1977, for an historical overview). Most of the methods concentrate directly on remedying or improving the speech disorder. If, however, one shares the view that stuttering has a neuropsychological basis which is significantly influenced by psychosocial factors, then it follows that speech training procedures address only a limited area of stuttering symptomatology. Speech techniques are meaningful only when they are integrated as elements in a comprehensive treatment plan. Such a plan should also adress the psychosocial disturbances which affect the stuttering and can seriously impair the stutterer's psychosocial well-being.

1. Speech Therapy and Fluency Training

Apparently there is no fluency training technique or speech therapy that can permanently eliminate stuttering (Andrews/Howie/Dozsa/Guitar 1982). Nevertheless, systematic practice of new speech habits and speech patterns are indispensable to speech disorder treatments. The form of speech training employed and its relative importance within the total treatment plan depends, among other factors, upon the severity of the stuttering. With regard to the introduction of new speech habits, it is important to distinguish between speech therapy and fluency training.

1.1. Speech Therapy

As subgroup of treatment methods *speech therapy methods* demand a controlled therapeutic setting and generally lead directly to noticeable improvement in speech. However, in most cases, these methods call for the support of another (trained) person, which makes the transfer of therapeutic progress into daily life difficult.

1.1.1. Simultaneous Speech and Shadowing

Here, the stutterer and the therapist (or another person) read a text aloud simultaneously. Alternatively, the stutterer repeats with a slight delay, material from a text that is read aloud or recited by another person (like a shadow). Simultaneous speaking is also known as the Unisono-method (already presented by Liebmann in 1914). The symptom reduction during such practice is considerable. It is not, however, significantly maintained outside of the experimental or practice setting. The efficacy of both methods can be explained by the hypothesis that stuttering is caused by a defect of perceptive awareness and that this kind of aid to speech diverts the attention of the stutterer from his/her own speech to that of the other person doing the talking (see Cherry/Sayers 1956). The application of these procedures is justified, for one, by the possibility of demonstrating to a severrely speech-disturbed stutterer that his/her stuttering can be influenced.

1.1.2. Masking

The presence of a strong sound (or strong white noise) over earphones, can prevent the stutterer from engaging in an auditory control of his/her articulation. Theoretically, this explains the considerable symptom reduction and supports the perceptive awareness hypothesis (Cherry/Sayers 1956; Van Riper 1973). A therapeutic goal of this procedure can also be the systematic practice of new speech pattern accompanied by white noise (the reestablishment of neuromotor autoregulation; Fiedler/Standop 1986). Of course, this method is impractical in daily life. This led to the development of aids which mask hearing and which can be worn in the ear outside of the therapy situation. Evidently, these masking devices help only very few stutterers; therefore, the effectiveness of using extremely costly speech aids must necessarily be thoroughly considered (see Ingham/Southwood/Horsburgh 1981).

1.1.3. Reinforcement and Feedback

In the 1970s many operant procedures were tried individually or in combination to treat stuttering. For example: response contingent positive and negative verbal reinforcement, as well as other operant techniques (such as time-out and token economy) were intended to have an effect on the frequency of stuttered verbal behavior (e. g. Ingham/Andrews 1973; Shames/Egolf 1976; James 1976). Likewise, biofeedback using electromyographic feedback for relaxation during reading and spontaneous speech, was introduced (e. g. Guitar 1975; Lanyon 1977). The application of operant techniques does lead to significant progress in speaking. Surprisingly, though, the successes that usually occur immediately do not follow the typical learning curves and thus cannot be explained in terms of classical learning theory. These results lead to the interesting assumption, among others, that attention must be brought back to a conscious concentration on speech and, above all, on an associated gradual slowing of the style of speaking (Becker/Kessler/Fuchsgruber 1975; Fiedler 1991). Unfortunately, the hoped-for therapeutic effect of this procedure does not last long outside of the therapy situation. Therefore, the application of operant techniques and biofeedback can only be recommended in conjunction with other methods.

1.2. Fluency Training

Systematic rehearsal of newly acquired fluency stands in the center of goal-directed fluency training. The wide variety of fluency training methods is almost impossible to thoroughly describe. Most of them, however, involve techniques and 'tricks' which were first 'discovered' by stutterers themselves during their attempts to overcome their speech difficulties. Subsequently they were systematically studied and further developed by therapists. These styles of speech are incompatible with stuttering and the majority of them help stutterers to speak fluently (in the therapy situation) within less than hours, sometimes after only minutes (e. g. Howie/Andrews 1984). Fluency techniques can usually be applied without mechanical devices and thus offer a good premise for the transfer of learning to daily situations. They should, therefore, take priority over speech therapy techniques in the treatment of stuttering.

1.2.1. Changing the Sound of the Voice: Gentle Onset

"Gentle onset" (changing the volume level of the voice) is a so-called "starter" (Widlak 1977) typically used in self-help techniques and at the same time is one of the most troublesome stuttering symptoms. Starters are parts of words that by and large can be produced without errors and are easy for the stutterer to pronounce. They serve as regular starting aids for articulation of difficult words and word-beginnings.

One type of the therapy using starters reqirers stutterers to concentrate on the modification of their breathing and their speech habits, as described by Schwartz (1976). In Schwartz's blowing technique aimed at preventing tension in the laryngeal region, in particular spasms of the vocal band (lanryngospasm), speaking is precede by an inaudible aspirate. This recalls the breathing method proposed by A. Gutzmann (1879).

In this procedure the client begins talking with 'audible' sigh which is gradually replaced by a voiceless 'blowing'. The aim of blowing is to set the vocal bands into vibration by 'gently' emitting a stream of air before starting to say difficult words and then to maintain it in speaking a sentence. Using a silent /h/ as a starting aspirate is the most common example of this technique. Also common is the 'bridging' of stuttering by means of sounds like /e/, /w/ or /m/. In therapy, this technique is first practiced with obvious exaggeration which is reduced until the client is able to employ the technique without listeners discerning it. Because the danger exists that this technique could lead to the development of a new secondary symptom in the stuttering syndrome, it should not be used as the sole treatment approach (see Van Riper 1973).

1.2.2. Changing the Prosody: Accentuation and Intonation

The key principle lies in the conscious addition of speech intonation features directed towards changing ones prosody (for rationale, e. g. Wingate 1979; Bergman 1987). Better known forms of this approach are:

(a) expanding vowels and "vocal" binding of successive words (until the whole sentence is articulated as one word; Bluemel 1913; H. Gutzmann, as early as 1898),
(b) the conscious emphasis of syllables ("syllable-timed-speech"; Andrews/Harris 1964), and
(c) monotonous speaking ("monotoned speech"; Adams/Sears/Ramig 1982).

We recommend the latter less because it belongs to the stuttering symptom constellation. In contrast, speech is accent optimally by introducing learned gestures to accompany speech (Calavrezo 1965; mimic exercises, Krause 1981; gesture exercises, Fiedler/Standop 1983; 1986).

1.2.3. Rhythmic Speaking

This procedure belongs to every approach that attempts the most obvious reduction of speech errors possible. Even though it is not exactly one of the most popular procedures due to its prosody-changing quality, it is nonetheless one of the central components of many behavior therapy programs (e. g. Beech/Fransella 1971; Andrews/Ingham 1972; Öst/Götesham/Melin 1976; Helps/Dalton 1979; Wendlandt 1980). Normally the pronunciation of syllables, words, or sentence parts follows acoustic (metronome, ear-metronome), tactile (haptometronome), or visual stimuli. The goal of the therapy exercises is to gradually move from a very slow speech rhythm, which is oriented towards errors-free speech, to a more normal speed and intonation.

1.2.4. Prolonged Speech

At this point, prolonged speech may be one of the most effective speech techniques (see Andrews/Guitar/Howie 1980). In practice, it is built into supposedly different approaches which are in fact similarly structured: for example, as "smooth motion speech" (Howie/Tanner/Andrews 1981), as "systematic slowed speech" (Resick/Wedinggesen/Ames/Meyer 1978), or within the well-known so called "Lagato"-technique (Gutzmann 1879). The previous use of delayed auditory feeedback (DAF) to support prolonged speech (e. g. Perkins 1973a; 1973b) is not necessary or helpful in every case. Today most authors work with prolonging-instructions and observation learning (e. g. Howie/Tanner/Andrews 1981). Typically, prolonged speech begins at a rate of 50 syllables per minute. When the stutterer can produce error-free speech at this rate, the tempo is increased in steps of 5 syllables per minute until it approaches that of normal speech.

1.3. Other Aspects of Speech Therapy and Fluency Training

At present, prolonged speech is one of the fluency training methods which can best be supported empirically and which has proven most reliable in short-term, as well as longitudinal, studies (Fiedler 1988). Experience has shown that if fluency training is to be effective in the long run, a very long period of systematic practice (significantly more than 50 practice hours) is necessary. Accomplishments through treatment can be maintained in various ways. Of these, the systematic construction of a training program seems particularly useful. Further suggested measures include:

– symptom recognition exercises (self-monitoring: Van Riper 1973, 245–265; Ingham 1982), – breathing exercises (e. g. "regulated breathing approach": Azrin/Nunn, 1974; for critique, see Rohjahn/Pesta 1977), – autogenic training (Krech 1963) and relaxation techniques (especially, the direct relaxation of the muscles and body parts involved in speaking; Lanyon 1977), and above all the use of
– sound and video recordings as speech feed-

back (Datiles 1977; Toups 1979; Fiedler/Standop 1986).

The adjunct use of *medication* in stuttering treatment, such as the occasionally recommended low dosage of a neuroleptic (Haloperidol), strikes us as counterindicated for numerous reasons (Andrews/Dosza 1977; Murray/Kelly/Campbell/Stefanik 1977; Prins/Mandelkern/Cerf 1980): First of all, the possible reduction in stuttering rate made possible with Haloperidol remains far behind the possibilities of other speech therapies and it contaminates their effectiveness. Furthermore, the use of neuroleptics can lead to serious side-effects (concentration disturbances, lethargy, extrapyramidal dyskinesia, nausea). Previous therapy studies have shown that this has regularly led to premature termination of therapy by over one third of the patients.

2. The Combination of Speech and Social Therapy Measures

By now it is accepted therapy practice to combine speech and fluency training with social therapy measures. Exactly when and to what degree this occurs in treatment depends upon the severity of the speech disturbance and the extent of the stigmatisation caused by the stuttering.

2.1. Training Social Skills and Assertiveness

Most authors agree that social training should begin as early as possible in the treatment. Role-playing of socially relevant skills is most often recommended (Van Riper 1973; Wendlandt 1980; 1984). Here, video and acoustic feedback play an important role. The goal in every case is to test the fluency training and new social strengths which were gained in the protected therapy setting under 'real-life' conditions.

2.2. Group Treatment

In general, it appears common to extend treatment to a group format at an appropriate time (Fiedler 1986; 1990): Fluency skills such as social competence are more easily gained in a group setting, to some extent through modeling without the therapist having to lead or prompt each individual. Overall, a group offers the most promising prerequisite for a transfer of therapeutic progress, especially when group members exchange their strategies with one another and support such a transfer. People who are similarly affected by stuttering can observe the outbreak of factors which may help to maintain stuttering: the secondary disturbances and anticipation anxiety (as well as the secondary gains which may possibly develop in these processes). The goal of social therapy often extends to an examination of the daily life of the stutterer.

Participation in group therapy can facilitate the establishment of a self-help group. The therapy can be continued by the clients more independent of therapists: the clients can mutually control and support their therapy regime; they can also maintain regular telephone contact, organize activities together outside of therapy, and found self-help groups for others who are affected.

3. Multimodal Therapy

Current therapy practice calls for the combination of speech and social therapy components in a thorough treatment program. Such multimodal treatment concepts generally emphasize the following four aspects (these examples are taken from the Fiedler/Standop 1986, 225–230, treatment program):

(1) *Speech therapy and accompanying measures:* The fluency training is pursued by prolonged speech (via direct instructions, modeling, and video-feedback). Additionally, the following are introduced: an exact self-evaluation of speech behavior via symptom-/self-monitoring, then specific relaxation of muscles in the head, neck and upper body, as well as speech variation exercises (such as intended fluent stuttering as in the nonavoidance approaches; see Sheehan 1970, 269ff).

(2) *Social skills training:* We prefer training social competency through role-play and the use of video-feedback. The use of one of the standard behavior therapy procedures is not meant here, rather the training is individually planned for each client specifically in regards to his/her particular social deficits in his/her private life and occupation.

(3) *Transfer:* This therapy step is primarily concerned with the transference of newly learned speech methods and social skills to daily life situations. Stuttering groups are formed in which the skills learned in therapy are practiced in the most realistic daily life situations possible (for example, executing important telephone conversations in front of a video-camera or the videotaping and subsequent evaluation of a therapeutic excursion

of the group in the city interviewing people; Fiedler 1990).

(4) *Self-modification and relapse prevention:* Since relapses amongst adults are still more the rule than the exception, the therapy group developes detailed plans to deal with possible crises and relapses, enabling individual clients to handle them independently. Criteria are also established for the event that renewed help from a therapist is advisable.

There has long been a selection of multimodal therapy programs, and recently concrete therapy manuals have appeared which well suit he needs of speech pedagogy (e. g. Perkins 1973a; b; Van Riper 1973; Böhme 1977; Ryan/Van Kirk 1978; Wendlandt 1984). They vary according to the technical execution of the speech therapy or the fluency training.

4. Therapy Success and Prognosis

Spontaneous remission, often observed in stuttering children, is noticeably less frequent as they age, rarely occuring in adults. Quarrington (1977) found that spontaneous remission in adults depends upon an arduous self-therapy by the stutterer. The success in such self-therapy efforts does not ever, however, occur 'spontaneously', rather, it was, as a rule, obtained after one to five years.

The number of *relapses* amongst adults has remained an unsolved problem. Although the speech therapy possibilities in the last decades have improved considerably, only few adult stutterers today dare hope to be completely 'cured' of their stuttering. This stands in marked contrast to the beginner's success that one often sees in stuttering treatment. Most of the measures described above lead within the controlled therapy situation to a near complete reduction of stuttering frequency — often after only a few hours of practice. Relapses usually arise first after therapy ceases, and unless a catamnesis takes place, they will remain hidden from the therapist. This problem, thus, earns special attention. Most of the therapy studies carried out up to now were based upon catamnesis studies from 6 to 12 months (see Jehle 1982). Based on available knowledge about the individual nature of relapses, however, it seems highly necessary that a follow-up catamnesis after at least 2 years take place (see Bloodstein 1975).

For several reasons, many of the success stories found in therapy reports should be viewed cautiously (Fiedler 1988): The number of *drop-outs* in therapy studies ranges at least between 4 and 25 percent, the problems associated with this rate are hardly discussed. Examinations of the maintained success of improved speaking behavior are usually administered under standardized conditions which do not greatly tax the speaker. The general transfer of the treatment effect to daily life is only seldom checked, even though this is exactly the area where the reasons for the variability of the speech disturbance are to be found. The findings of the simple follow-up measure via a telephone conversation only a few weeks after therapy termination (which is unfortunately too seldom executed), have been distinctly discouraging (e. g. Resick/Wediggensen/Ames/Meyer 1978).

Among other factors which influence the treatment process are the age and gender of the stutterer. In general, girls have better therapeutic prognosis than boys. In adulthood, however, this situation reverses: woman have significantly less success-chances than men (Case 1960). The length of treatment also plays a role. 100 sessions or more promise a better prognosis (Andrews/Guitar/Howie 1980). It appears to be of only secondary importance whether this treatment is stretched over several months or wether it is concentrated intramurally in a block of several weeks. Finally, unrealistic high and low success expectations appear to correlate with lower therapeutic success (Guitar/Bass 1978).

5. Conclusion

The majority of authors today feel that the treatment of stuttering in adult patients demands setting of multidimensional goals achieved by an eclectic treatment approach. Such an approach should carefully select treatment measures which take into consideration both the individual's unique speech impediments (stuttering, articulation, prosody, mimic, gesture, etc.), and his/her current conditions and resulting problems (above all, speech anxiety and possible limitations in behavior and performance within his/her private and occupational interpersonal relationships). The variation range and effectiveness of the possible treatment steps is now so diverse that a satisfactory impact on the current degree of speech disturbances may be made. In view of the persistent relapse rate, however, it appears advisable that the success prognosis in therapy of adult stutterers should be realistically modest, so that they can really be actualized within the therapy. Furthermore, 'freedom from symptoms' is rarely a realistic prognosis. In the therapy of the stuttering adult we find 'flowing speech' or "more fluent stuttering than at the beginning of therapy" to be much more realistic. Since there are almost no predictors of therapy success known as of yet, the beginning of therapy should not raise any inappropriate expectations, especially not too high or too low of success expectations, since these can impede therapy.

6. References

Adams, M. R., Sears, R. L., & Ramig, P. R. (1982). Vocal changes in stutterers and nonstutterers during monotoned speech. *Journal of Fluency Disorders, 7*, 21–35.

Andrews, G. & Dosza, M. (1977). Haloperidol and the treatment of stuttering. *Journal of Fluency Disorders, 2*, 217–224.

Andrews, G., Guitar, B., & Howie P. (1980). Meta-analysis of the effects of stuttering treatment. *Journal of Speech and Hearing Disorders, 45*, 287–307.

Andrews, G. & Harris, M. (1964). *The syndrome of stuttering*. London: Heinemann.

Andrews, G., Howie, P. M., Dozsa, M., & Guitar, B. E. (1982). Stuttering: Speech pattern characteristics under fluency-inducing conditions. *Journal of Speech and Hearing Research, 25*, 208–216.

Andrews, G. & Ingham, R. J. (1972). Stuttering: An evaluation of follow-up procedures for syllable-timed speech / token system therapy. *Journal of Communication Disorders, 5*, 307–319.

Azrin, N. H. & Nunn, R. G. (1974). A rapid method of eliminating stuttering by a regulated breathing approach. *Behavior Research & Therapy, 12*, 279–286.

Beech, H. R. & Fransella, F. (1971). *Research and experiments in stuttering* (2nd ed.). New York: Pergamon.

Becker, P., Keßler, B., & Fuchsgruber, K. (1975). Ein vergleichendes Therapieexperiment zur Theorie und Effizienz der Stotterbehandlung auf operanter Grundlage. *Archiv für Psychologie, 127*, 78–92.

Bergmann, G. (1987). Stuttering as a prosodic disturbance: A link between speech execution and emotional processes. In: H. F. M. Peters & W. Hulstijn (Eds.), *Speech motor dynamics in stuttering 393–407*. New York: Springer.

Bloodstein, O. (1975). *A handbook on stuttering* (2nd ed.). Chicago: National Easter Seal Society for Crippled Children and Adults.

Bluemel, C. S. (1913). *Stammering and cognate defects of speech* (Vol. 2). New York: Stechert.

Böhme, G. (1977). *Das Stotter-Syndrom:* Aetiologie, Diagnostik und Therapie. Bern: Huber.

Calavrezo, C. (1965). Die Behandlung des Stotterns durch die Sprachgebärden. *De Therapie Vocis et Loquelae, 1*, 399–401.

Case, H. W. (1960). Therapeutic methods in stuttering and speech blocking. In H. J. Eysenck (Ed.), *Behavior therapy and the neuroses. 207–220*. Oxford: Pergamon.

Cherry, E. C. & Sayers, B. M. (1956). Experiments upon the total inhibition of stammering by external control, and some clinical results. *Journal of Psychosomatic Research, 1*, 233–246.

Datiles, U. P. (1977). *The effects of videotape feedback on the modification of stuttering behavior through self-confrontation and analysis*. Educ. Diss. Illinois: Northern University.

Fiedler, P. (1986). Verhaltenstherapie in Gruppen: Überblick und Perspektiven. *Gruppendynamik, 17*, 341–360.

Fiedler, P. (1988). Sprechstunde oder Psychotherapie? Wege und Umwege in der erfolgreichen Behandlung erwachsener Stotternder. In F. Hinteregger & F. Meixner (Eds.), *Stottern – aus der Sicht der Betroffenen und der Therapeuten. 51–60*. Wien: Jugend & Volk.

Fiedler, P. (1990). Aktuelle Entwicklungen in der therapeutischen Gruppenarbeit: Konzepte, Wirkfaktoren und Indikationen. *Forum des Zentralverbandes für Logopädie, 2/90*, 1–6.

Fiedler, P. (1991). Neuropsychologische Grundlagen des Stotterns. In M. Grohnfeld (Ed.), *Handbuch der Sprachtherapie*. Band 5: Störungen der Redefähigkeit (43–60). Berlin: Edition Marhold.

Fiedler, P. & Standop, R. (1983). *Stuttering: integrating theory and practice*. Rockville, Maryland: Aspen.

Fiedler, P. & Standop, R. (1986). *Stottern, Ätiologie, Diagnose, Behandlung* (2nd ed.). München: Psychologie Verlags Union.

Guitar, B. (1975). Reduction of stuttering using analog electromyographic feedback. *Journal of Speech and Hearing Research, 18*, 672–685.

Guitar, B. & Bass, C. (1978). Stuttering therapy: the relation between attitude change and longterm outcome. *Journal of Speech and Hearing Disorders, 43*, 392–400.

Gutzmann, A. (1879). *Das Stottern und seine gründliche Beseitigung durch ein methodisch geordnetes und praktisch erprobtes Verfahren*. Berlin: Med. Diss..

Gutzmann, H. (sen.) (1898). *Das Stottern*. Eine Monographie für Ärzte, Pädagogen und Behörden. Frankfurt/M.: Rosenheim.

Helps, R. & Dalton, P. (1979). The effectiveness of an intensive group speech therapy programme for adult stutterers. *British Journal of Disorders of Communication, 14*, 17–30.

Howie, P. & Andrews, G. (1984). Treatment of adult stutterers: managing fluency. In: R. F. Curlee

& W. H. Perkins (Eds.), *Nature and treatment of stuttering: new directions. 425–446.* San Diego: College-Hill.

Howie, P. M., Tanner, S., & Andrews, G. (1981). Short- and long-term outcome in an intensive treatment program for adult stutterer. *Journal of Speech and Hearing Disorders, 46,* 104–109.

Ingham, R. J. (1982). The effects of self-evaluation training on maintenance and generalization during stuttering treatment. *Journal of Speech and Hearing Disorders, 47,* 289–301.

Ingham, R. J. & Andrews, G. (1973). Behavior therapy and stuttering: A review. *Journal of Speech and Hearing Disorders, 38,* 405–441.

Ingham, R. J., Southwood, H., & Horsburgh, G. (1981). Some effects of the Edinburgh Masker on stuttering during oral reading and spontaneous speech. *Journal of Fluency Disorders, 6,* 135–154.

James, J. E. (1976). The influence of duration on the effects of time-out from speaking. *Journal of Speech and Hearing Research, 19,* 206–215.

Jehle, P. (1982). Zur Problematik des Rückfalls in der Stottertherapie. In D. Nord-Rüdinger, I. Graudenz, N. Barth, R. S. Jäger, P. Jehle & R.Kühn (Eds.), *Beiträge zu Theorie und Praxis in Psychologie und Pädagogik. 51–74.* Frankfurt: Deutsches Institut für Internationale Pädagogische Forschung.

Krause, R. (1981). *Sprache und Affekt: Das Stottern und seine Behandlung.* Stuttgart: Kohlhammer.

Krech, H. (1963). Das Entspannungstraining. In H. Jacobi (Ed.), *Phoniatrie. 148–153.* Leipzig: Barth.

Lanyon, R. I. (1977). Effects of biofeedback-based relaxation on stuttering during reading and spontanous speech. *Journal of Consulting and Clinical Psychology, 45,* 860–866.

Liebmann, A. (1914). *Vorlesungen über Sprachstörungen.* (Heft 9: Die psychische Behandlung von Sprachstörungen). Berlin: Coblentz.

Motsch, H. J. (1983). *Problemkreis Stottern: Theoretische und therapeutische Neuorientierung* (2nd ed.). Berlin: Marhold.

Murray, T. J., Kelly, P., Campbell, L., & Stefanik, K. (1977). Haloperidol in the treatment of stuttering. *British Journal of Psychiatry, 130,* 370–373.

Öst, L., Götesham, K., & Melin, L. (1976). A controlled study of two behavioral methods in the treatment of stuttering. *Behavior Therapy, 7,* 587–592.

Perkins, W. H. (1973a). Replacement of stuttering with normal speech: I. Rationale. *Journal of Speech and Hearing Disorders, 38,* 283–294.

Perkins, W. H. (1973b). Replacement of stuttering with normal speech: II. Clinical procedures. *Journal of Speech and Hearing Disorders, 38,* 295–303.

Prins, D., Mandelkorn, T., & Cerf, F. A. (1980). Principal and differential effects of Haloperidol and placebo treatment upon speech disfluencies in stutterers. *Journal of Speech and Hearing Research, 23,* 614–629.

Quarrington, B. (1977). How do the various theories of stuttering facilitate our therapeutic approach? *Journal of Communication Disorders, 10,* 77–83.

Resick, P. A., Wendiggensen, P., Ames, S., & Meyer, V. (1978). Systematic slowed speech: A new treatment for stuttering. *Behavior Research and Therapy, 16,* 161–167.

Rieber, R. W. & Wollok, J. R. (1977). The historical roots of the theory and therapy of stuttering. *Journal of Communication Disorders, 10,* 3–24.

Rojahn, J. & Pesta, I. (1977). Die Sprechpause als Stotter-Inkompatible Reaktion: Therapeutische Abgrenzung und Einsatzmöglichkeiten bei Stotternden. *Zeitschrift für Klinische Psychologie, 6,* 281–302.

Ryan, B. & Van Kirk, B. (1978). *Monterey-Fluency-Program.* Palo Alto, Cal.: Monterey Learning Systems (German Edition 1982: Monterey Sprachtrainingsprogramm. Palo Alto, Cal.: Monterey Learning Systems).

Schwartz, M. (1976). *Stuttering solved.* Philadelphia: Lippincott.

Shames, G. H. & Egolf, D. B. (1976). *Operant conditioning and the management of stuttering.* Englewood Cliffs, N. J.: Prentice-Hall.

Sheehan, J. G. (1970). Role-Therapy. In J. G. Sheehan (Ed.), *Stuttering. Research and therapy. 260–311.* New York: Harper & Row.

Toups, F. (1979). *Empirische Untersuchungen zur Streßwirkung audiovisueller Selbstkonfrontation auf Stotternde.* Frankfurt: Lang.

Van Riper, C. (1973). *The treatment of stuttering.* Englewood-Cliffs: Prentice-Hall.

Wendlandt, W. (1980). *Verhaltenstherapie des Stotterns.* Weinheim: Beltz.

Wendlandt, W. (1984). *Zum Beispiel Stottern. Stolperdrähte, Sackgassen und Lichtblicke im Therapiealltag.* München: Pfeiffer.

Widlak, H. (1977). *Modifikation des Stotterns durch negative Praxis.* Phil. Diss. Münster: Westfälische Wilhelms-Universität.

Wingate; M. E. (1979). The loci of stuttering: grammer or prosody? *Journal of Communication Disorders, 12,* 283–290.

Peter Fiedler, Heidelberg (Germany)

87. Language Changes in Old Age

Old age is characterized by changes in many aspects of cognition, including memory, problem solving, and reasoning (Salthouse 1982). Until recently, however, it was believed that language was immune from the effects of aging found in other areas of cognition. For instance, less than 20 years ago, Riegel made the claim that "language functions remain highly stable and do not reveal any dramatic or 'interesting' changes in development" (Riegel 1973, 479) in old age. The thesis of this chapter is that such claims are only partly correct. Some aspects of language indeed remain stable and some change. In particular, despite the apparent preservation of semantic knowledge in old age, both comprehension and production of language show age-related changes consistent with the position that performance factors set limits on older adults' ability to understand and produce language. The chapter is divided into four sections. Research dealing with the representation of semantic knowledge in old age is reviewed in the first section. The second and third take up issues related to comprehension and production of language, respectively. The fourth and last section compares language in normal aging to that in aphasia and in Alzheimer's disease.

1. Organization of Semantic Information

Within the framework of network models of memory (Anderson 1983), both semantic and episodic information are represented by nodes, which stand for concepts or propositions, and these nodes are connected by associative pathways. When a concept is encountered, its node is activated, and activation also spreads along associative pathways to related nodes, increasing their availability for further processing. These activation processes, both automatic and attentional, have been implicated in virtually all aspects of natural language understanding and production, including perception of words in spoken or written form (McClelland/Rumelhart 1981), determining the syntactic structure of sentences (Tanenhaus/Dell/Carlson 1987), deriving the meaning of single sentences and entire discourses (Kintsch 1988), and producing discourse (Dell 1986). Activation of pragmatic or general world knowledge embodied in schemata is necessary for making inferences, for establishing the topic of a discourse, and for determining the antecedents of pronouns. Hence, differences across age in either the way knowledge is represented in memory or in the way that activation proceeds could result in both comprehension and production impairments. Evidence about possible age differences in the representation or activation of conceptual knowledge comes from a variety of sources, including word-finding difficulties, responses in word association tasks, representation of schemata, semantic priming in lexical decision and word naming, particularization of word meanings in discourse, and judgments of similarity or relatedness of concepts.

1.1. Word-Finding Difficulties

There is little evidence for a decline in vocabulary size as people grow older (e. g. Salthouse 1982). Older adults do nevertheless have more word-finding difficulties than young adults. These are shown in reduced verbal fluency in tasks in which people are given a fixed amount of time to generate as many words as they can that meet specific criteria, such as beginning with a particular letter or being members of particular categories (Howard 1980; McCrae/Arenberg/Costa 1987; Schaie/Parham 1977). Older adults are more prone than young adults to tip-of-the-tongue experiences in which familiar words are temporarily unretrievable (Burke/MacKay/Worthley/Wade 1991; Cohen/Faulkner 1986). There is increased difficulty in naming to definition in old age (Bowles/Poon 1985; Maylor 1990; but see Rissenberg/Glanzer 1987 for a counterexample). Picture naming errors are generally found to increase in old age, though perhaps not until the eighth decade of life (Albert/Heller/Milberg 1988; Borod/Goodglass/Kaplan 1980; Van Gorp/Satz/Kiersch/Henry 1986), but some investigators report no age difference on this task (Flicker/Ferris/Crook/Bartus 1987; Mitchell 1989).

In spontaneous speech, there is some evidence for increased frequency of pauses, which may signal word-finding problems, but the findings are not consistent across studies (cf. 3.3.). In retelling stories, older adults are more likely to use pronouns without mentioning their antecedents (Cohen 1979; Obler 1980; Pratt/Boyes/Robins/Manchester 1989; Ulatowska/Cannito/Hayashi/Fleming 1985) though this may signal a problem in remembering previously mentioned antecedents rather than a general deficit in word retrieval. There have also been reports of fewer proper nouns, increased frequency of general nouns, and less lexical variety of nouns in the speech of older adults (Ulatowska et al. 1985), though studies reporting type/token ratios or number of unique words do not usually find age declines in these measures of lexical variety (Bromley 1991; Cooper 1990; Kemper/Kynette/Rash et al. 1989; Kynette/Kemper 1986; Walker/Hardiman/Hedrick/Holbrook 1981; Walker/Roberts/Hedrick 1988).

Reduced verbal fluency, increased frequency of tip-of-the-tongue experiences, problems in confrontation naming and naming to definition, and word finding problems in spontaneous speech could all be symptomatic of changes in either the completeness or the organization of conceptual knowledge. That is, if semantic representations in old age contain fewer features or if the associations between concepts and their attributes have a different distribution of strengths than they do in younger individuals, then changes such as these would be expected. These changes, however, would also be consistent with problems in accessing the orthographic or phonological realizations of words even in the presence of an intact semantic system. There are a number of reasons for believing that the latter alternative provides a better account of the data.

(1) Older adults produce fewer phonological features (first letters, number of syllables) of targets than young adults when in a tip-of-the-tongue state (Burke/MacKay/Worthley/Wade 1991); this is more consistent with a transmission deficit in old age which reduces the availability of phonological information rather than a change in the structure of the semantic concepts themselves. (2) Phonemic cues are equally helpful as hints to young and older adults in confrontation naming tasks (Nicholas/Obler/Albert/Goodglass 1985) and orthographically similar primes are actually more helpful to the old than to the young in naming to definition (Bowles/Poon 1985). (3) An increase with age in the proportion of semantically related errors could indicate either a disruption (loss or disorganization) of information within specific semantic domains (if the errors are near synonyms or responses in the same category as the correct word) or of word finding problems (if the errors are circumlocutions such as *cutting the wood* for *sawing*). If anything, however, there is a drop in the proportion of semantically related errors and an increase in the proportion of circumlocutions (Albert/Heller/Milberg 1988; Bowles/Obler/Albert 1987; Nicholas/Obler/Albert/Goodglass 1985). Taken together, these results are more in keeping with lexical retrieval failures than with semantic deficits.

1.2. Word Associations

In free association tasks, the instructions are to give the first word that comes to mind when a stimulus word is presented. According to semantic network models, presentation of the stimulus word activates the node standing for this concept. Activation also spreads automatically from this node to all concepts having attributes in common with it and, hence, sharing pathways with it. The first word to come to mind should be the one whose concept has the most shared properties or whose semantic distance is the smallest. In controlled association tasks, further restrictions are placed on the response to be given. For instance, the task may be to produce a superordinate of the word or a physical characteristic of an object or an action that can be performed with the object. Here, network models would assume that there is a compound stimulus consisting of the word and the type of response to be produced. Activation from this compound stimulus may converge automatically on an appropriate response. Alternatively, all properties of the stimulus concept may be activated and the concept associated with the pathway labelled with the appropriate relation may be selected as the response.

The results of both free and controlled word association tasks argue for preservation of the semantic system in old age. (1) Young and older adults produce pretty much the same types of responses. For instance, both young and older adults typically produce paradigmatic rather than syntagmatic responses in free association tasks (Burke/Peters 1986; Lovelace/Cooley 1982). When asked to produce particular types of responses to words naming objects – a characteristic action, a distinctive physical feature, or a general associate – the percentage of acceptable responses does not differ reliably across age (Nebes/Brady 1988). When people are asked to produce properties for nouns, the breakdown of attributes into those referring to physical features, functional features, specifiers (elaborations on functions that specify their objects), category names, and exemplars is very similar for young and old (Stine 1986; see also Lovelace/Cooley 1982). Moreover, strong correlations are found between the frequencies with which young and older adults produce particular associates when generating members of taxonomic categories (Howard 1980) or properties of stimulus terms (Howard 1979).

(2) The variability of associative responses seems fairly constant across age. As noted by Burke/Peters (1986), response variability would be expected to increase if older adults have atypical associations or if features important to meaning were absent. Although it has been reported that normal older adults produce a greater number of different associates or more unique associates (Riegel/Riegel 1964), such differences are generally not observed when young and older adults are carefully equated on education or vocabulary (Bowles/Williams/Poon 1983; Burke/Peters 1986; Howard 1979, 1980; Lovelace/Cooley 1982). Overall, then, there is considerable stability in the types of responses that older adults make and in the production frequencies for particular associates.

1.3. Schemata

Our memories of experiences are organized in knowledge structures. Schemata are believed to play a central role in language comprehension and memory, guiding expectations about what will come next in a discourse, facilitating perception of individual words, and aiding in integration of old and new information (Sanford/Garrod 1981; Sharkey 1986). If young and older adults did not share knowledge structures or if there were age differences in accessing or modifying these structures, comprehension and communication could be severely impaired. Fortunately, however, there appears to be considerable similarity of conceptual organization across age. When asked to generate a sequence of actions that are typically performed by most people in carrying out some activity such as going to the doctor or writing a letter to a friend, young and older adults produce much the same actions (Hess 1985; Light/Anderson 1983). Correlations between age groups are also quite high when actions are rated for typicality or necessity for completion of an activity or likelihood of occurrence during an event sequence (Hess 1985; Light/Anderson 1983; List 1986). Young and older adults also agree on the order of actions in carrying out particular activities (Roman/Brownell/Potter/Seibold 1987).

1.4. Lexical Decision and Word Naming Tasks

It takes less time to decide whether a string of letters is a word or to name a target when it is preceded by a semantically related prime word or by an appropriate sentence context than when it is preceded by an unrelated prime (Meyer/Schvaneveldt 1971; Stanovich/West 1983). Such semantic priming effects are generally interpreted as evidence for spreading activation in a network and, therefore, similar patterns of semantic priming in young and older adults would constitute evidence for the integrity of the semantic system. That is, differences across age in the sensitivity of priming to variations in the associative strength of primes and targets, or to different prime-target semantic relationships, would suggest a semantic deficit. In addition, differences in the time course of activation could have consequences for the integration of information in a discourse.

The available evidence from semantic priming studies, however, points to the absence of such a deficit. The extent of priming is generally evaluated by comparing latencies when the target is preceded by a related prime to latencies when the target is preceded by an unrelated prime or by a neutral prime. Comparable priming effects have been obtained in young and old when the target is a cohyponym of the prime (Howard/McAndrews/Lasaga 1981), when the target names a descriptive property of the prime (Howard et al. 1981), when the target is an associate of the prime (Balota/Duchek 1988), and when the prime is a superordinate of the target (Balota/Duchek 1988; Burke/White/Diaz 1987). Both young and older adults also show facilitation in lexical decision and naming tasks when sentence rather than single word primes are used (Burke/Harrold 1988; Burke/Yee 1984; Cohen/Faulkner 1983; Madden

1986, 1988, 1989; Nebes/Boller/Holland 1986).

In lexical decision (the task most often used to assess age-related differences in priming) the results reveal similarity in the extent of priming and no evidence for reduced benefits or costs when latencies following related and unrelated primes are compared to latencies following neutral primes (Bowles/Poon 1985; Burke/Yee 1984; Chiarello/Church/Hoyer 1985; Howard 1983; Howard/McAndrews/Lasaga 1981; Howard/Shaw/Heisey 1986; Madden 1986, 1988, 1989). Benefits are believed to reflect a mix of automatic and attentional processes, while costs are thought to arise solely from attentional processes; these results, then, argue against age differences in either automatic or attentional components of activation. Indeed, a recent meta-analysis (Laver/Burke 1990) found generally larger semantic priming effects in the old than in the young.

As noted above, age differences in rate of activation could have consequences for both comprehension and production of language. If activation spreads more slowly in the old, less semantic priming should be obtained at very short prime-target asynchronies. This does not, however, appear to be the case (Balota/Duchek 1988; Burke/White/Diaz 1987; Madden 1989; Stern/Prather/Swinney/Zurif 1991; but see Howard et al. 1986, for a different outcome).

Some caution is nevertheless needed in evaluating studies of semantic priming in young and older adults. MacKay/Burke (1990) point out that older adults have more practice with semantically associated words, increasing the strength of their connections relative to younger adults, and that because of the many interconnections between nodes in a semantic network, there may be a summation of priming that masks age deficits in this domain. Moreover, because older adults have longer reaction times in semantic priming experiments, there is more time for activation to spread from prime to target. The evidence reviewed here thus does not constitute definitive proof of age constancy in the magnitude or rate of semantic activation. There is also reason to believe that intact semantic priming is at best weak evidence for preserved semantic structure because patients with aphasia or Alzheimer's disease who perform poorly on overt semantic judgment tasks nevertheless show priming (Chertkow/Bub/Seidenberg 1989; Warrington/Shallice 1984).

1.5. Particularization of Word Meanings in Sentences

The results of controlled association studies and judgments of similarity or relatedness (cf. 1.6.) suggest that young and older adults share beliefs about the properties and functions of objects. Different aspects of a word's meaning are not equally salient in all contexts. Although some core or central properties may always be activated regardless of context, particular linguistic contexts emphasize or highlight different aspects of meaning, with unemphasized properties being inhibited (Tabossi/Johnson-Laird 1980). If semantic structures were degraded in old age or if activation or inhibition processes were impaired, it would not be surprising to find that older adults were less precise in particularizing word meanings in discourse contexts. Hasher/Zacks (1988) have recently argued that inhibitory processes are less efficient in old age and would therefore predict less effective or slower particularization of word meanings. The available evidence, however, gives no support for this conclusion. Young and older adults both show inhibition of properties of objects that are inappropriate in particular sentence contexts (Burke/Harrold 1988), activation of instruments implied by verbs (Burke/Yee 1984), and instantiation of general terms with specific category exemplars (Light/Valencia-Laver/Zavis 1991).

1.6. Judgments of Similarity

Another approach to studying possible age differences in the structure of conceptual knowledge involves the use of tasks which require judgments about similarity between pairs of objects. For instance, people may be asked to judge whether two words mean approximately the same thing (Hertzog/Raskind/Cannon 1986; Madden 1985), to decide whether a word names a category member or whether two words belong to the same category (Hertzog et al. 1986; Mueller/Kausler/Faherty 1980), or just to decide whether two words are related, without the precise nature of the relation being specified (Byrd 1984; Nebes/Brady 1988). Although older adults are slower than younger adults to make semantic judgments, their error rates are no higher, suggesting the availability of information about the relationships queried or, when the judgment is about simple relatedness, the availability of information that an association exists. When category instances varying in production frequency or typicality are used, the extent to which typicality affects response latency is the same across age, suggesting that category structure is similar across age (Byrd 1984; Hertzog et al. 1986; Mueller et al. 1980).

Judgments of relatedness do not require that a basis for similarity be explicitly retrieved and judgments of the category membership or synonymity of two words do not require the production of these words. Older adults perform more poorly on tests in which particular relationships are explicitly queried. For instance, performance on the WAIS Similarities subtest, which requires the statement of how two things are related, declines with age (see Salthouse 1982 for a review). Riegel (1959) found that young and older adults equated on ability to select synonyms on a mutiple choice test had problems in choosing antonyms, in selecting salient properties, in choosing two coordinates for a target when a superordinate was not actually stated, and in solving verbal analogies which required computation of similarity relationships. These tasks are more specific in the knowledge they tap than tasks that involve production of properties or judgments of similarity or category membership; they require the abstraction and, in some cases, the verbalization of relationships between two objects. One hypothesis is that older adults are impaired in these processes, but that semantic structure is indeed intact. However, age differences are not observed when people are asked to select items that belong to a particular taxonomic category (Flicker/Ferris/Crook/Bartus 1986) or to explain why they categorized objects in particular ways (Smiley/Brown 1979).

1.7. Summary

Little evidence has surfaced for age-related changes in semantic organization. Although older adults have word finding difficulties, the simplest explanation for these is that lexical access is impaired. There is great consistency in the type of word associations produced by young and older adults and little indication that word associations are more variable or idiosyncratic in the old. The representation of schematic information is similar in young and old. Semantic priming appears to be preserved in old age and, in fact, there is evidence that older adults may show greater priming than young adults. Young and older adults are equally likely to particularize word meanings in sentences. Older adults are as accurate as young adults in deciding whether two concepts are related or whether they share particular aspects of meaning. Although the old do show declines on tasks which require the explicit statement or selection of the way in which words are related, it is not clear whether this result should be taken as signalling an alteration in semantic structures. The same result may be indicative of problems in accessing particular knowledge or even of shifts in the criteria for similarity without implicating a semantic deficit.

2. Language Comprehension

Much of the research on language comprehension in old age has been carried out within a processing resources framework. There are two very good reasons for this. First, working memory plays a central role in most models of sentence and discourse comprehension. Limitations in working memory capacity (the ability to store and manipulate information over short periods of time) affect comprehension of complex sentences (Bock 1982) and integrative processes responsible for establishing discourse coherence (Kintsch/van Dijk 1978; Sanford/Garrod 1981). Second, older adults are slower to carry out cognitive operations than young adults and also demonstrate reduced working memory capacity (Light/Anderson 1985; Salthouse 1990). Hence, increasing presentation rate or working memory load should have more deleterious effects on comprehension in the old. Much (but not all) of the available evidence from studies of speech perception, sentence comprehension, and integration of information within a discourse is consistent with this view.

2.1. Speech Perception

Evaluating the contribution of working memory or cognitive slowing to age-related impairments in comprehension is complicated by the fact that older adults also have impaired speech perception. Perception of words and sentences may be impaired to an extent greater than would be predicted from puretone audiometry (Jerger/Hayes 1977). Speech discrimination (assessed in terms of the proportion of words or sentences correctly identified at a given loudness) may be worse for sentences than for words in old age (Jerger/Hayes 1977). Also, age differences in speech perception are intensified when speech is presented under adverse listening conditions such as when speech is presented in noise or time-compressed by periodic deletions of small segments (Bergman 1980; Wingfield/Poon/Lombardi/Lowe 1985).

Age-related decrements in speech perception may be due to changes in peripheral portions of the auditory nervous system or to more central changes, such as reduced speed in integration of information, or both. Several findings implicate central processes. Although the performance of the elderly is more affected by speeded presentation than that of the young, the presence of semantic, syntactic, or prosodic information in the material to be perceived is more beneficial to the old than to the young (Wingfield et al. 1985; Wingfield/Lahar/Stine 1989). Age differences in perception of words and sentences in noise are also reduced by the availability of appropriate sentential context (Cohen/Faulkner 1983; Hutchinson 1989; Obler/Nicholas/Albert/Woodward 1985). Similarly, in a word-onset gating paradigm (in which increasing amounts of word onset information are presented until the target can be identified), age differences in correctly identifying the first phoneme of the target at very short gates are reduced when sentence context is more constraining (Wingfield/Aberdeen/Stine 1991). These results argue for a central locus of impaired speech perception in the elderly. They also suggest that the interaction of top-down processes with sensory information is important in old age. Finally, we note that tests of word and sentence perception are typically tests of short-term memory which require subjects to repeat the items they have heard out loud; age-related declines are generally found in memory span, so that a greater decline in memory for sentences than for single words is unsurprising.

2.2. Sentence Comprehension

Sensitivity to the syntactic constraints of language has been studied in a number of ways differing in the explicitness of the measures used. For instance, Wingfield/Poon/Lombardi/Lowe (1985) asked young and older adults to repeat 5- and 8-word strings that were normal sentences, syntactically correct but semantically anomalous strings, or random sequences presented at rates varying from 275 to 425 words per minute. The old showed relatively poorer performance than the young at fast rates, as first semantic and then syntactic redundancy were eliminated in the syntactically correct and random strings. When asked to segment either spoken or written prose for immediate recall, both young and old show respect for syntactic boundaries (Stine 1990; Wingfield/Lahar/Stine 1989). There is nonetheless some evidence that older adults allocate less time at sentence boundaries, suggesting that they do not engage in as much processing that integrates larger conceptual units as young adults; this would be consistent with a working memory deficit in old age (Stine 1990).

Studies which directly manipulate variables expected to be sensitive to working memory limitations show mixed results. Age differences are sometimes found on the Token Test on which a series of commands of increasing syntactic and semantic complexity are given for manipulating small pieces of plastic which vary in size, shape, and color (e. g. Bergman 1980; Emery 1985; Lesser 1976), and Lesser (1976) has shown that scores on the Token Test correlate negatively with measures of short-term memory; however, age differences on this test are not universally obtained (see Light 1988 for a review). Experimental studies of the effect of syntactic complexity on comprehension have generally found that increasing syntactic complexity differentially impairs the performance of older adults. Thus, age differences are greater for verbatim and gist repetition of left-branching or center-embedded sentences than for right-branching sentences (Bergman 1980; Kemper 1986; Norman/Kemper/Kynette et al. 1991). Although young and old are equally able to judge the well-formedness of simpler sentences and to correct errors in syntactically anomalous ones (Bayles/Tomoeda/Boone 1985), age differences are found in judgments of the grammaticality of syntactically well-formed strings if these involve complex constructions (Pye/Cheung/Kemper in press). Sentences containing center-embedded or left-branching clauses impose greater memory loads than those consisting of simple or right-branching clauses because of the greater separation of subject and predicate terms that belong together. Hence, there are greater concomitant risks of forgetting parts of the sentences or having difficulty in generating a reasonable interpretation of the constituents. In some cases, age differences in sentence comprehension may arise from the need to engage in fairly extensive problem solving. Emery (1985) found that pre-middle-aged high school graduates obtained higher scores than elderly aged 75 and over on a battery of sentence comprehension tests. It is not always clear whether it is syntactic complexity or exessive reasoning demands which produces the age difference. For instance, in *John runs faster than George but slower than Humphrey*, the subject must construct a three term series by figuring out that Humphrey is faster than George, and in *What is the relationship of my grandfather's son-in-law to me?*, reasoning about kinship terms is required. In both cases, working memory demands are high.

There are, nonetheless, variables which should produce age differences in comprehension, if these are due to reduced working memory capacity, but which in fact do not. Thus, increasing the propositional density of sentences of constant length does not differentially reduce gist recall in the old (Stine/Wingfield/Poon 1986) although greater propositional density may have more deleterious effects on recall of longer passages in the old (Stine/Wingfield 1990). Further, sentence complexity (whether a sentence is positive or negative) does not consistently interact with age in a sentence verification task (Craik/Morris/Gick 1990). Nor does varying the size of a concurrent memory load differentially affect young and old sentence verification latencies; this is contrary to predictions from hypotheses that working memory mediates sentence comprehension (Craik et al. 1990). Some studies have included measures of working memory as well as comprehension; these studies generally report that comprehension correlates positively with memory span (Feier/Gerstman 1980; Kemper/Kynette/Norman 1992; Norman/Kemper/Kynette et al. 1991). In Kemper et al. and Norman et al.'s studies, the data suggest that correlations between age and comprehension are reduced by controlling statistically for working memory capacity; however, the significance tests that would unambiguously demonstrate the role of working memory in producing differential age differences as a function of complexity are not given (cf. Salthouse 1985). Further, Stine/Wingfield (1987) reported that age differences on a working memory measure could not fully account for age differences in recall of word strings, so that variables other than working memory capacity must also contribute here.

2.3. Integration of Information in Discourse

As noted earlier, working memory is generally believed to play a major role in discourse comprehension. In Kintsch/van Dijk's (1978) model, construction of a coherent representation of a discourse proceeds in cycles. At the end of each cycle, there is too much information in the short-term buffer to be carried forward; only the most important and most recent propositions are maintained in the buffer for subsequent processing together with new inputs. The structure that evolves from this process is based on argument repetition. When there are no propositions remaining in the buffer that share arguments, it becomes necessary to either produce a bridging inference based on general world knowledge or to search all recently processed propositions to determine whether any contain arguments overlapping with those currently in the buffer. The final product is a coherent network of propositions which is organized hierarchically, with the most important propositions (i. e., those with the most argument repetitions) at the highest level. These more important propositions are known to be better recalled, a phenomenon called 'the levels effect'. Within this framework, there are many ways for discourse processing to be compromised in old age. Reduction of buffer size would reduce the number of propositions that could be processed simultaneously as well as the number of propositions that could be carried over from cycle to cycle. As a consequence, the necessity for both inference generation and memory search would be increased. Either or both of these processes may be impaired in old age (Anders/Fozard/Lillyquist 1972; Craik/Byrd 1982). As a result, the coherence of discourse representations should be lower in old age. This model permits a number of specific predictions with regard to aging.

(1) Older adults should show reduced recall of lower level propositions because fewer of these can be carried forward from previous cycles if buffer size is reduced. This result is sometimes obtained, but not always (cf. Cohen 1988). A recent meta-analysis found no consistent age difference in the magnitude of the levels effect (Zelinski/Gilewski 1988).

(2) Older adults should be more sensitive to distance effects. Increasing the number of irrelevant propositions intervening between propositions to be linked reduces the likelihood that these propositions will reside simultaneously in the buffer and therefore reduces the likelihood that they will be linked. Because the number of propositions that can be processed in one cycle depends on buffer size, thought to be reduced in old age, dis-

tance effects should be magnified in the old. Light/Capps (1986) found that young and older adults did not differ in ability to assign referents to ambiguous pronouns when memory load was low (i. e., when there was no material intervening between a sentence containing a pronoun and a sentence containing its possible antecedents) but older adults were less accurate when there were two intervening sentences. This result, however, was not replicated in a study using long passages (12 sentences) and many potential antecedents (Light/Anderson 1985); in this case young adults were better at answering questions about pronouns, but there was no interaction of age with distance.

(3) Topic change should have more deleterious consequences for discourse comprehension in the old than in the young. Van Dijk/Kintsch (1983) note that the importance of material is largely determined by the extent to which it is relevant to the current topic of a discourse. When the amount of material intervening between two sentences to be integrated is held constant, the likelihood that the initial information will be in working memory is smaller when there has been a topic change that backgrounds it. Under these conditions, successful integration depends on retrieval of recently processed propositions which may have been forgotten. Older adults are relatively less able than young adults to detect anomalies when relevant information is backgrounded, and the effect appears to be related to forgetting that relevant information (Light/Albertson 1988).

(4) If ability to draw inferences based on general world knowledge were impaired in old age, integration of discourse would be expected to suffer. It has been hypothesized that this should occur because of reduced working memory capacity in the old (Cohen 1979; Craik/Byrd 1982). Under most circumstances, however, older adults have no difficulty in generating pragmatic inferences. When comprehension is assessed during or immediately after a sentence is read, young and older adults give no evidence of differing in ability to draw inferences about the instruments with which actions are performed (Burke/Yee 1984), the instance of a category implied by a sentence context (Light/Valencia-Laver/Zavis 1991), the properties of nouns highlighted by sentences (Burke/Harrold 1988), the antecedents of noun-phrase anaphors (Light/Albertson 1988; Zelinski 1988; but see Hasher/Zacks 1988, for the suggestion that activation of antecedents takes longer in older adults), or the antecedents of pronouns (Light 1992; Light/Capps 1986).

Some studies do find age differences in ability to draw inferences, but these generally have not used on-line measures of comprehension and, therefore, confound processes occurring during comprehension with those dependent on storage and retrieval (Till/Walsh 1980) or use tasks involving heavy memory loads, leaving open the possibility that forgetting of relevant information or inability to activate previous information underlies problems in generation of inferences (Cohen 1979; Light/Anderson 1985; Light/Capps 1986; Hasher/Zacks 1988). Moreover, even with longer passages or delays between study and test, age differences in memory for inferences are not always found (cf. Light 1992).

In the studies reviewed thus far, inferences depended on general world knowledge where the literal meaning of sentences was involved. It is possible that access to general world knowledge in understanding more figurative language might be impaired in older adults. Some theorists have suggested that understanding figurative language requires two stages of processing, one in which a literal reading of an utterance is constructed and rejected and a second in which a contextually appropriate reading is produced (Searle 1979). The second process is viewed as more effortful and producing heavier demands on memory and, in the case of comprehending proverbs and metaphors, as requiring the computation of similarity relationships (Miller 1979). Hence, older adults, who may have difficulty in abstracting the basis of similarity between two concepts, might have greater difficulty than young adults in understanding proverbs and metaphors, though possibly not in understanding more formulaic indirect requests. The evidence in part favors this prediction, but in part does not. Bayles/Tomoeda/Boone (1985) found no age differences in ability to judge the literalness or directness of utterances or to identify the illocutionary intent of a speaker. On the other hand, interpretation of proverbs has been found less accurate in older adults (Albert/Duffy/Naeser 1987). This outcome may depend on the nature of the comprehension test used. Albert et al. used both free interpretation and forced-choice versions of Gorham's Proverb Interpretation Test. Light and Owens (cf.Light 1992) found evidence for age differences in comprehension of novel metaphors on a cued recall test but not on a more indirect sentence verification paradigm.

2.4. Summary

Some, but not all, predictions based on the hypothesis that working memory deficits underlie impaired language comprehension in the elderly receive empirical support. In general, the old are less accurate than the young in repeating sentences with complex syntactic structures and in answering questions based on them. Studies in which measures of working memory as well as sentence comprehension have been assessed suggest that age differences in working memory capacity explain age differences in comprehension but the data are by no means compelling. Specific predictions about age-related changes in integration of discourse are only partially confirmed. Older adults are more affected by topic change in building a coherent discourse representation, probably because they forget or do not carry forward for further processing information necessary to establish coherence. However, levels effects do not appear to vary with age. Nor are processes involved in online inference generation or comprehension of figurative language susceptible to aging effects. Moreover, older adults do not show greater sensitivity to propositional density effects in sentence comprehension, though a working-memory hypothesis predicts that they should.

Making sense of these findings is complicated by the fact that the role of working memory in sentence and discourse comprehension is not entirely understood. One approach is to treat working memory as a single pool of resources which can be assessed in a straightforward manner by obtaining an appropriate measure of working memory (Salthouse 1990). Although there is reason to believe that the operations underlying language comprehension draw upon resources distinct from those involved in other aspects of cognition (Baddeley/Logie/Nimmo-Smith/Brereton 1985), studies taking an individual difference approach to the role of working memory in age-related language impairment have been conducted within this single-pool framework. An alternate approach is that of Baddeley (1986) who has hypothesized that working memory consists of a central executive, together with a set of slave systems which have specialized storage functions. Within this framework two components, an articulatory loop and a phonological store, are important for language. A number of possible roles have been suggested for a phonological memory store – maintaining information until analysis of earlier portions of a sentence is completed, maintaining information for resolution of local syntactic ambiguities, keeping lexical items in the syntactic representation, maintaining a back-up record for use when postinterpretive processes are needed to resolve ambiguities, rehearsing difficult material for verbatim repetition (Caplan/Waters 1990; Martin 1990). Studies designed to tease apart these possibilities with respect to aging remain to be performed. Finally, patients suffering from focal brain damage whose short-term memory impairments are far more severe than those presented by normal older adults sometimes show quite good comprehension. A systematic comparison of such patients with normal elderly adults should reveal commonalities and differences in the nature of comprehension deficits in these populations.

3. Production of Discourse

Working memory is believed to play an important role in speech production (Bock 1982; Levelt 1989), and, as a consequence, age-related differences in language production paralleling those observed in language comprehension would be expected. Evidence germane to this question comes from examination of the syntactic complexity and coherence of discourse as well as analysis of the frequency of speech errors and repairs across age.

3.1. Syntactic Complexity

One clear prediction is that reduced working-memory capacity in old age should give rise to shorter and less syntactically complex spoken and written discourse. The evidence on this point suggests that this may be true but is not altogether consistent. Obler (1980) reported two studies of written descriptions of the cookie-theft picture from the Boston Diagnostic Aphasia Examination that suggested that older adults use more elaborate language. However, in both a naturalistic study of diaries and a laboratory study in which written language samples about a significant life event were obtained, Kemper (1987; Kemper/Kynette/Rash et al. 1989) found reliable declines in syntactic complexity; reductions were observed in the frequency of several clause types, including relative clauses, subordinates, gerunds, and double and triple embeddings. Similarly, Bromley (1991) reported a decrease in the use of subordinating conjunctions in older adults' self-descriptions.

The data are also somewhat equivocal with respect to speech. Walker/Hardiman/Hedrick/Holbrook (1981) computed the number of words in a T-unit (a main clause and any subordinate clauses attached or embedded in it) and found reliably shorter productions for older adults. Although the young had somewhat more words per clause and clauses per T-unit, these measures showed no age effects. In a second study, Walker/Roberts/Hedrick (1988) reported reliable age differences for both words per clause and words per T-unit, though not for clauses per T-unit, suggesting age differences in length but not complexity of discourse. An absence of reliable effects of age has also been reported for number of complex sentences (Shewan/Henderson 1988). Cooper (1990) found no decline across age in number of words produced, prepositional phrases per 100 words, or subordinate clauses per 100 words on a picture description task. In a study comparing the discourse of middle-aged and older nuns, Ulatowska/Cannito/Hayashi/Fleming (1985) found no difference across age in the complexity of expressions used to refer to entities within the discourse. These studies suggest that there are few changes across age in either the length or complexity of spoken discourse. However, Kemper and her colleagues have conducted a series of studies using more sensitive measures of syntactic complexity which challenge this conclusion. Although Kemper has found no age difference in mean length of utterance, the spontaneous speech of older adults shows a reduction in a variety of complex syntactic structures, especially left-branching constructions which tax working memory, and many of their grammatical errors were associated with attempts to use such structures (Kemper/Kynette/Rash et al. 1989; Kemper/Rash/Kynette/Norman 1990; Kynette/Kemper 1986).

Kemper has also amassed considerable evidence that working memory limitations are responsible for decreased use of complex syntactic structures in old age. Backward digit span, a measure of working memory, is an excellent predictor of mean clauses per utterance and per cent of left-branching clauses; adding age, education, and vocabulary does not improve prediction (Kemper et al. 1989). Drops in digit span over a three year period are also associated with a reduction in the use of left branching clauses (Kemper/Kynette/Norman 1992). Moreover, of 11 complexity metrics studied by Cheung/Kemper (1992), 8 showed age-related declines; these 8 also had strong correlations with digit span, whereas the the 3 metrics which did not show age drops were unrelated to digit span. Interestingly enough, one of the metrics which was insensitive to age was propositional density, a variable which has relatively little effect on age differences in discourse comprehension. Finally, there is some evidence that older adults trade syntactic complexity for structural complexity of narratives, perhaps because of working memory limitations (Kemper 1990; Kemper/Rash/Kynette/Norman 1990).

3.2. Discourse Coherence

Kemper (1990; Kemper/Rash/Kynette/Norman 1990) found that older adults' written diaries and oral stories are more structurally complex than those of young adults in that they include multiple episodes, embedded episodes, and codas which draw a moral lesson from the events being narrated. Though evaluated by external raters as higher in quality, more interesting, and technically better, older adults' narratives were less cohesive. With increasing age of the diarist, there was a concomitant decrease in the use of the more common cohesive devices, namely anaphora and conjunctions, though not in the use of lexical cohesion (repetition or synonyms), also a common device, or the less frequent devices of cataphora, exophora, ellipsis, and substitution of a nominal (e. g. one), a verbal (e. g. do it), or a clausal (e. g. so) in place of an item in the same grammatical class. Decreased cohesiveness was associated with increased structural complexity. A similar pattern of results was obtained for story telling, with the use of anaphora, conjunctions, and ellipsis declining with age and increased narrative complexity. Ambiguous reference also increases with age across a variety of discourse types including story retelling, story generating, answering questions, describing stereotypical action sequences, and making diary entries (Cohen 1979; Kemper 1990; Kemper/Rash/Kynette/Norman 1990; Pratt/Boyes/Robins/Manchester 1989; Ulatowska/Hayashi/Cannito/Fleming 1986). Ambiguous reference may be an accommodation to forgetting of proper names when retelling stories (Pratt et al. 1989) and is associated with lower performance on a memory test (Ulatowska/Cannito/Hayashi/Fleming 1985). In addition, there is evidence that working memory contributes to the incidence of referential errors. Together with the frequency of use of character names, memory span predicts referential errors in story retelling, with age of participant making no further significant contribution to prediction (Pratt et al. 1989). Digit symbol substitution, a measure of processing resources, is negatively related to ambiguous use of pronouns (Ulatowska et al. 1986), while backward digit span is positively related to the use of anaphora, ellipsis, lexical repetition, and conjunction as well as to the occurrence of left-branching clauses and greater structural complexity of narratives (Kemper et al. 1990). These findings suggest that working memory is needed to produce narrative structures, to construct syntactically complex sentences, and to establish text coherence.

3.3. Speech Errors and Disfluencies

Pauses and other disfluencies in speech may signal the need for time to plan what comes next in an utterance, to prepare to revise what has been said, or to emphasize a particular point; they may also stem from word-finding difficulties. The two prominent classes of theories of speech errors and repairs, monitoring theories and spreading activation theories (Levelt 1989; MacKay 1987), both make predictions about aging. Monitoring theories postulate an editor which can catch an error either before or after it is produced. Speech errors which actually occur represent monitoring failures, perhaps due to attentional lapses. Working memory deficits should increase attentional lapses and therefore result in greater numbers of speech errors and fewer repairs in the elderly. Moreover, increased planning time in old age might be associated with longer pauses. Spreading activation theories which posit transmission deficits also predict word finding difficulties in the old (cf. 1.1.) as well as poorer error detection (MacKay/Burke 1990). In MacKay's (1987) model of error detection, the production of a speech error sends priming to an uncommitted node in the network; if this node is activated, its contents become conscious. Inadequate transmission reduces the likelihood that an uncommitted node will become activated in the old and, hence, reduces the likelihood of error detection.

A number of studies have examined the frequency with which different types of disfluencies occur across age. Yairi/Clifton (1972) found an increase with age in total number of disfluencies (interjections, part-word repetitions, word repetitions, phrase repetitions, revisions of incomplete phrases, disrhythmic phonations, and tense pauses), but the pattern of speech errors was similar for high school seniors and older adults. Interpreting their study is complicated by the fact that their older sample included residents of a nursing home, raising the possibility that increased disfluency is associated with poorer health. Walker/Roberts/Hedrick (1988) found an increase in the proportion of older adults producing revisions and interjections (empty words or filled pauses) but not repetitions. Their study, however, is flawed because (a) the educational level attained by the older adults in their sample was considerably lower (9 years) than that of the young adults (14 years) and (b) no statistics are reported (see also Walker/Hardiman/Hedrick/Holbrook 1981). In other studies, including some which used the same set of measures as Yairi and Clifton, few reliable effects of age on rate of speech errors or repairs are reported (Cooper 1990; Duchin/Mysak 1987; Kemper 1992; Kemper et al. 1989, 1990; Kynette/Kemper 1986; Pratt et al. 1989; Shewan/ Henderson 1988) though Cooper (1990) has observed longer filled pauses in older adults. On balance, then, there is as yet little solid evidence for an increase in speech errors or a drop in repairs in old age. Nevertheless, Kemper (1992) has recently suggested that there is a shift in the nature of some kinds of disfluencies in adults aged 60–74 and 75–90. In a study of sentence fragments, old-old adults were more likely to produce filled pauses marking problems in noun retrieval. False starts which occur just before verbs index problems in processing syntax in complex sentences; because the old-old produce fewer complex sentences, they show fewer false starts than the young-old.

3.4. Summary

Spontaneous speech in old age is marked by reduced syntactic complexity and decreased use of certain cohesive devices, just as would be predicted by the hypothesis that language changes in old age arise from reduced working memory capacity. Moreover, there is some evidence from correlational studies that these effects are indeed the consequence of individual differences in working memory. Yet the narratives of older adults are more structurally complex and are rated as better than those of younger adults. These findings are unanticipated, but may reflect trade-offs between syntactic complexity and local cohesiveness with structural complexity. To some extent, also, they may reflect an increased concern on the part of older adults for clarity in communication. Use of simpler sentences and provision of the point or moral of a narrative result in listener-friendly discourse. On the other hand, ambiguous reference is certainly not considerate of listeners. At this time, then, the role of pragmatic considerations in the speech of older adults remains unclear. Another area of uncertainty is whether speech errors and monitoring failures increase with age as would be predicted by both working-memory and transmission deficit hypotheses.

4. Language in Normal Aging, Aphasia, and Alzheimer's Disease

Differentiating language changes which occur in normal aging from those in aphasia and senile dementia of the Alzheimer's type has both theoretical and clinical implications. In this section, language in normal aging is briefly compared to language in aphasia and in Alzheimer's disease.

4.1. Aphasia and Normal Aging

When young and old are compared on standard neuropsychological batteries used to assess language deficits following focal brain damage, systematic age differences favoring the young are sometimes, but not always, found (Bayles/Tomoeda/Boone 1985; Emery 1985); when age-related differences are found, they may be secondary to cohort differences in education or hearing problems (Borod/Goodglass/Kaplan 1980; Goldstein/Shelly 1984) when these are not controlled. When age differences are found on neuropsychological tests of language, they do not consistently resemble any one pattern of aphasia. The one possible area of similarity is that of word finding and confrontation naming. Many aphasics have confrontation naming problems (Goodglass 1980), and some residual anomia is common in patients who have otherwise recovered from aphasia. The lexical retrieval difficulty of healthy older adults shares some properties with at least some cases of anomic aphasia, though it is far less severe. That is, in both normal aging and anomic aphasia there may be problems in retrieving the phonological forms of words coupled with an intact conceptual system (cf. Kay/Ellis 1987). There is also some reason to believe that word-finding problems in anomic aphasia are more severe for nouns than for verbs, a pattern different from that found in agrammatism (Zingeser/Berndt 1990). Older adults, too, may show this asymmetry between nouns and verbs, though the evidence is far from conclusive. For instance, error rates on the Boston Naming Test show larger age differences than those on the Action Naming Test (Nicholas/Obler/Albert/Goodglass 1985). The pattern of speech disfluencies also suggests that the elderly have more difficulty in retrieving nouns than verbs, perhaps because of shifts in the syntactic complexity of their utterances (Kemper 1992). Finally, in a diary study, Burke/MacKay/Worthley/Wade (1992) found that older adults had more tip-of-the-tongue experiences for proper names and common objects than young adults, but in an induced tip-of-the-tongue experiment, only the age difference for proper names was reliable. In the diary study, there was some evidence that the young had proportionately more problems with abstract words (verbs and adjectives) than the old; however, the young were in a formal educational setting that encouraged greater use of abstract words and therefore afforded more opportunities for abstract word retrieval difficulties. The naming problem in aphasia also has properties different from that in normal aging. Patients with anomic aphasia and those with Wernicke's aphasia both tend to produce more pronouns without antecedents, deictic terms, paraphasias, and repetitions than age-matched controls; Wernicke's aphasics produce neologisms whereas normal controls do not (Glosser/Deser 1990; Nicholas/Obler/Albert/Helm-Estabrooks 1985).

There are few studies that explicitly compare language in aphasia and normal aging. Bayles/Boone/Tomoeda et al. (1989) compared normal elderly to fluent (Wernicke's, transcortical sensory, conduction, and anomic) and nonfluent (Broca's and transcortical motor) aphasics considerably younger than them in mean age but matched with them in education and estimated intelligence. Their test battery assessed oral object description, disambiguation of sentences containing lexical, structural, or logical ambiguities, word fluency, receptive vocabulary, reading comprehension of words, sentences, and paragraphs, expressive pantomime, and picture description (scored for number of idea units). Both aphasic groups scored lower on all tests than the normal elderly group. The only tests on which the differences between elderly and aphasic groups were not reliable were word reading comprehension and pantomime expression for the fluent aphasics and word reading comprehension for the nonfluent aphasics. Fluent aphasics produce fewer complex sentences in spontaneous speech; their spontaneous speech is not, however, rated as less coherent on either local or global levels (Glosser/Deser 1990). They also produce a greater number of sentence fragments and anacolutha (changes of syntactic construction or contaminations of two or more syntactic structures within an utterance) than do controls (Blanken/Dittmann/Haas/Wallesch 1987). Relative to controls, then, fluent aphasics show preserved macrostructure and impaired microstructure.

4.2. Alzheimer's Disease and Normal Aging

Language impairment is characteristic of Alzheimer's disease. Performance on neuropsychological tests is generally poorer and outside the normal range on almost all measures of language function though phonology appears to be well preserved – at least initially (Appell/Kertesz/Fisman 1982; Bayles 1982; Bayles/Boone/Tomoeda et al. 1989; Cummings/Benson/Hill/Read 1985). Not all aspects of language, however, are affected to the same degree. Early in the course of the disease, there is a dissociation between lexical-semantic impairment and syntax which is opposite to that shown by agrammatic aphasics. That is, early in Alzheimer's disease syntax is unaffected relative to the semantic system, whereas in agrammatism the reverse is true. For instance, in spontaneous speech, grammatical errors are few though utterances may be devoid of meaning (Bayles 1982; Hier/Hagenlocker/Shindler 1985). The relative frequency of different syntactic constructions is similar in Alzheimer's patients and in age-matched controls (Kempler/Curtiss/Jackson 1987). Detection and correction of grammatical anomalies in sentences is better for syntactic than for semantic errors (Bayles 1982). In writing to dictation, homophone spelling is more accurate in the context of syntactic cues (my nose) than semantic cues (mouth nose) (Kempler et al. 1987). This does not mean, however, that syntax is completely spared even early in Alzheimer's disease inasmuch as syntactic processing in comprehension is affected (Emery 1985; Tomoeda/Bayles/Boone et al. 1990). An increase in sentence fragments in spontaneous speech has also been reported (Hier et al. 1985; Ulatowska/Allard/Donnell et al. 1988), though this is not invariably found (Blanken et al. 1987). Thus, the emphasis must be on relative, rather than absolute, sparing of syntax in Alzheimer's disease.

The semantic deficit in Alzheimer's disease is manifested in numerous ways. Some of these suggest that the problem lies in word finding. Thus, performance is lower on tests of confrontation naming, naming to definition, and verbal fluency (Appell et al. 1982; Huff/Corkin/Growdon 1986; Martin/Fedio 1983; Rissenberg/Glanzer 1987). Also, spontaneous speech in Alzheimer's disease is noteworthy for its circumlocutions, ambiguous pronoun reference, excessive use of empty deictic terms and indefinite anaphora, and repetitions (Hier et al. 1985; Nicholas/Obler/Albert/Helm-Estabrooks 1985), all of which are consistent with word finding difficulties. Consonant with this conclusion, Nicholas/Obler/Albert/Helm-Estabrooks (1985) found a positive correlation between naming accuracy and number of content elements produced in a picture description task and a negative correlation between naming accuracy and number of indefinite terms; however, correlations of naming accuracy with other measures related to word-finding problems (deictic terms, pronouns without antecedents, comments on the task) were not statistically reliable. The fact that phonological cues benefit patients in confrontation naming tasks points to an impairment in accessing the phonological representations of words as the mechanism underlying such word-finding problems (Neils/Brennan/Cole et al. 1988), though Henderson/Mack/Freed et al. (1990) argue that it is also compatible with a disruption in the semantic system.

Other findings seem more in line with a disruption within the semantic system due to loss or disorganization of conceptual information. (1) Patients unable to name a picture are often unable to answer questions about the concept which it represents (Chertkow/Bub/Seidenberg 1989; Huff/Corkin/Growdon 1986) and there is evidence for greater consistency in errors than would be expected by chance when the same pictures are named on two occasions (Henderson/Mack/Freed et al. 1990). (2) Errors in confrontation naming are most often semantically related to targets, though in more severely affected patients there is an increase in unrelated responses (Bayles/Tomoeda 1983; Huff et al. 1986; Martin/Fedio 1983). (3) The word associations of patients are more idiosyncratic and show a reduction in the proportion of paradigmatic responses (though syntagmatic responding appears not to be affected – further evidence of preserved syntax), suggesting that features are lost (Gewirth/Shindler/Hier 1984; Santo Pietro/Goldfarb 1985). However, Abeysinghe/Bayles/Trosset (1990) found that patients who gave no response, unrelated responses, or stimulus repetition responses on a word association test were sometimes able to give meaningful definitions for these items; they caution against accepting word association data as evidence for loss of conceptual knowledge and argue that abnormal responding arises from a loss of associations rather than of conceptual information. (4) Knowledge of scripts is impaired in Alzheimer's disease; patients generate more actions which are implausible (though possible within script boundaries) and are less accurate in ordering pairs of actions (Grafman/Thompson/Weingartner et al. 1991). (5) Patients suffering from Alzheimer's disease are less accurate in generating actions, physical features, or associates of objects (Nebes/Brady 1988) and in judging how important an associate is to the meaning of a concept (Grober/Buschke/Kawas/Fuld 1985) or how strongly associated two words are (Abeysinghe et al. 1990). These tasks require retrieval of specific relationships or explicit judgments of degree of association. On tasks which measure knowledge of semantic relationships more indirectly and do not require a deep analysis of the nature of the relationsship between words, the performance of Alzheimer's patients appears pretty much normal. For instance, patients and normal elderly adults show the same pattern of response times to actions, physical features, and associates of objects when asked to judge whether they are related (Nebes/Brady 1988) and show equal sensitivity to the response dominance of attributes in a similar task (Nebes/Brady 1990). If anything, patients appear to show greater semantic priming effects in lexical decision and word naming tasks (cf. Nebes 1989).

4.3. Summary

In normal aging, many aspects of language, including both word-finding and comprehension and production of complex grammatical structures, show subtle changes which are not always detectable by standardized neuropsychological instruments. Although there is as yet no research that suggests a disproportionate impairment in one particular facet of language rather than another, such as might be expected in an aphasia resulting from focal brain damage, there is some similarity between word-finding difficulties in normal aging and anomic aphasia. In early Alzheimer's disease, however, there is severe impairment in most aspects of language accompanied by a dissociation between syntax and semantics. The available evidence does not permit a choice among alternative explanations of the semantic deficit in Alzheimer's disease. It seems likely that loss of conceptual information and problems in realizing the phonological representations of words both play a role. Two important questions that remain to be answered are whether the changes observed in normal aging presage those found in Alzheimer's disease (i. e., are similar but less severe) and which of the mechanisms discussed above (or others, see Nebes 1989) are responsible for the pattern of spared and impaired language function in Alzheimer's disease.

Author's Note:
Preparation of this chapter was supported by National Institute on Aging Grant R37 AG02452.

5. References

Abeysinghe, S. C., Bayles, K. A., & Trosset, M. W. (1990). Semantic memory deterioration in Alzheimer's subjects: Evidence from word association, definition, and associate ranking tasks. *Journal of Speech and Hearing Research*, *33*, 574–582.

Albert, M., Duffy, F. H., & Naeser, M. (1987). Nonlinear changes in cognition with age and their neuropsychologic correlates. *Canadian Journal of Psychology*, *41*, 141–157.

Albert, M. S., Heller, H. S., & Milberg, W. (1988). Changes in naming ability with age. *Psychology and Aging*, *3*, 173–178.

Anders, T. R., Fozard, J. L., & Lillyquist, T. D. (1972). Effects of age upon retrieval from short-term memory. *Developmental Psychology*, *6*, 214–217.

Anderson, J. A. (1983). A spreading activation theory of memory. *Journal of Verbal Learning and Verbal Behavior*, *22*, 261–295.

Appell, J., Kertesz, A., & Fisman, M. (1982). A study of language functioning in Alzheimer patients. *Brain and Language*, *17*, 73–91.

Baddeley, A. (1986). *Working memory*. Oxford: Oxford University Press.

Baddeley, A., Logie, R., Nimmo-Smith, I., & Brereton, N. (1985). Components of fluent reading. *Journal of Memory and Language, 24*, 119–131.

Balota, D. A. & Duchek, J. M. (1988). Age-related differences in lexical access, spreading activation, and simple pronunciation. *Psychology and Aging, 3*, 84–93.

Bayles, K. A. (1982). Language function in senile dementia. *Brain and Language, 16*, 265–280.

Bayles, K. A., Boone, D. R., Tomoeda, C. K., Slauson, T. J., & Kaszniak, A. W. (1989). Differentiating Alzheimer's patients from the normal elderly and stroke patients with aphasia. *Journal of Speech and Hearing Disorders, 54*, 74–87.

Bayles, K. A. & Tomoeda, C. K. (1983). Confrontation naming impairment in dementia. *Brain and Language, 19*, 98–114.

Bayles, K. A., Tomoeda, C. K., & Boone, D. R. (1985). A view of age-related changes in language function. *Developmental Neuropsychology, 1*, 231–264.

Bergman, M. (1980). *Aging and the perception of speech.* Baltimore: University Park Press.

Blanken, G., Dittmann, J., Haas, J.-C., & Wallesch, C.-W. (1987). Spontaneous speech in senile dementia and aphasia: Implications for a neurolinguistic model of language production. *Cognition, 27*, 247–274.

Bock, J. K. (1982). Toward a cognitive psychology of syntax: Information processing contributions to sentence formulation. *Psychological Review, 89*, 1–47.

Borod, J. C., Goodglass, H., & Kaplan, E. (1980). Normative data on the Boston Diagnostic Aphasia Examination, Parietal Lobe Battery, and the Boston Naming Test. *Journal of Clinical Neuropsychology, 2*, 209–215.

Bowles, N. L., Obler, L. K., & Albert, M. L. (1987). Naming errors in healthy aging and dementia of the Alzheimer type. *Cortex, 23*, 519–524.

Bowles, N. L. & Poon, L. W. (1985). Aging and retrieval of words in semantic memory. *Journal of Gerontology, 40*, 71–77.

Bowles, N. L., Williams, D., & Poon, L. W. (1983). On the use of word association norms in aging research. *Experimental Aging Research, 9*, 175–177.

Bromley, D. B. (1991). Aspects of written language production over adult life. *Psychology and Aging, 6*, 296–308.

Burke, D. M. & Harrold, R. M. (1988). Automatic and effortful semantic processes in old age: Experimental and naturalistic approaches. In L. L. Light & D. M. Burke (Eds.), *Language, memory, and aging. 100–116.* New York: Cambridge University Press.

Burke, D. M., MacKay, D. G., Worthley, J. S., & Wade, E. (1991). On the tip of the tongue: What causes word finding failures in young and older adults? *Journal of Memory and Language, 30*, 542–579.

Burke, D. M. & Peters, L. (1986). Word associations in old age: Evidence for consistency in semantic encoding during adulthood. *Psychology and Aging, 1*, 283–292.

Burke, D. M., White, H., & Diaz, D. L. (1987). Semantic priming in young and older adults: Evidence for age constancy in automatic and attentional processes. *Journal of Experimental Psychology: Human Perception and Performance, 13*, 79–88.

Burke, D. M. & Yee, P. L. (1984). Semantic priming during sentence processing by young and older adults. *Developmental Psychology, 20*, 903–910.

Byrd, M. (1984). Age differences in the retrieval of information from semantic memory. *Experimental Aging Research, 10*, 29–33.

Caplan, D. & Waters, G. S. (1990). Short-term memory and language comprehension: A critical review of the neuropsychological literature. In G. Vallar & T. Shallice (Eds.), *Neuropsychological impairments of short-term memory. 337–389.* Cambridge: Cambridge University Press.

Chertkow, H., Bub, D., & Seidenberg, M. (1989). Priming and semantic memory loss in Alzheimer's disease. *Brain and Language, 36*, 420–446.

Cheung, H. & Kemper, S. (1992). Competing complexity metrics and adults' production of complex sentences. *Applied Psycholinguistics, 13*, 53–76..

Chiarello, C., Church, K. L., & Hoyer, W. J. (1985). Automatic and controlled semantic priming: Accuracy, response bias, and aging. *Journal of Gerontology, 40*, 593–600.

Cohen, G. (1979). Language comprehension in old age. *Cognitive Psychology, 11*, 412–429.

Cohen, G. (1988). Age differences in memory for text: Production deficiency or processing limitations? In L. L. Light & D. M. Burke (Eds.), *Language, memory, and aging. 171–190.* New York: Cambridge University Press.

Cohen, G. & Faulkner, D. (1983). Word recognition: Age differences in contextual facilitation effects. *British Journal of Psychology, 74*, 239–251.

Cohen, G. & Faulkner, D. (1986). Memory for proper names: Age differences in retrieval. *British Journal of Developmental Psychology, 4*, 187-197.

Cooper, P. V. (1990). Discourse production and normal aging: Performance on oral picture description tasks. *Journal of Gerontology: Psychological Sciences, 45*, P210–214

Craik, F. I. M. & Byrd, M. (1982). Aging and cognitive deficits: The role of attentional resources. In F. I. M. Craik & S. Trehub (Eds.), *Aging and cognitive processes. 191–211.* New York: Plenum Press.

Craik, F. I. M., Morris, R. G., & Gick, M. L. (1990). Adult age differences in working memory.

In G. Vallar & T. Shallice (Eds.), *Neuropsychological impairments of short-term memory. 247–267.* Cambridge: Cambridge University Press.

Cummings, J. L., Benson, D. F., Hill, M. A., & Read, S. (1985). Aphasia in dementia of the Alzheimer type. *Neurology, 35*, 394–397.

Dell, G. S. (1986). A spreading-activation theory of retrieval in sentence production. *Psychological Review, 93*, 283–321.

Duchin, S. W. & Mysak, E. D. (1987). Disfluency and rate characteristics of young adult, middle-aged, and older males. *Journal of Communication Disorders, 20*, 245–257.

Emery, O. B. (1985). Language and aging. *Experimental Aging Research, 11*, 3–60.

Feier, C. D. & Gerstman, L. J. (1980). Sentence comprehension abilities throughout the adult life span. *Journal of Gerontology, 35*, 722–728.

Flicker, C., Ferris, S. H., Crook, T., & Bartus, R. T. (1986). The effects of aging and dementia on concept formation as measured on an object-sorting task. *Developmental Neuropsychology, 2*, 65–72.

Flicker, C., Ferris, S. H., Crook, T., & Bartus, R. T. (1987). Implications of memory and language dysfunction in the naming deficit of senile dementia. *Brain and Language, 31*, 187–200.

Gewirth, L. R., Shindler, A.G., & Hier, D. B. (1984). Altered patterns of word associations in dementia and aphasia. *Brain and Language, 21*, 307–317.

Glosser, G, & Deser, T. (1990). Patterns of discourse production among neurological patients with fluent language disorders. *Brain and Language, 40*, 67–88.

Goldstein, G. & Shelly, C. (1984). Relationships between language skills as assessed by the Halstead-Reitan battery and the Luria-Nebraska language-related factor scales in a nonaphasic patient population. *Journal of Clinical Neuropsychology, 6*, 143–156.

Goodglass, H. (1980). Disorders of naming following brain injury. *American Scientist, 68*, 647–655.

Grafman, J., Thompson, K., Weingartner, H., Martinez, R., Lawlor, B. A., & Sunderland, T. (1991). Script generation as an indicator of knowledge representation in patients with Alzheimer's disease. *Brain and Language, 40*, 344–358.

Grober, E., Buschke, H., Kawas, C., & Fuld, P. (1985). Impaired ranking of semantic attributes in dementia. *Brain and Language, 26*, 276–286.

Hasher, L. & Zacks, R. T. (1988). Working memory, comprehension, and aging: A review and a new view. In G. H. Bower (Ed.), *The psychology of learning and motivation* (Vol. 22). *193–225.* New York: Academic Press.

Henderson, V. W., Mack, W., Freed, D. M., Kempler, D., & Anderson, E. S. (1990). Naming consistency in Alzheimer's disease. *Brain and Language, 39*, 530–538.

Hertzog, C., Raskind, C. L. & Cannon, C. J. (1986). Age-related slowing in semantic information processing speed: An individual differences analysis. *Journal of Gerontology, 41*, 500–502.

Hess, T. M. (1985). Aging and context influences on recognition memory for typical and atypical script actions. *Development Psychology, 21*, 1139–1151.

Hier, D. B., Hagenlocker, K., & Shindler, A. G. (1985). Language disintegration in dementia: Effects of etiology and severity. *Brain and Language, 25*, 117–133.

Howard, D. V. (1979). *Restricted word association norms for adults between the ages of 20 and 80.* (Tech. Rep. NIA-79-2). Washington, DC: Georgetown University.

Howard, D. V. (1980). Category norms: A comparison of the Battig and Montague (1969) norms with the responses of adults between the ages of 20 and 80. *Journal of Gerontology, 35*, 225–231.

Howard, D. V. (1983). The effects of aging and degree of association on the semantic priming of lexical decisions. *Experimental Aging Research, 9*, 145–151.

Howard, D. V., Mc Andrews, M. P., & Lasaga, M. I. (1981). Semantic priming of lexical decisions in young and old adults. *Journal of Gerontology, 36*, 707–714.

Howard, D. V., Shaw, R. J., & Heisey, J. G. (1986). Aging and the time course of semantic activation. *Journal of Gerontology, 41*, 195–203.

Huff, F. J., Corkin, S., & Growdon, J. H. (1986). Semantic impairment and anomia in Alzheimer's disease. *Brain and Language, 28*, 235–249.

Hutchinson, K. M. (1989). Influence of sentence context on speech perception in young and older adults. *Journal of Gerontology: Psychological Sciences, 44*, P36–44.

Jerger, J. & Hayes, D. (1977). Diagnostic speech audiometry. *Archives of Otolaryngology, 103*, 216–222.

Kay, J. & Ellis, A. (1987). A cognitive neuropsychological case study of anomia. *Brain, 110*, 613–629.

Kemper, S. (1986). Imitation of complex syntactic constructions by elderly adults. *Applied Psycholinguistics, 7*, 277–288.

Kemper, S. (1987). Life-span changes in syntactic complexity. *Journal of Gerontology, 42*, 323–328.

Kemper, S. (1990). Adults' diaries: Changes made to written narratives across the life span. *Discourse Processes, 13*, 207–223.

Kemper, S. (1992). Adults' sentence fragments: Who, what, when, where, and why. *Journal of Communication Research, 19*, 332–346.

Kemper, S., Kynette, D., & Norman, S. (1992). Age differences in spoken language. In R. West & J. Sinnott (Eds.), *Everyday memory and aging: Current research and methodology. 138–152.* New York: Springer Verlag.

Kemper, S., Kynette, D., Rash, S., O'Brien, K., & Sprott, R. (1989). Life-span changes to adults' language: Effects of memory and genre. *Applied Psycholinguistics, 10*, 49–66.

Kemper, S., Rash, S., Kynette, D., & Norman, S. (1990). Telling stories: The structure of adults' narratives. *European Journal of Cognitive Psychology, 2*, 205–228.

Kempler, D., Curtiss, S., & Jackson, C. (1987). Syntactic preservation in Alzheimer's disease. *Journal of Speech and Hearing Research, 30*, 343–350.

Kintsch, W. (1988). The role of knowledge in discourse comprehension: A construction-integration model. *Psychological Review, 95*, 163–182.

Kintsch, W. & van Dijk, T. A. (1978). Toward a model of text comprehension and production. *Psychological Review, 85*, 363–394.

Kynette, D. & Kemper, S. (1986). Aging and the loss of grammatical forms: A cross-sectional study of language performance. *Language & Communication, 6*, 65–72.

Laver, G. D. & Burke, D. M. (1990). *Are semantic priming effects equivalent in young and older adults?* Unpublished manuscript available from the author, Department of Psychology, Claremont Graduate School, Claremont, CA.

Lesser, R. (1976). Verbal and non-verbal memory components in the Token Test. *Neuropsychologia, 14*, 79–85.

Levelt, W. J. M. (1989). *Speaking: From intention to articulation.* Cambridge, MA: MIT Press.

Light, L. L. (1988). Language and aging: Competence versus performance. In J. E. Birren & V. L. Bengtson (Eds.), *Emergent theories of aging. 177–213.* New York: Springer.

Light, L. L. (1992). The organization of memory in old age. In F. I. M. Craik & T. A. Salthouse (Eds.), *Handbook of aging and cognition. 111–165.* Hillsdale, NJ: Erlbaum.

Light, L. L. & Albertson, S. (1988). Comprehension of pragmatic implications in young and older adults. In L. L. Light & D. M. Burke (Eds.), *Language, memory, and aging. 133–153.* New York: Cambridge University Press.

Light, L. L. & Anderson, P. A. (1983). Memory for scripts in young and older adults. *Memory & Cognition, 11*, 435–444.

Light, L. L. & Anderson, P. A. (1985). Working-memory capacity, age, and memory for discourse. *Journal of Gerontology, 40*, 737–747.

Light, L. L. & Capps, J. L. (1986), Comprehension of pronouns in young and older adults. *Developmental Psychology, 22*, 580-585.

Light, L. L., Valencia-Laver, D., & Zavis, D. (1991). Instantiation of general terms in young and older adults. *Psychology and Aging, 6*, 337–351.

List, J. A. (1986). Age and schematic differences in the reliability of eyewitness testimony. *Developmental Psychology, 22*, 50–57.

Lovelace, E. A. & Cooley, S. (1982). Free associations of older adults to single words and conceptually related word triads. *Journal of Gerontology, 37*, 432–437.

MacKay, D. G. (1987). *The organization of perception and action.* New York: Springer-Verlag.

MacKay, D. G. & Burke, D. M. (1990). Cognition and aging: A theory of new learning and the use of old connections. In T. M. Hess (Ed.), *Aging and cognition: Knowledge organization and utilization. 213–264.* Amsterdam: North Holland.

Madden, D. J. (1985). Age-related slowing in the retrieval of information from long-term memory. *Journal of Gerontology, 40*, 208–210.

Madden, D. J. (1986). Adult age differences in visual word recognition: Semantic encoding and episodic retention. *Experimental Aging Research, 12*, 71–77.

Madden, D. J. (1988). Adult age differences in the effects of sentence context and stimulus degradation during visual word recognition. *Psychology and Aging, 3*, 167–172.

Madden, D. J. (1989). Visual word identification and age-related slowing. *Cognitive Development, 4*, 1–29.

Martin, A. & Fedio, P. (1983). Word production and comprehension in Alzheimer's disease: The breakdown of semantic knowledge. *Brain and Language, 19*, 124–141.

Martin, R. C. (1990). Neuropsychological evidence on the role of short-term memory in sentence processing. In G. Vallar & T. Shallice (Eds.), *Neuropsychological impairments of short-term memory. 390–427.* Cambridge: Cambridge University Press.

Maylor, E. A. (1990). Age, blocking and the tip of the tongue state. *British Journal of Psychology, 81*, 123–134.

McClelland, J. L. & Rumelhart, D. E. (1981). An interactive activation model of context effects in letter perception: Part 1. An account of basic findings. *Psychological Review, 88*, 375–407.

McCrae, R. R., Arenberg, D., & Costa, P. T. (1987). Declines in divergent thinking with age: Cross-sectional, longitudinal, and cross-sequential analyses. *Psychology and Aging, 2*, 130–137.

Meyer, D. E. & Schvaneveldt, R. W. (1971). Facilitation in recognizing pairs of words: Evidence of a dependence between retrieval operations. *Journal of Experimental Psychology, 90*, 227–234.

Miller, G. A. (1979). Images and models, similes and metaphors. In A. Ortony (Ed.), *Metaphor and thought*. *202–250*. Cambridge: Cambridge University Press.

Mitchell, D. B. (1989). How many memory systems? Evidence from aging. *Journal of Experimental Psychology: Learning, Memory, and Cognition*, *15*, 31–49.

Mueller, J. H., Kausler, D. H., & Faherty, A. (1980). Age and access time for different memory codes. *Experimental Aging Research*, *6*, 445–449.

Nebes, R. D. (1989). Semantic memory in Alzheimer's disease. *Psychological Bulletin*, *106*, 377–394.

Nebes, R. D., Boller, F., & Holland, A. (1986). Use of semantic context by patients with Alzheimer's disease. *Psychology and Aging*, *1*, 261–269.

Nebes, R. D. & Brady, C. B. (1988). Integrity of semantic fields in Alzheimer's disease. *Cortex*, *24*, 291–299.

Nebes, R. D. & Brady, C. B. (1990). Preserved organization of semantic attributes in Alzheimer's disease. *Psychology and Aging*, *5*, 574–579.

Neils, J., Brennan, M. M., Cole, M., Boller, F., & Gerdeman, B. (1988). The use of phonemic cueing with Alzheimer's disease patients. *Neuropsychologia*, *26*, 351–354.

Nicholas, M., Obler, L., Albert, M., & Goodglass, H. (1985). Lexical retrieval in healthy aging. *Cortex*, *21*, 595–606.

Nicholas, M., Obler, L. K., Albert, M. L., & Helm-Estabrooks, N. (1985). Empty speech in Alzheimer's disease and fluent aphasia. *Journal of Speech and Hearing Research*, *28*, 405–410.

Norman, S., Kemper, S., Kynette, D., Cheung, H., & Anagnopoulos, C. (1991). Syntactic complexity and adults' running memory span. *Journal of Gerontology: Psychological Sciences*, *46*, P346–351.

Obler, L. K. (1980). Narrative discourse style in the elderly. In L. K. Obler & M. L. Albert (Eds.), *Language and communication in the elderly*. *75–90*. Lexington, MA: D. C. Heath.

Obler, L. K., Nicholas, M., Albert, M. L., & Woodward, S. (1985). On comprehension across the life span. *Cortex*, *21*, 273–280.

Pratt, M. W., Boyes, C., Robins, S., & Manchester, J. (1989). Telling tales: Aging, working memory, and the narrative cohesion of story retellings. *Developmental Psychology*, *25*, 628–635.

Pye, C., Cheung, H., & Kemper, S. (in press). Islands at eighty. In H. Goodluck & M. Rochemont (Eds.), *Island constraints: Theory, acquisition, and processing*. Dordrecht: Reidel.

Riegel, K. F. (1959). A study of verbal achievements of older persons. *Journal of Gerontology*, *14*, 453–456.

Riegel, K. F. (1973). Language and cognition: Some life-span developmental issues. *Gerontologist*, *13*, 478–482.

Riegel, K. F. & Riegel, R. M (1964). Changes in associative behavior during later years of life: A cross-sectional analysis. *Vita Humana*, *7*, 1–32.

Rissenberg, M. & Glanzer, M. (1987). Free recall and word finding ability in normal aging and senile dementia of the Alzheimer's type: The effect of item concreteness. *Journal of Gerontology*, *42*, 318–322.

Roman, M., Brownell, H. H., Potter, H. H., & Seibold, M. S. (1987). Script-knowledge in right hemisphere-damaged and in normal elderly adults. *Brain and Language*, *31*, 151–171.

Salthouse, T. A. (1982). *Adult cognition: An experimental psychology of human aging*. New York: Springer-Verlag.

Salthouse, T. A. (1985). *A theory of cognitive aging*. Amsterdam: North Holland.

Salthouse, T. A. (1990). Working memory as a processing resource in cognitive aging. *Developmental Review*, *10*, 101–124.

Sanford, A. J. & Garrod, S. C. (1981). *Understanding written language: Explorations of comprehension beyond the sentence*. Chichester, England: John Wiley.

Santo Pietro, M. J. & Goldfarb, R. (1985). Characteristic patterns of word association responses in institutionalized elderly with and without senile dementia. *Brain and Language*, *26*, 230–243.

Schaie, K. W. & Parham, I. A. (1977). Cohort-sequential analyses of adult intellectual development. *Developmental Psychology*, *13*, 649–653.

Searle, J. R. (1979). Metaphor. In A. Ortony (Ed.), *Metaphor and thought*. *92–123*. Cambridge: Cambridge University Press.

Sharkey, N. E. (1986). A model of knowledge-based expectations in text comprehension. In J. A. Galambos, R. P. Abelson, & J. B. Black (Eds.), *Knowledge structures*. *49–70*. Hillsdale, NJ: Lawrence Erlbaum Associates.

Shewan, C. M. & Henderson, V. L. (1988). Analysis of spontaneous language in the older normal population. *Journal of Communication Disorders*, *21*, 139–154.

Smiley, S. S. & Brown, A. L. (1979). Conceptual preferences for thematic or taxonomic relations: A nonmonotonic age trend from preschool to old age. *Journal of Experimental Child Psychology*, *28*, 249–257.

Stanovich, K. E. & West, R. F. (1983). On priming by a sentence context. *Journal of Experimental Psychology: General*, *112*, 1–36.

Stern, C., Prather, P., Swinney, D., & Zurif, E. (1991). The time course of automatic lexical access and aging. *Brain and Language*, *40*, 359–372.

Stine, E. L. (1986). Attribute-based similarity perception in younger and older adults. *Experimental Aging Research*, *12*, 89–94.

Stine, E. A. L. (1990). On-line processing of written text by younger and older adults. *Psychology and Aging*, *5*, 68–78.

Stine, E. L. & Wingfield, A. (1987). Process and strategy in memory for speech among younger and older adults. *Psychology and Aging*, *2*, 272–279.

Stine, E. A. L. & Wingfield, A. (1990). How much do working memory deficits contribute to age differences in discourse memory? *European Journal of Cognitive Psychology*, *2*, 289–304.

Stine, E. L., Wingfield, A., & Poon, L. W. (1986). How much and how fast: Rapid processing of spoken language in later adulthood. *Psychology and Aging*, *1*, 303–311.

Tabossi, P. & Johnson-Laird, P. N. (1980). Linguistic context and the priming of semantic information. *Quarterly Journal of Experimental Psychology*, *32*, 595–603.

Tanenhaus, M. K., Dell, G. S., & Carlson, G. (1987). Context effects and lexical processing: A connectionist approach to modularity. In J. L. Garfield (Ed.), *Modularity in knowledge representation and natural-language understanding. 83–110.* Cambridge, MA: MIT Press.

Till, R. E. & Walsh, D. A. (1980). Encoding and retrieval factors in adult memory for implicational sentences. *Journal of Verbal Learning and Verbal Behavior*, *19*, 1–16.

Tomoeda, C. K., Bayles, K. A., Boone, D. R., Kaszniak, A. W., & Slauson, T. J. (1990). Speech rate and syntactic complexity effects on the auditory comprehension of Alzheimer patients. *Journal of Communication Disorders*, *23*, 151–161.

Ulatowska, H. K., Allard, L., Donnell, A., Bristow, J., Haynes, S.M., Flower, A., & North, A. J. (1988). Discourse performance in subjects with dementia of the Alzheimer type. In H. A. Whitaker (Ed.), *Neuropsychological studies of nonfocal brain damage. 108–131.* New York: Springer-Verlag.

Ulatowska, H. K., Cannito, M. P., Hayashi, M. M., & Fleming, S. G. (1985). Language abilities in the elderly. In H. K. Ulatowska (Ed.), *The aging brain: Communication in the elderly. 125–139.* San Diego, CA: College-Hill Press.

Ulatowska, H. K., Hayashi, M. M., Cannito, M. P., & Fleming, S. G. (1986). Disruption of reference in aging. *Brain and Language*, *28*, 24–41.

Van Dijk, T. A. & Kintsch, W. (1983). *Strategies of discourse comprehension.* New York: Academic Press.

Van Gorp, W., Satz, P., Kiersch, M. E., & Henry, R. (1986). Normative data on the Boston Naming Test for a group of normal older adults. *Journal of Clinical and Experimental Neuropsychology*, *8*, 702–705.

Walker, V. G., Hardiman, C. J., Hedrick, D. L., & Holbrook, A. (1981). Speech and language characteristics of an aging population. In N. J. Lass (Ed.), *Speech and language: Advances in basic research and practice. 143–202.* New York: Academic Press.

Walker, V. G., Roberts, P. M., & Hedrick, D. L. (1988). Linguistic analyses of the discourse narratives of young and aged women. *Folia Phoniatrica*, *40*, 58–64.

Warrington, E. K. & Shallice, T. (1984). Category specific semantic impairments. *Brain*, *107*, 829–854.

Wingfield, A., Aberdeen, J. S., & Stine, E. A. L. (1991). Word onset gating and linguistic context in spoken word recognition by young and elderly adults. *Journal of Gerontology: Psychological Sciences*, *46*, P127–129.

Wingfield, A., Lahar, C. J., & Stine, E. A. L. (1989). Age and decision strategies in running memory for speech: Effects of prosody and linguistic structure. *Journal of Gerontology: Psychological Sciences*, *44*, P106–113.

Wingfield, A., Poon, L. W., Lombardi, L., & Lowe, D. (1985). Speed of processing in normal aging: Effects of speech rate, linguistic structure, and processing time. *Journal of Gerontology*, *40*, 579–585.

Yairi, E. & Clifton, N. F., Jr. (1972). Disfluent speech behavior of preschool children, high school seniors, and geriatric persons. *Journal of Speech and Hearing Research*, *15*, 714–719.

Zelinski, E. M. (1988). Integrating information from discourse: Do older adults show deficits? In L. L. Light & D. M. Burke (Eds.), *Language, memory, and aging. 117–132.* New York: Cambridge University Press.

Zelinski, E. M. & Gilewski, M. J. (1988). Memory for prose and aging: A meta-analysis. In M. L. Howe & C. J. Brainerd (Eds.), *Cognitive development in adulthood. 133–158.* New York: Springer-Verlag.

Zingeser, L. G. & Berndt, R. S. (1990). Retrieval of nouns and verbs in agrammatism and anomia. *Brain and Language*, *39*, 14–32.

Leah L. Light, Claremont, California (USA)

VI. Indexes

88. Editors and Contributors

James H. Abbs
University of Wisconsin
Speech & Motor Control Laboratories
Waisman Center
Madison, Wisconsin
USA

William Badecker
The Johns Hopkins University
Department of Cognitive Science
Baltimore, Maryland
USA

Joseph Bayer
Universität Düsseldorf
Seminar für Allgemeine Sprachwissenschaft
Düsseldorf
Germany

Kathryn A. Bayles
University of Arizona
Department of Speech and Hearing Sciences
Tucson, Arizona
USA

Gerhard Blanken
Universität Freiburg/Br.
Forschungsschwerpunkt Neuropsychologie/
Neurolinguistik
Deutsches Seminar
Freiburg/Br.
Germany

Hugh W. Buckingham
Louisiana State University
Interdepartmental Linguistics Program
College of Arts and Sciences
Baton Rouge, Louisiana
USA

Brian Butterworth
University College
Department of Psychology
London
United Kingdom

Stefano F. Cappa
Università di Brescia
Clinica Neurologica
Brescia
Italy

Alfonso Caramazza
The Johns Hopkins University
Department of Cognitive Science
Baltimore, Maryland
USA

Sandra Chapman
The University of Texas
Callier Center for Communication
Disorders
Dallas, Texas
USA

Ria De Bleser
Rheinisch-Westfälische Technische
Hochschule Aachen
Neurologische Klinik
Aachen
Germany

Gérard Deloche
Hôpital de la Salpêtrière
Salle Racine, Service du Prof. Pierrot-
Desseilligny
Paris
France

Roxanne DePaul
University of Wisconsin
Departments of Neurology and
Neurophysiology
Medical School
Madison, Wisconsin
USA

Jürgen Dittmann
Universität Freiburg/Br.
Deutsches Seminar
Freiburg/Br.
Germany

Barbara Dodd
The University of Queensland
Department of Speech and Hearing
St. Lucia, Queensland
Australia

Christian Eggers
Rheinische Landes- und Hochschulklinik
Klinik für Kinder- und Jugendpsychiatrie
Essen
Germany

Susan Ellis Weismer
University of Wisconsin
Department of Communicative Disorders
Madison, Wisconsin
USA

Pierre Feyereisen
Université Catholique de Louvain
Département de Psychologie Expérimentale
Unité de Neuropsychologie Cognitive
Louvain-la-Neuve
Belgium

Peter Fiedler
Universität Heidelberg
Psychologisches Institut
Heidelberg
Germany

Marilyn Ford
Griffith University
C. I. T. Division of Science and Technology
Nathan, Brisbane
Queensland
Australia

Carol A. Fowler
Haskins Laboratories
New Haven, Connecticut
USA

Angela D. Friederici
Freie Universität Berlin
Institut für Psychologie
Berlin
Germany

Trian Fundudis
The Royal Free Hospital, School of
Medicine
London
United Kingdom

Merrill F. Garrett
University of Arizona
Faculty of Social and Behavioral Sciences
Cognitive Science
Tucson, Arizona
USA

Pierre Goulet
Centre Hospitalier Côte-des-Neiges
Centre de Recherche
Montréal, Québec
Canada

Hannelore Grimm
Universität Bielefeld
Fakultät für Psychologie und
Sportwissenschaft
Abteilung für Psychologie
Bielefeld
Germany

Berthold Gröne
Kliniken Schmieder
Neurologisches Rehabilitationskrankenhaus
Allensbach
Germany

Murray Grossman
University of Pennsylvania Medical Center
Department of Neurology
Philadelphia, Pennsylvania
USA

Jennifer M. Gurd
The Radcliffe Infirmary
Neuropsychology Unit
Oxford
United Kingdom

Curt Hamre
Texas Tech University
Department of Speech and Hearing Sciences
Lubbock, Texas
USA

Didier Hannequin
Hôpital Charles-Nicolle
Rouen
France

William Harn
Texas Tech University
Department of Speech and Hearing Sciences
Lubbock, Texas
USA

David E. Hartman
University of Wisconsin
Department of Neurology
Madison, Wisconsin
USA

Claus Heeschen
Max-Planck-Institut für
Psycholinguistik
Nijmegen
The Netherlands

Erika Hoff-Ginsberg
University of Wisconsin-Parkside
Division of Behavioral Science
Kenosha, Wisconsin
USA

Ralph E. Hoffman
Yale University
School of Medicine
New Haven, Connecticut
USA

Audrey L. Holland
University of Arizona
Department of Speech and Hearing Sciences
Tucson, Arizona
USA

Charles Hulme
University of York
Department of Psychology
Heslington, York
United Kingdom

Janis Costello Ingham
University of California Santa Barbara
Department of Speech and Hearing Sciences
Santa Barbara, California
USA

Yves Joanette
Centre Hospitalier Côte-des-Neiges
Centre de Recherche
Montréal, Québec
Canada

Helge S. Johannsen
Universität Ulm
Phoniatrische Ambulanz
Ulm
Germany

Helga Johannsen-Horbach
Schule für Logopäden
Freiburg/Br.
Germany

Judith R. Johnston
University of British Columbia
School of Audiology and Speech Sciences
Vancouver, British Columbia
Canada

Alan G. Kamhi
Memphis State University
Memphis Speech and Hearing Center
Memphis, Tennessee
USA

Marie-Louise Käsermann
Psychiatrische Universitätsklinik
Bern
Switzerland

Janice Kay
University of Exeter
Department of Psychology
Exeter
United Kingdom

J. A. Scott Kelso
Florida Atlantic University
Center for Complex Systems
Boca Raton, Florida
USA

Raymond D. Kent
University of Wisconsin Madison
Waisman Center
Madison, Wisconsin
USA

Andrew Kertesz
University of Western Ontario
Department of Clinical Neurological
Sciences
St. Joseph's Hospital
London, Ontario
Canada

Marcel Kinsbourne
Boston University
Behavioral Neurology Unit
Boston, Massachusetts
USA

Susan E. Kohn
Braintree Hospital
Department of Neurology
Braintree, Massachusetts
USA

Israel Kolvin
The Royal Free Hospital, School of Medicine
London
United Kingdom

M. Mary Konstantareas
University of Toronto
Clarke Institute of Psychiatry
Toronto, Ontario
Canada

Karen L. Landahl
University of Chicago
Department of Linguistics
Chicago, Illinois
USA

Yvan Lebrun
Vrije Universiteit Brussel
Faculteit Geneeskunde
Neurolinguistiek
Brussel
Belgium

André Roch Lecours
Centre Hospitalier Côte-des-Neiges
Centre de Recherche
Montréal, Québec
Canada

Laurence B. Leonard
Purdue University
Department of Audiology and Speech Sciences
West Lafayette, Indiana
USA

Ruth Lesser
University of Newcastle-upon-Tyne
Department of Speech
Newcastle-upon-Tyne
United Kingdom

Willem J. M. Levelt
Max-Planck-Institut für Psycholinguistik
Nijmegen
The Netherlands

Richard S. Lewis
Pomona College
Department of Psychology
Claremont, California
USA

Leah L. Light
Pitzer College
Claremont, California
USA

Fernando Lolas
Universidad de Chile
Facultad de Medicina
Santiago de Chile
Chile

Christy L. Ludlow
National Institute on Deafness and Other Communication Disorders
Voice and Speech Section
Bethesda, Maryland
USA

Donald G. MacKay
University of California Los Angeles
Department of Psychology
Los Angeles, California
USA

Brendan A. Maher
Harvard University
Department of Psychology
Cambridge, Massachusetts
USA

John C. Marshall
The Radcliffe Infirmary
Neuropsychology Unit
Oxford
United Kingdom

Harald Marx
Universität Bielefeld
Fakultät für Psychologie und Sportwissenschaft
Abteilung für Psychologie
Bielefeld
Germany

Lynn Mawhood
University of London
Institute of Psychiatry
De Crespigny Park
London
United Kingdom

Paula Menyuk
Boston University
School of Education
Literacy and Language Institute
Boston, Massachusetts
USA

Edward C. Merrill
The University of Alabama
Department of Psychology
Tuscaloosa, Alabama
USA

Anne E. Mills
Universiteit Amsterdam
Algemene Taalwetenschap
Amsterdam
The Netherlands

Kay Mogford-Bevan
University of Newcastle-upon-Tyne
Department of Speech
Newcastle-upon-Tyne
United Kingdom

Dave Müller
Suffolk College
Ipswich, Suffolk
United Kingdom

Michel Paradis
McGill University
Department of Linguistics
Montréal, Québec
Canada

Sally J. Peterson-Falzone
University of California San Francisco
Department of Growth and Development
San Francisco, California
USA

Klaus Poeck
Rheinisch-Westfälische Technische Hochschule Aachen
Neurologische Klinik
Aachen
Germany

Steven Z. Rapcsak
University of Arizona
Department of Neurology
Tucson, Arizona
USA

Friedel M. Reischies
Freie Universität Berlin
Psychiatrische Klinik und Poliklinik
Berlin
Germany

Donald A. Robin
The University of Iowa
Department of Speech Pathology and Audiology
Wendell Johnson Speech and Hearing Center
Iowa City, Iowa
USA

David P. Roeltgen
Hahnemann University
Department of Neurology
Philadelphia, Pennsylvania
USA

John C. Rosenbek
W. S. Middleton Memorial VA Medical Center
Audiology and Speech Pathology
Madison, Wisconsin
USA

J. Douglas Saddy
The University of Queensland
Psychology Department
Brisbane, Queensland
Australia

Paul Satz
University of California Los Angeles
The Neuropsychiatric Institute & Hospital
Los Angeles, California
USA

Gerheid Scheerer-Neumann
Am Gottesberg 59
Bielefeld
Germany

Paul W. Schönle
Kliniken Schmieder
Neurologisches Rehabilitationskrankenhaus
Allensbach
Germany

Hartmut Schulze
Universität Ulm
Phoniatrische Ambulanz
Ulm
Germany

Barbara B. Shadden
The University of Arkansas
Speech and Hearing Clinic
Fayetteville, Arkansas
USA

Helmut Skowronek
Universität Bielefeld
Fakultät für Psychologie und Sportwissenschaft
Abteilung für Psychologie
Bielefeld
Germany

Anne Smith
Purdue University
Department of Audiology and Speech Sciences
West Lafayette, Indiana
USA

Margaret J. Snowling
University of Newcastle-upon-Tyne
Department of Psychology
Newcastle-upon-Tyne
United Kingdom

Manfred Spitzer
Universität Heidelberg
Psychiatrische Klinik und Poliklinik
Heidelberg
Germany

Joseph P. Stemberger
University of Minnesota
Department of Communication Disorders
Minneapolis, Minnesota
USA

Yasufumi Tanaka
Jichi Medical School
Department of Neurology
Tochigi
Japan

Christine M. Temple
University of Essex
Department of Psychology
Colchester
United Kingdom

Cynthia K. Thompson
Northwestern University
Department of Communication Sciences and Disorders
Evanston, Illinois
USA

Betty Tuller
Florida Atlantic University
Center for Complex Systems
Boca Raton, Florida
USA

Hanna K. Ulatowska
The University of Texas
Callier Center for Communication Disorders
Dallas, Texas
USA

Diana Van Lancker
University of Southern California
Department of Veterans Affairs
Outpatient Clinic
Los Angeles, California
USA

Mathias Vogel
Städtisches Krankenhaus München-Bogenhausen
Neuropsychologische Abteilung
München
Germany

Claus-W. Wallesch
Neurologische Universitätsklinik
Freiburg/Br.
Germany

Sabine Weinert
Universität Bielefeld
Fakultät für Psychologie und Sportwissenschaft
Abteilung für Psychologie
Bielefeld
Germany

Marilyn C. Welsh
University of Northern Colorado
Department of Psychology
Greeley, Colorado
USA

Dorothea Weniger
Universitätsspital Zürich
Neuropsychologische Abteilung
Zürich
Switzerland

Klaus Willmes
Rheinisch-Westfälische Technische Hochschule Aachen
Neurologische Klinik
Aachen
Germany

Wolfram Ziegler
Städtisches Krankenhaus München-Bogenhausen
Entwicklungsgruppe Klinische Neuropsychologie
München
Germany

Gerald N. Zimmermann
Joe Johnston Law Firm P. C.
Iowa City, Iowa
USA

89. Index of Names

C

D

E

F

G

H

I

J

K

M

N

Q

R

S

T

U

V

W

Y

Z

90. Subject Index

The organization of the handbook allows readers to find their topics of interest by way of the volume's list of contents as well as the list of contents preceding each article. Accordingly, the subject index could be confined to include only the most important additional terms.

In compound terms the adjective is listed first (e.g. 'amnestic aphasia'). Specifying attributes follow the reference noun (e.g. 'aging, normal'). Explanatory supplements to terms are given in parentheses after the term (e.g. 'muteness (in autism)'). Recurring terms have received only one page reference per article.

A

H

I

J

K

L

R

T

U

V

W

X